ESSENTIAL SOURCES IN THE SCIENTIFIC STUDY OF CONSCIOUSNESS

ESSENTIAL SOURCES IN THE SCIENTIFIC STUDY OF CONSCIOUSNESS

edited by Bernard J. Baars, William P. Banks, and James B. Newman

A Bradford Book
The MIT Press
Cambridge, Massachusetts
London, England

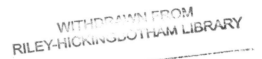

© 2003 Massachusetts Institute of Technology

This book was set in Times New Roman on 3B2 by Asco Typesetters, Hong Kong.
Printed and bound in the United States of America.

Library of Congress Cataloging-in-Publication Data

Essential sources in the scientific study of consciousness / edited by Bernard J. Baars, William P. Banks, and James B. Newman.
    p.   cm.
"A Bradford book."
Includes bibliographical references and index.
ISBN 0-262-02496-9 (hbk. : alk. paper)—ISBN 0-262-52302-7 (pbk. : alk. paper)
1. Consciousness—Physiological aspects. 2. Cognitive neuroscience. I. Baars, Bernard J. II. Banks, William P. III. Newman, James B.
QP411 .E85   2003
153—dc21   2002029376

Contents

Contents

Contents

Preface

Reliable scientific evidence about consciousness has often been difficult to find. This volume presents more than five dozen significant articles in the brain and cognitive sciences, all with a direct bearing on the subject. Our guiding idea has been to select studies that ask, "What *difference* does consciousness make? What are its properties, and what role could it play in the nervous system? How do conscious brain functions differ from unconscious ones?" Among the published articles that satisfy this standard we have aimed for the most definitive, the pioneering, the most articulate, and the briefest. We believe they are of fundamental importance.

We have thought especially about readers who are new to this fast-growing literature. Wherever possible we have looked for good introductory articles, and our own introductions are meant to highlight briefly why each one is important. We are painfully aware that we have had to omit many significant articles. Each selection should therefore be considered a point of entry to a larger body of published work.

Although we emphasize breadth, we have not covered neighboring topics such as voluntary control and self. A new literature is emerging there, such as the remarkable reconstruction by Hannah Damasio and coauthors of the brain of Phineas Gage, the nineteenth-century brain-injured patient who underwent a great change of personality when his frontal cortex was penetrated by an explosively driven railroad spike (1994). An equally important body of findings is now growing on voluntary control, including work by psychologists like Daniel Wegner on agency (Wenzlaff and Wegner 2000) and by neurologists on brain conditions that dissociate voluntary from involuntary control. Consciousness, self, and voluntary control are indeed sister issues, but they cannot be covered in depth in a single volume.

Finally, we omitted ideas that are unsupported by evidence at this time. There has been much discussion of quantum-theory claims about consciousness, for example, for which we have no direct evidence at present. Although no hypothesis can be excluded a priori, this volume presents ideas for which we have reasonably direct evidence today.

The Rediscovery of Consciousness

Because of the curious history of consciousness in the twentieth century, this most fundamental human question has been oddly neglected. Yet for decades now, the evidence has been mounting in quantity and quality. The scientific community has responded with rising interest. After almost a century of neglect, consciousness has become a major focus for research. Each month new findings appear in leading journals. In the coming century this new ferment is likely to reshape our understanding of mind and brain in the most basic way.

Consciousness has long been seen as central to the human condition, with a serious literature dating to the earliest written records from Asia and the Fertile Crescent. It interpenetrates all human functions. Sensory perception, attention, and language can be usefully divided into conscious and unconscious aspects. Many memory researchers now believe that consciousness partitions their field in crucial ways, in distinguishing between fundamental concepts like "recall" and "recognition," for example. Motivation, action control, emotion, learning, and development all interact with consciousness in fundamental ways.

With the advent of a body of scientific evidence bearing directly on the subject, a core study program seems to be emerging. In the brain sciences, psychology, and philosophy, new courses and seminars are being taught. Specialized doctoral programs have been organized in a few places, and many laboratories are refocusing their efforts. Even where the word "consciousness" is still treated with caution, the same questions are debated. We believe this volume can contribute to informed discussion by presenting the breadth and depth of the field, showing the strength of the scientific foundations and highlighting pathways for the future.

Our gratitude goes to the authors presented here and to those who deserved to be included, but for the limitations of space. We honor the pioneers, who often had to work in very difficult circumstances. All who care about understanding human consciousness are in their debt.

Note: After the manuscript of this book was essentially complete, James Newman died unexpectedly, to the great shock and regret of his friends. Jim was a pioneer in scientific studies of consciousness. He made noteworthy contributions to the interpretation of thalamocortical mechanisms, as well as to scientific organizations and activities in the field. He was affiliated with Colorado Neurological Institute. This book is gratefully dedicated to his memory.

References

Damasio, H., Grabowski, T., Frank, R., Galaburda, A. M., and Damasio, A. R. (1994) The return of Phineas Gage: Clues about the brain from the skull of a famous patient. *Science* 264: 1102–1105.

Gray, J. A., Wedderburn, A. A. I. (1960) Grouping strategies with simultaneous stimuli. *Quarterly Journal of Experimental Psychology* 12, 180–184.

Wenzlaff, R. M., Wegner, D. M. (2000) Thought suppression. *Annual Review of Psychology* 51: 59–91.

Bernard J. Baars*
The Neurosciences Institute

William P. Banks
Pomona College

*Supported by The Neurosciences Institute and The Neurosciences Research Foundation, which are gratefully acknowledged.

Sources

1. Bernard J. Baars. Introduction: Treating Consciousness as a Variable: The Fading Taboo. (Written for this volume.)

2. G. A. Mandler (1975) Consciousness: Respectable, useful, and probably necessary. In Solso, R. (ed.). (1975) *Information processing and cognition: The Loyola Symposium.* Hillsdale, N.J.: Erlbaum.

3. F. Crick and C. Koch (1998) Consciousness and neuroscience. *Cerebral Cortex*, 8, 97–107. Reprinted with permission of Oxford University Press and the authors.

4. A. Treisman (1998) Feature binding, attention, and object perception. *Philos. Trans. R. Soc. Lond. B Biol. Sci.*, 353, 1295–1306. Reprinted with permission of The Royal Society.

5. M. S. Livingstone and D. H. Hubel (1981) Effects of sleep and arousal on the processing of visual information in the cat. *Nature*, 291, 554–561. Reprinted with permission of *Nature.*

6. D. L. Sheinberg and N. K. Logothetis (1997) The role of temporal cortical areas in perceptual organization. *Proceedings of the National Academy of Sciences, USA*, 94, 3408–3413. Reprinted with permission of the National Academy of Sciences, USA.

7. G. Tononi, R. Srinivasan, D. P. Russell, and G. M. Edelman (1998) Investigating neural correlates of conscious perception by frequency-tagged neuromagnetic responses. *Proceedings of the National Academy of Sciences, USA*, 95, 3198–3203. Reprinted with permission of the National Academy of Sciences, USA.

8. A. K. Engel, P. Fries, P. R. Roelfsema, P. König, M. Brecht, and W. Singer (1999) Temporal binding, binocular rivalry, and consciousness. *Consciousness and Cognition*, 8, 128–151.

9. L. Weiskrantz (1991) Disconnected awareness for detecting, processing, and remembering in neurological patients. *J. Royal Society of Medicine*, 84, 466–470.

10. A. Cowey and P. Stoerig (1995) Blindsight in monkeys. *Nature*, 373, 247–249. Reprinted with permission of *Nature.*

11. R. W. Sperry (1968) Hemisphere deconnection and unity in conscious awareness. *American Psychologist*, 23, 723–733. Reprinted with permission of the American Psychological Association.

12. M. A. Goodale and A. D. Milner (1992) Separate visual pathways for perception and action. *Trends in Neurosciences*, 15, 20–25. Reprinted with permission of Elsevier Science.

13. S. E. Palmer (1999) Consciousness and isomorphism: Can the color spectrum really be inverted? Revised from S. Palmer (in press) *Behavioral and Brain Sciences.* Revised for this volume.

14. A. M. Treisman (1969) Strategies and models of selective attention. *Psychological Review*, 76, 282–299. Reprinted with permission of the American Psychological Association.

15. G. Rees, C. Russell, C. D. Frith, and J. Driver (1999) Inattentional blindness versus inattentional amnesia for fixated but ignored words. *Science*, 286, 2503–2507.

16. D. G. MacKay (1973) Aspects of a theory of comprehension, memory, and attention. *Quarterly Journal of Experimental Psychology*, 25, 22–40. Reprinted with the permission of the Psychology Press.

17. R. A. Rensink, J. K. O'Regan, and J. J. Clark (1997) To see or not to see: The need for attention to perceive changes in scenes. *Psychological Science*, 8, 368–373. Reprinted with the permission of Blackwell Publishers.

18. F. Crick (1984) Function of the thalamic reticular complex: The searchlight hypothesis. *Proceedings of the National Academy of Sciences, USA*, 81, 4586–4590. Reprinted with permission of the National Academy of Sciences, USA.

19. J. Moran and R. Desimone (1985) Selective attention gates visual processing in the extrastriate cortex. *Science*, 229, 782–784. Reprinted with the permission of *Science.*

20. M. I. Posner (1994) Attention: The mechanisms of consciousness. *Proceedings of the National Academy of Sciences, USA*, 91, 7398–7403. Reprinted with permission of the National Academy of Sciences, USA.

21. D. LaBerge (1997) Attention, awareness, and the triangular circuit. *Consciousness and Cognition*, 6, 149–181. Reprinted with permission of Academic Press.

22. G. Sperling (1960) The information available in brief visual presentations. *Psychological Monographs*, 74, 1–29. Reprinted with permission of the American Psychological Association. (public domain)

23. G. A. Miller (1956) The magical number seven, plus or minus two: Some limits on our capacity for processing information. *The Psychological Review*, 63, 81–97. Reprinted with permission of the American Psychological Association. (public domain)

24. R. C. Atkinson and R. M. Shiffrin (1971) The control of short-term memory. *Scientific American*,

225, 82–90. Reprinted with the permission of *Scientific American*.

25. A. D. Baddeley (1993) Verbal and visual subsystems of working memory. *Current Biology*, 3, 563–565.

26. P. S. Goldman-Rakic (1992) The prefrontal landscape: Implications of functional architecture for understanding human mentation and the central executive. *Philos. Trans. R. Soc. Lond. B., Biol. Sci.*, 351, 1445–1453. Reprinted with the permission of The Royal Society.

27. E. E. Smith and J. Jonides (1999) Storage and executive processes in the frontal lobes. *Science*, 283, 1657–1661.

28. E. R. John, P. Easton, and R. Isenhart (1997) Consciousness and cognition may be mediated by multiple independent coherent ensembles. *Consciousness and Cognition*, 6, 3–39. Reprinted with permission of Academic Press.

29. S. M. Kosslyn (1988) Aspects of a cognitive neuroscience of mental imagery. *Science*, 240, 1621–1626. Reprinted with the permission of *Science*.

30. M. J. Farah (1989) The neural basis of mental imagery. *Trends in Neuroscience*, 12, 395–399. Reprinted with permission of Elsevier Science.

31. J. L. Singer (1993) Experimental studies of ongoing conscious experience. In G. R. Bock and J. Marsh (eds.) *Experimental and theoretical studies of consciousness. CIBA Foundation Symposium*, 174, pp. 100–116. New York: Wiley. Reprinted with the permission of the Novartis Foundation.

32. K. A. Ericsson and H. A. Simon (1987) Verbal reports on thinking. In C. Faerch and G. Kasper (eds.) *Introspective methods in second-language acquisition*, pp. 24–53. Clevedon, U.K., Multilingual Matters, Ltd. Reprinted with permission of Multilingual Matters, Ltd. Copyright 1987, National Academy of Sciences, USA.

33. J. Cheesman and P. M. Merikle (1986) Distinguishing conscious from unconscious perceptual processes. *Canadian Journal of Psychology*, 40, 343–367.

34. H. Shevrin and S. Dickman (1980) The psychological unconscious: A necessary assumption for all psychological theory? *American Psychologist*, 35, 421–434. Reprinted with permission of the American Psychological Association.

35. B. Libet (1982) Brain stimulation in the study of neuronal functions for conscious sensory experiences.

Human Neurobiology, 1, 235–242. Reprinted with permission of Springer.

36. E. Tulving (1985) Memory and consciousness. *Canadian Psychology*, 26, 1–12. Reprinted with permission of the Canadian Psychological Association.

37. D. L. Schacter, N. M. Alpert, C. R. Savage, S. L. Rauch, and M. S. Albert (1996) Conscious recollection and the human hippocampal formation: Evidence from positron emission tomography. *Proceedings of the National Academy of Sciences, USA*, 93, 321–325. Reprinted with permission of the National Academy of Sciences, USA.

38. A. S. Reber (1989) Implicit learning and tacit knowledge. *Journal of Experimental Psychology: General*, 118, 219–235. Reprinted with permission of the American Psychological Association.

39. R. M. Shiffrin (1997) Attention, automatism, and consciousness. In J. D. Cohen and J. W. Schooler (eds.) *Scientific approaches to consciousness*, pp. 49–64. Hillsdale, NJ: Erlbaum.

40. E. J. Langer and L. G. Imber (1979) When practice makes imperfect: Debilitating effects of overlearning. *Journal of Personality and Social Psychology*, 37, 2014–2024. Reprinted with permission of the American Psychological Association.

41. M. E. Raichle (1998) The neural correlates of consciousness: An analysis of cognitive skill learning. *Phil. Trans. R. Soc. Lond. B*, 353, 1–14. Reprinted with permission of The Royal Society.

42. A. Tversky and D. Kahneman (1973) Availability: A heuristic for judging frequency and probability. *Cognitive Psychology*, 5, 207–232.

43. J. M. Gardiner, C. Ramponi, and A. Richardson-Klavehn (1998) Experiences of remembering, knowing, and guessing. *Consciousness and Cognition*, 7, 1–26. Reprinted with permission of Academic Press.

44. L. L. Jacoby (1994) Measuring recollection: Strategic versus automatic influences of associative context. In C. Umilta and M. Moscovitch (eds.) *Attention and Performance, vol. 15: Conscious and nonconscious information processing*. Cambridge, MA: MIT Press. Pp. 661–680. Reprinted with permission of The MIT Press.

45. B. Mangan. The conscious "fringe": Bringing William James up to date. (Written for this volume.)

46. B. J. Baars (1988) The fundamental role of context: Unconscious shaping of conscious information. In B. J. Baars (ed.) *A cognitive theory of consciousness.*

New York: Cambridge University Press. Reprinted with permission of the author.

47. J. F. Kihlstrom (1987) The cognitive unconscious. *Science*, 237, 1445–1452.

48. E. R. Hilgard, A. H. Morgan, and H. Macdonald (1975) Pain and dissociation in the cold pressor test: A study of hypnotic analgesia with "hidden reports" through automatic key pressing and automatic talking. *J. Abnormal Psychol.*, 84, 280–289. Reprinted with permission of the American Psychological Association.

49. V. S. Ramachandran (1995) Anosognosia in parietal lobe syndrome. *Consciousness and Cognition*, 4, 22–51. Reprinted with permission of Academic Press.

50. D. Galin (1974) Implications for psychiatry of left and right cerebral specialization: A neurophysiological context for unconscious processes. *Arch. Gen. Psychiatr.*, 31, 572–583. Reprinted with permission of the American Medical Association.

51. G. Moruzzi and H. W. Magoun (1949) Brain stem reticular formation and activation of the EEG. *EEG Clin. Neurophysiol.*, 1, 455–473.

52. A. B. Scheibel (1980) Anatomical and physiological substrates of arousal. In J. A. Hobson and M. A. B. Brazier (eds.) *The reticular formation revisited*, pp. 55–66. New York: Raven Press. Reprinted with permission of Raven Press–Lippincott Press.

53. J. E. Bogen (1995) On the neurophysiology of consciousness: An overview. *Consciousness and Cognition*, 4, 52–62. Reprinted with permission of Academic Press.

54. H. Flohr (1995) An information processing theory of anaesthesia. *Neuropsychologia*, 9, 1169–1180. Reprinted with permission of Elsevier Science.

55. M. T. Alkire, R. J. Haier, J. H. Fallon (2000) Toward a unified theory of narcosis: Brain imaging evidence for a thalamocortical switch as the neurophysiologic basis of anesthetic-induced unconsciousness. *Consciousness and Cognition*, 9, 370–386. Reprinted with permission of Academic Press.

56. W. Dement and N. Kleitman (1957) The relation of eye movements during sleep to dream activity: An objective method for the study of dreaming. *J. Exp. Psychol.*, 53, 339–346. Reprinted with permission of the American Psychological Association. (public domain)

57. J. A. Hobson and R. W. McCarley (1977) The brain as a dream state generator: An activation-synthesis hypothesis of the dream process, *The American Journal of Psychiatry*, 134, 1335–1348. Reprinted with permission of the American Psychiatric Association.

58. S. P. LaBerge, L. E. Nagel, W. C. Dement, and V. P. Zarcone, Jr (1981) Lucid dreaming verified by volitional communication during REM sleep. *Perceptual and Motor Skills*, 52, 727–732.

59. R. Llinás and D. Paré (1991) Commentary: Of dreaming and wakefulness. *Neuroscience*, 44, 512–535. Reprinted with permission of Elsevier Science.

60. G. Tononi and G. M. Edelman (1998) Consciousness and complexity. *Science*, 282, 1846–1851. Reprinted with the permission of *Science*.

61. S. Grossberg (1999) The link between brain learning, attention, and consciousness. From *Consciousness and Cognition*, 8, 1–44. Reprinted with permission of Academic Press.

62. J. Taylor and F. N. Alavi (1993) A global competitive network for attention. *Neural Network World*, 5, 477–502. Reprinted with the permission of International Science Publishers and *Neural Network World*.

63. A. R. Damasio (1989) Time-locked multiregional retroactivation: A systems-level proposal for the neural substrates of recall and recognition. *Cognition*, 33, 25–62.

64. W. Singer and C. M. Gray (1995) Visual feature integration and the temporal correlation hypothesis. *Annual Review of Neuroscience*, 18, 555–586. Reprinted with permission of Annual Reviews.

65. B. J. Baars (1998) Metaphors of consciousness and attention in the brain. *Trends in Neurosciences*, 21, 58–62. Reprinted with permission of Elsevier Science.

66. B. J. Baars (1993) How does a serial, integrated, and very limited stream of consciousness emerge from a nervous system that is mostly unconscious, distributed, parallel, and of enormous capacity? In G. R. Bock and J. Marsh (eds.) *Experimental and theoretical studies of consciousness*, pp. 282–303. Chichester, U.K.: Wiley. CIBA Foundation Symposium 174.

67. J. Newman, B. J. Baars, and S.-B. Cho (1997) A Neural Global Workspace model for conscious attention. *Neural Networks* (Special issue), 10, 1195–1206. Reprinted with permission of Elsevier Science.

68. S. Franklin and A. Graesser (1999) A software agent model of consciousness. *Consciousness and Cognition*, 8, 285–301. Reprinted with permission of Academic Press.

1 Introduction: Treating Consciousness as a Variable: The Fading Taboo

Bernard J. Baars

Consciousness is both the most obvious and the most hotly debated topic in psychology and brain science. All healthy humans are conscious of sights and sounds, of some mental images, of inner speech and emotional feelings, and of some of our goals and beliefs. Essentially all biopsychological experiments involve consciousness in one way or another. Yet for most of this century, scientists have been hesitant to explore the issue directly.

This hesitation is historically new. More than two millenia ago, philosophers in Asia and Greece began the written record of human thought by exploring conscious experiences. Most of our basic mental concepts have their origin in this long tradition. Modern scientific psychology and neurology began in about 1800 with the study of human conscious experience, and some works from that era, such as William James's *Principles of Psychology* (1890/1983) are still widely read today. Until the twentieth century, scientists were deeply involved in efforts to understand consciousness.

That receptive attitude changed radically in the years just after 1900, when a great shift occurred toward scientific physicalism—the idea that all human activities must be explained by physical brain processes or by physical stimuli and responses. In brain science this philosophy was popularized by I. P. Pavlov, and in the new discipline of psychology, by behaviorists like John B. Watson and later B. F. Skinner and many others. Although consciousness did not go away, so little physical evidence was known about it that serious scientists tended to avoid it altogether. The universal fact of human consciousness came to resemble a scientific taboo.

The neglect of consciousness is now fading rapidly. After almost a century, an accelerating series of significant papers has begun to appear in leading journals such as *Science* and *Nature*, reporting marked progress in understanding conscious vision in the cortex, conscious memories mediated by the hippocampus, and more. In all cases, conscious events are compared to unconscious ones: conscious vision is contrasted with unconscious visual activity, and conscious (explicit) memories with unconscious ones. But that is only the tip of the iceberg. Since the early 1980s, thousands of studies of conscious and unconscious processes have appeared in the brain and psychological literature, under various headings. There is little doubt that we are again looking at questions that were familiar to William James and his generation, but now with better evidence and theory than ever before.

Evidence

Many scientists question whether there is any evidence about conscious experience *as such*. In this volume we approach this issue by selecting studies that *treat consciousness as a variable*. They include the following comparisons:

Between conscious and unconscious streams of stimulation

Between conscious and unconscious elements in memory

Between forms of brain damage that selectively impair conscious processes and those that do not

Between wakefulness compared to deep sleep, coma, and anesthesia

Between new and habituated events

Many comparison cases like these have been studied. In each of them, consciousness is treated as an experimental variable, just as in any other topic of scientific study. We believe that such comparisons are the key to the evidence.

Although many studies explore consciousness in this way, this fact may not be obvious because the word "consciousness" is

Table 1.1

Some widely studied polarities between matched conscious and unconscious phenomena

Conscious	Unconscious
1. Explicit cognition	Implicit cognition
2. Immediate memory	Longer term memory
3. Novel, informative, and significant events	Routine, predictable, and nonsignificant events
4. Attended information	Unattended information
5. Focal contents	Fringe contents (e.g., familiarity)
6. Declarative memory (facts, etc.)	Procedural memory (skills, etc.)
7. Supraliminal stimulation	Subliminal stimulation
8. Effortful tasks	Spontaneous/automatic tasks
9. Remembering (recall)	Knowing (recognition)
10. Available memories	Unavailable memories
11. Strategic control	Automatic control
12. Grammatical strings	Implicit underlying grammars
13. Intact reticular formation and bilateral intralaminar thalamic nuclei	Lesioned reticular formation, or bilateral intralaminar nuclei
14. Rehearsed items in Working Memory	Unrehearsed items
15. Wakefulness and dreams (cortical arousal)	Deep sleep, coma, sedation (cortical slow waves)
16. Explicit inferences	Automatic inferences
17. Episodic memory (autobiographical)	Semantic memory (conceptual knowledge)
18. Autonoetic memory	Noetic memory
19. Intentional learning	Incidental learning
20. Normal vision	Blindsight (cortical blindness)

sometimes still avoided. Instead, investigators talk about "explicit" versus "implicit" cognition, or "attended" versus "unattended" stimulation. Table 1.1 shows some of the popular substitutes for "conscious" and "unconscious."

Notice, by the way, that any theory of the conscious component of human cognition must somehow explain all of these contrasts. The problem is therefore very strongly bounded. One cannot simply make up a theory to explain one of the contrasts and expect it to explain the others. (See Baars 1988, 1997, and 2002 for many detailed examples).

This profusion of terms tends to hide underlying similarities. All words on the left side of table 1.1 refer to reportable, broadly conscious processes. All those on the right side refer to very similar processes that are not reportable and not conscious. This simple fact is easily lost in the great variety of technical synonyms. But it is now increasingly being recognized. One aim of this volume is to call attention to such fundamental similarities.

It is relatively easy to scour any major research literature for studies that compare conscious and unconscious events. For this volume we did not find it difficult to find seventy seminal articles that do just that. Indeed, our problem was to winnow down hundreds of candidate articles to a more practical number; many excellent articles had to be left out. Contrary to traditional opinion, therefore, our empirical knowledge about consciousness is quite extensive. (See Baars 1988, 1997, and in press.)

It Has Been Historically Difficult to Think of Consciousness as a Variable

Scientifically it seems obvious that we can only study something as an empirical variable, comparing more of it to less of it. A number of historic breakthroughs in science emerged from the realization that some previously assumed constant, like atmospheric pressure or gravity, was actually a variable. The first step is always to find at least one comparison condition: earth gravity compared to near-zero gravity in space, or sea-level air pressure compared to an artificial vacuum. Discovering comparison conditions is often a wrenching process. In the case of gravity, it required a great leap of imagination for natural philosophers in the seventeenth century to understand that all objects in the universe need not fall toward the center of the earth. It was Newton's ability to imagine variable amounts and directions of gravitational force that led to the solution of the ancient puzzle of planetary motion. Likewise, the reality of atmospheric pressure was not recognized until variations in air pressure could be observed with barometers, which were invented only a few hundred years ago. Gravity and atmospheric pressure were simply taken for granted before they were found to be variable in the sixteenth and seventeenth centuries. Most of these conceptual advances were vigorously opposed.

Yet discovering comparison conditions is often the key to new insights. Biology as a science emerged from Darwin's revolutionary idea that species are not fixed, but variable over geologic time. Modern earth sciences emerged from the key idea that the world's continents are not stable, but are floating fragments of earth crust. Relativistic physics and quantum theory provide other familiar examples. Perhaps all the sciences have their origins in such moments of insight, when an apparent constant is suddenly revealed to be variable. When new comparison conditions emerge, facts long hidden from view may suddenly become visible and salient.

Historically, however, consciousness seemed to be different from all other scientific concepts. It has been extraordinarily difficult to see it as a variable. The persistent pattern over centuries has been to see our own experience as the *only* psychological domain that can be conceived, one that has no conceivable comparison condition. The notion that conscious experience is incommensurable with any other event may be a con-

sequence of our inability to compare our own private experience with other things. We cannot vary our own consciousness from the inside; as soon as we decrease it, we lose the ability to observe anything. And the consciousness of others is simply invisible as a direct datum.

What are the natural comparison conditions for conscious events? To study consciousness as a variable, the events to be compared must be similar enough to make comparison meaningful. The evidence that unconscious brain events are often comparable to conscious ones is now extensive (Baars 1988, 1997, in press). Most readings in this book present more support for this claim. The notion that consciousness can be studied with natural comparison conditions, which cast light on the fundamental question, has now emerged in many different places in mind and brain science. As a result, we have a burgeoning scientific literature with much to tell us. After many years of neglect and confusion, the topic has come back into focus.

Some of our existing knowledge about consciousness now seems so obvious that we rarely bother to make it explicit. There is good evidence, for example, that waking consciousness is both widespread and biologically adaptive. Sleep-waking cycles occur throughout the vertebrate phylum, associated with characteristic neuronal activity and such behavioral activities as goal-directed seeking and avoidance. Outside of the waking state, vertebrates do not feed, mate, reproduce, defend their territory or young, migrate, or carry out any other purposeful survival or reproductive activity. Physiologically, consciousness has pervasive effects: its characteristic electrical signature (fast, low voltage, and irregular) can be found throughout the waking brain, and in unconscious states like deep sleep and coma, slow and coherent waves are equally widely distributed. In these respects, consciousness is not some subtle or hard-to-observe phenomenon. It is hard to avoid.

Brain and cognitive scientists all over the world have come to similar conclusions in recent years, so that today a new race to understand consciousness is in full swing. Most articles in this volume were published in the last decade, and the trend toward more research in consciousness appears to be accelerating.

Consciousness as a Construct Indexed by Behavioral Report

Many observers have pointed out that science is obliged to treat consciousness not as an observable datum but as an inferred concept based on public evidence. To *each of us* conscious sights and sounds appear as primary events, but as researchers dealing with public evidence, we can confirm only the *reports* people make about their conscious experience. Scientifically, therefore, consciousness is not something we know directly; it is a theoretical construct based on shared, public observations.

Edwin G. Boring (1933) summarized this view several decades ago,

... that human consciousness is an inferred construct, a capacity as inferential as any of the other psychological realities, and that literally immediate observation, the introspection that cannot lie, does not exist. All observation is a process that takes time and is subject to error in the course of its occurrence. (p. 23)

This is a familiar strategy in science. We now have three decades of research showing that we can make useful inferences about constructs like selective attention, working memory, imagery, and the like, based on robust observable evidence. Consciousness can be viewed as another theoretical construct, one that has the remarkable feature of *reportability* across a vast range of contents. In most cases this objective construct also coincides with our own experience.

It cannot be overemphasized that inferred constructs are not unique to psychology and brain science. All sciences make inferences that go beyond the observations. The atom was highly inferential in its first modern century; so was the gene; so was the vastness of geological time, a necessary assumption for Darwinian evolution; and other scientific constructs too numerous to list. Cognitive neuroscience applies this common-sense epistemology more explicitly than in everyday life. We can speak of meaning, thought, imagery, attention, memory, and recently, conscious and unconscious processes—all inferred concepts that have been tested in careful experiments and stated in increasingly adequate theories.

Operational Definitions

Our standard behavioral index for consciousness is the ability people have to report their experiences, often in ways that can be checked for accuracy. More than a century of investigation into sensory processes is based on this fundamental fact. Indeed our knowledge of the senses comes largely from psychophysical research, in which we ask people to report their conscious experiences of precisely controlled sensory stimuli. Under well-defined conditions, such reports are exquisitely sensitive.

Conscious processes can be operationally defined as events that:

1. can be reported and acted upon,
2. with verifiable accuracy,
3. under optimal reporting conditions,
4. and which are reported as conscious.

These conditions fit standard practice in the study of perception, immediate memory, problem-solving, imagery, and many other phenomena. "Optimal reporting conditions" implies a minimum delay between the event and the report, freedom from distraction, and the like. The fourth condition is helpful to differentiate focal conscious contents from other events that meet the first three conditions but that are not typically reported as conscious. A noteworthy example is William James's "fringe conscious" events, such as the feeling of knowing that something is familiar or beautiful or true, without being able to pinpoint the conscious event that is the source of such feelings. (See section VIII, and below.)

Reportability as an operational criterion seems to generalize to other primates. This has been studied especially well in the macaque monkey. Blindsight (cortical blindness) is a condition in which the first cortical projection area (V1) of the primary visual pathway is damaged. In the occluded part of the visual field, humans report a loss of conscious visual qualities like color, motion, and object identity. Yet there is excellent evidence that such properties of the visual stimulus are still processed by the visual brain. In forced-choice tasks, blindsight patients can point to a visual object, name it, and detect motion and color, while strongly denying that they have a conscious visual experience of the object. This makes blindsight an ideal case for studying visual consciousness (Weiskrantz 1986; Cowey and Stoerig, chap. 10, this volume).

The macaque's visual brain resembles the human one in many ways. Careful lesion studies show that the macaque behaves much like a human blindsighted subject when parts of area V1 are removed. But how can we be sure that the "blindsighted" macaque has lost conscious visual qualities, the "qualia" discussed by philosophers, such as color, motion, and texture? A remarkable experiment by Cowey and Stoerig (chap. 10, this volume) makes this case, using a behavioral index called the "commentary key," which allows the macaque not merely to choose between two stimuli but also to make a metacognitive comment about its own response. Like a human blindsight subject, the blindsighted macaque can choose accurately between colors, for example. The commentary key allows it to signal whether a chosen stimulus in the occluded visual field can also be *distinguished from a blank trial* in the intact field. Cowey and Stoerig were able to show that macaques could do the first task but not the second one. In effect, the mon-

key was saying, "Yes, I can discriminate behaviorally between the two colors, but I don't really *experience* the difference between colored and blank slides." The analogous human case is to perform a successful discrimination task while denying visual qualitative experience of the stimuli. Such results strengthen the case that macaques have conscious visual experiences not unlike ours.

In sum, behavioral reports of conscious experience have proved to be quite reliable. Although more direct measures are desirable, reportability provides a useful public criterion for brain studies of consciousness in humans and some animals.

Unconscious Events

If we are to treat consciousness as a variable, we also need a way to operationally define the unconscious comparison condition. Operationally, an event can be defined as unconscious if:

1. knowledge of its presence can be verified, even if

2. that knowledge is not claimed to be conscious;

3. and it cannot be voluntarily reported, acted on, or avoided;

4. even under optimal reporting conditions.

There is again a reasonable fit between this definition and existing scientific practice. The simplest example is the great multitude of memories that are currently unconscious. You may recall this morning's breakfast—but what happened to that memory before it was brought to mind? We believe it was still extant in the nervous system, though not consciously. We know, however, that unconscious memories can influence other processes without ever coming to mind. If you had orange juice for breakfast today, you may want milk tomorrow, even without bringing today's orange juice to mind. The observation that unconscious memories can influence behavior without becoming conscious goes back to Hermann Ebbinghaus, who noticed that repeatedly memorizing the same word in a list produces improvements in recall, without conscious recall of earlier efforts to memorize the word. Any systematic behavioral change like this, without reportability, can be used as evidence for unconscious processes.

Note that both conscious and unconscious processes involve inferences from publicly observable behavior. But although it is easy to infer consciousness from accurate reports of events, inferring unconscious ones is much trickier. Can we really be sure that an unreported event is necessarily unconscious? In some cases, apparently unconscious events may be momentarily conscious, but so quickly or vaguely that we cannot recall them even a few seconds later (e.g., Sperling, chap. 22, this volume). William James understood this problem very well and suggested in response that there may be no unconscious psychological processes at all! (See James 1890/ 1983, Baars 1988.)

This is one of those tricky cases wherein the evidence for unconsciousness could retreat ever further and further beyond the grasp of diligent experimenters. Jacoby and Kelley (1992) suggest an attractive answer—a criterion for unconscious events that does not *solve* the problem exactly, but which does give a reasonable basis for consensus. Suppose, they suggest, that we ask a subject to consciously *avoid* reporting certain memories when they are evoked? If people can avoid reporting specific memories on cue, they must have some knowledge of the memory and must be conscious of it. If they *cannot* suppress a particular memory, it is presumably because they do not consciously know that it is to be avoided. As an example, take Ebbinghaus's discovery that repeated words show improved recall even when we are not conscious that they were encountered before (Ebbinghaus 1885/1913). One way to test this "unconscious savings" hypothesis is to ask subjects to avoid saying repeated material.

If they cannot avoid repeating previously seen words, they were plausibly unconscious of the difference between old and new material.

This may not be the ultimate solution; the Jacoby and Kelley criterion only taps into what might be called "functional consciousness"—the ability to act on, report, and avoid reporting a fleeting mental event. But it does provide an empirical standard for separating conscious from other mental events. This may be the best we can do for the time being. In due course, improved brain measures may bring us a step closer.

Fringe Conscious Events

There is an interesting class of phenomena that is neither quite conscious nor unconscious, but that is nevertheless central to normal mental functioning. William James believed that such "fringe conscious" events were at least as important as focal conscious experiences. Fringe events include feelings of rightness, beauty, coherence, anomaly, familiarity, attraction, repulsion, and so on. Fringe states seem to be very useful. There is evidence that they are involved in accurate decision-making, predict resolution of tip-of-the-tongue states, and give a sense of availability of a memory even before it comes to mind (Mangan 1993; chap. 45, this volume).

When people experience a melody as beautiful they may be quite confident of their judgment. But is the experience of beauty specifiable in detail, like the sight of a red plastic toothbrush? Surely not. The combination of high confidence and low experienced detail defines a "fringe conscious" state. Mangan (1993) has developed James's ideas about fringe consciousness in modern terms, suggesting that fringe phenomena may not be subject to the classical capacity limitations of consciousness. As we listen to a song, we can feel moved by it, know that it is familiar, and have a sense of rightness and fit, seemingly at the same instant in time. Given that focal conscious capacity is notoriously limited to one consistent event at any moment, Mangan sees fringe experience as a means of circumventing that limitation. The fringe may be, in Mangan's terms, a "radical condensation" of unconscious information in near-consciousness.

Research on fringe consciousness is still in its early stages. We can, however, suggest a useful operational definition for fringe conscious events—for instance, the feeling of familiarity created by a well-known song or cliche. The fringe experience of familiarity:

1. is reported with verifiable accuracy and high confidence,

2. and can be voluntarily acted on,

3. but is not reported to have differentiated conscious contents,

4. even under optimal reporting conditions.

Note that the ability to report conscious contents as conscious (3) differentiates these fringe criteria from those for focal conscious contents, as well as unconscious events, as described above.

But Is It Really Consciousness? The Question of Subjectivity

Although "reportability" is the best operational measure available today, we cannot forget that it is only a behavioral index to the entire rich world of subjective experience. Many philosophers and scientists have pointed out that it is subjective experience that constitutes the core of the issue. As David Chalmers has recently written:

We can say that a being is conscious if there is something it is like to be that being, to use a phrase made famous by the philosopher Thomas Nagel. Similarly, a mental state is conscious if there is something it is like to be in that mental state. To put it another way, we can say that a mental state is conscious if it has a qualitative feel—an associated quality of experience. Those qualitative feels are also known as phenomenal qualities, or qualia for short. The problem of explain-

ing these phenomenal qualities is just the problem of explaining consciousness. This is the really hard part of the mind-body problem. (Chalmers 1996, p. 4).

Philosophers like Thomas Nagel, Ned Block, and David Chalmers have argued that scientists can address some aspects of consciousness, but that subjectivity, the experience of redness or the grittiness of wet sand, may be inherently beyond scientific study (Nagel 1974, Block 1995). Notice that the stated definition of subjectivity does not treat consciousness as a variable. It claims that subjectivity is incommensurable with any comparison condition, except perhaps the subjective experience of others. Yet when we treat consciousness as a variable, subjectivity is necessarily included. After all, there is no serious question that all the events on the left side of table 1.1 are experienced subjectively by human beings. We can point out, therefore, that science routinely makes use of subjectivity as a source of information.

Consider the following example. If you, the reader, focus fixedly on a single letter on this page from about 12 inches away, you may be conscious of neighboring letters within a few degrees of visual arc of your fixation point, but of no letters in your visual periphery, although we know the peripheral field needs to process printed words in order to aim accurate eye movements in reading. There is no question that your experience of the focal contents of vision is indeed a genuine subjective experience. But it also has natural unconscious comparison conditions in the visual periphery, outside the visual focus. For another example, you were very probably unaware of the nine alternative meanings of the word "focus" in the previous sentence. Yet there is good evidence that some additional meanings of ambiguous words tend to be processed unconsciously in normal reading. It therefore makes sense to compare conscious and unconscious meaning representations of the same word. This comparison involves genuine subjectivity on the conscious side, but it also enables us to study the entire dimension empirically. From this perspective there is no conflict between the deep philosophical questions about subjectivity, and standard scientific practice. We are addressing the same issue.

In cognitive neuroscience we always supplement subjective reports with objectively verifiable methods. For scientific purposes we prefer to use public reports of conscious experiences. But there is generally such a close correlation between objective reports and the subjective experiences they refer to, that for all intents and purposes we can talk of *phenomenology*, of consciousness as experienced. Thus in modern science we are practicing a kind of verifiable phenomenology.

The strategy of treating consciousness as a variable provides a useful empirical basis. No longer are we exclusively dependent on plausible intuitions, thought experiments, or rhetorical brilliance, the bread and butter of traditional thought. We can actually test hypotheses, and the results have a plausible bearing on long-standing questions of consciousness.

Accurate reports of conscious experiences are used every day in scientific studies of sensory perception and have been for almost two centuries. The results have been wholly reliable and cumulative, just like other scientific efforts, and they often converge well with our rapidly increasing understanding of the brain. Surely there is something important in the fact that you and I can be conscious of the words in front of us right now and that we can come to substantial agreement on those experiences. In many tasks, this human rule of thumb seems to work for science as well.

Limits of Consciousness Reports

Sometimes reports of subjective experiences are remarkably fruitful, but sometimes they lead to predictable failure. Nisbett and Wilson (1977) have pointed out that introspective reports are not very accurate in finding out why people make decisions. Human beings often misattribute their reasons for doing things. Yet such errors rarely occur in sensory perception, in reporting inner speech during problem solving, or in vivid mental imagery. Reports of those "inner and outer senses" yield extremely useful data (Ericsson and Simon 1984/1993, Farah 1989, Kosslyn 1980). Scientifically this is quite normal. All operational indices have their limits. Mercury thermometers are useless for measuring the heat of the stars, and yardsticks do not help to measure the altitude of clouds. Part of the job of science is to specify such measurement limits.

Under the proper conditions, objective indices of conscious events often fit our own experience. This is exactly what we would expect of an empirical construct, a convergence between objective and subjective evidence when conditions are optimal. That is why perception researchers often use their own experience to understand objective experiments. Sometimes we can even serve as our own formal subjects, in randomly controlled psychophysical studies, for example. That can work very well; but in other experiments, being one's own subject guarantees bad results. Whether our own experience is a useful guide is an empirical question.

The frequent convergence between subjective experience and objective measures raises questions about the behavioristic taboo against taking our own conscious experiences into account. We could even turn behavioristic skepticism about consciousness on its head—we could ask, "By what scientific authority do we know that our conscious experience is useless at all times? Who is it that laid down the law against considering our own reliable, conscious experiences of color, texture, visual images, inner speech, and the like?"

And of course there is no such authority. The taboo against using one's own experience seems to come from the methods of physics and biology, reinforced by a debatable critique of "introspectionism" about 1900 (see Blumenthal 1979). In ordinary science, such issues are treated as purely pragmatic.

Nothing I have claimed here proves that subjectivity is understandable. It is an open question that has inspired scientists since Fechner and Helmholtz. Subjectivity may forever be unknowable. But it seems more sensible to go on asking testable questions than to speculate about impassable barriers. If empirical investigation runs into a solid wall, we'll know it very quickly.

Summary

Contrary to past beliefs, many aspects of consciousness are not untestable at all, as shown by productive research traditions on topics like attention, perception, psychophysics, problem-solving, thought monitoring, imagery, dream research, and so on. All of these efforts meet the most widely used operational criterion of conscious experience—namely, verifiable report of some event described as conscious by an observer. The key, I would suggest, is to study consciousness as a variable, by seeing whether it is a difference that *makes* a difference. But do the results tell us about real consciousness? Could it be just a behavioral response, without subjectivity? In fact, most objective reports correspond well to our own experience. Investigations into conscious processes like sensation continue to cumulate well after two centuries, which suggests that they have not yet run into some insurmountable barrier. I suggest that consciousness should be treated like any other fundamental scientific question.

Acknowledgment

With thanks to The Neurosciences Institute and The Neurosciences Research Foundation.

References

Baars, B. J. (1986) *The cognitive revolution in psychology.* New York: Guilford Press.

Baars, B. J. (1988) *A cognitive theory of consciousness.* New York: Cambridge University Press. Second edition in press with MIT Press, Cambridge, Mass.

Baars, B. J. (1997) *In the theater of consciousness: The workspace of the mind.* Oxford: Oxford University Press.

Baars, B. J. (2002) *The conscious access hypothesis: origins and recent evidence. Trends in Cognitive Sciences, 6* (1): 47–52.

Block, N. (1995) On a confusion about the function of consciousness. *Behavioral and Brain Sciences, 18,* 227–287.

Blumenthal, A. L. (1979) Wilhelm Wundt, the founding father we never knew. *Contemporary Psychology, 24* (7), 547–550.

Boring, E. G. (1933) *The physical dimensions of consciousness.* New York: Century.

Boring, E. G. (1950) *A history of experimental psychology.* New York: Appleton-Century-Crofts.

Chalmers, D. (1996) *The conscious mind: In search of a fundamental theory.* Oxford: Oxford University Press.

Cowey, A., and P. Stoerig. (1995) Blindsight in monkeys. *Nature, 373* (6511): 247–249.

Crick, F. (1984) Function of the thalamic reticular complex: The searchlight hypothesis. *Proceedings of the National Academy of Sciences USA, 81*: 4586–4590.

Dennett, D. C. (1992) *Consciousness explained.* New York: Basic Books.

Ebbinghaus, H. (1885/1913) *Memory: A contribution to experimental psychology.* (H. A. Ruger and C. E. Bussenius, trans.) New York: Teachers College.

Edelman, G. (1989) *The remembered present: A biological theory of consciousness.* New York: Basic Books.

Jacoby, L. L., and C. M. Kelley. (1992) A process-dissociation framework for investigating unconscious influences: Freudian slips, projective tests, subliminal perception, and signal detection theory. *Current Directions in Psychological Science, 1* (6): 174–179.

James, W. (1890/1983) *The principles of psychology.* New York: Holt. Republished by Harvard University Press, Cambridge, Mass.

Leopold, D. A., and N. K. Logothetis. (1996) Activity changes in early visual cortex reflect monkey's percepts during binocular rivalry. *Nature, 379*: 549–553.

Mangan, B. (1993) Taking phenomenology seriously: The "fringe" and its implications for cognitive research. *Consciousness and Cognition, 2* (2): 89–108.

Nagel, T. (1974) What is it like to be a bat? *Philosophical Review, 4,* 435–450.

Nisbett, R. E., and T. D. Wilson. (1977) Telling more than we can know: Verbal reports on mental processes. *Psychological Review, 84,* 231–259.

Sperling, G. (1960) The information available in brief visual presentations. *Psychological Monographs, 74* (498): 1–29.

Watson, J. B. (1913) Psychology as the behaviorist sees it. *Psychological Review, 20*: 158–177.

Weiskrantz, L. (1986) *Blindsight: A case study and implications.* Oxford: Clarendon Press.

I OVERVIEW

A classic paper by George Mandler states the problem of consciousness with traditional caution: It is "respectable, useful, and probably necessary." Specifically,

I hope to show that consciousness is respectable in the sense that it has become the object of serious and impressive experimental research; it is useful because it avoids circumlocutions as well as [artificial] constructions . . . that are more easily addressed by an appeal to consciousness as part of the apparatus of cognition; and it is probably necessary because it serves to tie together many disparate but obviously related mental concepts. . . .

Mandler speaks as a cognitive scientist emerging from a strong neobehavioristic tradition. He speaks in part "to undo the harm that consciousness suffered during 50 years (approximately 1910 to 1960) in the oubliettes of behaviorism. It is additionally needed because so many of us have a history of collaboration with the keepers of the jail and to speak freely of the need for a concept of consciousness still ties the tongues of not a few cognitive psychologists." Some decades later that is still true, but it is clearly changing.

Crick and Koch (1998) provide a broad introduction to several recent methods and results. Although their article is addressed to neuroscientists, it is of interest to a wider audience. Francis Crick has indeed been one of the great proponents of neuroscientific research into consciousness for many years. Crick and Koch have proposed several influential hypotheses (see Crick 1984). One of them is the notion that sensory consciousness must involve *binding* of widely separated sensory feature neurons for color, motion, shading, and so forth, into a single coherent representation, perhaps involving temporally coordinated oscillations (see Singer and Gray, chap. 64). Another is that in visual cortex, the first projection area V1 may not be the locus of visual consciousness, although damage to V1 does abolish visual experience (see Weiskrantz, chap. 9). Yet perhaps their most important contribution has been simply to encourage scientists to take a serious look at a formerly taboo problem.

References for each section introduction do not include chapters in this volume.

Consciousness: Respectable, Useful, and Probably Necessary

George Mandler

I welcome this opportunity to act as *amicus curiae* on behalf of one of the central concepts of cognitive theory—consciousness. Another statement, however imperfect, may be useful to undo the harm that consciousness suffered during fifty years (approximately 1910 to 1960) in the oubliettes of behaviorism. It is additionally needed because so many of us have a history of collaboration with the keepers of the jail and to speak freely of the need for a concept of consciousness still ties the tongues of not a few cognitive psychologists.

I hope to show that consciousness is respectable in the sense that it has become the object of serious and impressive experimental research; it is useful because it avoids circumlocutions as well as constructions, such as short-term memory and focal attention, that are more easily addressed by an appeal to consciousness as part of the apparatus of cognition; and it is probably necessary because it serves to tie together many disparate but obviously related mental concepts, including attention, perceptual elaboration, and limited capacity notions.

The Revival of Consciousness

The history of consciousness is strewn with philosophical, theological, and pedestrian semantic debris; the history of unconscious concepts has, by inherited contrast, suffered similarly. Having made the decision to recall the concept of consciousness to service, it is useful to start baldly with the distinction between conscious and unconscious processes. I do so with some sense of embarrassment vis-à-vis the contributions of others. Freud, in particular, has contributed much to the finer distinctions among shadings of the unconscious. However, if we are to make a fresh start within the experimental investigation of consciousness, we shall probably also have

to rediscover these distinctions within the new realm of discourse. For present purposes the distinction among preconscious, preattentitive, primary processes, and unconscious are premature. It suffices to distinguish those processes that are accessible to consciousness and those that are not. We shall note that Neisser, for example, assumes that the product of preattentive (preconscious) processes are holistic, vague, and unelaborated. It is not at all certain that current research on reading and language production and comprehension will bear out this assumption. Miller (1962), following Freud, set a distinct boundary between preconscious and unconscious processes, implying that the latter are inaccessible. The evidence suggests that accessibility of unconscious processes shades from the readily accessible to the inaccessible. In what follows I shall have repeated occasions to use the various different terms of consciousness as they occur in context. However, the intent, from my vantage point, is—at this time—to distinguish only between the contents of consciousness and unconscious processes. The latter include these that are no available to conscious experience, be they feature analyzers, deep syntactic structures, affective appraisals, computational processes, language production systems, action system of many kinds, or whatever.

Much of what we know and say today about consciousness has been known and said by others before us, in the past hundred years by Wundt, the Würzburgers, Lashley, and many others. I only want to summarize here the high points of a modern view of consciousness as it has developed, or rather revived, during the development of a disciplined and highly structured new view of cognitive psychology.

The development of this viewpoint was tentative, as one would expect it to be against the background of the established dogma of behaviorism in the United States. In 1962, George A.

Miller, one of the prophets of the new mentalism of the 1970s, started off his discussion of consciousness by suggesting that we "ban the word [consciousness] for a decade or two until we can develop more precise terms for the several uses which 'consciousness' now obscures" (p. 25). More than a decade has passed and we seem to be doing as prescribed without any intervening banishment. Most current thought on the topic was, as a matter of fact, well summarized by Miller.

Following William James, Miller stressed the selective functions of consciousness—the notion that only some part of all the possible experiences that are available at any point in time and space is selected for conscious expression. Miller also noted what we will stress again later, namely that "the selective function of consciousness and the limited span of attention are complementary ways of talking about the same thing" (p. 49). And, with Lashley, he reminds us that "[it] is the *result* of thinking, not the process of thinking that appears spontaneously in consciousness" (p. 56).

It is well to keep that last statement in mind, because it is an important part of the new mentalism, of modern cognitive psychology, of the human information processing approach. "Thinking" or cognition or information processing for the psychologist is a term that refers to theoretical processes, complex transformations on internal and external objects, events, and relations. These processes are not conscious; they are, in the first instance, constructions generated by the psychological theorist. By definition the conscious individual cannot be conscious—in any acceptable sense of the term—of theoretical processes involved to explain his actions. In the same sense, the term *mind* refers to the totality of theoretical processes that are ascribed to the individual. To accept this point of view avoids the solipsisms and sophisms of philosophies of mind.

The important advances in our excursions into consciousness must come through the usual in-

terplay of empirical investigation and imaginative theory. The functions of consciousness are slowly being investigated and the beginnings of theoretical integrations of the concept of consciousness into cognitive models are emerging.

As a prolegomena to theory and better understanding of private knowledge, Natsoulas (1970) has examined the content of "introspective awareness." Although he does not present us with any conclusions, Natsoulas has provided a partial list of the problems that psychologists and philosophers encounter when they want to deal directly with these contents. We have, in general, not gone far beyond such a listing since it is obviously too early to argue for a specific model of private experience or consciousness—it does not exist, not even in the broadest outline. However, some of the necessary first steps have been taken to build some of the components that such a theory must accommodate. At the same time, psychologists are becoming sensitive to the need for a critical evaluation of common sense and philosophical notions about consciousness. Many phenomenologically oriented philosophers and psychologists are still wedded to a Wundtian idea that psychology should be the study of conscious mental events, whereas unconscious (mental) mechanisms are to be left to some other world such as physiology.

In modern theory, one of the most influential books, Neisser's *Cognitive psychology* (1967), is strangely circumspect about the problem of consciousness. Was it too early then to talk openly about the Imperial Psychology's clothes? Not that Neisser avoids the subject—he clearly talks about consciousness though one comes upon it in circuitous ways. In his final chapter Neisser tackles the relationship between iconic memory and consciousness; he comes to consciousness via the attentive processes in visual perception and thence to memory. He notes that the constructive processes in memory "themselves never appear in consciousness, their products do" (Neisser 1967, p. 301). And in rational problem solving the executive processes "share many of the properties of focal attention in vision and of analysis-by-synthesis in hearing" (p. 302). Noting the distinction between primary and secondary processes (see also Garner 1974), he asserts that rational and therefore presumably conscious thought operates as a secondary process—elaborating often unconscious, probably unlearned primary process operations in the Freudian sense. The products of the primary process alone, preceding consciousness and attention, are only "fleetingly" conscious unless elaborated by secondary processes. By implication the elaboration by secondary processes is what produces fully conscious events. By tentative implication primary processes are "like" preattentive processes in vision and hearing, the conscious processes are "like" focal attention. The secondary processes elaborate and select. We shall hear similar arguments from Posner and Shallice shortly. However, Neisser's contribution to the study of consciousness is in his discussion of preattentive processes and focal attention. When we turn to these processes, the clues from the final chapter open up a major contribution to the theory of consciousness. I apologize for the talmudic exegesis before coming to this point, but it does, I believe, illustrate the gingerly and skitterish way in which psychologists, up until very recently, have permitted themselves to talk about consciousness.

In chapter 4, Neisser starts by taking the term "focal attention" straight from Schachtel (1959), a psychoanalyst whose history has not prevented a frank discussion of these forbidden topics. If you will, in what follows, permit the free translation of "attention" into consciousness, you will note why Neisser's contribution is important.

First, "attention ... is an allotment of analysing mechanisms to a limited region of the field" (p. 88). In other words, consciousness is a limited capacity mechanism. On the other hand, preattentive processes, that is, processes that are not in attention but precede it, have the function of forming the objects of attention. Some of these preattentive processes (the primary processes of the final chapter) are innate. Many actions are under such preattentive control. Walking, driving, and many others are "made without the use of focal attention" (p. 92). There are processes that run off outside of consciousness (unconsciously) while others do not: "More permanent storage of information requires an act of attention" (p. 93). Transfer to permanent storage requires consciousness. As apparently do some decisional processes. Harking back to another ear, "the processes of attentive synthesis often lead to an internal verbalization" (p. 103). We often talk about the contents of consciousness.

In brief summary, then, Neisser's interpretation is in concord with much modern speculation about the role of consciousness. It is a limited-capacity mechanism, often synonymous with the notion of attention. The processes that make up consciousness are secondary processes, secondary in elaboration and time to primary, preattentive processes that are unconscious, sometimes innate and often the result of automatization. Consciousness is an area that permits decision processes of some types to operate, where the outputs from different systems may be integrated, and where transfers to long term storage systems take place.[1]

Among the important attempts specifically to incorporate awareness notions into contemporary cognitive theory, Shallice (1972) has argued for the necessity of studying phenomena of consciousness if for no other reasons than that there exist a number of concepts in current psychological theory that require the implicit or explicit postulation of some consciousness mechanisms. Among these are the postulation of conscious rehearsal in primary memory and the frequent equation of attention and consciousness (see, e.g., Mandler 1974); others are methodological, as in experiments which require subjects to monitor private experiences (e.g., Sperling 1967). In his theoretical development Shallice argues for an isomorphism between phenomenal experience and information-processing concepts.

Specifically he develops in some detail the notion that the content of consciousness can be identified with a selector input that determines first what particular action system will become dominant, and, second, sets the goal for the action system.

Another approach, derived from problems of attention, has been mounted by Posner and his associates. They have focused on those mental operations which are characterized by interference effects or in other words, by a limited capacity mechanism which may be related to the "subjective experience of the unity of consciousness" (Posner and Keele 1970). By studying the processes that interfere one with another and showing how limited capacity is assigned to different functions, one can "connect the operations of this limited capacity mechanism to intention, awareness, storage and other traditional functions of consciousness" (Posner and Keele 1970).

Both Shallice and Posner deny any attempt to specify a mechanism of consciousness or private experience that is coextensive with common language uses of the concept. The attempt is, so to speak, from the bottom up, trying to specify with some rigor some of the mechanisms that may be isomorphic with consciousness and learn more about their operation within theoretical systems.

Posner and Boise (1971) in their ingenious study of the components of attention have noted that "attention in the sense of central processing capacity is related to mental operations of which we are conscious, such as rehearsing or choosing a response ..." (p. 407). Conversely, they noted that the contact between input and long-term memory is not part of this attentional (conscious) process, and in fact, the conscious component of the processing mechanism occurs, as a result, rather late in the sequence of "attentional" events.

Posner and Klein (1973) have summarized this interpretation of the use of "consciousness" within the context of experimental investigations. They suggest that it refers to operations such as rehearsal or priming that require access to a limited capacity system. Although the conscious processes are usually late in the processing sequence and follow "habitual" or preattentive encoding, they are flexible and may occur early under time pressure. Also, in a bridge to other similar views these processes are seen as setting up required responses "without depending upon the actual release of the motor program" (Posner and Klein 1973, p. 34).[2]

The recurrent theme of readiness for and choices among actions has also been invoked by Festinger et al. (1967). They have suggested that, in part, the conscious aspect of some perceptual phenomena depends on preprogrammed sets of efferent (action) programs that a particular input puts into a state of readiness for immediate use.

The limited evidence from the experimental studies as well as from informed theory points to extensive preconscious processing which is, under some circumstances, followed by conscious processing. Much of behavior, however, is automatic and does not require conscious attention. Typically such actions are called habitual, automatic, or preprogrammed. Typically also they tend to be ballistic in form and run off with little variation.

It is far beyond the scope of this paper to discuss the problem of automaticity and the kinds of structures that occur automatically in contrast with those that require attentional, conscious work. In reference to response sequences—or actions systems as I prefer to call them now—I have discussed the notion that cognitive structures or symbolic analogues of discrete actions systems develop during overlearning (Mandler 1962). It is well known in the integration that occurs during skill learning, for example, driving. I allude to the probem here simply to note that much of "learned" behavior and actions can be integrated into new central structures, which then become functional units represented cognitively as single chunks and manipulable consciously in the constructions of new plans and new actions. At the action side of consciousness relatively little work has been done to describe how the limited capacity system is used in integrating representation of overt actions into larger units. Just as consciousness deals with chunks of incoming information, so must it deal with chunks of efferent actions.

In the arena of perceptual events the topic of automatic processing or encoding confronts us repeatedly as the converse of conscious processing. Posner and Warren (1972) have discussed the variety of such automatic processes involved in coding mechanisms. Generally what is automatic is very much like what Neisser calls preattentive, parallel processes. In contrast, Posner and Warren note that conscious processes are more variable and that conscious constructions provide the new mnemonic devices needed to store material in long-term representations. It is here that we face the insistence that new encodings for long-term storage depend on a functioning conscious system.

LaBerge (1974) has addressed the issue of automatization in a novel way—asking not only about the relation between automatization and attention, but also about the process whereby certain coding systems become automatized. He concludes that during postcriteria performance there occurs a gradual withdrawal of attention from the particular components of a task. Under this process of decreasing attention (consciousness?) the part of the processing involved in coding the particular perceptual material is being made automatic. Eventually much of the perceptual processing can "be carried out automatically, that is prior to the focussing of attention on the processing." LaBerge also implies that this postcriterial, overlearning process produces the integration of new, higher order units or chunks. He is obviously addressing the development of preattentive processes, and also the functional unity and autonomy of these units, particularly when he notes that often "one cannot prevent the processing once it starts." There is a useful similarity between these propositions about the development of automatic encodings

and my previous discussion on the representation of overlearned action patterns.

We have here a possible distinction between two kinds of unconscious (preattentive, primary) processes. Those that are innate or preprogrammed or dependent primarily on some structural characteristics of the organism; those that, though initially conscious, become, by some process such as overlearning, automatic and unconscious. Although the latter are easily brought into consciousness it is also intuitively likely that this might be difficult, if not impossible, for the former.

It seems to be agreed that consciousness is a clearing house that enters into the flow of processing under certain specifiable, but at present still not specified, conditions. Certain processes operate on conscious information generaged by nonconscious (preattentive) processes. However, it bears repeating that there are important nonconscious postattentive processes that are operative subsequent to information generated by conscious processes. Many of these involve actions (which my older colleagues in psychology have inadequately called "behavior") that operate often without conscious attention. These actions and their representation systems are as complex and as finely structured as the preattentive perceptual systems. Unfortunately, partly by accidents of history, cognitive psychologists tend to be somewhat careless about specifying how organisms come to act. However, the hierarchic, structural view of action has an honorable and creative history. I would draw your attention to the most recent and important exposition of this view proposed by Gallistel (1974).

In summary, current thought has concentrated on the consciousness of the perceptual or encoding side of information flow. Some attention has been given to its functions in memory storage and retrieval. Much is still to be done at the output side. Current notions have focussed on the functions of consciousness as selecting encoded sensory information and preparing choices among appropriate action or response alternatives. Many other functions of consciousness still await detailed analyses or may be incorrect assignments to this particular system.

Conscious Contents and Processes

My own interest in consciousness arose in part out of a long-term project on the relation between mind and emotion, and more immediately out of some recent considerations of the limits of attention and consciousness (Mandler 1974). In that presentation I argued for a direct translation between focal attention and consciousness. I suggested that some of the so-called short-term memory phenomena are best assigned to the limited capacity mechanism of consciousness and that the limitations of that single conscious system in terms of dimensional analyses may serve as a bridging concept for George A. Miller's puzzle about the similar limitations he noted for both short term memory and absolute judgment.

The limited capacity of "short-term" memory, the immediate memory span, as well as the limitation in absolute judgment task to some seven values or categories, can usefully be assigned to the limited capacity of conscious content. The limitation refers to the limited number of values on any single dimension (be it physical, acoustic, semantic, or whatever) that can be kept within the conscious field.

The main points of the argument relevant to the present topic concern certain distinctions among the concepts of attention, consciousness and short-term memory. In the first instance, I want to restrict the concept of consciousness to events and operation within a limited capacity system, with the limitation referring to number of functional units or chunks that can be kept in consciousness at any one point in time. This concept has much in common with what has been called *focal attention*. Attentional processes are those mechanisms that deal with the selection of objects or events that occur in consciousness. Second, I want to assert a distinction between short-term memory and consciousness. The limited reach of consciousness has a respectable history, going back at least 200 years (see Mandler 1974). However, it is not a memory system—it does not involve any retrieval. What is in the momentary field of consciousness is not remembered, it is psychologically present.

None of the foregoing denies the utility of the conception of different memory systems, whether long term, working, or operational. It is probably most reasonable to consider these different "systems" on a continuum of depth of processing, as proposed by Craik and Lockhart (1972). Different types of analyses require different processing depths and different processing times. But the information that, so to speak, can be "read off" the contents of consciousness is not memorial as such. Depth of processing determines how and what can be remembered. If processing time is short, or encoding "superficial," and if the code decays rapidly, it will be short; if processing is extended or if encoding is "complex," information adequate for long term retrieval or reconstruction will be stored. Within certain limits, the storage processes—at whatever depths—can only take place on conscious material; conversely, retrieval usually implies retrieval into the conscious field. However, the memory *mechanisms* and the contents of consciousness are two very distinct kinds of mental events.

Posner, who has contributed much to recent investigations of the structure of the limited capacity system of conscious events, suggested as early as 1967 that "operational" and "short-term" memories should be considered as different systems. The operating systems may vary à la Craik and Lockhart in their time course and their products, but they should not be confounded with the immediately given content of consciousness. The confounding of these two systems in early investigations and theories is understandable, given the very brief time course of some memory processes and the rapid changes in the focus of consciousness (attention). However, within consciousness many different kinds of operations may be performed—consciousness is not limited in the complexity of the information it draws on, only in the amount. Consciousness is modality independent, and, depending on the task facing the individual, many involve very complex and abstract operations. In general then, I will prefer to use the term *consciousness* to focal attention (although they may have to be interchanged) but differentiate strictly between consciousness and short-term memory processes, which deal with storage and retrieval (cf. Craik and Lockhart 1972).

I do not intend to invoke a separate processing stage or system to accommodate the concept of consciousness. Consciousness, in the first instance, refers to a state of a structure. Certain operations and processes act on these structures which constitute conscious content. Cognitive structures, or schemas, may, under certain circumstances, become conscious, that is, enter the conscious state; when they do not, they are by definition unconscious. Limited capacity refers to the number of such unitary structures that may be conscious at any one point in time. There is no separate system, however, that contains the conscious contents. Rather conscious structures differ from others in that certain operations, such as storage, retrieval, and choice (see below), may be performed on them.

It is beyond the intent of this chapter to discuss the origins of consciousness. It is a characteristic of the organism that certain structures can become conscious, but it is a function of human interactions with the environment that determines which structures do in fact become conscious. Piaget (1953) has discussed extensively these interactions and stressed the transactions among perceptions of the self, the environment, and the development of consciousness. The development of consciousness is not, from my view, some magical burgeoning of internal awareness but rather dependent on specific organism-environment interactions. These

involve, to a large part, the internalizations of actions (see also Mandler 1962). More important, however, the conditions of personal and social development determine what can and what cannot be represented in consciousness. Depending on these conditions, different individuals, groups, and cultures will have different conscious contents—different social and cultural consciousness, different realities. However, the primary purpose of the present chapter is to discuss how these conscious contents operate, not what they are or how they might be established.

Finally, conscious contents can be spoken about. I shall discuss later the lack of any one-to-one correspondence between consciousness and language, but this should not obscure the important relationship between private conscious events and language. It is by the use of the latter that we primarily communicate our own private view of reality, and it is in turn by the use of language that, in the adult at least, many conscious structures are manipulated and changed.

With these primarily definitional problems out of the way, I want to address first some of the ancient and admittedly complex and very special problems that the concept of consciousness poses for any psychological theory. I shall not propose any radical solutions but rather that the problem of the private datum can be approached reasonably and analytically, rather than frantically or mystically. Next, I want to sketch some of the possible uses of consciousness in cognitive theory, followed by some suggestions for the adaptive functions of consciousness. Finally, in the last section, I want to address the broader problem of the flow of consciousness and its relations to limited capacity, with particular attention to special states of consciousness.

Consciousness: A Special Problem for Mental Theory

The individual experiences feelings, attitudes, thoughts, images, ideas, beliefs, and other contents of consciousness, but these contents are not accessible to anyone else. Briefly stated, that is the special problem facing psychologists. There are no evasions possible. It is not possible to build a phenomenal psychology that is shared. A *theory* of phenomena may be shared but the private consciousness, once expressed in words, gestures, or in any way externalized is necessarily a transformation of the private experience. No theory external to the individual, that is, one that treats the organism as the object of observation, description, and explanation, can at the same time be a theory that uses private experiences, feelings, and attitudes as data (see Gray 1971). Events and objects in consciousness can never be available to the observer without having been restructured, reinterpreted, and appropriately modified by structures that are specific to the individual doing the reporting. These structures may even be specific to the kinds of experiences, feelings, and attitudes that are reported. The content of consciousness, as philosophers and psychologists have told us for centuries, is not directly available as a datum in psychology.

How then are we to deal with the contents of consciousness? Can the perennial problem of private datum and public inference at least be stated concisely in order to indicate the magnitude of the problem and possible directions for future development?

We are faced with a phenomenon that might be called the uncertainty principle of psychology. Adrian (1966) for example, noted: "The particular difficulty that the questioner may influence the answer recalls the uncertainty principle in physics, which limits the knowledge we can gain about any individual particle" (p. 242).

There are two related problems in the study of consciousness. The first is more fundamental than the question that Adrian addresses. It is not only the case that the nature of the interrogation may affect the reported content of consciousness, but, more basically, the act of examination itself may affect the individually observable conscious contents. This conjecture is reasonable even at the level of processing capacity, since the con-

scious act of interrogating one's conscious content must occupy some part of the limited capacity. As a result the available content is altered by the process of interrogation.

Given that the act of interrogation changes the content of consciousness, the source of that inquiry becomes of secondary importance. The second problem to be faced is the fact that the contents of consciousness are not simply reproducible by some one-to-one mapping into verbal report. Even if these contents were always couched in language, which they surely are not, some theory of transmission would be required. As a result we are faced with the individual's observation of the contents of his consciousness on the one hand, and on the other with the psychologist's theoretical inference about those contents, based on whatever data, including introspective reports, are available. Both of these knowledges may be used as relevant to the construction of a psychology of cognition, though it may in principle be impossible to determine, in any exact sense, the relation between these two interpretations of consciousness.

Private experiences are important aspects of the fully functioning mental system. It is possible to get transformed reports about those events and it should be possible to develop appropriate theories that relate contents of consciousness, their transformations, and their report. However, it is not possible to build a theory that makes direct predictions about private experience since the outcome of those predictions cannot be inspected by the psychologist/observer.

This position does admit the development of private theories, by the individual—about himself. To the individual his experience *is* a datum, and as a consequence his theories about his own structures are, within limits, testable by direct experience. These individual, personal theories of the self are both pervasive and significant in explaining human action, but they cannot, without peril, be generalized to others or to the race as a whole (see Mandler and Mandler 1974).

We note, therefore, that people's reports about their experiences, their behavior, and their actions are very frequently, and may always be, fictions or theories about those events. However, it is only those reports that are available to us. Even the introspecting individual who says that his experience conforms to certain predicted aspects is making statements about derived correspondences resulting from mental transformations. Indirect scientific predictions about experiences are possible, but the test of those predictions is one step removed from the actual experiences, as are all predictions about the values of theoretical entities. If the behaviorist revolution, with all the negative influences it has had on the development of a fully theoretical psychology, has had one positive effect, it is this realization that even the complete acceptance of the importance of private experience does not thereby make it a possible end point for a scientific theory.

Some Uses of Consciousness

One of the important processes in which consciousness intervenes is in the testing of potential action choices and the appraisal of the situational givens. The relation between choice and consciousness, as we have seen, has motivated much of the recent research. The analysis of situations and appraisal of the environment, on the other hand, goes on mainly at the nonconscious level, which will be discussed in greater detail later. In any case, the outcomes of these analyses may be available in consciousness and the effect of potential actions on the present situation can be estimated and evaluated. Consciousness is a field in which potential choices are given the opportunity to be evaluated against potential outcomes. This delay produces reflective consideration and may in fact be responsible for greater "freedom" of action (see Mandler and Kessen 1974).

Much of what is often considered to be the meaning of the common sense term "thinking" is

what takes place in consciousness when the outcome of different structures, and even in some cases their composition, are evaluated and decisions are made. It is possible for the cognitive system to call for the testing of specific outcomes while temporarily blocking output from the system as a whole, to compare the consequences of different outcomes and to choose outcomes which produce one or another desired alternative. The notion of choice would be entirely within the context of modern choice theories (e.g., Luce 1959, Tversky 1972), and the choice itself, of course, would go through some "unconscious" cognitive structures before a "decision" is made. However, consciousness permits the comparison and inspection of various outcomes so that the choice systems which may in fact be "unconscious" can operate on these alternatives.

It appears that one of the functions of the consciousness mechanism is to bring two or more (previously unconscious) mental contents into direct juxtaposition. The phenomenal experience of choice, as a matter of fact, seems to demand exactly such an occurrence. We usually do not refer to a choice unless there is a "conscious" choice between two or more alternatives. The attribute of "choosing" is applied to a decision process between two items on a menu, several possible television programs, or two or more careers, but not to the decision process that decides whether to start walking across a street with the right or left foot, whether to scratch one's ear with a finger or the ball of the hand, or whether to take one or two sips from a cup of hot coffee. I would argue that the former cases involve the necessity of deciding between two or more choices presented to a choice mechanism at the same time, whereas the latter involve only the situationally predominant action. However, these cases may be transferred to the conscious choice state if and when certain conditions of possible consequences and immediate adaptability supervene. Given a hot cup of coffee so labeled, I may "choose" to take one very small sip, or I may "choose" to start with my right foot in a 100-meter race, given certain information on its advantage to my time in the distance. In other words, consequences and social relevance determine which choices are conscious. More important, however, the mechanisms of choice (including the various theories of choice behavior) are not conscious. It is presumably the operation of these mechanisms on material in the conscious state that give the epiphenomenal experience of free choice, the appearance that someone (the agent) is doing the choosing. He or she is, but by the operation of unconscious mechanisms, which therefore give the appearance of voluntary choice among the conscious alternatives. Mental mechanisms "choose" among both conscious and unconscious events.

It might be noted that the so-called mentalism that philosophers talk about often refers to these "thought" processes, the outcome of unconscious mental processes that are evaluated in the "conscious" system. However, to mistake conscious mental events for much more complex nonconscious structures is surely in error and leads to the kind of naive mentalism shown in the works of some philosophers of the mind.

Evaluative activities often act on conscious content, but evaluative activities also may take place at an "unconscious" level. Clearly many cognitive structures that lead to certain outcomes and the anticipation of these outcomes (a scanning ahead of a particular structure) may switch the system from one structure to another. However, these changes are not available to inspection, and are only available to indirect inspection by the process of hypothesizing their constitution and testing these hypotheses.

If the only difference between these two kinds of evaluative actions and choices is that some take place in consciousness and others do not, the end result would be a rather puny achievement for so imposing a mechanism as consciousness. I would propose initially two arguments for the distinction between conscious and unconscious evaluations and choices. First,

many relational processes operate primarily, if not exclusively, on conscious content. I have already indicated this particular argument in the case of simple choice. However, there are other relational operators that seem to do their work primarily on conscious content. In addition to choice, these include evaluation, comparison, grouping, categorization, and serial ordering. In short, practically all novel relational orderings require that the events to be ordered must be simultaneously present in the conscious field. This applies to choice, as well as to relational concepts stored in memory, for example. Needless to say, there are many relational judgments that do not require conscious comparisons. To say that "a dog is an animal" makes uses of established structures and does not require a new relational operation. However, to say that "Rex looks like a cross between a dachshund and a spaniel" would presumably require conscious juxtaposition. Once relations (by they superordinate, subordinate, opposites, or whatever) have been established and stored, subsequent evaluations are frequently unconscious.

The second argument for the importance of consciousness suggests that choice and other processes that operate on conscious content are dependent on those structures that can enter the conscious state. Only those structures that can become conscious can be subjected to choice activities. Thus, situational and social relevance determine the content of consciousness and the "ideational' operations that can be performed on the individual's reality.

The Possible Adaptive Functions of Consciousness

One may look at some of these uses also from the point of view of their adaptive significance. Probably because of the unpleasantness of the past 50 or 60 years relatively little has been said about the adaptive functions of consciousness. Miller (1962) has described them in general terms and Gray (1971) has called for a more intensive look at the evolutionary significance of conscious systems. In general, however, American psychologists particularly have shied away from looking at the functional significance of consciousness. This is at least surprising, since we are faced with a characteristic of the human species that is without exception. Given the rather weak evidence that psychologists have accepted as indicants for the evolutionary significance of such vague concepts as aggression and intelligence, why avoid a phenomenon as indisputably characteristic of the species as consciousness? Partly, the answer lies in the behaviorist dogma that consciousness is epiphenomenal and, by implication, has no adaptive significance. It is in part in opposition to that dogma that I want to suggest some possible directions in which speculations and investigations about the adaptiveness of consciousness might go.

There is a variety of functions that the consciousness system may perform, all of which may be said to have evolutionary significance and all of which have varying degrees of evidence for their utility and theoretical significance:

1. The first, and most widely addressed function of consciousness considers it as a scratch pad for the choice and selection of actions systems. Decisions are made often on the basis of possible outcomes, desirable outcomes, and appropriateness of various actions to environmental demands. Such a description comes close to what is often called "covert trial and error" behavior in the neobehaviorist literature. This function permits the organism more complex considerations of action-outcome contingencies than does the simple feedback concept of reinforcement, which alters the probability of one or another set of actions. It also permits the consideration of possible actions that the organisms has never before performed, thus eliminating the overt testing of possible harmful alternatives. In this sense the process is similar to the TOTE system of Miller, Galanter, and Pribram (1960).

2. Within the same general framework as the first function, consciousness is used to modify and interrogate long-range plans, rather than immediate-action alternatives. In the hierarchy of actions and plans in which the organism engages, this slightly different function makes it possible to organize disparate action systems in the service of a higher plan. For example, in planning a drive to some new destination one might consider subsets of the route, or, in devising a new recipe, the creative chef considers the interactions of several known culinary achievements. Within the same realm, consciousness is used to retrieve and consider modifications in long-range planning activities. These, in turn, might be modified in light of other evidence, either from the immediate environment or from long term storage.

3. In considering actions and plans consciousness participates in retrieval programs from long-term memory, even though these retrieval programs and strategies themselves are usually not conscious. Thus, frequently, though not always, the retrieval of information from long-term storage is initiated by relatively simple commands—in program language, rather than machine language. These may be simple instructions such as, "What is his name?" or, "Where did I read about that?" or more complex instructions, such as, "What is the relation between this situation and previous ones I have encountered?" This process has the adaptive function of permitting simple addresses to complex structures.

4. Comments on the organism's current activities occur in consciousness and use available cognitive structures to construct some storable representation of current activity. Many investigators have suggested that these new codings and representations always take place in consciousness. Such processes as mnemonic devices and storage strategies apparently require the intervention of conscious structures. Certainly many of them, such as categorization and mental

images, do. Once this new organization of information is stored, it may be retrieved for a variety of important purposes.

First, in the social process consciousness provides access to the memory bank which, together with an adequate system of communication, such as human language, has tremendous benefit to cooperative social efforts. Other members of the species may receive solutions to problems, thus saving time if nothing else; they may be appraised of unsuccessful alternatives, or, more generally, participate in the cultural inheritance of the group. This process requires selection and comparison among alternatives retrieved from long-term storage, all of which apparently takes place in consciousness.

Second, both general information, as well as specific sensory inputs, may be stored in either propositional or analogue form. The rerepresentation at some future time makes possible decision processes that depend on comparisons between current and past events, and the retrieval of relevant or irrelevant information for current problem solving.

5. Another aspect that consciousness apparently permits is a "troubleshooting" function for structures normally not represented in consciousness. There are many systems that cannot be brought into consciousness, and probably most systems that analyze the environment in the first place have that characteristic. In most of these cases only the product of cognitive and mental activities are available to consciousness; among these are sensory analyzers, innate action patterns, language-production systems, and many more. In contrast, many systems are generated and built with the cooperation of conscious processes, but later become nonconscious or automatic. These latter systems may apparently be brought into consciousness, particularly when they are defective in their particular function (see also Vygotsky 1962). We all have had experiences of automatically driving a car, typing a letter, or even handling cocktail party conversation, and being suddenly brought up short

by some failure such as a defective brake, a stuck key, or a "You aren't listening to me." At that time, the particular representations of actions and memories involved are brought into play in consciousness, and repair work gets under way. Thus, structures that are not species specific and general but are the result of experience can be inspected and reorganized more or less easily.

Many of these functions permit the organism to react reflectively rather than automatically, a distinction that has frequently been made between humans and lower animals. All of them permit more adaptive transactions between the organism and its environment. Also, in general, the functions of consciousness permit a focusing upon the most important and species relevant aspects of the environment. The notion that attentional mechanisms select personally relevant materials and events is commonplace in attentional research. The processes that define such relevance are generally unknown, although we can assume that an adaptive function of selection into consciousness exists. However, there remains the unexplored mystery of the processes of information reduction that select some aspect of the surround.

The need for a rapid reduction of all the sensory information available to an organism at any given point in time and space is obvious. If we were conscious of all the information available at the sensory surface, we would never escape from the confusion generated by our environment. Consciousness (or attention) is highly selective. The sensory systems themselves are, of course, selective in the first instance. The evolutionary process has generated organisms that register only a limited amount of the information available in their environment. How these limitations from the environment to the sensory surface have developed has been the subject of some biological speculations. The reduction from the sensory surface to consciousness is even more spectacular, but we have few clues for the evolutionary reason of this reduction. We know that it exists (e.g. Miller 1956, Mandler 1974), and attention theorists have been concerned primarily with the filtering mechanisms that reduce the sensory information to the few chunks of information that reach consciousness. However, why that number should be 5 or 6 or 7, rather than 3 or 12, is still shrouded in mystery.

The Limitation of Conscious Capacity and the Flow of Consciousness

One of the most perplexing results of experimental studies of consciousness has been the counterintuitive notion that consciousness seems to be discrete, relatively short, and quite transient. How does this contrast with consciousness in the common discourse? It seems to be continuous, flowing, extending without break throughout our waking hours, and just as flowing and continuous in our dreams. William James aptly called it "the stream of thought, of consciousness, or of subjective life." How can we reconcile these two impressions?

Before tackling that particular problem, consider the role of consciousness in our perception of time, or better, duration. For this purpose, I shall adopt the theory of time duration proposed by Ornstein (1969). This review relates the time experience to "the mechanisms of attention, coding, and storage" (Ornstein 1969, p. 48). Ornstein's central thesis is that storage size is the basis for the construction of the duration of an interval. The notion of storage size derives directly from recent organizational theory that emphasizes the compact organization of information in memory and experience. The more different unrelated units the greater the storage size, the more highly organized the units, objects, or events are, the fewer are the units or chunks and the smaller is the storage size. As storage size of the material in consciousness increases, the duration experience lengthens. What changes storage size are increases or decreases in the amount of information received, changes in the coding or chunking of input, or, as Ornstein has

shown experimentally, influencing the memory of the interval after it has passed. As Ornstein summarized in a later book (1972) "the more organized ... the memory ... the shorter the experience of duration" (p. 87).

Generally, then, the experience of duration (in consciousness) is one possible construction drawing on immediately pressing factors (such as attentiveness) but primarily on our stored long-term memory. Duration is constructed—first in the momentary consciousness, and second in the retrieval of events and codes that are recalled during the "construction" of a past interval. The contents of consciousness thus determine the experience of duration. Restricting these contents shortens duration, expanding them, for example, by increasing the complexity of an experience lengthens duration. Viligance, which increases expectancy of some event, lengthens duration; Ornstein uses the example of the "watched pot." On the other hand, condensing some experience into a very brief code ("I made breakfast") condenses the duration. Ornstein notes, as have others, that our Western linear mode of constructing duration is not the only mode and that present centeredness is not only possible but, in fact, the mode for other cultures than ours. The concatenation of limited conscious capacity, on the one hand, and the same consciousness serving as a vehicle for constructing experience of duration, on the other, brings us back to the disjunction between discrete consciousness and the flow of consciousness.

There is in principle no objection to constructing a flow model of consciousness out of the discrete units of attention or consciousness. The metaphor that comes to mind is a simplistic view of modern conceptions of light, which may be described either in terms of particles or in terms of waves. Again borrowing from physics, we then may metaphorically speak of the quantum of consciousness on the one hand and the flow of consciousness on the other. Another possible metaphor is that of the illusion of moving pictures that consist of individual frames.

Neither metaphor probably does justice to the phenomenon, as no metaphor ever does. In particular, it is likely that instead of individual quanta or frames, the flow of consciousness frequently may involve the successive sampling of materials across a continuous retrieval of connected material from long-term storage. Such a phenomenon would depend on the retrieval strategies being used on long-term storage as well as on the nature of the material being sampled. In the case of consciousness of externally generated events, for example, somebody else's speech, the overlapping moving model may be the most appropriate, whereas in attempting the retrieval of a specific chunk of knowledge, the retrieval may be discontinuous.

Because of the limited capacity characteristics of discrete consciousness, I shall use the figure of speech of the conscious frame. We still carry with us the unsolved problem of the content of that slice of consciousness. For the time being we can only allude to the probability that it involves units or chunks of unitary aggregates of information.

Regardless of one's view of the conscious frame as sampling discrete, overlapping, or continuous elements of mental content or environmental input, our view requires a continuous interchange between long-term storage and the conscious state. In the case of an exclusively internal dialogue between the two, material is brought into consciousness and then returned to long-term storage either in essentially unchanged form or after some operations may have been performed on it while in consciousness. Thus, the memory of a friend brought into consciousness may be combined with a new insight that he resembles a recent acquaintance, and then the information is returned with the new relationship coded with it. Or information from storage is brought (within consciousness) in conjunction with new information currently being processed from the environment, for example, "Joe has grown a beard" and then returned to storage newly coded. Many experimental studies of memory require exactly this retrieval from storage and combination, in consciousness, with new information, such as that the word belongs to a particular list or category, or occurs at a particular serial position. I should note, of course, that the distinction between internal and external information is not a very clean one. Clearly, external events do not enter into consciousness as "pure" perceptions, rather they are coded and identified in terms of existing preattentive structures before they enter consciousness.

In general this position joins the long tradition of cognitive and phenomenological psychologists in asserting the importance of the role of consciousness in developing knowledge of oneself and the environment. I do not think that consciousness is primary or sufficient; it is one mode of processing. Just because some evaluation or knowledge does not enter consciousness does not permit a pejorative evaluation of such "automatic" or "unconscious" processing.

Conscious Stopping

One special reason why the view of the conscious frame is useful is that it permits a consideration of the special conditions when the flow of consciousness stops, single frames enter into consciousness, and remain there. Experimental psychologists have paid some attention to this phenomenon, as in the concept of maintaining or primary rehearsal, in which material is repeated but does not enter into long-term storage (Craik and Watkins 1973, Woodward, Bjork, and Jongeward 1973). However, the major source of knowledge of this phenomenon comes from esoteric psychologies and meditative methods.

The best objective presentation of these methods is once again provided by Ornstein (1972). He reviews meditation techniques dispassionately and positively. However, in reading Ornstein's description of these methods, a recurrent theme may be discerned. The achievement of the special kinds of conscious states that are claimed to occur seem to depend, without exception, on the unique attempt to stop the flow of ordinary consciousness—to concentrate on the frame, to hold it fixed in the focus of consciousness. The very difficulty of achieving the initial, apparently trivial, exercises of these techniques suggest the difficulty of stopping the flow. It requires total attention to a single, restricted set of limited thoughts or perceptions. In Zen, the exercises start with counting breaths, and then go on to concentrate on the process of breathing. Yogic meditation uses the *mantra*, "sonorous, flowing words which repeat easily." Some of the Sufi practices are seen as an "exercise for the brain based on repetition." The Christian mystic St. John of the Cross says (quoted in Ornstein 1972): "Of all these forms and manners of knowledge the soul must strip and void itself and it must strive to lose the imaginary apprehension of them, so that there may be left in it no kind of impression of knowledge, nor trace of thought.... This cannot happen unless the memory can be annihilated in all its forms,..." (pp. 119–120). Or, as Ornstein points out, many prayers are monotonous, repetitive chants. In summary, "[The] common element in these diverse practices seems to be the active restriction of awareness to one single, unchanging process, and the withdrawal of attention from ordinary thought" (Ornstein 1972, p. 122). Again: "The specific object used for meditation is much less important than the maintenance of the object as the single focus of awareness during a long period of time ..." (p. 122).

I suggest that the "object of the single focus" must be no more than a frame of consciousness, that in fact it is restricted by the very limits that the limited capacity mechanism has been shown to exhibit. One could not mediate on an event that, at first, contains more than five to seven chunks. The observations that Ornstein and many others have reported suggest that it is in fact possible to stop the flow of consciousness to keep a single frame of consciousness in focus for extended periods of time. However, such an experience should in fact be a very *different* form

of consciousness; the normal form is the flow. We thus become aware of this new consciousness, though only after the extensive practice it requires. However, we must also experience a very different content of consciousness. Given that the single "object" is held in consciousness, many new and different aspects of it then may be discovered.

Consider the possibility that at first any such object consists of several related qualities (or chunks). Presumably as these various attributes are related one to the other, the new relations form a more compact perception; the number of chunks, as it were, is reduced. In turn, this opens up the possibility of new chunks or attributes entering into the single frame. New relationships are discovered and again coalesce. Under these circumstances we may go through a process of structuring and restructuring, of discovering aspects of objects or events that would not normally be available during the flow of consciousness. Once this ability has been achieved, one should, in principle, be able to use the special consciousness to stop the flow of events, examine new nuances, and then continue. Thus, a limited set of attributes within a single frame is available at first; then new aspects enter and old ones drop away. The complexities of a rose, a face, or a cake "become conscious." This seems, in fact, to be taking place in what Ornstein calls the "opening up" of awareness, which follows the "turning off" phase and which provides the individual with a different state of comprehension of ongoing actions and events. Again, to quote Ornstein (1972): "The concentrative form turns off the normal mode of operation and allows a sensitivity to subtle stimuli which often go unnoticed in the normal mode.... It also produces an *aftereffect* of 'fresh' perception when the practitioner returns to his usual surroundings" (p. 136). All I wish to add to Ornstein's insightful discussion is the possibility that modern psychology may define the process wherein this attentiveness occurs and also the processes which generate new perceptions and sensitivities. Meditative techniques provide us, in this fashion, with new insights into a mechanism that otherwise seems rather mundane and restrictive. There need not be anything mysterious about meditation, nor anything pedestrian about an information processing analysis of consciousness.

The enriching of knowledge though meditative experiences or, as we might call it, conscious stopping, should be put into the proper context of the ordinary, normal means of enriching experience. Without doubt, we enrich our experience and knowledge about the world around us without resorting to meditation. We can, without special preparation, perceive new facets about the world, about other people, even about ourselves as we gain new perspectives, new ways of structuring out experience. One of the main differences between the normal and the meditative enrichment is that the former deals with an open system; the latter deals with a closed one. Our enrichment in knowledge and appreciation of a lover, a novel, a science, an occupation occurs always in new contexts, sometimes widely different, sometimes only minutely so. However, the relationship between the object or event and ourselves is changed continuously by our mutual relations with the rest of the world. The new information, in a way, is always acquired in new contexts. What seems to distinguish this usual accretion from the meditative one is that the latter is a closed system; we are restricted to those relationships among qualities and attributes that are given in that object or situation. This restriction of possible relations presumably provides not only the illusion but possibly also the reality of depth of perception which the special experience provides. In contrast, artists and scientists, for example, apparently achieve the same depth of perception of special objects or events without the meditative experience.

Ornstein's notion that the experience of duration is constructed, based on the storage size of the cognitive structures that constitute an interval, may be applied directly to the flow and frame aspects of consciousness. In the open-system flow, time experience is constructed across frames out of cognitive structures that will, to varying degrees, occupy the capacity of the limited-capacity frame. Consider listening to a lecture on difficult, but interesting material. As the speaker proceeds, information is transmitted at a great rate, taking up the full capacity of each frame of consciousness. In Ornstein's terms, storage of information is near a maximum. As a result, the duration experience increases. In contrast, the redundant speaker makes fewer demands on each frame, the very ability to approach a difficult subject slowly and cumulatively permits us to use less of the full capacity of the frame, or, as another possibility, the capacity is filled less frequently in physical time and fewer frames are expended. In any case, the experience of duration is more extended in the former than in the latter case.

It is interesting to speculate that Ornstein's storage metaphor may be directly translated into the frame locution. Since consciousness is necessary for the transfer of information to long-term storage, complex (many chunks and relations) information requires more frames for the transfer function, as does rapidly presented information (more chunks per unit physical time). It appears that the storage metaphor is quite consistent with the frame-flow notion of consciousness. In the latter mode the construction of time depends on the sheer number of frames of consciousness activated or utilized during a specified interval. Parenthetically this position also indicates the independence of the conscious frame from physical time. The specious present, the limited-capacity mechanism, does not have a time constant. Frames are replaced under a variety of conditions, all of which seem to depend on using up their capacity, a new perceptual dimension, another class of stimulation, a sudden demand for focusing (attention), and many others will demand a shift to another content of consciousness, which is perceived as another *moment* of consciousness.

Finally, we may note the rather drastic changes in time perception that take place as a result of meditative experience. Given that the flow of frames is radically altered, one would naturally expect a similar and unusual change in duration experiences. The direction can be either way. Holding a single unit of consciousness and impeding the flow may collapse the duration experience, whereas the eventual ability to manipulate the flow of consciousness may change the usual duration experience with its apparently rather constant rate of change into a more variable ebb and flow of "short" and "long" durations. Instead of the flow of frames during normal states, during meditation the change from one conscious content to another occurs infrequently in physical time. The slow changes in perceptual structures which I suggested earlier for the meditative phase thus produce unusual duration experiences.

It is intriguing to speculate that the action of hallucinogenic or "mind-expanding" drugs has a similar locus and effect. Changes in perceptual processes coexist with changes in the experience of duration. It has been argued that these drugs often produce in the instant the experiences that meditative methods generate with extensive practice. It is possible that some drugs in fact slow the flow of conscious frames, and that some of the lasting effects of these drugs may be due to structural changes in control of the flow of consciousness.

Conclusion

The concept of consciousness was abandoned as a proper object of experimental study some 60 years ago. The reasons were manifold. The introspective method erred in assuming that consciousness could be made the datum of psychology or that verbal report was a royal road to its exploration. The failure of introspection both engendered behaviorism and failed to provide any viable alternatives. Others, like the Gestalt

school and the French and English enclaves, successfully defended their views of the conscious organism, but had, for theoretical reasons, little grounds to mount a major analytic attack. The return of American psychology to a theory-rich as well as experimentally rigorous stance has given us the opportunity to develop the proper theoretical tools to return consciousness to its proper place in a theory of thought, mind, and actions. Most of the early steps that have been taken have been necessarily preliminary models and developments of experimental methods. My primary aim in these pages has been to try to point to the directions that these preliminary steps are taking. Granted that this has been a personal view at the current stage, it will have been successful if it generates discussion and investigation and, eventually, theory, which will define and specify the role that consciousness plays in man's transactions with his world.

Acknowledgments

The preparation of this chapter was supported in part by grants from the National Science Foundation (GB 20798) and the National Institute of Mental Health (MH-15828). I am indebted to my students and colleagues at the Center for Human Information Processing for listening and reacting to my preliminary meanderings on the topic of consciousness. I am in great debt to my colleague Jean M. Mandler, whose patient and insightful critiques went far beyond the requirements of connubial duty. Both Ulric Neisser and C. R. Gallistel critically and creatively reacted to an earlier version—and I hope that this chapter does justice to their valuable assistance.

Notes

1. In a personal communication Neisser has indicated that he does *not* believe that consciousness is a useful concept for a stage of mental processing and that his

avoidance of the concept has been deliberate rather than unconscious.

2. Posner has extended these views most instructively in this volume.

References

Adrian, E. D. Consciousness. In J. C. Eccles (Ed.), *Brain and conscious experience*. New York: Springer Publ., 1966.

Craik, F. I. M., & Lockhart, R. S. Levels of processing: A framework for memory research. *Journal of Verbal Learning and Verbal Behavior*, 1972, 11, 671–684.

Craik, F. I. M., & Watkins, M. J. The role of rehearsal in short-term memory. *Journal of Verbal Learning and Verbal Behavior*, 1973, 12, 599–607.

Festinger, L., Burnham, C. A., Ono, H., & Bamber, D. Efference and the conscious experience of perception. *Journal of Experimental Psychology Monograph*, 1967, 74, No. 4.

Gallistel, C. R. Motivation as central organizing process: The psychophysical approach to its functional and neurophysiological analysis. In *Nebraska symposium on motivation: 1974*. Lincoln, Nebraska: University of Nebraska Press, 1974.

Garner, W. R. *The processing of information and structure*. Hillsdale, New Jersey: Lawrence Erlbaum Associates, 1974.

Gray, J. A. The mind-brain identity theory as a scientific hypothesis. *Philosophical Quarterly*, 1971, 21, 247–252.

LaBerge, D. Acquisition of automatic processing in perceptual and associative learning. In P. M. A. Rabbitt & S. Dornic (Eds.), *Attention and performance V*. London: Academic Press, 1974.

Luce, R. D. *Individual choice behavior: A theoretical analysis*. New York: Wiley, 1959.

Mandler, G. From association to structure. *Psychological Review*, 1962, 69, 415–427.

Mandler, G. Memory storage and retrieval: Some limits on the reach of attention and consciousness. In P. M. A. Rabbitt & S. Dornic (Eds.), *Attention and performance V*. London: Academic Press, 1974.

Mandler, G., & Kessen, W. The appearance of free will. In S. C. Brown (Ed.), *Philosophy of psychology*. London: Macmillan, 1974.

Mandler, J. M., & Mandler, G. Good guys vs. bad guys: The subject-object dichotomy. *Journal of Humanistic Psychology*, 1974, 14, 63–87.

Miller, G. A. The magic number seven, plus or minus two: Some limits on our capacity for processing information. *Psychological Review*, 1956, 63, 81–97.

Miller, G. A. *Psychology: The science of mental life*. New York: Harper and Row, 1962.

Miller, G. A., Galanter, E. H., & Pribram, K. *Plans and the structure of behavior*. New York: Holt, 1960.

Natsoulas, T. Concerning introspective "knowledge." *Psychological Bulletin*, 1970, 73, 89–111.

Neisser, U. *Cognitive psychology*. New York: Appleton-Century-Crofts, 1967.

Ornstein, R. E. *On the experience of time*. Harmondsworth: Penguin, 1969.

Ornstein, R. E. *The psychology of consciousness*. San Francisco: Freeman, 1972.

Piaget, J. *The origin of intelligence in the child*. London: Routledge & Kegan Paul, 1953.

Posner, M. I. Short-term memory systems in human information processing. *Acta Psychologica*, 1967, 27, 267–284.

Posner, M. I., & Boies, S. J. Components of attention. *Psychological Review*, 1971, 78, 391–408.

Posner, M. I., & Keele, S. W. Time and space as measures of mental operations. Paper presented at the Annual Meeting of the American Psychological Association, 1970.

Posner, M. I., & Klein, R. M. On the functions of consciousness. In S. Kornblum (Ed.), *Attention and performance IV*. New York: Academic Press, 1973.

Posner, M. I., & Warren, R. E. Traces, concepts, and conscious constructions. In A. W. Melton & E. Martin (Eds.), *Coding processes in human memory*. Washington, D.C.: Winston, 1972.

Schachtel, E. G. *Metamorphosis*. New York: Basic Books, 1959.

Shallice, T. Dual functions of consciousness. *Psychological Review*, 1972, 79, 383–393.

Sperling, G. Successive approximations to a model for short-term memory. *Acta Psychologica*, 1967, 27, 285–292.

Tversky, A. Elimination by aspects: A theory of choice. *Psychological Review*, 1972, 79, 281–299.

Vygotsky, L. S. *Thought and language.* Cambridge, Mass.: MIT Press, 1962.

Woodward, A. E., Jr., Bjork, R. A., & Jongeward, R. H., Jr. Recall and recognition as a function of primary rehearsal. *Journal of Verbal Learning and Verbal Behavior*, 1973, 12, 608–617.

3 Consciousness and Neuroscience

Francis Crick and Christof Koch

Clearing the Ground

We assume that when people talk about "consciousness," there is something to be explained. While most neuroscientists acknowledge that consciousness exists, and that at present it is something of a mystery, most of them do not attempt to study it, mainly for one of two reasons:

1. They consider it to be a philosophical problem, and so best left to philosophers.

2. They concede that it is a scientific problem, but think it is premature to study it now.

We have taken exactly the opposite point of view. We think that most of the philosophical aspects of the problem should, for the moment, be left on one side, and that the time to start the scientific attack is now.

We can state bluntly the major question that neuroscience must first answer. It is probable that at any moment some active neuronal processes in your head correlate with consciousness, while others do not: *what is the difference between them*? In particular, are the neurons involved of any particular neuronal type? What is special (if anything) about their connections? And what is special (if anything) about their way of firing? The neuronal correlate of consciousness is often referred to as the NCC. Whenever some information is represented in the NCC it is represented in consciousness.

In approaching the problem, we made the tentative assumption (Crick and Koch 1990) that all the different aspects of consciousness (pain, visual awareness, self-consciousness, and so on) employ a basic common mechanism or perhaps a few such mechanisms. If one could understand the mechanism for one aspect, then, we hope, we will have gone most of the way towards understanding them all.

We made the personal decision (Crick and Koch 1990) that several topics should be set aside or merely stated without further discussion, for experience had shown us that valuable time can be wasted arguing about them without coming to any conclusion.

1. Everyone has a rough idea of what is meant by being conscious. For now, it is better to avoid a precise definition of consciousness because of the dangers of premature definition. Until the problem is understood much better, any attempt at a formal definition is likely to be either misleading or overly restrictive, or both. If this seems evasive, try defining the word "gene." So much is now known about genes that any simple definition is likely to be inadequate. How much more difficult, then, to define a biological term when rather little is known about it.

2. It is plausible that some species of animals—in particular the higher mammals—possess some of the essential features of consciousness, but not necessarily all. For this reason, appropriate experiments on such animals may be relevant to finding the mechanisms underlying consciousness. It follows that a language system (of the type found in humans) is not essential for consciousness—that is, one can have the key features of consciousness without language. This is not to say that language does not enrich consciousness considerably.

3. It is not profitable at this stage to argue about whether simpler animals (such as octopus, fruit flies, nematodes) or even plants are conscious (Nagel 1997). It is probable, however, that consciousness correlates to some extent with the degree of complexity of any nervous system. When one clearly understands, both in detail and in principle, what consciousness involves in humans, then will be the time to consider the problem of consciousness in much simpler animals. For the same reason, we will not ask

whether some parts of our nervous system have a special, isolated, consciousness of their own. If you say, "Of course my spinal cord is conscious but it's not telling me," we are not, at this stage, going to spend time arguing with you about it. Nor will we spend time discussing whether a digital computer could be conscious.

4. There are many forms of consciousness, such as those associated with seeing, thinking, emotion, pain, and so on. Self-consciousness—that is, the self-referential aspect of consciousness—is probably a special case of consciousness. In our view, it is better left to one side for the moment, especially as it would be difficult to study self-consciousness in a monkey. Various rather unusual states, such as the hypnotic state, lucid dreaming, and sleep walking, will not be considered here, since they do not seem to us to have special features that would make them experimentally advantageous.

Visual Consciousness

How can one approach consciousness in a scientific manner? Consciousness takes many forms, but for an initial scientific attack it usually pays to concentrate on the form that appears easiest to study. We chose visual consciousness rather than other forms, because humans are very visual animals and our visual percepts are especially vivid and rich in information. In addition, the visual input is often highly structured yet easy to control.

The visual system has another advantage. There are many experiments that, for ethical reasons, cannot be done on humans but can be done on animals. Fortunately, the visual system of primates appears fairly similar to our own (Tootell et al. 1996), and many experiments on vision have already been done on animals such as the macaque monkey.

This choice of the visual system is a personal one. Other neuroscientists might prefer one of the other sensory systems. It is, of course,

important to work on alert animals. Very light anaesthesia may not make much difference to the response of neurons in macaque V1, but it certainly does to neurons in cortical areas like V4 or IT (inferotemporal).

Why Are We Conscious?

We have suggested (Crick and Koch 1995a) that the biological usefulness of visual consciousness in humans is to produce the best current interpretation of the visual scene in the light of past experience, either of ourselves or of our ancestors (embodied in our genes), and to make this interpretation directly available, for a sufficient time, to the parts of the brain that contemplate and plan voluntary motor output, of one sort or another, including speech.

Philosophers, in their carefree way, have invented a creature they call a "zombie," who is supposed to act just as normal people do but to be completely *un*conscious (Chalmers 1995). This seems to us to be an untenable scientific idea, but there is now suggestive evidence that part of the brain does behave like a zombie. That is, in some cases, a person uses current visual input to produce a relevant motor output, without being able to say what was seen. Milner and Goodale (1995) point out that a frog has at least two independent systems for action, as shown by Ingle (1973). These may well be unconscious. One is used by the frog to snap at small, prey-like objects, and the other for jumping away from large, looming discs. Why does not our brain consist simply of a series of such specialized zombie systems?

We suggest that such an arrangement is inefficient when very many such systems are required. Better to produce a single but complex representation and make it available for a sufficient time to the parts of the brain that make a choice among many different but possible plans for action. This, in our view, is what seeing is about. As pointed out to us by Ramachandran and

Hirstein (1997), it is sensible to have a *single* conscious interpretation of the visual scene, in order to eliminate hesitation.

Milner and Goodale (1995) suggest that in primates there are two systems, which we shall call the on-line system and the seeing system. The latter is conscious, while the former, acting more rapidly, is not. The general characteristics of these two systems and some of the experimental evidence for them are outlined below in the section on the on-line system. There is anecdotal evidence from sports. It is often stated that a trained tennis player reacting to a fast serve has no time to see the ball; the seeing comes afterwards. In a similar way, a sprinter is believed to start to run before he consciously hears the starting pistol.

The Nature of the Visual Representation

We have argued elsewhere (Crick and Koch 1995a) that to be aware of an object or event, the brain has to construct a multilevel, explicit, symbolic interpretation of part of the visual scene. By multilevel, we mean, in psychological terms, different levels such as those that correspond, for example, to lines or eyes or faces. In neurological terms, we mean, loosely, the different levels in the visual hierarchy (Felleman and Van Essen 1991).

The important idea is that the representation should be explicit. We have had some difficulty getting this idea across (Crick and Koch 1995a). By an explicit representation, we mean a small-ish group of neurons which employ coarse coding, as it is called (Ballard et al. 1983), to represent some *aspect* of the visual scene. In the case of a particular face, all of these neurons can fire to somewhat face-like objects (Young and Yamane 1992). We postulate that one set of such neurons will be all of one type (say, one type of pyramidal cell in one particular layer or sublayer of cortex), will probably be fairly close together, and will all project to roughly the same place. If

all such groups of neurons (there may be several of them, stacked one above the other) were destroyed, then the person would not see a face, though he or she might be able to see the parts of a face, such as the eyes, the nose, the mouth, etc. There may be other places in the brain that explicitly represent other aspects of a face, such as the emotion the face is expressing (Adolphs et al. 1994).

Notice that while the *information* needed to represent a face is contained in the firing of the ganglion cells in the retina, there is, in our terms, no explicit representation of the face there.

How many neurons are there likely to be in such a group? This is not yet known, but we would guess that the number to represent one aspect is likely to be closer to 10^2-10^3 than to 10^4-10^6.

A representation of an object or an event will usually consist of representations of many of the relevant aspects of it, and these are likely to be distributed, to some degree, over different parts of the visual system. How these different representations are bound together is known as the binding problem (von der Malsburg 1995).

Much neural activity is usually needed for the brain to construct a representation. Most of this is probably unconscious. It may prove useful to consider this unconscious activity as the computations needed to find the best interpretation, while the interpretation itself may be considered to be the *results* of these computations, only some of which we are then conscious of. To judge from our perception, the results probably have something of a winner-take-all character.

As a working hypothesis we have assumed that only some types of specific neurons will express the NCC. It is already known (see the discussion under "Bistable Percepts") that the firing of many cortical cells does not closely correspond to what the animal is currently seeing. An alternative possibility is that the NCC is necessarily global (Greenfield 1995). In one extreme form this would mean that, at one time or another, any neuron in cortex and associated structures could express the NCC. At this point we feel it more fruitful to explore the simpler hypothesis—that only particular types of neurons express the NCC—before pursuing the more global hypothesis. It would be a pity to miss the simpler one if it were true. As a rough analogy, consider a typical mammalian cell. The way its complex behavior is controlled and influenced by its genes could be considered to be largely global, but its genetic instructions are localized, and coded in a relatively straightforward manner.

Where Is the Visual Representation?

The conscious visual representation is likely to be distributed over more than one area of the cerebral cortex and possibly over certain subcortical structures as well. We have argued (Crick and Koch 1995a) that in primates, contrary to most received opinion, it is not located in cortical area V1 (also called the striate cortex or area 17). Some of the experimental evidence in support of this hypothesis is outlined below. This is not to say that what goes on in V1 is not important, and indeed may be crucial, for most forms of vivid visual awareness. What we suggest is that the neural activity there is not directly correlated with what is seen.

We have also wondered (Crick 1994) whether the visual representation is largely confined to certain neurons in the lower cortical layers (layers 5 and 6). This hypothesis is still very speculative.

What Is Essential for Visual Consciousness?

The term 'visual consciousness' almost certainly covers a variety of processes. When one is actually looking at a visual scene, the experience is very vivid. This should be contrasted with the much less vivid and less detailed visual images produced by trying to remember the same scene.

(A vivid recollection is usually called a hallucination.) We are concerned here mainly with the normal vivid experience. (It is possible that our dimmer visual recollections are mainly due to the back pathways in the visual hierarchy acting on the random activity in the earlier stages of the system.)

Some form of very short-term memory seems almost essential for consciousness, but this memory may be very transient, lasting for only a fraction of a second. Edelman (1989) has used the striking phrase 'the remembered present' to make this point. The existence of iconic memory, as it is called, is well-established experimentally (Coltheart 1983; Gegenfurtner and Sperling 1993).

Psychophysical evidence for short-term memory (Potter 1976; S. Subramaniam, I. Biederman and S. A. Madigan, submitted) suggests that if we do not pay attention to some part or aspect of the visual scene, our memory of it is very transient and can be overwritten (masked) by the following visual stimulus. This probably explains many of our fleeting memories when we drive a car over a familiar route. If we do pay attention (e.g., a child running in front of the car) our recollection of this can be longer lasting.

Our impression that at any moment we see all of a visual scene very clearly and in great detail is illusory, partly due to ever-present eye movements and partly due to our ability to use the scene itself as a readily available form of memory, since in most circumstances the scene usually changes rather little over a short span of time (O'Regan 1992).

Although working memory (Baddeley 1992; Goldman-Rakic 1995) expands the time frame of consciousness, it is not obvious that it is *essential* for consciousness. It seems to us that working memory is a mechanism for bringing an item, or a small sequence of items, into vivid consciousness, by speech, or silent speech, for example. In a similar way, the episodic memory enabled by the hippocampal system (Zola-Morgan and Squire 1993) is not essential for consciousness, though a person without it is severely handicapped.

Consciousness, then, is enriched by visual attention, though attention is not essential for visual consciousness to occur (Rock et al. 1992; Braun and Julesz 1997). Attention is broadly of two types: bottom-up, caused by the sensory input; and top-down, produced by the planning parts of the brain. This is a complicated subject, and we will not try to summarize here all the experimental and theoretical work that has been done on it.

Visual attention can be directed to either a location in the visual field or to one or more (moving) objects (Kanwisher and Driver 1992). The exact neural mechanisms that achieve this are still being debated. In order to interpret the visual input, the brain must arrive at a *coalition* of neurons whose firing represents the best interpretation of the visual scene, often in competition with other possible but less likely interpretations; and there is evidence that attentional mechanisms appear to bias this competition (Luck et al. 1997).

Recent Experimental Results

We shall not attempt to describe all the various experimental results of direct relevance to the search for the neuronal correlates of visual consciousness in detail but rather outline a few of them and point the reader to fuller accounts.

Action without Seeing

Classical Blindsight
This will already be familiar to most neuroscientists. It is discussed, along with other relevant topics, in an excellent book by Weiskrantz (1997). It occurs in humans (where it is rare) when there is extensive damage to cortical area V1 and has also been reproduced in monkeys (Cowey and Stoerig 1995). In a typical case, the patient can indicate, well above chance level, the direction of movement of a spot of light over a certain range of speed, while denying that he sees anything at all. If the movement is less salient, his performance falls to chance; if more salient (that is, brighter or faster), he may report that he had some ill-defined visual percept, considerably different from the normal one. Other patients can distinguish large, simple shapes or colors. (For Weiskrantz's comments on Gazzaniga's criticisms, see pp. 152–153; and on Zeki's criticisms, see pp. 247–248.)

The pathways involved have not yet been established. The most likely one is from the superior colliculus to the pulvinar and from there to parts of visual cortex; several other known weak anatomical pathways from the retina and bypassing V1 are also possible. Recent functional magnetic resonance imaging of the blindsight patient G. Y. directly implicates the superior colliculus as being active *specifically* when G. Y. correctly discriminates the direction of motion of some stimulus without being aware of it at all (Sahraie et al. 1997—this paper should be consulted for further details of the areas involved).

The On-line System
The broad properties of the two hypothetical systems—the on-line system and the seeing system—are shown in table 3.1, following the account by Milner and Goodale in their book, *The visual brain in action* (1995), to which the reader is referred for a more extended account. For a recent review, see Boussaoud et al. 1996. The on-line system may have multiple subsystems (for eye movements, for arm movements, for body posture adjustment, and so on). Normally, the two systems work in parallel, and indeed there is evidence that in some circumstances the seeing system can interfere with the on-line system (Rossetti 1998).

One striking piece of evidence for an on-line system comes from studies on patient D. F. by Milner, Perrett, and their colleagues (1991). Her brain has diffuse damage produced by carbon

Table 3.1
Comparison of the hypothetical on-line system and the seeing system (based on Milner and Goodale, 1995)

	On-line system	Seeing system
Visual inputs handled	must be simple	can be complex
Motor outputs produced	stereotyped responses	many possible responses
Minimum time needed for response	short	longer
Effect of a few seconds' delay	may not work	can still work
Coordinates used	egocentric	object-centered
Certain perceptual illusions	not effective	seen
Conscious	no	yes

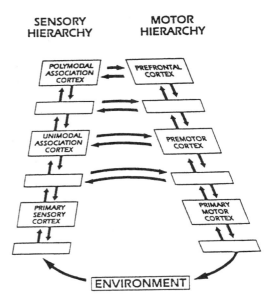

Figure 3.1
Fuster's figure (reproduced with permission by Lippincott-Raven Publishers) showing the fiber connections between cortical regions participating in the perception-action cycle. Empty rhomboids stand for intermediate areas or subareas of the labeled regions. Notice that there are connections between the two hierarchies at several levels, not just at the top level.

monoxide poisoning. She is able to see color and texture very well but is very deficient in seeing orientation and form. In spite of this, she is very good at catching a ball. She can "post" her hand or a card into a slot without difficulty, though she cannot report the slot's orientation.

It is obviously important to discover the difference between the on-line system, which is unconscious, from the seeing system, which is conscious. Milner and Goodale (1995) suggest that the on-line system mainly uses the dorsal visual stream. They propose that rather than being the "where" stream, as suggested by Ungerleider and Mishkin (1982), it is really the "how" stream. This might imply that all activity in the dorsal stream is unconscious. The ventral stream, on the other hand, they consider to be largely conscious. An alternative suggestion, due to Steven Wise (personal communication and Boussaoud et al. 1996), is that direct projections from parietal cortex into premotor areas are unconscious, whereas projections to them via prefrontal cortex are related to consciousness.

Our suspicion is that while these suggestions about two systems are on the right lines, they are probably oversimple. The little that is known of the neuroanatomy would suggest that there are likely to be *multiple* cortical streams, with numerous anatomical connections between them (Distler et al. 1993). This is implied in figure 3.1, a diagram often used by Fuster (Fuster 1997: see his fig. 8.4). In short, the neuroanatomy does not suggest that the sole pathway goes up to the highest levels of the visual system, and from there to the highest levels of the prefrontal system and then down to the motor output. There are numerous pathways from most intermediate levels of the visual system to intermediate frontal regions.

We would therefore like to suggest a general hypothesis: that the brain always tries to use the *quickest appropriate* pathway for the situation at hand. Exactly how this idea works out in detail remains to be discovered. Perhaps there is competition, and the fastest stream wins. The postulated on-line system would be the quickest of these hypothetical cortical streams. This would be the zombie part of you.

Bistable Percepts

Perhaps the present most important experimental approach to finding the NCC is to study the behavior of single neurons in the monkey's brain when it is looking at something that produces a bistable percept. The visual input, apart from minor eye movements, is constant; but the subject's percept can take one of two alternative forms. This happens, for example, when one looks at a drawing of the well-known Necker cube.

It is not obvious where to look in the brain for the two alternative views of the Necker cube. Allman suggested a more practical alternative: to study the responses in the visual system during binocular rivalry (Myerson et al. 1981). If the visual input into each eye is different, but perceptually overlapping, one usually sees the visual input as received by one eye alone, then by the other one, then by the first one, and so on. The input is constant, but the percept changes. Which neurons in the brain mainly follow the input, and which the percept?

This approach has been pioneered by Logothetis and his colleagues working on the macaque visual system. They trained the monkey to report which of two rival inputs it saw. The experiments are difficult, and elaborate precautions had to be taken to make sure the monkey was not cheating. The fairly similar distribution of switching times strongly suggests that monkeys and humans perceive these bistable visual inputs in the same way.

The first set of experiments (Logothetis and Schall 1989) studied neurons in cortical area MT (medial temporal, also called V5), since they preferentially respond to movement. The stimuli were vertically drifting horizontal gratings. Only the first response was recorded. Of the relevant neurons, only ~35% were modulated according to the monkey's reported percept. Surprisingly, half of these responded in the opposite direction to the one expected.

The second set of experiments (Leopold and Logothetis 1996) used stationary gratings. The orientation was chosen in each case to be optimal for the neuron studied, and orthogonal to it in the other eye. They recorded how the neuron fired during several alterations of the reported percept. The neurons were in foveal V1/V2 and in V4. The fraction following the percept in V4 was similar to that in MT, but a rather smaller fraction of V1/V2 neurons followed the percept. Also, here, but not in V4, none of the cells were anticorrelated with the stimulus.

The results of the third set of experiments (Sheinberg and Logothetis 1997) were especially striking. In this case the visual inputs tried included images of humans, monkeys, apes, wild animals, butterflies, reptiles, and various manmade objects. The rival image was usually a sunburst-like pattern (see figure 3.2). If a new image was flashed into one eye while the second eye was fixating another pattern, the new stimulus was the one that was always perceived ("flash suppression"). Recordings were made in the upper and lower banks of the superior temporal sulcus (STS) and inferior temporal cortex (IT). Overall, ~90% of the recorded neurons in STS and IT were found to reliably predict the perceptual state of the animal. Moreover, many of these neurons responded in an almost all-or-none fashion, firing strongly for one percept, yet only at noise level for the alternative one.

More recently, Bradley et al. (1998) have studied a different bistable percept in macaque MT, produced by showing the monkey, on a television screen, the two-dimensional projection of a transparent, rotating cylinder with random dots on it, without providing any stereoscopic disparity information. Human subjects

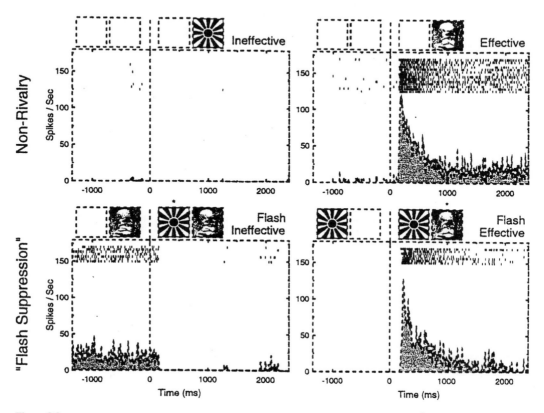

Figure 3.2
The activity of a single neuron in the superior temporal sulcus (STS) of a macaque monkey in response to different stimuli presented to the two eyes (taken from Sheinberg and Logothetis 1997). In the upper left panel a sunburst pattern is presented to the right eye without evoking any firing response ("ineffective" stimulus). The same cell will fire vigorously in response to its "effective" stimulus, here the image of a monkey's face (upper right panel). When the monkey is shown the face in one eye for a while, and the sunburst pattern is flashed onto the monitor for the other eye, the monkey signals that it is "seeing" this new pattern and that the stimulus associated with the rival eye is perceptually suppressed ("flash suppression"; lower left panel). At the neuronal level, the cell shuts down in response to the ineffective yet perceptual dominant stimulus following stimulus onset (at the dotted line). Conversely, if the monkey fixates the sunburst pattern for a while, and the image of the face is flashed on, it reports that it perceives the face, and the cell will now fire strongly (lower right panel). Neurons in V4, earlier in the cortical hierarchy, are largely unaffected by perceptual changes during flash suppression.

exploit structure-from-motion and see a three-dimensional cylinder rotating around its axis. Without further clues, the direction of rotation is ambiguous and observers first report rotation in one direction, a few seconds later, rotation in the other direction, and so on. The trained monkey responds as if it saw the same alternation. In their studies on the monkey, about half the relevant MT neurons Bradley et al. recorded from followed the percept (rather than the "constant" retinal stimulus).

These are all exciting experiments, but they are still in the early stages. Just because a particular neuron follows the percept, it does not automatically imply that its firing is part of the NCC. The NCC neurons may be mainly elsewhere, such as higher up in the visual hierarchy. It is obviously important to discover, for each cortical area, *which* neurons are following the percept (Crick 1996). That is, what type of neurons are they, in which cortical layer or sublayer do they lie, in what way do they fire, and, most important of all, *where do they project*? It is, at the moment, technically difficult to do this, but it is essential to have this knowledge, or it will be almost impossible to understand the neural nature of consciousness.

Electrical Brain Stimulation

An alternative approach, with roots going back to Penfield (1958), involves directly stimulating cortex or related structures in order to evoke a percept or behavioral act. Libet and his colleagues (Libet 1993) have used this technique to great advantage on the somatosensory system of patients. They established that a stimulus, at or near threshold, delivered through an electrode placed onto the surface of somatosensory cortex or into the ventrobasal thalamus required a minimal stimulus duration (between 0.2 and 0.5 s) in order to be consciously perceived. Shorter stimuli were not perceived, even though they could be detected with above-chance probability, using a two-alternative, forced-choice

procedure. In contrast, a skin or peripheral sensory-nerve stimulus of very short duration could be perceived. The difference appears to reside in the amount and type of neurons recruited during peripheral stimulation versus direct central stimulation. Using sensory events as a marker, Libet also established (1993) that events caused by direct cortical stimulation were back-dated to the beginning of the stimulation period.

In a series of classical experiments, Newsome and colleagues (Britten et al. 1992) studied the macaque monkey's performance in a demanding task involving visual motion discrimination. They established a quantitative relationship between the performance of the monkey and the neuronal discharge of neurons in its medial temporal cortex (MT). In 50% of all the recorded cells, the psychometric curve—based on the behavior of the entire animal—was statistically indistinguishable from the neurometric curve—based on the averaged firing rate of a single MT cell. In a second series of experiments, cells in MT were directly stimulated via an extracellular electrode (Salzman et al. 1990) (MT cells are arranged in columnar structure for direction of motion). Under these conditions, the performance of the animal shifted in a predictable manner, compatible with the idea that the small brain stimulation caused the firing of enough MT neurons, encoding for motion in a specific direction, to influence the final decision of the animal. It is not clear, however, to what extent visual consciousness for this particular task is present in these highly overtrained monkeys.

The V1 Hypothesis

We have argued (Crick and Koch 1995a) that one is not directly conscious of the features represented by the neural activity in primary visual cortex. Activity in V1 may be necessary for vivid and veridical visual consciousness (as is activity in the retinae), but we suggest that the firing of none of the neurons in V1 directly correlates with what we consciously see. (For a critique of our hypothesis, see Pollen 1995, and our reply, Crick and Koch 1995b.)

Our reasons are that at each stage in the visual hierarchy the explicit aspects of the representation we have postulated are always recoded. We have also assumed that any neurons expressing an aspect of the NCC must project directly, without recoding, to at least some of the parts of the brain that plan voluntary action—that is what we have argued seeing is for. We think that these plans are made in some parts of frontal cortex (see below).

The neuroanatomy of the macaque monkey shows that V1 cells do not project directly to any part of frontal cortex (Crick and Koch 1995a). Nor do they project to the caudate nucleus of the basal ganglia (Saint-Cyr et al. 1990), the intralaminar nuclei of the thalamus (L. G. Ungerleider, personal communication), the claustrum (Sherk 1986) nor to the brainstem, with the exception of a small projection from peripheral V1 to the pons (Fries 1990). It is plausible, but not yet established, that this lack of connectivity is also true for humans.

The strategy to verify or falsify this and related hypotheses is to relate the receptive field properties of individual neurons in V1 or elsewhere to perception in a quantitative manner. If the structure of perception does not map to the receptive field properties of V1 cells, it is unlikely that these neurons directly give rise to consciousness. In the presence of a correlation between perceptual experience and the receptive field properties of one or more groups of V1 cells, it is unclear whether these cells just correlate with consciousness or directly give rise to it. In that case, further experiments need to be carried out to untangle the exact relationship between neurons and perception.

A possible example may make this clearer. It is well known that the color we perceive at one particular visual location is influenced by the wavelengths of the light entering the eye from surrounding regions in the visual field (Land and McCann 1971, Blackwell and Buchsbaum 1988).

This form of (partial) color constancy is often called the Land effect. It has been shown in the anesthetized monkey (Zeki 1980, 1983; Schein and Desimone 1990) that neurons in V4, but *not* in V1, exhibit the Land effect. As far as we know, the corresponding information is lacking for alert monkeys. If the same results could be obtained in a behaving monkey, it would follow that it would not be *directly* aware of the "color" neurons in V1.

Some Experimental Support

In the last two years, a number of psychophysical, physiological and imaging studies have provided some support for our hypothesis, although this evidence falls short of proving it (He et al. 1995, Kolb and Braun 1995, Cumming and Parker 1997, summarized in Koch and Braun 1996; but see Morgan et al. 1997). Let us briefly discuss two other cases.

When two isoluminant colors are alternated at frequencies beyond 10 Hz, humans perceive only a single fused color with a minimal sensation of brightness flicker. In spite of the perception of color fusion, color opponent cells in primary visual cortex of two alert macaque monkeys follow high-frequency flicker well above heterochromatic fusion frequencies (Gur and Snodderly 1997). In other words, neuronal activity in V1 can clearly represent certain retinal stimulation yet is not perceived. This is supported by recent fMRI studies on humans by Engel et al. (1997).

The study by He et al. (1996) is based on a common visual aftereffect (see figure 3.3a). If a subject stares for a fraction of a minute at a horizontal grating, and is then tested with a faint grating at the same location to decide whether it is oriented vertically or horizontally, the subject's sensitivity for detecting a horizontal grating will be reduced. This adaptation is orientation specific—the sensitivity for vertical gratings is almost unchanged—and disappears quickly. He and colleagues projected a single patch of grating onto a computer screen some

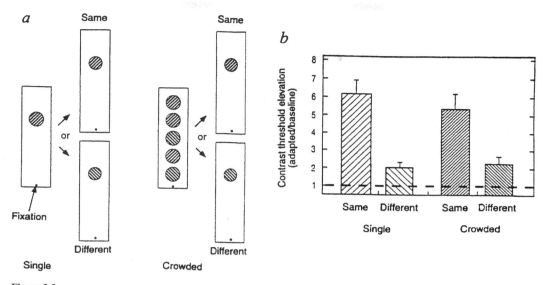

Figure 3.3
Psychophysical displays (schematic) and results pertaining to an orientation-dependent aftereffect induced by "crowded" grating patches (reproduced with permission from He, Cavanagh, and Intriligator 1996). (*a*) Adaptation followed by contrast threshold measurement for a single grating (left) and a crowded grating (right). In each trial, the orientation of the adapting grating was either the same or orthogonal to the orientation of the test grating. Observers fixated at a distance of ~25° from the adapting and test gratings. (*b*) Threshold contrast elevation after adaptation relative to baseline threshold contrast before adaptation. Data are averaged across four subjects. The difference between same and different adapt-test orientations reflects the orientation-selective aftereffect of the adapting grating. The data show that this aftereffect is comparable for a crowded grating (whose orientation is not consciously perceived) and for a single grating (whose orientation is readily perceived).

25° from the fixation point. It was clearly visible and their subjects showed the predictable orientation-selective adaptation effect. Adding one or more similar patches of gratings to either side of the original grating—which remained exactly as before—removed the lines of the grating from visibility; it was now "masked." Subjectively, one still sees "something" at the location of the original grating, but one is unable to make out its orientation, even when given unlimited viewing time. Yet despite this inability to "see" the adapting stimulus, the aftereffect was as strong and as specific to the orientation of the 'invisible' grating as when the grating was visible (see figure 3.3b). What this shows, foreshadowed by earlier

experiments (Blake and Fox 1974), is that visual awareness in such cases must occur at a higher stage in the visual hierarchy than orientation-specific adaptation. This aftereffect is thought to be mediated by oriented neurons in V1 and beyond, implying that at least in this case the neurons which mediate visual awareness must be located past this stage.

Our ideas regarding the absence of the NCC from V1 are not disproven by positron emission tomography experiments showing that in at least some people V1 is activated during visual imagery tasks (Kosslyn et al. 1995), though severe damage to V1 is compatible with visual imagery in patients (Goldenberg et al. 1995). There is no obvious reason why such top-down effects should not reach V1. Such V1 activity would not, by itself, prove that we are *directly* aware of it, any more than the V1 activity produced there when our eyes are open proves this. We hope that further neuroanatomical work will make our hypothesis plausible for humans, and that further neurophysiological studies will show it to be true for most primates. If correct, it would narrow the search to areas of the brain farther removed from the sensory periphery.

The Frontal Lobe Hypothesis

As mentioned several times, we hypothesize that the NCC must have access to explicitly encoded visual information and directly project into the planning stages of the brain, associated with the frontal lobes in general and with prefrontal cortex in particular (Fuster 1997). We would therefore predict that patients unfortunate enough to have lost their entire prefrontal cortex on both sides (including Broca's area) would not be visually conscious, although they might still have well-preserved, but unconscious, visual-motor abilities. No such patient is known to us (not even Brickner's famous patient; for an extensive discussion of this, see Damasio and Anderson 1993). The visual abilities of any such "frontal lobe" patient would need to be carefully evaluated using a battery of appropriate psychophysical tests.

The fMRI study of the blindsight patient G. Y. (Sahraie et al. 1997) provides direct evidence for our view by revealing that prefrontal areas 46 and 47 are active when G. Y. is visually aware of a moving stimulus.

Large-scale lesion experiments carried out in the monkey suggest that the absence of frontal lobes leads to complete blindness (Nakamura and Mishkin 1980, 1986). One would hope that future monkey experiments reversibly inactivate specific prefrontal areas and demonstrate the specific loss of abilities linked to visual percep-

tion while visual-motor behaviors—mediated by the on-line system—remain intact.

It will be important to study the pattern of connections between the highest levels of the visual hierarchy—such as inferotemporal cortex—and premotor and prefrontal cortex. In particular, does the anatomy reveal any feedback loops that might sustain activity between IT and prefrontal neurons (Crick and Koch 1998)? There is suggestive evidence (Webster et al. 1994) that projections from prefrontal cortex back into IT might terminate in layer 4, but these need to be studied directly.

Gamma Oscillations

Much has been made of the presence of oscillations in the gamma range (30–70 Hz) in the local-field potential and in multi-unit recordings in the visual and sensory-motor system of cats and primates (Singer and Gray 1995). The existence of such oscillations remains in doubt in higher visual cortical areas (Young et al. 1992). We remain agnostic with respect to the relevance of these oscillations to conscious perception. It is possible that they subserve attention or figure-ground in early visual processing.

Philosophical Matters

There is, at the moment, no agreed philosophical answer to the problem of consciousness, except that most living philosophers are not Cartesian dualists—they do not believe in an immaterial soul which is distinct from the body. We suspect that the majority of neuroscientists do not believe in dualism, the most notable exception being the late Sir John Eccles (1994).

We shall not describe here the various opinions of philosophers, except to say that while philosophers have, in the past, raised interesting questions and pointed to possible conceptual confusions, they have had a very poor record, historically, at arriving at valid scientific answers. For this reason, neuroscientists should listen to the questions philosophers raise but should not be intimidated by their discussions. In recent years the amount of discussion about consciousness has reached absurd proportions compared to the amount of relevant experimentation.

The Problem of Qualia

What is it that puzzles philosophers? Broadly speaking, it is qualia—the blueness of blue, the painfulness of pain, and so on. This is also the layman's major puzzle. How can you possibly explain the vivid visual scene you see before you in terms of the firing of neurons? The argument that you cannot explain consciousness by the action of the parts of the brain goes back at least as far as Leibniz (1686, trans. 1965). But compare an analogous assertion: that you cannot explain the "livingness" of living things (such as bacteria, for example) by the action of "dead" molecules. This assertion sounds extremely hollow now, for a number of reasons. Scientists understand the enormous power of natural selection. They know the chemical nature of genes and that inheritance is particulate, not blending. They understand the great subtlety, sophistication and variety of protein molecules, the elaborate nature of the control mechanisms that turn genes on and off, and the complicated way that proteins interact with, and modify, other proteins. It is entirely possible that the very elaborate nature of neurons and their interactions, far more elaborate than most people imagine, is misleading us, in a similar way, about consciousness.

Some philosophers (Searle 1984, Dennett 1996) are rather fond of this analogy between "livingness" and "consciousness," and so are we; but, as Chalmers (1995) has emphasized, an analogy is only an analogy. He has given philosophical reasons why he thinks it is wrong. Neuroscientists know only a few of the basics of neuroscience, such as the nature of the action potential and the chemical nature of most synapses. Most important, there is not a comprehensive, overall theory of the activities of the brain. To be shown to be correct, the analogy must be filled out by many experimental details and powerful general ideas. Much of these are still lacking.

This problem of qualia is what Chalmers (1995) calls "The Hard Problem": a full account of the manner in which subjective experience arises from cerebral processes. As we see it, the hard problem can be broken down into several questions, of which the first is the major problem: How do we experience anything at all? What leads to a particular conscious experience (such as the blueness of blue)? What is the function of conscious experience? Why are some aspects of subjective experience impossible to convey to other people (in other words, why are they private)?

We believe we have answers to the last two questions (Crick and Koch 1995c). We have already explained, in the section "Why Are We Conscious," what we think consciousness is for. The reason that visual consciousness is largely private is, we consider, an inevitable consequence of the way the brain works. (By "private," we mean that it is inherently impossible to communicate the exact nature of what we are conscious of.) To be conscious, we have argued, there must be an explicit representation of each aspect of visual consciousness. At each successive stage in the visual cortex, what is made explicit is recoded. To produce a motor output, such as speech, the information must be recoded again, so that what is expressed by the motor neurons is related, but not identical, to the explicit representation expressed by the firing of the neurons associated with, for example, the color experience at some level in the visual hierarchy.

It is thus not possible to convey with words the exact nature of a subjective experience. It is possible, however, to convey a *difference* between subjective experiences—to distinguish between red and orange, for example. This is possible because a difference in a high-level visual cortical area can still be associated with a difference at the motor stage. The implication is that we can never explain to other people the nature of any conscious experience, only, in some cases, its relation to other ones.

Is there any sense in asking whether the blue color you see is subjectively the same as the blue color I see? If it turns out that the neural correlate of blue is exactly the same in your brain as in mine, it would be scientifically plausible to infer that you see blue as I do. The problem lies in the word "exactly." How precise one has to be will depend on a detailed knowledge of the processes involved. If the neural correlate of blue depends, in an important way, on my past experience, and if my past experience is significantly different from yours, then it may not be possible to deduce that we both see blue in exactly the same way (Crick 1994).

Could this problem be solved by connecting two brains together in some elaborate way? It is impossible to do this at the moment, or in the easily foreseeable future. One is therefore tempted to use the philosopher's favorite tool, the thought experiment. Unfortunately, this enterprise is fraught with hazards, since it inevitably makes assumptions about how brains behave, and most of these assumptions have so little experimental support that conclusions based on them are valueless. For example, how much is a person's percept of the blue of the sky due to early visual experiences?

The Problem of Meaning

An important problem neglected by neuroscientists is the problem of meaning. Neuroscientists are apt to assume that if they can see that a neuron's firing is roughly correlated with some aspect of the visual scene, such as an oriented line, then that firing must be part of the neural correlate of the seen line. They assume that because they, as outside observers, are conscious of the correlation, the firing must be part

of the NCC. This by no means follows, as we have argued for neurons in V1.

But this is not the major problem, which is: How do other parts of the brain know that the firing of a neuron (or of a set of similar neurons) produces the conscious percept of, say, a face? How does the brain know what the firing of those neurons represents? Put in other words, how is meaning generated by the brain?

This problem has two aspects. How is meaning expressed in neural terms? And how does this expression of meaning arise? We suspect (Crick and Koch 1995c) that meaning derives both from the correlated firing described above and from the linkages to related representations. For example, neurons related to a certain face might be connected to ones expressing the name of the person whose face it is, and to others for her voice, memories involving her and so on, in a vast associational network, similar to a dictionary or a relational database. Exactly how this works in detail is unclear.

But how are these useful associations derived? The obvious idea is that they depend very largely on the consistency of the interactions with the environment, especially during early development. Meaning can also be acquired later in life. The usual example is a blind man with a stick. He comes to feel what the stick is touching, not merely the stick itself. For an ingenious recent demonstration along similar lines, see Ramachandran and Hirstein 1997.

Future Experiments

Although experiments on attention, short-term and working memory, the correlated firing of neurons, and related topics may make finding the NCC easier, at present the most promising experiments are those on bistable percepts. These experiments should be continued in numerous cortical and thalamic areas and need extending to cover other such percepts. It is also important to discover *which* neurons express the NCC in each case (which neuronal subtype, in what layer, and so on), how they fire (e.g., do they fire in bursts) and, especially, to where they project. To assist this, more detailed neuroanatomy of the connectivity will be needed. This is relatively easy to do in the macaque but difficult in humans (Crick and Jones 1993). It is also important to discover how the various on-line systems work, so that one can contrast their (unconscious) neuronal activity with the NCC.

To discover the exact role (if any) of the frontal cortex in visual perception, it would be useful to inactivate it reversibly by cooling and/or the injection of GABA agonists, perhaps using the relatively smooth cortex of an owl monkey.

Inevitably, it will be necessary to compare the studies on monkeys with similar studies on humans, using both psychophysical experiments as well as functional imaging methods such as PET or fMRI. Conversely, functional imaging experiments on normal subjects or patients, showing, for instance, the involvement of prefrontal areas in visual perception (Sahraie et al. 1997, Weiskrantz 1997), can provide a rationale for appropriate electrophysiological studies in monkeys. It would help considerably if there were more detailed architectonic studies of cortex and thalamus, since these can be done postmortem on monkeys, apes and humans. The extremely rapid pace of molecular biology should soon provide a wealth of new markers to help in this endeavor.

To understand a very complex nonlinear system, it is essential to be able to interfere with it both specifically and delicately. The major impact of molecular biology is likely to be the provisions of methods for the inactivation of all neurons of a particular type. Ideally, this should be done reversibly on the mature animal (see, for example, No et al. 1996, Nirenberg and Meister 1997). At the moment this is only practical on mice, but in future one may hope for methods that can be used on mature monkeys (perhaps using a viral vector), as such methods are also needed for the medical treatment of humans.

As an example, consider the question of whether the cortical feedback pathways—originating in a higher visual area (in the sense of Felleman and Van Essen 1991) and projecting into a lower area—are essential for normal visual consciousness. There are at least two distinct types of back pathways (Salin and Bullier 1995): one, from the upper cortical layers, goes back only a few steps in the visual hierarchy; the other, from the lower cortical layers, can also go back over longer distances. We would like to be able to selectively inactivate these pathways, both singly and collectively, in the mature macaque. Present methods are not specific enough to do this, but new methods in molecular biology should, in time, make this possible.

It will not be enough to show that certain neurons embody the NCC in certain—limited— visual situations. Rather, we need to locate the NCC for all types of visual inputs, or at least for a sufficiently large and representative sample of them. For example, when one blinks, the eyelids briefly (30–50 ms) cover the eyes, yet the visual percept is scarcely interrupted (blink suppression; Volkmann et al. 1980). We would therefore expect the NCC to be also unaffected by eye blinks (e.g., the firing activity should not drop noticeably during the blink) but not to blanking out of the visual scene for a similar duration due to artificial means. Another example is the large number of visual illusions. For instance, humans clearly perceive, under appropriate circumstances, a transient motion aftereffect. On the basis of fMRI imaging it has been found that the human equivalent of cortical area MT is activated by the motion aftereffect (in the absence of any moving stimuli; Tootell et al. 1995). The timecourse of this illusion parallels the timecourse of activity as assayed using fMRI. In order to really pinpoint the NCC, one would need to identify individual cells expressing this, and similar, visual aftereffects. We have assumed that the visual NCC in humans is very similar to the NCC in the macaque, mainly because of the similarity of their visual systems. Ultimately, the link between neurons and perception will need to be made in humans.

The problem of meaning and how it arises is more difficult, since there is not, as yet, even an outline formulation of this problem in neural terms. For example, do multiple associations depend on transient priming effects? Whatever the explanation, it would be necessary to study the developing animal to show how meaning arises: in particular, how much is built in epigenetically and how much is due to experience.

In the long run, finding the NCC will not be enough. A complete theory of consciousness is required, including its functional role. With luck this might illuminate the hard problem of qualia. It is likely that scientists will then stop using the term consciousness except in a very loose way. After all, biologists no longer worry whether a seed or a virus in "alive"; they just want to know how it evolved, how it develops, and what it can do.

Finale

We hope we have convinced the reader that the problem of the neural correlate of consciousness (the NCC) is now ripe for direct experimental attack. We have suggested a possible framework for thinking about the problem, but others may prefer a different approach; and, of course, our own ideas are likely to change with time. We have outlined the few experiments that directly address the problem and mentioned briefly other types of experiments that might be done in the future. We hope that some of the younger neuroscientists will seriously consider working on this fascinating problem. After all, it is rather peculiar to work on the visual system and not worry about exactly what happens in our brains when we "see" something. The explanation of consciousness is one of the major unsolved problems of modern science. After several thousand years of speculation, it would be very gratifying to find an answer to it.

Acknowledgments

For helpful comments we thank David Chalmers, Leslie Orgel, John Searle, and Larry Weiskrantz. We thank the J. W. Kieckhefer Foundation, the National Institute of Mental Health, the Office of Naval Research, and the National Science Foundation.

References

Adolphs R, Tranel D, Damasio H, Damasio A (1994) Impaired recognition of emotion in facial expressions following bilateral damage to the human amygdala. Nature 372:669–672.

Baddeley A (1992) Working memory. Science 255:556–559.

Ballard DH, Hinton GE, Sejnowski TJ (1983) Parallel visual computation. Nature 306:21–26.

Blackwell KT, Buchsbaum G (1988) Quantitative studies of color constancy. J Opt Soc Am A5:1772–1780.

Blake R, For R (1974) Adaptation to invisible gratings and the site of binocular rivalry suppression. Nature 249:488–490.

Boussaoud D, di Pellegrino G, Wise SP (1996) Frontal lobe mechanisms subserving vision-for-action versus vision-for-perception. Behav Brain Res 72:1–15.

Bradley DC, Chang GC, Andersen RA (1998) A link between kinetic depth perception and neural activity in primate cortical area MT. Nature 392:714–717.

Braun J, Julesz B (1997) Dividing attention at little cost. Percept Psychophys 60:1–23.

Britten KH, Shadlen MN, Newsome WT, Movshon JA (1992) The analysis of visual motion: a comparison of neuronal and psychophysical performance. J Neurosci 12:4745–4765.

Chalmers D (1995) The conscious mind: in search of a fundamental theory. Oxford: Oxford University Press.

Coltheart M (1983) Iconic memory. Phil Trans R Soc Lond B 302:283–294.

Cowey A, Stoerig P (1995) Blindsight in monkeys. Nature 373:247–249.

Crick F (1994) The astonishing hypothesis. New York: Scribner's.

Crick F (1996) Visual perception: rivalry and consciousness. Nature 379:485–486.

Crick F, Jones E (1993) Backwardness of human neuroanatomy. Nature 361:109–110.

Crick F, Koch C (1990) Towards a neurobiological theory of consciousness. Semin Neurosci 2:263–275.

Crick F, Koch C (1995a) Are we aware of neural activity in primary visual cortex? Nature 375:121–123.

Crick F, Koch C (1995b) Cortical areas in visual awareness—reply. Nature 377:294–295.

Crick F, Koch C (1995c) Why neuroscience may be able to explain consciousness. Scient Am 273:84–85.

Crick F, Koch C (1998) Constraints on cortical and thalamic projections. The no-strong-loops hypothesis. Nature 391:245–250.

Cumming BG, Parker AJ (1997) Responses of primary visual cortical neurons to binocular disparity without depth perception. Nature 389:280–283.

Damasio AR, Anderson SW (1993) The frontal lobes. In: Clinical neuropsychology, 3rd edn (Heilman KM, Valenstein E, eds), pp. 409–460. Oxford: Oxford University Press.

Dennett D (1996) Kinds of minds: toward an understanding of consciousness. New York: Basic Books.

Distler C, Boussaoud D, Desimone R, Ungerleider LG (1993) Cortical connections of inferior temporal area TEO in macaque monkeys. J Comp Neurol 334:125–150.

Eccles JC (1994) How the self controls its brain. Berlin: Springer-Verlag.

Edelman GM (1989) The remembered present: a biological theory of consciousness. New York: Basic Books.

Engel S, Zhang X, Wandell B (1997) Colour tuning in human visual cortex measured with functional magnetic resonance imaging. Nature 388:68–71.

Felleman DJ, Van Essen D (1991) Distributed hierarchical processing in the primate cerebral cortex. Cereb Cortex 1:1–47.

Fries W (1990) Pontine projection from striate and prestriate visual cortex in the macque monkey: an anterograde study. Vis Neurosci 4:205–216.

Fuster JM (1997) The prefrontal cortex: anatomy, physiology, and neuropsychology of the frontal lobe, 3rd edn. Philadelphia: Lippincott-Raven.

Gegenfurtner KR, Sperling G (1993) Information transfer in iconic memory experiments. J Exp Psychol Hum Percept Perform 19:845–866.

Goldenberg G, Müllbacher W, Nowak A (1995) Imagery without perception—a case study of anosognosia for cortical blindsight. Neuropsychologia 33:1373–1382.

Goldman-Rakic PS (1995) Cellular basis of working memory. Neuron 14:477–485.

Greenfield SA (1995) Journey to the centers of the mind. New York: Freeman.

Gur M, Snodderly DM (1997) A dissociation between brain activity and perception: chromatically opponent cortical neurons signal chromatic flicker that is not perceived. Vis Res 37:377–382.

He S, Cavanagh P, Intriligator J (1996) Attentional resolution and the locus of visual awareness. Nature 383:334–337.

He S, Smallman H, MacLeod D (1995) Neural and cortical limits on visual resolution. Invest Opthal Vis Sci 36:2010.

Ingle D (1973) Two visual systems in the frog. Science 181:1053–1055.

Kanwisher N, Driver J (1992) Objects, attributes, and visual attention: which, what, and where. Curr Dir Psychol Sci 1:26–31.

Koch C, Braun J (1996) On the functional anatomy of visual awareness. Cold Spring Harbor Symp Quant Biol 61:49–57.

Kolb FC, Braun J (1995) Blindsight in normal observers. Nature 377:336–339.

Kosslyn SM, Thompson WL, Kim IJ, Alpert NM (1995) Topographical representations of mental images in primary visual cortex. Nature 378:496–498.

Land EH, McCann JJ (1971) Lightness and retinex theory. J Opt Soc Am 61:1–11.

Leibniz GW (1965) Monadology and other philosophical essays (Schrecker P, Schrecker AM, trans). Indianapolis: Bobbs-Merrill.

Leopold DA, Logothetis NK (1996) Activity changes in early visual cortex reflect monkeys' percepts during binocular rivalry. Nature 379:549–553.

Libet B (1993) Neurophysiology of consciousness: selected papers and new essays by Benjamin Libet. Boston: Birkhäuser.

Logothetis N, Schall J (1989) Neuronal correlates of subjective visual perception. Science 245:761–763.

Luck SJ, Chelazzi L, Hillyard SA, Desimone R (1997) Neural mechanisms of spatial selective attention in areas V1, V2, and V4 of macaque visual cortex. J Neurophysiol 77:24–42.

Milner D, Goodale M (1995) The visual brain in action. Oxford: Oxford University Press.

Milner AD, Perrett DI, Johnston RS, Benson PJ, Jordan TR, Heeley DW et al. (1991) Perception and action in "visual form agnosia." Brain 114:405–428.

Morgan MJ, Mason AJS, Solomon JA (1997) Blindsight in normal subjects? Nature 385:401–402.

Myerson J, Miezin F, Allman J (1981) Binocular rivalry in macaque monkeys and humans: a comparative study in perception. Behav Anal Lett 1:149–156.

Nakamura RK, Mishkin M (1980) Blindness in monkeys following nonvisual cortical lesions. Brain Res 188:572–577.

Nakamura RK, Mishkin M (1986) Chronic blindness following lesions of nonvisual cortex in the monkey. Exp Brain Res 62:173–184.

Nagel AHM (1997) Are plants conscious? J Consc Stud 4:215–230.

Nirenberg S, Meister M (1997) The higher response of retinal ganglion cells is truncated by a displaced amacrine circuit. Neuron 18:637–650.

No D, Yao T-P, Evans RM (1996) Ecdysone-inducible gene expression in mammalian cells and transgenic mice. Proc Natl Acad Sci USA 93:3346–3351.

O'Regan JK (1992) Solving the "real" mysteries of visual perception: the world as an outside memory. Can J Psychol 46:461–488.

Penfield W (1958) The excitable cortex in conscious man. Liverpool: Liverpool University Press.

Pollen DA (1995) Cortical areas in visual awareness. Nature 377:293–294.

Potter MC (1976) Short-term conceptual memory for pictures. J Exp Psychol Hum Learn Mem 2:509–522.

Ramachandran VS, Hirstein W (1997) Three laws of qualia: what neurology tells us about the biological functions of consciousness. J Consc Stud 4:429–457.

Rock I, Linnett CM, Grant P, Mack A (1992) Perception without attention: results of a new method. Cogn Psychol 24:502–534.

Rossetti Y (1998) Implicit perception in action: short-lived motor representations of space evidenced by brain-damaged and healthy subjects. In: Finding consciousness in the brain (Grossenbacher PG, ed.) pp. 131–178. Philadelphia: Benjamins.

Sahraie A, Weiskrantz L, Barbur JL, Simmons A, Williams SCR, Brammer MJ (1997) Pattern of neuronal activity associated with conscious and unconscious processing of visual signals. Proc Natl Acad Sci USA 94:9406–9411.

Saint-Cyr JA, Ungerleider LG, Desimone R (1990) Organization of visual cortex inputs to the striatum and subsequent outputs to the pallidonigral complex in the monkey. J Comp Neurol 298:129–156.

Salin P-A, Bullier J (1995) Corticocortical connections in the visual system: structure and function. Physiol Rev 75:107–154.

Salzman CD, Britten KH, Newsome WT (1990) Cortical microstimulation influences perceptual judgements of motion direction. Nature 346:174–177.

Scalaidhe SPO, Wilson FAW, Goldman-Rakic PS (1997) Areal segregation of face-processing neurons in prefrontal cortex. Science 278:1135–1138.

Schein SJ, Desimone R (1990) Spectral properties of V4 neurons in the macaque. J Neurosci 10:3369–3389.

Searle J (1984) Minds, brains, and science. The Reith Lectures, 101–102. London: British Broadcasting Corporation.

Sheinberg DL, Logothetis NK (1997) The role of temporal cortical areas in perceptual organization. Proc Natl Acad Sci USA 94:3408–3413.

Sherk H (1986) The claustrum and the cerebral cortex. In: Cerebral cortex, vol. 5: Sensory-motor areas and aspects of cortical connectivity (Jones EG, Peters A, eds), pp. 467–499. New York: Plenum Press.

Singer W, Gray CM (1995) Visual feature integration and the temporal correlation hypothesis. Annu Rev Neurosci 18:555–586.

Tootell RBH, Dale AM, Sereno MI, Malach R (1996) New images from human visual cortex. Trends Neurosci 19:481–489.

Tootell RBH, Reppas JB, Dale AM, Look RB, Sereno MI, Malach R, Brady TJ, Rosen BR (1995) Visual motion aftereffect in human cortical area MT revealed by functional magnetic resonance imaging. Nature 375:139–141.

Ungerleider LG, Mishkin M (1982) Two cortical visual systems. In: Analysis of visual behavior (Ingle DJ, Goodale MA, Mansfield RJW, eds), pp. 549–586. Cambridge, MA: MIT Press.

Volkmann FC, Riggs LA, Moore RK (1980) Eye-blinks and visual suppression. Science 207:900–902.

von der Malsburg C (1995) Binding in models of perception and brain function. Curr Opin Neurobiol 5:520–526.

Webster MJ, Bachevalier J, Ungerleider LG (1994) Connections of inferior temporal areas TEO and TE with parietal and frontal cortex in macaque monkeys. Cereb Cortex 5:470–483.

Weiskrantz L (1997) Consciousness lost and found. Oxford: Oxford University Press.

Young MP, Yamane S (1992) Sparse population coding of faces in the inferotemporal cortex. Science 256:1327–1331.

Young MP, Tanaka K, Yamane S (1992) On oscillating neuronal responses in the visual cortex of the monkey. J Neurophysiol 67:1464–1474.

Zeki S (1980) The representation of colours in the cerebral cortex. Nature 284:412–418.

Zeki S (1983) Colour coding in the cerebral cortex: the reaction of cells in monkey visual cortex to wavelengths and colours. Neurosci 9:741–765.

Zola-Morgan S, Squire LR (1993) Neuroanatomy of memory. Annu Rev Neurosci 16:547–563.

Note Added in Proof (*Cerebral Cortex*, March 1998)

The recent discovery of neurons in the inferior pre-frontal cortex (IPC) of the macaque that respond selectively to faces—and that receive direct input from regions around the superior temporal sulcus and the inferior temporal gyrus that are well known to contain face-selective neurons—is of considerable interest (Scalaidhe et al. 1997). It raises the questions of why would face cells be represented in *both* IT and IPC. Do they differ in some important aspect?

II CONSCIOUSNESS IN VISION

The senses seem to present the most richly detailed domain of conscious experience. In perceptual studies we always ask people to report what they experience under optimal report conditions, and we generally build in verification checks. Most of these studies therefore meet the standard operational criteria for consciousness reports. A number of perceptual studies allow a close comparison between conscious and unconscious sensory functions. (See Introduction, chap. 1.) Of all the senses, vision has been most intensively explored, giving us some of the best examples of scientific studies of consciousness today.

Conscious Visual Features

The first chapter by Anne Treisman (1998; chap. 4, this volume) provides psychological evidence for visual feature analysis in the brain. She points out that visual perception is typically effortless and holistic, a process in which people have rapid access to figural Gestalts like objects and events, rather than to subordinate features of color, light edges, shadows, motion, and the like. Nevertheless, there is both psychological and brain evidence that the visual stream is initially decomposed into such elementary features in the cortex, only to be recombined into higher-level units at an anatomically later point in the flow.

Before Livingstone and Hubel's 1981 article (see chap. 5), single-cell recording in the visual brain almost always involved unconscious animals. Whether the cat or monkey was awake and conscious simply did not seem relevant to the search for visual feature cells. Thus no comparison could be made between conscious and unconscious visual processes. Livingstone and Hubel made history simply by pinching the tail of their anesthetized cat, thereby waking it up, and observed that the same visual neurons now fired differently. By treating consciousness as a variable, Livingstone and Hubel were able to

observe increased firing in visual feature neurons during waking consciousness. A variable that was taken for granted—consciousness of visual stimuli—suddenly emerged as figure from ground.

Binocular Rivalry, the New Methodology of Choice?

Some of the most revealing recent studies have used binocular rivalry, in which two incompatible images are presented to the two eyes, so that normal binocular fusion cannot occur. Instead, one eye's input dominates visual consciousness for some time, while the other is unconscious. Each eye may be dominant for seconds or longer. Binocular rivalry has now become so effective a tool for studying visual consciousness that it deserves special attention.

Binocular rivalry has many advantages. For one, we can now track both the conscious and the unconscious input stream well into visual cortex, as shown by Sheinberg and Logothetis (1997; chap. 6, this volume). By counterbalancing conditions (right vs. left eye, conscious vs. unconscious, one stimulus vs. the other), we can tease out which effects are due to consciousness as such, and which are dependent on the particular eye or stimulus. Further, rivalrous pairs of stimuli can be designed to trigger activity at any level of specific feature neurons in the brain. As William James pointed out in 1890, a set of left-slanting diagonal lines in one eye will compete against right-slanting lines in the other eye. Today we know that the cortical neurons that detect line orientation are found early in the visual feature fields of the temporal cortex. On the other hand, a face presented to one eye will also compete against a picture of a coffee cup presented to the other eye, and such object rivalry apparently cannot be resolved until rather late in the visual feature hierarchy, near the tip of the lower temporal cortex. Thus different kinds of binocular rivalry seem to "poll" different levels of visual analysis. Because one eye is always conscious while the other is unconscious, rivalry allows us to compare conscious and unconscious neuronal activity at many different levels of the visual cortex.

Some remarkable research has now been carried out using this approach. For more than a decade Logothetis and colleagues have compared single-cell activity in response to conscious versus unconscious visual input in macaque monkeys, whose visual brain resembles the human one in many ways. Their work on binocular rivalry now constitutes our most detailed source of knowledge about conscious neuronal processing in visual cortex. Earlier work showed that binocular rivalry activates small numbers of cells in early visual cortex, where single visual features are represented, such as color, motion, line orientation, and spatial frequency. Some of these early cells respond to the "conscious eye," at the same time that others respond to the unconscious input in the other eye. More than half of the cells at any level of early visual analysis do not respond to either stream. However, Sheinberg and Logothetis (chap. 6, this volume) demonstrated that this pattern changes dramatically toward the anterior end of the visual ventral stream, where whole objects are represented in inferotemporal cortex (area IT). There 90% of neurons respond to conscious, but not to unconscious input (1997).

Area IT therefore appears to be the best current candidate for a distinctive locus of visual consciousness, because it clearly distinguishes between the conscious and unconscious input stream, and unlike earlier regions it massively favors the conscious stream. Because IT represents whole objects, it involves by definition the integration of many specific features into a single, integrated representation. However, whereas IT appears to be the single best candidate for a neuronal correlate of visual consciousness, consciousness still appears to be crucially dependent on other parts of the brain, including subcortical regions (see section 10).

The chapter by Tononi, Srinivasan, Russell, and Edelman (1998; chap. 7, this volume) extends the use of binocular rivalry to the human brain and to much larger volumes of brain tissue. It applies a clever technique pioneered by E. R. John and Robert Thatcher some 20 years ago, using flickering stimuli to drive frequency-matched neuronal firing in the brain, which can be tracked using time-sensitive brain measures like EEG and MEG (Thatcher and John 1977). The flickering input therefore creates a neuronal tag, which can be easily detected in regions throughout the brain. Tononi et al. presented a slightly different flickering stimulus to each eye in a binocular rivalry situation. Neurons driven by the two flickering inputs were detected by MEG. The resulting signal-to-noise ratio of the brain response is remarkably high, 25 to one or more, and can be detected far beyond the visual cortex. Tononi et al. found clear differences between neurons responding to the conscious and unconscious input streams, with the conscious one having more widespread and higher amplitude effects. This appears to be the first study to break through some of the practical limits of previous studies, extending the binocular method to humans and to much larger amounts of brain tissue than before.

The role of temporal correlation in binding diverse neurons into a single visual percept has been much discussed (see Crick and Koch 1998; chap. 3, this volume; Singer and Gray 1995; chap. 64, this volume). It is attractive to suppose that neurons distant from each other may "sing in harmony" by way of pacing rhythms, so that all the different features of a visual percept can combine into a single conscious event. The next study, by Engel, Fries, Roelfsema, König, Brecht, and Singer (1999), describes the use of binocular rivalry to study temporal correlation in strabismic cats, that is, animals with eye deviations that block normal binocular fusion. They found that the conscious input stream "increased the synchronicity and the regularity of their oscillatory patterning," whereas the unconscious stream decreased such patterns.

In sum, binocular rivalry seems to be an attractive and broadly applicable technique for studying visual consciousness in the intact brain. It is currently one of the most revealing and convenient methods available and can be used for studying humans as well as animals, for single neurons as well as large regions of brain tissue. Rivalry allows us to "treat consciousness as a variable" by comparing the fate of two identical stimuli, one of which is conscious and the other not (see chap. 1). There is now reliable evidence that the unconscious stimulus is still analyzed well into visual cortex and that the conscious input may only begin to be dominant toward the end of the ventral visual pathway. Analogues of visual rivalry can be found in hearing and the body senses. In sum, this may be one of our most promising tools so far.

Brain Damage That Selectively Impairs Conscious Vision

Although methods like binocular rivalry are useful for studying consciousness in the intact brain, there is much to be learned from a variety of brain lesions that impair conscious but not unconscious processes (see Weiskrantz 1991; chap. 9, this volume). Cortical blindness or "blindsight" has now been studied intensively for 30 years. It involves lesions to the first visual projection area (V1), where the main optic tract first reaches cortex. A considerable amount of accurate vision goes on without area V1, but victims of blindsight vigorously disavow any qualitative conscious experience in the lesioned field. They claim not to be conscious of objects or colors, all the "obvious" parts of a normal visual scene. Nevertheless, indirect evidence shows clearly that blindsight subjects can respond accurately to visual objects, location, color, motion, and so on. Blindsight thus presents another opportunity for making close comparisons between conscious and unconscious visual processing.

The great philosophical question about visual consciousness is whether there can ever be an objective method to assess individual qualitative experience. Is your experience of the color green is the same as mine? Can we ever know the answer? Or is it true, as John Locke claimed in the seventeenth century, that some people might perceive reds for greens, but that no one could ever know as long as they called their unique experiences "red" and "green," according to the usual social convention? If visual qualities like color are utterly private, we could never know whether others experience color the way we do. Cowey and Stoerig (1995; chap. 10, this volume) developed a brilliant way to address the philosophical question of visual qualia in animals. They asked whether a blindsighted macaque monkey would lose qualities like color, shape, and motion when part of V1 was lesioned as in human blindsight subjects. People with blindsight complain of their inability to see colors and objects, though they will respond accurately when they are cajoled into doing so. But monkeys only seem to respond by pushing button or pulling a lever, rather than telling us about their experiences. Cowey and Stoerig made use of a behavioral index called the "commentary key," which allows the macaque to signal whether a stimulus in the cortically blind part of the visual field *can be distinguished from a blank trial* in the intact part of the field. That is, they asked the monkey, in effect, whether having a V1 lesion is like looking at a blank screen? As it turned out, the macaques could not tell the difference. Thus V1-lesioned macaques resemble human blindsight patients, who tell us they do not really experience visual qualitative events, even though they make accurate behavioral distinctions. Such results strengthen the case that macaques have conscious visual experiences much like our own.

The most famous type of brain damage that dramatically changes consciousness is the "split brain," the case of patients whose corpus callosum has been sectioned, thereby blocking the constant flow of neuronal impulses between the two cerebral hemispheres. Sperry (1968; chap. 11, this volume) received a Nobel Prize for his work on these patients, which revealed that the two hemispheres could have a surprising degree of autonomy, at least in these special cases. Split-brain patients challenge the notion of subjective unity of consciousness more profoundly perhaps than any other source of evidence. That does not mean that conscious unity is an artifact, given that it is a subjective perception and such perceptions are never entirely veridical. Rather, conscious unity appears to be a basic assumption of our subjective universe, not just in perception, but in the unity of personal experience over seconds, days, and years. Such a sense of unity is always constructed by the brain, and the split-brain preparation is a remarkable challenge to our intuitive assumptions in that respect.

Another surprising finding shows that visually guided motor tasks, like reaching for an object, have a significant unconscious component. The conscious and unconscious aspects of vision can be dissociated by brain damage, but even in sighted subjects there seems to be a separate system situated in the "dorsal stream" of the visual system, involved with motor aspects of vision, in contrast to the "ventral stream," which runs along the lower temporal lobe, and which seems to represent the visual features and objects that can become conscious. The work by Goodale, Milner, and co-authors represents this body of research (Goodale, Milner, Jakobson, and Carey 1991; Goodale and Milner, chap. 12, this volume).

Visual Qualia

Stephen Palmer (chap. 13, this volume) approaches the philosophical problem of visual qualia from another angle. As previously noted, the philosopher John Locke first claimed that the colors of the spectrum could be inverted without changing anything that could be observed objectively. Someone who perceives green instead of red presumably learns by convention to call reds "green." Thus color perception, the argument goes, is a purely private event, a *quale* (plural: *qualia*) that can make no publically observable difference. Based on an extensive analysis of color vision, Palmer challenges the claim of color equivalence. This chapter is a scientific answer to the common philosophical claim that conscious experiences are essentially private and "incorrigible" by objective evidence.

In sum, this section presents scientific studies that seem to be making significant progress toward solving problems that have long been debated. Remarkably, much of this progress has occurred in the last decade, though the foundations were laid over many years.

Is There a Special Link between Consciousness and the Senses?

The problem of consciousness is not limited to sensory perception, but perception seems to have a special relationship to consciousness. A rough comparison of major input, output, and intermediate systems suggests that consciousness is closely allied with the *input* side of the nervous system. Although perceptual processes are obviously not conscious in detail, the end product of perception is a very rich domain of information to which we seem to have exquisitely detailed conscious access. By comparison, imagery seems less richly conscious, as are inner speech, bodily feelings, and the like. Action control seems even less conscious—indeed, many observers have argued that the most obviously conscious components of action consist of feedback from actions performed and anticipatory images of actions planned. But of course, action feedback is itself perceptual, and imagery is quasi-perceptual. Thus the conscious components of action and imagery resemble conscious perception.

Likewise, thought and memory seem to involve fewer conscious details than perception. Even in working memory we are only conscious of the item that is currently being rehearsed, not of others; and the conscious rehearsed item in working memory often has a near-perceptual quality. We are clearly not conscious of information in long-term memory or in the semantic, abstract component of memory. In thinking and problem-solving we encounter phenomena like problem incubation, to remind us that the details of problem solving are often carried out unconsciously. The most obviously conscious components in thinking and memory involve imagery or inner speech—and these resemble perceptual events. The thoughts that come to mind after incubation often have a perceptual or imaginal quality. In sum, when we compare input events (perception and imagery) with output (action) and mediating events (thought and memory), it is the input side that seems most clearly conscious in its details. This kind of comparison is very rough indeed, but it does suggest that the senses have a special relationship to consciousness.

Reference

Thatcher, R. W. and John, E. R. (1977) *Foundations of cognitive processes*. New York: Harper & Row.

4 Feature Binding, Attention, and Object Perception

Anne Treisman

1 The Binding Problem

The binding problem in perception deals with the question of how we achieve the experience of a coherent world of integrated objects, and avoid seeing a world of disembodied or wrongly combined shapes, colours, motions, sizes, and distances. In brief, how do we specify what goes with what and where? The problem is not an intuitively obvious one, which is probably a testimony to how well, in general, our brains solve it. We simply are not aware that there is a problem to be solved. Yet findings from neuroscience, computer science and psychology all imply that there is.

There is considerable evidence that the visual system analyses the scene along a number of different dimensions in various specialized modules. Both anatomical and physiological evidence (reviewed, for example, by Cowey 1985 and Zeki 1993) suggests the existence of several maps of the visual scene laid out in different visual areas of the brain. Recordings from single or multiple neurons in animals have shown different specializations. Ungerleider and Mishkin (1982) distinguished a dorsal pathway, coding motion and space, and a ventral pathway, coding colour, shape and other features in extrastriate areas and eventually objects in the inferior temporal (IT) area. Consistent with this inferred modularity, localized brain damage in human patients leads to selective losses in perceptual abilities. For example, colour vision can be lost in achromatopsia, without any impairment in shape or motion perception (Meadows 1974, Damasio et al. 1980); the ability to perceive motion can also be independently lost in akinetopsia, resulting in perception of frozen stills (Zihl et al. 1983, Zeki 1991); so can the ability to discriminate orientations or simple shapes (Goodale and Milner 1992). Finally, in humans

with intact brains, positron emission tomography (PET) and functional magnetic resonance imaging (fMRI) have shown focal activity shifting to different brain areas as subjects are asked to respond to different aspects of the same displays—the shapes, colours and directions of motion (see Corbetta et al. 1991, Gulyas and Roland 1991, Sereno et al. 1995).

These findings, suggesting that specialized areas code different aspects of the visual scene, raise the question of how we get from dispersed brain representations to the unified percepts that we experience. If the world contained only one object at a time, this need not be a problem: there is nothing to demand that a unitary percept must depend on a unitary localized neural code. However, the binding problem is raised in a more acute form when we realize two facts: first, that we typically do not look at scenes with only one object in them. The world around us is a crowded place, full of objects. Second, receptive fields in many of the specialized visual areas are quite large—up to 30° in temporal areas. Beyond the earliest stages of visual processing, single neurons respond across areas that would certainly hold several objects in crowded displays. If two objects with potentially interchangeable properties are detected by the same units, the potential for miscombining is present. For example, if a unit responding to red is active at the same time as a unit responding to motion, we need some way of distinguishing whether their receptive fields contain a moving red object, or a moving green object together with a stationary red object.

Which mechanisms could resolve this ambiguity? One possibility is that single units directly code conjunctions of features at earlier levels where receptive fields are small enough to isolate single objects. Certainly most cells in both early and late visual areas are selective along more than one dimension. Tanaka (1993) has shown single units in IT area that respond to relatively complex combinations of features. But in these experiments the animals were typically shown one object at a time, so the binding problem did not arise. The cells in IT could be coding the output of the binding process. There must be limits to the use of direct conjunction coding as a solution to the binding problem. We can see an essentially unlimited number of arbitrary conjunctions, immediately, the first time we are shown them. A purple giraffe with wings would look surprising but it would not be invisible. There are certainly too few neurons to code individually the combinatorial explosion of arbitrary conjunctions that we are capable of seeing.

A suggestion that is currently arousing interest in both neuroscience and computer modelling is that binding might depend on synchronized neural activity. Units that fire together would signal the same object. Gray et al. (1989) and Singer and Gray (1995) have collected evidence showing the presence of stimulus-dependent synchrony between units in quite widely separated areas of the brain. It is an interesting hypothesis, but I don't think it solves the same binding problem that I raised at the beginning of this paper. Synchrony is a possible way of holding on to the solution, of tagging the units that are responding to the same object once they have been identified, but we still need a way of finding which those are. The Gestalt psychologists identified a number of perceptual cues, such as collinearity, proximity, similarity, which determine perceptual grouping within dimensions such as colour, orientation, and common motion. Facilitatory connections between cells responding to the same or related features within dimensions might mediate this grouping by helping to synchronize their firing across different locations see, for example, Hummel and Biederman 1992), but risk also leading to false bindings when different objects share the same features. Furthermore, they would not bind the different features like orientation, motion, and colour, that happen to belong to the same object. This paper suggests a possible mechanism for binding across dimensions through shared locations, and also for using similarity to bind within dimensions across locations.

2 A Role for Spatial Attention?

Psychologists have been interested for many years in a spatially selective mechanism of visual attention. For example, Posner (1980) showed that giving a spatial cue, such as a momentary brightening of one of two frames, would speed responses to a target object that subsequently appeared in that frame, even when the subject's eyes remained fixated centrally. We use the analogy of a "window" of attention for this unitary, spatially selective mechanism. Other experiments have investigated visual search by asking subjects to find a target object in a display of nontargets (we call them distractors). We measure how long it takes to find the target as a function of how many distractors there are in the display. In some search tasks, the search time increases linearly with the number of distractors, as though subjects used a serial process of checking objects to find the target. Perhaps the same attention window must be centred on each object in turn. There is evidence that the attention window can be scaled—its size can adjust to fit the objects or groups of objects that are relevant to the task. For instance, in a display containing a global letter made of smaller local letters, we can attend to the global letter or to any one of the local ones, and it takes time to switch between these two states (Navon 1977, Ward 1982). In search, we process homogeneous groups of items in parallel (Treisman 1982).

Some years ago, I suggested that spatially selective attention may play a role in binding (Treisman and Gelade 1980, Treisman 1988). The idea, a very simple one, was that we code one object at a time, selected on the basis of its location at an early level where receptive fields are small. By temporarily excluding stimuli

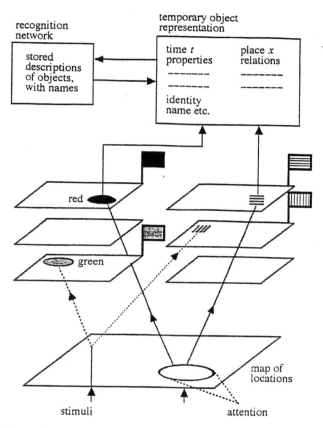

recognition
network

temporary object
representation

stored
descriptions
of objects,
with names

time *t*
properties

place *x*
relations

----

identity
name etc.

red

green

map of
locations

stimuli

attention

Figure 4.1
Model suggesting the relation between feature coding, spatial attention, and binding in object perception.

from other locations, we can simply bind whatever properties are currently attended. Figure 4.1 shows the model I proposed to relate the early parallel stages of vision to later attentional stages. It includes a master map of locations, that registers the locations of regions without giving access to the features that define them—for example, whether they represent discontinuities in luminance, colour, depth, or motion—and a separate set of feature maps. The feature maps contain two kinds of information: a "flag" signalling whether the feature is present anywhere in the field, and some implicit information about the current spatial layout of the feature. Not all tasks require binding. If a task can be done simply by checking the flag for the presence of activity within a single feature map, it should not depend on attention. So, for example, the information that there is something red out there can be accessed directly from the feature maps, but the location of the red thing and its other features cannot.

The hypothesis is that locating and binding the features requires retrieval of their connections to the master map of locations. To put "what" and "where" together, an attention window moves within the location map and selects from the feature maps whatever features are currently linked to the attended location, temporarily excluding the features of all other objects from the object perception level. The attended features can then be entered, without risk of binding errors, into the currently active object representation where their structural relations can be analysed. At the instant shown in the figure, the information explicitly available would be a detailed specification of the object currently in the attentional window, plus the fact that green and vertical are present elsewhere. There might also be surviving representations of previously attended objects, although, surprisingly, there is some evidence that the bindings are lost as soon as attention is withdrawn (Wolfe 1998). Once a unitary object has been set up, it can be matched to stored models and identified, and actions such as reaching or grasping it can be programmed.

3   Evidence from Illusory Conjunctions

Next, I will outline some behavioural evidence that seems consistent with this hypothesis. Perhaps the most dramatic comes from a patient who seems to have severe problems in binding features (Friedman-Hill et al. 1995, Robertson et al. 1997). They illustrate what can happen when binding breaks down. We showed R. M. some very simple displays containing just two coloured letters selected from T, X, and O in red, blue, or yellow, and asked him to tell us the first letter he saw (figure 4.2). The exposure durations ranged from 0.5 to 10 s. In some sessions, even with exposures as long as 10 s, he made binding errors, reporting one letter in the colour of the other, in more than 35% of trials. He reported a feature that was not in the display in less than 10% of trials. If he were guessing, these two

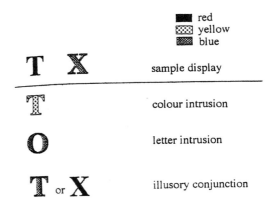

Figure 4.2
Stimuli used to test feature binding in patient R. M.

kinds of errors would be equally likely, as there was always one other colour or shape in the display and one not presented, so we can infer that one-quarter to one-third of his responses were binding errors. Clearly something had gone very wrong with his ability to bind. He had lost the ability that we all rely on to see stable well-integrated objects, and he now lives in a troubling world in which the binding problem is one he must constantly confront. I will return later to discuss other aspects of his perceptual problems.

Are there any conditions in which normal people have similar problems? As the hypothesis was that spatial attention is involved, we tried to prevent people from focusing attention by giving them a brief presentation and requiring them to spread their attention globally over the whole display (Treisman and Schmidt 1982). In one experiment, the displays contained four shapes varying in colour, size, shape, and format (filled or outline) arranged at the corners of a square, flanked on each side by two smaller black digits (figure 4.3a). Subjects were asked to give priority to noting the digits and to report them first. In addition they were to report all the features they could of the shape in one of the four locations, cued by a bar marker which appeared 200 ms

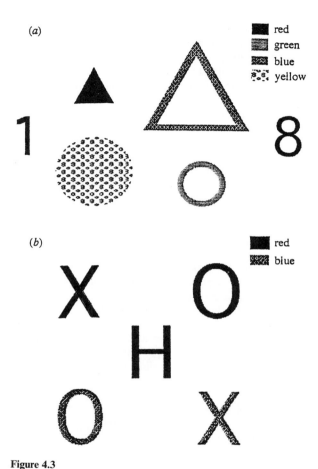

Figure 4.3
(*a*) Display illustrating task to test the role of attention in binding in normal subjects. The task is the report the identity of the two digits first and then as many features as are confidently seen for the object in the cued location, indicated by the bar marker. (*b*) Display illustrating same-different matching task that reveals binding errors without a load on memory.

after the display. The prediction is that they too should then make binding errors, putting features together in the wrong conjunctions. Subjects did in fact make many conjunction errors recombining the shape, size, format and colour. These occurred in 18% of trials, compared with only 6% intrusion errors. Again, we would expect equal numbers of each if subjects were guessing or misperceiving the individual features. Instead they seemed to form illusory conjunctions recombining features that in fact characterized separate objects. In another experiment with coloured letters, there were more than 30%. We called these errors "illusory conjunctions," implying that they are real perceptual illusions. Having frequently experienced them myself, although I had not expected to, I do think they are real illusions. Some are seen with high confidence. Also several subjects reported seeing coloured digits—even though they were not asked to report the colour of the digits and in fact had been told that they would always be black. Some binding errors may arise in memory; for example, a subject might remember seeing some red but forget where it was. But we still get a substantial number of illusory conjunctions when the task is simply to report whether there are two identical items in a display like that in figure 4.3b, where you can recombine the colour of the red H with the shape of the blue O to create an illusory red O, matching the one that is actually present.

Can we tie these binding errors more closely to the fact that we prevented subjects from focusing attention? In the experiment I described, where the relevant item was cued only after the display, subjects had no time to focus down to each coloured shape in turn in the brief exposures we gave them (around 200 ms). Using the same displays with another group of subjects, we cued the relevant item 150 ms before the display, and allowed subjects to ignore the digits, so that they could focus attention on the target item. We matched the overall accuracy by using a briefer exposure. As predicted, the binding errors dis-

appeared: there were about as many intrusions (10% compared with 12%), which means that all the errors could be accounted for as misperceptions of the target feature or guesses. So it does seem that spatial attention plays a role specifically in the binding process.

In other experiments we have recorded similar errors that recombine parts of shapes, like lines and Ss that recombine to form dollar signs in displays like those in figure 4.4a,b, even when the lines must be taken from apparently holistic perceptual units like triangles (figure 4.4c). We get illusory arrows from lines and angles (figure 4.4d), but not illusory triangles (figure 4.4e), at least not until we add some circles to the display (figure 4.4f; Treisman and Paterson 1984). The explanation we proposed here is that triangles have the extra visual feature, closure, that also has to be present in the display before an illusory triangle can be generated.

The theory predicts that illusory conjunctions are created on the basis of the flags that signal the presence of particular features. If this is the case, the number of binding errors should not be affected by the similarity of the objects on other attributes. This is what we found. Differences in the shape or size of the objects made little difference to the probability of a binding error involving colour, as though the features are detected independently of each other and then bound. In generating the resulting percept, the spatial distribution of colour is selected to fit the shape with which it has been bound, whether correctly or erroneously.

Some researchers (see, for example, Cohen and Ivry 1989) have shown spatial proximity effects on illusory conjunctions, such that features are more likely to be wrongly bound if they are close in space than if they are distant. Cohen and Ivry suggested that features have "coarse" location tags that are preattentively available. Proximity effects on binding errors could be a problem if we assume that locations are not available within the feature maps. However, it is very difficult to distinguish coarse coding of lo-

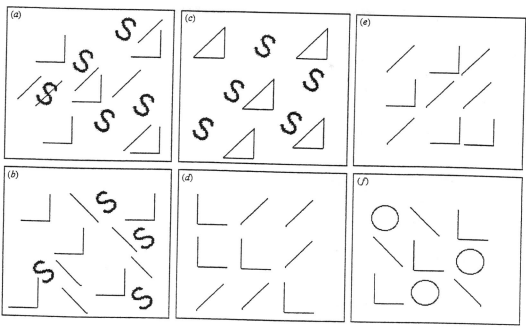

Figure 4.4
Examples of displays used to look for illusory conjunctions of parts of shapes. Subjects report illusory dollar signs in
4.4a, illusory arrows in 4.4b, and illusory triangles in 4.4d but not 4.4c.

cation from the idea that attention can rapidly
zoom in to define a general area (like the upper
left quadrant), but that it takes longer to focus
more finely on one of two adjacent items. When
the task prevented this zooming in by focusing
attention narrowly at the fovea, our normal
subjects showed no more illusory conjunctions
between adjacent than between distant items
(Treisman and Schmidt 1982). The Balint's patient, R. M., showed no effect of distance on his
binding error rates, consistent with the suggestion (see chapter 5) that he had lost his map of
locations.

Another prediction is that the number of
binding errors should also be independent of
the number of instances of particular features
because the claim is that all we have before the

binding has occurred is information about the
presence of features (the "flags" in figure 4.1),
not their individual instantiations. In an experiment (A. Treisman, unpublished data), we varied
the number of instances of particular features in
a display of four bars varying in orientation,
format (filled, outline or dotted) and colour. To
minimize memory errors, we cued subjects immediately after the display whether to report the
digits (on 20% of trials) or one of the bars (on
80% of trials), giving high priority to accuracy in
reporting the digits whenever they were cued. In
displays with three instances of one feature (e.g.,
red) and only one of another (e.g., green), we
found little difference in the number of illusory
conjunctions involving migrations of the feature
with three instantiations and of those with only

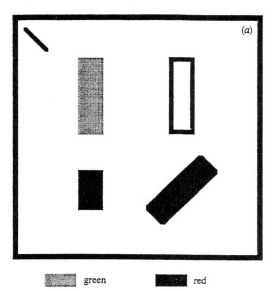

green red

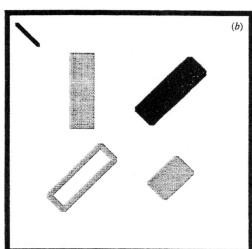

Figure 4.5
Examples of displays to test whether feature tokens or feature types migrate when binding errors are formed. In reporting the colour of the cued bar, the token hypothesis predicts three times as many illusory migrations of red in (a) as in (b).

one. The ratio was 1.5:1, rather than the 3:1 ratio that would be predicted if individuated tokens of the features were migrating. For example, in figure 4.5, reports of an illusory red bar in panels (a) and (b) were made on 15% and 10% of trials, respectively, although there are three times as many red objects in panel (a). In another experiment varying just colour and orientation the ratio was even lower, 1.2:1. Note that to the extent that the amount of red present affects the chance of detecting it, quite apart from the number of instances of red, we would expect the ratio to exceed 1:1.

The evidence from illusory conjunctions supports four claims: (i) that features are separately coded, otherwise they could not recombine; (ii) that the binding problem is therefore a real one; (iii) that focused attention is involved in solving it; and (iv) that attention is not required for the simple detection of separate features (although it is often attracted by the prior detection of a unique feature).

4 Visual Search and Binding

Search tasks offer another source of information on the role of attention in binding. We can define a target so that it either does or does not require binding. In displays of green Xs and brown Ts, a target specified only by a conjunction of features, for example a green T, should require focused attention to each item in turn, whereas a target specified by either of two unique features, a blue letter or a curved letter, should not involve binding and might therefore be detected independently of attention. If attention must be focused on each item in turn to find conjunction targets, we predict a linear increase in search times with the number of items in the display. This is what we found (Treisman and Gelade 1980). On the other hand, feature targets, signalled by flags on the feature maps, showed no effect of the number of items. They simply popped out of the displays.

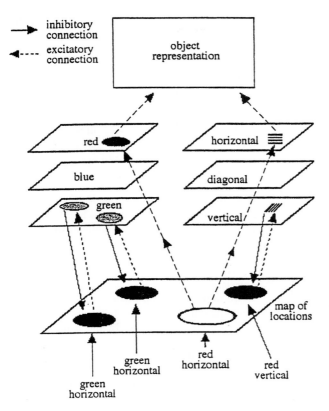

Figure 4.6
Modified model to allow control of selective attention from one or more feature maps as well as through a serial scan by a spatial window.

In some conjunction search tasks, there are other strategies besides the serial scan with focused attention, that can be used. We and others (see, for example, Treisman 1988, Wolfe et al. 1989, Nakayama 1990, Treisman and Sato 1990) have shown that when the target features are known in advance and when the relevant features are highly discriminable, subjects can use a feature-based grouping strategy to bypass the binding process. Essentially in looking for a red O among red Xs and blue Os, they may inhibit any location that contains blue and any location that contains an X. The red O would then emerge unscathed, without any need to bind distractor features. In the model, this would be implemented by reverse connections between the feature maps and the location map, selectively inhibiting all locations that contain unwanted features, and leaving only the target location to be checked (see figure 4.6).

5   Evidence from Parietal Lesions

So far this paper has been mostly behavioural. The model was developed from perceptual experiments. Can we tie it more closely to the brain? A classic experiment by Moran and Desimone (1985) seems consistent with the idea that attention selects by narrowing an attention window around the relevant object. Recording from cells in monkeys' area V4, they showed receptive fields essentially shrinking to exclude an unattended object when it fell into the same receptive field as the object to which the animal was trained to attend. What areas might control the attentional window? The parietal lobes are certainly involved in spatial attention. Unilateral damage to one parietal lobe produces a marked attentional deficit in the contralateral area of space. Particularly with right parietal damage, patients often show severe neglect of the left side of the visual field or the left side of an object. Investigations involving the patient I described earlier, who had such severe binding problems, may lead to a greater understanding of the brain areas involved. R. M. was unfortunate enough to suffer two successive strokes which destroyed both his parietal lobes, one after the other. He has normal acuity, contrast sensitivity, colour vision, stereopsis, and visual fields as tested formally by an ophthalmologist. However, he was left with a severe set of perceptual disabilities, some of which I've already outlined. Our hypothesis is that the master map of locations depends on parietal function. If this is correct, we can predict the set of deficits that the model would predict from his lesions.

1. Like any other theory, it would predict severe difficulties in conscious access to spatial information. The ability to point, reach for, or verbally label locations would be lost.

2. If individuating objects depends on binding them to separate locations, only one should be visible at a time.

3. If space is the medium in which attention binds features, there is a risk of illusory conjunctions whenever more than one object is present.

4. Conjunction search should be abnormally difficult or impossible; however, in feature search tasks, there should be no difficulty in detecting the presence of a target feature, even when it is embedded in several nontargets, as feature detection does not depend on binding.

I have already described data from R. M. confirming prediction 3—the illusory conjunctions. It is important to note that R. M. has no difficulty in binding the features of single objects presented sequentially. When we presented two coloured letters successively for 3 s each (instead of simultaneously for a total of 10 s), the estimate of binding errors was 0. So R. M. does not have a general deficit in binding features or a memory problem in remembering them; his difficulty is specifically in the ability to bind simultaneously presented features to the correct objects.

We tested R. M. on prediction 4, and found a dramatic difference in his ability to do the tasks. The target was a red X. In the feature search condition, the distractors differed either in shape (red Os) or in colour (blue Xs). In the conjunction search task, he looked for a red X among red Os and blue Xs. He had no difficulty with the feature targets. He detected the unique colour or shape in almost every trial, and independently of the number of items in the display, but he was unable to do the conjunction search, even with displays of only three to five items. He took up to 5 s and had error rates of 25%.

What about the first two predictions? These are the classic symptoms that Balint described in 1909. The spatial difficulties and the inability to see more than one object (simultanagnosia) are usually assumed to be separate and unrelated deficits, except that they cooccur with parietal damage. However, feature integration theory suggests that the simultanagnosia may actually be caused by the loss of space, simply because attention uses space to bind features to objects. R. M. did show severe deficits in his ability to localize. We asked him to report whether an X was at the top, bottom, left or right of the screen, or whether it was to the right, left, above or below an O. He was at chance in judging the relative locations of a widely separated X and O on the computer screen, and only slightly better at saying whether a single X was at the top, bottom, left or right of the screen. He seemed to have lost his representation of space almost completely. The confusion was not with the meaning of the words: he performed almost perfectly when asked to localize a touch on his back as up or down, or left or right. His somatosensory spatial functions were intact, and his spatial difficulties were specific to the visual modality.

R. M. also conformed to the second prediction. His simultanagnosia was as striking as his localization failures, at least in the early days after his stroke. When we held up two objects, say, a comb and a pair of scissors, he typically saw only one of them. When we asked him to count dots in displays of one to five, in an early session he saw at most two dots, even when we presented five. In later sessions, he guessed higher numbers but was still very inaccurate. We think he switched to attending more globally, to the group of dots as a whole, but this made him unable to access any individual dot and count it. R. M.'s simultanagnosia makes his normal performance in feature search all the more surprising. At a time when he could typically see only one or two objects, he had no difficulty detecting a unique colour or shape, regardless of how many other items were present.

An intriguing incident throws more light on R. M.'s perceptual experience. One morning he told us he had found a good way to improve his vision. With the help of his granddaughter, he had made a tube through which he looked at whatever he wanted to see more clearly. For someone suffering from simultanagnosia, one would think that a tube restricting the angle of vision would be the last thing they needed. However, on reflection, it makes more sense. If the damage to his brain prevents the normal

binding of features without preventing their detection at early levels of visual processing, the features of different objects should tend to coalesce into a single object, producing confusing mixtures of several features in the one object that is seen. R. M. did complain of such illusions. For example, he said "When I first look at it, it looks blue and it changes real quick to red. I see both colours coming together.... Sometimes one letter is going into the other one. I get a double identity. It kind of coincides." His descriptions sound as though he has no perceptual space in which to separate the letters and bind colours to shapes. The tube he invented may have helped by restricting the early detection of features to those of a single object. Essentially, he constructed an external window of attention to supplement a defective internal window. The findings with R. M. are consistent with the predictions that follow if he has lost the location map that controls spatial attention.

Further support for a parietal role, both in shifting spatial attention and in binding, comes from two recent studies of PET activation by Corbetta, Petersen, and others (Petersen et al. 1994, Corbetta et al. 1995; see also Corbetta 1998). They compared activation in a conjunction search task and in a task that required active shifting of attention between locations to track a target. They found similar activation in the superior parietal cortex in both tasks, consistent with the prediction that the binding process required in conjunction search does involve scanning with spatial attention, and that the parietal area is involved in its control. Ashbridge and coworkers (1997) found that transcranial magnetic stimulation to the right parietal lobe slowed conjunction search but left feature search unaffected. Taken together, these data suggest that we need an explicit representation of space for accurate conscious binding of features to objects. Thus, the dorsal parietal pathway interacts with the ventral pathway in mediating the perception of simultaneously presented objects. There might be "reentrant" connections from the parietal lobes, perhaps via the pulvinar, to selected locations in visual areas V1 or V2.

6 Binding in Feature Search

Having shown a possible link between the model and the brain, I will describe next some further behavioural findings with normal subjects that led us to elaborate the theory. One challenge to the feature integration account of search came from a suggestion that the pattern of linearly increasing search times with increasing number of distractors might result when targets are difficult to discriminate from distractors because they are similar to them, and when the distractors are sufficiently different from each other to prevent good grouping and segregation from the target (Duncan and Humphreys 1989). This could account for the difficulty of conjunction search, in which the target shares one or other feature with all the distractors while the two distractor types differ in both features from each other. It also predicts that search for feature targets could be equally difficult if they closely resemble the distractors, although no feature binding should be involved. One can certainly get steep and linear search functions with targets defined by a small unidimensional difference (see, for example, Treisman and Gormican 1988). However, the critical question is what counts as a feature for the visual system. The answer must be determined empirically. The challenge led to some further research which pointed to a new version of the binding problem that might explain these data.

When I drew the model in figure 4.1, I put in three feature maps per dimension, mainly because drawing 50 was beyond my artistic capabilities. But there is some evidence that the visual system does use coarse coding, representing different values on each dimension by ratios of activity in only a few separate populations of detectors (for example, vertical, diagonal, and horizontal for orientation, or red, green, blue,

and yellow for colour). Stimuli differing only slightly along a single dimension would not activate separate populations of feature detectors and would not be expected to pop out. They would pose a somewhat different binding problem—binding to location—so that the small differences in activation between areas containing only distractors and an area containing the target as well could be discriminated.

We have observed large asymmetries in search difficulty with many different pairs of stimuli, depending on which is the target and which the distractors (Treisman and Gormican 1988). A tilted line pops out among vertical lines, a curved line among straight ones, a circle with a gap among closed circles, an ellipse among circles, whereas the reverse pairings—a vertical line among tilted ones, a straight line among curves, a closed circle among circles with gaps, and a circle among ellipses—give search that is much slower and seems to require focused attention to each item in turn. The targets that pop out behave as though they have a unique perceptual feature, like a red dot among green dots, whereas the others do not. We also find a marked search asymmetry when we compare search for a shape with an added feature (like a Q among Os) and search for a shape that lacks the same feature (like an O in a display of Qs; Treisman and Souther 1985). Note that detecting an O among Qs also requires binding. To find the one circle which lacks a tail, we must locate all the tails and bind them to the Qs. On the other hand, to find a Q among Os, we can simply check for the presence of a tail anywhere in the display. There is no need to bind the tail to know that a Q is present. In this example, the same discrimination poses very different problems for the visual system, depending on whether or not the task requires binding.

Can we find an analogy in the case of the search asymmetries with apparently unidimensional stimuli like the targets defined by orientation or curvature? Here is where the coarse coding of features becomes relevant. A slightly tilted line might be coded by activity mainly in the detectors for vertical, with some additional activity in the diagonal detectors, just as a Q can be described as an O plus an extra tail. A slightly curved line could be coded as basically straight, plus some additional activity in detectors for curvature. The hypothesis is that the presence of this extra activity is detected without any need to bind it to the object, and this is enough to signal that the target is present. On the other hand, when the target is the one vertical line in a display in which all the lines but one are slightly tilted, both vertical and tilted detectors would be active everywhere except in the one location where the vertical target leaves the tilt detectors silent.

If this hypothesis is correct, we should be able also to prevent popout for a tilted target by turning its detection into a task that requires binding. The assumption is that a tilted target pops out among verticals because of the additional unique activity it evokes in the detectors for diagonals. If we now mix diagonal distractors with the vertical ones, activity in the vertical and diagonal detectors must be bound together to identify the target by its particular ratio of activation levels in the two detector populations. This changes the task into search for a conjunction target, and we should expect to switch from parallel popout to serial search with focused attention. Similarly a purple target will pop out among either blue or red distractors alone, but among a mixture of blue and red distractors it will require binding of activity in blue and red detectors that share the same location and should therefore depend on serial attentive scanning. I tested search for purple targets tilted 27° in displays of blue vertical bars and pink bars tilted 63°, and found that search indeed looked serial, even though the colour and orientation of the target were objectively unique in the display and easily discriminable from either type of distractor alone (Treisman 1991). Furthermore, when we briefly flashed displays with the same stimuli, subjects made a large number of false

alarms, detecting illusory targets. They saw far more illusory conjunctions in these displays in which I suggest that within-dimension binding is required than in displays where the target, although equated for similarity, was defined by a colour and orientation that would be directly coded by standard feature detectors, for example a blue vertical bar among purple and turquoise bars tilted 27° left and right. Thus, coarse coding by ratios of firing in different populations of feature detectors does seem to create another kind of binding problem.

The features that are preattentively detected are probably not those of the retinal image. Enns and Rensink (1991) and He and Nakayama (1992) have shown rapid or parallel detection of simple three-dimensional (3D) features of surfaces and illumination. The shading that results from 3D shape can produce segregation of a group of convex objects among concave ones, assuming lighting from above (Ramachandran 1988). This segregation is much clearer than with supposedly simpler black and white patterns. Although these might seem like conjunctions of shape and texture or luminance, the critical question is whether they are directly sensed by separate populations of neural detectors. Lehky and Sejnowski (1988) showed that simple neural networks, when trained to respond to gradients of shape from shading, evolve hidden units (i.e., units intermediate between the input and the output units) that look very similar to the simple cells that Hubel and Wiesel (1968) identified in area V1 and that have normally been assumed to be bar or grating detectors. The features that are directly coded by the visual system may actually be features that characterize 3D surfaces. It seems harder to find plausible candidates for featurehood in the geometric line arrangements of the cubes whose 3D orientations define the target in some of Enns and Rensink's (1991) experiments. However, what they find are asymmetries of search rather than the flat search functions associated with popout. Search is much faster for some target-distractor combina-

Table 4.1
Visual search studies

Serial search (attention required)	Parallel search (automatic pop-out)
Conjunction targets (e.g., green T in green Hs and brown Ts)	Feature targets (e.g., blue or S in green Hs and brown Ts)
Os in Qs	Qs in Os
Vertical line in tilted lines	Tilted line in vertical lines
Straight line in curved lines	Curved line in straight lines
Parallel lines in converging lines	Converging lines in parallel lines
Circle with gap in closed circles	Closed circle in circles with gaps
Purple bar tilted 27° in blue 0° (vertical) bars and red bars tilted 63°	Blue 0° (vertical) bar in purple bars tilted 27° left and turquoise bars tilted 27° right

tions than for others but not usually parallel unless shading is also present. Table 4.1 summarizes the results I have described on search and binding.

7   Implicit Processing of Conjunctions

For the last part of the paper, we move to another line of research which opens up issues in three new directions: so far I have discussed binding under a fairly narrow definition: it has been measured by conscious reports rather than by implicit indices; it has been manifested in immediate perceptual tests rather than in memory; and finally the information has concerned only stimulus features and locations, not the binding of actions to perceived events. Yet these are also aspects of a more general binding problem. We need to retain bindings in memory after the objects disappear, and we need to bind appropriate responses to the objects we identify. The experiments I have been pursuing recently extend the research in these three directions by comparing implicit with explicit measures of visual memory and specifying the choice of which object requires a response. The results have surprised us, and seem to have important implications for a more general understanding of binding.

First the question whether any implicit binding can be revealed, which we are unable to access consciously. There is increasing evidence that explicit reports may not exhaust all the information available to the visual system. Understanding what makes some information accessible and some not is an intriguing challenge. In particular, it is important to determine whether binding imposes a real computational limitation, or whether it is just a problem for conscious representation?

First, we did get a few surprising results with the patient R. M., when we used indirect measures to probe for implicit information about locations. We presented the word "UP" or "DOWN" at the top or bottom of a vertical rectangle. In any given trial, the semantics of the word and its location could be consistent (e.g., the word "UP" in the upper location), or inconsistent (e.g., the word "UP" in the lower location). R. M. read the words rapidly and correctly (note that binding was not necessarily involved in this reading task because the two words to be discriminated differed in all their letters and also in length), but his response times were 142 ms slower when the word was in an inconsistent location. So the locations interfered with his reading at a time when he was at chance in voluntarily locating the words. We were also able to show unconscious priming of spatial selection by a cross-modal cue although R. M. was unable voluntarily to select the cued item. We presented two visual letters, one on each side of the screen, at the same time as tapping his right or left shoulder. When we asked him to name the letter on the side that we had tapped, he was at chance, but when we simply asked him to name the first (or only) letter he saw, he reported significantly more from the tapped side. It seems that some implicit representation of space remains despite the loss of parietal function, perhaps in extrastriate areas of the ventral pathway, although this information is not consciously accessible. Finally, Egly and colleagues (1995) ran another experiment that also revealed implicit information about the spatial distribution of elements. Their displays consisted of a global letter made of local letters. When asked what he saw, R. M. never reported the global letter. He seemed to see only one of the local letters. Yet when asked to classify the local letter as one of two possible targets, he was significantly slower when the global letter was inconsistent with the local one than when it was consistent. Again, he seemed to have implicit information—this time about the whole, even though he could only respond to a part.

DeSchepper and I have explored implicit visual processing in normal subjects as well. We found indirect evidence that fairly complex patterns can be registered, bound and stored implicitly without conscious attention. However, it is important to add that this seems to be true only for one unattended object. When more are added, the evidence for implicit binding disappears (Neumann and DeSchepper 1992). The measure we used is known as negative priming. Subjects are typically shown two objects and asked to respond to one of the two, selected by some simple distinguishing feature like its colour. So, for example, Tipper and Cranston (1985) asked subjects to name pictures of familiar objects selecting the red one in each overlapped pair. Their responses were slower when the unattended green object on one trial became the attended red one on the next, relative to when two new objects were shown. A plausible account was that subjects inhibited the green object to avoid naming it instead of the red. When it then became the relevant object, on the next trial, they had to overcome the inhibition. As a result, the response was slightly delayed. This

negative priming implies: (i) that subjects formed and retained a memory trace of the picture, even when it was the unattended member of a pair; and (ii) that an action tag was bound to the memory, specifying whether it should be responded to or ignored.

DeSchepper and I wondered whether novel patterns would also produce negative priming. If so, this would be evidence that a representation of their shape was formed, even in the absence of attention. We used overlapped pairs of 270 nonsense shapes that the subjects had never seen before, similar to those in figure 4.7 (DeSchepper and Treisman 1996). The task was to decide whether the green shape on the left matched a single white shape to the right of the display, ignoring the red shape. We gave subjects some practice with a set of 12 shapes that we used repeatedly, and then we introduced new shapes mixed with the old. We found a clear negative priming effect of about 30 ms, which was actually larger on the first trial in which a new shape was presented than it was for the familiarized shapes. Subjects apparently set up a new representation for the unattended as well as the attended shape and attached an inhibitory action tag to it, specifying that it should be rejected. On the other hand, they had no conscious memory at all for the unattended shape. Their recognition was at chance, even when probed immediately after a pair was presented. We infer that attention is needed at the time of encoding if objects are to be explicitly retrieved.

Can we say any more about the nature of these implicit memory traces? How detailed and specific are they? How well bound are their parts and properties? With two other students, Alex Kulczycki and Xuexin Zhang, I asked what happens if we change either a feature or a component of the unattended prime before presenting it again as the attended probe (Zhang et al. 1996). In one experiment, we either kept the size the same, or changed it to larger or smaller. Surprisingly, when we changed the size, the result was not inhibition but facilitation. Subjects

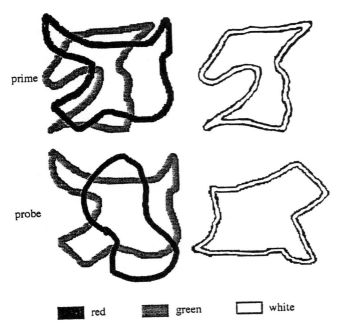

prime

probe

red   green   white

Figure 4.7
Examples of a prime and a probe trial testing negative priming with novel nonsense shapes. Subjects attended to the green shape in each trial and decided whether it matched the white one. They ignored the red shape, which on negative priming trials reappears as the attended shape in green, resulting in slower responses.

were slightly quicker to respond to the previously unattended shape when its size was changed than to respond to a new shape. In another experiment, we presented only half of the prime shape combined with half a new shape, to see if the inhibition was attached only to the whole or separately to each component part. Figure 4.8 shows three successive trials in which subjects matched the two outside shapes and ignored the central shape. Two trials later, half of the first ignored central shape appeared as half of the relevant outside shapes, combined with half of the second ignored shape. We got negative priming as usual when the shapes were identical, but again there was facilitation when we recombined two previously unattended halves from two different

trials to form a new whole, and also when we presented only half the prime shape combined with a new half shape. Khurana and coworkers (1994) looked at negative priming for faces and got a similar result: when the prime and the probe face were identical, they got inhibition, but when they reversed the contrast on the probe trial, they got facilitation.

Thus, the action tag that produces negative priming seems to be bound to a very specific conjunction of shape with size or contrast and of the parts of a shape with each other. But in addition we form a more abstracted representation which is size and contrast-invariant, and which may have separate articulated parts. This representation is not linked to the specific responses

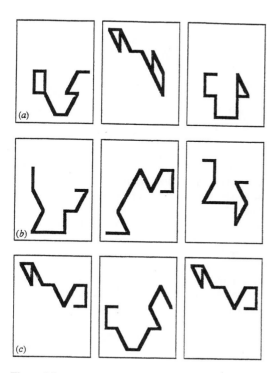

Figure 4.8
Examples of two prime trials and a probe trial. The task was to decide as quickly as possible whether the shapes in the two outside positions were the same or different. The third (probe) trial recombines two previously unattended half primes to form the attended shape. Instead of negative priming, facilitation was observed relative to a new shape that had not been previously presented.

required in the context in which it was seen, and it can facilitate later perception of similar or related objects.

We wondered how long these implicit memory traces for novel unattended shapes would linger in our subjects' brains. So we looked for negative priming, not only in the next trial, but after 10, 100, or 200 intervening trials with up to 400 different intervening shapes. To our considerable

surprise, we found that the inhibition was undiminished 200 trials later. The binding here seems quite persistent even though it is formed in a single unattended trial. We also tested intervals of a day, a week, and a month and found significant priming even at those long delays, but with some indication of a shift from inhibition to facilitation. The survival of these memory traces for novel shapes in our experiments suggests a surprising combination of visual plasticity and persistence. The newly formed representations remain available, separate and distinct from each other, for days or even weeks. If we had to speculate about where the representations are formed and stored, the temporal lobes in the ventral pathway seem a likely neural basis. Single unit recordings in monkeys, and brain imaging studies in humans, suggest that this is the area where objects are perceptually coded and form the memory traces that mediate subsequent priming. For explicit memory, on the other hand, the hippocampus and adjacent cortical areas are likely to be involved.

8   Conclusions

It is time to try to pull things together, both the different results described here, and their relation to the different view of attention proposed by Duncan (1998). The results on tasks requiring explicit binding, both from normal subjects and from the patient R. M., suggested that attention is needed to bind features together, and that without attention, the only information recorded is the presence of separate parts and properties. Yet both the negative priming results in normals and the interference from global letters in R. M. suggest that there are conditions in which wholes are registered automatically, without attention or conscious awareness.

I think there is no real contradiction between these results. Binding failures typically occur with high load displays when several objects must be processed under high time pressure.

When there is only one unattended object, its features must belong together, so there should be no problem determining what goes with what. Indeed, when the number of unattended objects in a negative priming task was increased from one to two or three, Neumann and DeSchepper (1992) found that negative priming disappears. Attention here plays a different role: the unattended object may be suppressed to prevent response conflict and to ensure that conscious experience is coherent and consistent with our behavioural responses.

The patient R. M. makes binding errors with only two objects present because he is unable to separate them spatially to select one for attention and ignore the other. His implicit knowledge about locations that he cannot consciously locate may come from the ventral pathway where it is not normally accessible for conscious perception. As Humphreys (1998) suggests, spatial relations within objects may be coded by separate systems from the spatial relations between objects. The arrangement of parts within an object may be coded holistically in order to identify the object rather than to relate the two parts as separate entities in space. We might explain the spatial Stroop interference shown by R. M., if his ventral pathway coded the rectangle together with its word as a consistent or inconsistent whole. In the location naming task, on the other hand, R. M. was asked to relate the position of the word as an object to the rectangle as another object, presumably requiring the use of his damaged parietal lobes to label these between-object relations.

The hypothesis outlined in this chapter about the role of attention in binding appears to conflict with Duncan's view of attention as integrated competition between objects (Desimone and Duncan 1995, Duncan 1998; see also Bundesen 1998). In Duncan's language, attention is a state into which the system settles through global competition between objects for dominance over experience and action, rather than a selective process that helps create those objects. He denies

the need for any external selective mechanism. However, for the features of the same object to cooperate in competition with others and to benefit from each other's ascendancy in the competition, it seems as though they would already need to be bound. Duncan's suggestion is that binding is achieved through detectors directly coding conjunctions of pairs of attributes. An alternative is that the competition postulated in Duncan's framework could arise at a later level than the binding mechanism proposed here, and could have evolved to determine selection for the control of actions. Attention need not be a unitary process simply because a single word is used in everyday language.

One of the findings supporting Duncan's account is the long duration that he and his colleagues observed for the "attentional blink" (the interference with detecting a second target caused by detecting the first in a rapid visual sequence of items (Duncan et al. 1994)). The interference lasts for about 500 ms after the first target has been detected, suggesting an "attentional dwell time" of half a second rather than the 60 or so milliseconds implied when one interprets the slope of search times against the number of items simultaneously presented as a serial scanning rate. However, there are a number of ways of reconciling these findings. One is that scanning items that are simultaneously present amd unmasked may allow some parallel preprocessing to occur at the same time as the serial attentional binding, whereas each item in a sequential display interrupts the processing of its predecessor and must itself be processed from scratch. With a presentation rate of 150 ms instead of 90 ms per item, we found little evidence of a blink, suggesting that when the processing is not interrupted by the early onset of a new item or mask, an upper limit to the dwell time is 100–200 ms rather than 500 ms. Another contrast with most attentional blink experiments is that processing in search displays is serial across distractors, not targets, if it is serial at all. Processing of targets is likely to take longer than processing of distractors, as it requires commitment to a response. Finally, if processing in search is serial across pairs or small groups of homogeneous distractors rather than single items, observed slopes of 60 ms per item would imply dwell times of 120 or 180 ms (Treisman and Sato 1990), reducing the apparent discrepancy between sequential and simultaneous presentation.

As must be clear, this is work in progress and there is much that is not yet understood. The use of implicit priming measures opens new perspectives. The intriguing dissociations that we and others are finding between conscious experience and indirect priming suggest that the binding problem may be intimately bound up with the nature of consciousness, but that is a story that I think no one is yet ready to tell.

Acknowledgments

This work was supported by NSF, grant numbers SBR-9511633 and SBR-9631132. I thank D. Kahneman for helpful comments on the manuscript.

References

Ashbridge, E., Walsh, V. & Cowey, A. 1997 Temporal aspects of visual search studied by transcranial magnetic stimulation. *Neuropsychologia* 35, 1121–1131.

Bundesen, C. 1998 A computational theory of visual attention. *Philos. Trans. R. Soc. Lond. B. Biol. Sci.* 353, 1271–1281.

Cohen, A. & Ivry, R. 1989 Illusory conjunctions inside and outside the focus of attention. *J. Exp. Psychol. Hum. Percept. Perf.* 15, 650–663.

Corbetta, M., Miezin, F., Dobmeyer, S., Shulman, G. & Petersen, S. 1991 Selective and divided attention during visual discrimination of shape, colour and speed: functional anatomy by positron emission tomography. *J. Neurosci.* 11, 2383–2402.

Corbetta, M. & Shulman, G. L. 1998 Human cortical mechanisms of visual attention during orienting and search. *Philos. Trans. R. Soc. Lond. B. Biol. Sci.* 353, 1353–1362.

Corbetta, M., Shulman, G. L., Miezin, F. M. & Petersen, S. E. 1995 Superior parietal cortex activation during spatial attention shifts and visual feature conjunction. *Science* 270, 802–805.

Cowey, A. 1985 Aspects of cortical organization related to selective attention and selective impairments of visual attention. In *Attention and performance XI* (ed. M. P. & O. Marin), pp. 41–62. Hillsdale, NJ: Lawrence Erlbaum.

Damasio, A., Yamata, T., Damasio, H., Corbetta, J. & McKee, J. 1980 Central achromatopsia: behavioral, anatomic, and physiologic aspects. *Neurology* 30, 1064–1071.

DeSchepper, B. & Treisman, A. 1996 Visual memory for novel shapes: implicit coding without attention. *J. Exp. Psychol. Learn. Mem. Cogn.* 22, 27–47.

Desimone, R. & Duncan, J. 1995 Neural mechanisms of selective visual attention. *A. Rev. Neurosci.* 18, 193–222.

Duncan, J. 1998 Converging levels of analysis in the cognitive neuroscience of visual attention. *Philos. Trans. R. Soc. Lond. B. Biol. Sci.* 353, 1307–1317.

Duncan, J. & Humphreys, G. W. 1989 Visual search and stimulus similarity. *Psychol. Rev.* 96, 433–458.

Duncan, J., Ward, R. & Shapiro, K. 1994 Direct measurement of attentional dwell time. *Nature* 369, 313–315.

Egly, R., Robertson, L. C., Rafal, R. & Grabowecky, M. 1995 Implicit processing of unreportable objects in Balint's syndrome. Los Angeles: Psychonomic Society Abstracts.

Enns, J. & Rensink, R. A. 1991 Preattentive recovery of three-dimensional orientation from line drawings. *Psychol. Rev.* 98, 335–351.

Friedman-Hill, S. R., Robertson, L. C. & Treisman, A. 1995 Parietal contributions to visual feature binding: evidence from a patient with bilateral lesions. *Science* 269, 853–855.

Goodale, M. A. & Milner, A. D. 1992 Separate visual pathways for perception and action. *Trends. Neurosci.* 15, 20–25.

Gray, C. M., Konig, P., Engel, A. & Singer, W. 1989 Oscillatory responses in cat visual cortex exhibit inter-columnar synchronization which reflects global stimulus properties. *Nature* 338, 334–337.

Gulyas, B. & Roland, P. E. 1991 Cortical fields participating in form and colour discrimination in the human brain. *NeuroReport* 2, 585–588.

He, Z. J. & Nakayama, K. 1992 Surfaces versus features in visual search. *Nature* 359, 231–233.

Hubel, D. H. & Wiesel, T. N. 1968 Receptive fields and functional architecture of monkey striate cortex. *J. Physiol.* 195, 215–243.

Hummel, J. E. & Biederman, I. 1992 Dynamic binding in a neural network for shape recognition. *Psychol. Rev.* 99, 480–517.

Humphreys, G. W. 1998 Neural representation of objects in space: a dual coding account. *Philos. Trans. R. Soc. Lond. B. Biol. Sci.* 353, 1341–1351.

Khurana, B., Smith, W. C., Baker, M. T. & Huang, C. 1994 Face representation under conditions of inattention. *Invest. Ophthalmol. Vis. Sci.* 35 (Suppl. 4), Abstract No. 4135.

Lehky, S. R. & Sejnowski, T. J. 1988 Network model of shape-from-shading: neural function arises from both receptive and projective fields. *Nature* 332, 154–155.

Meadows, J. C. 1974 Disturbed perception of colours associated with localized cerebral lesions. *Brain* 97, 615–632.

Moran, J. & Desimone, R. 1985 Selective attention gates visual processing in the extra-striate cortex. *Science* 229, 782–784.

Nakayama, K. 1990 The iconic bottleneck and the tenuous link between early visual processing and perception. In *Vision: coding and efficiency* (ed. C. Blakemore), pp. 411–422. Cambridge University Press.

Navon, D. 1977 Forest before trees: the precedence of global features in visual perception. *Cogn. Psychol.* 9, 353–383.

Neumann, E. & DeSchepper, B. G. 1992 An inhibition-based fan effect: evidence for an active suppression mechanism in selective attention. *Can. J. Psychol.* 46, 1–40.

Petersen, S. E., Corbetta, M., Miezin, F. M. & Shulman, G. L. 1994 PET studies of parietal involvement in spatial attention: comparison of different task types. *Can. J. Exp. Psychol.* 48, 319–338.

Posner, M. I. 1980 Orienting of attention. *Q. J. Exp. Psychol.* 32, 3–26.

Ramachandran, V. S. 1988 Perceiving shape from shading. *Sci. Am.* 259, 76–83.

Robertson, L., Treisman, A., Friedman-Hill, S. & Grabowecky, M. 1997 The interaction of spatial and object pathways: evidence from Balint's syndrome. *J. Cogn. Neurosci.* 9, 254–276.

Sereno, M. I., Dale, A. M., Reppas, J. B., Kwong, K. K., Belliveau, J., Brady, T. J., Rosen, B. R. & Tootell, R. B. H. 1995 Borders of multiple visual areas in humans revealed by functional magnetic resonance imaging. *Science* 268, 889–893.

Singer, W. & Gray, C. M. 1995 Visual feature integration and the temporal correlation hypothesis. *A. Rev. Neurosci.* 18, 555–586.

Tanaka, K. 1993 Neuronal mechanisms of object recognition. *Science* 262, 685–688.

Tipper, S. P. & Cranston, M. 1985 Selective attention and priming: inhibitory and facilitatory effects of ignored primes. *Q. J. Exp. Psychol. A* 37, 591–611.

Treisman, A. 1982 Perceptual grouping and attention in visual search for features and for objects. *J. Exp. Psychol. Hum. Percept. Perf.* 8, 194–214.

Treisman, A. 1988 Features and objects: the Fourteenth Bartlett Memorial Lecture. *Q. J. Exp. Psychol. A* 40, 201–237.

Treisman, A. & Gelade, G. 1980 A feature integration theory of attention. *Cogn. Psychol.* 12, 97–136.

Treisman, A. & Gormican, S. 1988 Feature analysis in early vision: evidence from search asymmetries. *Psychol. Rev.* 95, 15–48.

Treisman, A. & Paterson, R. 1984 Emergent features, attention and object perception. *J. Exp. Psychol. Hum. Percept. Perf.* 10, 12–21.

Treisman, A. & Sato, S. 1990 Conjunction search revisited. *J. Exp. Psychol. Hum. Percept. Perf.* 16, 459–478.

Treisman, A. & Schmidt, H. 1982 Illusory conjunctions in the perception of objects. *Cogn. Psychol.* 14, 107–141.

Treisman, A. & Souther, J. 1985 Search asymmetry: a diagnostic for preattentive processing of separable features. *J. Exp. Psychol. Gen.* 114, 285–310.

Ungerleider, L. G. & Mishkin, M. 1982 *Two cortical visual systems*. Cambridge, MA: MIT Press.

Ward, L. 1982 Determinants of attention to local and global features of visual forms. *J. Exp. Psychol. Hum. Percept. Perf.* 8, 562–581.

Wolfe, J. M. 1998 Inattentional amnesia. In *Fleeting memories* (ed. V. Coltheart). Cambridge, MA: MIT Press. (In the press.)

Wolfe, J. M., Cave, K. R. & Franzel, S. L. 1989 Guided search: an alternative to the feature integration model for visual search. *J. Exp. Psychol. Hum. Percept. Perf.* 15, 419–433.

Zeki, S. M. 1991 Cerebral akinetopsia (visual motion blindness). *Brain* 114, 811–824.

Zeki, S. 1993 *A vision of the brain.* Oxford: Blackwell.

Zihl, J., von Cramon, D. & Mai, N. 1983 Selective disturbance of movement vision after bilateral brain damage. *Brain* 106, 313–340.

5 Effects of Sleep and Arousal on the Processing of Visual Information in the Cat

Margaret S. Livingstone and David H. Hubel

Subjectively it seems obvious that the way in which the brain handles sensory information must change radically between sleeping and waking. To examine these changes it is important to be able to influence the firing of neurones along a sensory pathway by natural stimulation. We have chosen the visual system to study neural activity as a function of the state of arousal because, in the pathway from the retina through the lateral geniculate body (LGB) to the primary visual cortex, the properties of the cells are well understood in terms of their optimum visual stimuli. In an animal that closes its eyes when asleep, additional mechanisms for blocking visual messages during sleep might seem unnecessary but, beyond the retina, such mechanisms do seem to exist. In the cat, spontaneous firing patterns of cells in the LGB[1,2] and primary visual cortex[3-6] show marked differences between sleeping and waking. In the LGB Coenen and Vendrik[7] have shown that responses to light stimulation are strongly enhanced on arousal in lightly anaesthetized cats. In the present study we have recorded from single cells in the LGB and striate cortex,[8] examining the effects of the state of wakefulness on both the vigour and specificity of responses. We have also compared sleep and arousal using the 2-deoxyglucose method for labelling neurones according to activity.[9,10]

Single-Cell Recording

We compared spontaneous and visually evoked firing in sleeping and waking states in 130 cortical cells in 15 cats, and in 14 geniculate neurones in 2 cats.

Each cat was first sleep deprived overnight in a slowly revolving (0.5 r.p.m.) drum, and then prepared as if for chronic recording,[1,4] under halothane anaesthesia. Four chlorided silver electroencephalogram (EEG) electrodes were cemented over the dura and a pedestal for holding a hydraulic microelectrode advancer was cemented to the skull. For cortical recording we positioned the pedestal over the postlateral gyrus. For geniculate recording the animal's head was put in a Horsley–Clarke headholder and the pedestal cemented stereotaxically above the LGB. The head was then freed, well before terminating the anaesthesia. We infiltrated skin incisions with Xylocaine, intubated the trachea, paralysed the animal with continuous intravenous succinylcholine, and monitored levels of expired CO_2. The head was held firmly with adhesive tape and gauze pads. Pupils were dilated with homatropine, contact lenses were fitted so that images on a screen at 1.5 m distance produced a focused image on the retina, and the optic disk and area centralis of each eye were mapped by optical projection. When necessary we used an adjustable prism to bring the two centres of gaze into superposition.

The halothane was then discontinued, and in the EEG irregular high-voltage activity of the anaesthetized state gave way, in a few minutes, to the low-voltage rapid activity of the waking state. Most of the cats then slept spontaneously and frequently, as indicated by high-voltage slow waves. Arousal from slow-wave sleep was spontaneous or could be produced by a noise or tactile stimulus. Rapid eye movement (REM) sleep was recognized by episodes of large monophasic potentials recorded from the visual cortex (ponto-geniculo-occipital (PGO) waves), which could be suppressed by arousing the animal.

For each cell we first mapped receptive fields on the screen with a hand-held slide projector. For cortical cells a computer-driven optic bench was adjusted to produce moving-slit stimuli which were tailored for optimal position, orientation, shape and rate of movement. The stimuli for geniculate cells were stationary circular spots

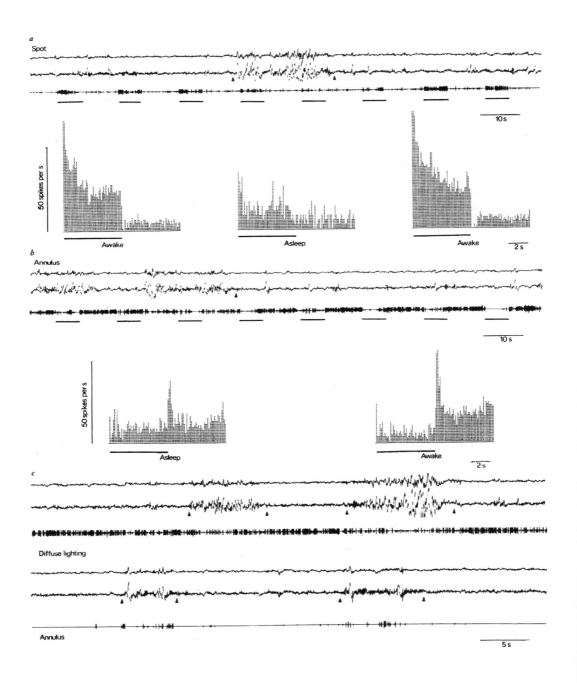

or annuli. Action potentials, EEGs, and traces representing the presentations of the stimuli were recorded on a Grass polygraph and on magnetic tape for subsequent averaging. Every cell included in the series was followed over several transitions between waking and high-voltage slow-wave sleep.

Recordings from Lateral Geniculate Body

With the screen diffusely lit, geniculate cells showed an increase in spontaneous firing rate when the animal was aroused from slow-wave sleep, as expected from previous studies.[7,11–13] Moreover, the pattern of firing changed from high-frequency bursts of two to eight spikes to more regular firing.[1,3,14]

In all 14 geniculate cells there were marked changes also in responsiveness to visual stimuli, as illustrated in figure 5.1. In figure 5.1a, during an otherwise wakeful period, there was a brief episode of high-voltage slow-wave sleep lasting about 30 s and ending spontaneously. The stimulus, which was repeated throughout, was a small (1/4°) spot of light covering the receptive field centre. During the slow waves there was a depression of the on-response, obvious in both the spike record and the average-response histograms. This change is most easily explained by supposing that the efficacy of optic nerve fibres in triggering the geniculate cell is enhanced on arousal.[7] All the effects of arousal cannot be explained in this way, however. In figure 5.1b, the stimulus was an annulus covering the surround of the cell's receptive field. Now spontaneous arousal was accompanied not only by an increase in the off-discharge, but also by an enhanced suppression of firing while the annulus was on.

Figure 5.1c shows the enhancement of suppression for the same on-centre cell, in a slightly different way. In figure 5.1c, upper half, the screen was lit steadily and diffusely by a low-level background light. The tonic firing of the cell was obviously decreased during each of the two bursts of slow waves. In the lower half, an annulus covering the receptive field surround tonically suppressed the firing. The suppression was almost complete when the EEG was flat, but during the slow waves there were bursts of impulses. Thus arousal could depress or elevate the cell's firing rate, depending on the visual stimulus used.

Figure 5.1

(a) and (b), Responses of an on-centre cell from layer A of the lateral geniculate nucleus in a drowsy cat. In each polygraph record the upper two traces are the bipolar EEGs from anterior and posterior head regions; the third trace shows the spikes from the geniculate cell, converted into pulses, in these and subsequent polygraph records, by a Schmitt trigger circuit. Each record lasts ~2 min. Brief periods of sleep, which end spontaneously, are indicated by the slow waves in the middle of record (a) and (roughly) the left half of (b). The approximate transitions between the flat waking EEG record and periods of slow-wave sleep are indicated by arrowheads. In (a) a spot covering the receptive field centre is flashed on and off. The relative weakness of the on responses during periods of slow waves can be seen in the record of spikes and in the three histograms. The left histogram is the average of 13 responses, of which the last 3 are shown. The middle histogram is an average of the 2 responses during the burst of slow waves, and the right histogram the average of the next 16 responses. In (b) the stimulus is an annulus covering the receptive-field surround. Both the suppression of firing during the stimulus and the off-discharge are weaker during sleep. Histograms are the average of nine responses each, before and after the arrowhead. (c) Effects of slow-wave sleep on steady-state firing of the same cell. In the upper set of three traces (50 s) the screen is diffusely lit by the background light. At each burst of slow waves in the cortical EEG (upper two traces) the rate of firing declines. In the lower set an annulus covers the receptive-field surround. In the aroused periods the discharges are almost completely suppressed, but each episode of slow waves is accompanied by bursts of impulses. Onset and end of slow-wave bursts are indicated by arrowheads.

For off-centre cells there was a similar enhancement, both in the suppression of firing and off-discharge to a spot covering the receptive field centre, and in the on-response to an annulus. In both on-centre and off-centre cells diffuse light was less effective than a spot confined to the receptive field centre. This is characteristic of geniculate cells. The diffuse light responses of both on-centre and off-centre cells showed little or no enhancement on arousal from slow-wave sleep, presumably because the increase in the response from the field centre was counterbalanced by an increased opponent response from the surround. To understand the significance of this one must recall that a weaker response to a large spot than to a small one just covering the field centre is characteristic also of retinal ganglion cells.[15,16] But geniculate cells receiving their main excitatory optic input from a single retinal ganglion cell show a more pronounced reduction in response to stimuli including the field surround than do the retinal ganglion cells[14,17]: indeed, this is the main known contribution of the lateral geniculate to the processing of visual information. If the response enhancement on arousal were greater for a large spot than for a small one, one would have to conclude that arousal led to an impairment of this function.

Arousal from slow-wave sleep produced no obvious changes in geniculate receptive field sizes as mapped by small spots. As visual acuity is presumably related in geniculate cells to receptive field centre size, an increase in centre size on arousal[18] would have been perplexing if not dismaying.

In summary, arousal from slow-wave sleep increased the spontaneous firing rate of lateral geniculate cells and reduced or eliminated the high-frequency bursts (not resolved in the slow time scale of figure 5.1); both the excitatory and inhibitory components of responses to spatially restricted visual stimuli were enhanced; and, finally, responses from the receptive field centre and the antagonistic surround were both enhanced.

Presumably the mechanism of these effects depends on nonretinal projections to the LGB because in mammals there do not seem to be projections from brain to retina, and firing of retinal ganglion cells is unaffected by arousal.[1] The increase in the on- or off-discharges on arousal is known to reflect an increase in the proportion of optic nerve impulses that succeed in triggering geniculate impulses (the firing index).[7] The enhanced suppression of discharge seen on arousal may reflect enhanced inhibition from other geniculate neurones that are excited by the stimulus and whose firing index is increased by arousal; or arousal may lead to an enhancement of both excitatory and inhibitory synapses. An increased firing during sleep might also be somehow related to the high-voltage cortical slow waves, which, if present in thalamus and cortex concurrently, could be associated with swings in membrane potential capable of triggering bursts of impulses. Suppressing these slow waves, on arousal, could then abolish the discharges.

Visual Cortex

In contrast to geniculate cells, cortical cells varied greatly from one to the next in the degree to which they were influenced by changes in arousal level. Marked differences were often seen between two cells simultaneously recorded from two electrodes spaced 1 mm or less apart, or between two cells simultaneously recorded from one electrode. Nevertheless, each individual cell showed a consistent type of change over several cycles of sleeping and waking. Usually (in two-thirds of the 130 cells studied) an irregular burst of spontaneous firing in slow-wave sleep was reduced in overall rate and replaced by a smoother, more regular pattern on awakening. In 10 cells there was an increased firing rate and a smoothing. The rest of the cells showed no difference in spontaneous activity between sleeping and waking. Visually evoked responses were either unaffected or enhanced by awakening: in no cells were responses diminished. Roughly one-third of all cells showed an increase in evoked response that was obvious on the polygraph record; many more cells showed an enhancement of responses that were detected only by histogram averaging. Even in cells showing no increase in evoked response, the response was usually easier to observe against the more regular or reduced background firing.

Figure 5.2 shows an example of the effects of arousal on the responses of a cortical cell. The stimulus was an optimally oriented moving slit of light. The responses, which were weak and capricious during slow-wave sleep, became stronger and more consistent after arousal by a noise. Despite the increase in response to the optimum direction of movement (up and to the right), the reverse direction remained ineffective.

Figure 5.3 shows six extracts from a record of another cell, taken over a 15-min. period during which the cat repeatedly slept and awoke. The visually evoked responses were drastically changed, from vigorous while awake to almost completely absent during sleep. The increase in the response in the awake state was especially obvious because the background firing was reduced.

Four of the cells showed a transient burst of smooth steady firing lasting for about 30 s when the animal awoke spontaneously or was aroused by a noise or touch. After the burst the firing remained regular, usually stabilizing at a rate about the same as that during sleep or slightly higher. Had these cells not been clearly and specifically driven by particular visual stimuli, they might have been classed as multimodal, given their tendency to respond to any stimulus capable of arousing the animal. We saw no cells in striate cortex that responded to sense modalities other than visual, except in association with arousal.

A fall in both orientation specificity and movement-direction selectivity has been reported following stimulation of the menencephalic reticular formation.[19] Our preliminary results with natural arousal do not, however, point to a loss of specificity; on the contrary there may sometimes be an improvement. Figure 5.4 shows that the response to an optimally oriented slit was clearly, though not dramatically, improved after arousal, caused in this case by a loud noise, while the background firing was reduced and smoother. Directional selectivity was slightly improved, in that the response to the less effective direction of movement declined. For most directionally selective cells, however, the responses to the two opposite directions changed roughly in proportion. If, as in figure 5.2, one direction of movement failed to evoke a response in sleep, the same was so after arousal. No cell lost directional selectivity after arousal from sleep.

In testing orientation selectivity with a hand-held visual stimulator, we usually found no change. A few cells showed a slight improvement, but to be certain of this it will be necessary to compare orientation tuning curves.

Finally, in several cells we studied the effects of awakening on end stopping—the decline in response that occurs in some cells, termed hypercomplex, when a slit, edge, or dark bar is made longer than optimal[20]; the degree of stopping did not vary with level of arousal. The enhanced excitation from the activating part of the receptive field is therefore presumably offset by an enhanced inhibition from the outlying areas.

These observations are consistent with previous ones[20-22] that deepening barbiturate anaesthesia suppresses responses but does not change their specificity or lead to other qualitative changes. They also confirm the finding of Wurtz[23] that cells in area 17 recorded from awake alert monkeys with chronic recording techniques show responses that are not obviously different from responses obtained under barbiturate anaesthesia.

Most of the cells we studied were complex in type. The few simple cells examined showed

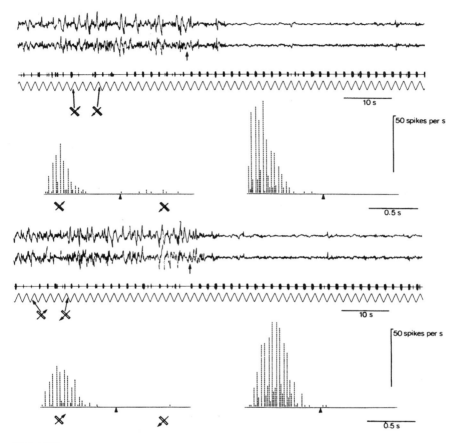

Figure 5.2
Effects of arousal on the responses of a cell in layer 6 of striate cortex. The record is 85 s long. Near the middle a noise (arrow) arouses the cat, as shown by the suppression of the EEG slow waves in the upper pairs of traces. Responses of the cell (third trace) are to a $1/2° \times 5°$ stimulus oriented 45° anticlockwise to vertical and swept up and to the right and down to the left (indicated in the fourth trace by up-and-down deflections). On arousal the responses are more consistent and on the whole stronger, as can be seen in the average response histograms. Each histogram is the average of 40 responses. The arrowhead below each histogram indicates when the stimulus reversed direction.

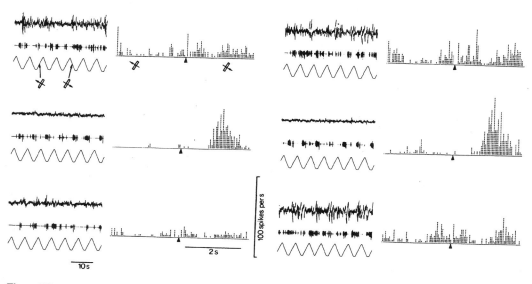

Figure 5.3

Responses of a cell in the striate cortex with the cat in various levels of arousal. Each record lasts 45 s, and ~3 min. elapse between records. As indicated by the EEG (upper trace), the three records on the left side are taken, from above downwards, in slow-wave sleep, awake and slow-wave sleep; those on the right are in slow-wave sleep, awake and slow-wave sleep. The middle trace shows impulse discharges, and lower trace indicates by up-and-down deflections left and right movements of a $1/4° × 2°$ slit oriented 30° clockwise to vertical. In the alert state the cell responds briskly to rightward movement, but hardly at all to leftward movement. In drowsiness and sleep spontaneous firing is greatly increased, and responses to the moving slits are almost completely absent. Each histogram is the average of 12 responses.

the same types of changes as the complex cells. Though we have too few cells to make reliable comparisons of laminar distribution, the most striking changes in responses seemed to be in deeper-layer cells.

2-Deoxyglucose Studies

We examined deoxyglucose uptake as a function of waking state in eight cats. Four cats, two awake and two in slow-wave sleep, were stimulated with moving vertical stripes confined to the right visual field. The other four cats were half the time awake and half the time asleep (see

below). The cats studied in slow-wave sleep were sleep deprived on a treadmill.

Cats were prepared in the same way as those used for physiological recordings, except that the microelectrode advancer was not installed. After discontinuing the anaesthetic we waited until the arrhythmic slow-wave pattern of halothane anaesthesia gave way to the low-voltage rapid activity characteristic of arousal. In the sleep-deprived animals this waking activity was soon replaced by the high-voltage slow waves of slow-wave sleep. A noise or tactile stimulus was sufficient to arouse the animals.

The visual stimulus was a moving set of irregularly spaced vertical black and white stripes

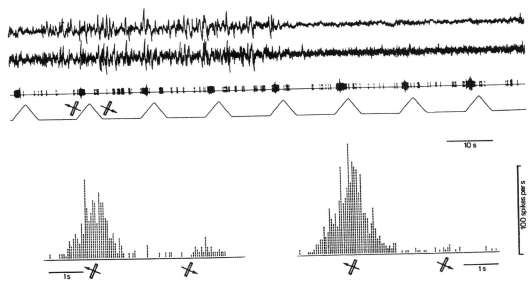

Figure 5.4
Effects of arousal from slow-wave sleep on responses and response selectivity of a cell in layer 2 of striate cortex. About halfway through the 2-min. record the cat is aroused by a noise. An optimal slit, $1/2° \times 3°$, oriented 25° clockwise to vertical, evokes a response (third trace) that is much greater to movement up and to the left than down and to the right. Arousal results in a moderate increase in the response to leftward movement, and a virtual elimination of the response to rightward movement (see the histograms). Arousal also produces suppression and smoothing of the spontaneous firing.

projected on a screen by a slide projector and a motor-driven mirror, which produced a back-and-forth movement at $2° \ s^{-1}$. Stripe width was about $1/4°$ near the vertical midline, gradually increasing to $2-3°$ in the periphery. The stripes were confined to the right field of vision, and did not include the vertical midline but extended from 2° to 3° to the right of the midline, out to $\sim45°$. The diffusely lit part of the screen (0.5 log cd m^{-2}) covered the vertical meridian and left visual field. We injected ^{14}C-2-deoxyglucose in a single pulse over 5–10 s, began the stimulus immediately and continued it for 45 min.

The cats were then deeply anaesthetized with thiopental and perfused with normal saline followed by formol-saline. The brains were re-moved, frozen in liquid N$_2$–cooled Freon-25 at $-100°$C and sectioned on a cryostatat at $-30°$C. Sections were mounted on glass coverslips, heated to 75°C to drive off water and exposed against X-ray film. We sometimes combined autoradiographs of 2–4 successive cortical sections by making enlargements on film and superimposing them, so that we could average the patterns seen in several single sections and obtain an enhancement of the overall pattern.

Though the two waking brains differed consistently from the two sleeping ones, we were worried that the differences might be due to variability between individual cats rather than to differences in their arousal state. In our first attempt to demonstrate differences in a single animal we alternated the stimuli, presenting stripes to the left visual field when the cat was awake and to the right field when it was asleep. The result was unsatisfactory, perhaps because each hemisphere was stimulated only half the time and any label associated with visual stimuli would be seen against a background representing both states of wakefulness.

To overcome these problems (and also with an eye to countless other applications), we developed a double-label 2-deoxyglucose technique, exploiting the differential sensitivity to ^{14}C and ^{3}H β-emissions of standard X-ray film and LKB Ultrofilm ^{3}H. In standard X-ray film the emulsion is protected by a gelatin layer, ~1 μm thick, which acts as a partial barrier to the low-energy ^{3}H emissions. The LKB film lacks this coating and is roughly 20 times more sensitive than X-ray film to ^{3}H, whereas the two films are about equally sensitive to ^{14}C. These ratios were determined by exposing both types of film to standards made by soaking pieces of filter paper in serial dilutions of ^{3}H and ^{14}C. In the autoradiographs shown here we increased the ratio of sensitivity to ^{14}C to sensitivity to ^{3}H of the X-ray film to about 100:1 by interposing an additional 10-μm layer of polyethylene film.

In the injections of deoxyglucose we tried to achieve a $^{14}C/^{3}H$ ratio that would allow the ^{3}H to overpower the ^{14}C on the LKB film, and the ^{14}C to predominate on the X-ray film.

Both double-label cats were sleep deprived on a treadmill and prepared as described for the single-label (^{14}C) cats. After the halothane was discontinued we waited until the EEG had shifted to a normal slow-wave sleep pattern from which the animal could easily be aroused. We then injected the ^{14}C-2-deoxyglucose and stimulated the left visual field with vertical black and white stripes for 45 min., all the while praying that the animal would stay asleep. Next we aroused the cat, injected the ^{3}H-deoxyglucose and stimulated the right visual field for 45 min., keeping the cat awake by a general uproar and tactile stimuli as needed. To be certain of con-

fining the stimulus to the contralateral hemisphere we avoided stimulating a strip of visual field 2–3° to either side of the vertical midline. The cat was perfused and the brain sectioned as already described. The histological sections (together with a set of filter paper standards) were exposed first to X-ray film protected by polyethylene film and then to LKB film.

Lateral Geniculate Autoradiography

In the two single-label animals whose right visual fields were stimulated when awake, the left LGBs were heavily labelled. The region of dense label was confined to the part of the geniculate corresponding to the area of visual field stimulated, extending on coronal sections medially almost to the medial border, which corresponds to the vertical meridian, and laterally over half to two-thirds of the geniculate's width, corresponding to the 45° lateral extent of the stimulus (figure 5.5a). The right (unstimulated) LGB showed label only at background levels. In one of the two animals stimulated while in slow-wave sleep, both sides showed label only at background levels; in the other animal there was only very faint labelling on the stimulated side (not shown). In the double-label cat (figure 5.5b) only the ^{3}H-sensitive film showed a left-right difference in geniculate labelling, and again the region with increased label (in the left geniculate) corresponded exactly to the part of the visual field stimulated. No difference was seen between the two sides on the polyethylene-protected X-ray film, except for slightly heightened labelling on the left, in exactly the same place as the label on the ^{3}H film and doubtless due either to some unfiltered ^{3}H or to some ^{14}C-deoxyglucose still in the cat's bloodstream 45 min. after the first injection, when the second, waking, ^{3}H stimulus was begun. That the lack of ^{14}C label on the right side was not due to failure of uptake of ^{14}C is clear from the cortical autoradiographs in the same animal (see below). Considering the pro-

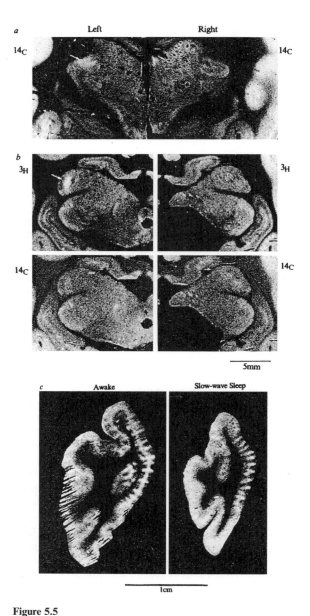

Figure 5.5
(*a*) 2-Deoxyglucose labelling of lateral geniculate nucleus in an awake cat by a moving grating of vertical black and white stripes. Stimulus was confined to the right field of vision, coming to within 2° or 3° of the vertical midline. Label in the left LGB is indicated by the arrow. Another waking cat gave a similar result. Figs 5.5 and 5.6 are

found effects of slow-wave sleep on responses of the individual cells we studied, the pronounced differences in the autoradiography are not too surprising.

Cortical Autoradiography

A consistent and marked difference was also seen in the pattern of labelling in the visual cortex. Figure 5c shows representative overlaid sections from two single-label (^{14}C) cats, awake and in slow-wave sleep. These animals both had had their right visual fields stimulated, and in each there were conspicuous columns in the left hemisphere, and no hint of any periodic labelling pattern in the right hemisphere. In the awake animal the columns extended through the full thickness of cortex (except for layer 1) with roughly uniform density. In the cats stimulated during slow-wave sleep, the columns in the upper layers (above layer 4) were labelled about as densely as in the waking cats, but below layer 4 they were in most sections hardly visible against the background. In some cats layer 4 was continuously and densely labelled, whereas in other cats it was not. These differences in layer 4 labelling did not consistently correlate with sleep state and we cannot account for them.

The double-label cat gave the same result (figure 5.6). The upper pair of autoradiograph

overlays are made from the same sets of sections as the lower pair, the only differences being in the type of film used and the interposition of a sheet of polyethylene film in the lower (^{14}C) set. Columns extended through the full thickness of cortex in the waking, ^{3}H-labelled side, and for the most part only halfway down on the sleeping, ^{14}C side. The figure also demonstrates how effectively this technique can distinguish between two different stimuli, as in each case only the appropriate hemisphere shows columns.

Discussion

One might have imagined that when an animal awakens the neurones in its brain would simply become more active, as suggested by Sherrington.[24] While this may apply to some areas of the brain, for example to parts of the brain stem reticular formation, it does not fit well with what we know of the cerebral cortex. The EEG does not elucidate this question, because although it is a sensitive indicator of arousal, its interpretation in terms of underlying neuronal activity is equivocal: a flattening on arousal from slow-wave sleep can be due to a reduction of activity or a desynchronization; the waves themselves may represent summation of impulses or of graded potentials. Recordings from single cortical neurones have shown that the flattening of

negatives; labelled regions show as bright areas. (*b*) Four autoradiographs showing results of the sleep-waking double-label experiment. After the ^{14}C-2-deoxyglucose injection (100 μCi kg^{-1}), the cat was stimulated while in slow-wave sleep for 45 min., the stimulus being confined to the left visual field. ^{3}H-2-deoxyglucose (5 μCi kg^{-1}) was then given, and followed by 45 min. of stimulation to the right visual field during which the cat was kept aroused. The same sets of sections were exposed to LKB Ultrofilm (^{3}H) and to polyethylene-protected X-ray film (^{14}C). The ^{14}C autoradiographs of coronal sections show no obvious labelling; the ^{3}H autoradiographs by contrast show a dense patch of label in the appropriate part of the left LGB. (*c*) Deoxyglucose labelling of visual cortex in two cats, awake and in slow-wave sleep, stimulated with vertical stripes confined to the right visual field. Each part consists of three superimposed successive sections. Columns are labelled on the medial surface (to the right) in both coronal section through the left hemispheres; the vertical midline projection (postlateral gyrus, at the top) is, as expected, not labelled. In the waking cat the columns (which appear bright in these negatives) extend through the full cortical thickness; in the slow-wave sleep cat they are well labelled in the superficial half of the cortex, but below that they are faint or absent.

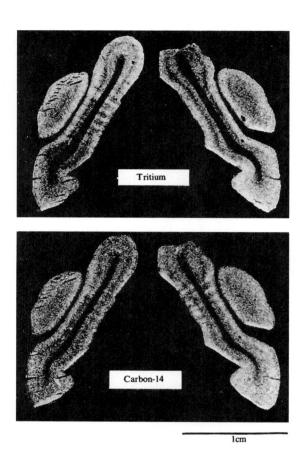

1cm

Figure 5.6
Double-label deoxyglucose labelling of cortex; three successive sections exposed to LKB film (^{3}H) and to protected X-ray film (^{14}C) are superimposed. In the upper, waking, ^{3}H-labelled autoradiograph, columns are seen only in the left hemisphere and extend through the full cortical thickness. In the lower, sleeping, ^{14}C-labelled autoradiograph they are more densely labelled in the upper layers than in the lower ones.

the EEG on arousal from slow-wave sleep is most often associated with a lowered rate of spontaneous neuronal firing.[4,5,25] Some cells, in our experience a minority, show a transient increase in firing rate. Usually high-frequency bursts are replaced by more regular firing.

Early studies of the effects of arousal on responses from the primary visual cortex used direct electrical stimulation at various points along the pathway, or diffuse light flashes. These stimuli have the disadvantage (compared with stimulation by small spots or lines) that they may evoke competing excitatory and inhibitory mechanisms with consequent loss of effectiveness. Nevertheless the responses they do evoke are facilitated by arousal from slow-wave sleep.[26-28] In studies much farther along in the visual pathway, in the inferotemporal region of nitrous oxide-anaesthetized monkeys, neurones have been observed to respond to complex stimuli more vigorously when the EEG is flat than during periods of high-voltage slow waves.[29]

Our results suggest that arousal brings about an improvement in signal-to-noise ratio: geniculate cells showed enhanced evoked discharges and most cortical cells showed enhanced responses against a lowered or less chaotic background. (Similar effects were seen in somatosensory cortex of monkeys by Gücer.[30]) But more than that, all components of the response were enhanced, suppression of firing as well as increases. Arousal may thus be attended by either depression or elevation of firing rate, depending on stimulus conditions. A cell in an awake animal is more the slave of incoming sensory inputs; in sleep it is more independent, less fettered by sensory constraints, but more at the mercy of events related to the still all-too-mysterious slow waves.

In normal life, even with the eyes open and surveying a complex scene, only a small fraction of cells in the visual cortex is likely to be engaged at any given instant because, for example, a light-dark contour can have only one orientation, can move only in one direction and at one velocity. For a few cells the discharge rate will probably be increased by the stimulus, but the remainder will continue to fire at their spontaneous rate, which will on the whole be depressed by arousal. If the visual cortex is representative of the rest of the brain, then in wakefulness most cells are not active but held in quiet readiness.

The effects of arousal in the small sample of geniculate cells studied were surprisingly strong, in contrast with the effects on cortical cells, most of which showed only a modest increase in response. This suggests that for some cortical cells the enhanced responsiveness of geniculate cells may be transmitted not as more vigorous firing but as more selective firing. Several cells showed a relatively greater enhancement to an optimal stimulus than to a suboptimal one, and consequently an improved selectivity for orientation or movement direction. We never saw a decline in selectivity.

In the cat the transition from the awake state to slow-wave sleep may be gradual, characterized in the EEG by bursts of high-voltage slow waves similar to those seen in continuous full-blown slow-wave sleep, alternating every few seconds with the low-voltage fast activity of arousal. The EEG alone cannot tell us whether this represents repeated transitory changes in arousal level or instead is a steady-state level of low arousal (drowsiness) characterized by a fluctuating EEG. Our single-cell recordings from geniculate and cortex support the former alternative, given the often tight correlation, within a few seconds, between a cell's behaviour and the onset or termination of an episode of slow waves.

Certain brain-stem neurones have long been known to show firing patterns that are closely correlated with levels of arousal.[31-39] Recently attention has focused increasingly on two monoaminergic brain-stem regions, the raphé nuclei and the locus coeruleus. Neurones in both these structures fire more rapidly during periods of increased alertness.[40-43] Like visual neurones, the brainstem neurones show a remarkably close correlation with the EEG, but in the brain stem, changes in firing rate usually precede the EEG changes by several seconds.[43,44] As both pharmacological and physiological studies have suggested that monoaminergic brain-stem neurones are important in controlling arousal, we compared, in a few cats, the effects on visual neurones of stimulating the locus coeruleus to the effects of spontaneous arousal and awakening induced by sensory stimuli. In each case they were the same. The effects of natural arousal from slow-wave sleep on spontaneous and evoked activity could be further exaggerated in an already awake animal by a loud noise or pinch; here again locus coeruleus stimulation had the same effect as a loud noise or a pinch.

The deoxyglucose autoradiographs showed clearly that the depression of activity in slow-wave sleep is different in different layers, being especially profound in 5 and 6. (This is consistent with an observation by Singer et al.,[19] that cortical cells that could be antidromically activated from tectum or geniculate were particularly likely to be activated by brain-stem stimulation.) Our single-cell recordings had hinted at laminar differences, but it was certainly not true that in sleep suppression of responses occurred in all of the deeper-layer cells, or in none of the upper-layer cells. The autoradiographic differences may not be due entirely to cell-body labelling: only electron microscopy will show whether the radioactivity is in cell bodies, axon terminals, dendrites, or all three.

The fact that some cells in layers 5 and 6 shut down in slow-wave sleep is pertinent to the functioning of the superior colliculus and LGB, for they are the respective major targets of these two layers. One guess might be that the source of the arousal effects observed in the LGB is the brain stem, because the locus coeruleus is known to send strong projections to the geniculate, and the dorsal raphé nucleus probably does.[45,46] Arousal could also act on the geniculate indirectly by reviving some otherwise dormant cells in layer 6 (ref. 19). This could be tested by cortical cooling or injection of local anaesthetics during examination of arousal effects in geniculate cells. It will be especially interesting to compare the responses of cells in the superior colliculus during waking and sleeping, because cooling and ablation of the visual cortex are known to abolish directionally selective responses to moving visual stimuli.[47] Our physiological findings imply either that the responses of many visual neurones in the central nervous system are enhanced on arousal, or that in sleep the responses are dulled. As the function of sleep is unknown, it is, of course, not clear whether a muffling of sensory input during sleep serves to insulate the animal from its environment to permit uninterrupted sleep or whether sensory systems also need to rest and the decreased responsiveness we see reflects whatever recuperative process the brain undergoes during sleep.

Acknowledgments

David Freeman did the computer programming and electronics, the histology was done by Birthe Storai, Suzanne Fenstemaker, and Debra Hamburger, and the photography by Marc Peloquin. We thank David Ferster for interesting criticisms. Simon LeVay suggested the technique of overlaying adjacent autoradiographs. Some of the early work on developing the double label was done with Dr Gary Blasdel. The work was supported by NIH grant R01 EY00605, grants from the Rowland Foundation and the Klingenstein Fund and by NIH grant R01 NS 07848 to E. A. Kravitz.

Notes

1. Hubel, D. H. *J. Physiol.*, Lond. 150, 91–104 (1960).

2. Singer, W. *Physiol. Rev.* 57, 386–420 (1977).

3. Hubel, D. H. *Am. J. Ophthal.* 46, 110–122 (1958).

4. Hubel, D. H. *J. Physiol.*, Lond. 147, 226–238 (1959).

5. Evarts, E. V. in *The Nature of Sleep* (eds Wolstenholme, G. E. W. & O'Connor, M.) 171–182 (Churchill, London, 1961).

6. Evarts, E. V., Bental, E., Bihari, B. & Huttenlocher, P. R. *Science* 135, 726–728 (1962).

7. Coenen, A. U. L. & Vendrik, A. J. H. *Expl Brain Res.* 14, 227–242 (1972).

8. Hubel, D. H. & Livingstone, M. S. *Neurosci. Abstr. 10th a. Meet.*, Cincinnati, No. 113.3 (1980).

9. Sokoloff, L. et al. *J. Neurochem.* 28, 897–916 (1979).

10. Livingstone, M. S. & Hubel, D. H. *Neurosci. Abstr. 10th a. Meet.*, Cincinnati, No. 113.4 (1980).

11. Singer, W. & Dräger, U. C. *Brain Res.* 41, 214–220 (1972).

12. Maffei, L. & Rizzolatti, C. T. *Arch. ital. Biol.* 103, 609–622 (1965).

13. Sakakura, H. *Jap. J. Physiol.* 18, 23–42 (1968).

14. Hubel, D. H. & Wiesel, T. N. *J. Physiol., Lond.* 155, 385–398 (1961).

15. Kuffler, S. *J. Neurophysiol.* 16, 37–68 (1953).

16. Barlow, H. B. *J. Physiol., Lond.* 119, 69–88 (1953).

17. Cleland, B. G., Dubin, M. W. & Levick, W. R. *Nature new Biol.* 231, 191–192 (1971).

18. Meulders, M. & Godfraind, J. M. *Expl Brain Res.* 9, 201–220 (1969).

19. Singer, W., Tretter, F. & Cynader, M. *Brain Res.* 102, 71–90 (1976).

20. Hubel, D. H. & Wiesel, T. N. *J. Neurophysiol.* 28, 229–289 (1965).

21. Hubel, D. H. & Wiesel, T. N. *J. Physiol., Lond.* 160, 106–154 (1962).

22. Hubel, D. H. & Wiesel, T. N. *J. Physiol., Lond.* 195, 215–243 (1968).

23. Wurtz, R. H. *J. Neurophysiol.* 32, 727–742 (1969).

24. Sherrington, C. S. *Man on His Nature*, 183–184 (Doubleday, New York, 1953).

25. Murata, K. & Kameda, K. *Arch. ital. Biol.* 101, 306–331 (1963).

26. Akimoto, H., Saito, Y. & Nakamura, Y. *Neurophysiologie und Psychophysik des visuellen Systems* (eds Jung, R. & Kornhuber, H.) 363–374 (Springer, Berlin, 1961).

27. Evarts, E. V. *J. Neurophysiol.* 26, 229–248 (1963).

28. Evarts, E. V. in *Colloque International sur les Aspects Anatomo-fonctionnels de la Physiologie du Sommeil*, 189–212 (Éditions du Centre National de la Recherche Scientifique, Paris, 1965).

29. Gross, C. G., Rocha-Miranda, C. E. & Bender, D. B. *J. Neurophysiol.* 35, 96–111 (1972).

30. Gücer, G. *Expl Brain Res.* 34, 287–298 (1979).

31. Mollica, A., Moruzzi, G. & Naquet, R. *EEG J.* 5, 571–584 (1953).

32. Machne, X., Calma, I. & Magoun, H. W. *J. Neurophysiol.* 18, 547–558 (1955).

33. Strumwasser, F. *Science* 127, 469–470 (1958).

34. Schlag, J. *L'activité Spontanée des Cellules du Système Nerveux Central* (Editions Arscia, Bruxelles, 1959).

35. Huttenlocher, P. R. *J. Neurophysiol.* 24, 451–568 (1961).

36. Beniot, O. *J. Physiol., Paris* 56, 259–262 (1964).

37. Kasamatsu, T. *Brain Res.* 14, 506–509 (1969).

38. Kasamatsu, T. *Expl Neurol.* 28, 450–470 (1970).

39. Hobson, J. A., McCarley, R. W., Pivik, R. T. & Freedman, R. *J. Neurophysiol.* 37, 497–511 (1974).

40. Chu, N.-S. & Bloom, F. E. *Science* 179, 908–910 (1973).

41. McGinty, D. J., Harper, R. M. & Fairbanks, M. K. *Serotonin and Behavior* (eds Barchas, S. & Usdinin, E.) 267–279 (Academic, New York, 1973).

42. McGinty, D. J. & Harper, R. M. *Brain Res.* 101, 569–575 (1976).

43. Foote, S. L., Aston-Jones, G. & Bloom, F. E. *Proc. natn. Acad. Sci. U.S.A.* 77, 3033–3037 (1980).

44. Trulson, M. E. & Jacobs, B. L. *Brain Res.* 163, 135–150 (1979).

45. Moore, R. Y. & Bloom, F. E. *A. Rev. Neurosci.* 2, 113–168 (1979).

46. Moore, R. Y., Halaris, A. E. & Jones, B. E. *J. comp. Neurol.* 180, 417–438 (1978).

47. Wickelgren, B. G. & Sterling, P. *J. Neurophysiol.* 32, 16–32 (1969).

The Role of Temporal Cortical Areas in Perceptual Organization

D. L. Sheinberg and N. K. Logothetis

Neurons in the visual areas of the anterior temporal lobe of monkeys exhibit pattern-selective responses that are modulated by visual attention and are affected by the stimulus in memory, suggesting that these areas play an important role in the perception of visual patterns and the recognition of objects (1, 2). To understand the role of these areas in perception and object vision, we conducted combined psychophysical and electrophysiological experiments in monkeys experiencing binocular rivalry. Binocular rivalry refers to the stochastic changes of perception when one is viewing two different patterns dichoptically. We have recently shown that the perceived image during rivalry is independent of which eye it is seen through (3), a finding that suggests that binocular rivalry may be the result of competition between different stimulus representations throughout the visual cortex, rather than between the two monocular channels early in striate cortex (for review see ref. 4). The study of cell activity during binocular rivalry may therefore provide us with significant insights regarding the neural sites and mechanisms underlying the perceptual multistability experienced when one is viewing any ambiguous figures, such as the well-studied figure–ground reversals, and may lead to a better understanding of the principles of perceptual organization.

Methods

Two animals (*Macaca mulatta*) participated in the experiments reported in this paper. After the monkeys were familiarized with the laboratory environment and the experimenter, they underwent an aseptic surgery (5, 6). After recovery, the monkeys were trained to fixate a light spot and to perform a categorization task by pulling one of two levers attached to the front of their primate chair. They were taught to pull and hold the left lever whenever a sunburst-like pattern (left-object) was displayed and to pull and hold the right lever upon presentation of other figures, including images of humans, monkeys, apes, wild animals, butterflies, reptiles, and various manmade objects (right-objects). In addition, they were trained not to respond or to release an already pulled lever upon presentation of a physical blend of different stimuli (mixed-objects).

Example stimuli are shown in figure 6.1. The patterns were generated using a graphics computer (Indigo2, Silicon Graphics) and were presented on a display monitor placed 97 cm away from the animal. Stereoscopic presentations were accomplished using a liquid crystal polarizer (NuVision SGS19S) that allowed alternate transmission of images with circularly opposite polarization at the rate of 120 frames per second (60 frames per second for each eye). Polarized glasses were worn to allow the passage of only every other image to each eye.

During the behavioral task, individual observation periods consisted of random transitions between presentations of left-, right-, and mixed-objects. Juice reward was delivered only after the successful completion of an entire observation period. However, negative feedback was always given to the monkeys in the form of aborting an observation period following an incorrect response. Once the animals had learned to classify the different object types rapidly and accurately, periods of rivalrous stimulation (7–20 s) were introduced in observation periods lasting 15–30 s. During rivalrous periods, no feedback was given to the monkeys. Eye position was constantly monitored and stored. Excursions of the eyes outside of a $\pm 0.75°$ window surrounding the fixation spot automatically aborted the observation period.

Single-cell activity was recorded in both monkeys in the upper and lower banks of superior temporal sulcus (STS) and the inferior temporal

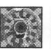 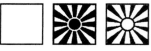

"Left" Objects   "Mixed" Objects   "Right" Objects

Figure 6.1
Example stimuli used during the experiments. Stimuli consisted of geometrical sunburst patterns (left-objects), images of animate objects (right-objects), and physical blends of images that were used to mimic piecemeal rivalry (mixed-objects). The monkeys were trained to pull the left lever whenever the left-objects were visible, the right-lever whenever right-objects were visible, and neither lever when mixed-objects were visible.

cortex (IT) using of a chamber consisting of a ball-and-socket joint with a 18-gauge stainless steel tube passing through its center (7). The base of the well was secured to the skull using small skull-screws and bone cement. The position of the guide-tube could be varied before each experimental session in any direction using a calibration device, attachable to the outer part of the ball-and-socket joint. The placement of the chambers was aided by a set of X-ray images combined with a set of magnetic resonance images (2.4-Tesla Magnet; Bruker, Billerica, MA) acquired before the head-post surgery of each monkey. We recorded from three hemispheres in two monkeys with the chambers placed at AP = 20, L = 20; AP = 19, L = 20; and AP = 19, L = 19, respectively. By swiveling the guide tube, different sites could be accessed within an $\approx 8 \times 8$ mm^2 cortical region. Since both monkeys are still alive and participating in similar experiments, the recording areas were estimated from the stereotaxic coordinates of the guide tube and the white-to-gray matter transitions expected from magnetic resonance images. According to these estimates, the recording sites were probably in areas TPO1, TPO2, and TEa and in the gyral portion of IT, most likely areas TEm, TE1, and TE2.

Results

Because the interpretation of the neurophysiological data of this study strongly depended on the reliability of the animals' behavioral responses, special care was taken to ensure that the monkeys were reporting their perceptions accurately, rather than alternately pulling the levers in a random fashion. To encourage reliable performance, each observation period consisted of randomly intermixed periods of rivalrous and nonrivalrous stimulation, during which left-objects and right-objects were displayed monocularly. The slightly lustrous appearance of a monocularly viewed image served to maximize the similarity of percepts elicited by nonrivalrous and rivalrous stimulation and to reduce the chances of the monkey adopting different behavioral strategies in the two different stimulation conditions. Moreover, to train the monkey to report only exclusive visibility of a figure, mixed-objects, mimicking piecemeal rivalry, were randomly intermixed within each observation period. The monkeys reliably withheld response during these mixed periods, even when such periods constituted an entire observation period.

Finally, we systematically compared the monkeys' psycho-physical performance with that of humans in the same tasks. During binocular rivalry, the time for which different stimuli are perceived depends strongly on the images' relative stimulus strength, a term specifying the combined effect of such stimulus parameters as luminance, contrast, spatiotemporal frequency, and amount of contour per stimulus area (8). For our task, we varied stimulus strength by changing the spatial frequency content of one image in the stimulus pair by lowpass filtering it. In humans, limiting the spatial frequency content of an image has been shown to decrease the stimulus' predominance (9), where predominance of a stimulus is typically defined as the percentage of the total viewing time during which this stimulus is perceived (8). Since our stimuli were large enough ($2.5 \times 2.5°$) to often instigate piecemeal rivalry, predominance of the stimulus was defined to be the ratio of the time for which one stimulus was exclusively visible to the total time for which either stimulus was exclusively visible.

Figure 6.2 shows the remarkable similarity in the dependency of predominance of a visual pattern on its spatial frequency content in both monkeys and humans. We take the consistency in both sets of data as strong evidence for the reliability of the monkeys' behavior.

Following the initial behavioral training, we began the combined psychophysical-physiological experiments. We isolated 159 visually responsive single units. Responsiveness was determined by presenting stimuli from a battery of hundreds of visual images. The selectivity of these cells was tested by repeatedly presenting a subset of the available visual stimuli in pseudo-random order in search of one or more effective stimuli, while the monkey fixated a central light spot.

Example responses of an IT neuron are shown in figure 6.3a. The cell discharges action potentials upon presentation of the effective stimuli, here images of particular butterflies, and responds minimally to all other tested stimuli (including the sunburst pattern). Of the visually responsive neurons, 50 were found to be selective enough to be tested during the object classification task under both nonrivalrous and rivalrous conditions. The rivalry stimuli were created by presenting the effective stimulus to one eye and the ineffective stimulus (i.e., the sunburst) to the other. Figure 6.3b shows two observation periods during this task, one from each monkey.

Each plot illustrates the stimulus configuration, the neuron's activity, and the monkey's reported percept throughout the entire observation period. In both cases, the neuron discharged only before and during the periods in which the monkey reported seeing the effective stimulus. During rivalrous stimulation, the stimulus configuration remained constant, but significant changes in cell activity were accompanied by subsequent changes in the monkeys' perceptual report.

The neural activity was further analyzed by constructing average spike density functions (SDFs), sorted by the monkey's perceptual reports. Figure 6.4a shows these data for the same cell depicted in the figure 6.3b Upper. Figure 6.4a Upper and Lower show responses in nonrivalrous and rivalrous conditions, respectively. As shown in figure 6.3a, this neuron fired vigorously when the monkey reported seeing the cell's preferred pattern in both the nonrivalrous and rivalrous conditions. However, when the monkey reported seeing the ineffective stimulus, the cell response was almost eliminated, even when the effective stimulus was physically present during rivalry.

To increase the instances of exclusive visibility of one stimulus, and to further ensure that the monkey's report accurately reflected which stimulus he perceived at any given time, we also tested the psychophysical performance of the monkeys and the neural responses of STS and IT cells using the flash suppression paradigm (10). In this condition, one of the two stimuli used to instigate rivalry is first viewed monocularly for 1–2 s. Following the monocular preview, rivalry is induced by presenting the second image to the contralateral eye. Under these conditions, human subjects invariably perceive only the newly presented image and the previewed stimulus is rendered invisible. Previous studies have shown that the suppression of the previewed stimulus is not due to forward masking or light adaptation (10) and that instead it shares much in common with the perceptual suppression experienced

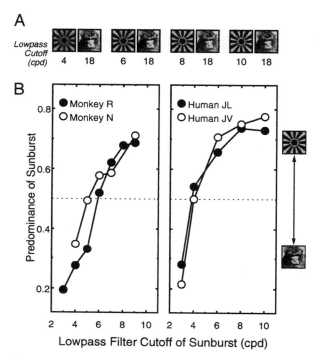

Figure 6.2

Behavioral verification of monkey's performance during rivalry. (*a*) Each pair of images depicts a stimulus condition, wherein the image of the face remained unchanged while that of the sunburst was blurred, to various degrees, by lowpass filtering. Filtering was achieved by multiplying the amplitudes of forward Fourier transformed images by an exponential gain and then converting back to the space domain. The lowpass cutoffs shown below each image refer to the frequency at which the exponential filter was equal to $1/e$. (*b*) Predominance of a stimulus as function of spatial frequency bandwidth. Predominance is defined here as $T_{sunburst}/(T_{sunburst} + T_{face})$, where $T_{sunburst}$ and T_{face} are the time durations for which the sunburst and the face were exclusively visible. (*Left*) Data from monkeys and (*Right*) data from experimentally naïve human subjects. Note that predominance is systematically related to the spatial frequency content of the sunburst pattern for both monkeys and humans; as the sunburst is blurred to greater extents, it is perceived dominant for decreasing proportion of time.

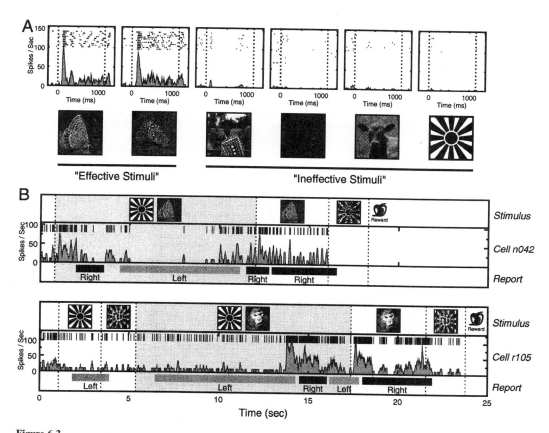

Figure 6.3

Neural responses during passive viewing and during the behavioral task. (*a*) Response selectivity of an IT neuron. Effective stimuli were the two butterfly images, while almost all other tested images (30 tests, 4 shown) elicited little or no response from the cell. Each plot shows aligned rasters of spikes collected just before, during, and after the presentation of the image depicted below the graph. The smooth filled lines in each plot are the mean SDFs for all trials. The dotted vertical lines mark stimulus onset and stimulus removal. (*b*) Example observation periods taken from the behavioral task for individual cells from monkey N (*Upper*) and monkey R (*Lower*). Observation periods during behavioral testing consisted of random combinations of nonrivalrous stimuli and rivalous periods. Dotted vertical lines mark transitions between stimulus conditions. Rivalry periods, which could occur at any time during an observation period, are shown by the filled gray background. The horizontal light and dark bars show the time periods for which the monkey reported exclusive visibility of the left-lever (sunburst) and right-lever (e.g., butterfly or monkey face) objects. Note that during rivalry the monkey reports changes in the perceived stimulus with no concomitant changes of the displayed images. Such perceptual alternations regularly followed a significant change in the neurons' activity, as shown by the individual spikes in the middle of each plot and by the SDFs below the spikes. Note the similarity of the responses elicited by the unambiguous presentation of the effective and ineffective stimuli (white regions) with those responses elicited before either stimulus becomes perceptually salient during rivalrous stimulation (gray region).

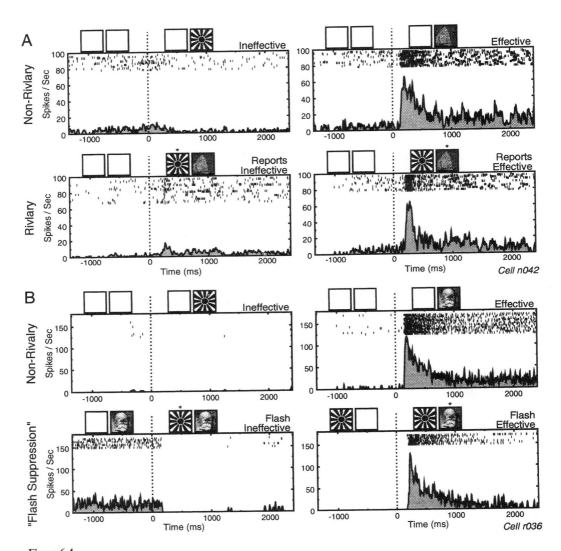

Figure 6.4
Cell activity sorted by the dominant percept during nonrivalrous and rivalrous conditions. (*A Upper*) Averaged responses to the monocularly presented ineffective and effective stimuli. Above each graph is a pictorial representation of the visual stimuli presented. At time zero, depicted by the dotted line, the stimulus changed from either a blank screen or a mixed-object (data not shown) to the ineffective (*Left*) or effective (*Right*) stimulus. The cell fired only in response to the butterfly pattern. Presentation of the sunburst had little or no effect on the neuron's activity. (*Lower*) Response of the cell just before and after the onset of rivalrous stimulation, with the effective stimulus presented to one eye and the ineffective to the other. The data are sorted based on the monkey's perceptual report: trials in which the monkey first reported seeing the ineffective stimulus (*Left*) and those for which the monkey first

during binocular rivalry (11). In our experiments, the monkeys, just like the human subjects, consistently reported seeing the stimulus presented to the eye contralateral to the previewing eye during the flash suppression trials.

To confirm that the animals responded only when a flashed stimulus was exclusively dominant, catch trials were introduced in which mixed stimuli were flashed, after which the monkey was required to release both levers. Performance for both animals was consistently >95% for this task. Figure 6.4b shows the activity of an STS neuron in the flash suppression condition. Figure 6.4b Upper shows the cell responses for monocular presentations, and the figure 6.4b Lower shows the neuron's activity at the end of the monocular preview (to the left of the dotted vertical line) and when perceptual dominance is exogenously reversed as the rival stimulus is presented to the other eye (to the right of dotted vertical line). The cell fires vigorously when the effective stimulus dominates perception and ceases firing entirely when the ineffective stimulus is made dominant. To better understand the differences between the temporal areas and the prestriate areas, recordings were also performed in area V4 using the flash suppression paradigm (D. Leopold and N. K. L., unpublished observations). V4 neurons were largely unaffected by the perceptual changes during flash suppression. Presenting the ineffective stimulus after priming with the effective one caused no alteration in the firing rate of any of the cells; presenting the effective stimulus after

priming with the other had an weak effect on a small percentage of V4 neurons.

Across the population of cells from which we recorded, we found significant differences in the temporal structure of individual neural responses. Some neurons responded in a sustained fashion, while others exhibited a periodic burst or very transient response (figure 6.5a). We were concerned that typical methods of characterizing cell response, such as counting the number of spikes occurring within a fixed time window, would ignore these potentially informative variations. We thus characterized the entire spike waveforms for each trial using a well established method of dimensionality reduction and then applied multivariate statistical tests on the data to test for differences in cell response between the ineffective and effective trials (13). A detailed description of the analysis methods is given elsewhere (14). Briefly, the spike train for each trial was defined as a discrete function over the interval $[0, N - 1]$, where N was the number of points in the peristimulus time window (for population analysis, 800 points spaced 1 ms apart). The spike function takes the value 1 if a spike occurs at point t, with $t \in [0, N - 1]$, and zero otherwise. Each trial's SDF was computed using the adaptive-kernel estimation process (15). These SDFs were subjected to principal components analysis (16), which is an orthogonal transform that typically results in a description of the data in a response space with strongly reduced dimensionality, and whose basis vectors, called the principal components, are uncorre-

reported seeing the effective stimulus (*Right*). In these conditions, the stimuli presented are identical, but the recorded cell response correlates well with the monkey's reported percept. (*B*) Data collected using the suppression paradigm. The nonrivalrous trials (*Upper*) show that this cell consistently responded to the effective stimulus and not at all to the ineffective stimulus. The flash suppression trials are similar to the rivalry trials shown in *A*, except that preceding the rivalrous stimulation, either the effective stimulus (*Lower left*) or ineffective stimulus (*Lower right*) was previously presented monocularly. Rivalry onset, marked by the dotted vertical line, thus consisted of adding either the ineffective or effective stimulus to the rivalrous pair. Following rivalry onset, the monkey's reported percept consistently switched to the newly presented stimulus, and the previewed stimulus was perceptually suppressed. Using this paradigm, phenomenal suppression was especially effective, and cell activity during the onset of rivalrous stimulation closely mirrored that during the nonrivalrous controls.

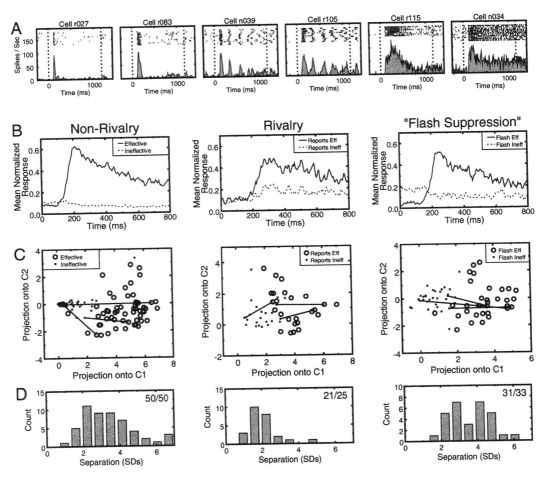

Figure 6.5

(*A*) Examples of different response types of neurons in STS and IT. While some cells elicited relatively sustained responses to visual stimuli (e.g., cells r115 and n034), others exhibited a periodic bursting behavior (e.g., n039 and r105), or a highly transient response (e.g., r027 and r083). (*B*) Mean normalized cell responses in the nonrivalrous (50 cells), rivalrous (24 cells), and flash suppression (33 cells) conditions, for the effective (solid line) and ineffective (dotted line) trials. In all conditions, average cell response in the effective trials was elevated over response during the ineffective trials. (*C*) Scatter diagram of average cell responses for all tested neurons. For visualization purposes, only projections of the response vectors onto the two first components, C1 and C2, are presented. Each marker represents the mean of all ineffective (•) and effective (○) trials for a given cell. The distance (exemplified by the solid lines for three of the cells) between almost all pairs of reponses are statistically significant (see below). (*D*) Separation of mean responses to the perceived effective and ineffective stimuli for the three stimulation conditions. Each individual response is represented by an eight-element vector. Separation is given by the Mahalanobis distance (12), $D = \sqrt{((\mu_1 - \mu_2)' \Sigma^{-1} (\mu_1 - \mu_2))}$, where μ_1 and μ_2 are the mean response vectors for the effective and ineffective lated (and can thus be studied independent of one another) and ordered to represent decreasing proportions of the total variance of the data. In this study, the principal components of cell responses were extracted using the variances and covariances of subsampled (every 5 ms) SDFs, after centering the data (the mean SDF for a stimulus or report condition was subtracted from individual SDFs). Response vectors for individual trials were calculated by projecting a given SDF onto each of the leading principal components. For these data, a maximum of eight components was required to explain at least 75% of the cumulative response variance, and thus an eight-dimensional space was used to represent each cell's response to the two different perceptual conditions.

Figure 6.5b shows that, on average, cell response was consistently higher for those trials in which the effective stimulus dominated perception compared with trials in which the ineffective stimulus dominated. Figure 6.5c depicts each cell's mean response for the ineffective and effective trials, as projected into the first two dimensions of the eight-dimensional space used to analyze the data. In these graphs, each cell is represented twice, once for effective trials and once for ineffective trials. The separation of these populations at the individual cell level is further quantified in figure 6.5d, which shows a histogram of separations, in units of standard de-

viation, of each cell's ineffective and effective response vectors. Overall, ≈90% of the recorded cells in STS and IT were found to reliably predict the perceptual state of the animal. The proportion of cells showing statistically significant separations between the effective and ineffective conditions are shown in the top right of each plot in figure 6.5d.

The reliability of a given response pattern in predicting the animal's perceived stimulus was also tested by comparing the performance of a statistical pattern classifier with that of the monkey. Two eight-dimensional subspaces were generated by extracting the principal components of the responses to the effective and ineffective stimulus in the nonrivalrous trials. Individual responses in the rivalry trials were then assigned to one or the other subspace by using a minimum-distance statistical pattern classifier. On average, 78.5% (range = 66–91%) of the monkey's reported percept was predicted by this trial by trial classification method.

Discussion

These results show that the activity of the vast majority of studied temporal cortex neurons is contingent upon the perceptual dominance of an effective visual stimulus. Neural representations in these cortical areas appear, therefore, to

trials, respectively, and Σ is the covariance matrix of the eight-dimensional response vectors. Because the two response types usually had different variances, Σ was replaced by its unbiased estimate, $S_u = (n_1 S_1 + n_2 S_2)/(n - 2)$, where S_1 and S_2 are the covariance matrices for responses to the effective and ineffective stimulus, respectively, n_1 and n_2 are the number of presentations of each stimulus type, and $n = n_1 + n_2$. The significance of this variance-weighted distance was assessed by means of the Hotelling T^2 statistic (13) given by $(n_1 n_2/n)D^2 = (n_1 n_2/n)(\mu_1 - \mu_2)'\Sigma^{-1}(\mu_1 - \mu_2)$, which relates to the F distribution by $[n_1 n_2(n - p - 1)/n(n - 2)p]D^2 \sim F_{p,n-p-1}$, where p stands for the dimensionality of the response space. The numbers in the top right of each plot show the proportion of cells for which the response in the ineffective and effective trials was significantly different at the $\alpha = 0.05$ level. It should be noted that the high percentages of modulating neurons reported here was not due to the specific multivariate analysis. Similar results, in terms of proportions of significantly modulating cells, were obtained by the more traditional analysis of counting the number of spikes occurring in individual trials. Computing mean rates, however, requires arbitrary decisions pertaining the time window over which these rates must be computed when neurons show highly variable temporal modulations.

be very different from those in striate and early extrastriate cortex. Only 18% of the sample in striate cortex (5) and ≈20% and 25% of the cells in areas MT and V4, respectively (5, 6), were found to increase their firing rate significantly when their preferred stimulus was perceived. Moreover, one-fifth of the studied MT neurons and 13% of V4 neurons responded only when the effective stimulus was phenomenally suppressed, while other cells showed response selectivity only during perceptual rivalry and not while the animal was involved in passive fixation. The different response types in these areas may be the result of the feedforward and feedback cortical activity that underlies the processes of grouping and segmentation—processes that are probably perturbed when ambiguous figures are viewed. If so, the areas reported here may represent a stage of processing beyond the resolution of ambiguities, where neural activity reflects the integration of constructed visual percepts into those subsystems responsible for object recognition and visually guided action.

It is worth considering how the present data can be interpreted in light of the growing body of literature concerning so-called attentional modulation of cortical activity (1, 17, 18). Indeed, paradigms employed in studies of visual selective attention bear great similarity to be rivalry paradigm, in that more than one competing stimuli is generally presented to the subject and the effects of this competition are closely monitored. These experiments have often found that the activity of cells in visual cortex is both a function of the visual stimulus and of the animal's set or state, indicating that other neural processes—generally referred to as attention—can influence cell activity above and beyond that which can be explained by the visual stimulus alone. Our view is that the phenomenon of binocular rivalry is also a form of visual selection, but that this selection occurs between competing visual patterns even in the absence of explicit instructions to attend to one stimulus or the other. Decades of research have failed to reliably demonstrate

that the perceptual alternations experienced during rivalry are under the direct control of voluntary attention. As such, we believe that rivalry accentuates the selective processing that underlies basic perceptual processes including image segmentation, perceptual grouping, and surface completion. In this view, the modulation of cortical activity reported here may be of distinct origin from the modulatory effects reported for tasks in which attention is overtly directed to one stimulus or another. Nonetheless, it is striking that both the effects of modulation due to rivalry and to attention have been reported in many of the same visual cortical areas. It will be of great interest to see if and how the same neurons participate in both phenomena.

Acknowledgments

We thank David Leopold for many useful suggestions and comments on the manuscript. This research was supported by the National Institutes of Health Grants NIH 1R01EY10089-01 to N. K. L. and NRSA 1F32EY06624 to D. L. S.

Notes

1. Desimone, R. & Duncan, J. (1995) *Annu. Rev. Neurosci.* 18, 193–222.

2. Logothetis, N. K. & Sheinberg, D. L. (1996) *Annu. Rev. Neurosci.* 19, 577–621.

3. Logothetis, N. K., Leopold, D. A. & Sheinberg, D. L. (1996) *Nature (London)* 380, 621–624.

4. Blake, R. R. (1989) *Psychol. Rev.* 96, 145–167.

5. Leopold, D. A. & Logothetis, N. K. (1996) *Nature (London)* 379, 549–553.

6. Logothetis, N. K. & Schall, J. D. (1989) *Science* 245, 761–763.

7. Schiller, P. H. & Koerner, F. (1971) *J. Neurophysiol.* 34, 920–936.

8. Levelt, W. J. M. (1965) *On Binocular Rivalry* (Royal VanGorcum, Assen, The Netherlands).

9. Fahle, M. (1982) *Vision Res.* 22, 787–800.

10. Wolfe, J. (1984) *Vision Res.* 24, 471–478.

11. Baldwin, J. B., Loop, M. S. & Edwards, D. J. (1996) *Invest. Ophthalmol. Visual Sci.* 37, Suppl., 3016.

12. Mahalanobis, P. C. (1936) *Proc. Natl. Inst. Sci. India* 12, 49–55.

13. Mardia, K. V. (1972) *Statistics of Directional Data* (Academic, New York).

14. Richmond, B. J., Optican, L. M., Podell, M. & Spitzer, H. (1987) *J. Neurophysiol.* 57, 132–146.

15. Richmond, B. J., Optican, L. M. & Spitzer, H. (1990) *J. Neurophysiol.* 64, 351–369.

16. Jolliffe, I. T. (1986) *Principal Component Analysis* (Springer, New York).

17. Colby, C. L. (1991) *J. Child Neurol.* 6, S90–S118.

18. Maunsell, J. H. R. (1995) *Science* 270, 764–769.

7 Investigating Neural Correlates of Conscious Perception by Frequency-Tagged Neuromagnetic Responses

Giulio Tononi, Ramesh Srinivasan, D. Patrick Russell, and Gerald M. Edelman

Binocular rivalry is a useful experimental paradigm for identifying aspects of neural activity that are correlated with conscious experience (1, 2). If two incongruent visual stimuli are simultaneously presented one through each eye, only one stimulus at a time is consciously perceived, and the two percepts alternate every few seconds. It was thought initially that rivalry might reflect competition between monocular neurons in primary visual cortex or at earlier stages. However, recent psychophysical studies have demonstrated that perceptual rivalry can occur even when both stimuli are presented through the same eye or when they are alternated between the eyes (2). Furthermore, single-unit recordings during binocular rivalry in monkeys indicate that, while the firing of most neurons in primary visual cortex correlates with the stimulus but not with the percept (3), the firing of cortical units in higher visual areas, such as inferior temporal cortex and superior temporal sulcus (4), is highly correlated with the visual percept.

Human subjects are the referent of choice for investigating conscious perception (5). However, brain activity associated with rivalry is difficult to study in humans with techniques such as positron emission tomography and functional MRI because of their limited temporal resolution. Unit recordings, on the other hand, while offering high temporal resolution as well as neuronal specificity, are typically performed in overtrained animals and are not practical for providing global coverage of neural responses. At the expense of spatial resolution, magnetoencephalograms (MEGs) and electroencephalograms (EEGs) offer the advantage of high temporal resolution and reflect the synchronous activity of large populations of neurons (6, 7). In this study, we made use of a 148-channel MEG array to compare whole-head, steady-state-evoked responses when subjects viewing a stimulus were consciously perceiving it and when they were not. Rivalry was produced by presenting red vertical gratings to one eye and blue horizontal gratings to the other eye. The subjects signaled which of the two stimuli was consciously perceived (perceptual dominance) by activating right- or left-hand switches. To evaluate brain responses specific to each reported percept a method of "frequency tagging" was employed. Each of the two stimuli was flickered at a different frequency in the range of 7–12 Hz, and steady-state evoked responses at the tag frequency specific to each stimulus were detected in many MEG channels. These responses allowed us to assess how stimulus-related signals were distributed over the whole head when a particular stimulus was consciously perceived and when it was not. They also allowed us to establish whether such responses were modulated in relation to conscious perception, and to determine whether such modulation was global or regionally specific.

Methods

Seven right-handed subjects (five males and two females) of ages 25–49 participated in this study. Each had a corrected visual acuity of 20/20 and could see large-disparity random-dot stereograms. All subjects gave informed consent. Neuromagnetic data were collected using a Magnes 2500WH MEG system from Biomagnetic Technologies (San Diego). This consists of an array of 148 magnetometer coils (1-cm diameter) spaced ≈3 cm apart and providing coverage of the entire scalp. The MEG array was in a magnetically shielded room, and computer-generated stimuli were projected through a porthole and a single mirror onto a screen in front of the subjects.

In each trial, subjects viewed high-contrast (>95%) square-wave gratings of 1.7 cycles per degree in a square field subtending a visual angle of 13° at the fovea over a uniform dark gray background. The size and intensity of the stimulus were adjusted to generate complete or near-complete rivalry, with sufficiently long episodes of dominance (mean of 2 s), and a high signal-to-noise-ratio (SNR) in the recorded signal. A vertical red grating was presented to one eye and a horizontal blue grating to the other eye by having subjects wear correspondingly colored goggles. The intensity of the red stimulus was adjusted such that, under conditions of rivalry, the subjects reported that the two stimuli were of comparable brightness. To aid convergence, subjects viewed a dim gray fixation point at the center of each grating.

In rivalry trials, one stimulus (s1) was flickered continuously at one frequency (f1) and the other stimulus (s2) was flickered at a different frequency (f2). For each f1–f2 pair, two of the following frequencies were used: 7.41 Hz (one grating-on frame every 9 video frames, at 67 frames/s), 8.33 Hz, 9.50 Hz, or 11.12 Hz. A photodiode recorded in real time the flicker of s1 and s2 on a computer screen driven in parallel with the projector. Subjects were asked to activate one switch with their left index finger whenever the red stimulus was perceptually dominant and another switch with the right index finger whenever the blue stimulus was dominant. They were instructed to activate neither switch if neither of the two percepts was clearly dominant, that is, when they saw a mixture of red vertical and blue horizontal gratings. The activation of the switches was recorded by an additional channel.

After a brief exposure to the stimuli, subjects had no trouble categorizing the percepts as red, blue, or mixed, and the alternation of perceptual dominance between the percepts became quite stable. If asked, the subjects reported perceiving the stimulus flicker, but they did not comment on any difference in frequency between f1 and f2. During the experiments, stimuli were presented for 30–60 s before recording to establish a steady-state response. Neuromagnetic data were

then recorded for 315 s, resulting in a frequency resolution of 0.0032 Hz. Data were bandpass filtered at 1–50 Hz and digitized at 254 Hz. For each channel, the power spectrum of the entire recording interval was calculated by using a fast Fourier transform algorithm (MATLAB, Natick, MA). The peaks corresponding to f1 and f2 were identified in the spectrum of the photodiode signal, and the presence of peaks in the MEG data at the corresponding frequencies was verified. These peaks were contained within a single bin of 0.0032-Hz width. The recording of the behavioral response yielded two response functions r1 and r2, which were set to 1 during the intervals when the subject signaled that stimulus s1 or s2, respectively, was perceptually dominant, and to 0 otherwise. The values of r1 and r2 for episodes lasting less than 250 msec were set to 0.

To obtain the power corresponding to the periods when the subject was consciously perceiving s1 (perceptual dominance), the MEG data were multiplied by r1 prior to the Fourier transform. The power corresponding to the periods when the subject was not conscious of s1 (perceptual nondominance, defined as the periods when the subject was conscious of s2) was calculated by multiplying the MEG data by r2 before the fast Fourier transform. The power values at f1, normalized by the total duration of positive intervals in r1 and r2, were subtracted to yield the difference at f1 between perceptual dominance and perceptual nondominance. Multiplying MEG time data by the response function corresponds to convolving the respective frequency spectra and results in some smearing. Numerical simulations indicated, however, that the contamination of the signal peak was negligible compared with the size of the effects observed in this study.

To emphasize the effect of perceptual dominance/nondominance over stimulus-specific factors, stimulus-frequency pairings and stimulus-eye pairings were counterbalanced for each subject so that, for each frequency pair, each stimulus was presented at each frequency and to each eye for a total of four trials. Two different frequency pairs were used successively in the rivalry condition, with one frequency common to both pairs, yielding eight trials at that frequency. The average power difference at the common frequency across the eight rivalry trials was calculated.

To compare power differences between perceptual dominance and nondominance due to binocular rivalry with power differences due to the physical presence or absence of the stimulus, stimulus-alternation trials were used. In such trials, stimulus s1 alone was presented to one eye at frequency f1 for a random interval of time, after which stimulus s2 alone was presented to the other eye at frequency f2 for another random interval, and so on for 315 s. The time intervals were drawn from a γ distribution (2) with a mean of 2 s and a SD of 1 s. Stimulus-alternation trials were performed with only one frequency pair. A total of 12 trials were performed in a session that lasted 2–3 hr.

A randomization test (8) was employed to assess the statistical dependence of the power difference between perceptual dominance and nondominance on the response functions r1 and r2. For each subject, bootstrap samples were computed by systematically permuting the pairing between the MEG data for the eight rivalry trials and their response functions. A total of $8! = 40,320$ possible pairings were available, including the observed pairing. For each bootstrap sample, the power difference was computed for each trial in the same manner as for the observed data but by using the randomly assigned response functions. The sum of squared power differences across all the sensors was used as an omnibus statistic. The significance of the observed omnibus power difference was established by comparing it with the distribution of the omnibus power differences obtained from the bootstrap samples. After establishing the significance of whole-array (global) differences, power-difference values were plotted topographically to examine regional contributions.

Results

The average duration of the episodes of perceptual dominance in rivalry trials was 2.1 ± 1.1 s. In most subjects, the number and length of intervals in which the red and blue gratings were perceived were comparable (on average, 54 episodes for the red grating and 55 for the blue grating in each trial). For 5–25% of the total recording time neither stimulus was perceptually dominant.

High-resolution power spectra of steady-state evoked potentials recorded over posterior and anterior regions during a rivalry trial are shown in figure 7.1 Upper left. Two peaks are clearly visible, one at 7.41 Hz and the other at 9.50 Hz. Note that each peak occupies just one bin (bin size = 0.0032 Hz). Note also that the magnitude of each peak is much higher than the average power in nearby frequency bins, corresponding to a SNR of 25–50. Finally, the amplitude of the peak at 9.5 Hz is higher at posterior channels (e.g., channel 103), corresponding to occipital cortex, than at anterior channels (e.g., channel 128). These narrow peaks elicited by each stimulus served as frequency tags to identify neural activity that was directly or indirectly related to each stimulus. Steady-state responses completely disappeared when the corresponding eye was occluded.

Figure 7.1 (Lower) shows the topographic distribution of power at the peak frequency of 7.41 Hz for stimulus-alternation and rivalry trials of one subject (O. S.). The power values were obtained by averaging all trials in which a stimulus flicker frequency of 7.41 Hz was presented. In both stimulus-alternation and rivalry trials, a horseshoe-shaped distribution of the peak at 7.41 Hz was observed, with maximum amplitude over posterior regions.

The power at 7.41 Hz (f1) when s1 was perceptually dominant and when it was perceptually nondominant (defined as when s2 was perceptually dominant) was calculated for each channel by multiplying the MEG data by the response

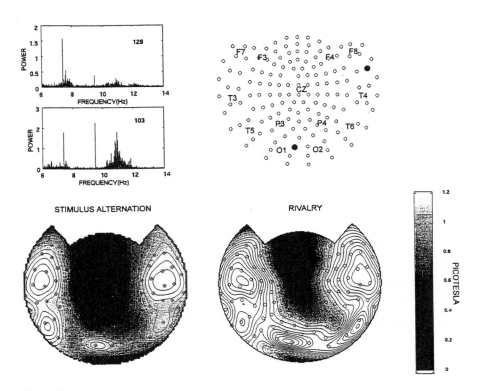

Figure 7.1

(*Upper left*) High-resolution power-frequency spectra for steady-state evoked potentials recorded over an anterior channel (128) and over a posterior channel (103) during rivalry trials (subject O. S.). Note the sharp peak at 7.41 Hz (f1), the flicker frequency of s1, as well as at 8.33 Hz (f2), the flicker frequency of s2. The peak is confined to 1 frequency bin (0.0032 Hz). The SNR, defined as the ratio of the power at the peak and the average power in a 0.06 Hz band (40 bins) surrounding it, is 25.0 (7.41 Hz, anterior channel), 29.7 (8.33 Hz, anterior channel), 39.2 (7.41 Hz, posterior channel), and 48.9 (8.33 Hz, posterior channel). A broad-band peak in the alpha range is visible at the posterior channel. (*Upper right*) Schematic topographic representation of the 148 channels in the MEG array. For convenience, a few points designated based on the ten-twenty electrode placement system are superimposed: F, frontal; C, central; P, parietal; O, occipital; and T, temporal. The locations of channels 128 and 103 are indicated by filled blue circles. (*Lower*) Topographic display of signal power at the stimulus flicker frequency of 7.41 Hz. The topographic maps were generated by interpolating the amplitude values (square root of power) at 148 sensors on a best-fit sphere with a three-dimensional spline. The sensor positions on the best-fit sphere are indicated by dots. The map is then projected from the sphere onto a plane. Channels meeting an SNR criterion of at least 2 are indicated by an open circle. (*Left*) Stimulus-alternation trials. In this and the subsequent figures, the values represent an average of four trials. (*Right*) Rivalry trials. In this and the subsequent figures, the values represent an average of eight trials in which the stimulus flicker frequency 7.41 Hz was associated with either the red vertical grating or the blue horizontal grating and presented to either the right or the left eye (see *Methods*). Note the typical horseshoe distribution of the peak in power at 7.41 Hz, which is similar under stimulus-alternation and rivalry conditions (subject O. S.). Solid contour lines begin at 1 picotesla in steps of 0.1 picoteslas. Dashed contour lines range from 0 to 0.9 picoteslas.

functions r1 and r2, respectively, and subtracted to yield a power difference value. The power difference values at 7.41 Hz were calculated with the response function offset from the neuro-magnetic data by an offset time τ ranging from -2.5 to $+2.5$ s in steps of 250 ms. The offsets were introduced to take into account the variable relationship between the motor output and the establishment of the steady-state response. The former depends upon the reaction time and the strategy used for perceptual decision, while the latter depends on the speed at which the steady-state response is modulated, all of which may vary across subjects.

For stimulus-alternation trials, the power differences at 7.41 Hz between the periods during which the stimulus flickering at that frequency was being presented and during which the other stimulus was being presented are shown in figure 7.2 (Left) as a function of offset time τ. In the figure, the contour lines in magenta indicate a positive difference in power, while green lines indicate a negative difference in power. The figure shows a strong positive power difference for most channels that starts at $\tau = -250$ ms and lasts until $\tau = +1.5$ s; the response peak is at $\tau = -0.25$ s. A negative difference, of reduced amplitude, is noticeable at earlier and later offsets. Such negative differences occur because on average, a 2-s interval in which s1 is dominant is preceded and followed, at $\tau = \pm 2$ s, by a 2-s interval during which s2 is dominant (and hence s1 is nondominant). Correspondingly, the interval between positive and negative peaks is ≈ 2 s. Note that the time course of the amplitude difference suggests that the steady-state response takes time to develop and that its peak value can occur after the onset of the behavioral response.

In figure 7.2 Right a similar plot is shown for the rivalry condition in the same subject. The plot represents the average of eight trials in which the stimulus was presented at a flicker frequency of 7.41 Hz. In this case there is again a positive power difference in many channels,

straddling $\tau = 0$ and surrounded by negative differences. Note, however, that both the magnitude of the difference and the number of channels involved are reduced with respect to stimulus-alternation trials. Furthermore, the maximum positive difference occurs at a longer time offset than in stimulus-alternation trials ($\tau = 0.75$ rather than $\tau = 0.25$). As in stimulus-alternation trials, the presence of negative differences is due to a degree of periodicity manifested by the intervals of perceptual dominance (mean alternation interval $= 2.9$ s). In different subjects, the peak positive differences occurred at different times, presumably reflecting differences between subjects in reaction time as well as in the strategy adopted in deciding when a percept was dominant. However, within each subject the peaks occurred at the same offset τ across trials. All subsequent analyses were performed with the reference functions offset at each subject's characteristic offset time.

Figure 7.3 shows topographic maps of the power at 7.41 Hz corresponding to the episodes of perceptual dominance, the power corresponding to the episodes of perceptual nondominance, and the difference in power between dominance and nondominance. In stimulus-alternation trials (figure 7.3 Left), the distribution of power differences was approximately coextensive with the distribution of the steady-state power during dominance. During nondominance there was no stimulus at that frequency and, as expected, there was no power contribution.

For rivalry trials (figure 7.3 Right), the steady-state responses at 7.41 Hz during perceptual dominance and nondominance were distributed in a similar way. However, a marked difference in power was observed according to whether the stimulus was consciously perceived or not. In many channels, the power was 50–85% lower during perceptual nondominance than during perceptual dominance, while in some channels the opposite was true. The difference in power was statistically significant ($P < 0.05$) using a

Tononi et al.

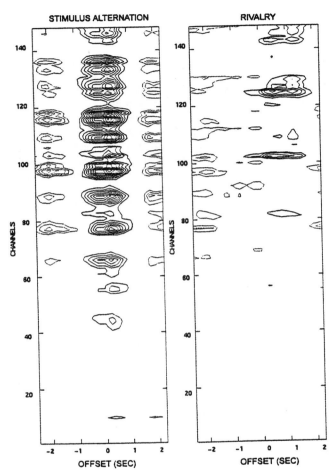

Figure 7.2
Power difference values between perceptual dominance and nondominance for all channels at different offsets (τ) of the response function. (*Left*) Stimulus-alternation trials. The contour lines in magenta indicate a positive difference in power, while green lines indicate a negative difference in power. The magnitude of the power difference is indicated by the number of contour lines. Contour lines begin at 0.05 picotesla^2 in steps of 0.025 picotesla^2. (*Right*) Rivalry trails (subject O. S.). Note that for most channels the maximum power difference occurs at $\tau = 0.25$ s for stimulus-alternation trials, and at $\tau = 0.75$ s for rivalry trials.

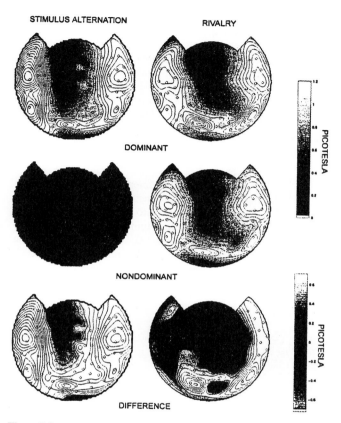

Figure 7.3

Topographic display of power at 7.41 Hz corresponding to perceptual dominance (*Top*), to perceptual non-dominance (*Middle*), and to the difference in power between dominance and nondominance (*Bottom*), at the offset for which the difference was maximal. Amplitude values (square root of power) are plotted. (*Left*) Stimulus-alternation trials. During nondominance, there is no amplitude contribution at the frequency of the absent stimulus. The difference in amplitude is coextensive with the distribution of stimulus-related responses. (*Right*) Rivalry trials. Note that the distribution of stimulus-related responses during nondominance is similar to that during dominance. Many channels show, however, amplitude values that are lower by 50–85% during nondominance. A positive difference in amplitude between perceptual dominance and nondominance is observed bilaterally at occipital, temporal, and frontal channels (subject O. S.). The omnibus significance of the map was computed as described in *Methods* ($P < 0.05$).

conservative randomization test. It is evident from the figure that the difference in power between dominance and nondominance extends to many but not all the channels showing a stimulus-related response. For the subject shown in figure 7.3 Right, a positive difference is observed bilaterally over occipital, frontal, and temporal regions. Smaller negative differences are observed in fewer channels over central and frontal regions. Several channels in which a consistent stimulus-related response was observed (SNR ≥ 2), did not show any modulation. Power difference values between perceptual dominance and nondominance for four other subjects are shown in figure 7.4. All subjects showed a marked power differences as a function of perceptual dominance at occipital, temporal, and frontal regions, although the particular set of modulated channels varied across subjects.

Discussion

In this study, visual steady-state neuromagnetic responses to two rivalrous stimuli presented at different frequencies were simultaneously recorded over many cortical areas. These neuromagnetic responses, labeled by frequency tags, were used to determine how brain activity differs, under rivalry conditions, when a human subject is conscious of a stimulus and when the subject is not.

The present experiments resulted in several significant observations. A first observation is that neural responses to rivalrous visual stimuli occurred in a large number of cortical regions both when the subject consciously perceived the stimuli and when he did not. Moreover, such evoked responses extended to anterior areas, the activity of which has not previously been exam-

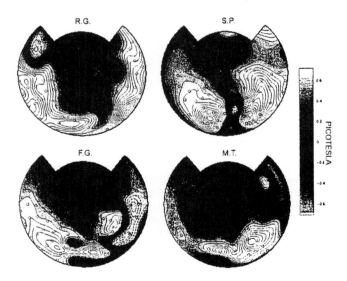

Figure 7.4
Topographic display of power differences between perceptual dominance and nondominance in four other subjects. Amplitude values (square root of power) are plotted. The frequency tested for each subject was: R. G. (8.33 Hz), S. P. (7.41 Hz), L. G. (7.41 Hz), and M. T. (7.41 Hz). The values are based on eight runs counterbalanced across eyes and color. The omnibus significance of the maps was P < .0005 for all subjects.

ined during binocular rivalry. The flickering stimuli used in this study activated primary visual areas directly through thalamocortical inputs. The recording of stimulus-related responses in other cortical areas, including anterior regions, is presumably due to neural circuits linking visual cortex to anterior regions through direct or indirect connections (6). It cannot be ruled out, however, that subcortical inputs may also have contributed to the signals recorded in anterior areas (9).

The second main finding of this study is that the neuromagnetic responses evoked by a stimulus over a large portion of the scalp were stronger when the subjects were conscious of it than when they were not. Interestingly, the sign of this effect was opposite in a subset of the channels. The magnitude of the modulation due to rivalry was of the order of 50–85%, to be compared with the 100% modulation due to the physical presence/absence of the stimulus in stimulus-alternation trials. The specific subset of channels showing such modulation, which varied from subject to subject, included occipital channels but was not restricted to them. Examination of single trials suggests that variations in the topography of such modulation depends on experimental variables such as frequency, eye, and color and these, as well as significant intersubject variances, deserve further investigation.

Previous EEG studies using a few occipital electrodes have reported that visual evoked potentials recorded over occipital cortex were suppressed when a rivalrous stimulus was introduced (10–12). Studies using orthogonal gratings that were modulated in counterphase (13) or tagged with different flicker frequencies (14) also reported that the amplitude of the visual evoked potential generated by the perceptually dominant stimulus was larger that that of the suppressed stimulus. In a recent study using the latter approach, the amplitude of the visual evoked potential induced by a stimulus presented to one eye was positively correlated with its perceptual dominance in real time (15). The finding of a strong modulation of evoked responses over occipital areas in the present experiments and in previous EEG studies contrasts with the results of single-unit recordings. In monkeys, only a small fraction of neurons in early visual areas showed activity that correlated with perceptual dominance, in sharp contrast with units in higher visual areas (4). This apparent discrepancy may be accounted for in part by differences in the experimental protocol, such as the use of flickering versus nonflickering stimuli. Most importantly, the steady-state responses recorded in the present study are sensitive to the synchronous activation of a large number of synapses rather than to the firing levels of individual units. Changes in synchronization among large populations of neurons due to reentrant interactions (16, 17) are a prerequisite for the modulation of electrical and magnetic potentials recorded at the scalp (6, 17). Consistent with this interpretation, it has recently been reported that, in strabismic cats, perceptual dominance under conditions of binocular rivalry is associated with increased synchronization in early visual areas, while perceptual suppression is associated with reduced synchronization (18).

In the present study, the analysis of steady-state responses at 148 MEG sensors covering the whole head allowed us to detect stimulus-related signals with high SNR in many brain areas in addition to visual cortex. The results obtained here show that the modulation of the evoked responses by perceptual dominance extends to a large subset of the brain areas that respond to the stimulus, including lateral and anterior regions that are not part of visual cortex. A possible interpretation is that the modulation in response amplitude in early visual areas indirectly affects the responses of other areas to which visual areas are functionally connected (19). Irrespective of the specific mechanisms, these findings indicate that neural correlates of the conscious perception of visual stimuli extend to areas beyond visual cortex.

When the stimulus was consciously perceived, the corresponding frequency tag was distributed almost as widely in rivalry trials as in stimulus-alternation trials. As expected, in stimulus-alternation trials the stimulus-related response disappeared at every channel when the stimulus was not physically present. In rivalry trials, by contrast, when the stimulus was not consciously perceived the stimulus-related response was modulated at many but not all the sensors where it was detected. Thus, the present findings show that neural responses that correlate with conscious experience are not global but are distributed to a subset of brain regions. Nevertheless, the widespread modulation of neuromagnetic responses observed here implies that changes in the synchronous firing of large, distributed populations of neurons are associated with changes in perceptual dominance.

Some intrinsic limitations of the present study should be pointed out. A precise correspondence between signals recorded at different channels and neural activity in underlying cortical areas cannot be established unless further assumptions are made, for example by applying source models of neuromagnetic field generation. Previous studies achieving whole-head coverage with dense arrays of EEG electrodes have demonstrated, however, that steady-state visual evoked responses in areas other than occipital visual areas are in part due to local generators and are not far-field potentials (6). Similarly, it is likely that MEG steady-state responses recorded at anterior channels reflect significant anterior sources. Another methodological limitation is that, unlike single-unit recordings, neuromagnetic recordings cannot disentangle the responses of individual neurons that have different stimulus preferences but are spatially intermingled within a brain region. For example, the activity of neurons that fire when their preferred stimulus is not perceptually dominant could be confounded with that of neurons that fire to the competing stimulus when it is dominant. Such neurons have in fact been recorded in area MT

(2). Furthermore, steady-state responses are insensitive to neural activity that is correlated with perceptual rivalry but is either sustained without being time locked to the flickering stimulus, or is present only transiently at the perceptual switch and therefore does not contribute sufficient power.

Despite these limitations, there are obvious advantages to the use of steady-state evoked responses. Frequency tagging provides the ability to sharply differentiate stimulus-related responses from background neuronal activity with high temporal resolution (20). In combination with whole-head MEG, it permits the investigation of the distribution of stimulus-related signals beyond sensory projection areas. Unlike single-unit recordings, which are not practical for global coverage of neural activity and are generally performed in overtrained animals, steady-state evoked responses permit one to sample the synchronous activity of large populations of neurons in human subjects who are not overtrained (6, 7). Frequency tagging also offers great potential for generalization, because it can be applied to stimuli in any sensory modality, provided that the frequencies used elicit widespread stimulus-related responses. As shown here, frequency tagging can be used to study neural correlates of conscious experience in human subjects who can directly report their conscious states. Further studies using the frequency tag methodology under conditions of rivalry or attentional modulation may help in delineating the cortical regions that contribute to conscious experience.

Acknowledgments

We thank Lacey Kurelowech for her expert contribution and Fellows of The Neurosciences Institute for useful comments. This work was carried out as part of the theoretical neurobiology program at The Neurosciences Institute, which is supported by Neurosciences Research

Foundation. The Foundation receives major support for this program from Novartis Pharmaceutical Corporation.

Notes

1. Miezin, F. M., Myerson, J., Julesz, B. & Allman, J. M. (1981) *Vision Res.* 21, 177–179.

2. Logothetis, N. K., Leopold, D. A. & Sheinberg, D. L. (1996) *Nature (London)* 380, 621–624.

3. Leopold, D. A. & Logothetis, N. K. (1996) *Nature (London)* 379, 549–553.

4. Sheinberg, D. L. & Logothetis, N. K. (1997) *Proc. Natl. Acad. Sci. USA* 94, 3408–3413.

5. Edelman, G. M. (1989) *The Remembered Present: A Biological Theory of Consciousness* (BasicBooks, New York).

6. Nunez, P. L. (1995) *Neocortical Dynamics and Human EEG Rhythms* (Oxford Univ. Press, New York).

7. Srinivasan, R., Nunez, P. L. & Silberstein, R. B. (1998) *IEEE Trans. Biomed. Eng.* 45, 805.

8. Efron, B. & Tibshirani, R. J. (1993) *An Introduction to the Bootstrap* (Chapman & Hall, New York).

9. Robinson, D. L. & Petersen, S. E. (1992) *Trends in Neurosci.* 15, 127–132.

10. Lansing, R. W. (1964) *Science* 146, 1325–1327.

11. MacKay, D. M. (1968) *Nature (London)* 217, 81–83.

12. Wright, K. W., Ary, J. P., Shors, T. J. & Eriksen, K. J. (1986) *J. Pediatr. Ophthalmol. Strabismus* 23, 252–257.

13. Cobb, W. A., Morton, H. B. & Ettlinger, G. (1967) *Nature (London)* 216, 1123–1125.

14. Lawwill, T. & Biersdorf, W. R. (1968) *Invest. Ophthalmol.* 7, 378–385.

15. Brown, R. J., Norcia, A. M. (1997) *Vision Res.* 37, 2401–2408.

16. Lumer, E. D., Edelman, G. M. & Tononi, G. (1997) *Cereb. Cortex* 7, 228–236.

17. Tononi, G., Sporns, O. & Edelman, G. M. (1992) *Cereb. Cortex* 2, 310–335.

18. Fries, P., Roelfsema, P. R., Engel, A. K., Koenig, P. & Singer, W. (1997) *Proc. Natl. Acad. Sci. USA* 94, 12699–12704.

19. Tononi, G., McIntosh, A. R., Russell, D. P. & Edelman, G. M. (1998) *NeuroImage* 7, 133.

20. Regan, D. (1989) *Human Brain Electrophysiology* (Elsevier, New York).

8 Temporal Binding, Binocular Rivalry, and Consciousness

Andreas K. Engel, Pascal Fries, Pieter R. Roelfsema, Peter König, Michael Brecht, and Wolf Singer

Introduction

This chapter intends to contribute to the ongoing debate about the neural correlate(s) of consciousness from the viewpoint of a particular experimental approach: the study of distributed neuronal processing and of dynamic interactions that implement specific "bindings" in neural network architectures. The now-classical notion of binding and the search for potential binding mechanisms has received increasing attention during the past decade. Having been introduced first in the psychological discourse (for review, see Treisman 1986, 1996), the issue of binding has now advanced into the focus of research also in other disciplines within cognitive science such as neural network modeling (e.g., Hinton, McClelland, and Rumelhart 1986; Smolensky 1990; Hummel and Biederman 1992; Schillen and König 1994), philosophy of mind (e.g., Fodor and Pylyshyn 1988; van Gelder 1990; Fodor and McLaughlin 1990) and cognitive neuroscience (e.g., von der Malsburg 1981, 1995; Crick 1984; Sejnowski 1986; Damasio 1990; Engel et al. 1992; Engel et al. 1997; Singer 1993; Singer and Gray 1995; Roelfsema, Engel, König, and Singer 1996).

In all these domains, the problem has been identified that encoding and retrieval of information in neuronal networks requires some sort of binding mechanism that allows the expression of specific relationships between elementary processors. This "binding problem" arises for several reasons: First, information processing underlying cognitive functions is typically distributed across many network elements and, thus, one needs to identify those neurons or network nodes that currently participate in the same cognitive process (Hinton et al. 1986). Second, perception of and action in a complex environment usually requires the parallel processing of infor-

mation related to different objects or events that have to be kept apart to allow sensory segmentation and goal-directed behavior. Thus, neuronal activity pertaining, for example, to a particular object needs to be distinguished from unrelated information in order to avoid confusion and erroneous conjunctions (von der Malsburg 1981). Third, it has been claimed that specific yet flexible binding is required within distributed activation patterns to allow the generation of syntactic structures and to account for the systematicity and productivity of cognitive processes (Fodor and Pylyshyn 1988). Fourth, many cognitive functions imply the context-dependent selection of relevant information from a richer set of available data. It has been suggested that appropriate binding may be a prerequisite for the selection and further joint processing of subsets of information (Singer and Gray 1995; Singer et al. 1997). These arguments suggest that cognitive functions require the implementation of binding mechanisms in the distributed networks subserving these functions.

In what follows, we want to focus on the idea that some kind of binding mechanism may also be critical for the establishment of conscious mental states. In recent years, several authors have emphasized a close link between binding and consciousness, following the intuition that consciousness requires some kind of integration, or coherence, of mental contents (von der Malsburg 1997). Damasio (1990) has suggested that conscious recall of memory contents requires the binding of distributed information stored in spatially separate cortical areas. In various publications, Crick and Koch have discussed the idea that binding may be intimately related to the neural mechanisms of sensory awareness (Crick and Koch 1990a,b, Koch and Crick 1994, Crick 1994). According to their view, only appropriately bound neuronal activity can enter short-term memory and, hence, become available for access to phenomenal consciousness. Llinás, Ribary, Joliot, and Wand (1994) have proposed that arousal and awareness require binding of sensory information that is implemented by interactions between specific and nonspecific thalamocortical loops. Recently, Metzinger (1995) has extended this discussion by speculating that binding mechanisms might not only account for low-level properties of phenomenal consciousness like the holistic character of perceptual objects, but also for the formation of a phenomenal self-model and its embedding into a global world-model. Pöppel (1997) has suggested that binding is required for conscious time perception and establishment of subjective time frames.

Our discussion of the consciousness issue will be restricted to one particular aspect, namely, sensory awareness. With many authors, we share the view that sensory awareness is one of those facets of consciousness that is (probably) most easily accessible both in terms of experimental quantification and theoretical explanation (Crick and Koch 1990a, Farber and Churchland 1995). Furthermore, there can be little doubt that we have this basic form of phenomenal consciousness in common with many other species (presumably with at least most other higher mammals). Thus, it is conceivable that research on animals can contribute substantially to explaining this aspect of consciousness, which may not hold for many higher-order features of consciousness which, for instance, require a language system or an elaborated self-model.

There seems to be wide agreement that awareness as the basic form of phenomenal consciousness has the following prerequisites: First, generating sensory awareness seems to involve some form of attentional mechanism, that is, a mechanism that selects relevant information and enhances its impact on subsequent processing stages (Crick and Koch 1990a, Newman and Baars 1993, Crick 1994, Desimone and Duncan 1995). Second, awareness presumably requires working memory, which allows the short-term

storage of episodic contents (Goldman-Rakic 1992, Moscovitch 1995). Third, awareness seems to presuppose the capacity for structured representation, that is, the ability to achieve coherence of the contents of mental states and to establish specific relationships between representational items. Our basic assumption is that all three capacities are, on the one hand, closely related to each other and, on the other hand, strongly dependent on binding mechanisms implemented in sensory systems. This is probably most obvious for the third capacity mentioned, the establishment of coherence in mental states. As will be further discussed below, attentional selection may also depend on appropriate binding of neuronal responses. Similarly, there is evidence that binding is important for inducing changes of synaptic efficacy and hence, for the transfer of information into memory structures (for review, see Singer 1993). With these issues in mind, we will discuss one particular candidate mechanism, namely, dynamic binding by transient and precise synchronization of neuronal discharges. As we will argue, there is now empirical evidence suggesting that such "temporal binding" may be crucial for generating functionally efficacious representational states and for the selection of perceptually or behaviorally relevant information.

The Concept of Temporal Binding

The concept of dynamic binding by synchronization of neuronal discharges has been developed mainly in the context of perceptual processing. One source of inspiration for this model has come from the insight that perception, like most other cognitive functions, is based on highly parallel information processing carried out by numerous brain areas. A paradigmatic case is provided by visual processing, which shows a highly distributed organization (Livingstone and Hubel 1988, Zeki and Shipp 1988, Felleman and Van Essen 1991). In monkeys, anatomical and physiological studies have led to the identification of more than 30 distinct visual areas in the cortex. This parcellation is assumed to reflect some kind of functional specialization because neurons in each of these visual areas are, at least to some degree, selective for characteristic subsets of object features. Thus, for instance, some areas contain cells responding to the color of objects, whereas others primarily process information about the form of an object or its direction of motion in the visual field. As a consequence of this functional specialization, any object present in the field of view will activate neurons in many cortical areas simultaneously. The highly complex organization of visual processing naturally raises the question of how distributed neuronal responses can be integrated, which seems necessary to enable the brain to represent and store information about the external world in a useful way.

It has been suggested that the binding problem arising in distributed sensory networks may be solved by a mechanism which exploits the temporal aspects of neuronal activity (von der Malsburg 1981, 1995; for review, see Engel et al. 1992, 1997; Singer 1993; Singer and Gray 1995; Singer et al. 1997). The prediction is that neurons that respond to the same sensory object might fire their action potentials in temporal synchrony with a precision in the millisecond range (see figure 8.1). However, no such synchronization should occur between cells that are activated by different objects appearing in sensory space. Such a temporal integration mechanism would provide an elegant solution to the binding problem because, on the one hand, the synchrony would selectively tag the responses of neurons that code for the same object and demarcate their responses from those of neurons activated by other objects. This highly selective temporal structure would allow to establish a distinct representational pattern (a so-called assembly) for each object and, thus, would enable the visual system to achieve figure-ground segregation. On the other hand, such a temporal

binding mechanism could also serve to establish relationships between neuronal responses over large distances and, thus, solve the problems imposed by the anatomical segregation of specialized processing areas.

This strategy of temporal binding exhibits a number of crucial advantages. First, it preserves the general advantages of distributed coding schemes such as robustness against loss of network elements and "richness" of representations which contain explicit information about object features and do not only signal the presence of the object (like a small set of "cardinal cells" would do; see Barlow 1972). Second, this strategy enhances processing speed because binding can, in principle, occur using the very first spikes of a response (Singer et al. 1997; Fries, Roelfsema, Singer, and Engel 1997a). Third, temporal binding alleviates superposition problems that occur in conventional distributed systems that operate solely on the basis of average firing rates (von der Malsburg 1981). The reason is that using synchrony as an additional coding dimension allows the dissociation of the binding code from the feature code (object features being signaled by firing rates). This allows multiple assemblies to coactivate without confusion, because the temporal relationship between neuronal discharges permits the unambiguous distinction of subsets of functionally related responses. Fourth, temporal binding provides an efficient mechanism for selection of assemblies for further processing (Singer and Gray 1995, Singer et al. 1997), because precisely synchronized spikes constitute highly salient events which can be detected by coincidence-sensitive neurons in other brain areas (Abeles 1982; König, Engel, and Singer 1996; Alonso, Usrey, and Reid 1996).

It should be noted at this point that, although the temporal binding model has mainly been elaborated with respect to the visual modality, it can be generalized because binding problems similar to those described here for vision have to be coped with by other systems as well. Obviously, the problem of perceptual integration

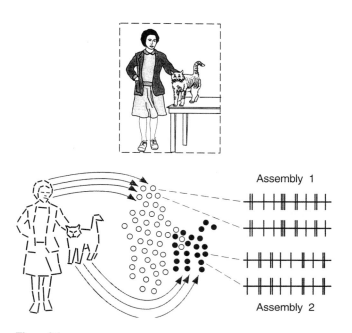

Figure 8.1

Establishment of coherent representational states by temporal binding. The model assumes that objects are represented in the visual cortex by assemblies of synchronously firing neurons. In this example, the lady and her cat would each be represented by one such assembly (indicated by open and filled symbols, respectively). These assemblies comprise neurons that detect specific features of visual objects (such as, for instance, the orientation of contour segments) within their receptive fields (Lower left). The relationship between the features can then be encoded by temporal correlation among these neurons (Lower right). The model assumes that neurons that are part of the same assembly fire in synchrony whereas no consistent temporal relation is found between cells belonging to different object representations. (From Engel et al. 1997)

just exemplifies a much more general problem of integration that always occurs in neuronal networks operating on the basis of coarse coding and distributed representation (Sejnowski 1986, Damasio 1990). Because information processing in other sensory modalities and in the motor system is also highly parallel, the needs to organize and bind distributed responses are similar to those encountered in the visual system. Furthermore, information must be flexibly coordinated both across sensory modalities as well as between sensory and motor processes in order to allow for adaptive behavior of the organism

(Roelfsema et al. 1996). The hypothesis pursued here predicts, therefore, that temporal binding mechanisms should exist not only in the visual system but in other cortical systems as well and, moreover, that synchrony should occur between different systems.

In the present context, the most radical extension of the concept of temporal binding has been its application to the issue of consciousness by Crick and Koch. As has been mentioned already, they have argued for a close relationship between binding and sensory awareness (Crick and Koch 1990a,b). Beyond that, they were the first to suggest that a temporal binding mechanism of precisely the kind discussed here could be required for the establishment of awareness. Inspired by the finding that visual stimuli can elicit synchronized oscillatory activity in the visual cortex (Eckhorn et al. 1988; Gráy and Singer 1989; Gray, König, Engel, and Singer 1989; Engel, König, Gray, and Singer 1990), they proposed that an attentional mechanism could induce synchronous oscillations in selected neuronal populations, and that this temporal structure would facilitate transfer of the encoded information to working memory. The provocative scent of this hypothesis comes from the authors' implicit assumpion that these are not just necessary, but indeed sufficient conditions for the occurrence of awareness. At the time it was published, Crick and Koch's speculative proposal was not supported by experimental evidence. In the present contribution, we will discuss more recent results that suggest that temporal binding may indeed be a prerequisite for the access of information to phenomenal consciousness. However, although largely in line with Crick and Koch's hypothesis, the present data do not seem to support the conclusion that synchronization of assemblies would constitute a *sufficient* condition for production of awareness.

Evidence for Temporal Binding

By now, the synchronization phenomena predicted by the temporal binding hypothesis are well documented for a wide variety of neural systems. It is well established that neurons in both cortical and subcortical centers can synchronize their discharges with a precision in the millisecond range (for review, see Engel et al. 1992, 1997; Singer 1993; Singer and Gray 1995; König and Engel 1995; Singer et al. 1997). This has been demonstrated in particular for the visual system, but similar observations have been made for the other sensory systems, for the motor system, and for cortical association areas.

In the following, we will focus on experimental data suggesting that the observed synchrony does indeed serve for the binding and selection of functionally related responses. These data have been obtained mainly in experiments on cats and monkeys, but presumably the results can be generalized to the human brain where recent EEG and MEG studies have provided evidence for similar synchronization phenomena (see Sauve).

For the case of the visual system, the temporal binding model predicts a synchronization of spatially separate cells within individual visual areas to account for the integration of perceptual information across different locations in the visual field. Additionally, synchrony should occur across large distances in the cortex to allow for binding between visual areas involved in the analysis of different object features. According to the temporal binding model, this would be required for the full representation of objects. Both predictions have been confirmed experimentally. In cats and monkeys (both in the anesthetized and awake preparation) synchrony has been observed within striate and extrastriate visual areas (Ts'o, Gilbert, and Wiesel 1986; Ts'o and Gilbert 1988; Eckhorn et al. 1988; Gray et al. 1989; Engel et al. 1990; Kreiter and Singer 1992; Brosch, Bauer, and Eckhorn 1995; Livingstone 1996; Gray and Viana Di Prisco 1997). Moreover, it has been shown that response synchronization can extend well beyond the borders of a single visual area. Thus, for instance, correlated firing has been observed between neurons located in different cerebral hemispheres (Engel, König, Kreiter, and Singer 1991a; Nowak et al. 1995). In terms of the temporal binding hypothesis, this result is important because interhemispheric synchrony is required to bind the features of objects extending across the midline of the visual field. Temporal correlations have also been studied for neurons located in different areas of the same hemisphere (Eckhorn et al. 1988; Engel, Kreiter, König, and Singer 1991b; Nelson et al. 1992; Roe and Ts'o 1992; Frien et al. 1994;

Roelfsema et al. 1997). Finally, recent evidence shows that synchronous firing is not confined to the cortex but occurs also in subcortical visual structures such as the retina, the lateral geniculate nucleus and the superior colliculus (Meister, Lagnado, and Baylor 1995; Neuenschwander and Singer 1996; Alonso, Usrey, and Reid 1996; Brecht, Singer, and Engel 1996, 1998). It is important to note that, at the cortical and subcortical level, synchrony can occur both internally generated (non-stimulus-locked) as well as externally imposed (stimulus-locked). Most of the studies cited above have focussed on the former type, which occurs predominantly with smoothly changing stimuli or during tonic response phases, and is generated by lateral interactions within the respective structures (Engel et al. 1991a; Munk, Nowak, Nelson, and Bullier 1995). In contrast, externally imposed synchrony is characterized by phase-locking to the stimulus, occurs in response to rapid stimulus transients (Kruse and Eckhorn 1996; Rager and Singer 1998) and is presumably mostly due to feedforward signal flow from the periphery.

Studies in nonvisual sensory modalities and in the motor system have provided evidence for very similar synchronization phenomena. Synchronization is well known to occur in the olfactory system of various vertebrate and invertebrate species, where these phenomena have been related to the processing of odor information (Freeman 1988, Laurent 1996). Moreover, in both the auditory (Eggermont 1992, deCharms and Merzenich 1996) and the somatosensory cortex (Murthy and Fetz 1992; Nicolelis, Baccala, Lin, and Chapin 1995; Steriade, Amzica, and Contreras 1996) precise neuronal synchronization has been observed. Furthermore, neuronal interacitons with a precision in the millisecond range have been described in the hippocampus (Bragin et al. 1995; Buzsáki and Chrobak 1995) and in the frontal cortex (Abeles et al. 1993; Vaadia et al. 1995). Finally, similar evidence is available for the motor system, where neural synchronization has been discovered both

during preparation and execution of movements (Murthy and Fetz, 1992, 1996a,b; Sanes and Donoghue 1993; Kristeva-Feige et al. 1993; Riehle, Grün, Diesmann, and Aertsen 1997).

Although the temporal binding model offers an attractive conceptual scheme for understanding the binding and selection of distributed neuronal responses, definitive evidence that the brain actually uses synchronization in exactly this way has not yet been obtained. However, a number of findings strongly suggest that the synchrony is indeed functionally relevant. One important result supporting the temporal binding model is that neuronal synchronization in the visual system depends on the stimulus configuration. Thus, it could be demonstrated that spatially separate cells show strong synchronization only if they respond to the same visual object. However, if responding to two independent stimuli moving in different directions, the cells fire in a less correlated manner or even without any fixed temporal relationship. This effect has been documented for the synchrony within (Gray et al. 1989; Engel, König, and Singer 1991c; Freiwald, Kreiter, and Singer 1995; Livingstone 1996; Kreiter and Singer 1996; Brosch, Bauer, and Eckhorn 1997) as well as across visual areas (Engel et al. 1991b, 1995). Along the same lines, it has recently been shown that precise synchronization in striate cortex is weakened if textures composed of spatially discontinuous elements (moving random-dot patterns) are applied as stimuli, rather than patterns comprising continous contours (Engel, Fries, Goebel, and Neuenschwander 1998). In such cases, precise neuronal synchronization disappears completely if the texture elements move incoherently (i.e., if the dot patterns contain substantial fractions of noise). Taken together, these experiments demonstrate that Gestalt criteria such as continuity or coherent motion, which have psychophysically been shown to support perceptual grouping, are important for the establishment of precise synchrony among neurons in the visual cortex. These data strongly support the

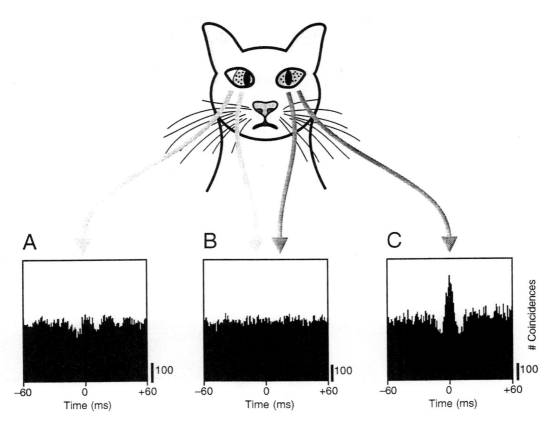

Figure 8.2
Neuronal synchronization in the primary visual cortex of cats with strabismic ambylopia. The lower panel shows examples of cross correlograms between cells driven by the normal eye, by the amblyopic eye, and between cells dominated by different eyes. Temporal correlation is strong if both recording sites are driven by the normal eye (*C*). Synchronization is, on average, much weaker between cells dominated by the amblyopic eye (*A*) and is in most cases negligible if the recording sites receive their input from different eyes (*B*). (Modified from Roelfsema et al. 1994)

A

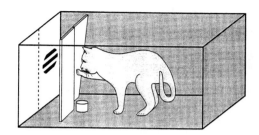

B

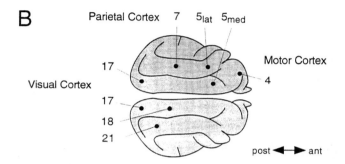

Parietal Cortex   7   5_{lat}   5_{med}

Visual Cortex

Motor Cortex

17

17

18

21

4

post ◄───► ant

C

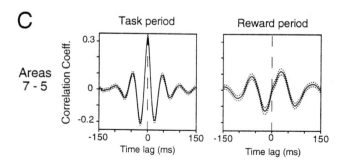

Areas
7 - 5

Task period

Reward period

Correlation Coeff.

0.3

0

-0.2

-150   0   150
Time lag (ms)

-150   0   150
Time lag (ms)

D

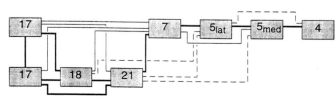

17   7   5_{lat}   5_{med}   4

17   18   21

hypothesis that correlated firing provides a dynamic mechanism for feature binding and response selection.

Additional evidence that neuronal synchronization is indeed functionally relevant and related to the animal's perception is provided by experiments on cats with convergent squint (Roelfsema et al. 1994). Subjects with this type of strabismus often use only one eye for active fixation. The nonfixating eye then develops a syndrome of perceptual deficits called strabismic amblyopia. Symptoms of strabismic amblyopia include a reduced acuity of the affected eye, temporal instability and spatial distortions of the visual image, and the so-called crowding phenomenon, that is, discrimination of details deteriorates further if other contours are nearby. Clearly, at least some of these deficits indicate a reduced capacity of integrating visual information and an impairment of the mechanisms responsible for feature binding. The results of the correlation study by Roelfsema et al. (1994) indicate that these perceptual deficits may be due to a disturbance of intracortical interactions (see figure 8.2). Thus, clear differences were observed in the synchronization of cells driven by the normal and the amblyopic eye, respectively. In the primary visual cortex, responses of neurons activated through the amblyopic eye showed a much weaker correlation than the discharges of neurons driven by the normal eye. Surprisingly, however, in terms of average firing rates the responses of neurons driven by the normal and amblyopic eye were indistinguishable. These results indicate that strabismic amblyopia is accompanied by a selective impairment of intracortical interactions that synchronize neurons responding to coherent stimuli. As mentioned above, most of the problems in amblyopic vision result from an improper segregation of features and the formation of false conjunctions. Therefore, the fact that the only measurable abnormality correlating with the perceptual deficit was the reduced synchronicity is in good agreement with the hypothesis that synchronization is employed for feature binding and serves to disambiguate distributed response patterns.

Evidence for a functional role of neural synchrony is also provided by recent studies of sensorimotor interactions. Synchronization between sensory and motor assemblies has been investigated in a recent study on awake behaving cats that were trained to perform a visuomotor coordination task (see figure 8.3) (Roelfsema

Figure 8.3
Synchronization between visual, parietal, and motor cortex in awake, behaving cats. Local field potentials were recorded with electrodes chronically implanted in several areas of the visual and parietal cortex as well as in the primary motor cortex. (*A*) The cats were situated unrestrained in a testing box and had to watch a screen through a transparent door. At the beginning of each trial, a grating was projected onto the screen. The cat had to respond by pressing the door with the forepaw and had to hold it until the grating was rotated. Upon change of the visual stimulus, the animal had to release the door. After correct trials, a reward was presented in a food well at the bottom of the box. (*B*) Location of the recording sites. Electrodes were implanted in area 17, 18, and 21 of the visual cortex, in areas 5 and 7 of parietal cortex, and in area 4 of the motor cortex where the forepaw is represented that the cat used for pressing the door. (*C*) Example of synchronization between area 7 and 5 of the parietal cortex during the task period, that is, the epoch where the cat was watching the grating and waiting for its rotation (left) and the reward period (right). The interactions are dependent on the behavioral context. Thus, during the task, zero-phase synchrony occurs between the areas. However, during the reward period the synchrony is lost and a large phase-shift appears in the correlogram. (*D*) Summary of temporal correlation between the recorded area during the task period. Thick lines indicate strong correlation (correlation coefficients large than 0.10), thin and hatched lines show weak, but still significant interactions (correlation coefficients smaller than 0.10 or smaller than 0.05, respectively). Area have been placed according to their position in the processing stream that links the visual cortex to the motor cortex. The diagram shows that precise synchrony is a global cortical phenomenon and is not restricted to the visual cortex. (Modified from Roelfsema et al. 1997)

et al. 1997). In these animals, neural activity was recorded with electrodes chronically implanted in various areas of the visual, parietal, and motor cortex. The results of this study show that synchronization of neural responses does not only occur within the visual system but also between visual and parietal areas as well as between parietal and motor cortex. Importantly, the interareal interactions changed dramatically in different behavioral situations. Precise neuronal synchronization between sensory and motor areas occurred specifically in those task epochs where the animal had to process visual information attentively to direct the required motor response. The observations of this study suggest that synchrony may indeed be relevant for visuomotor coordination and may serve for the linkage of sensory and motor aspects of behavior. The specificity of such interactions might allow, for instance, the selective channeling of sensory information to different motor programs that are concurrently executed (Roelfsema et al. 1996). Similar conclusions are suggested by recent studies in monkeys, where synchronization between sensory and motor cortical areas has also been reported (Murthy and Fetz 1992, 1996a,b).

Complementing these animal experiments, supportive evidence for the notion of temporal binding comes from psychophysical studies in humans, where the role of external timing for buildup of coherent percepts has been investigated. Thus, it has been shown that small temporal offsets can induce figure-ground segregation (Leonards, Singer, and Fahle 1996). As demonstrated in this study, a subset of elements in a flickered texture can be perceptually segregated if there is a temporal lag between figure and ground elements of more than 10 ms. Very similar effects of external timing on grouping of texture elements and on detection of colinear contours have recently been observed by Usher and Donnelly (1998). Moreover, it has been shown that perception of globally coherent motion is strongly enhanced if the contrast of stim-

ulus components is synchronously modulated (Alais, Blake, and Lee 1998). Finally, external timing can enhance visual feature binding also if the temporal cue is not present in the target display itself but, rather, in a priming stimulus consisting of synchronously flickered figural elements (Elliott and Müller 1998). In such cases, the detection of coherent features is facilitated in those locations where the synchronously flickered prime had been presented. The conclusion from these studies is that external timing cues can impose, via phase-locking of neuronal discharges to the respective stimulus transients, significant temporal structure on visual assemblies. Given that the timing differences were on the order of 10–20 ms, these data clearly support the notion that sensory systems can exploit precise temporal structure (whether internally generated or externally imposed) for perceptual integration and the selection of coherent information. An important point is that in these experiments, the external timing cues leading to binding and figure-ground segregation *themselves* are usually not consciously perceived (Usher and Donnelly 1998, Elliott and Müller 1998).

Binding and Phenomenal Consciousness

The experimental data discussed in the preceding section clearly argue for the importance of precise neuronal synchrony in the establishment of coherent sensory representations and for sensorimotor integration. Recent evidence indicates that these synchronization phenomena may also be relevant for the buildup of phenomenal states and the selection of visual information for access to awareness. This is suggested by experiments in which we recorded neuronal responses from the visual cortex of strabismic cats under conditions of binocular rivalry (Fries et al. 1997b). Binocular rivalry is a particularly interesting case of dynamic response selection, which occurs when the images in the two eyes are incongruent and cannot be fused into a coherent percept. In this case, only signals from one of the two eyes are selected and perceived, whereas those from the other eye are suppressed (Blake 1989). In normal subjects, perception alternates between the stimuli presented to left and right eye, respectively. The important point is that this shift in perceptual dominance can occur without any change of the physical stimulus. Obviously, this experimental situation is particularly revealing for the issue at stake, because neuronal responses to a given stimulus can be studied either with or without being accompanied by awareness (Crick and Koch 1990a, Farber and Churchland 1995) and, thus, there is a chance of revealing the mechanisms leading to the selection of perceptual information.

Previous studies have examined the hypothesis that response selection in binocular rivalry is achieved by a modulation of firing rate. In these experiments, a number of different visual cortical areas were recorded in awake monkeys experiencing binocular rivalry (Logothetis and Schall 1989, Leopold and Logothetis 1996, Sheinberg and Logothetis 1997). With respect to early processing stages (visual areas V1, V2, V4, MT), the results of these investigations were not conclusive. The fraction of neurons that decreased their firing rates upon suppression of the stimulus to which they responded was about the same as the fraction of cells that increased their discharge rate, and altogether response amplitudes changed in less than 50% of the neurons when eye dominance switched (Logothetis and Schall 1989, Leopold and Logothetis 1996). A clear and positive correlation between firing rate and perception was found only in inferotemporal cortex, that is, at a relatively late stage of visual processing (Sheinberg and Logothetis 1997).

In our study (Fries et al. 1997b) we investigated the hypothesis that response selection in early visual areas might be achieved by modulation of the synchronicity rather than the rate of discharges. These measurements were performed in awake cats with wire electrodes chronically implanted in areas 17 and 18 (see figure 8.4). The

animals were subjected to dichoptic visual stimulation—that is, patterns moving in different directions were simultaneously presented to the left and the right eye, respectively. Perceptual dominance for a given set of stimuli was inferred from the direction of eye movements induced by the drifting gratings (the so-called optokinetic nystagmus) recorded by periorbital electrodes (during correlation measurements, however, precautions were taken to minimize eye movements; for details, see Fries et al. 1997b). As a baseline, neuronal responses were also recorded under monocular stimulation conditions. The results obtained with this experimental approach show that visual cortical neurons driven by the selected and the suppressed eye, respectively, do neither differ in the strength nor in the synchronicity of their response to monocular visual stimulation. They show, however, striking differences with respect to their synchronization behavior when exposed to the rivalry condition. Neurons representing the stimulus that wins in rivalry and is perceived increase their synchrony, whereas cells processing the suppressed visual pattern decrease their temporal correlation. However, no differences were noted under the rivalry condition for the discharge rates of cells responding to the selected and the suppressed eye, respectively.

These results show that, in areas 17 and 18 of awake, strabismic cats, dynamic selection and suppression of sensory signals are associated with modifications of the synchrony rather than the rate of neuronal discharges. This suggests that at an early level of visual processing, it is the degree of synchronicity rather than the amplitude of responses that determines which of the input signals will be processed further and then support perception and oculomotor responses. Changes in synchronicity at early stages of processing are bound to result in changes of discharge rate at later stages. Thus, the rate changes observed with perceptual rivalry in higher cortical areas (Sheinberg and Logothetis 1997) could be secondary to modifications of neuronal syn-

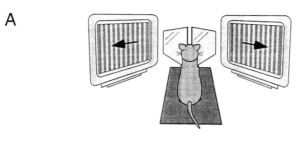

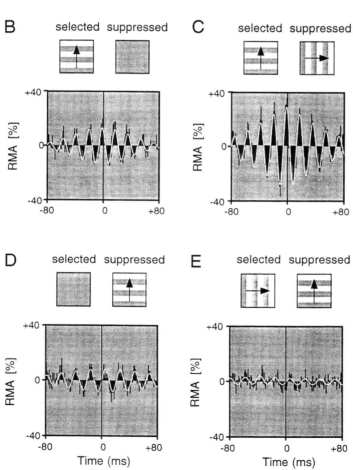

A

B   selected   suppressed

C   selected   suppressed

D   selected   suppressed

E   selected   suppressed

RMA [%]

Time (ms)

chronization at lower levels of processing. An interesting aspect of our results is that the synchronicity of responses representing the dominant stimulus even increased when the rivalry condition was introduced, which suggests the action of a mechanism that enhances the saliency of the selected responses. One possibility is that both the increase in synchronicity of the selected and the reduced synchronicity of the suppressed signals are due to local competition among the populations of neurons responding to the right and left eye, respectively. However, it is also conceivable that attention-related top-down processes contribute to the selection of input signals by controlling their synchronicity. The possibility that attentional mechanisms act not only by modulating the rate but also the synchronicity of responses is supported by the evidence that neuronal synchronization increases during states characterized by arousal and focused attention (see next section).

In the present context, the important conclusion from these experiments is that only strongly synchronized neuronal responses can contribute to awareness and conscious phenomenal states. The data suggest that activation of feature-detecting cells is, as such, not sufficient to grant access of the encoded information to consciousness (note that the cells representing the suppressed stimulus are still well responding). Rather, to be functionally effective and to be selected for perception, neurons have to be strongly synchronized and bound into assemblies. In this respect, our data support the proposal by Crick and Koch (1990a,b) that neuronal synchronization may be a necessary condition for the occurrence of awareness. Admittedly, our conclusion rests on the assumption that sensory awareness of the stimulus correlates well with the oculomotor behavior that we have used as an indirect measure of the cat's perceptual state. However, this correspondence has been well established in humans, where a nearly perfect correlation has been found between the direction of the pursuit phase of the optokinetic nystagmus and the perceived direction of motion (Enoksson 1963; Fox, Todd, and Bettinger 1975), meaning that it is impossible, in the rivalry situation, to track one of the patterns with the eyes but consciously perceive the other.

At this point, we wish to add a brief comment on the issue of oscillations. As in many studies on correlated activity in visual cortex, the synchrony observed in our rivalry experiments was associated with a strong oscillatory modulation of the responses at frequencies in the gamma range, that is, between 30 and 80 Hz (Fries et al. 1997b; for a review on gamma-oscillations, see Engel et al. 1992, 1997; Singer and Gray 1995). Under rivalry conditions, these oscillations show the same changes as the synchrony across recording sites—that is, the power in the gamma

Figure 8.4
Neuronal synchronization under binocular rivalry. (*A*) Cats were placed on a recording table and their head fixed by means of an implanted bolt. In front of the animal's head two mirrors were mounted such that each eye was viewing a separate monitor. Panels (*B–E*) show normalized cross correlograms for two pairs of recording sites activated by the selected (*B, C*) and the suppressed eye (*D, E*), respectively. Insets above the correlograms indicate stimulation conditions. (*B, C*) Synchronization among neurons driven by the eye that is selected under rivalry conditions. Under monocular stimulation applied as a control (*B*), the cells showed a significant temporal correlation. Under rivalry conditions (*C*) these cells, which were representing the perceptually selected stimulus, increased their synchrony. (*D, E*) Correlation among cells driven by the nonperceived stimulus. In the monocular control condition (*D*), these neurons also showed significant synchronization. However, under dichoptic stimulation (*E*) the cells (which were responding to the suppressed stimulus) decreased their temporal correlation. The white continuous line superimposed on the correlograms represents a damped cosine function fitted to the data. RMA, relative modulation amplitude of the center peak in the correlogram, computed as the ratio of peak amplitude over offset of correlogram modulation. (Modified from Fries et al. 1997b)

band increases for neurons representing the dominant stimulus, whereas it decreases for cells responding to the suppressed stimulus. At present, the function of these oscillations is unresolved and it seems possible that selection of perceptually relevant information could also occur on the basis of nonoscillatory synchronized activity. However, as discussed in detail elsewhere, the oscillations may at least be of indirect relevance for response selection because they seem to facilitate the establishment of synchrony among distributed neurons (Engel et al. 1992, 1997; Singer 1993; König, Engel, and Singer 1995; Singer et al. 1997).

Relation to Arousal and Attention

The data on the changes of neuronal synchronization under rivalry conditions seem to provide, at this point, the most direct evidence for a relation between synchrony and perceptual awareness. However, a number of other studies also support the idea that synchronization is related to awareness and to attentive processing of information. These studies suggest that neuronal synchronization increases during states characterized by arousal and focused attention, and moreover, that high-frequency (gamma) oscillations are also particularly prominent during epochs of higher vigilance. Thus, experiments in rats (Franken, Dijk, Tobler, and Borbély 1994) and cats (Steriade et al. 1996, Steriade 1997) have shown that gamma-band synchronization is enhanced during REM sleep and waking as compared to deep sleep. Moreover, electrical activation of the midbrain reticular formation (one of the structures responsible for change of vigilance states) has been shown to induce a shift from low to high oscillation frequencies and an increase of stimulus-induced synchronization in the visual cortex (Munk et al. 1996). Also, studies in awake, behaving animals demonstrate that precise neuronal synchronization and fast oscillations are enhanced in the cortex during

epochs of focussed attention (Rougeul, Bouyer, Dedet, and Debray 1979, Roelfsema et al. 1997).

Further support for a relationship between temporal binding and attentional mechanisms comes from recent work on the superior colliculus, a midbrain structure with important integrative functions which mediates orienting responses towards a target of interest (Stein and Meredith 1993). Lesions of the colliculus lead to neglect, that is, a severe impairment of spatial attention and phenomenal awareness for events in the space contralateral to the lesion. Based on lesion studies and other physiological evidence, it has been assumed that the colliculus is involved in shifting of attention to new locations (Posner and Petersen 1990, Kustov and Robinson 1996). Recent experiments suggest that temporal structure in collicular activity patterns may play a crucial role for the target selection performed by this structure. In the cat, it could be shown that neurons in visual cortical areas can synchronize, via the corticotectal pathway, with cells in the superficial layers of the colliculus (Brecht, Singer, and Engel 1998). Moreover, synchrony occurs within the colliculus itself if the neurons are responding to a coherent visual stimulus (Brecht, Singer, and Engel 1996). These findings suggest that potential targets for attentional shifts and associated orienting behavior may be represented in the colliculus by assemblies of synchronously firing cells. More recent experiments have attempted a more direct test of the idea that temporal binding may play a role for target selection in the colliculus (Brecht, Singer, and Engel 1997). In these experiments, it was investigated how electrically evoked saccadic eye movements were affected by varying the temporal relation between microstimulation trains applied at two different sites in the colliculus. As shown in figure 8.5, small temporal phase-shifts lead to a motor output radically different from that evoked by synchronous stimulation. Thus, these data strongly suggest that synchrony in the millisecond range is an important determinant for target selection in the corticotectal pathway

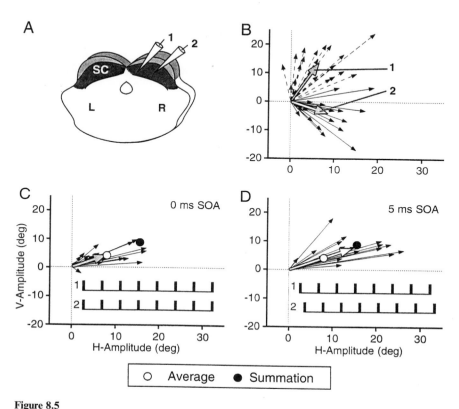

Figure 8.5
Effects of time-varied microstimulation in the superior colliculus on saccade vectors with different directions.
(*A*) Position of the stimulation electrodes. Both electrodes were located in the deep layers of the right superior colliculus (SC). (*B*) Saccade vectors evoked by stimulating the two sites individually. Small dashed arrows refer to the individual saccades evoked by electrical microstimulation at site 1, whereas the continuous arrows refer to effects of stimulating site 2. The thick arrows indicate the respective mean vectors. (*C, D*) Saccade vectors obtained with different microstimulation timing protocols. Small arrows display the vectors of individual saccades, the thick arrow represents the mean vector, and the pattern of microstimulation bursts is schematically indicated below each set of saccades. (*C*) Synchronous microstimulation of the two sites leads to vector averaging—that is, to movements along a vector corresponding to the mean of the saccades evoked by stimulating the two sites individually (white dot indicates the averages of vectors 1 and 2; cf. *B*). (*D*) Slight temporal offsets of, for example, 5 ms between the microstimulation pulses delivered to the two sites result in a completely different movement pattern: in this case, the saccades correspond to the sum, rather than the average, of the individual vectors (black dot indicates the sum of vectors 1 and 2 as shown in *B*); that is, they have the same direction as those evoked by synchronous pulse trains but show approximately double amplitude. SOA, stimulus onset asynchrony. (From Brecht et al. 1997)

and, hence, also for the role of this system in directing spatial attention.

Specific changes of neural synchronization with arousal and attention are also demonstrated by EEG and MEG studies in humans. Thus, high-frequency components of sensory evoked potentials, which indicate precise neuronal synchronization when recorded in the awake state, have been shown to disappear under deep anesthesia (Schwender et al. 1994; note that under such conditions the neurons are—in terms of their average firing rate—still responding well to sensory stimuli). Furthermore, EEG measurements have provided clear evidence that synchronization in the gamma band is enhanced during arousal and during focused attention (Sheer 1989, Desmedt and Tomberg 1994). Finally, recent results suggest that gamma synchronization is correlated with conscious perception of distinct auditory events (Joliot, Ribary, and Llinás 1994) and with perception of coherent visual stimuli (Tallon, Bertrand, Bouchet, and Pernier 1995; Müller, Junghöfer, Elbert, and Rockstroh 1997), in particular during attentive visual search (Tallon-Baudry, Bertrand, Delpuech, and Pernier 1997). Taken together, these data demonstrate that arousal (as one of the prerequisites for awareness) and selective attention (as a focussed form of sensory awareness) are characterized by an enhancement of synchrony in the relevant neuronal populations. This evidence seems to agree well with our results on binocular rivalry, further corroborating the notion that temporal binding may be required to grant access of information to phenomenal consciousness (Crick and Koch 1990a,b).

Conclusions

In this paper, we have discussed the concept of temporal binding and its application to the issue of sensory processing and perceptual awareness. The basic assumption is that synchrony is introduced as an additional coding dimension that complements the conventional rate code. Whereas the latter serves for the coarse coding of representational contents, the former may permit the dynamic expression of specific relations within a network. In this way, the combination of two different coding strategies could allow the multiplexing of different types of information within the same activity patterns and, thus, could enhance the representational power of distributed systems. As discussed, the available data suggest that a temporal binding mechanism may indeed exist in the brain. Rather than being a futile epiphenomenon of network connectivity, precise synchronization of neuronal discharges seems to be functionally relevant for the binding of distributed responses in a wide variety of neural systems. In sensory systems, temporal binding may serve for perceptual grouping and, thus, constitute an important prerequisite for scene segmentation and object recognition. Moreover, temporal binding may be involved in sensorimotor integration, that is, in establishing selective links between sensory and motor aspects of behavior.

The crucial advantage of temporal binding is that it could permit the rapid and reliable selection of perceptually or behaviorally relevant information. Because precisely synchronized discharges have a high impact on the respective postsynaptic cells, the information tagged by such a temporal label could be rapidly and preferentially relayed to other processing centers (Singer and Gray 1995, Singer et al. 1997). We propose that such a process of response selection, which is based on temporal correlation among subsets of activated neurons, may be an integral part of the mechanisms responsible for perceptual awareness. As shown by our experiments on binocular rivalry, selection of visual information for perception is associated with an enhanced synchronization of the respective neuronal populations. Therefore, temporal binding may indeed be a necessary condition for the occurrence of awareness and the establishment of conscious phenomenal states.

In the present context, a question of obvious interest is why selection based on temporal binding would lead to awareness in some cases but not in others. Thus, for instance, both the attentive search for a particular object as well as the visuomotor coordination in a frequently practiced task like driving require context-dependent selection that, according to our hypothesis, may be implemented by synchronization of appropriate neural assemblies. However, although in the former case the selection process usually leads to awareness, this does not necessarily hold for the latter. What makes the difference, and what would be a *sufficient* condition for the instigation of awareness? A suggestion that we would like to make at this point is that the difference may relate to the "routing" (or targeting) of the selected information to processing centers downstream of the visual system. It might be, for instance, that sensory contents reach awareness only if the perceptual information is transferred to prefrontal areas and, thus, becomes part of short-term memory and is available for extended action planning. In contrast, if the "loop" leading to action is different, mainly involving a direct coupling of the sensory information to premotor/motor areas or to subcortical centers, then the same information might be less available for global control and, thus, less accompanied by awareness (Newman and Baars 1993). Clearly, further studies are required that elaborate on the "readout" of temporally bound sensory information and on the routing of selected information in different behavioural contexts.

Other unresolved problems relate to the mechanisms leading to a specific enhancement of synchrony in subsets of distributed neuronal populations. Presumably, multiple factors can contribute to such an enhancement as a prerequisite for selection. First, the binding criteria implemented in the network architecture of sensory areas and, in addition, reentrant interactions between different modules in a sensory system are of basic importance. If binding criteria residing in different areas are consistently met, this may lead—via mutual augmentation—to a high degree of coherence within distributed assemblies (Tononi, Sporns, and Edelman 1992; Schillen and König 1994). Second, sensorimotor interactions and modification of the processing by sensorimotor loops may be important (for a more detailed discussion, see Roelfsema et al. 1996). We suggest that attentional selection of information for awareness is never "purely sensory" but is always determined by the integral sensorimotor state of the system. Third, central modulatory systems can contribute to enhancement by upregulation of synchronizing influences (Munk et al. 1996). Fourth, as previously discussed, synchronization is very likely subject to attentional influences (Crick and Koch 1990a,b). Finally, interactions with memory structures will very likely have a profound influence on selection. Thus, for instance, dynamic interactions with working memory (Goldman-Rakic 1992, Moscovitch 1995, Desimone and Duncan 1995), implemented by assemblies in prefrontal areas, are conceivable. These considerations indicate that an enhancement of synchronization leading to selection of neuronal populations may be based on a combination of both bottom-up as well as top-down influences, but further studies are required here as well to fully resolve the nature of these mechanisms.

In summary, we wish to suggest that studying the dynamics of neuronal interactions may be particularly rewarding in search for the neural correlates of consciousness. The important point of the results presented here is that, at least at early stages of sensory processing, the degree of synchronicity predicts reliably whether neural activity will contribute to conscious experience or not. We propose that experiments designed to investigate neuronal synchronization may help to identify the selection mechanisms that are required for phenomenal consciousness. At this point, we have deliberately restricted our discussion to the issue of awareness because it seems that, based on the present data, one can hardly argue about a relevance of binding mechanisms for other forms of consciousness. However, it has been speculated that temporal binding may also account for higher-order properties of phenomenal consciousness (Metzinger 1995)—an exciting possibility that clearly awaits future research.

Acknowledgments

Financial support by the Max-Planck-Society, by the Deutsche Forschungsgemeinschaft (grants En203/4-1, En203/5-1, En203/5-2), and by the Minna-James-Heineman-Foundation is gratefully acknowledged. A. Engel is obliged to the Institute for Advanced Study Berlin, where most of this paper has been written, for providing excellent working facilities during the academic year 1997–98. At the Institute for Advanced Study A. Engel has been supported by a Daimler-Benz fellowship.

References

Abeles, M. (1982) Role of the cortical neuron: Integrator or coincidence detector? *Israel Journal of Medical Sciences* 18: 83–92.

Abeles, M., Vaadia, E., Bergman, H., Prut, Y., Haalman, I., and Slovin, H. (1993) Dynamics of neuronal interactions in the frontal cortex of behaving monkeys. *Concepts in Neuroscience* 4: 131–158.

Alais, D., Blake, R., and Lee, S.-H. (1998) Visual features that vary together over time group together over space. *Nature Neuroscience* 1: 160–164.

Alonso, J.-M., Usrey, W. M., and Reid, R. C. (1996) Precisely correlated firing in cells of the lateral geniculate nucleus. *Nature* 383: 815–819.

Barlow, H. B. (1972) Single units and sensation: A neuron doctrine for perceptual psychology? *Perception* 1: 371–394.

Blake, R. (1989) A neural theory of binocular rivalry. *Psychological Review* 96: 145–167.

Bragin, A., Jandó, G., Nádasdy, Z., Hetke, J., Wise, K., and Buzsáki, G. (1995) Gamma (40–100 Hz) oscillation in the hippocampus of the behaving rat. *Journal of Neuroscience* 15: 47–60.

Brecht, M., Singer, W., and Engel, A. K. (1996) Temporal coding in the cat superior colliculus. *Society for Neuroscience Abstracts* 22: 1446.

Brecht, M., Singer, W., and Engel, A. K. (1997) Collicular saccade vectors defined by synchronization. *Society for Neuroscience Abstracts* 23: 843.

Brecht, M., Singer, W., and Engel, A. K. (1998) Correlation analysis of cortico-tectal interactions in the cat visual system. *Journal of Neurophysiology* 79: 2394–2407.

Brosch, M., Bauer, R., and Eckhorn, R. (1995) Synchronous high-frequency oscillations in cat area 18. *European Journal of Neuroscience* 7: 86–95.

Brosch, M., Bauer, R., and Eckhorn, R. (1997) Stimulus-dependent modulations of correlated high-frequency oscillations in cat visual cortex. *Cerebral Cortex* 7: 70–76.

Bullier, J., and Nowak, L. G. (1995) Parallel versus serial processing: New vistas on the distributed organization of the visual system. *Current Opinion in Neurobiology* 5: 497–503.

Buzsáki, G., and Chrobak, J. J. (1995) Temporal structure in spatially organized neuronal ensembles: A role for interneuronal networks. *Current Opinion in Neurobiology* 5: 504–510.

Crick, F. (1984) Function of the thalamic reticular complex: The searchlight hypothesis. *Proceedings of the National Academy of Sciences USA* 81: 4586–4590.

Crick, F. (1994) *The astonishing hypothesis*. New York: Simon and Schuster.

Crick, F., and Koch, C. (1990a) Towards a neurobiological theory of consciousness. *Seminars in Neurosciences* 2: 263–275.

Crick, F., and Koch, C. (1990b) Some reflections on visual awareness. *Cold Spring Harbor Symposia on Quantitative Biology* 55: 953–962.

Damasio, A. R. (1990) Synchronous activation in multiple cortical regions: A mechanism for recall. *Seminars in Neurosciences* 2: 287–296.

deCharms, R. C., and Merzenich, M. M. (1996) Primary cortical representation of sounds by the coordination of action-potential timing. *Nature* 381: 610–613.

Desimone, R., and Duncan, J. (1995) Neural mechanisms of selective visual attention. *Annual Review of Neuroscience* 18: 193–222.

Desmedt, J. E., and Tomberg, C. (1994) Transient phase-locking of 40 Hz electrical oscillations in prefrontal and parietal human cortex reflects the process of conscious somatic perception. *Neuroscience Letters* 168: 126–129.

Eckhorn, R., Bauer, R., Jordan, W., Brosch, M., Kruse, W., Munk, M., and Reitboeck, H. J. (1988) Coherent oscillations: A mechanism for feature linking in the visual cortex? *Biological Cybernetics* 60: 121–130.

Eggermont, J. J. (1992) Neural interaction in cat primary auditory cortex: Dependence on recording depth, electrode separation, and age. *Journal of Neurophysiology* 68: 1216–1228.

Elliott, M. A., and Müller, H. J. (1998) Synchronous information presented in 40 Hz flicker enhances visual feature binding. *Psychological Science* 9: 277–283.

Engel, A. K., Fries, P., Goebel, R., and Neuenschwander, S. (1998) Synchronization induced by moving random-dot patterns in cat striate cortex. *Society for Neuroscience Abstracts* 24.

Engel, A. K., König, P., Gray, C. M., and Singer, W. (1990) Stimulus-dependent neuronal oscillations in cat visual cortex: Inter-columnar interaction as determined by crosscorrelation analysis. *European Journal of Neuroscience* 2: 588–606.

Engel, A. K., König, P., Kreiter, A. K., Schillen, T. B., and Singer, W. (1992) Temporal coding in the visual cortex: New vistas on integration in the nervous system. *Trends in Neurosciences* 15: 218–226.

Engel, A. K., König, P., Kreiter, A. K., and Singer, W. (1991a) Interhemispheric synchronization of oscillatory neuronal responses in cat visual cortex. *Science* 252: 1177–1179.

Engel, A. K., König, P., Roelfsema, P. R., Munk, M. H. J., and Singer, W. (1995) Interhemispheric synchronization in cat visual cortex is comparable to synchrony within hemispheres. *Society for Neuroscience Abstracts* 21: 1649.

Engel, A. K., König, P., and Singer, W. (1991c) Direct physiological evidence for scene segmentation by temporal coding. *Proceedings of the National Academy of Sciences USA* 88: 9136–9140.

Engel, A. K., Kreiter, A. K., König, P., and Singer, W. (1991b) Synchronization of oscillatory neuronal responses between striate and extrastriate visual cortical areas of the cat. *Proceedings of the National Academy of Sciences USA* 88: 6048–6052.

Engel, A. K., Roelfsema, P. R., Fries, P., Brecht, M., and Singer, W. (1997) Role of the temporal domain for response selection and perceptual binding. *Cerebral Cortex* 7: 571–582.

Enoksson, P. (1963) Binocular rivalry and monocular dominance studied with optokinetic nystagmus. *Acta Ophthalmologica* 41: 544–563.

Farber, I. B., and Churchland, P. S. (1995) Consciousness and the neurosciences: philosophical and theoretical issues. In M. S. Gazzaniga (Ed.), *The cognitive neurosciences*, pp. 1295–1306. Cambridge: MIT Press.

Felleman, D. J., and Van Essen, D. C. (1991) Distributed hierarchical processing in the primate cerebral cortex. *Cerebral Cortex* 1: 1–47.

Fodor, J., and McLaughlin, B. P. (1990) Connectionism and the problem of systematicity: Why Smolensky's solution doesn't work. *Cognition* 35: 183–204.

Fodor, J. A., and Pylyshyn, Z. W. (1988) Connectionism and cognitive architecture: A critical analysis. *Cognition* 28: 3–71.

Fox, R., Todd, S., and Bettinger, L. A. (1975) Optokinetic nystagmus as an objective indicator of binocular rivalry. *Vision Research* 15: 849–853.

Franken, P., Dijk, D.-J., Tobler, I., and Borbély, A. A. (1994) High-frequency components of the rat electrocorticogramm are modulated by vigilance states. *Neuroscience Letters* 167: 89–92.

Freeman, W. J. (1988) Nonlinear neural dynamics in olfaction as a model for cognition. In E. Basar (Ed.), *Dynamics of sensory and cognitive processing by the brain*, pp. 19–29. Berlin: Springer.

Freiwald, W. A., Kreiter, A. K., and Singer, W. (1995) Stimulus dependent intercolumnar synchronization of single unit responses in cat area 17. *Neuroreport* 6: 2348–2352.

Frien, A., Eckhorn, R., Bauer, R., Woelbern, T., and Kehr, H. (1994) Stimulus-specific fast oscillations at zero phase between visual areas V1 and V2 of awake monkey. *Neuroreport* 5: 2273–2277.

Fries, P., Roelfsema, P. R., Engel, A. K., König, P., and Singer, W. (1997b) Synchronization of oscillatory responses in visual cortex correlates with perception in interocular rivalry. *Proceedings of the National Academy of Sciences USA* 94: 12699–12704.

Fries, P., Roelfsema, P. R., Singer, W., and Engel, A. K. (1997a) Correlated variations of response latencies due to synchronous subthreshold membrane potential fluctuations in cat striate cortex. *Society for Neuroscience Abstracts* 23: 1266.

Goldman-Rakic, P. S. (1992) Working memory and the mind. *Scientific American* 9/92: 73–79.

Gray, C. M., König, P., Engel, A. K., and Singer, W. (1989) Oscillatory responses in cat visual cortex exhibit inter-columnar synchronization which reflects global stimulus properties. *Nature* 338: 334–337.

Gray, C. M., and Singer, W. (1989) Stimulus-specific neuronal oscillations in orientation columns of cat visual cortex. *Proceedings of the National Academy of Sciences USA* 86: 1698–1702.

Gray, C. M., and Viana Di Prisco, G. (1997) Stimulus-dependent neuronal oscillations and local synchronization in striate cortex of the alert cat. *Journal of Neuroscience* 17: 3239–3253.

Hinton, G. E., McClelland, J. L., and Rumelhart, D. E. (1986) Distributed representations. In D. E. Rumelhart, J. L. McClelland, and the PDP Research Group (Eds.), *Parallel distributed processing.* Vol. 1, pp. 77–109. Cambridge: MIT Press.

Hummel, J. E., and Biederman, I. (1992) Dynamic binding in a neural network for shape recognition. *Psychological Review* 99: 480–517.

Joliot, M., Ribary, U., and Llinás, R. (1994) Human oscillatory brain activity near 40 Hz coexists with cognitive temporal binding. *Proceedings of the National Academy of Sciences USA* 91: 11748–11751.

Koch, C., and Crick, F. (1994) Some further ideas rearding the neuronal basis of awareness. In C. Koch, and J. L. Davis (Eds.), *Large-scale neuronal theories of the brain,* pp. 93–109. Cambridge: MIT Press.

König, P., and Engel, A. K. (1995) Correlated firing in sensory-motor systems. *Current Opinion in Neurobiology* 5: 511–519.

König, P., Engel, A. K., and Singer, W. (1995) The relation between oscillatory activity and long-range synchronization in cat visual cortex. *Proceedings of the National Academy of Sciences USA* 92: 290–294.

König, P., Engel, A. K., and Singer, W. (1996) Integrator or coincidence detector? The role of the cortical neuron revisited. *Trends in Neurosciences* 19: 130–137.

Kreiter, A. K., and Singer, W. (1992) Oscillatory neuronal responses in the visual cortex of the awake macaque monkey. *European Journal of Neuroscience* 4: 369–375.

Kreiter, A. K., and Singer, W. (1996) Stimulus-dependent synchronization of neuronal responses in the visual cortex of awake macaque monkey. *Journal of Neuroscience* 16: 2381–2396.

Kristeva-Feige, R., Feige, B., Makeig, S., Ross, B., and Elbert, T. (1993) Oscillatory brain activity during a motor task. *Neuroreport* 4: 1291–1294.

Kruse, W., and Eckhorn, R. (1996) Inhibition of sustained gamma oscillations (35–80 Hz) by fast transient responses in cat visual cortex. *Proceedings of the National Academy of Sciences USA* 93: 6112–6117.

Kustov, A. A., and Robinson, D. L. (1996) Shared neural control of attentional shifts and eye movements. *Nature* 384: 74–77.

Laurent, G. (1996) Dynamical representation of odors by oscillating and evolving neural assemblies. *Trends in Neuroscience* 19: 489–496.

Leonards, U., Singer, W., and Fahle, M. (1996) The influence of temporal phase differences on texture segmentation. *Vision Research* 36: 2689–2697.

Leopold, D. A., and Logothetis, N. K. (1996) Activity changes in early visual cortex reflect monkey's percepts during binocular rivalry. *Nature* 379: 549–553.

Livingstone, M. S. (1996) Oscillatory firing and interneuronal correlations in squirrel monkey striate cortex. *Journal of Neurophysiology* 75: 2467–2485.

Livingstone, M., and Hubel, D. (1988) Segregation of form, colour, movement, and depth: Anatomy, physiology, and perception. *Science* 240: 740–749.

Llinás, R., Ribary, U., Joliot, M., and Wand, X.-J. (1994) Content and context in temporal thalamocortical binding. In G. Buzsaki et al. (Eds.), *Temporal coding in the brain,* pp. 251–272. Berlin: Springer.

Logothetis, N. K., and Schall, J. D. (1989) Neuronal correlates of subjective visual perception. *Science* 245: 761–763.

Meister, M., Lagnado, L., and Baylor, D. A. (1995) Concerted signaling by retinal ganglion cells. *Science* 270: 1207–1210.

Metzinger, T. (1995) Faster than thought: Holism, homogeneity and temporal coding. In T. Metzinger (Ed.), *Conscious experience,* pp. 425–461. Paderborn: Schöningh.

Moscovitch, M. (1995) Models of consciousness and memory. In M. S. Gazzaniga (Ed.), *The cognitive neurosciences,* pp. 1341–1356. Cambridge: MIT Press.

Müller, M. M., Junghöfer, M., Elbert, T., and Rockstroh, B. (1997) Visually induced gamma-band responses to coherent and incoherent motion: A replication study. *Neuroreport* 8: 2575–2579.

Munk, M. H. J., Nowak, L. G., Nelson, J. I., and Bullier, J. (1995) Structural basis of cortical synchronization: II. Effects of cortical lesions. *Journal of Neurophysiology* 74: 2401–2414.

Munk, M. H. J., Roelfsema, P. R., König, P., Engel, A. K., and Singer, W. (1996) Role of reticular activation in the modulation of intracortical synchronization. *Science* 272: 271–274.

Murthy, V. N., and Fetz, E. E. (1992) Coherent 25- to 35-HZ oscillations in the sensorimotor cortex of awake behaving monkeys. *Proceedings of the National Academy of Sciences USA* 89: 5670–5674.

Murthy, V. N., and Fetz, E. E. (1996a) Oscillatory activity in sensorimotor cortex of awake monkeys: Synchronization of local field potentials and relation to behavior. *Journal of Neurophysiology* 76: 3949–3967.

Murthy, V. N., and Fetz, E. E. (1996b) Synchronization of neurons during local field potential oscillations in sensorimotor cortex of awake monkeys. *Journal of Neurophysiology* 76: 3968–3982.

Nelson, J. I., Salin, P. A., Munk, M. H. J., Arzi, M., and Bullier, J. (1992) Spatial and temporal coherence in cortico-cortical connections: A cross-correlation study in areas 17 and 18 in the cat. *Visual Neuroscience* 9: 21–37.

Neuenschwander, S., and Singer, W. (1996) Long-range synchronization of oscillatory light responses in the cat retina and lateral geniculate nucleus. *Nature* 379: 728–733.

Newman, J., and Baars, B. J. (1993) A neural attentional model for access to consciousness: A global workspace perspective. *Concepts in Neuroscience* 4: 255–290.

Nicolelis, M. A. L., Baccala, L. A., Lin, R. C. S., and Chapin, J. K. (1995) Sensorimotor encoding by synchronous neural ensemble activity at multiple levels of the somatosensory system. *Science* 268: 1353–1358.

Nowak, L. G., Munk, M. H. J., Nelson, J. I., James, A. C., and Bullier, J. (1995) Structural basis of cortical synchronization: I. Three types of interhemispheric coupling. *Journal of Neurophysiology* 74: 2379–2400.

Pöppel, E. (1997) A hierarchical model of temporal perception. *Trends in Cognitive Sciences* 1: 56–61.

Posner, M. I., and Petersen, S. E. (1990) The attention system of the human brain. *Annual Review of Neuroscience* 13: 25–42.

Rager, G., and Singer, W. (1998) The response of cat visual cortex to flicker stimuli of variable frequency. *European Journal of Neuroscience* 10: 1856–1877.

Riehle, A. Grün, S., Diesmann, M., and Aertsen, A. (1997) Spike synchronization and rate modulation differentially involved in motor cortical function. *Science* 278: 1950–1953.

Roe, A. W., and Ts'o, D. Y. (1992) Functional connectivity between V1 and V2 in the primate. *Society for Neuroscience Abstracts* 18: 11.

Roelfsema, P. R., Engel, A. K., König, P., and Singer, W. (1996) The role of neuronal synchronization in response selection: A biologically plausible theory of structured representation in the visual cortex. *Journal of Cognitive Neuroscience* 8: 603–625.

Roelfsema, P. R., Engel, A. K., König, P., and Singer, W. (1997) Visuomotor integration is associated with zero time-lag synchronization among cortical areas. *Nature* 385: 157–161.

Roelfsema, P. R., König, P., Engel, A. K., Sireteanu, R., and Singer, W. (1994) Reduced synchronization in the visual cortex of cats with strabismic amblyopia. *European Journal of Neuroscience* 6: 1645–1655.

Rougeul, A., Bouyer, J. J., Dedet, L., and Debray, O. (1979) Fast somato-parietal rhythms during combined focal attention and immobility in baboon and squirrel monkey. *Electroencephalography and Clinical Neurophysiology* 46: 310–319.

Sanes, J. N., and Donoghue, J. P. (1993) Oscillations in local field potentials of the primate motor cortex during voluntary movement. *Proceedings of the National Academy of Sciences USA* 90: 4470–4474.

Schillen, T. B., and König, P. (1994) Binding by temporal structure in multiple feature domains of an oscillatory neuronal network. *Biological Cybernetics* 70: 397–405.

Schwender, D., Madler, C., Klasing, S., Peter, K., and Pöppel, E. (1994) Anesthetic control of 40-Hz brain activity and implicit memory. *Consciousness and Cognition* 3: 129–147.

Sejnowski, T. R. (1986) Open questions about computation in cerebral cortex. In J. L. McClelland and D. E. Rumelhart (Eds.), *Parallel distributed processing.* Vol. 2, pp. 372–389. Cambridge: MIT Press.

Sheer, D. E. (1989) Sensory and cognitive 40-Hz event-related potentials: Behavioral correlates, brain function, and clinical application. In E. Basar and T. H. Bullock (Eds.), *Springer Series in brain dynamics.* Vol 2, pp. 339–374. Berlin: Springer.

Sheinberg, D. L., and Logothetis, N. K. (1997) The role of temporal cortical areas in perceptual organization. *Proceedings of the National Academy of Sciences USA* 94: 3408–3413.

Singer, W. (1993) Synchronization of cortical activity and its putative role in information processing and learning. *Annual Review of Physiology* 55: 349–374.

Singer, W., Engel, A. K., Kreiter, A. K., Munk, M. H. J., Neuenschwander, S., and Roelfsema, P. R. (1997) Neuronal assemblies: Necessity, significance, and detectability. *Trends in Cognitive Sciences* 1: 252–261.

Singer, W., and Gray, C. M. (1995) Visual feature integration and the temporal correlation hypothesis. *Annual Review of Neuroscience* 18: 555–586.

Smolensky, P. (1990) Tensor product variable binding and the representation of symbolic structures in connectionist systems. *Artificial Intelligence* 46: 159–216.

Stein, B. E., and Meredith, M. A. (1993) *The merging of the senses.* Cambridge: MIT Press.

Steriade, M. (1997) Synchronized activities of coupled oscillators in the cerebral cortex and thalamus at different levels of vigilance. *Cerebral Cortex* 7: 583–604.

Steriade, M., Amzica, F., and Contreras, D. (1996) Synchronization of fast (30–40 Hz) spontaneous cortical rhythms during brain activation. *Journal of Neuroscience* 16: 392–417.

Tallon, C., Bertrand, O., Bouchet, P., and Pernier, J. (1995) Gamma-range activity evoked by coherent visual stimuli in humans. *European Journal of Neuroscience* 7: 1285–1291.

Tallon-Baudry, C., Bertrand, O., Delpuech, C., and Pernier, J. (1997) Oscillatory γ-band (30–70 Hz) activity induced by a visual search task in humans. *Journal of Neuroscience* 17: 722–734.

Tononi, G., Sporns, O., and Edelman, G. M. (1992) Reentry and the problem of integrating multiple cortical areas: Simulation of dynamic integration in the visual system. *Cerebral Cortex* 2: 310–335.

Treisman, A. (1986) Properties, parts, and objects. In K. Boff, L. Kaufman, and I. Thomas (Eds.), *Handbook of perception and human performance*, pp. 35.1–35.70. New York: Wiley.

Treisman, A. (1996) The binding problem. *Current Opinion in Neurobiology* 6: 171–178.

Ts'o, D. Y., and Gilbert, C. D. (1988) The organization of chromatic and spatial interactions in the primate striate cortex. *Journal of Neuroscience* 8: 1712–1727.

Ts'o, D. Y., Gilbert, C. D., and Wiesel, T. N. (1986) Relationships between horizontal interactions and functional architecture in cat striate cortex as revealed by cross-correlation analysis. *Journal of Neuroscience* 6: 1160–1170.

Usher, M., and Donnelly, N. (1998) Visual synchrony affects binding and segmentation in perception. *Nature* 394: 179–182.

Vaadia, E., Haalman, I., Abeles, M., Bergman, H., Prut, Y., Slovin, H., and Aertsen, A. (1995) Dynamics of neuronal interactions in monkey cortex in relation to behavioural events. *Nature* 373: 515–518.

van Gelder, T. (1990) Compositionality: A connectionist variation on a classical theme. *Cognitive Science* 14: 355–384.

von der Malsburg, C. (1981) *The correlation theory of brain function.* Internal Report 81-2. Göttingen: Max-Planck-Institute for Biophysical Chemistry. Reprinted (1994) in E. Domany, J. L. van Hemmen, and K. Schulten (Eds.), *Models of neural networks.* Vol. 2, pp. 95–119. Berlin: Springer.

von der Malsburg, C. (1995) Binding in models of perception and brain function. *Current Opinion in Neurobiology* 5: 520–526.

von der Malsburg, C. (1997) The coherence definition of consciousness. In M. Ito, Y. Miyashita, and E. T. Rolls (Eds.), *Cognition, computation, and consciousness*, pp. 193–204. Oxford: Oxford University Press.

Zeki, S., and Shipp, S. (1988) The functional logic of cortical connections. *Nature* 335: 311–317.

Disconnected Awareness for Detecting, Processing, and Remembering in Neurological Patients

L. Weiskrantz

I write here about some modern neuropsychological evidence that can be brought full turn into relationship with Jackson's own percipient views on levels of organization, advanced by him so influentially. For the past 20 years or so, neuropsychology and cognitive neuroscience have been otherwise occupied—with discovering and analysing dissociations between *systems* or *sub*-systems: for example, the different modes of processing in dyslexia, such as word-form versus phonemic modes; or the different memory systems, such as short-term, episodic, semantic; or specific categories of agnosia; or multiple visual systems; and so forth.[1] From such evidence a very rich harvest has been reaped of what we might call "*vertical* dissociations," that is, between vertically organized systems or modules. But in the past few years there has been something of an epidemic of discoveries of *horizontal* dissociations between *levels*, and it is some of these that I wish to discuss here. All of them concern dissociations between intact function and acknowledged awareness of such function. Some of these discoveries, as we shall see, exemplify Jackson's views about hierarchical organization, and some do not.

Blindsight

I start with what might be the most surprising and counterintuitive example—namely, stimulus detection in the absence of awareness. Actually, there is an already familiar example of such a dissociation which reflects, literally, a disconnexion of levels, namely the preservation of spinal reflexes in paraplegia, in which there can be a vigorous response to stimuli that are not felt as such. In Sherrington's magisterial language, "A needle-prick causes invariably the drawing up of the limb... The nervous arcs of pain-nerves, broadly speaking, dominate the spinal centres ... *where pain is, of course non-existent.*" (italics added).[2] This example is usually not thought to be surprising, because it is assumed to be a disconnexion of the spine from the brain, which is the organ of conscious sensation. But there is already a paradox: neurones are neurones, full stop. Why should the collection of neurones in the spinal column not suffice for awareness, whereas other collections of neurones, in the brain, do? (Indeed, some nineteenth-century physiologists *did* declare the isolated frog spinal cord to be conscious.)

A more direct approach to the question is to consider disconnexions within to the brain itself, which is what I shall do for the rest of the lecture. The best studied example of such a dissociation of *detection* and awareness is "blindsight."[3,4] Occipital lesions in man, typically, cause field defects which are blind to the patient. This is surprising in its own right, for two reasons. The first is that in other primates striate cortex lesions still allow a range of visual discriminations to occur, albeit changed quantitatively and qualitatively. The second is that the pathway to the striate cortex via the lateral geniculate nucleus is but one of 10 pathways from the retina to targets in the brain. Admittedly the geniculate-striate pathway is the largest, but the *non-striate* pathways taken together are five times larger than the whole of the auditory nerve—not a trivial capacity.

We normally test human subjects by asking them what they "see." Even if this is not explicit, it is usually implicit. Of course, we cannot do that with an animal—we must use forced-choice discriminations in which a particular response to a particular stimulus leads to a particular outcome. Surprisingly, when this same approach was used with human subjects, as Warrington, Marshall, and Sanders and I did in 1974,[5] in some of them at least they could make discriminative responses like those of monkeys with striate cortex lesions. But, and here was the surprise, they said that they did not "see" the stimuli. They thought they were guessing, or under certain restricted conditions had a gut-feeling and "knew" that stimuli were present, but it was not visual, not "seeing." Hence, their field defects *were* blind experientially, but not visually disconnected.

Several examples of "blindsight" are available (see references 3 and 4 for reviews). Some subjects generate a saccade (first reported by Poppel et al. in 1974)[5] or point[6] to the location of randomly placed flashes. Discrimination of orientation in the frontal plane have also been found. Visual acuity can be assessed by varying the spacing of gratings which are discriminated from homogeneous equal-energy patches. Differential responses to direction of movement has also been studied. A threshold of detection *qua* detection, can be measured. Perhaps the most remarkable recent evidence concerns the measurement of detection thresholds by Stoerig and Cowey[7] to determine spectral sensitivity and wavelength discrimination, together with evidence for opponent process colour discrimination in some subjects, in the total absence of any acknowledged experience of the stimuli.[8]

Anatomical and physiological evidence is available to permit reasonable hypotheses about just which visual attributes will be detectable.[4,9] Neurones in V4 are primarily sensitive to wavelength. Those in MT, or V5, on the other hand are primarily sensitive to movement. Both of these areas have retinal inputs that by-pass striate cortex, and we know that the neurones in MT continue to show the same response properties even with total removal of V1—striate cortex—in the monkey. Hence, it is becoming clear why some subjects but not others might be sensitive to wavelength differences, and others to direction of movement.

Vision is by far the most thoroughly studied sensory system in this regard, but reports of "blind touch"[10] and also of "deaf hearing"[11] have also appeared in association with relevant cortical lesions. Much remains to be done in all modalities, including vision, but research should be helped by the devising of testing methods that are less tedious than administering the thousands of forced-choice trials in which a subject is required to guess about nonexperienced stimuli to determine psychophysical limits of capacity. The general strategy with these newer methods bypasses any need whatever to ask the subject what he sees, in blindsight, for example, to measure how stimuli in the blind field *modulate* or interact with responses to seen stimuli in the intact field. I have reviewed the area elsewhere,[4] but a recent paper to appear in *Science* by Rafal and colleagues[12] provides a nice illustration. Their subjects were simply instructed to saccade as quickly as possible to an eccentrically-located stimulus. What Rafal et al. demonstrated was that an "unseen" stimulus presented to the *blind* temporal hemi-field of hemianopic subjects 0–50 ms prior to a stimulus to the intact field inhibited the latency of a saccade to the seen stimulus in the intact field. (The bias favouring the temporal hemi-field was predicted from the stronger crossed projection of the optic nerve to the superior colliculus.) An earlier study by Marzi and colleagues[13] used the same approach but with reaction times to key press rather than saccade latency. In such examples, the subject never need be asked to guess about the unseen stimuli—the effect is measured directly by its effect on the response to seen stimuli. Such methods also allow comparative studies to be carried out on animals or young children. Another alternative is to use autonomic responses such as galvanic skin response to unseen stimuli in the blind field—and here the pupillary response is turning out to be of potential great value.

To turn to a higher level of control of detection: as the "search-light of attention" focuses upon different parts of the visual scene, some regions are highlighted and others ignored. An extreme form of bias in attention is seen in parietal lobe lesions, typically right hemisphere, causing unilateral left-sided hemi-neglect. By definition this must be neglect rather than hemi-blindness because it can occur in the presence of full visual fields. A recent rather graphic example of detection in the neglected field given by Marshall and Halligan[14] appeared in *Nature*, labelled as an example of "blindsight in visuo-spatial neglect." The neglect patient was asked to make a same-different judgement between two simultaneously presented pictures, one of a house, the other of the same house but with its left side in flames. As the left side was neglected, the subject consistently responded "same." But when then asked to select the house she would *prefer to live in*, she chose the non-inflamed one over the other, at a high level of statistical significance, but remarking that it was a silly question as the two were identical.

Aphasia

On encountering phenomena of detection without acknowledged awareness, it is natural to consider them to be a kind of disconnexion syndrome in which stimulus reception is somehow disconnected from verbal encoding or communicating, and to think of superficially similar phenomena reported for the right hemisphere of "split-brain" patients—in other words, to consider the problem not one of detection as such, but of processing at a later stage. Such an interpretation, in fact, in terms of faulty access to verbal processing, will not work for "blindsight," for reasons spelled out elsewhere.[3] But even within the dominant left hemisphere itself, and with that capacity which is usually reckoned to be the most highly developed and *the* uniquely human sill, namely, linguistic comprehension, a dissociation can be found between covert and overt processing. A study by Lorraine Tyler at Cambridge[15] provides a striking example. She studied a Wernicke's aphasic patient, who had a severe impairment of verbal comprehension. In formal language tests, such as matching a sentence to a picture, or in the Token test, he was no better than at chance. Tyler showed that nevertheless the patient was normally sensitive to the nuances of the English language. One way she demonstrated this was to instruct the subject to respond as quickly as possible to a particular target word in English. She then buried this word in correct or degraded sentences. The degradation could be either to the semantics or the syntax or to the "pragmatic" appropriateness of the sentence. The key comes from the fact that normal subject spot a target word faster when it is in a normal linguistic structure than when it is anomalous. And so does the aphasic patient. He is somewhat slower, not surprisingly than controls, but his pattern of reactions times is very similar.

Other variations of the same theme were carried out by Tyler, with comparable results: the reactions reflected the semantic and syntactic structure, even though the subject was at chance in identifying whether a sentence as "correct" or not.

Thus, in the realms of detection, attention, and verbal processing, we can find neuro-psychological evidence of intact processing together with a failure of awareness or comprehension of that processing or of its results. But it is perhaps in the field of memory that the oldest and most numerous researches can be found.

Amnesia

The amnesic syndrome refers to patients who apparently cannot remember experiences from minute to minute: they have severe anterograde amnesia. The causes are varied—bilateral temporal lobe surgery, herpes simplex encephalitis, alcohol, carbon monoxide—all acting upon a system of limbic lobe brain structures that are currently under intense scrutiny by anatomists, pathologists, physiologists, and neuro-psychologists. The patients' immediate memory are typically normal, for example in reciting back strings of digits or in performing more formal short-term memory tests. They can solve problems if these do not require bridging an interval of time. There need be no loss of cognitive and perceptual capacities or well-established verbal or other skills. Their vocabularies are intact, and their IQs can be quite normal. But the anterograde amnesia is severe and crippling, reflected in failure of recognition of an experience after an interval of a minute or so, but also with some considerable retrograde amnesia for events prior to the brain damage.

Over the past 20 years a remarkable set of findings has been produced.[16] It gradually has become clear that these patients are very well capable of learning a large variety of new tasks, and they retain them over very long times—weeks, or even months—and often as well as normal persons. This first became clear from studies of motor skill learning, such as sustained performance of tracking tasks or mirror drawing[17] even though the patients deny having any memory for the tasks on each new occasion. But even with verbal material they can be shown to have good retentive powers. For example, in a series of experiments by Professor Warrington and me at the National Hospital initiated more than 20 years ago, we showed amnesic patients long lists of words. A few minutes later the subjects firmly denied having any memory for any of the words, and were at chance in a test of forced-choice recognition of them. But if we showed them the first few letters of the words, or fragmented versions of the words, and simply asked them to guess what words they stood for, they were greatly helped by having seen the word in a list before. Needless to say, they were not helped if the word had not been in the list. The same technique can be used with pictures. With it one can study learning and forgetting in a systematic way.[18] A large number of variations have now been produced, all of which show intact learning and retention by such patients. The general phenomenon is called "priming" and is practically a research industry both with patients and with normal subjects in experimental psychology.

Other examples can be found in perceptual learning,[19] for example, for specific jigsaw puzzles. The meaning of anomalous sentences[20] or pictures[21] can be acquired and retained. New associations can be established by classical conditioning,[22] as can the applications of rules to paired-associate learning[23] or arithmetic.[24]

Despite all of these examples of good learning and retention, the only person who remains unconvinced that they occur is the amnesic patient. The newly stored items do not have the quality of being "remembered." You may have noticed that all of the sensitive tasks are carried out in such a way that it is not necessary to *ask* the patient whether he remembers—instead one just presents the relevant stimulus and asks for the relevant response. The amnesic patient does not remember if he is asked to remember. He literally loses the experience of *remembering*, as such.

Agnosia

There is another memory system that does not carry this quality of experience, as such: it is for the vast store of knowledge that we all possess—a capacity that is sometimes called semantic memory. Neurological disturbances also occur to categories or items of acquired knowledge, constituting the various types of agnosias. Such patients do not lose the experience of memory as such, instead they lose the meaning in relevant categories. Indeed, they can readily recall a previous occasion when they were equally unable to identify the meaning of the same object.

Here, too, in this type of memory disturbance, a dissociation can be found between the agnosic explicit loss of meaning and an intact level of processing that is covert and unavailable to the patient's awareness. Prosopagnosia, an agnosia for familiar faces, is an area in which research has been especially focused. It has been shown, for example, by Bauer[25] and Tranel and Damasio[26] that at least some prosopagnosic patients have an electrical skin conductance response to familiar faces that is different from that to unfamiliar faces. That is, even if the patient cannot recognize familiar faces, his autonomic nervous system can. But it is not only the autonomic system that is privy to such knowledge. More surprisingly, as shown by Young and his colleagues, if the patients are asked to make judgements about the professions of well-known persons' faces or, for example, to learn names that go with the faces, they are slower to learn name-face or profession-face pairings when the name or profession is incorrectly paired with a familiar face than when it is correctly paired with it, even though they display no recognition of the familiar faces—all seem equally unfamiliar to them.[27] Some part of them "knows" the familiar face.

Dissociation, Fractionation, and Levels of Organization

And so, in every major realm of cognitive achievement—perception, recognition memory and recall, language, problem solving, meaning, motor skill learning—robust hidden processes can be found that are relatively immune to neurological brain dysfunction. There are striking dissociations between what can be processed and what aspect of that process is available to awareness. The strength and duration of these covert reactions can be equal to those shown by normal control subjects—they are not just pale Humean images. A related but opposite condition also exists: there can be an excess of awareness in relation to reality in the condition of anosagnosia, when patients deny their loss of function, for example, blindness or loss of tactile sensitivity. Even here there have been claims of covert *non*-denial.[28] The evidence from neuropsychology has also stimulated research for similar dissociations in normal functioning, for which there is now a large literature but about which I am going to say nothing here.

My examples of disconnected awareness from intact function are by no means exhaustive—there are also reports in dyslexia[28] and other agnosic states[28]—and the research epidemiology is so vigorous that I suspect that there will probably be no cognitive neuropsychological dysfunction that will be immune. But are all of these logically the same type of dissociation? The answer appears to be no. In an anatomical arrangement such as that underlying blindsight, where we have a number of parallel and independent pathways from the retina into the cerebrum, it is reasonable to analyse the outcome in terms of fractionation. Where one finds *double* dissociations of function, with convergent evidence of independent pathways, one has both a necessary and a sound basis for inferring independent components or biases. Warrington and I found just this type of *double* dissociation in a blindsight patient.[3] The blindsight field was more biased towards detection than the intact "seeing" field, and *just* the opposite bias for form discrimination. In that sense, the evidence was consistent with earlier theories of "two visual systems," the geniculo-striate for identification and the midbrain system for detection and orientation. Even beyond the striate cortex, we have multiple and parallel outputs, and so independent components of vision are becoming clear (e.g., movement and form), together with mutually independent varieties of blindsight. Similarly, in the area of memory disorders, it is often considered that brain damage can cause a fractionation into functionally different memory systems—for example, declarative versus procedural, short-term versus long-term, episodic versus semantic, and so forth—some of which are accompanied by awareness, and others of which are not.

Varieties of fractionation cannot be easily accommodated in a Jacksonian *hierarchy* of levels. But some of the other examples I have cited appear to fit such a scheme quite easily and compellingly. The logical requirement for the Jacksonian view is a *single*, rather than a double dissociation. That is, the higher level can be disrupted without disrupting the lower but not vice versa. The evidence from aphasia almost certainly follows that pattern. It would be difficult to consider an outcome such that implicit processing of grammar and semantics would be damaged without the explicit operation also being damaged, although as we have seen from Tyler's work, the opposite can and does occur. Jackson's view of the structure of the hierarchy ascending from the most automatic and most tightly organized to the voluntary and loosely organized maps onto that situation well. Indeed, his description of the outcome in aphasia, "as the loss of the most voluntary service or words, with a persistence of a more automatic service of words" is close to Tyler's own account, although her results elevate semantics and syntactical structure to the service of the "automatic." (Indeed, we all know that elaborate ritualistic verbal exchanges occur that are wholly automatic and often unconscious.)

Some Implications

Leaving taxonomic questions aside, are there any general implications that emerge from the body of research taken as a whole? One implication is obvious: the profile and severity of dysfunction, in one sense, cannot be judged from verbal intercourse with a patient alone, including formal tests or procedures that themselves are simply translations of putative explicit verbal exchanges into test scores. So long as the patient is asked to respond when he "sees," residual blindsight evidence will not be found. Similarly tests of memory based on recognition or recall, no matter how elegantly constructed will never reveal powerful but hidden retention based on priming. The conventional clinical interview, of course, will fall very far short. Unfortunately, alternative procedures for expanding the profile to include covert as well as overt function are sometimes tedious, but procedures are evolving that will make that task easier.

Another practical implication might also follow, although it is still early days: therapy might be based on building upon covert residual function. We already know that visual field defects in the monkey can be made to shrink significantly with particular methods of specialized training that "push" the extra-striate pathways. Application of the same methods to hemianopia human has led to claims of a similar modest expansion of intact fields. Similarly, some researchers are trying to teach new verbal associations to severely amnesic patients, using priming methodology.

If therapy based on covert processing turns out to be practicable, it carries its own paradox: it is that patients cannot live on implicit processing alone. The amnesic patient is severely crippled and requires permanent custodial care, despite a rich crop of retained facilitations induced through priming. The prosopagnosic patient may show a healthy galvanic skin response to a familiar face, but he will be deeply embarrassed by the inability in everyday life to recognize the face of his spouse or close friends until they speak. The blindsight patient will fail to identify or see objects and bump into them in his hemianopic field. The aphasic patient will not be helped in his comprehension or communication by virtue of intact sensitivity, at a lower level, to syntax and semantics. And so forth. In short, none of these patients can *think* or imagine in the terms or on the basis of the processes of which they are unaware, and they all suffer severe handicaps as a result. If therapy is to occur, it must build upon, but emerge from the level of implicit processing to one that allows explicit awareness of residual function to occur. How to do so is the challenge.

Finally, of course, there are theoretical and philosophical implications concerning the neurological basis of awareness, in some ways the most challenging.[29] Jackson uncompromisingly endorsed a dualistic position that was commonly held in his time, of psychophysical parallelism. This now sits very uncomfortably with the evidence I have cited, although it cannot be refuted by evidence alone. But, philosophy aside, the more abiding message from Jackson concerned the *organization* of the nervous system, cast in terms of hierarchical levels of increasing complexity but decreasing strength. Perhaps such a seminal hierarchical approach in terms of levels of covert and overt processing can now also be put to the service of the neurology of awareness itself.

References

1. Shallice T. *From neuropsychology to mental structure*. Cambridge: Cambridge University Press, 1988

2. Sherrington CS. Spinal cord. *Encyclopaedia Britannica*, vol 21. London: Encyclopaedia Britannica Ltd, 1957:227–8

3. Weiskrantz L. *Blindsight. A case study and implications*. Oxford: Oxford University Press, 1986

4. Weiskrantz L. Outlooks for blindsight: explicit methodologies for implicit processes. *Proc R Soc London* 1990;239:247–78

5. Poppel E, Held R, Frost D. Residual visual function after brain wounds involving the central visual pathways in man. *Nature* 1973;243:295–6

6. Weiskrantz L, Warrington EK, Sanders MD, Marshall JC. Visual capacity in the hemianopic field following a restricted occipital ablation. *Brain* 1974;97:709–28

7. Stoerig P, Cowey A. Wavelength sensitivity in blindsight. *Nature* 1990;324:916–18

8. Stoerig P, Cowey A. Increment-threshold spectral sensitivity in blindsight: evidence for colour opponency. *Brain* 1991;114, Pt3, 1487–512

9. Cowey A, Stoerig P. The neurobiology of blindsight. *Trends Neurosci* 1991;14:140–5

10. Paillard J, Michel F, Stelmach G. Localization without content: a tactile analogue of "blind sight." *Arch Neurol* 1983;40:548–51

11. Michel F, Peronnet F. A case of cortical deafness: clinical and electrophysiological data. *Brain and Language* 1980;10:367–77

12. Rafal R. Extrageniculate vision in hemianopic humans. *Science* 1990;250:118–21

13. Marzi CA, Tassinari G, Aglioti S, Lutzemberger L. Spatial summation across the vertical meridian in hemianopics: a test of blindsight. *Neuropsychologia* 1986;24:749–58

14. Marshall JC, Halligan PW. Blindsight and insight in visuo-spatial neglect. *Nature* 1988;336:766–7

15. Tyler LK. Spoken language comprehension in a fluent aphasic patient. *Cognitive Neuropsychology* 1988;5:375–400

16. Cermak LS, ed. *Human memory and amnesia*. Hillsdale, New Jersey: Erlbaum, 1982

17. Corkin S. Acquisition of motor skill after bilateral medial temporal-lobe excision. *Neuropsychologia* 1968;6:255–65

18. Shimamura AP. Priming effects in amnesia: evidence for a dissociable memory function. *Q J Exp Psychol* 1986;38A:619–44

19. Brooks DN, Baddeley AD. What can amnesic patients learn? *Neuropsychologia* 1976;14:111–22

20. McAndrews MP, Glisky EL, Schacter DL. When priming persists: long-lasting implicit memory for a single episode in amnesic patients. *Neuropsychologia* 1987;25:497–506

21. Warrington EK, Weiskrantz L. An analysis of short-term and long-term memory defects in man. In: Deutsch JA, ed. *The physiological basis of memory*. New York: Academic Press, 1973:365–95

22. Weiskrantz L, Warrington EK. Conditioning in amnesic patients. *Neuropsychologia* 1979;17:187–94

23. Winocur G, Weiskrantz L. An investigation of paired-associate learning in amnesic patients. *Neuropsychologia* 1976;14:97–110

24. Kinsbourne M, Wood F. Short-term memory and the amnesic syndrome. In: Deutsch DD, Deutsch JA, eds. *Short-term memory*. New York: Academic Press, 1975:258–91

25. Bauer RM. Autonomic recognition of names and faces in prosopagnosia: a neuropsychological application of the guilty knowledge test. *Neuropsychologia* 1984;22:457–69

26. Tranel D, Damasio AR. Knowledge without awareness: an autonomic index of facial recognition by prosopagnosics. *Science* 1985;228:1453–4

27. De Haan EHF, Young A, Newcombe F. Faces interfere with name classification in a prosopagnosic patient. *Cortex* 1987;23:309–16

28. Schacter DL, McAndrews MP, Moscovitch M. Access to consciousness: dissociations between implicit and explicit knowledge in neuropsychological syn-

dromes. In: Weiskrantz L, ed. *Thought without language*. Symposium of the Fyssen Foundation. Oxford: Oxford University Press, 1988:242–78

29. Weiskrantz L. Some contributions of neuropsychology of vision and memory to the problem of consciousness. In: Marcel AJ, Bisiach E, eds. *Consciousness in contemporary science*. Oxford: Oxford University Press, 1988:183–99

10 Blindsight in Monkeys

Alan Cowey and Petra Stoerig

Blindsight, the visually evoked voluntary responses of patients with striate cortical destruction that are demonstrated despite a phenomenal blindness, has attracted attention from neuroscientists and philosophers interested in problems of perceptual consciousness and its neuronal basis.[1-3] It is assumed to be mediated by the numerous extra-geniculostriate cortical retinofugal pathways whose properties are studied primarily in monkeys.[4] Like patients with blindsight,[4-7] monkeys with lesions of the primary visual cortex can learn to detect, localize and distinguish between visual stimuli presented within their visual field defects.[4,8-11] Although the patients deny seeing the stimuli they can nevertheless respond to (by forced-choice guessing) in their phenomenally blind fields, it is not known whether the monkeys experience the same absence of phenomenal vision. To determine whether they too have blindsight, or whether they actually see the stimuli in their field defects, monkeys who showed excellent detection in tasks where a visual stimulus was presented on every trial, albeit at different positions, were tested in a signal-detection task[12] in which half the trials were blank trials, with no visual stimulus. They classified the visual stimuli presented in the field defect as blank trials, demonstrating, like patients, blindsight rather than degraded real vision.

If we want to understand why blindsight is blind, we need to know whether the monkeys, like patients, lose phenomenal vision as a result of striate cortical destruction. To answer this question, we studied four macaque monkeys. One, called Rosie, a female (*Macaca mulatta*) aged 8 years, had normal vision. The other three, Dracula, Lennox, and Wrinkle, were older males (two *M. mulatta* and one *M. fascicularis*) who had had the striate cortex of the left cerebral hemisphere surgically removed and the splenium of the corpus callosum severed several years be-

fore the present experiment. All monkeys are still being studied behaviourally, but histological evidence from the excised tissue and a magnetic resonance scan showed that the ablation was complete (see figure 10.1).

For three years their ability to detect and localize brief visual stimuli was studied while the monkey looked at the display shown in figure 10.2b. Eye movements were monitored (figure 10.2a) and a touchscreen recorded where the monkey touched the display. When a 2° white square of intensity 40 cd m^{-2} appeared at the bottom centre of the white screen (0.6 cd m^{-2}) and the monkey fixated and touched it, the square disappeared and was followed instantaneously by a brief (10–200 ms) 2° stimulus at one of the four positions 19° off the vertical midline. If the monkey touched the position at which the target had appeared, he/she was rewarded with a peanut or raisin. Two of these positions were within the normal left hemifield, the other two were in the right hemifield affected by the striate cortical lesion. Random responding would yield about 50% correct responses in either hemifield. By varying the intensity of the stimulus, we determined the increment thresholds for 75% correct performance. Compared with the normal side, they were elevated by 0.5 (Dracula and Lennox) to 1.5 log units (Wrinkle) in the affected hemifield. Note that a visual stimulus appeared on every trial, and that all monkeys performed at levels approaching 100% correct with stimuli 0.7 log units above threshold (figure 10.2c). When we conducted an entire session without presenting a visual stimulus (all blank trials), they usually failed to respond or scored no better than 25% correct when they did respond.

Having shown that monkeys respond to targets in the affected hemifield, we modified the task by presenting blank trials intermingled with stimulus trials, and required a different response

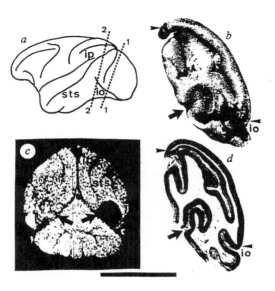

Figure 10.1

(*A*) Outline drawing of a side view of the left hemisphere of a macaque monkey, *Macaca mulatta*. Dashed line 1 shows the position of the occipital lobectomy just behind the rostral border of the lateral striate cortex. (*B*), Photograph of an excised lobe seen from in front. The arrowheads indicate the limits of the striate cortex on the lateral surface. The arrow shows the striate cortex in the calcarine fissure. (*C*), Magnetic resonance image in the coronal plane, at approximately the position marked by dashed line 2 in *A*. The most rostral part of the calcarine fissure, arrowed and corresponding to the representation of peripheral vision, is intact in the right hemisphere (shown on the left) but is missing in the left hemisphere. The image is from a spin echo sequence with parameters. Echo time (TC), 38 ms; repetition rate (TR), 1.5 s; field of view (FOV), 12.5 cm^2; data matrix = 256 × 256. The magnet was a 2-T, 1-m bore (Oxford Magnet Technology) interfaced to a Brüker (Karlsruhe, Germany) Biospec spectrometer. (*D*), Photomicrograph of a Nissl-stained section of the excised lobe shown in (*B*), several millimetres behind the cut. Abbreviations: ip, intraparietal sulcus; sts, superior temporal sulcus; io, inferior occipital sulcus. Scale bar: (a) 45 mm; (b) 20 mm; (c) 30 mm; (d) 20 mm.

to each. The display shown in figure 10.3a was used. On half the trials, a longer (750 ms) 2° white visual stimulus of supra-threshold luminance appeared randomly in one of five positions in the upper (or lower) left quadrant of the display, in which case the monkey had to touch it or its remembered position. This quadrant is in the normal hemifield of all four animals. If no visual stimulus (a blank) was presented, the animal obtained reward by pressing instead the black outlined rectangle permanently present in the lower (or upper) quadrant. They rapidly mastered this new task. Then a stimulus was presented on every twentieth trial at an eccentricity of ~20° in the right half of the display, that is, in the hemianopic field of three of the monkeys. On these probe trials, Rosie (normal), Lennox, and Wrinkle were rewarded whether they pressed the probe or the outline square, whereas Dracula was never rewarded, that is, he was tested in extinction. Would the hemianopic monkeys now classify a stimulus in the affected hemifield as a stimulus or as a blank? The answer is shown in figure 10.3b. The normal monkey consistently responded to the stimulus in the right hemifield in the same manner as to the targets on the left. In contrast, the three hemianopic monkeys almost always responded by signalling "blank." They touched the probe on only 2–8% of probe trials, and when they did the video monitor revealed that they had moved their eyes to it, allowing them to see it with their normal hemifield.

If physically identical stimuli appear much dimmer in the hemianopic field, the monkeys might categorize them as blanks even though they do in fact see them, that is, even though they have a weak phenomenal perception, like patients with partially recovered relative field defects.[13] To test this possibility, we repeated the tests (1,000 trials; 50 probes) with stimuli that were 0.3 log units above threshold in the normal left visual hemifield and 1.0 log unit above threshold in the right (hemianopic) hemifield.

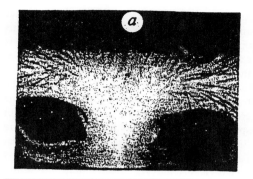

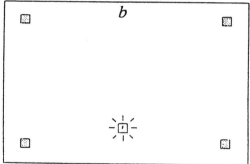

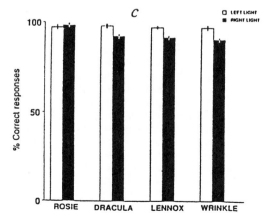

The hemianopic monkeys Lennox and Dracula touched the position of the probe on only 0 and 2%, respectively, whereas the control monkey Rosie reported all probe trials regardless of the luminance difference. She was additionally tested with 40-cd m^{-2} targets on the left and 1-cd m^{-2} targets on the right. This had no effect on her performance. Finally, to test the possibility that the low percentage of probe trials influenced their classification, we tested the third hemi-anopic monkey, Wrinkle, for 200 trials where the probability for probes was 25%. He signalled all 50 of them as blanks.

These results show that monkeys with unilateral striate cortical ablations classify stimuli briefly flashed in their hemianopic field as blank trials when given this option, even though they

mounted above the monitor provided an on-line image of the eyes in the distant control room. The infrared light sources directed at the eyes from the edges of the VDU produced three specular reflections which allowed us to monitor eye position and to ensure that the monkeys looked at the starting light at the centre bottom of the screen when they touched it. (*B*), Diagram of the visual display used in the first part of the experiment in order to determine detection thresholds in the left and right hemifields. The monkey's faced a 14-inch colour VDU (Microvitech 895) subtending 51° × 39°. The visual stimuli were generated by a Pluto II graphics device (Electronic Graphics) controlled by a microcomputer. The overall lighting conditions were low photopic provided by a white screen background of 0.6 cd m^{-2} and adjacent white walls of 1–4 cd m^{-2}. The front of the VDU was scanned by infrared lights which recorded where the monkey touched the display. F is fixation and starting light. (*C*), Percentage correct responses for 10 testing sessions, each with 100 or more trials, with a green or white 200-ms target about 0.7 log units above the psychophysically determined threshold in both half-fields of the normal monkey (Rosie) and in the impaired right half-field of the other monkeys. All monkeys detected and correctly localized the target at better than 90% correct in both half-fields. □, Left light; ■, right light.

Figure 10.2

(*A*) Video picture of the eyes of monkey Wrinkle viewing the stimulus display. The monkey's head was restrained with plastic baffles and a video camera

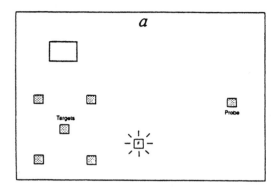

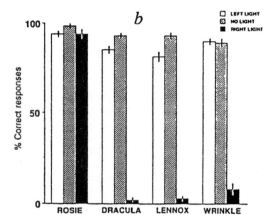

can detect and localize these same or even briefer and dimmer stimuli in experiments lacking this option. This paradigm-dependent dissociation is reminiscent of patients with blindsight who claim that they do not see the stimuli they can nonetheless respond to in their hemianopic fields. The results show that the consequences of striate cortical lesions are likely to be similar in both species, contrary to some assertions,[14] and are therefore helpful in determining the neuronal basis of phenomenal vision. Whether monkeys would classify moving visual stimuli in a different way, like at least one patient,[14–16] remains to be tested.

Acknowledgments

The work was supported by the MRC and the Deutsche Forschungsgemeinschaft. We thank N. Brown for testing the monkeys and in devising the software, P. Styles and D. Taylor for making the magnetic resonance images of two monkeys' brains; and the Oxford McDonnell-Pew Centre for a network travel grant.

Figure 10.3

(A) Diagram of the visual display when using blank trials and probes. The monkey started the trial by pressing the bright small fixation square (F) near the bottom. On light trials the visual stimulus (7 cd m^{-2} for two monkeys and 40 cd m^{-2} for the other two) appeared for 750 ms at one of the five positions shown in the bottom left quadrant of the display. These positions were not permanently marked, so that whenever the monkey did not respond promptly it had to touch the remembered position of the target. On blank trials no visual stimulus was presented and the monkey had to touch the outlined rectangle that was permanently present in the upper left quadrant. On probe trials the visual stimulus appeared on the right at the position marked "Probe." For three of the four monkeys the task was subsequently repeated with the rectangle in the bottom quadrant and the visual stimuli appearing at five positions in the top left quadrant. (B), Percentage correct responses for the four monkeys during 10 (Wrinkle) or 20 (others) testing sessions. For each monkey the first bar indicates percentage correct when a visual stimulus appeared in the left hemifield, the second bar indicates percentage correct on blank trials, when no visual stimulus was presented, and the third bar indicates percentage correct for 50 (Wrinkle) or 100 (others) probe trials where a visual stimulus, known from the initial experiments to be well above detection threshold, appeared in the right hemifield. Note that all monkeys made errors even in the normal visual field. Almost always this occurred when the monkey reached out to the light, or to its remembered position, was slightly off target, and promptly reached instead for the rectangle appropriate for blank trials. This never occurred on probe trials with the hemianopic monkeys.

References

1. Crick, F. & Koch, C. *Semin. Neurosci.* 2, 263–275 (1990).

2. Nelkin, N. *Phil. Sci.* 60, 419–434 (1993).

3. Stoerig, P. & Brandt, S. *Theor. Med.* 14, 117–135 (1993).

4. Cowey, A. & Stoerig, P. *Trends Neurosci.* 14, 140–145 (1991).

5. Weiskrantz, L. *Blindsight: A Case Study and Implications* (Clarendon, Oxford, 1986).

6. Blythe, I. M., Kennard, C. & Ruddock, K. H. *Brain* 110, 887–905 (1987).

7. Weiskrantz, L. *Proc. R. Soc. Lond.* B239, 247–278 (1990).

8. Klüver, H. *J. Psychol.* 11, 23–45 (1941).

9. Cowey, A. & Weiskrantz, L. *Q. J. exp. Psychol.* 15, 91–115 (1963).

10. Mohler, C. W. & Wurtz, R. H. *J. Neurophysiol.* 40, 74–94 (1977).

11. Pasik, P. & Pasik, T. *Contrs sens. Physiol.* 7, 147–200 (1982).

12. Swets, J. A. & Pickett, R. M. *Evaluation of Diagnostic Systems* (Academic, New York, 1982).

13. Stoerig, P. & Cowey, A. *Brain* 114, 1489–1512 (1991).

14. Fendrich, R., Wessinger, C. M. & Gazzaniga, M. S. *Science* 258, 1489–1491 (1992).

15. Barbur, J. L., Ruddock, K. H. & Waterfield, V. A. *Brain* 103, 905–928 (1980).

16. Barbur, J. L., Watson, J. D. G., Frackowiak, R. S. J. & Zeki, S. *Brain* 116, 1293–1302 (1993).

R. W. Sperry

The following article is a result of studies my colleagues and I have been conducting with some neurosurgical patients of Philip J. Vogel of Los Angeles. These patients were all advanced epileptics in whom an extensive midline section of the cerebral commissures had been carried out in an effort to contain severe epileptic convulsions not controlled by medication. In all these people the surgical sections included division of the corpus callosum in its entirety, plus division also of the smaller anterior and hippocampal commissures, plus in some instances the massa intermedia. So far as I know, this is the most radical disconnection of the cerebral hemispheres attempted thus far in human surgery. The full array of sections was carried out in a single operation.

No major collapse of mentality or personality was anticipated as a result of this extreme surgery: earlier clinical observations on surgical section of the corpus callosum in man, as well as the results from dozens of monkeys on which I had carried out this exact same surgery, suggested that the functional deficits might very likely be less damaging than some of the more common forms of cerebral surgery, such as frontal lobotomy, or even some of the unilateral lobotomies performed more routinely for epilepsy.

The first patient on whom this surgery was tried had been having seizures for more than 10 years with generalized convulsions that continued to worsen despite treatment that had included a sojourn in Bethesda at the National Institutes of Health. At the time of the surgery, he had been averaging two major attacks per week, each of which left him debilitated for another day or so. Episodes of *status epilepticus* (recurring seizures that fail to stop and represent a medical emergency with a fairly high mortality risk) had also begun to occur at 2- to 3-month intervals. Since leaving the hospital following his

surgery over 5 1/2 years ago, this man has not had, according to last reports, a single generalized convulsion. It has further been possible to reduce the level of medication and to obtain an overall improvement in his behavior and well being (see Bogen and Vogel 1962).

The second patient, a housewife and mother in her 30s, also has been seizure-free since recovering from her surgery, which was more than 4 years ago (Bogen, Fisher, and Vogel 1965). Bogen related that even the EEG has regained a normal pattern in this patient. The excellent outcome in the initial, apparently hopeless, last-resort cases led to further application of the surgery to some nine more individuals to date, the majority of whom are too recent for therapeutic evaluation. Although the alleviation of the epilepsy has not held up 100% throughout the series (two patients are still having seizures, although their convulsions are much reduced in severity and frequency and tend to be confined to one side), the results on the whole continue to be predominantly beneficial, and the overall outlook at this time remains promising for selected severe cases.

The therapeutic success, however, and all other medical aspects are matters for our medical colleagues, Philip J. Vogel and Joseph E. Bogen. Our own work has been confined entirely to an examination of the functional outcome, that is, the behavioral, neurological, and psychological effects of this surgical disruption of all direct cross-talk between the hemispheres. Initially we were concerned as to whether we would be able to find in these patients any of the numerous symptoms of hemisphere deconnection that had been demonstrated in the so-called split-brain animal studies of the 1950s (Myers 1961; Sperry 1967a,b). The outcome in man remained an open question in view of the historic Akelaitis (1944) studies that had set the prevailing doctrine of the 1940s and 1950s. This doctrine maintained that no important functional symptoms are found in man following even complete surgical section of the corpus callosum and anterior commissure, provided that other brain damage is excluded.

These earlier observations on the absence of behavioral symptoms in man have been confirmed in a general way to the extent that it remains fair to say today that the most remarkable effect of sectioning the neocortical commissures is the apparent lack of effect so far as ordinary behavior is concerned. This has been true in our animal studies throughout, and it seems now to be true for man also, with certain qualifications that we will come to later. At the same time, however—and this is in contradiction to the earlier doctrine set by the Akelaitis studies—we know today that with appropriate tests one can indeed demonstrate a large number of behavioral symptoms that correlate directly with the loss of the neocortical commissures in man as well as in animals (Gazzaniga 1967; Sperry 1967a,b; Sperry, Gazzaniga, and Bogen 1968). Taken collectively, these symptoms may be referred to as the syndrome of the neocortical commissures or the syndrome of the forebrain commissures or, less specifically, as the syndrome of hemisphere deconnection.

One of the more general and also more interesting and striking features of this syndrome may be summarized as an apparent doubling in most of the realms of conscious awareness. Instead of the normally unified single stream of consciousness, these patients behave in many ways as if they have two independent streams of conscious awareness, one in each hemisphere, each of which is cut off from and out of contact with the mental experiences of the other. In other words, each hemisphere seems to have its own separate and private sensations; its own perceptions; its own concepts; and its own impulses to act, with related volitional, cognitive, and learning experiences. Following the surgery, each hemisphere also has thereafter its own separate chain of

memories that are rendered inaccessible to the recall processes of the other.

This presence of two minds in one body, as it were, is manifested in a large number and variety of test responses which, for the present purposes, I will try to review very briefly and in a somewhat streamlined and simplified form. First, however, let me take time to emphasize that the work reported here has been very much a team project. The surgery was performed by Vogel at the White Memorial Medical Center in Los Angeles. He has been assisted in the surgery and in the medical treatment throughout by Joseph Bogen. Bogen has also been collaborating in our behavioral testing program, along with a number of graduate students and postdoctoral fellows, among whom M. S. Gazzaniga, in particular, worked closely with us during the first several years and managed much of the testing during that period. The patients and their families have been most cooperative, and the whole project gets its primary funding from the National Institute of Mental Health.

Most of the main symptoms seen after hemisphere deconnection can be described for convenience with reference to a single testing setup—shown in figure 11.1. Principally, it allows for the lateralized testing of the right and left halves of the visual field, separately or together, and the right and left hands and legs with vision excluded. The tests can be arranged in different combinations and in association with visual, auditory, and other input, with provisions for eliminating unwanted stimuli. In testing vision, the subject with one eye covered centers his gaze on a designated fixation point on the upright translucent screen. The visual stimuli on 35-mm transparencies are arranged in a standard projector equipped with a shutter and are then back-projected at 1/10 of a second or less—too fast for eye movements to get the material into the wrong half of the visual field. Figure 11.2 is merely a reminder that everything seen to the left of the vertical meridian through either eye is

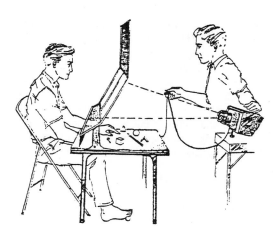

Figure 11.1
Apparatus for studying lateralization of visual, tactual, lingual, and associated functions in the surgically separated hemispheres.

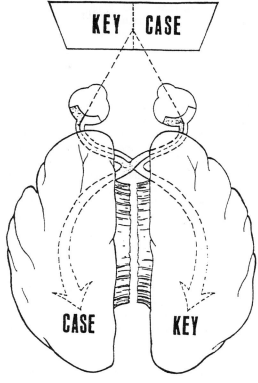

Figure 11.2
Things seen to the left of a central fixation point with either eye are projected to the right hemisphere and vice versa.

projected to the right hemisphere and vice versa. The midline division along the vertical meridian is found to be quite precise without significant gap or overlap (Sperry 1968).

When the visual perception of these patients is tested under these conditions the results indicate that these people have not one inner visual world any longer, but rather two separate visual inner worlds, one serving the right half of the field of vision and the other the left half—each, of course, in its respective hemisphere. This doubling in the visual sphere shows up in many ways: For example, after a projected picture of an object has been identified and responded to in one half field, we find that it is recognized again only if it reappears in the same half of the field of vision. If the given visual stimulus reappears in the opposite half of the visual field, the subject responds as if he had no recollection of the previous exposure. In other words, things seen through the right half of the visual field (i.e., through the left hemisphere) are registered in mental experience and remembered quite sepa-

rately from things seen in the other half of the field. Each half of the field of vision in the commissurotomized patient has its own train of visual images and memories.

This separate existence of two visual inner worlds is further illustrated in reference to speech and writing, the cortical mechanisms for which are centered in the dominant hemisphere. Visual material projected to the right half of the field—left-hemisphere system of the typical right-handed patient—can be described in speech and writing in an essentially normal manner. However, when the same visual material is projected into the left half of the field, and hence to the right hemisphere, the subject consistently insists that he did not see anything or that there was only a flash of light on the left side. The subject acts as if he were blind or agnostic for the left half of the visual field. If, however, instead of asking the subject to tell you what he saw, you instruct him to use his left hand to point to a matching picture or object presented among a collection of other pictures or objects, the subject has no trouble as a rule in pointing out consistently the very item that he has just insisted he did not see.

We do not think the subjects are trying to be difficult or to dupe the examiner in such tests. Everything indicates that the hemisphere that is talking to the examiner did in fact not see the left-field stimulus and truly had no experience with, nor recollection of, the given stimulus. The other, the right or nonlingual hemisphere, however, did see the projected stimulus in this situation and is able to remember and recognize the object and can demonstrate this by pointing out selectively the corresponding or matching item. This other hemisphere, like a deaf mute or like some aphasics, cannot talk about the perceived object and, worse still, cannot write about it either.

If two different figures are flashed simultaneously to the right and left visual fields, as for example a "dollar sign" on the left and a "question mark" on the right and the subject is asked to draw what he saw using the left hand out of sight, he regularly reproduces the figure seen on the left half of the field, that is, the dollar sign. If we now ask him what he has just drawn, he tells us without hesitation that the figure he drew was the question mark, or whatever appeared in the right half of the field. In other words, the one hemisphere does not know what the other hemisphere has been doing. The left and the right halves of the visual field seem to be perceived quite separately in each hemisphere with little or no cross-influence.

When words are flashed partly in the left field and partly in the right, the letters on each side of the midline are perceived and responded to separately. In the "key case" example shown in figure 11.2 the subject might first reach for and select with the left hand a key from among a collection of objects indicating perception through the minor hemisphere. With the right hand he might then spell out the word "case" or he might speak the word if verbal response is in order. When asked what kind of "case" he was thinking of here, the answer coming from the left hemisphere might be something like "in *case* of fire" or "the *case* of the missing corpse" or "a *case* of beer," and so on, depending upon the particular mental set of the left hemisphere at the moment. Any reference to "key case" under these conditions would be purely fortuitous, assuming that visual, auditory, and other cues have been properly controlled.

A similar separation in mental awareness is evident in tests that deal with stereognostic or other somesthetic discriminations made by the right and left hands, which are projected separately to the left and right hemispheres, respectively. Objects put in the right hand for identification by touch are readily described or named in speech or writing, whereas, if the same objects are placed in the left hand, the subject can only make wild guesses and may often seem unaware that anything at all is present. As with vision in the left field, however, good perception, comprehension, and memory can be demonstrated for these objects in the left hand when the tests are so designed that the subject can express himself through nonverbal responses. For example, if one of these objects which the subject tells you he cannot feel or does not recognize is taken from the left hand and placed in a grab bag or scrambled among a dozen other test items, the subject is then able to search out and retrieve the initial object even after a delay of several minutes is deliberately interposed. Unlike the normal subject, however, these people are obliged to retrieve such an object with the same hand with which it was initially identified. They fail at cross-retrieval. That is, they cannot recognize with one hand something identified only moments before with the other hand. Again, the second hemisphere does not know what the first hemisphere has been doing.

When the subjects are first asked to use the left hand for these stereognostic tests they commonly complain that they cannot "work with that hand," that the hand "is numb," that they "just can't feel anything or can't do anything with it," or that they "don't get the message from that hand." If the subjects perform a series of successful trials and correctly retrieve a group of objects which they previously stated they could not feel, and if this contradiction is then pointed out to them, we get comments like "Well, I was just guessing," or "Well, I must have done it unconsciously."

With other simple tests a further lack of cross-integration can be demonstrated in the sensory and motor control of the hands. In a "symmetric handpose" test the subject holds both hands out of sight symmetrically positioned and not in contact. One hand is then passively placed by the examiner into a given posture, such as a closed fist, or one, two, or more fingers extended or crossed or folded into various positions. The subject is then instructed verbally or by demonstration to form the same pose with the other hand, also excluded from vision. The normal subject does this quite accurately, but the commissurotomy patient generally fails on all but the very simplest hand postures, like the closed fist or the fully extended hand.

In a test for crossed topognosis in the hands, the subject holds both hands out of sight, forward and palm up with the fingers held apart and extended. The examiner then touches lightly a point on one of the figures or at the base of the fingers. The subject responds by touching the same target point with the tip of the thumb of the same hand. Cross-integration is tested by requiring the patient to use the opposite thumb to find the corresponding mirror point on the

opposite hand. The commissurotomy patients typically perform well within either hand, but fail when they attempt to cross-locate the corresponding point on the opposite hand. A crude cross-performance with abnormally long latency may be achieved in some cases after practice, depending on the degree of ipsilateral motor control and the development of certain strategies. The latter breaks down easily under stress and is readily distinguished from the natural performance of the normal subject with intact callosum.

In a related test the target point is presented visually as a black spot on an outline drawing of the hand. The picture is flashed to the right or left half of the visual field, and the subject then attempts as above to touch the target spot with the tip of the thumb. The response again is performed on the same side with normal facility but is impaired in the commissurotomy patient when the left visual field is paired with a right-hand response and vice versa. Thus the duality of both manual stereognosis and visuognosis is further illustrated; each hemisphere perceives as a separate unit unaware of the perceptual experience of the partner.

If two objects are placed simultaneously, one in each hand, and then are removed and hidden for retrieval in a scrambled pile of test items, each hand will hunt through the pile and search out selectively its own object. In the process each hand may explore, identify, and reject the item for which the other hand is searching. It is like two separate individuals working over the collection of test items with no cooperation between them. We find the interpretation of this and of many similar performances to be less confusing if we do not try to think of the behavior of the commissurotomy patient as that of a single individual, but try to think instead in terms of the mental faculties and performance capacities of the left and the right hemispheres separately. Most of the time it appears that the major, that is, the left, hemisphere is in control. But in some tasks, particularly when these are forced in testing procedures, the minor hemisphere seems able to take over temporarily.

It is worth remembering that when you split the brain in half anatomically you do not divide in half, in quite the same sense, its functional properties. In some respects cerebral functions may be doubled as much as they are halved because of the extensive bilateral redundancy in brain organization, wherein most functions, particularly in subhuman species, are separately and rather fully organized on both sides. Consider for example the visual inner world of either of the disconnected hemispheres in these patients. Probably neither of the separated visual systems senses or perceives itself to be cut in half or even incomplete. One may compare it to the visual sphere of the hemianopic patient who, following accidental destruction of an entire visual cortex of one hemisphere, may not even notice the loss of the whole half sphere of vision until this has been pointed out to him in specific optometric tests. These commissurotomy patients continue to watch television and to read the paper and books with no complaints about peculiarities in the perceptual appearance of the visual field.

At the same time, I want to caution against any impression that these patients are better off mentally without their cerebral commissures. It is true that if you carefully select two simple tasks, each of which is easily handled by a single hemisphere, and then have the two performed simultaneously, there is a good chance of getting better than normal scores. The normal interference effects that come from trying to attend to two separate right and left tasks at the same time are largely eliminated in the commissurotomized patient. However, in most activities that are at all complex the normally unified cooperating hemispheres still appear to do better than the two disconnected hemispheres. Although it is true that the intelligence, as measured on IQ tests, is not much affected and that the personality comes through with little change, one gets the impression in working with these people that their intellect is nevertheless handicapped in ways that

are probably not revealed in the ordinary tests. All the patients have marked short-term memory deficits, which are especially pronounced during the first year, and it is open to question whether this memory impairment ever clears completely. They also have orientation problems, fatigue more quickly in reading and in other tasks requiring mental concentration, and presumably have various other impairments that reduce the upper limits of performance in functions that have yet to be investigated. The patient that has shown the best recovery, a boy of 14, was able to return to public school and was doing passing work with B to D grades, except for an F in math, which he had to repeat. He was, however, a D student before the surgery, in part, it would seem, for lack of motivation. In general, our tests to date have been concerned mostly with basic cross-integrational deficits in these patients and the kind of mental capacities preserved in the subordinate hemisphere. Studied comparisons of the upper limits of performance before and after surgery are still needed.

Much of the foregoing is summarized schematically in figure 11.3. The left hemisphere in the right-handed patients is equipped with the expressive mechanisms for speech and writing and with the main centers for the comprehension and organization of language. This "major" hemisphere can communicate its experiences verbally and in an essentially normal manner. It can communicate, that is, about the visual experiences of the right half of the optic field and about the somesthetic and volitional experiences of the right hand and leg and right half of the body generally. In addition, and not indicated in the figure, the major hemisphere also communicates, of course, about all of the more general, less lateralized cerebral activity that is bilaterally represented and common to both hemispheres. On the other side we have the mute aphasic and agraphic right hemisphere, which cannot express itself verbally, but which through the use of nonverbal responses can show that it is not agnostic; that mental processes are indeed present

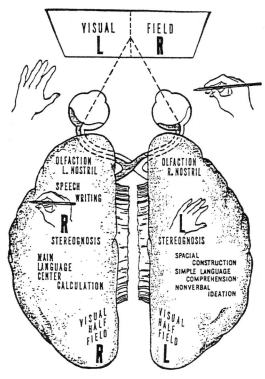

Figure 11.3
Schematic outline of the functional lateralization evident in behavioral tests of patients with forebrain commissurotomy.

of the field in order to prevent compensation by eye movements. The defects in manual stereognosis are not apparent unless vision is excluded; nor is doubling in olfactory perception evident without sequential occlusion of right and left nostril and elimination of visual cues. In many tests the major hemisphere must be prevented from talking to the minor hemisphere and thus giving away the answer through auditory channels. And, similarly, the minor hemisphere must be prevented from giving nonverbal signals of various sorts to the major hemisphere. There is a great diversity of indirect strategies and response signals, implicit as well as overt, by which the informed hemisphere can be used to cue in the uninformed hemisphere (Levy-Agresti 1968).

Normal behavior under ordinary conditions is favored also by many other unifying factors. Some of these are very obvious, like the fact that these two separate mental spheres have only one body, so they always get dragged to the same places, meet the same people, and see and do the same things all the time and thus are bound to have a great overlap of common, almost identical, experience. Just the unity of the optic image—and even after chiasm section in animal experiments, the conjugate movements of the eyes—means that both hemispheres automatically center on, focus on, and hence probably attend to, the same items in the visual field all the time. Through sensory feedback a unifying body schema is imposed in each hemisphere with common components that similarly condition in parallel many processes of perception and motor action onto a common base. To get different activities going and different experiences and different memory chains built up in the separated hemispheres of the bisected mammalian brain, as we do in the animal work, requires a considerable amount of experimental planning and effort.

In motor control we have another important unifying factor, in that either hemisphere can direct the movement of both sides of the body, including to some extent the movements of the

centered around the left visual field, left hand, left leg, and left half of the body; along with the auditory, vestibular, axial somatic, and all other cerebral activities that are less lateralized and for which the mental experiences of the right and left hemispheres may be characterized as being similar but separate.

It may be noted that nearly all of the symptoms of cross-integrational impairment that I have been describing are easily hidden or compensated under the conditions or ordinary behavior. For example, the visual material has to be flashed at 1/10 of a second or less to one half

HEMISPHERE DECONNECTION

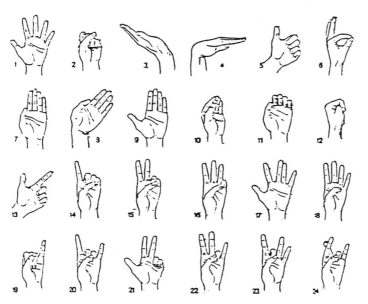

Figure 11.4
In tests for ipsilateral motor control, different hand postures in outline drawing are projected one at a time to left right visual field (see figure 11.1). Subject attempts to copy the sample hand pose with the homolateral and contralateral hand.

ipsilateral hand (Hamilton 1967). Insofar as a response involves mainly the axial parts and proximal limb segments, these patients have little problem in directing overall response from sensory information restricted to either single hemisphere. Control of the distal limb segments and especially of the finer finger movements of the hand ipsilateral to the governing hemisphere, however, are borderline functions and subject to considerable variation. Impairments are most conspicuous when the subject is given a verbal command to respond with the fingers of the left hand. The absence of the callosum, which normally would connect the language processing centers in the left hemisphere to the main left-hand motor controls in the opposite hemisphere,

is clearly a handicap, especially in the early months after surgery. Cursive writing with the left hand presents a similar problem. It may be accomplished in time by some patients using shoulder and elbow rather than finger movement. At best, however, writing with the left hand is not as good after as before they surgery. The problem is not in motor coordination per se, because the subject can often copy with the left hand a word already written by the examiner when the same word cannot be written to verbal command.

In a test used for more direct determination of the upper limits of this ipsilateral motor control, a simple outline sketch of a finger posture (see figure 11.4) is flashed to a single hemisphere, and the subject then tries to mimic the posture with the same or the opposite hand. The sample posture can usually be copied on the same side (i.e., through the main, contralateral control system) without difficulty, but the performance does not go so easily and often breaks down completely when the subject is obliged to use the opposite hand. The closed fist and the open hand with all fingers extended seem to be the two simplest responses, in that these can most often be copied with the ipsilateral hand by the more adept patients.

The results are in accord with the thesis (Gazzaniga, Bogen, and Sperry 1967) that the ipsilateral control systems are delicate and marginal and easily disrupted by associated cerebral damage and other complicating factors. Preservation of the ipsilateral control system in varying degree in some patients and not in others would appear to account for many of the discrepancies that exist in the literature on the symptoms of hemisphere deconnection, and also for a number of changes between the present picture and that described until 2 years ago. Those acquainted with the literature will notice that the present findings on dyspraxia come much closer to the earlier Akelaitis observations than they do to those of Liepmann or of others expounded more recently (see Geschwind 1965).

To try to find out what goes on in that speechless agraphic minor hemisphere has always been one of the main challenges in our testing program. Does the minor hemisphere really possess a true stream of conscious awareness or is it just an agnostic automaton that is carried along in a reflex or trancelike state? What is the nature, the quality, and the level of the mental life of this isolated subordinate unknown half of the human brain—which, like the animal mind, cannot communicate its experiences? Closely tied in here are many problems that relate to lateral dominance and specialization in the human brain, to the functional roles mediated by the neocortical commissures, and to related aspects of cerebral organization.

With such in mind, I will try to review briefly some of the evidence obtained to date that pertains to the level and nature of the inner mental life of the disconnected minor hemisphere. First, it is clear that the minor hemisphere can perform intermodal or cross-modal transfer of perceptual and mnemonic information at a characteristically human level. For example, after a picture of some object, such as a cigarette, has been flashed to the minor hemisphere through the left visual field, the subject can retrieve the item pictured from a collection of objects using blind touch with the left hand, which is mediated through the right hemisphere. Unlike the normal person, however, the commissurotomy patient is obliged to use the corresponding hand (i.e., the left hand, in this case) for retrieval and fails when he is required to search out the same object with the right hand (see figure 11.5). Using the right hand the subject recognizes and can call off the names of each object that he comes to if he is allowed to do so, but the right hand or its hemisphere does not know what it is looking for, and the hemisphere that can recognize the correct answer gets no feedback from the right hand. Hence, the two never get together, and the performance fails. Speech and other auditory cues must be controlled.

It also works the other way around: that is, if the subject is holding an object in the left hand, he can then point out a picture of this object or the printed name of the object when these appear in a series presented visually. But again, these latter must be seen through the corresponding half of the visual field; an object identified by the left hand is not recognized when seen in the right half of the visual field. Intermodal associations of this sort have been found to work between vision, hearing and touch, and, more recently, olfaction in various combinations within either hemisphere but not across from one hemisphere to the other. This perceptual or mnemonic transfer from one sense modality to another has special theoretical interest in that it is something that is extremely difficult or impossible for the

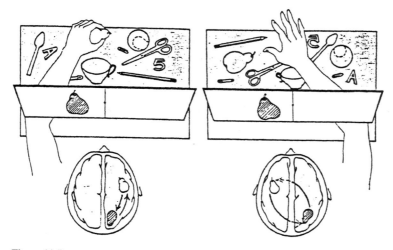

Figure 11.5
Visuo-tactile associations succeed between each half of the visual field and the corresponding hand. They fail with crossed combinations in which visual and tactual stimuli are projected into opposite hemispheres.

monkey brain. The right hemisphere, in other words, may be animallike in not being able to talk or write, but in performances like the foregoing and in a number of other respects it shows mental capacities that are definitely human.

Other responses from the minor hemisphere in this same testing situation suggest the presence of ideas and a capacity for mental association and at least some simple logic and reasoning. In the same visuo-tactual test described above, the minor hemisphere, instead of selecting objects that match exactly the pictured item, seems able also to select related items or items that "go with" the particular visual stimulus, if the subject is so instructed. For example, if we flash a picture of a wall clock to the minor side and the nearest item that can be found tactually by the left hand is a toy wrist watch, the subjects significantly select the watch. It is as if the minor hemisphere has an idea of a timepiece here and is not just matching sensory outlines. Or, if the picture of a dollar sign is flashed to the minor side, the subject searches through the list of items with the left

hand and finally selects a coin such as a quarter or a 50¢ piece. If a picture of a hammer is presented, the subject may come up with a nail or a spike after checking out and rejecting all other items.

The capacity to think abstractly with symbols is further indicated in the ability of the minor hemisphere to perform simple arithmetical problems. When confronted with two numerals each less than 10, the minor hemisphere was able in four of six subjects so tested to respond with the correct sum or product up to 20 or so. The numbers were flashed to the left half of the visual field or presented as plastic block numerals to the left hand for identification. The answer was expressed by pointing to the correct number in columns of seen figures, or by left-hand signals in which the fingers were extended out of the subject's sight, or by writing the numerals with the left hand out of sight. After a correct left-hand response had been made by pointing or by writing the numeral, the major hemisphere could then report the same answer verbally, but the verbal report could not be made prior to the left-hand response. If an error was made with the left hand, the verbal report contained the same error. Two different pairs of numerals may be flashed to right and left fields simultaneously and the correct sum or products signaled separately by right and left hands. When verbal confirmation of correct left-hand signals is required under these conditions, the speaking hemisphere can only guess fortuitously, showing again that the answer must have been obtained from the minor and not from the major hemisphere. This has been demonstrated recently in a study still in progress by Biersner and the present writer. The findings correct an earlier impression (Gazzaniga and Sperry 1967) in which we underestimated the capacity for calculation on the minor side. Normal subjects and also a subject with agenesis of the callosum (Saul and Sperry 1968) were able to add or to multiply numerals shown one in the left and one in the right field under these conditions. The commissurotomy subjects, however, were able to perform such calculations only when both numerals appeared in the same half of the visual field.

According to a doctrine of long standing in the clincial writings on aphasia, it is believed that the minor hemisphere, when it has been disconnected by commissural or other lesions from the language centers on the opposite side, becomes then "word blind," "word deaf," and "tactually alexic." In contradiction to this, we find that the disconnected minor hemisphere in these commissurotomy patients is able to comprehend both written and spoken words to some extent, although this comprehension cannot be expressed verbally (Gazzaniga and Sperry 1967, Sperry 1966, Sperry and Gazzaniga 1967). If the name of some object is flashed to the left visual field, like the word "eraser," for example, the subject is able then to search out an eraser from among a collection of objects using only touch with the left hand. If the subject is then asked what the item is after it has been selected correctly, his replies show that he does not know

what he is holding in his left hand—as is the general rule for left-hand stereognosis. This means of course that the *talking* hemisphere does not know the correct answer, and we concluded accordingly that the minor hemisphere must, in this situation, have read and understood the test world.

These patients also demonstrate comprehension of language in the minor hemisphere by being able to find by blind touch with the left hand an object that has been named aloud by the examiner. For example, if asked to find a "piece of silverware," the subject may explore the array of test items and pick up a fork. If the subject is then asked what it is that he has chosen, he is just as likely in this case to reply "spoon" or "knife" as fork. Both hemispheres have heard and understood the word "silverware," but only the minor hemisphere knows what the left hand has actually found and picked up. In similar tests for comprehension of the spoken word, we find that the minor hemisphere seems able to understand even moderately advanced definitions like "shaving instrument" for razor or "dirt remover" for soap and "inserted in slot machines" for quarter.

Work in progress shows that the minor hemisphere can also sort objects into groups by touch on the basis of shape, size, and texture. In some tests the minor hemisphere is found to the superior to the major, for example, in tasks that involve drawing spatial relationships and performing block design tests. Perceptive mental performance in the minor hemisphere is also indicated in other situations in which the two hemispheres function concurrently in parallel at different tasks. It has been found, for example, that the divided hemispheres are capable of perceiving different things occupying the same position in space at the same time, and of learning mutually conflicting discrimination habits, something of which the normal brain is not capable. This was shown in the monkey work done some years ago by Trevarthen (1962) using a system of polarized light filters. It also required section of the optic chiasm, which of course is not included in the human surgery. The human patients, unlike normal subjects, are able to carry out a double voluntary reaction-time task as fast as they carry out a single task (Gazzaniga and Sperry 1966). Each hemisphere in this situation has to perform a separate and different visual discrimination in order to push with the corresponding hand the correct one of a right and left pair of panels. Whereas interference and extra delay are seen in normal subjects with the introduction of the second task, these patients with the two hemispheres working in parallel simultaneously perform the double task as rapidly as the single task.

The minor hemisphere is also observed to demonstrate appropriate emotional reactions as, for example, when a pinup shot of a nude is interjected by surprise among a series of neutral geometric figures being flashed to the right and left fields at random. When the surprise nude appears on the left side the subject characteristically says that he or she saw nothing or just a flash of light. However, the appearance of a sneaky grin and perhaps blushing and giggling on the next couple of trials or so belies the verbal contention of the speaking hemisphere. If asked what all the grinning is about, the subject's replies indicate that the conversant hemisphere has no idea at this stage what it was that had turned him on. Apparently, only the emotional effect gets across, as if the cognitive component of the process cannot be articulated through the brainstem.

Emotion is also evident on the minor side in a current study by Gordon and Sperry (1968) involving olfaction. When odors are presented through the right nostril to the minor hemisphere the subject is unable to name the odor but can frequently tell whether it is pleasant or unpleasant. The subject may even grunt, make aversive reactions or exclamations like "phew!" to a strong unpleasant smell, but not be able to state verbally whether it is garlic, cheese, or some decayed matter. Again it appears that the affec-

tive component gets across to the speaking hemisphere, but not the more specific information. The presence of the specific information within the minor hemisphere is demonstrated by the subject's correct selection through left-hand stereognosis of corresponding objects associated with the given odor. The minor hemisphere also commonly triggers emotional reactions of displeasure in the course of ordinary testing. This is evidenced in the frowning, wincing, and negative head shaking in test situations where the minor hemisphere, knowing the correct answer but unable to speak, hears the major hemisphere making obvious verbal mistakes. The minor hemisphere seems to express genuine annoyance at the erroneous vocal responses of its better half.

Observations like the foregoing lead us to favor the view that in the minor hemisphere we deal with a second conscious entity that is characteristically human and runs along in parallel with the more dominant stream of consciousness in the major hemisphere (Sperry 1966). The quality of mental awareness present in the minor hemisphere may be comparable perhaps to that which survives in some types of aphasic patients following losses in the motor and main language centers. There is no indication that the dominant mental system of the left hemisphere is concerned about or even aware of the presence of the minor system under most ordinary conditions except quite indirectly as, for example, through occasional responses triggered from the minor side. As one patient remarked immediately after seeing herself make a left-hand response of this kind, "Now I know it wasn't me did that!"

Let me emphasize again in closing that the foregoing represents a somewhat abbreviated and streamlined account of the syndrome of hemisphere deconnection as we understand it at the present time. The more we see of these patients and the more of these patients we see, the more we become impressed with their individual differences, and with the consequent qualifications that must be taken into account. Although the general picture has continued to hold up in the main as described, it is important to note that, with respect to many of the deconnection symptoms mentioned, striking modifications and even outright exceptions can be found among the small group of patients examined to date. Where the accumulating evidence will settle out with respect to the extreme limits of such individual variations and with respect to a possible average "type" syndrome remains to be seen.

Acknowledgments

Invited address presented to the American Psychological Association in Washington, D.C., September 1967, and to the Pan American Congress of Neurology in San Juan, Puerto Rico, October 1967. Original work referred to in the text by the writer and his co-workers was supported by Grant MH-03372 from the National Institute of Mental Health, United States Public Health Service, and by the Hixon Fund of the California Institute of Technology.

References

Akelaitis, A. J. A study of gnosis, praxis, and language following section of the corpus callosum and anterior commissure. *Journal of Neurosurgery*, 1944, 1, 94–102.

Bogen, J. E., Fisher, E. D., and Vogel, P. J. Cerebral commissurotomy: A second case report. *Journal of the American Medical Association*, 1965, 194, 1328–1329.

Bogen, J. E., and Vogel, P. J. Cerebral commissurotomy: A case report. *Bulletin of the Los Angeles Neurological Society*, 1962, 27, 169.

Gazzaniga, M. S. The split brain in man. *Scientific American*, 1967, 217, 24–29.

Gazzaniga, M. S., Bogen, J. E., and Sperry, R. W. Dyspraxia following division of the cerebral commissures. *Archives of Neurology*, 1967, 16, 606–612.

Gazzaniga, M. S., and Sperry, R. W. Simultaneous double discrimination following brain bisection. *Psychonomic Science*, 1966, 4, 262–263.

Gazzaniga, M. S., and Sperry, R. W. Language after section of the cerebral commissures. *Brain*, 1967, 90, 131–148.

Geschwind, N. Disconnexion syndromes in animals and man. *Brain*, 1965, 88, 237–294, 584–644.

Gordon, H. W., and Sperry, R. W. Olfaction following surgical disconnection of the hemispheres in man. In, *Proceedings of the Psychonomic Society*, 1968.

Hamilton, C. R. Effects of brain bisection on eye-hand coordination in monkeys wearing prisms. *Journal of Comparative and Physiological Psychology*, 1967, 64, 434–443.

Levy-Agresti, J. Ipsilateral projection systems and minor hemisphere function in man after neocommissurotomy. *Anatomical Record*, 1968, 160, 384.

Myers, R. E. Corpus callosum and visual gnosis. In J. F. Delafresnaye (Ed.), *Brain mechanisms and learning.* Oxford: Blackwell, 1961.

Saul, R., and Sperry, R. W. Absence of commissurotomy symptoms with agenesis of the corpus callosum. *Neurology*, 1968, 18 (3), 307.

Sperry, R. W. Brain bisection and mechanisms of consciousness. In J. C. Eccles (Ed.), *Brain and conscious experience.* New York: Springer-Verlag, 1966.

Sperry, R. W. Mental unity following surgical disconnection of the hemispheres. *The Harvey lectures.* Series 62. New York: Academic Press, 1967. (a)

Sperry, R. W. Split-brain approach to learning problems. In G. C. Quarton, T. Melnechuk, and F. O. Schmitt (Eds.), *The neurosciences: A study program.* New York: Rockefeller University Press, 1967. (b)

Sperry, R. W. Apposition of visual half-fields after section of neocortical commissures. *Anatomical Record*, 1968, 160, 498–499.

Sperry, R. W., and Gazzaniga, M. S. Language following surgical disconnection of the hemispheres. In C. H. Milikan (Ed.), *Brain mechanisms underlying speech and language.* New York: Grune & Stratton, 1967.

Sperry, R. W., Gazzaniga, M. S., and Bogen, J. E. Function of neocortical commissures: Syndrome of hemisphere deconnection. In P. J. Vinken and G. W. Bruyn (Eds.), *Handbook of neurology.* Amsterdam: North Holland, 1968.

Trevarthen, C. B. Double visual learning in split-brain monkeys. *Science*, 1962, 136, 258–259.

12 Separate Visual Pathways for Perception and Action

Melvyn A. Goodale and A. David Milner

In an influential article that appeared in *Science* in 1969, Schneider[1] postulated an anatomical separation between the visual coding of the location of a stimulus and the identification of that stimulus. He attributed the coding of the location to the ancient retinotectal pathway, and the identification of the stimulus to the newer geniculostriate system; this distinction represented a significant departure from earlier monolithic descriptions of visual function. However, the notion of 'localization' failed to distinguish between the many different patterns of behaviour that vary with the spatial location of visual stimuli, only some of which turn out to rely on tectal mechanisms.[2-4] Nevertheless, even though Schneider's original proposal is no longer generally accepted, his distinction between object identification and spatial localization, between "what" and "where," has persisted in visual neuroscience.

Two Cortical Visual Systems

In 1982, for example, Ungerleider and Mishkin[5] concluded that "appreciation of an object's qualities and of its spatial location depends on the processing of different kinds of visual information in the inferior temporal and posterior parietal cortex, respectively." They marshalled evidence from a number of electrophysiological, anatomical and behavioural studies suggesting that these two areas receive independent sets of projections from the striate cortex. They distinguished between a "ventral stream" of projections that eventually reaches the inferotemporal cortex, and a "dorsal stream" that terminates finally in the posterior parietal region. The proposed functions of these two streams were inferred largely from behavioural evidence derived from lesion studies. They noted that monkeys with lesions of the inferotemporal

cortex were profoundly impaired in visual pattern discrimination and recognition,[6] but less impaired in solving "landmark" tasks, in which the location of a visual cue determines which of two alternative locations is rewarded. Quite the opposite pattern of results was observed in monkeys with posterior parietal lesions.[7-9]

So, according to Ungerleider and Mishkin's 1982 version of the model of two visual systems, the inferotemporal lesions disrupted circuitry specialized for identifying objects, while the posterior parietal lesions interfered with neural mechanisms underlying spatial perception. Thus, within the visual domain, they made much the same functional distinction between identification and localization as Schneider, but mapped it onto the diverging ventral and dorsal streams of output from the striate cortex. Since 1982, there has been an explosion of information about the anatomy and electrophysiology of cortical visual areas[10,11] and, indeed, the connectional anatomy among these various areas largely confirms the existence of the two broad "streams" of projections proposed by Ungerleider and Mishkin (see figure 12.1).[12,13]

It has recently been suggested[14] that these two streams can be traced back to the two main cytological subdivisions of retinal ganglion cells: one of these two subdivisions terminates selectively in the parvocellular layer, while the other terminates in the magnocellular layer of the lateral geniculate nucleus (LGN).[14-16] Certainly, these "parvo" and "magno" subdivisions remain relatively segregated at the level of the primary visual cortex (V1) and in the adjacent visual area V2. They also appear to predominate, respectively, the innervation of area V4 and the middle temporal area (MT), which in turn provide the major visual inputs to the inferotemporal and posterior parietal cortex, respectively. However, it is becoming increasingly clear that the separa-

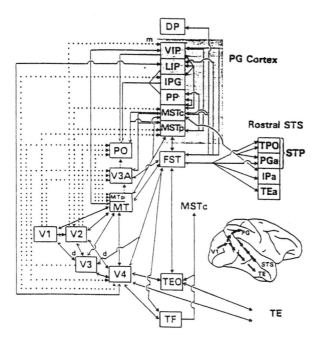

Figure 12.1

The 1982 version of Ungerleider and Mishkin's[5] model of two visual systems is illustrated in the small diagram of the monkey brain inset into the larger box diagram. In the original model, V1 is shown sending a dorsal stream of projections to the posterior parietal cortex (PG), and a ventral stream of projections to the inferotemporal cortex (TE). The box diagram illustrates one of the most recent versions of the interconnectivity of the visual cortical areas, showing that they can still be broadly segregated into dorsal and ventral streams. However, there is crosstalk between the different areas in the two streams, and there may be a third branch of processing projecting into the rostral superior temporal sulcus (STS) that is intimately connected with both the dorsal and ventral streams. (This is illustrated in both the brain and box diagrams.) Thus, the proposed segregation of input that characterized the dorsal and ventral streams in the original model is not nearly as clear cut as once was thought. (Modified, with permission, from reference 11.)

tion between magno and parvo information in the cortex is not as distinct as initially thought. For example, there is recent evidence for a parvo input into a subset of MT neurones[17] as well as for a large contribution from the magno pathway to V4 neurones[18] and to the "blobs" in V1 (Ref. 19). In short, it now appears that the dorsal and the ventral streams each receive inputs from both the magno and the parvo pathways.

Two Visuomotor Systems: "What" versus "How"

Our alternative perspective on modularity in the cortical visual system is to place less emphasis on input distinctions (e.g., object location versus object qualities) and to take more account of output requirements.[20,21] It seems plausible from a functional standpoint that separate processing modules would have evolved to mediate the different uses to which vision can be put. This principle is already generally accepted in relation to "automatic" types of behaviour such as saccadic eye movements,[22] and it is possible that it could be extended to other systems for a range of behavioural skills such as visually guided reaching and grasping, in which close coordination is required between movements of the fingers, hands, upper limbs, head, and eyes.

It is also our contention that the inputs and transformations required by these skilled visuomotor acts differ in important respects from those leading to what is generally understood as "visual perception." Indeed, as has been argued elsewhere, the functional modules supporting perceptual experience of the world may have evolved much more recently than those controlling actions within it.[21] In this article, it is proposed that this distinction ("what" versus "how")—rather than the distinction between object vision and spatial vision ("what" versus "where")—captures more appropriately the functional dichotomy between the ventral and dorsal projections.

Dissociation between Prehension and Apprehension

Neuropsychological studies of patients with damage to one projection system but not the other have also been cited in support of the model proposed by Ungerleider and Mishkin.[5,23] Patients with visual agnosia following brain damage that includes, for example, the occipitotemporal region, are often unable to recognize or describe common objects, faces, pictures, or abstract designs, even though they can navigate through the everyday world—at least at a local level—with considerable skill.[24] Conversely, patients suffering from optic ataxia following damage to the posterior parietal region are unable to reach accurately towards visual targets that they have no difficulty recognizing.[25]

Such observations certainly appear to provide support in humans for an occipitotemporal system mediating object vision but not spatial vision, and a parietal system mediating spatial vision but not object vision.

Closer examination of the behaviour of such patients, however, leads to a different conclusion. Patients with optic ataxia not only have difficulty reaching in the right direction, but also in positioning their fingers or adjusting the orientation of their hand when reaching toward an object that can be oriented at different angles.[25] Such patients may also have trouble adjusting their grasp to reflect the size of the object they are asked to pick up.

Visually guided grasping was recently studied in a patient who had recovered from Balint's syndrome, in which bilateral parietal damage causes profound disorders of spatial attention, gaze and visually guided reaching.[26] While this patient had no difficulty in recognizing line drawings of common objects, her ability to pick up such objects remained quite impaired. For example, when she reached out for a small wooden block that varied in size from trial to trial, there was little relationship between the magnitude of the aperture between her index finger and thumb and the size of the block as the movement unfolded. Not only did she fail to show normal scaling of the grasping movement; she also made a large number of adjustments in her grasp as she closed in on the object—adjustments rarely observed in normal subjects. Such studies suggest that damage to the parietal lobe can impair the ability of patients to use information about the size, shape and orientation of an object to control the hand and fingers during a grasping movement, even though this same information can still be used to identify and describe the objects. Clearly, a "disorder of spatial vision" fails to capture this range of visuomotor impairments.

There are, of course, other kinds of visuospatial disorders, many of which are associated with parietal lobe damage, while others are associated with temporal lobe lesions.[27,28] Unfortunately, we lack detailed analyses of the possible specificity of most such disorders: in many, the deficit may be restricted to particular behavioural tasks. For example, a recently described patient with a parietal injury performed poorly on a task in which visual guidance was needed to learn the correct route through a small ten-choice maze by moving a hand-held stylus.[23] However, he was quite unimpaired on a locomotor maze task in which he was required to move his whole body through space when working from a two-dimensional visual plan. Moreover, he had no difficulty in recalling a complex geometrical pattern, or in carrying out a task involving short-term spatial memory.[29] Such dissociations between performance on different "spatial" tasks show that after parietal damage spatial information may still be processed quite well for some purposes, but not for others. Of course, the fact that visuospatial deficits can be fractionated in humans does not exclude combinations of such impairments occurring after large lesions, nor would it exclude possible selective input disorders occurring after smaller deafferentation lesions close to where the dorsal stream begins.

Complications also arise on the opposite side of the equation (i.e., in relation to the ventral stream), when the behaviour of patients with visual agnosia is studied in detail. The visual behaviour of one patient (DF) who developed a profound visual-form agnosia following carbon monoxide poisoning was recently studied. Although MRI revealed diffuse brain damage consistent with anoxia, most of the damage in the cortical visual areas was evident in areas 18 and 19, with area 17 apparently remaining largely intact. Despite her profound inability to recognize the size, shape and orientation of visual objects, DF showed strikingly accurate guidance of hand and finger movements directed at the very same objects.[30,31] Thus, when she was presented with a pair of rectangular blocks of the same or different dimensions, she was unable to distinguish between them. When she was asked to indicate the width of a single block by means of her index finger and thumb, her matches bore no relationship to the dimensions of the object and showed considerable trial to trial variability (figure 12.2a). However, when she was asked simply to reach out and pick up the block, the aperture between her index finger and thumb changed systematically with the width of the object, just as in normal subjects (figure 12.2b). In other words, DF scaled her grip to the dimensions of the objects she was about to pick up, even though she appeared to be unable to "perceive" those dimensions.

A similar dissociation was seen in her responses to the orientation of stimuli. Thus, when presented with a large slot that could be placed in one of a number of different orientations, she showed great difficulty in indicating the orientation either verbally or manually (i.e., by rotating her hand or a hand-held card). Nevertheless, she was as good as normal subjects at reaching out and placing her hand or the card into the slot, turning her hand appropriately from the very onset of the movement.[30,31]

These disparate neuropsychological observations lead us to propose that the visual projection system to the human parietal cortex provides action-relevant information about the structural characteristics and orientation of objects, and not just about their position. On the other hand, projections to the temporal lobe may furnish our visual perceptual experience, and it is these that we postulate to be severely damaged in DF.

Dorsal and Ventral Systems in the Monkey

How well do electrophysiological studies of the two projection systems in the visual cortex of the monkey support the distinction we are making? While any correlations between human neuropsychology and monkey neurophysiology should only be made with caution, it is likely that humans share many features of visual processing

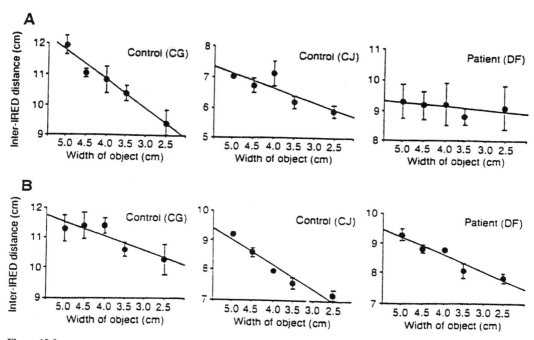

Figure 12.2

In both (*A*) the manual matching task and (*B*) the grasping task, five white plaques (each with an overall area of 25 cm² on the top surface, but with dimensions ranging from 5 × 5 cm to 2.5 × 10 cm) were presented, one at a time, at a viewing distance of approximately 45 cm. Diodes emitting infrared light (IREDs) were attached to the tips of the index finger and thumb of the right hand and were tracked with two infrared-sensitive cameras and stored on a WATSMART computer (Northern Digital Inc., Wateloo, Canada). The three-dimensional position of the IREDs and the changing distance between them were later reconstructed off line. (*A*) In the manual matching task, DF and two control subjects were instructed to indicate the width of each plaque over a series of randomly ordered trials by separating the index finger and thumb of their right hand. In DF, unlike the controls (CG and CJ), the aperture between the finger and thumb was not systematically related to the width of the target. DF also showed considerable trial-to-trial variability. (*B*) In contrast, when they were instructed to reach out and pick up each plaque, DF's performance was indistinguishable from that of the control subjects. The maximum aperture between index finger and thumb, which was achieved well before contact, was systematically related to the width of plaques in both DF and the two control subjects. In interpreting all these graphs, it is the slope of the function that is important rather than the absolute values plotted, since the placement of the IREDs and the size of the hand and fingers varied somewhat from subject to subject. Bars represent means ±SE. (Modified, with permission, from reference 31.)

with our primate relatives—particularly with the Old World monkeys in which most of the electrophysiology has been carried out. Furthermore, lesion studies of the two projection systems in the monkey should show parallels with the results of work done on human patients.

It was noted earlier that although there are differences in the major retinal origins of inputs to the dorsal and ventral systems in the monkey brain, there is subsequently a good deal of pooling of information. Moreover, there are convergent similarities in what is extracted within the two systems. For example, both orientation and disparity selectivity are present in neurones in both the magno and parvo systems within cortical areas V1 and V2.[15]

Nevertheless, there are special features in the properties of individual neurones in the posterior parietal cortex (and in its major input areas V3A and MT) that are not found in the ventral system. The most striking feature of neurones in the posterior parietal region is not their spatial selectivity (indeed, like those of inferotemporal cells, their receptive fields are typically large), but rather the fact that their responses depend greatly on the concurrent behaviour of the animal with respect to the stimulus. Separate subsets of cells in the posterior parietal cortex have been shown to be implicated in visual fixation, pursuit and saccadic eye movements, eye-hand coordination, and visually guided reaching movements.[32] Many cells in the posterior parietal region have gaze-dependent responses; that is, where the animal is looking determines the response amplitude of the cell (although not the retinal location of its receptive field).[33] In reviewing these studies, Andersen[32] emphasizes that most neurones in this area "exhibit both sensory-related and movement-related activity." In a particularly interesting recent development, Taira et al.[34] have shown that some parietal cells are sensitive to those visual qualities of an object that determine the posture of the hand and fingers during a grasping movement. They studied

neurones selectively associated with hand movements made by the monkey in reaching and picking up solid objects. Many of these cells were selective for the visual appearance of the object that was to be manipulated, including its size and in several cases its orientation.

The posterior parietal cortex may receive such form information from one or both of the areas V3 or V4, both of which project to area MT.[35] Other visual inputs pass through area MT and the adjacent medial superior temporal (MST) area, both of which contain cells variously selective for object motion in different directions, including rotation and motion in depth.[32] Thus, the posterior parietal cortex appears to receive the necessary inputs for continually updating the monkey's knowledge of the disposition and structural qualities of objects in its three-dimensional ego-space. Also, many motion-sensitive cells in the posterior parietal cortex itself appear to be well suited for the visual monitoring of limb position during reaching behaviour;[36] in contrast, motion-sensitive cells in the temporal lobe have been reported not to respond to such self-produced visual motion.[37] As for the output pathways, the posterior parietal region is strongly linked with those pre-motor regions of the frontal cortex directly implicated in ocular control,[33,38] reaching movements of the limb,[39] and grasping actions of the hand and fingers.[39]

Thus, the parietal cortex is strategically placed to serve a mediating role in the visual guidance and integration of prehensile and other skilled actions (see reference 40 for a detailed account of this argument). The results of behavioural analyses of monkeys with posterior parietal damage support this further. Like patients with optic ataxia, such animals fail to reach correctly for visual targets,[41] and they also have difficulty in shaping and orienting their hands when attempting to retrieve food.[42,43] Their reaching impairment is, therefore, one symptom of a wider visuomotor disorder, and most of the deficits that have been reported on "maze" tasks following posterior parietal damage may also be visuomotor in nature.[9,40]

Nonetheless, neurones in the dorsal stream do not show the high-resolution selectivity characteristic of neurones in the inferotemporal cortex, which are strikingly sensitive to form, pattern, and colour.[10] In this and in neighbouring temporal lobe areas, some cells respond selectively to faces, to hands, or to the appearance of particular actions in others.[44] Therefore, it is unsurprising that monkeys with inferotemporal lesions have profound deficits in visual recognition; however, as noted by Pribram,[45] they remain highly adept at the visually demanding skill of catching flies!

A further peculiarity of many visual cells in the temporal cortex is that they continue to maintain their selective responsiveness over a wide range of size, colour, optical, and viewpoint transformations of the object.[44,46] Such cells, far from providing the momentary information necessary for guiding action, specifically ignore such changing details. Consistent with this, behavioural studies have shown that by lesioning the inferotemporal cortex (but not the posterior parietal cortex), a monkey is less able to generalize its recognition of three-dimensional shape across viewing conditions.[47,48]

Visual and Attentional Requirements for Perception and Action

As DeYoe and Van Essen[15] have suggested, "parietal and temporal lobes could both be involved in shape analysis but associated with different computational strategies." For the purposes of identification, learning and distal (e.g., social) transactions, visual coding often (though not always[44,46]) needs to be "object-centred"; that is, constancies of shape, size, colour, lightness, and location need to be maintained across different viewing conditions. The above evidence from behavioural and physiological studies supports the view that the ventral stream of processing plays an important role in the computation of such object-specific descriptions. In contrast, *action* upon the object requires that the location of the object and its particular disposition and motion with respect to the observer is encoded. For this purpose, coding of shape would need to be largely "viewer-centred,"[49] with the egocentric coordinates of the surface of the object or its contours being computed each time the action occurs. We predict that shape-encoding cells in the dorsal system should predominantly have this property. Nevertheless, certain constancies, such as size, would be necessary for accurate scaling of grasp aperture, and it might therefore be expected that the visual properties of the manipulation cells found by Taira et al.[34] in the posterior parietal region would have this property.

It is often suggested that the neuronal properties of the posterior parietal cortex qualify it as the prime mediator of visuospatial attention.[50] Certainly, many cells (e.g., in area 7a) are modulated by switches of attention to different parts of the visual field.[51] (Indeed, the "landmark" disorder that follows posterior parietal damage in monkeys may be primarily due to a failure to attend or orient rather than a failure to localize.[9,40,52]) However, it is now known that attentional modulation occurs in neurones in many parts of the cortex, including area V4 and the inferotemporal region within the ventral stream.[53,54] This might explain the occurrence of landmark deficits after inferotemporal as well as posterior parietal damage.[7,8]

In general terms, attention needs to be switched to particular locations and objects whenever they are the targets either for intended action[51,55] or for identification.[54] In either case, this selection seems typically to be spatially based. Thus, human subjects performing manual aiming movements have a predilection to attend to visual stimuli that occur within the "action space" of the hand.[56] In this instance the attentional facilitation might be mediated by mechanisms within the dorsal projection system; in other instances it is probably mediated by the ventral system. Indeed, the focus of lesions causing the human attentional disorder of "unilateral neglect" is parietotemporal (unlike the superior parietal focus for optic ataxia[25]), as is the focus for object constancy impairments.[57] We conclude that spatial attention is physiologically non-unitary,[55] and may be as much associated with the ventral system as with the dorsal.

A Speculation about Awareness

The evidence from the brain-damaged patient DF described earlier suggests that the two cortical pathways may be differentiated with respect to their access to consciousness. DF certainly appears to have no conscious perception of the orientation or dimensions of objects, although she can pick them up with remarkable adeptness. It may be that information can be processed in the dorsal system without reaching consciousness, and that this prevents interference with the perceptual constancies intrinsic to many operations within the ventral system that do result in awareness. Intrusions of viewer-centred information could disrupt the continuity of object identities across changing viewpoints and illumination conditions.

If this argument is correct, then there should be occasions when normal subjects are unaware of changes in the visual array to which their motor system is expertly adjusting. An example of such a dissociation has been reported in a study on eye-hand coordination during visually guided aiming.[58] Subjects were unable to report, even in forced-choice testing, whether or not a target had changed position during a saccadic eye movement, although correction saccades and manual aiming movements directed at the target showed near-perfect adjustments for the unpredictable target shift. In other words, an illusory perceptual constancy of target position was maintained in the face of large amendments in visuomotor control. In another recent example,

it has been reported that the compelling illusion of slowed motion of a moving coloured object that is experienced at equiluminance does not prevent accurate ocular pursuit under the same conditions (see reference to Lisberger and Movshon, cited in reference 59). Such observations may illustrate the independent functioning of the ventral and dorsal systems in normal humans.

We do not, however, wish to claim that the division of labour we are proposing is an absolute one. In particular, the above suggestion does not imply that visual inputs are necessarily blocked from awareness during visuomotor acts, although that may be a useful option to have available. Rather, we assume that the two systems will often be simultaneously activated (with somewhat different visual information), thereby providing visual experience during skilled action. Indeed, the two systems appear to engage in direct crosstalk; for example, the posterior parietal and inferotemporal cortex themselves interconnect[33,60] and both in turn project to areas in the superior temporal sulcus.[11-13] There, cells that are highly form selective lie close to others that have motion specificity,[44] thus providing scope for cooperation between the two systems (see figure 12.1). In addition, there are many polysensory neurons in these areas, so that not only visual but also cross-modal interaction between these networks may be possible. This may provide some of the integration needed for the essential unity and cohesion of most of our perceptual experience and behaviour, although overall control of awareness may ultimately be the responsibility of superordinate structures in the frontal cortex.[61] Nevertheless, it is feasible to maintain the hypothesis that a *necessary condition* for conscious visual experience is that the ventral system be activated.

Concluding Remarks

Despite the interactions between the dorsal and ventral systems, the converging lines of evidence reviewed above indicate that each stream uses visual information about objects and events in the world in different ways. These differences are largely a reflection of the specific transformations of input required by perception and action. Functional modularity in cortical visual systems, we believe, extends from input right through to output.

Acknowledgments

The authors are grateful to D. Carey, L. Jakobson, and D. Perrett for their comments on a draft of this paper.

Selected References

1. Schneider, G. E. (1969) *Science* 163, 895–902

2. Ingle, D. J. (1982) in *Analysis of Visual Behavior* (Ingle, D. J., Goodale, M. A. and Mansfield, R. J. W., eds), pp. 67–109, MIT Press

3. Goodale, M. A. and Murison, R. (1975) *Brain Res.* 88, 243–255

4. Goodale, M. A. and Milner, A. D. (1982) in *Analysis of Visual Behavior* (Ingle, D. J., Goodale, M. A. and Mansfield, R. J. W., eds), pp. 263–299, MIT Press

5. Ungerleider, L. G. and Mishkin, M. (1982) in *Analysis of Visual Behavior* (Ingle, D. J., Goodale, M. A. and Mansfield, R. J. W., eds), pp. 549–586, MIT Press

6. Gross, C. G. (1973) *Prog. Physiol. Psychol.* 5, 77–123

7. Pohl, W. (1973) *J. Comp. Physiol. Psychol.* 82, 227–239

8. Ungerleider, L. G. and Brody, B. A. (1977) *Exp. Neurol.* 56, 265–280

9. Milner, A. D., Ockleford, E. M. and Dewar, W. (1977) *Cortex* 13, 350–360

10. Desimone, R. and Ungerleider, L. G. (1989) in *Handbook of Neuropsychology*, Vol. 2 (Boller, F. and Grafman, J., eds), pp. 267–299, Elsevier

11. Boussaoud, D., Ungerleider, L. G. and Desimone, R. (1990) *J. Comp. Neurol.* 296, 462–495

12. Morel, A. and Bullier, J. (1990) *Visual Neurosci.* 4, 555–578

13. Baizer, J. S., Ungerleider, L. G. and Desimone, R. (1991) *J. Neurosci.* 11, 168–190

14. Livingstone, M. and Hubel, D. (1988) *Science* 240, 740–749

15. DeYoe, E. A. and Van Essen, D. C. (1988) *Trends Neurosci.* 11, 219–226

16. Schiller, P. H. and Logothetis, N. K. (1990) *Trends Neurosci.* 13, 392–398

17. Maunsell, J. H. R., Nealy, T. A. and De Priest, D. D. (1990) *J. Neurosci.* 10, 3323–3334

18. Nealey, T. A. and Maunsell, J. H. R. (1991) *Invest. Ophthalmol. Visual Sci.* 32 (Suppl.) 1117

19. Ferrera, V. P., Nealey, T. A. and Maunsell, J. H. R. (1991) *Invest. Ophthalmol. Visual Sci.* 32 (Suppl.) 1117

20. Goodale, M. A. (1983) in *Behavioral Approaches to Brain Research* (Robinson, T. E., ed.), pp. 41–61, Oxford University Press

21. Goodale, M. A. (1988) in *Computational Processes in Human Vision: An Interdisciplinary Perspective* (Pylyshyn, Z., ed.), pp. 262–285, Ablex

22. Sparks, D. L. and May, L. E. (1990) *Annu. Rev. Neurosci.* 13, 309–336

23. Newcombe, F., Ratcliff, G. and Damasio, H. (1987) *Neuropsychologia* 25, 149–161

24. Farah, M. (1990) *Visual Agnosia*, MIT Press

25. Perenin, M.-T. and Vighetto, A. (1988) *Brain* 111, 643–674

26. Jakobson, L. S., Archibald, Y. M., Carey, D. and Goodale, M. A. (1991) *Neuropsychologia* 29, 803–809

27. Milner, B. (1965) *Neuropsychologia* 3, 317–338

28. Smith, M. L. and Milner, B. (1989) *Neuropsychologia* 27, 71–81

29. Ettlinger, G. (1990) *Cortex* 26, 319–341

30. Milner, A. D. et al. (1991) *Brain* 114, 405–428

31. Goodale, M. A., Milner, A. D., Jakobson, L. S. and Carey, D. P. (1991) *Nature* 349, 154–156

32. Andersen, R. A. (1987) in *Higher Functions of the Brain, Part 2 (The Nervous System, Vol. V, Handbook of Physiology, Section 1)* (Mountcastle, V. B., Plum, F. and Geiger, S. R., eds), pp. 483–518, American Physiological Association

33. Andersen, R. A., Asanuma, C., Essick, G. and Siegel, R. M. (1990) *J. Comp. Neurol.* 296, 65–113

34. Taira, M., Mine, S., Georgopoulos, A. P., Murata, A. and Sakata, H. (1990) *Exp. Brain Res.* 83, 29–36

35. Felleman, D. J. and Van Essen, D. C. (1987) *J. Neurophysiol.* 57, 889–920

36. Mountcastle, V. B., Motter, B. C., Steinmetz, M. A. and Duffy, C. J. (1984) in *Dynamic Aspects of Neocortical Function* (Edelman, G. M., Gall, W. E. and Cowan, W. M., eds), pp. 159–193, Wiley

37. Perrett, D. I., Mistlin, A. J., Harries, M. H. and Chitty, A. J. (1990) in *Vision and Action: The Control of Grasping* (Goodale, M. A., ed.), pp. 163–180, Ablex

38. Cavada, C. and Goldman-Rakic, P. S. (1989) *J. Comp. Neurol.* 287, 422–445

39. Gentilucci, M. and Rizzolatti, G. (1990) in *Vision and Action: The Control of Grasping* (Goodale, M. A., ed.), pp. 147–162, Ablex

40. Milner, A. D. and Goodale, M. A. (1993) *Prog. Brain Res.*

41. Bates, J. A. V. and Ettlinger, G. (1960) *Arch. Neurol.* 3, 177–192

42. Faugier-Grimaud, S., Frenois, C. and Stein, D. G. (1978) *Neuropsychologia* 16, 151–168

43. Haaxma, R. and Kuypers, H. G. J. M. (1975) *Brain* 98, 239–260

44. Perrett, D. I., Mistlin, A. J. and Chitty, A. J. (1987) *Trends Neurosci.* 10, 358–364

45. Pribram, K. H. (1967) in *Brain Function and Learning* (Lindsley, D. B. and Lumsdaine, A. A., eds), pp. 79–122, University of California Press

46. Perrett, D. I. et al. (1991) *Exp. Brain Res.* 86, 159–173

47. Humphrey, N. K. and Weiskrantz, L. (1969) *Quart. J. Exp. Psychol.* 21, 225–238

48. Weiskrantz, L. and Saunders, R. C. (1984) *Brain* 107, 1033–1072

49. Marr, D. (1982) *Vision*, Freeman

50. Goldberg, M. E. and Colby, C. L. (1989) in *Handbook of Neuropsychology* (Vol. 2) (Boller, F. and Grafman, J., eds), pp. 301–315, Elsevier

51. Bushnell, M. C., Goldberg, M. E. and Robinson, D. L. (1981) *J. Neurophysiol.* 46, 755–772

52. Lawler, K. A. and Cowey, A. (1987) *Exp. Brain Res.* 65, 695–698

53. Fischer, B. and Boch, R. (1981) *Exp. Brain Res.* 44, 129–137

54. Moran, J. and Desimone, R. (1985) *Science* 229, 782–784

55. Rizzolatti, G., Gentilucci, M. and Matelli, M. (1985) in *Attention and Performance XI* (Posner, M. I. and Marin, O. S. M., eds), pp. 251–265, Erlbaum

56. Tipper, S., Lortie, C. and Baylis, G. (1992) *J. Exp. Psychol. Human Percept. Perform.* 18 (4), 891–905

57. Warrington, E. K. and Taylor, A. M. (1973) *Cortex* 9, 152–164

58. Goodale, M. A., Pelisson, D. and Prablanc, C. (1986) *Nature* 320, 748–750

59. Sejnowski, T. J. (1991) *Nature* 352, 669–670

60. Cavada, C. and Goldman-Rakic, P. S. (1989) *J. Comp. Neurol.* 287, 393–421

61. Posner, M. I. and Rothbart, M. K. (1991) in *The Neuropsychology of Consciousness* (Milner, A. D. and Rugg, M. D., eds), pp. 91–111, Academic Press

13 Consciousness and Isomorphism

Stephen E. Palmer

In this chapter I consider a fascinating problem about consciousness that has intrigued philosophers and scientists since ancient times. Simply put, the question is whether your conscious experiences of color are the same as mine when we both look at the same environmental objects under the same physical conditions. I will call this ontological problem the "color question." I will also consider the important epistemological follow-up question: "... and how could we possibly know?"

The color question is related to an equally old philosophical issue called "the problem of other minds." Here one asks whether organisms or beings other than one's self are conscious or not, ... and how one could know. The color question is not the same as the problem of other minds, in part because the standard position in the color question is to grant that the other being has conscious experiences of color, and to ask only whether those color experiences are the same as one's own under the same conditions. More radical versions of the color question can also be framed—such as the possibility that I have qualitatively different color experiences or even none at all—and I will consider them as well.

The reader may already be wondering why color should be the focus of such a discussion. Why not ask the "pitch question" about sounds or the "saltiness question" about tastes, or whatever might be one's own favorite aspects of sensory experience? Indeed, all of these are perfectly good versions of the same underlying question, which we can call the "qualia question": are my sensory experiences (or qualia) the same as yours or not, ... and how can we know?

Different people have different reasons for focusing on color. My own reason is that we actually know an enormous amount about color perception, and this background of scientific knowledge makes it a good domain in which to ask such questions. I exploited this knowledge in my book (Palmer 1999), in which color vision plays a central role. I use it as the best example of why an interdisciplinary approach to vision is a good idea. Chapter 3 goes through the whole "color story" in detail, all the way from photon wavelengths and retinal cone types to how people in different cultures name colors using basic color terms. It really is a beautiful example. So, when I finally reached the last chapter, which is about visual awareness, I thought an analysis of color might shed some light on the problem of consciousness. And I think it does, in large part because of the huge base of facts that have accumulated over years of scientific research.

Others favor color for historical reasons. In particular, there is a very well known and persuasive argument in the philosophical literature, called the "inverted spectrum argument," that claims to show that we simply cannot know whether or not your color experiences are the same as mine. John Locke advanced this argument in 1690, and it has the following form. There isn't any way you could know whether my experiences of colors are the same as yours or whether they are spectrally inverted. For example, the spatial ordering of my color experiences on viewing the rainbow, going from top to bottom, might literally be inverted relative to yours. If this were the case, you would experience the rainbow with red at the top and violet at the bottom, but I would experience it with violet at the top and red at the bottom. We would both call the top color "red" and the bottom color "violet," of course, because that is what we have all been taught by our parents, teachers, and society at large. Everyone calls blood, ripe tomatoes, and Macintosh apples "red," so we all associate our internal color experiences on viewing these objects—and similarly colored ones—with this verbal label. But might not my internal experiences of color be inverted in just the way

Locke (1690/1987) suggested without its having any effect on how I behave in naming colors? Indeed, Locke claimed that such a spectral inversion of color experience could exist without there being *any* external manifestation, through naming or other observable behavior. It seems there just isn't any way to tell, because I cannot "get inside your head," and "have your experiences," nor can you have mine.

In this chapter I claim that there are ways of rejecting this particular argument without getting inside each other's heads and having each other's experiences. In fact, there is good, solid empirical evidence from behavioral psychology that at least this literal interpretation of Locke's argument is surely false. Once we see why, we can go on to ask whether there is any other transformation of your color experience that I might have without it being detectable in my behavior. There is an interesting generalization revealed by this line of reasoning that leads to an important distinction—which I call the *isomorphism constraint*—between what can and cannot be known about the correspondence of our experiences from behavioral evidence. But before we get to the isomorphism constraint, we need to go back and ground the discussion about color experience in scientific fact to evaluate Locke's argument rigorously.

To begin, we must ask how we could possibly get a scientific handle on a question that asks about the relation between our color experiences. It is pretty obvious that we cannot carry out the thought experiment Locke suggested with real people. What we can do instead is to analyze the inverted spectrum argument from what we know about color science and to see whether any known behavioral data would reveal such an inversion, if it existed.

Color Spaces

One important thing we can measure behaviorally about color experiences is their relative similarities. Everybody with normal color vision

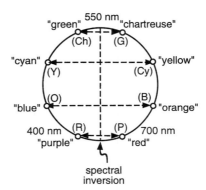

Figure 13.1
Newton's color circle and spectral inversion. Colors are arranged along the perimeter of a color circle, as indicated by the names on the outside of the circle. The dashed diameter indicates the axis of reflection corresponding to literal spectral inversion (rainbow reversal), and the dashed arrows indicate corresponding experiences under this transformation. Letters in parentheses inside the circle indicate the color experiences a spectrally inverted individual would have with the same physical stimuli a normal individual would experience as the colors indicated on the outside of the circle.

agrees, for example, that red is more similar to orange than it is to green. These relative similarities can be obtained for a large sample of triples of colors. It turns out that the results of measuring these three-way similarities can be summarized quite neatly in a geometric model of color experiences known as a *color space*. Each point in a color space corresponds to a color experience, and proximities between points correspond to similarities between colors. This means that nearby points in color space correspond to similar color experiences, and distant points in color space correspond to different color experiences.

Perhaps the simplest and best known color space is Newton's color circle, which is represented in figure 13.1. The saturated colors of the rainbow are arrayed around most of the perimeter of the circle. A few wavelengths of light that give rise to these colors are indicated around the outside of the circle, together with English names for a small sample of these colors. This color circle is not the most complete or accurate representation of human color experiences, but it is a good starting point for understanding how behavioral data can constrain the answer to the color question.

One of the interesting things about this geometrical representation of color similarities is that it allows a simple and transparent way to determine whether inverting the spectrum could be detected by behavioral measurements of color similarities. Within the color circle, inverting the spectrum is simply a reflection about the diameter passing through 550 nm, which is approximately the midpoint of the visible spectrum that ranges from 400 to 700 nm. Figure 13.1 illustrates this idea. The color experiences you have are indicated by abbreviations around the outside of the circle, and the ones I have are indicated around the inside. When you experience red (on the outside of this circle), I experience purple (on the inside of this circle); when you experience yellow (outside the circle), I experience cyan (inside the circle); and so forth. So there really is a difference between our color experiences. The dashed arrows in figure 13.1 indicate how our color experiences correspond to each other, a transformation that can be modeled simply by reflection about the indicated spectral inversion axis in color space.

But would these differences be detectible through measures of color similarities? You would say that red is more similar to orange than to green (because the outside point for red is closer to the outside point for orange than it is to the outside point for green). But I would say the same thing, even though, for me, it would correspond to experiencing purple as more similar to blue than to chartreuse (as reflected by proximities of the same points on the inside of the circle). And in fact, all the color similarity judgments you and I would make would be out-

wardly the same, even though our experiences would be inwardly different. This is just what Locke expected, and it supports his conclusion that spectral inversion would not be detectable.

The reason such differences could not be detected by similarity measures is that the color circle is symmetric with respect to reflection about this axis. We can therefore conclude that so-called spectral inversion of color experiences could not be detected by measurements of color similarity. Furthermore, we can see that this particular transformation is only one of many ways that my color experiences might differ from yours without the difference being detected by measuring color similarities. Any reflection about an axis passing through the center of the color circle would do as well, and so would any rotation about the center. In all these cases, our color experiences would indeed differ, but all our statements about the relative similarities of color samples would be the same.

But there is a great deal more that we can measure behaviorally about color experiences than just their similarities. Among the most important additional factors are relations of color composition, some of which are illustrated in figure 13.2. Most colors look like they are composed of other more primitive colors. Orange, for example, looks like it contains both red and yellow. Purple looks like it contains both red and blue. But there is a particular shade of red that is pure in the sense that it contains no traces of yellow or blue or any other color—it looks "just plain red." And people with so-called normal color vision agree about this fact. Nobody claims, for example, that red actually looks like a mixture of orange and purple, even though it lies between these two colors in color space. Color scientists call these experientially pure colors "unique colors," and there are four of them: unique red, unique yellow, unique green, and unique blue. They are indicated in figure 13.2 by the shaded boxes on the outside of the circle and the color names with boxes around them. All the rest are so-called binary colors.

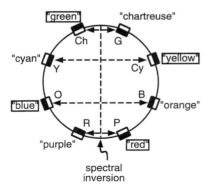

Figure 13.2
Detecting rainbow reversal via unique colors. Shaded rectangles on the outside of the circle represent the four compositionally pure colors (unique red, green, blue, and yellows) for a "normal" trichromat. Shaded rectangles on the inside represent the corresponding pure colors to a rainbow reversed individual, who would perceive unique colors at orange, purple, cyan (blue-green), and chartreuse (yellow-green).

The existence of these four unique colors provides another behavioral tool for detecting color transformations. Consider spectral inversion again, this time from the perspective of unique hues. Figure 13.2 shows unique color experiences as gray rectangles. You will designate unique hues at red, blue, green, and yellow (where the gray rectangles are on the outside of the circle), but I will designate them at what we call orange, purple, cyan, and chartreuse (where the gray rectangles are on the inside of the circle). The reason is simply that the experience of mine that is the same as your experience of unique red, results from my looking at color samples that we all call "purple." So for me, "purple" is a unique hue and "red" is not, whereas for you, "red" is a unique hue and "purple" is not. This behavioral difference can thus be used to unmask a rainbow-reversed individual, if such a person existed.

This example shows that unique hues and other relations of color composition further con-

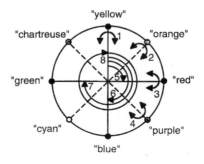

Symmetries of the Color Circle

Reflectional:
    1. yellow-blue axis
    2. orange-cyan axis
    3. red-green axis
    4. purple-chartreuse axis

Rotational:
    5. 90 degrees
    6. 180 degrees
    7. 270 degrees
    8. 360 degrees (identity)

Figure 13.3
Symmetries of the color circle with respect to color similarities and color composition. This diagram indicates the four central reflections and four central rotations over which the structure of the color circle is transformationally invariant.

strain the set of color transformations that can escape detection. We can now rule out literal spectral inversion in the sense of simply reversing the rainbow. Even so, there are still eight color transformations that will pass all behavioral tests of color similarity and composition with respect to the color circle. They are indicated in figure 13.3 as the four central reflections about the unique hue axes (red-green and blue-yellow) and their bisectors (Transformations 1–4 and the four central rotations of 90, 180, 270, and 360 degrees (Transformations 5–8). All have the crucial property that they map unique hues into other unique hues in addition to preserving relative similarity relations among colors.

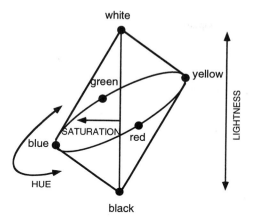

Figure 13.4
Three-dimensional color space. Colors are represented as points in a three-dimensional space according to the dimensions of hue, saturation, and lightness. The positions of the six unique colors (or Hering primaries) within this space are shown by filled circles.

By now, the reader can probably see where this argument is leading. Color transformations that can escape behavioral detection correspond to symmetries in an empirically constrained color space. The important issue for answering Locke's version of the color question, then, boils down to whether there are any symmetries in human color space. If there are, then my color experiences might differ from yours by the corresponding symmetry transformation.

Until now I have been pretending that the color circle, as augmented by the distinguished set of unique hues, is sufficient to represent what is known about human color experience. But there is a great deal more we know about color that is relevant to answering the color question. Most importantly, human color space is actually three-dimensional rather than two-dimensional. The three dimensions are usually called hue, saturation, and lightness, and together they define the lopsided spindle structure diagrammed in figure 13.4. The important fact about the three-

dimensional color spindle for purposes of this discussion is that it breaks many of the symmetries in the color circle.

Of most relevance is the fact that highly saturated yellows are quite a bit lighter than highly saturated blues. This asymmetry makes some further color transformations detectable by purely behavioral means. Any transformation in which your experience of yellow is supposed to be the same as my experience of blue (or vice versa) will be detectable because you will say that yellow is lighter than blue, whereas I will say that blue is lighter than yellow (because yellow looks to me like blue does to you, and vice versa). This difference can certainly be detected behaviorally—unless the lightness dimension of my color experience is *also* reversed, so that what looks black to you looks white to me, and what looks white to you looks black to me.

The upshot of such considerations is that if human color space has approximately the structure shown in figure 13.4, there are just three possible color transformations that might escape detection in experiments that assess color similarity and composition relations. They correspond to the three approximate symmetries of human color space shown in figure 13.5. Relative to the so-called normal space in figure 13.4, one transformation (figure 13.5a) reverses just the red-green dimension. The second (figure 13.5b) reverses blue-for-yellow and black-for-white, but not red-for-green. The third (figure 13.5c) is the composition of the other two, which calls for reflecting all three dimensions: red-for-green, blue-for-yellow, and black-for-white.

Although all three are logically possible, the simplest and by far the most plausible is reflecting just the red-green dimension. Indeed, it is so plausible that a good argument can be made that such red-green reversed perceivers actually exist in the population of so-called normal trichromats (Nida-Rümelin 1996). The argument, in a nutshell, goes like this. As figure 13.6 indicates, normal trichromats have three different pigments in their three cone types. Some people are

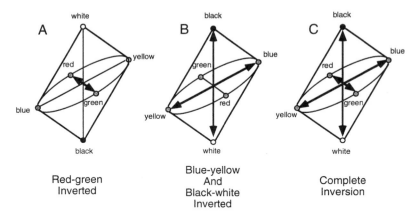

Figure 13.5
Three approximate symmetries of color space. The color space depicted in figure 13.4 has three approximate symmetries: reversal of the red-green dimensions only (*A*), reversal of both the blue-yellow and black-white dimensions (*B*), and reversal of all three dimensions (*C*).

red-green color blind because they have a gene that causes their long-wavelength cones to have the same pigment as their medium-wavelength cones. These people are called protanopes, and their M and L cones are colored gray to indicate that they have the M-pigment in both. Other people have a different form of red-green color blindness because they have a different gene that causes their medium-wavelength cones to have the same pigment as their long-wavelength cones. These people are called deuteranopes, and their M and L cones are colored black to indicate that they both have the L-pigment. In both cases, people with these genetic defects lose the ability to experience both red and green because the visual system codes both by taking the difference between the outputs of these two cone types. But suppose that someone had the genes for both forms of red-green color blindness simultaneously. Their L-cones would have the M-pigment and their M-cones would have the L-pigment. Such people would therefore not be red-green color blind at all, but simply red-green reversed trichromats. They should exist, and if

they do, they are proof that this color transformation is either undetectable or very difficult to detect by purely behavioral means because nobody has ever managed to find one!

There is a great deal more that can be said about the behavioral detectability of color transformations. One key issue for the existence of symmetries in color space is the possible relevance of the basic color terms and basic color categories discovered by Berlin and Kay (1969) in their ground-breaking cross-linguistic studies of color naming. To explain their relevance, I will have to make a brief digression to summarize their findings and theories.

Berlin and Kay made enormous headway in understanding how people describe colors linguistically by restricting their analysis to a basic core of terms. In doing so, they uncovered a very small number of words across all languages that can be used to name all possible colors. They called these words basic color terms (BCTs). BCTs are single, frequently used words that refer exclusively or primarily to colors rather than objects. In English, for example, there are 11

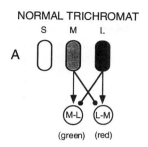

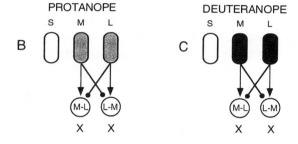

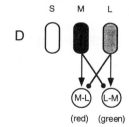

Figure 13.6

A biologically plausible mechanism for red-green inversion. Part *A* shows the "normal" photopigments for short (S), medium (M), and long (L) wavelength sensitive cones. Part *B* shows the result of one form of genetically determined red-green color blindness (both M and L cones have the normal M-cone pigment). Part *C* shows the result of the other form of genetically determined red-green color blindness (both M and L cones have the normal L-cone pigment). Part *D* shows the hypothetical result of both forms of red-green color blindness, which should lead to red-green color reversal.

BCTs: RED, GREEN, BLUE, YELLOW, BLACK, WHITE, GRAY, ORANGE, PURPLE, BROWN, and PINK. (Words like TURQUOISE and SILVER are not included because they refer primarily to substances and only secondarily to colors, and words like CHARTREUSE and CYAN are ruled out because they are not frequent enough.) Still, there are some BCTs that do not appear in English. In Russian, for example, there is a putative BCT (GOLUBOI) for light blue, analogous to PINK in English. In other languages with less fully developed color terms, there are four BCTs that do not appear in English. They can be translated roughly as WARM (yellows, oranges, and reds), COOL (blues and greens), LIGHT-WARM (warm colors plus whites), and DARK-COOL (cool colors plus blacks).

Kay and McDaniel (1978) further analyzed these 16 BCTs into three different types of basic color categories (BCCs), which they called *primary*, *derived*, and *composite*. The most basic are the six primary categories: RED, GREEN, BLUE, YELLOW, BLACK, and WHITE—which they modeled as fuzzy sets with a degree of membership that varies continuously from zero to unity (Zadeh 1965). From these, Kay and McDaniel derived six more categories by the fuzzy-logical AND-ing of two primary color categories:

GRAY is derived from WHITE AND BLACK,

ORANGE is derived from RED AND YELLOW,

PURPLE is derived from RED AND BLUE,

BROWN is derived from BLACK AND YELLOW,

PINK is derived from WHITE AND RED,

GOLUBOI (a Russian word) is derived from WHITE AND BLUE.

Notice that this set does not include all possible combinations of primary BCCs. Some are ruled out by the structure of color space itself: red-

green and blue-yellow cannot exist because they simply do not overlap and therefore would have no exemplars in the their fuzzy-logical intersection. Other combinations could exist as BCTs but do not for as-yet-unknown reasons. The combinatorially "missing" BCTs would refer to blue-green, yellow-green, light-green, light-yellow, dark-blue, dark-green, and dark-red.

The other four "composite" color categories are formed by the fuzzy-logical OR-ing of two or more primary color categories:

WARM is composed of RED OR YELLOW,

COOL is composed of GREEN OR BLUE,

LIGHT-WARM is composed of WHITE OR WARM which can be defined as WHITE OR RED OR YELLOW,

DARK-COOL is composed of BLACK OR COOL, which can be defined as BLACK OR GREEN OR BLUE.

Again, not all possible combinations of primary BCCs exist as composite BCTs. It seems reasonable that they be restricted to combinations of nearby primary BCCs in color space, ruling out RED OR GREEN and BLUE OR YELLOW. But it is not clear why there are few or no composite BCTs for RED OR BLUE, GREEN OR YELLOW, WHITE OR COOL, or BLACK OR WARM. These and other mysteries remain to be solved.

The relevance of basic color terms to the inverted spectrum argument is that they may place further behavioral constraints on what color transformations can escape behavioral detection. Many researchers believe that the existence of basic color terms reflects a corresponding set of underlying BCCs into which color experience is naturally partitioned. Because BCTs appear to be linguistically universal, it seems likely that there is something in the underlying structure of human color experience that supports these partitions rather than others that are equally logical. Why are there BCTs for

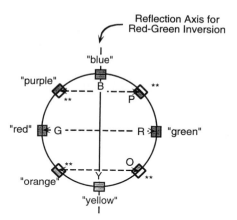

Figure 13.7
Detecting red-green reversal via basic color terms.
Shaded rectangles on the outside of the circle represent focal colors of BCTs for a "normal" trichromat, and open rectangles (**) indicate the lack of BCT. The shading of rectangles on the inside of the circle indicates corresponding BCTs for red-green reversed trichromats.

ORANGE and PURPLE, for instance, but not for BLUE-GREEN or YELLOW-GREEN?

Let us now consider the implications of these facts and theories about BCTs for the detection of color transformations via asymmetries in color space. No symmetry problems arise for the six primary BCTs—RED, GREEN, BLUE, YELLOW, BLACK, and WHITE—because they are the same as the six unique colors we have already considered in discussing color composition relations. But if the other ten of Berlin and Kay's basic color terms also arise from singularities in the structure of human color space, then all possible symmetries are broken. Consider, for example, how a red-green invertomat might be detected using the derived BCTs. If I am red-green inverted, I should find it implausible that there are basic color terms for orange and purple, but not for blue-green and yellow-green, as illustrated in figure 13.7. The

reason is that my experience of orange is like yours of yellow-green (and vice versa), and my experience of purple is like yours of blue-green (and vice versa). If this asymmetry in basic color categories is rooted in corresponding asymmetries in color experience, I should prefer there to be BCTs for mixtures of what we all call "greens," like cyan and chartreuse (which for me, remember, are experienced as what you would call purple and orange) than for the mixtures of reds (which for me are blue-greens and yellow-greens).

Another asymmetry in BCCs that would unmask a red-green invertomat is the fact that there is a BCT for light-red (PINK) and not for light-green. If I were a red-green invertomat, I should also find this strange, if indeed there is some corresponding asymmetry in color experience. The other two candidate symmetries of color space discussed earlier—complete inversion and blue-yellow plus black-white inversion—are similarly broken by other contrasts where BCTs are not symmetrically arranged in color space.

I am personally not totally convinced that these experiential asymmetries, assuming they exist, would be easily detected in behavior. They seem to be fairly subtle distinctions, and it is conceivable that cultural learning might be strong enough to overpower them. Even if I were a red-green invertomat, the fact that I had been trained all my life with color categories for ORANGE and PURPLE, but not blue-green or yellow-green, might have so firmly changed my thinking about colors that I would not find this way of carving up color experience at all strange, even though I should, at least in principle. Perhaps this is why no red-green invertomats have ever been found, even though they presumably exist.

In any event, the main point of my presentation to this point is that the symmetries of an empirically constrained color space are the key issue in the scientific evaluation of Locke's inverted spectrum argument. I have further argued that good solid behavioral evidence can be brought to bear on this old philosophical question, and that it rules out all or all-but-three possible transformations, depending on whether one includes BCTs or not. The question I want to turn to now is *why* symmetries of color space are crucial in this argument. This will lead to the second main point of this chapter, which is to identify what I call the "isomorphism constraint" and to discuss its role in the scientific analysis of the color question.

The Isomorphism Constraint

Symmetries have two important structural properties. First, they are what mathematicians call *automorphisms*: they map a given domain onto itself in a one-to-one fashion. This is important for the inverted spectrum argument because one of the ground rules is that both you and I have the same set of color experiences; they are just differently hooked up to the external world. Automorphism is not all that important for the more general color question or other forms of the qualia question, however, because my experience in response to stimulation by wavelengths of light might not be automorphically related to yours. My color space, for example, might be a somewhat shrunken version of yours, such that you would experience colors as more vivid and highly saturated than I do. One might think this would be detectable by the number of jnd's (just noticeable differences) between color pairs, but it wouldn't be if I were simply more sensitive to small differences in my experience than you were, thus compensating for the smaller size of my color space.

More radically, however, we can drop the requirement of automorphism entirely, for my color experiences might be nothing at all like yours. You and I could live in entirely different dimensions of experiential space, so to speak, and it would not matter with respect to what could be inferred about our color experiences

from purely behavioral measures. Still more radically, I might have no color experiences at all! I might be a color zombie who processes information about wavelengths of light, yet has no experiences of color whatsoever. (In fact, I know this to be quite untrue of myself, but it might conceivably be true to you!) In any case, if non-automorphic transformations of color experience are allowed, the presence or absence of symmetries within color space becomes irrelevant, and only the other structural property of symmetry matters.

This other property of symmetries is that they are what mathematicians call *isomorphisms*. Isomorphisms are functions that map a source domain onto a target domain in such a way that relational structure among elements in the source domain is preserved by relational structure among corresponding elements in the target domain. In the case of symmetries, the source and target domains are the same (because symmetries are automorphic isomorphisms), but this is not the case for isomorphisms in general. Figure 13.8 illustrates the basic requirements for an isomorphism to hold, using color space as an example. The objects of the source domain (in this case, color experiences) are mapped into those of the target domain (in this case, points in three-dimensional space) so that experiential relations between colors are preserved by corresponding spatial relations between points in color space. This is why spatial models work so well for color experience: They have the same intrinsic structure.

I want to argue that it is isomorphism— "having the same structure"—that is crucial for behavioral equivalence of conscious experiences. This means that as long as two people have the same structure of relations among their color experiences—whatever those experiences might be, in and of themselves—they will always give the same behavioral responses and therefore be behaviorally indistinguishable.

There appears to be a behaviorally defined brick wall, which I will call the subjectivity bar-

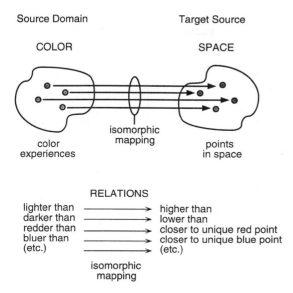

Source Domain   Target Source

COLOR   SPACE

isomorphic mapping

color experiences   points in space

RELATIONS

lighter than ———————→ higher than
darker than ———————→ lower than
redder than ———————→ closer to unique red point
bluer than ———————→ closer to unique blue point
(etc.) ———————→ (etc.)

isomorphic mapping

Figure 13.8
The color/space isomorphism. Color experiences are mapped into points in a multidimensional space (see figure 13.4) such that color relations (e.g., *lighter-than, redder-than*) are preserved by corresponding spatial relations (e.g., *higher-than, closer-to-unique-red-point*).

rier, that limits which aspects of aspects of our experience we can share and which we cannot, no matter how hard we might try. The importance of the isomorphism constraint is that it provides a clear dividing line: the part we can share is the structure in the relations; the part we cannot share is the nature of the experiences themselves. In the case of color experience, this means that we share relational facts such as that red is more like orange than it is like green, that gray is intermediate between black and white, that purple looks like it contains both red and blue, and that there is a shade of red that is compositionally pure. We can share them because they are about the relational structure of experiences. We may implicitly (or even explicitly) believe that we share the experiences too, at least in the sense of supposing that everyone else's are the same as ours, but that does not make it true!

Such arguments suggest to me, as figure 13.9 attempts to depict, that the subjectivity barrier divides shared relations from private experiences and thus coincides exactly with the condition of isomorphism. What I am calling the isomorphism constraint is simply the conjecture that behavior is sufficient to specify experience to the level of isomorphism and not beyond.

The picture that emerges is that the nature of individual color experiences cannot be uniquely fixed by behavioral means, but their structural interrelations can be. In case anyone feels disappointed in this, I hasten to point out that structural relations are absolutely crucial to the fabric of our mental life. Without them, redness would be as much like greenness as it is like orangeness ... or whiteness, or squareness, or middle C, or the taste of pumpkin pie. Without them, perceptual qualities would just be so many equally different experiences, and this certainly is

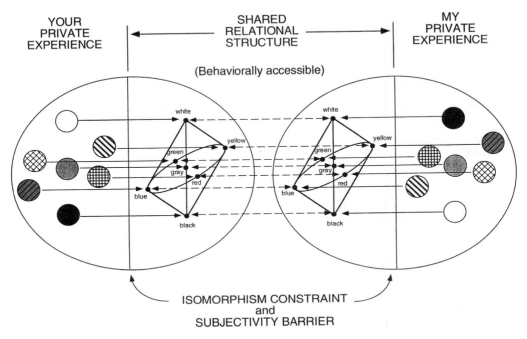

Figure 13.9
The proposed relations among private experiences, shared relational structure, the isomorphism constraint, and the subjectivity barrier in the domain of color perception. Relational structure is publically accessible via observable behavior only to the level of isomorphism. Beyond this level lies the qualitative nature of private experiences.

not so. But, by the same token, structural relations do not reflect everything one would like to know about experiences, for the isomorphism constraint implies that, logically speaking, any set of underlying experiences will do for color, provided they relate to each other in the required way. The same argument can be extended quite generally to other perceptual and conceptual domains, although both the underlying experiential components and their relational structure will obviously be different.

Behavioral scientists are not alone in working within the constraint of isomorphism, for it also exists in mathematics. In classical mathematics, a domain is formalized by specifying a set of primitive elements (e.g., points, lines, planes, and

three-dimensional spaces in geometry) and a set of axioms that specify the relations among them (e.g., two points uniquely determine a line, three noncollinear points a plane, etc.). Given a set of primitive elements, a set of axioms, and the rules of mathematical deduction, mathematicians can prove theorems that specify many further relations among mathematical objects within the domain. These theorems are guaranteed to be true if the axioms are true.

But the elements to which all the axioms and theorems refer cannot be fixed in any way except by the nature of the relations among them; they refer equally to any entities that satisfy the set of axioms. That is why mathematicians sometimes discover that there is an alternative interpreta-

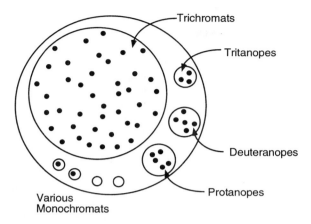

Figure 13.10
Equivalence classes of color perceivers. These Venn diagrams indicate the behaviorally defined equivalence classes of color perceivers who have isomorphic color experiences, but not necessarily equivalent color experiences.

tion of the primitive elements, called a *dual system*, in which all the same statements hold. For example, the points lines, planes, and spaces of projective geometry in three dimensions can be reinterpreted as spaces, planes, lines, and points, respectively, because all the same relations hold when the elements in the latter system are substituted systematically for their corresponding dual elements in the former system. All the same axioms hold, and therefore all the same theorems are true. An axiomatic mathematical system can therefore be conceived as a complex structure of mathematical relations on an underlying, but otherwise underfined, set of primitives that are free to vary in any way.

The brilliant French mathematician Poincaré (1952) put the situation very clearly. "Mathematicians do not study objects," he said, "but the relations between objects. To them it is a matter of indifference if these objects are replaced by others, provided that the relations do not change" (p. 20). The same can be said about behavioral scientists with respect to consciousness: we do not study experiences, but the relations among experiences. The isomorphism constraint therefore tells us exactly how far behavioral science can go in specifying experiences.

The Appeal to Biology

If the isomorphism constraint defines the limits of what can be known by behavioral means, figure 13.10 shows where this leaves us with respect to color. Based on psychophysical measures of color science, we can define the standard behavioral equivalence classes of color perception: so-called normal trichromats, three varieties of dichromats (protanopes and deuteranopes, who have slightly different forms of "red-green" color blindness, plus tritanopes, who have "blue-yellow" color blindness), and four types of monochromats. There are some further behavioral classes of so-called color weakness among trichromats that are not represented here, but this classification will do for now.

I have called these behaviorally defined equivalence classes, but with respect to statements about color experiences, it would be more accurate to call them "difference classes." Pairs of individuals who are in different classes certainly have different color experiences to the same stimulation. Beyond that, we cannot say. There may be many varieties of color experience within the set of normal trichromats, many others within the set of protanopes, and so forth. We just cannot tell on the basis of behavior alone, unless we make some pretty strong further assumptions, such as automorphism, which is difficult to justify at this point in our understanding of color science, given all the differences between different people's visual nervous systems.

This raises the important question of whether there is any way we can go beyond the level of isomorphism by applying biological methods, either alone or in concert with behavioral ones. It is tempting to believe that if consciousness is fundamentally a biological phenomenon, the answer must be, "Of course we can!" I am somewhat less optimistic, but I do not see the situation as completely hopeless, at least in principle, for reasons I will now try to explain.

It seems at first blush that one should be able to study subisomorphic differences in color experiences between two individuals by identifying relevant neurobiological differences and correlating them with differences in color experience, but this will not work. The problem is not in finding biological differences. We will presumably be able to identify the neural differences at whatever level current technology allows. The problem is that, try as we might, we won't be able to identify any subisomorphic differences in experience to correlate with the biological differences. The reason is simply that the subjectivity barrier is still very much in place. Whenever we try to asses how two people's experiences might differ, we can get no further than the isomorphism constraint.

Even so, quite a different line of thought suggests that biology must provide important constraints on the answer to the color question. It seems highly plausible, for example, that two clones, who have identical nervous systems, should have the same color experiences in response to the same stimulation. This is, in effect, a corollary of Kim's (1984) *principle of supervenience*: If the biology is the same, the experiences will be the same. (The converse is not necessarily true, however: If the experiences of two people are the same, the underlying biological processes might be the same, or they might be different.) Most cognitive scientists and neuroscientists ascribe to something like supervenience these days, although it is logically possible that the nature of experience depends on sub-biological facts about quarks, quantum gravity, or some even more esoteric physical entity that has yet to be conceived. I am not going to take such hypotheses seriously until I have to, and will therefore push on with conventional biological approaches, based on the assumption that clones have the same color experiences.

So, assuming the clone assumption to be well founded, is there any way this presumed subisomorphic level of conscious experience can be tapped? The only effective route I can see is one that avoids the subjectivity barrier to some extent by using within-subject designs. The idea is quite simple. Use a biological intervention on an individual and ask for reports about any changes in color experience from before to after the intervention. Suppose, for instance, there were a drug called invertacillin that exchanged the light-sensitive pigments in two classes of retina receptors. Let us also assume that the drug acts reasonably quickly, that it does not mysteriously alter people's long-term memories for object colors, and that it does not disturb the associations between internal experiences and color names. Then it seems plausible to suppose that subjects would indeed notice, and could reliably report, changes in their color experiences after taking the drug. If invertacillin swapped pigments in the medium- and long-wavelength cones, for example, they would presumably report that blood now looks green and grass now looks red. These are extreme examples, and subtler changes in experience would hopefully also

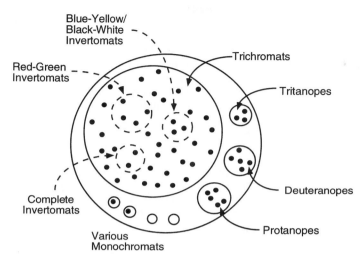

Figure 13.11
Hypothetical subisomorphic classes of color perceivers. Dashed circles indicate the possible existence of three classes of trichromats with color experiences that differ from those of "normal" trichromats at a subisomorphic level, corresponding to the three symmetries of color space indicated in figure 13.5.

be detectable. But the crucial point is that the same subisomorphic color transformations that are difficult or impossible to detect between individuals seem, in principle, quite easy to detect within individuals. Notice that we, as experimenters, have still not penetrated anyone's subjectivity barrier, for we don't actually know how blood or grass appeared to the subject either before or after the change. We only know that it reversed the red-green dimension of color experience, whatever that dimension might be like for that particular observer.

For the sake of argument, let us now suppose that we can figure out what the biological effects of the drug are and that it affects everyone's color experiences in the same way: namely, by reversing the red-green dimension of color space. Armed with this information, we can then divide the set of behaviorally defined trichromats into those who normally have the biological structure associated with the result of the invertacillin in-

tervention (labeled "Red-Green Invertomats" in figure 13.11) and those who do not. Notice that this biologically defined equivalence class does not imply equivalent color experiences for individuals within it. With respect to color experiences, they constitute a difference class, just like behaviorally defined difference classes. People in different difference classes have different color experiences, but people in the same difference class may or may not have the same color experiences. We cannot know whether people in the same class have the same experiences until we exhaust the set of all the relevant biological factors and all their possible interactions, which is a very large set indeed.

But suppose, for the sake of argument, that we could determine the complete catalog of the biological factors that are relevant to color experience in this way. Then we could, in principle, define real equivalence classes of people who presumably have the same color experiences.

Notice that such statements would always be inferences about two people having the same experiences based on certain assumptions, much like our earlier inference that two clones would have the same experiences based on knowledge that their biology is the same. We have plausible scientific reasons to believe that they would, but no way of testing it directly because of the subjectivity barrier. The clones themselves can neither confirm nor deny the conjecture, of course, because the subjectivity barrier exists for them as much as for everyone else.

But, if we were able to carry out this research program—and that may be too big an "if" for anyone but philosophers to swallow—it seems that we would, in principle, be able to infer what colors look like to at least some other people with reasonable certainty. People who are in the same biological equivalence class as yourself would experience the world pretty much as you do, within some reasonable margin of error. And people who are in at least some different equivalence classes might be inferred to have color experiences that differ from yours by identified transformations. If I am a red-green invertomat, for example, and you are a "normal trichromat"—and if the corresponding physiological difference were the only one in our chromatic neurobiology—then our experiences would differ specifically by the red-green inversion transformation caused by the invertacillin drug. You could then know what my color experiences of the world were like simply by taking invertacillin yourself.

But it is important to remember that the possibility that these color-transformed experiences enable you to know what the world looks like to me is necessarily based on inferences. You cannot have my experiences in any direct fashion because of the subjectivity barrier. The inference is based on at least two important assumptions. One is that any differences in experience result from standard biological differences. The other is that all relevant biological variables have been correctly taken into account. If either is false,

then the conclusion that you know what it is like to have my color experience by taking invertacillin is also false. Given the dubious nature of at least one of these assumptions, the chances of being able to bring this project off in reality are vanishingly small, even in the long run. Even so, I find the very possibility intriguing.

Acknowledgment

This chapter is based on an article to appear in *The Behavioral and Brain Sciences*. Its writing has been facilitated by grant R01-MH46141 from the National Institute of Mental Health to the author.

References

Berlin, B., and Kay, P. (1969) *Basic color terms: Their universality and evolution.* Berkeley: University of California Press.

Kay, P., and McDaniel, C. K. (1978) The linguistic significance of the meanings of basic color terms. *Language*, 54, 610–646.

Kim, J. (1984) Concepts of supervenience. *Philosophy and Phenomenological Research*, 65, 153–176.

Locke, J. (1690/1987) *An essay concerning human understanding.* Oxford: Clarendon Press.

Nida-Rümelin, M. (1996) Pseudonormal vision: An actual case of qualia inversion? *Philosophical Studies*, 82, 145–157.

Palmer, S. E. (1999) *Vision science: Photons to phenomenology.* Cambridge, MA: MIT Press.

Poincaré, H. (1952) *Science and hypothesis.* New York: Dover.

Zadeh, L. A. (1965) Fuzzy sets. *Information and Control*, 8, 338–353.

III ATTENTION: SELECTING ONE CONSCIOUS STREAM AMONG MANY

Consciousness is remarkably limited in capacity at any given moment. This is easy to show by asking people to pay attention to two incompatible things at the same time: typically, only one will become conscious at any given moment in time. In psychology, the first return to consciousness in modern times can be credited to Donald E. Broadbent, who adapted a simple and instructive experimental technique for the purpose, and suggested a basic theoretical metaphor to explain it (Broadbent 1958, Cherry 1953). Broadbent and colleagues presented people with two competing streams of speech. They asked subjects to "shadow" one stream—to say each word immediately, even while waiting for the next word. Rapid shadowing is a demanding task, and if one stream of speech is fed into one ear, it is not possible to experience much more than a vague vocal quality in the other ear. At the time, this seemed to indicate that human beings can fully process only one channel of information at a time. The role of attention, therefore, seemed to be to select one among the multiplicity of messages that may be coming to the senses at any given time (Broadbent 1958, James 1890/1983).

Given the behavioristic tenor of those times, consciousness was not seen as a source of limited capacity effects. Experiments were:

designed to be essentially objective and behavioristic; that is, the "subject" under test (the listener) is regarded as a transducer whose responses are observed when various stimuli are applied, whereas his subjective impressions are taken to be of minor importance. (Cherry 1953)

However, competing input tasks have two aspects: a selective one and an experiential one. The process of selecting one or another source of input is fundamental. But people in these experiments are also *conscious* of the selected stream: They report all its rich perceptual qualities, the timbre of the spoken voice, its rhythm, quality, and dialect, its location in space and distribution over time, its meanings and imme-

diate associations. All these features of the input come to consciousness as soon as it is selected. By contrast, any nonselected stream is unconscious, though it may be processed to quite a high level of analysis. Any competing input task therefore creates an opportunity to compare closely matched conscious and unconscious events; inherently, it allows us to "treat consciousness as a variable." (See Introduction.)

Yet the facts about consciousness in selective attention tasks has not received much research emphasis. Attention research has much to say about selection, but it is still very reluctant to acknowledge the conscious experience of selected input (e.g., Pashler 1997; on the distinction between attention and consciousness, see Baars 1998, 1999). Nevertheless, the same literature provides much incidental evidence on consciousness as such (e.g., Baars 1988, 1997, in press).

Psychological Evidence on Selective Attention

Much research has focused on whether selection occurs peripherally or centrally. Do neurons in the inner ear "turn down the volume" when attention shifts elsewhere? Or does selection take place in auditory cortex? Such debates are about "early versus late selection." The chapter by Treisman (1969; chap. 14, this volume) is a classic exploration of these positions.

The dominant theoretical metaphor of the time was the notion of a selective "filter" to weed out unneeded information in order to simplify input to the brain. Initially, the presumed filter was considered to be tuned to physical stimulus characteristics like sound frequency and source location. However, a little-known experiment by Gray and Wedderburn (1960) had profound implications for a richer conception of selective attention and consciousness. Gray and Wedderburn performed a standard dichotic shadowing experiment, with two streams of auditory information, one to each ear. One input stream consisted of spoken numbers and the other contained short, meaningful phrases like "Mice eat cheese." They alternated the two input channels between the ears at a rather rapid rate, a half second for each alternation—yet subjects still heard the meaningful phrases as a whole, regardless of the fact that the sound source alternated between the ears. Gray and Wedderburn's results are a major challenge to any physical filter theory of selective attention. If selective attention worked as a filter, it could not be a source location filter, because location of the input had negligible effects compared to meaning. The principle that conscious (attended) input in humans has a strong preference for meaningful coherence appears to be fundamental.

There is considerable evidence that the unconscious stream in a competing input task is processed to quite a high level of analysis. MacKay's (1973) article (chap. 16, this volume) provided an influential demonstration of this point. He showed that ambiguous words in the conscious channel could be resolved by semantic information on the unconscious side. When a conscious sentence was presented with an ambiguous word, such as "They were standing near the *bank* ...", simultaneous presentation of the word "water" in the unconscious ear would lead subjects to interpret "bank" as "river bank." When the simultaneous unconscious word was "money," the interpretation of "bank" would shift to "financial bank." This requires, of course, that the unconscious input be analyzed to the level of the meaning of the words "money" and "river." It seems that the unconscious side does not merely shut off input; some higher level of content analysis must be involved. MacKay also showed that more complex ambiguities, such as Chomskyan deep and surface structure ambiguities, are unaffected by resolving information in the unattended ear. This may be because such ambiguities involve integration over multiple words in a phrase or sentence, and unconscious input may not allow such multisecond integration (see Section 6).

MacKay's (1973) results present yet another challenge to the filter concept, because it implies that much analysis takes place in the nonselected auditory channel. Broadbent's filter hypothesis was predicated on the notion that selection saves processing capacity; but if even the unattended channel is analyzed, what capacity is being saved? As Broadbent himself noted:

If there were really sufficient machinery available in the brain to perform such an exhaustive analysis for every stimulus, and then use the results to decide which should be selected, it is difficult to see why any selection at all should occur. The obvious utility of a selective system is to produce an economy of mechanisms. If a complete analysis were performed even of the neglected message, there seems to be no reason for selection at all. (Broadbent 1971, p. 147)

Although hundreds of articles have been published on selective processes since these findings were published, these paradoxes have not been resolved. One possibility is that selection does not occur for immediate input as such, but rather over internal distribution in the brain (Baars 1988). It may be that all inputs are analyzed for meaning but that only one is distributed within the brain at any given moment. One can compare consciousness to a news agency that may receive and briefly analyze many sources of information, though only one coherent tale will be told to its audience. This is the "theater metaphor" of consciousness (Baars 1997; Baars, section 10, this volume). A related hypothesis suggests that the deciding factor in selection is not an input filter but an internal coherence constraint. MacKay's unconscious resolving words contributed to the understanding of the conscious input stream by making an ambiguous word unambiguous; Gray and Wedderburn's subjects were able to analyze the input from both ears in spite of rapid alternation of the input, because they were able to impose coherence on sentences like "Mice eat cheese" more easily than on sets of random numbers. In both cases, moment-to-moment internal coherence in the conscious input may have been the decisive ingredient in the selection process.

A similar insight comes from the chapter by Rees, Russell, Frith, and Driver (1999; chap. 15, this volume). They asked subjects to gaze at a single fixation point on a screen but to attend to either green pictures or red letter strings superimposed on each other at the fixation point for a quarter of a second, separated by half-second intervals (see figure 15.1). To ensure that subjects selected only one stream, they were asked to signal when two succeeding pictures or letter strings were identical, and in the case of words, to distinguish between real words and meaningless strings of consonants. Although both pictures and letter strings appeared exactly at the center of gaze, under these circumstances the observers were conscious of only one stream, either pictures or letters, but not both. This is another remarkable demonstration of "inattentional blindness," the fact that looking straight at an object is not enough to become conscious of it, if one is also tracking another stream of conscious events at the same time. It shows again that the conscious stream is not fully determined by its stimulus source, but is heavily dependent on moment-to-moment predictions made by the brain. Rees et al. showed from simultaneous fMRI brainscans that being conscious of pictures activated entirely different parts of the brain than being conscious of letter strings.

One remaining question is whether the results are due to "inattention" or "blindness"? That is, are the results due to selective exclusion prior to consciousness (inattention), or due to a failure of the input to become visually conscious (blindness)? The answer at this point is not known.

Rensink, O'Regan, and Clark (1997; chap. 17, this section) have recently discovered a surprising phenomenon called "change blindness." Subjects are shown two consecutive photos that differ in some detail, such as a jet plane with four engines, followed by a momentary blank field, and then by the identical airplane with only two

engines. Surprisingly, viewers rarely notice the change. The philosopher Daniel Dennett has used change blindness to argue that conscious experience may not be what we think it is, that our apparent awareness of a visual scene is illusory. Rensink, O'Regan, and Clark argue rather that selective attention may be a necessary condition for consciousness, a hypothesis that is currently of great interest (see Treisman, chap. 4, this volume). It is a complementary idea, in a sense, to the coherence notion mentioned above: Rensink, O'Regan, and Clark suggest that selective attention may shape consciousness, whereas the coherence hypothesis suggests that selectivity may itself be shaped by the coherence constraint on conscious perception. Both could be true.

The Brain Basis of Selectivity

Psychological studies of selective attention reflect brain mechanisms that are only beginning to come to light. The thalamus is an obviously tempting part of the brain to study for selective attention, given that it is situated as a kind of gateway or "traffic cop" on the way from nearly all sensory surfaces to the corresponding sensory cortices (see section 2). Indeed, the thalamus can be viewed as a kind of mini-cortex, mirroring the major regions of the cerebral cortex in sizable nuclei that project to those areas, and receiving reverse projections from in return. The thalamus is therefore the most natural strategic road-junction for selective control of sensory experience.

Francis Crick (1984; chap. 18, this volume) has suggested a searchlight hypothesis to account for thalamocortical interaction. He suggested that some parts of cortex are actively selected by thalamic nuclei in much the way a spotlight in a theater might select a part of the stage to light up. The idea of a conscious "bright spot" in cortex goes back at least to Pavlov (Crick, chap. 18, this volume; see also Baars 1998; chap. 65, this volume).

Moran and Desimone (1985; chap. 19, this volume) present direct evidence that paying attention to specific aspects of a stimulus actually makes a difference to the firing of neurons. Training monkeys to select some aspects of a visual stimulus increases the firing of stimulus-sensitive cells; training them to ignore it decreases neuronal firing. This is some of the first evidence that voluntary attentional selection has specifiable brain effects at the level of single cells. In general, a number of sources suggest that selective attention and consciousness increase firing neuronal firing rates, whereas deselection and unconscious brain representation appear to decrease nerve cell activity. (See Raichle 1998; chap. 41, this volume).

Based on a number of brain imaging studies of visual selective attention Posner (1994; chap. 20, this volume) suggests that several parts of the brain play a role in effortful selection. Posner places particular emphasis on an anterior attention network, including the anterior portion of the cingulate gyrus and the prefrontal cortex. The role of anterior cortex in selecting stimuli suggests an anatomical difference between selective attention and sensory consciousness. Posterior cortex is preeminently sensory, and work from Logothetis's group (chap. 6, this volume) suggests that some posterior neurons in temporal and occipital cortex fire selectively to conscious visual stimuli. There are many selective mechanisms, including subcortical ones, but voluntary selection of stimuli seems to require prefrontal cortex; particularly effortful selection seems to also involve the anterior cingulate. Baars (1999) has suggested a set of principled distinctions between selective visual attention and visual consciousness, on the basis of such anatomical, behavioral, and phenomenal differences.

David LaBerge (1997; chap. 21, this volume) has developed a parallel view that the function of the thalamocortical relay nuclei is to *amplify* selected sensory input to the corresponding cortices, under prefrontal control. In LaBerge's perspective, visual cortex involves visual con-scious experience, anterior mechanisms are involved in voluntary selection, and the thalamus serves to select and amplify cortical neurons that are selected. (See Section IX).

There is reliable evidence for each of the brain mechanisms described in these papers; a complete account of the brain basis of selective attention is likely to require all of them.

References

Baars, B. J. (1988) *A cognitive theory of consciousness.* New York: Cambridge University Press.

Baars, B. J. (1997) *In the theater of consciousness: The workspace of the mind.* Oxford: Oxford University Press.

Baars, B. J. (1998) Metaphors of consciousness and attention in the brain. *Trends Neurosci* 21: 58–62. [See Section 10.]

Baars, B. J. (1999) Attention versus consciousness in the visual brain: Differences in conception, phenomenology, behavior, neuroanatomy, and physiology. *Journal of General Psychology* 126, 224–233.

Broadbent, D. E. (1958) *Perception and communication.* New York: Pergamon Press.

Broadbent, D. E. (1971) *Decision and stress.* New York: Aademic Press.

Cherry, C. (1953) Some experiments on the recognition of speech, with one and two ears. *J. Acoustic. Soc. Am.* 25, 975–979.

James, W. (1890/1983). *The principles of psychology.* Cambridge, MA, Harvard University Press.

Pashler, H. E. (1997) *The psychology of attention.* Cambridge, MA: MIT Press.

14 Strategies and Models of Selective Attention

Anne M. Treisman

Work on attention raises problems of definition and of the interpretation and choice of experimental procedures. This review attempts to outline a coherent classification for attention tasks and to relate common experimental procedures to it. Discussion is restricted to tasks requiring immediate perception and response, in which subjects (Ss) are presented with more information than they can handle. It will not consider the role of attention in memory, discrimination learning, vigilance, or habituation, nor its relations with arousal or motivation. Even within this restricted area, a large variety of different experiments have been designed to throw light on the mechanisms of selective attention often with the assumption that all these tasks converged on a single, unitary process. How far is this assumption of a single mechanism justified?

In 1958 Broadbent summarized a large area of research and attempted to provide a unified explanation in his "filter" theory of selective attention. He assumed that, when several messages reach the senses, they are initially processed in parallel, but must at some central stage converge on a perceptual or decision channel of limited capacity. To reduce the load on this "p" system, a selective filter blocks irrelevant messages before they reach the bottleneck. Thus only a limited number of signals can be identified, stored in long-term memory or used to control behavior in any short period. Broadbent assumed that the information content, defined as bits per second, would be critical in determining how many stimuli could be perceived and he gave considerable evidence supporting this conclusion (e.g., Broadbent 1956, Webster and Thomson 1954). This model has proved very fruitful in stimulating further ideas and experiments. We may now, 11 years later, ask what changes or amplifications have become necessary.

Here are two examples of results which are not immediately explained by Broadbent's model.

(a) If two passages of prose are presented at normal speed, one to each ear, Ss are able to follow only one of the two (Cherry 1953). But if a single passage is given at twice the normal rate, it is almost as intelligible as before (Fairbanks, Guttman, and Miron 1957). Similarly if the information content of the passage is doubled by using a low-order approximation to English (Moray and Taylor 1958, Treisman 1965a), Ss achieve shadowing scores considerably higher than 50% of their original performance. The limit here seems to lie not in the overall information rate as such, but either in the number of physically separate inputs we can handle or in the number of separate sequences of interdependent items we can follow. (b) When Ss are asked to repeat back one of two dichotic auditory messages, the other produces negligible interference (Cherry 1953). But if they are asked to name the colors of printed words which themselves name other colors, they find it extremely difficult to attend selectively to the colors and the words cause severe interference (Stroop 1935). While Broadbent achieved an impressive and large-scale synthesis of a variety of different results by showing the features they had in common, we may now need to draw some logical distinctions between attention tasks and discuss their implications for explanatory models of attention.

A General Model of Perception

Attention can be defined as the selective aspect of perception and response. Any theory about attention therefore presupposes some general framework of ideas on the nature of the perceptual system. How can we best characterize the mechanisms converting physical stimuli, described objectively in terms like intensity, frequency, or wavelength, into the sights and sounds we experience? Like physical stimuli, our percepts appear to vary along a number of independent dimensions, such as color, size, and loudness, although these are not usually perfectly correlated with single physical dimensions (e.g., the wavelengths of light which alone are seen as red and green, in combination are seen as yellow). A plausible theory is that there are a number of different perceptual "analyzers," each of which provides a set of mutually exclusive descriptions for a stimulus (Sutherland 1959). For example, a given area cannot have more than one of the range of alternative colors, but it can also have values on the dimensions of size, brightness, and shape. Judgments about the different dimensions, although not fully additive in the information transmitted, appear to be made independently with little or no interaction (Beebe-Center, Rogers, and O'Connell 1955, Garner 1962, Pollack and Ficks 1954). These independent perceptual dimensions suggest the existence of separate analyzers.

However, the operation of independent analyzers giving one output for each value on single dimensions would not suffice to explain the perception of complex or multidimensional patterns, like letters, faces, or spoken words. Different shapes may be composed of common elements, such as curves, straight lines, and intersections, differing only in the way they are combined. One shape may constitute part of another; for example, "P" is contained in "R." In such cases the perceptual system might operate by detecting conjunctions of particular criterial attributes. Computer programs using this principle have been developed for the task of character recognition (e.g., Selfridge and Neisser 1960, Uhr 1963). Perception of shape may thus depend on two or more levels of analyzers, those at a higher level grouping and classifying the outputs of those at a lower level to give another mutually exclusive set of complex percepts, such as the letters of the alphabet or the words of the English language. Although the outputs of any single analyzer at one level may be mutually exclusive (a curved line cannot also be straight),

the outputs of different analyzers at one level could join in a variety of different combinations as inputs to the next level, in a way that is not possible within a simpler dimension like color.

The different perceptual analyzers may be arranged in series, in parallel, or in a hierarchy, but one assumes that the outputs of analyzers at any level, or any combination of outputs, may potentially be both stored in memory and used to control the overt response. It may also be possible at any stage to store not only the outputs but also the inputs to later analyzers, that is, to store for a short time in sensory form the data for subsequent analysis. Thus a single external "stimulus" may be held in two forms at once: (a) the results of analysis already made and (b) the sensory data for further analysis. We may already know that a particular sound was a word whispered by John and also retain a sensory "tape recording" which could allow us then to decide that the word was "Good-bye." This raises the question how the outputs of analyzers are recombined and in particular how they are correctly related to a common source or to different sources. For example, how does one know that it is the "H" that is large and red while the "G" is small and black and not some other combination? One suggestion is that the sensory inputs are labeled by the results of some early stage of analysis, for example, with their spatial location or their time of occurrence, and retain this label throughout analysis.

Although there may be some difficulty in determining empirically just what constitutes an independent analyzer for any particular organism, this conceptual framework may be useful in exploring some functional distinctions between different types of selective attention.

A Classification of Attention Tasks

An example of a complex visual search task may help to illustrate some different strategies or models for selective attention. We might ask *S* to decide whether a display of colored letters in different sizes and orientations contains the letter "G" or not. To do this he must first direct his attention to the display and not elsewhere in the room, that is, he must select the class of sensory data coming from one particular area as the *input* to the perceptual system. Second, he must attend to the shapes of the letters and not their colors, sizes, or orientations, that is, he must select the *analyzers* for shape and reject those for color, and so on. Next he must identify the *target* letter "G" if it is present, and if possible ignore differences between the other letters. To do this he may be able to modify the function of the shape analyzers so that they perform only the subset of *tests* for those critical features necessary to identify "G." He would therefore distinguish among the other letters only those which also differed by one or more of the critical features in "G." Finally, he must select the appropriate *output* of the shape analyzers to control the response, "G," giving a positive response and all other outputs a negative one.

In another form of the experiment S might be told that the target letter "G" will be red if it is present at all. This might enable him further to restrict the *inputs* to the shape analyzers by selecting only red items for analysis. To do this, of course, he would have to use the color analyzer at some earlier stage to distinguish red items from others, but he could still reject *analyzers* for size and orientation, and perhaps also reject *tests* for colors other than red and so ignore the differences between green and black letters. With this extra cue for input selection, Smith (1962) found that search was much more efficient.

This example shows that four functionally different types of selection could play a role in determining attention, one affecting only response and memory and the other three restricting perception. (a) We could select which *outputs* of the perceptual analyzers are stored and used to control our responses; (b) we could select which *inputs* (which set of sensory data) to

send to the analyzers; (c) we could select which *analyzers* to use; (d) we could select within the analyzers which *tests* to make or which *target* values to identify (red as opposed to green or black, "G" as opposed to "H" or "N"). These four types of attention shall be called (a) output selection, (b) input selection, (c) analyzer selection, and (d) test or target selection; the next section describes them in more detail.

Selection of Outputs

This model of attention assumes full analysis of all inputs by all analyzers and matches selected outputs to the appropriate actions. It assumes that there is some limit to the responses we can make and to the information we can store, and that simultaneous outputs of perceptual analysis compete for access to the limited capacity motor systems and memory. Competition might be between the outputs of different analyzers given the same input or between outputs of a single analyzer given different inputs. Deutsch and Deutsch (1963, 1967) and Reynolds (1964) have made the strong claim that all attention tasks can be explained simply in terms of selection of outputs with no restrictions at all on perceptual processing.

Selection of Inputs or Sets of Sensory Data for Analysis

This type of attention restricts perception by selecting which set of sensory data to analyze. The selected set could logically (though perhaps not in practice) be labeled by any property which has been analyzed at some earlier stage of perceptual processing, whether this property is as simple as the receptor stimulated (visual vs. auditory stimuli) or the spatial position (top vs. bottom of the page), or as complex as voice quality (John's voice vs. Peter's) or language (English vs. French). This type of attention necessarily implies at least two successive stages of analysis, so that the decision taken by the first analyzer can be used to label the sensory data wanted for analysis by the second analyzer. The selected set of sensory data might also be defined by a combination of outputs from earlier analyzers; for example, we might want to read the words written in large red letters only, ignoring the small red and large black letters. This type of attention defines the data we look *at* and listen *to*, and not the properties we look or listen *for*. It is analogous to Broadbent's attention to particular "channels" of information and is the type of attention to which his "filter" theory seems best to apply.

Selection of Analyzers

With this type of attention we select one or more dimensions or properties of stimuli to analyze and ignore other dimensions or properties. It specifies the complete set of mutually exclusive values between which we will discriminate, leaving other sets unanalyzed. This form of selection has been studied primarily in the context of discrimination learning, for example, by Sutherland (1959, 1960), Mackintosh (1965), and Zeaman and House (1963). However, since these experiments have been concerned with the effects of attention on learning rather than on immediate perception and response, they will not be further discussed in this paper. An example of an experiment measuring immediate responses rather than learning is the Stroop test, described earlier, in which *S*s are required to select the analyzer for color and reject those used in reading words.

Selection of Tests and Targets

With this type of attention we select particular targets or goals of perceptual analysis, particular items we wish to identify, where the items are defined by one or a specified set of critical features. Each of these critical features would constitute one value on a dimension identified by some particular analyzer. The target items might be defined in very general terms, for example, "human speech" as opposed to "bird song" or "traffic noise," or much more specifically, for example, "John's voice saying good-bye." The target items might be detected by one analyzer only (e.g., the color red) or by several (e.g., "a large red H"). Test selection differs from analyzer selection in that it specifies the desired end result of analysis, while analyzer selection specifies only the set of possible end results between which we will discriminate. It differs from input selection in that it selects a specific test or subset of tests to be made, while input selection selects one set of sensory data to analyze, using the results of an earlier test or set of tests to label the selected class. With both test and input selection "John's voice" may be the object of attention, but in different senses of the word: while test selection allows us to listen *for* John's voice (to see if *he* is speaking rather than Peter), input selection allows us to listen *to* John's voice (to see what he is saying or how loudly he is speaking, and to ignore what Peter is saying or how loudly).

Figure 14.1 shows two examples of tasks illustrating these four different types of attention; the first is the visual search task discussed earlier and the second is part of a selective listening task investigated by Lawson (1966). The cross-hatched areas do not necessarily imply positive inhibitory blocks to prevent analysis, but simply show which data are not further analyzed or which analyses and tests are not carried out. The actual mechanisms of selection are not discussed in this paper.

Some Experimental Tests of These Models

Selection of Outputs

Is response competition a sufficient explanation for attention limits in all cases? Since there

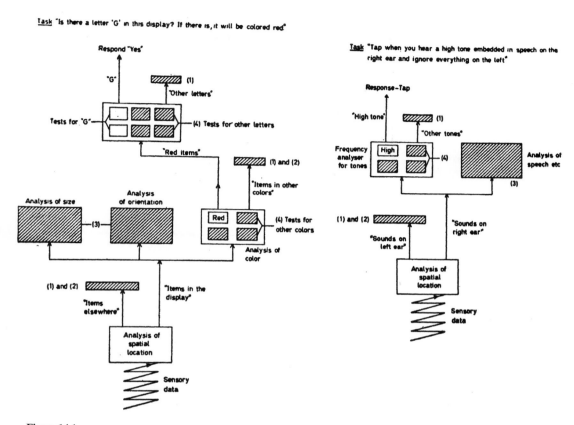

Figure 14.1
Different strategies for selective attention. (1. Rejection of outputs for response and memory; 2. rejection of inputs from further analysis; 3. rejection of irrelevant analyzers; 4. rejection of tests for nontarget items.)

is little point in examining the perceptual strategies, if all the findings can be explained by this mechanism alone, it seems important to test it first. In a recent experiment, Treisman and Geffen (1967) tried to equate response competition for the two messages in a selective listening task. The Ss were given the primary task of attending to and repeating back the message reaching one ear. They were also asked to make the same manual tapping response whenever they heard a

particular target word in either ear. Any asymmetry in the number of tapping responses to the "attended" and "unattended" message and in the interference these caused with shadowing would therefore indicate a perceptual rather than a response limit. On the other hand, any interference between tapping to and repeating back the target words in the "attended" message would show the effects of response competition. The result clearly indicated a perceptual limit

Table 14.1
Examples of the different ways attention can affect perception

	Divided attention			Focused attention	
Type	Object of attention	Example of task	Type	Object of attention	Example of task
1_D	Two or more sensory inputs	Listen to messages on both right and left ears	1_F	One sensory input	Listen to message on left ear only; ignore message on right ear
2_D	Two or more dimensions to analyze	Analyze both spatial location and loudness	2_F	One dimension	Analyze loudness, ignore spatial location
3_D	Two or more targets defined by critical features	Listen for the words "one," "five," and "eight"	3_F	One target or set of critical features	Listen for the word "eight"; ignore other words

(87% taps to target words in the "attended" message and only 8% to those in the "unattended" message). The degree of response competition between tapping to and repeating back the same "attended" target words was much less marked: of those words that received one correct response (and so had been correctly perceived) only 9% failed to elicit the other.

Another form of *perceptual* selection was shown by LaBerge and Tweedy (1964) and LaBerge, Tweedy, and Ricker (1967). They demonstrated that expectancy and motivation can both bias perception as well as response, by showing a decrease in the latency of an identical response to the more frequent or valued of two colors in a choice reaction-time task.

These experiments (among others) demonstrate that selective attention *can* affect perception, not, of course, that response competition is always unimportant. In experiments on discrimination learning and on habituation, where the decision time is less limited, selection for response or memory may well play the major role. But it seems clear that there are also perceptual limits restricting the amount of attention which simultaneous stimuli can receive. The remainder of the paper will discuss the relative importance and efficiency of the three types of perceptual attention.

An Important Experimental Variable: Division versus Focusing of Attention

There are two distinct procedures we can adopt in examining the role of attention in perception. The S can either divide his attention between two or more stimuli, or select one and focus his attention on it, rejecting the others. With divided attention tasks we investigate how necessary a selective system is. How far can we efficiently (a) handle two or more sensory inputs, (b) use two analyzers, or (c) test for two targets in parallel? In which type of task is the brain more vulnerable to overloading, forcing restrictions on our attention despite instructions to divide it? With focused attention tasks, on the other hand, we ask how efficiently we *can* select or focus on (a) a single sensory input, (b) a single analyzer, or (c) a single target, when the task requires us to ignore competing inputs, dimensions, or targets? Which is more efficient at rejecting irrelevant material—input-selective, analyzer-selective, or test-selective attention?

Table 14.1 summarizes and illustrates how the distinction between division and focusing applies to the three types of attention. Notice that these forms of attention can be combined in different ways for particular tasks: for example, the combination 1_D3_F might involve monitoring the inputs from both ears for the occurrence of the word "eight"; 1_F2_D might involve monitoring the left ear only for both the verbal content and the loudness of the speech items reaching it. Analyzer and test selection could be combined in the double task 2_F3_F, for example, by asking Ss to respond both to variations in the loudness of the items and to the word "eight." The response in input selection is made to some feature other than that defining the relevant input; in analyzer and test selection it is made to the dimension or targets specified in the table.

Notice also that there is no implication in these logical distinctions of any fixed hierarchy of analyzers or selective systems. Any of these strategies could be used at any level of analysis. The question of how far the order of perceptual processes and selective systems is fixed or variable is an empirical one, which should be decided experimentally, for example, by seeing which types of analysis can be made conditional on others, so giving economies of time or increased efficiency. We are here making logical distinctions between strategies, without prejudice to the levels of analysis at which they are usually applied.

Divided Attention

How far, then, can we (a) attend in parallel to two inputs, (b) use two analyzers at once, and (c) test for two targets at once? It has been argued against the existence of a perceptual limit that, since we possess the necessary analyzing systems anyway, no economy can be achieved by leaving some unused. This might be true of analyzer selection, but it does not apply to input selection in which a single analyzer receives inputs from two or more physical sources or to target selection where the targets may involve overlapping sets of tests within one analyzer. Perhaps then attention tasks might show more perceptual interference when competition is between inputs

or targets than when it is between different analyzers discriminating along dimensions which vary independently. It seems likely also, that the parallel use of several analyzers is biologically the most useful form of divided attention, since we typically need to recognize and respond to objects defined by values along a number of dimensions. Selective attention to inputs or targets often requires divided attention to different analyzers and tests.

Two different measures have been used to investigate how far perceptual processing can be done in parallel with divided attention, or must be done serially, requiring focused attention. The first measures *accuracy* and the second *latency*. The first method compares the accuracy of responses in tasks requiring attention to two inputs, dimensions, or targets with those requiring attention only to one. The second method measures differences in reaction time resulting from different numbers of inputs, dimensions, or targets to be matched or identified. A comprehensive review of all the evidence so far available shall not be attempted, but as examples some experiments shall be given which illustrate certain important points under each heading.

Tests Measuring Accuracy with Divided Attention

Competing Inputs

This is the main method which has been used in the growing body of research on selective listening. The experiments by Cherry (1953), by Treisman and Geffen (1967) described earlier, and by Moray (1959) have shown that division of attention between two auditory inputs to the speech analyzers is very limited. The Ss are able to recall or respond to very little of the verbal content of a secondary message when attending to and repeating back a primary message. When asked explicitly to divide their attention between two strings of auditory digits to detect some letters embedded in them, Ss did considerably less well on either input than when they focused their attention on one of the two (Moray and O'Brien 1967). In particular when two target letters occurred simultaneously, Ss succeeded in detecting both on only 17% of occasions.

When the two eyes receive different inputs, binocular rivalry usually results, which may be taken as one limit on divided attention. However, unlike selection between dichotic auditory inputs, the choice is not normally under voluntary control, and division of attention in vision is usually tested with inputs differing in spatial location. Webster and Haslerud (1964) showed a decrement in detection of the same peripheral lights when Ss were asked at the same time to count either foveal flashes or clicks. Most other visual experiments have used the tachistoscopic technique of single brief exposures. The span of apprehension, which is typically only four or five items, was taken to reflect the limits of divided attention with a single brief display. However, Sperling's (1963) experiments showing increases in letters detected (from 1 to 4) when a masking field was introduced at different intervals after the display, and Kinsbourne's (1968) experiment, showing changes in the latency of the subitizing response with different numbers of items, suggest that even below the span, items may be handled serially rather than in parallel, that is, that in these tasks attention may in fact not be divided but rather rapidly shifted.

There has been little investigation of divided attention to two continuous strings of visual items presented sequentially in two different positions, (which would be a closer parallel to the auditory experiments). In an unpublished pilot experiment, Treisman and Birch compared monitoring performance with two inputs when these were both auditory, both visual, or one auditory and one visual. With equal presentation rates, the visual-visual condition was considerably more efficient than the auditory-auditory, but it too revealed marked limits to the ability to divide attention when the target for which Ss

were set was any sequence of two consecutive digits (for example "23" or "78") rather than a single digit. Under these conditions accuracy was only 28%. The Ss did appreciably better when dividing their attention between a visual and an auditory list, although they still got only 44% correct. While two inputs to the same modality must share the same analyzers throughout, the two inputs to different modalities would be at least partly analyzed by independent systems.

This last result raises a point which may be of some importance. Most experiments so far have tested the accuracy of divided attention between two inputs to the same set of analyzers, while also forcing S to distinguish between the inputs (e.g., making him shadow one of the two). They have therefore not determined whether the difficulty arises in the shared use of one set of analyzers for two simultaneous sets of tests, or whether it comes in handling two inputs at once, taking them in and labeling them correctly by some preliminary analysis. One way around this would be to ask for the same response to both inputs, so that S need not first distinguish and label them. One could then compare three different conditions: (a) two inputs to a single analyzer (e.g., monitor two auditory strings of digits for one verbal target); (b) two inputs to two different analyzers (e.g., monitor one auditory string for a verbal target and another for a change of loudness or position); (c) one input to two analyzers (e.g., monitor a single auditory string for both a verbal target and a change of loudness) in all cases using the same single positive response.

Comparison of Accuracy with Inputs and Analyzers in Divided Attention

Although these tests have not been tried in exactly this form, two experiments suggest that the main limit is set by the double use of a single analyzer (Condition (a) is harder than Condition (b)), but that handling two inputs may also cause some difficulty (Condition (b) is harder than

Condition (c)). Treisman and Riley (1969) asked Ss to repeat a string of digits heard in one ear while listening to either ear for a letter, which was sometimes in the same voice as the digits and sometimes in a different voice. The Ss were therefore carrying out Task (a) when the target letter was in the same voice on the nonshadowed ear, Task (b) when it was in the different voice on the nonshadowed ear, and Task (c) when it was in the different voice on the shadowed ear. They detected virtually all targets in Conditions (b) and (c) and this monitoring produced no interference with the shadowing task. Thus a simple change of speaker can be detected in parallel with analysis of verbal content either of the same input or of a different input. On the other hand, the target letters in the same voice (which could only be distinguished by analysis of their verbal content) were detected much less often in the nonshadowed message (Task (a)), suggesting that the main difficulty arises in the shared use of a single analyzer for two inputs.

However, the two tasks also differed in complexity: discrimination of speakers was between only two voices, while the verbal targets had to be distinguished from 10 other words (the digits). In one condition of a similar experiment by Lawson (1966), Ss were asked to make a discriminative response to one of two possible tones embedded in a shadowed and a nonshadowed message; their performance was worse than with a single tone and now showed a greater decrement on the nonrepeated message. Thus although handling two inputs is easier when they are sent to different analyzers, (tones or voices vs. words), it may also be harder to use these different analyzers on two different inputs than on the same input, at least when the two inputs must be distinguished from each other. At least part of the overloading in divided attention tasks may therefore be due to the reception and labeling of inputs from two different sources, as well as to the double use of a single analyzer.

An experiment by LaBerge and Winokur (1965) confirms the relative ease of dividing attention between two analyzers with one input. The Ss were asked to name the colors in which digits were printed and at the same time to note and recall a letter which was embedded at some variable point in the lists. They therefore had two dimensions, color and shape, to analyze for the same physical inputs, and a complex discrimination to make in the monitoring task. With a single target letter in the last list position they found 100% recall; with consonant digrams or trigrams they found about 85% recall, but this was probably a failure of memory rather than perception, since the first consonant of the trigram also received 100% recall at the zero delay.

Another recent experiment in vision directly compares these three attention tasks. Lappin (1967) compared report of tachistoscopically presented circles varying in size, color, and angle of line through the center, when Ss were asked to report the three dimensions of one item, one dimension of three items, or a different dimension of three different items. The particular stimuli and the responses made were directly comparable, since the experimental conditions changed only the relations between them. The first condition was easiest and the last slightly harder than the second. In the present framework, the first required the use of three analyzers on one input, the second the use of one analyzer on three inputs, and the third the use of three analyzers on three different inputs. Division of attention between different inputs was again the main source of difficulty, and limits on the use of different analyzers only appeared when they were used for different inputs which S had to distinguish by their spatial location. Lappin also found that the responses to the three dimensions were essentially uncorrelated and independent, which would support the suggestion of parallel analysis. However, he found a large serial order effect on response accuracy, when the different dimensions belonged to different input items, the third dimension being worst reported and the first best. Lappin felt this cast doubt on the parallel-processing model.

With a single input, however, there was no decrease in accuracy from first to third dimension. The results could therefore be explained on the assumption of parallel processing by different *analyzers*, combined with serial intake of different *inputs* and serial processing of these inputs within any one analyzer, the rate varying with the analyzer (as shown by the different slopes of the serial order curves). The rate of serial intake did not appear to vary with spatial separation of the inputs. It may reflect the time taken to select and label the appropriate subset of inputs for analysis, rather than a spatial scan or shift of attention.

Another test of these suggestions might be to compare the use of two input modalities with one in the presentation of verbal material. It seems plausible to suppose that there is some central stage of analysis for verbal material which is shared between words presented auditorily and visually—the stage at which the syntax and meaning are identified—as well as a stage which is not shared, at which the words are identified through analysis of the visual or the auditory patterns of stimulation. Informal "experiments" in reading aloud to children suggest that it is perfectly possible to read aloud accurately (or to the children's satisfaction) while listening to another conversation, provided one ignores the meaning of the story one is reading. The same does not seem to be true when one repeats back one auditory message while attempting to listen to another. Thus two-input tasks using two analyzers seem easy, while two-input tasks with one analyzer are not. If this hypothesis is correct, one should be able to find tasks using identical inputs which in one case involve the use of the same central analyzer as well as the separate visual and auditory word analyzers, and in the other case only the use of separate modality-specific analyzers. For example, the monitoring task used by Treisman and Birch in one condition required S to detect a single target digit presented either visually or auditorily and in the other to detect an ascending sequence of two digits. The first might allow the S to bypass the shared central analyzers for symbolic information and to monitor in parallel for the specific patterns of sound and sight, while the second, which involved a symbolic aspect of the targets, would require analysis of both inputs by the central analyzer for meaning and so might prevent divided attention to vision and hearing. On the other hand, two inputs in the same modality would share not only the same central or symbolic analyzers but also the modality-specific pattern analyzers and so might rule out divided attention even in the nonsymbolic task. The results of the preliminary study were inconclusive because the particular display used for the visual stimuli made the visual-visual monitoring for the specific target too easy compared to the auditory-auditory. The problem is being explored further.

Accuracy of Divided Attention to Competing Targets

Rather more clear-cut limits to the division of attention have been shown in tasks requiring the identification of varied numbers of targets, where the targets are detected by overlapping sets of tests within the same group of analyzers. Treisman and Geffen (1967), for example, showed that accuracy of monitoring in a selective listening task decreased as the range of targets increased. The Ss detected fewer targets in both shadowed and nonshadowed passages when these were defined as "any digit" or "any color" than when they were defined as specific single words like "night" or "hot."

A rather different type of evidence for serial operation of different perceptual tests comes from ambiguous stimuli, such as auditory homophones or visual figures like the Necker cube. With these stimuli it is not usually possible to be aware of both versions at once; perception appears to alternate or to select one dominant version of the word or picture. In binocular rivalry, Treisman (1962) showed that suppression of one input takes place only within analyzers for the property on which they differ. Information about position and shape from both eyes could be used to give stereoscopic depth for stimuli whose colors were rivaling, so that only one color was visible at a time.

Most other tasks varying the number of targets attended to have used the latency measure and will be discussed later.

Tests Assessing Divided Attention by Response Latencies

Measures of reaction time have been used to study whether analysis of two or more stimuli or properties is carried out in series or in parallel. If the analysis can be shown to be serial, this implies that attention cannot be divided between the items analyzed serially. On the other hand, efficient division of attention cannot be inferred directly from parallel analysis, since it is possible for parallel processes to interfere with one another. One might then say that division of attention was possible but inefficient. One indication of serial processing is a linear increase in reaction time with the number of items analyzed. Parallel analysis without interference might also result in increased latencies as the number of items increases if there is some variance in the processing time for these items, but there would be a nonlinear upper bound on the increase to be expected in this case (see Sternberg 1966). Interference between parallel processes would further increase response latencies. Thus, if one found a linear or a marked and steep effect of number of items on latency of response, one could conclude that division of attention was either impossible (serial processing) or inefficient (parallel processing with interference).

Latency and Number of Inputs

Probably the clearest example of this type of task is one by Sternberg (1967), in which Ss

were asked to search through a visual display of varying size for a particular target letter. The reaction time increased linearly with the number of items in the display, strongly suggesting that visual items in different spatial locations must be identified serially. A further experiment also suggesting that different inputs are handled serially is one by Davis (1964), in which Ss made a same/different judgment about two visual stimuli presented successively with a varying interstimulus interval. When the interval was short, the repsonse was delayed, as though Ss could identify the second stimulus only after completing analysis of the first. Thus serial perception of inputs may be involved in the so-called psychological refractory period. Experiments by Kristofferson (1967) on judgments of successiveness similarly suggest some minimum time for identifying one stimulus before another stimulus can be accepted by the perceptual system.

Latency and Number of Analyzers

The evidence from reaction times for serial processing of different perceptual *dimensions* is more equivocal. Egeth (1966) compared latencies when Ss matched stimuli on one, two, or three dimensions (shape, color, and tilt) and found that the time to respond "different" decreased with the number of dimensions which were different and increased with the number which were relevant (when the number which were different was constant). However, the time to respond "same" did not increase monotonically with the number of relevant dimensions, as the serial model would predict. Nickerson (1966) did a similar experiment, using a classification rather than a matching task, and also got equivocal results. One possible factor affecting the results in both cases is that focused attention may not be possible, so that some analyses are carried out automatically whether they are relevant to the task or not. The irrelevant decisions then might interfere with the response and have to be suppressed. Another point is that latencies might be determined not only by the number of decisions to be taken but also by the process of evaluating the relevance of these decisions to the response. For example, where a match on any one of three dimensions is required, Ss might be slower in deciding to say "yes" if they have also detected a mismatch on one or more other dimensions.

Latency and Number of Targets

Many experiments have shown that choice reaction time to single stimuli increases with the number of possible alternatives (Bricker 1955, Hick 1952) unless the stimulus-response connection is highly compatible (Leonard 1959) or highly overlearned (Davis, Moray, and Treisman 1961, Mowbray and Rhoades 1959). This suggests a change from some form of serial search (perhaps the sequential binary decisions implied by the optimal coding of information theory) or from a parallel analysis where the overall capacity is limited and shared between the different stimulus-response channels, to a truly independent testing in parallel once the stimulus-response connections have grown very familiar.

Parallel testing for practiced and familiar targets was also suggested by experiments on visual search by Neisser (1964). His Ss searched for varying numbers of target letters in lines of printed letters; while the search time increased with the number of items per line to be looked at (i.e., the number of inputs) it did not increase with the number of items looked for (between one and 10 targets), with highly practiced Ss. However, he allowed high error rates, which may have changed the nature of the task to some extent. Very similar experiments (Kaplan and Carvellas 1965, Kaplan, Carvellas, and Metlay 1966) have shown serial rather than parallel functioning. Neisser's task also showed an effect of the number of targets when Ss were asked to search for their absence ("which line has no Q or H") as if they had to check the presence of each of the set of targets serially, while in the earlier

tasks their absence could be noted in parallel for the whole set.

Sternberg (1967) found strong evidence for serial search through a set of memorized targets. He measured reaction times to match one or more visual digits with a varying number of memorized digits, and found that the response latency increased linearly with the number of comparisons to be made, suggesting that looking for and looking at an additional target letter required equal processing capacity. Of course this equivalence between targets and inputs might hold only where the task requires an equally detailed analysis of items looked for and at. Some search tasks might allow only partial analysis of nontarget items in the display, using a subset of the critical features which normally define them: for example, Ss searching for a "Z" in a context of curved letters and "As" might discard the curved letters in the display on the basis of a single property (curvature), while fully indentifying the target "Z" and the nontarget "A." In this case, increasing the set of items looked for to include "A" as well as "Z" might actually reduce the perceptual load and the response time. As Rabbitt (1964) has pointed out, the range of features to be extracted or tests to be made may be more important than the range of letters.

In summary then, there is quite strong evidence that true division of attention is difficult or impossible and serial processing necessary, both with two or more inputs and with tests for two or more targets (unless these are highly familiar and practiced), while divided attention to different dimensions seems more efficient and serial processing in reaction-time tasks more dubious, at least with some of the dimensions so far tested.

Experimental Tests of Focused Attention

The second way of comparing these three forms of perceptual attention is to look at the relative efficiency of tasks which require attention to be focused on a single input, dimension, or set of tests. In tasks requiring focused attention, *S*'s failure to shut out irrelevant inputs, dimensions, or features can again be assessed either by a reduction in accuracy or by an increased latency of response to the selected stimuli. The accuracy measure will reveal how far *S* has *exclusive* access to the relevant stimuli and the latency measure how far he also has *direct* access to them, assuming they are analyzed serially. However, these measures will only be meaningful in tasks where division of attention is imperfect: if two inputs, dimensions, or targets can be analyzed in parallel with no interference, it is more difficult to discover how exclusively *S*s can focus at the perceptual level on one of the two. Some possible tests are (a) to use tasks where the two inputs, dimensions, or targets elicit conflicting responses, so that interference at the response level can reveal a failure to focus at the perceptual level; (b) to test incidental perception by asking *S*s after the focused attention task what, if anything, they can report about the irrelevant stimuli (Cherry 1953, Treisman 1965b); in this case, of course, the results depend not only on *S*s' perceiving the irrelevant variables but also on their storing them in memory. The results with divided attention suggest that these indirect tests may only be necessary to investigate selection of analyzers. For input or target-selection, measures of perceptual interference from irrelevant inputs or targets should be sufficient.

Focused Attention to One Input

In vision different inputs must inevitably come from different spatial locations. The most obvious and important method of focusing attention on one input is by peripheral control of the direction of gaze and of the degree of convergence and accommodation. But it may also be possible to demonstrate selectivity at some more central stage in situations where eye movements are excluded. An example of such an experiment is one by Sperling (1960). He asked *S*s to re-

port either a whole display of letters presented tachistoscopically or a subset of these defined immediately *after* the presentation by their positions in the display (a single row or column). Since the same shape analyzers would be used for many of the letters to be identified, a reduction in the number of items to be analyzed would presumably be beneficial. The *S*s in fact reported a much larger proportion of the selected subset than of the total display. Here the selective cue must have affected perceptual analysis rather than the order of report, since a different cue which itself required analysis of each shape (report of only digits from a display of digits and letters) did not show the same increase in accuracy of report. An experiment by Von Wright (1968) has shown that input-selection may also use other input-defining properties besides spatial position; his *S*s showed savings over total report with partial report of letters selected by their color.

Input selection in hearing may be easier to investigate, since peripheral adjustments play a less important role in focusing attention on stimuli from one particular source. Here the efficiency with which attention can be focused on one of two or more inputs varies both with the discriminability of the inputs to be selected and rejected, and with the number of inputs to be rejected. When two passages of speech are played separately to the two ears, selection is very efficient, as we have seen. There is negligible interference, since *S*s can repeat back about as many words correctly as with a single passage after a few trials of practice. When the inputs differ in apparent location (separated by differences in the ratio of intensities at the two ears), selection remains efficient until the apparent locations are very close together (Treisman 1961). When the inputs are distinguished only by voice quality, the repeating response is rather less efficient (74% correct words compared to 95%; Treisman 1964b), although there are no overt intrusions from the wrong passage. When the two passages differ only in average speech rate, efficiency is even less (51% correct and 8% intrusions; Treisman 1961).

Treisman (1964c) asked Ss always to attend to and repeat back the message reaching the right ear. The irrelevant material in the left ear was then varied in a number of different ways: (a) the number of irrelevant speech messages; (b) the number of different dimensions on which the irrelevant messages differed (i.e., spatial locations only or spatial location and voice quality); (c) the difference between the irrelevant messages on one of these dimensions (their apparent spatial separation); (d) the information content and meaningfulness of the words and sentences. She found that the interference varied not with the number of irrelevant messages (word sequences), nor with the number (above one) of dimensions on which they varied, nor with the difficulty of separating them on one dimension, nor with their verbal content, but rather with the number of different inputs, distinguished by one or more physical characteristics (location or voice quality).

Another essential requisite for focused attention to one input is, of course, that the analyzer used to distinguish the selected and rejected inputs precede the analyzer for the features controlling the response. For example, it would be impossible to select which sentences to identify on the basis of their meaning, since the meaning could not be known before the sentences had been identified. In other cases the task may not be logically impossible, but may be empirically so. It might be, for example, that spatial position is always identified at some very early stage, so that one cannot select for analysis of their spatial position, a subset of words distinguished by the speaker's voice, the meaning of the words or any other feature that is analyzed more centrally than the spatial position. Or it might in some cases be possible to reverse the order in which the analyzers are arranged to fit the demands of the task; thus, for example, while Ss can select a subset of shapes to identify by their color (iden-

tify the red letters and ignore the blue or green), they may also be able to select a subset of colors to identify by their shapes ("what colors are the 'Fs'; ignore the 'Ds' and 'Ys'"). Preliminary unpublished results by Treisman and Turner suggest that this particular reversal may be possible.

Focused Attention to One Analyzer

The evidence on selection of analyzers so far seems less conclusive. Many of the traditional experiments on selectivity in visual perception (see Egeth 1967, Haber 1966) come under this heading, since they required attention to be focused on particular dimensions rather than particular sources of stimuli. For example, Ss were told to attend to color and ignore shape, and their accuracy of report was compared when the dimension was specified before and after presentation (Chapman 1932, Harris and Haber 1963, Lawrence and LaBerge 1956). The Ss were usually more accurate on the selected dimension, but these experiments suggested that much, if not all, of the selective effect could be attributed to the order of report or of encoding for memory. For example, Ss did better on the selected dimension only when they verbally described the items dimension by dimension (red, green, square, circle) rather than input by input (red square, green circle).

Biederman (1966) gives evidence that irrelevant dimensions are analyzed and cause delays in reaction time. He compared response latencies in a contingent task (where the value of a stimulus on a primary dimension determined which of two secondary dimensions would control the response), a filtering task (where one dimension was always irrelevant), and a condensation task where the values on all three dimensions were relevant to the response. He found that intertrial changes on the irrelevant dimension delayed the response in both filtering and contingent tasks, the delay varying with discriminability. His main aim was to demonstrate that selective and serial processing of different dimensions is possible, and he argues that this is demonstrated by the facts that (a) reaction time was faster in the contingent than the condensation task, (b) intertrial repetitions and discriminability both had more effect when they involved the primary dimension than the secondary, and (c) errors were more frequent on the secondary dimension. Some of these findings, however, could also be explained on the assumption that all dimensions were analyzed in parallel, but the response was initiated as soon as the relevant information had been obtained. Then the slowest dimension (the least discriminable) would determine reaction times only when it was relevant to the tasks in the contingent condition, but would always be completed for the condensation task.

A task in which Ss clearly fail to reject an irrelevant analyzer is the Stroop test mentioned earlier, in which they are asked to name the colors of printed words which themselves name other colors (Stroop 1935). The irrelevant printed names interfere considerably with the color-naming task. Another is an experiment by Montague (1965) in which variations on a dimension which was sometimes relevant to responses interfered more with the identification of multidimensional sounds than variations on a dimension which was always irrelevant. A failure to select between more complex groups of higher level analyzers was found by Treisman (1964b). Two competing messages were spoken in the same voice, intensity, and position, but in different languages, to see how far selection could take the form of focusing on the analyzers for a particular language. If a bilingual S could refrain from "asking questions" which would lead him to identify French words when his task was to repeat back the English, he should do better with the irrelevant message in French than in English. This did not appear to be the case: An irrelevant message in a known foreign language caused as much interference with the relevant English

as another English passage, differentiated only by its subject matter, while an unknown foreign language (for which no analyzer was available to S) caused appreciably less interference.

These findings suggest that focusing on particular perceptual analyzers while excluding others may be difficult or impossible. It certainly appears to be less efficient than focusing on a selected input. Can one explain the marked interference in these focused attention tasks without casting doubt on the earlier conclusion that divided attention to different analyzers was relatively efficient? There are two possible sources of interference other than a direct perceptual limit on the number of analyzers which can operate simultaneously: (a) Interference may arise at the response level when the outputs of two analyzers evoke conflicting responses. Using the Stroop test, for example, Klein (1964) found that Ss did better if they were allowed first to read the words and suggested that allowing Ss first to "unload" the competing response facilitated their performance on the color-naming task. Another test would be to see if one could reduce the interference by using a nonverbal response, which should conflict less with the irrelevant but dominant reading response.

(b) Irrelevant analyzers may indirectly produce perceptual as well as response interference by effectively increasing the number of irrelevant *inputs* to be rejected. If the use of certain analyzers is obligatory, Ss may be forced to distinguish irrelevant sets of incoming data, so producing two or more irrelevant inputs to later analyzers instead of one. The experiment described earlier by Treisman (1964c) gives an example of this: Two irrelevant messages in different voices or different positions interfered more with attention to a third than two irrelevant messages which did not differ in voice quality or position. If Ss had been able, for example, to "switch out" the analyzers distinguishing the man's from the woman's voice, the two irrelevant messages which differed only in voice quality (like the two irrelevant messages in the same voice) would have acted as a single competing input to the speech analyzers instead of as two competing inputs.

Focused Attention to One Target

The ability to select voluntarily a single target or subset of features to look for is demonstrated by the same experiments which were used as evidence of serial rather than parallel processing in divided attention. If Ss were unable to set themselves for particular targets in a search task, the number of relevant targets should have no effect on search time. Since such an effect has been clearly demonstrated, for example, by Sternberg (1966) and by Kaplan et al. (1966), we must conclude that Ss can restrict their analysis to features relevant to the task. The ability to do this often improves considerably with practice, provided that the target chosen makes it possible potentially to select a subset of tests for critical features (Rabbitt 1964). LaBerge et al. (LaBerge and Tweedy 1964, LaBerge et al. 1967) showed similar selective effects on response latency with simpler targets defined as single values on a dimension—red versus other colors, for example. With ambiguous figures, however, and in binocular rivalry, the selection does not appear to be under direct voluntary control, although it may be influenced indirectly by expectancy or motivation (e.g., Engel 1956, Schafer and Murphy 1943).

Conclusions

These findings suggest that division of attention between two or more inputs and between two or more targets is difficult or impossible, when no time is allowed for alternating attention or serial analysis, and that selective focusing is both efficient and frequently used with inputs reaching a single analyzer from different physical sources or with target items identified by the same analyzer

or by overlapping groups of shared analyzers. However, the experiments requiring attention to different dimensions are less conclusive, partly because experiments testing focused attention have often assumed that divided attention is impossible and looked for perceptual interference from irrelevant analyzers, while experiments testing divided attention have often assumed that focused attention is possible and measured decrements with divided attention. The evidence on the whole suggests that *focusing* on a particular dimension is difficult, at least when it involves selecting one of two independent aspects of a single set of stimuli (i.e., when it cannot be combined with input-selective attention), while *division* of attention between analyzers is relatively efficient at least compared to division of attention between inputs. There may be some degree of perceptual interference, particularly when discriminability is poor and Ss are asked to make judgments of near threshold variations on two dimensions at once (see Lindsay, in press), but most decrements with two compared to one analyzer can be attributed to response interference or indirectly to an increase in the number of inputs.

Why then should focusing on a particular analyzer be more difficult than focusing on one input or one target? It is not simply that certain analyzers are located very peripherally in the nervous system (e.g., the three types of color receptors in the retina) and so are less subject to central control, since the failure to select can also occur between more central groups of analyzers like those for different languages. Analyzer selection is probably less practiced than input or target selection, since far fewer tasks require selective attention to single dimensions. But there may be a more fundamental reason: It may be that the nervous system is forced to use whatever discriminative systems it has available, *unless* these are already fully occupied with other tests or inputs, so that we tend to use our perceptual capacity to the full on whatever sense data reach the receptors. If we are correct in assuming the existence of independent analyzers, it would then follow that all dimensions of a stimulus input would be analyzed unless the analyzers were already engaged on some other input.

These conclusions and suggestions are of course very tentative. They may well be refuted by future results, or by existing data of which the author is not aware. The main object of this paper was to raise questions rather than propose answers. This brief general review has shown how many problems remain and how scanty is the evidence so far available. Words like "attention," "stimulus," or "input" have been used to cover a variety of logically different concepts. Clarifying these may help to explain the conflicting experimental results and to throw light on the underlying mechanisms. Even in these general terms the processes are very incompletely described. For example, little has been said about how the outputs of two analyzers are related when they refer to a single external source. Does mismatching sometimes occur in selective attention, so that, for example, a particular word may be heard or remembered in the wrong voice or position? The model might predict this type of error and subjectively one does sometimes experience it.

Another unanswered question is what the actual mechanisms of selection are for each type of attention. In selection of inputs is some positive blocking or reduction is signalto-noise ratio of rejected sensory data necessary, or can one choose simply not to analyze them further? Some discussion and evidence on this point are given by Treisman (1964a, 1965b, 1967), by Broadbent and Gregory (1963), and by Lindsay (1967, 1968). Similarly, in target selection and analyzer selection (if this occurs) does attention simply determine in an all-or-nothing fashion which features or dimensions are analyzed and which are not, or does it vary the decision criteria and/or the fineness of discrimination adopted in analyzing particular features or dimensions, or is there some positive blocking or reduction in signal-to-noise ratio of all sensory inputs reaching irrelevant test points or analyzers? It is possible that the three types of perceptual attention work through the same underlying mechanism and differ only in the range either of data or of tests to which they apply it. Current and future research may help to answer some of these questions.

Acknowledgments

Preparation of this paper was begun at Bell Telephone Laboratories, Murray Hill, New Jersey, and completed at Oxford University with the support of a grant from the Medical Research Council. The author is grateful to M. Treisman, S. Sternberg, G. Cohen, and J. Brand for helpful discussions of various points, and to D. E. Broadbent for his criticisms of an earlier draft.

References

Beebe-Center, J. G., Rogers, M. S., and O'Connell, D. M. Transmission of information about sucrose and saline solutions through the sense of taste. *Journal of Psychology*, 1955, 39, 157–160.

Biederman, I. Human performance in contingent information processing tasks. Technical Report No. 3, 1966, Human Performance Center, University of Michigan.

Bricker, P. D. Information measurement and reaction time: A review. In H. Quastler (Ed.), *Information theory in psychology*. Glencoe, Ill.: Free Press, 1955.

Broadbent, D. E. Listening between and during practised auditory distractions. *British Journal of Psychology*, 1956, 47, 51–60.

Broadbent, D. E. *Perception and communication*. London: Pergamon Press, 1958.

Broadbent, D. E., and Gregory, M. Division of attention and the decision theory of signal detection. *Proceedings of the Royal Society* (London), Series B, 1963, 158, 222–231.

Chapman, D. W. Relative effects of determinate and indeterminate aufgaben. *American Journal of Psychology*, 1932, 44, 163–174.

Cherry, E. C. Some experiments on the recognition of speech with one and with two ears. *Journal of the Acoustical Society of America*, 1953, 25, 975–979.

Davis, R. The combination of information from different sources. *Quarterly Journal of Experimental Psychology*, 1964, 16, 332–339.

Davis, R., Moray, N., and Treisman, A. M. Imitative responses and the rate of gain of information. *Quarterly Journal of Experimental Psychology*, 1961, 13, 78–89.

Deutsch, J. A., and Deutsch, D. Attention: Some theoretical considerations. *Psychological Review*, 1963, 70, 80–90.

Deutsch, J. A., and Deutsch, D. Comments on "Selective attention: Perception or response?" *Quarterly Journal of Experimental Psychology*, 1967, 19, 362–363.

Egeth, H. E. Parallel versus serial processes in multidimensional stimulus discrimination. *Perception and Psychophysics*, 1966, 1, 245–252.

Egeth, H. E. Selective attention. *Psychological Bulletin*, 1967, 67, 41–57.

Engel, E. The role of content in binocular resolution. *American Journal of Psychology*, 1956, 69, 87–94.

Fairbanks, G., Guttman, N., and Miron, M. S. Effects of time compression upon the comprehension of connected speech. *Journal of Speech and Hearing Disorders*, 1957, 22, 10–19.

Garner, W. R. *Uncertainty and structure as psychological concepts*. New York: Wiley, 1962.

Haber, R. N. Nature of the effect of set on perception. *Psychological Review*, 1966, 73, 335–351.

Harris, C. S., and Haber, R. N. Selective attention and coding in visual perception. *Journal of Experimental Psychology*, 1963, 65, 328–333.

Hick, W. E. On the rate of gain of information. *Quarterly Journal of Experimental Psychology*, 1952, 4, 11–26.

Kaplan, I. T., and Carvellas, T. Scanning for multiple targets. *Perceptual and Motor Skills*, 1965, 21, 239–243.

Kaplan, I. T., Carvellas, T., and Metlay, W. Visual search and immediate memory. *Journal of Experimental Psychology*, 1966, 71, 488–493.

Kinsbourne, M. Serial "count-out" from a fading visual trace. Paper presented at the meeting of the Psychonomic Society, St. Louis, October 1968.

Klein, G. S. Semantic power of words measured through the interference with color naming. *American Journal of Psychology*, 1964, 77, 576–588.

Kristofferson, A. B. Attention and psychophysical time. *Acta Psychologica*, 1967, 27, 93–100.

LaBerge, D., and Tweedy, J. R. Presentation probability and choice time. *Journal of Experimental Psychology*, 1964, 68, 477–481.

LaBerge, D., Tweedy, J. R., and Ricker, J. Selective attention: Incentive variables and choice time. *Psychonomic Science*, 1967, 8, 341–342.

LaBerge, D., and Winokur, S. Short-term memory using a visual shadowing procedure. *Psychonomic Science*, 1965, 3, 239–240.

Lappin, J. S. Attention in the identification of stimuli in complex visual displays. *Journal of Experimental Psychology*, 1967, 75, 321–328.

Lawrence, D. H., and LaBerge, D. L. Relationship between recognition accuracy and order of reporting stimulus dimensions. *Journal of Experimental Psychology*, 1956, 51, 12–18.

Lawson, E. A. Decisions concerning the rejected channel. *Quarterly Journal of Experimental Psychology*, 1966, 18, 260–265.

Leonard, J. A. Tactual choice reactions: I. *Quarterly Journal of Experimental Psychology*, 1959, 11, 76–83.

Lindsay, P. H. Comments on "Selective attention: Perception or response?" *Quarterly Journal of Experimental Psychology*, 1967, 19, 363–364.

Lindsay, P. H. Multichannel processing in perception. In D. E. Mostofsky (Ed.), *Attention: A behavioral analysis*. New York: Appleton-Century-Crofts, in press.

Mackintosh, N. Selective attention in animal discrimination learning. *Psychological Bulletin*, 1965, 64, 124–150.

Montague, W. E. Effect of irrelevant information on a complex auditory discrimination task. *Journal of Experimental Psychology*, 1965, 69, 230–236.

Moray, N. Attention in dichotic listening: Affective cues and the influence of instructions. *Quarterly Journal of Experimental Psychology*, 1959, 11, 56–60.

Moray, N., and O'Brien, T. Signal detection theory applied to selective listening. *Journal of the Acoustical Society of America*, 1967, 42, 765–772.

Moray, N., and Taylor, A. M. The effect of redundancy in shadowing one of two dichotic messages. *Language and Speech*, 1958, 1, 102–109.

Mowbray, G. H., and Rhoades, M. V. On the reduction of choice reaction times with practice. *Quarterly Journal of Experimental Psychology*, 1959, 11, 16–23.

Neisser, U. Visual search. *Scientific American*, 1964, 210, No. 6, 94–102.

Nickerson, R. S. Response times with a memory-dependent decision task. *Journal of Experimental Psychology*, 1966, 72, 761–769.

Pollack, I., and Ficks, L. Information of multidimensional auditory displays. *Journal of the Acoustical Society of America*, 1954, 26, 155–158.

Rabbitt, P. M. Ignoring irrelevant information. *British Journal of Psychology*, 1964, 55, 403–414.

Reynolds, D. Effects of double stimulation: Temporary inhibition of response. *Psychological Bulletin*, 1964, 62, 333–347.

Schafer, R., and Murphy, G. The role of autism in a visual figure-ground relationship. *Journal of Experimental Psychology*, 1943, 32, 335–343.

Selfridge, O. G., and Neisser, U. Pattern recognition by machine. *Scientific American*, 1960, 203, No. 8, 60–68.

Smith, S. L. Color coding and visual search. *Journal of Experimental Psychology*, 1962, 64, 434–440.

Sperling, G. The information available in brief visual presentations. *Psychological Monographs*, 1960, 74 (11, Whole No. 498).

Sperling, G. A model for visual memory tasks. *Human Factors*, 1963, 5, 19–31.

Sternberg, S. High speed scanning in human memory. *Science*, 1966, 153, 652–654.

Sternberg, S. Scanning a persisting visual image versus a memorized list. Paper presented at the meeting of the Eastern Psychological Association, Boston, April 1967.

Stroop, J. R. Studies of interference in serial verbal reactions. *Journal of Experimental Psychology*, 1935, 18, 643–662.

Sutherland, N. S. Stimulus analysing mechanisms. In, *Mechanisation of thought processes*. Vol. 2. London: Her Majesty's Stationery Office, 1959.

Sutherland, N. S. Visual discrimination in animals. *British Medical Bulletin*, 1964, 20, 54–59.

Treisman, A. M. Attention and speech. Unpublished doctoral dissertation, Oxford University, 1961.

Treisman, A. M. Binocular rivalry and stereoscopic depth perception. *Quarterly Journal of Experimental Psychology*, 1962, 14, 23–36.

Treisman, A. M. Selective attention in man. *British Medical Bulletin*, 1964, 20, 12–16. (a)

Treisman, A. M. Verbal cues, language and meaning in selective attention. *American Journal of Psychology*, 1964, 77, 206–219. (b)

Treisman, A. M. The effect of irrelevant material on the efficiency of selective listening. *American Journal of Psychology*, 1964, 77, 533–546. (c)

Treisman, A. M. The effects of redundancy and familiarity on translating and repeating back a foreign and a native language. *British Journal of Psychology*, 1965, 56, 369–379. (a)

Treisman, A. M. Monitoring and storage of irrelevant messages in selective attention. *Journal of Verbal Learning and Verbal Behavior*, 1965, 3, 449–459. (b)

Treisman, A. M. Reply to comments on "Selective Attention: Perception or Response?" *Quarterly Journal of Experimental Psychology*, 1967, 19, 364–367.

Treisman, A. M., and Geffen, G. Selective attention: Perception or response? *Quarterly Journal of Experimental Psychology*, 1967, 19, 1–17.

Treisman, A. M., and Riley, J. G. A. Is selective attention selective perception or selective response? A further test. *Journal of Experimental Psychology*, 1969, 79, 27–34.

Uhr, L. "Pattern recognition" computers as models for form perception. *Psychological Bulletin*, 1963, 60, 40–73.

Von Wright, J. M. Selection in visual memory. *Quarterly Journal of Experimental Psychology*, 1968, 20, 62–68.

Webster, R. G., and Haslerud, G. M. Influence on extreme peripheral vision of attention to a visual or auditory task. *Journal of Experimental Psychology*, 1964, 68, 269–272.

Webster, J. C., and Thomson, P. O. Responding to both of two overlapping messages. *Journal of the Acoustical Society of America*, 1954, 26, 396–402.

Zeaman, D., and House, B. J. The role of attention in retardate discrimination learning. In N. R. Ellis (Ed.), *Handbook in mental deficiency: Psychological theory and research*. New York: McGraw-Hill, 1963.

15 Inattentional Blindness Versus Inattentional Amnesia for Fixated but Ignored Words

Geraint Rees, Charlotte Russell, Christopher D. Frith, and Jon Driver

The extent of processing for unattended objects has been debated for over four decades (1). Recognition of unattended words is considered a crucial test case (1–3), because for these visual stimuli the processing of higher order cognitive properties (such as identity and meaning) can be dissociated from mere visual appearance. Early findings of little awareness or memory for ignored words (4) were taken to support the hypothesis that word recognition depends on attention. However, other studies suggested that word recognition still may take place unconsciously or implicitly for ignored words (5, 6), which led to proposals that word recognition is fully automatic (2, 7).

Functional imaging provides a way to measure unattended processing, but until now it has not been applied to the classic issue of the level of processing for unattended words. Recent data show that attention can modulate the activity evoked by visual stimuli within early brain areas (8), but all the stimuli used were meaningless or unfamiliar (for example, flashes, colored grids, or moving dots) and so cannot resolve the issue of unattended processing for meaningful familiar stimuli such as ignored words. Moreover, existing brain imaging data suggest that unattended processing may be attenuated rather than completely eliminated at early levels of processing, so processing of an unattended stimulus still may proceed through to higher levels beyond a rudimentary analysis of physical features (9). Here we resolve these issues by showing that brain activity in response to familiar visual words, versus random letters, wholly depends on attention.

We created a situation in which people could look directly at a word without attending to it (10). Brain activity was measured with functional magnetic resonance imaging (fMRI) (11) as participants viewed displays of a rapid stream of letter strings superimposed on a rapid stream of pictures (figure 15.1). The letter stream either consisted of meaningless strings of random consonants or contained a high proportion of meaningful familiar words. At any one time, participants attended only the stream of letters or only the superimposed stream of pictures in order to detect any immediate repetition of a stimulus within the attended stream. We arranged the stimulus parameters so that monitoring one stream for repetition was sufficiently demanding to preclude any attention to the other stream (10), even though both were superimposed at fixation. When the stream of letters was attended, we expected meaningful words within it to activate the extensive left-hemisphere network identified in previous imaging studies of word processing (12). The new question was whether meaningful words would similarly produce differential brain activation when the letter strings were ignored, with the superimposed pictures being attended instead. If true inattentional blindness can arise for ignored words, then activation for words versus nonwords should no longer be found. By contrast, if word processing is fully automatic, as is often argued to be the case (2, 7, 13), then differential activation still should be found even for ignored words because they are automatically perceived, with any effects of inattention being more akin to inattentional amnesia (14) than to inattentional blindness (15).

Immediately after scanning, participants underwent surprise recognition memory tests for the meaningful words they had been shown (16). Although recognition memory was excellent for those words that appeared in an attended stream, ignored words were not distinguished from new words (figure 15.1, bottom). This confirms that our manipulation of attention was psychologically effective and agrees with previous findings that people cannot recognize the identity of unattended stimuli retrospectively (17).

A

Picture stream target

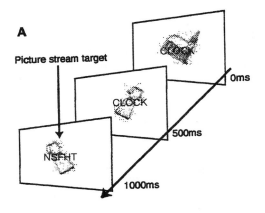

B

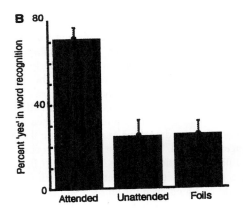

Figure 15.1
(*a*) Schematic illustration of stimulus configuration [see (*10*) for details]. (*b*) Performance in the surprise recognition memory test for words [see (*16*) for procedure]. Bar graph shows interparticipant mean and standard deviation of percent "yes" responses when judging whether a word had been shown in the imaging part of the experiment. Attended and unattended words refer to physically equivalent displays but with attention directed to the letter stream and to the picture stream, respectively. Foils refer to words that were never presented to a particular participant before, thus providing a measure of the tendency to answer falsely in the affirmative. Participants recognized almost all the attended words but did not differentiate unattended words from foils they had never seen before.

First we compared brain activations when participants were attending to the picture streams versus the letter streams overall (*18*). The stimuli were identical for these comparisons, as were the motor responses when detecting repetition, so any differential brain response must be due to what was attended. Attending to pictures compared with letter strings activated an extensive network of ventral visual areas bilaterally (figure 15.2a, green), whereas attending to letter strings compared with pictures activated a left occipital region (figure 15.2a, red) previously associated with letter perception (*19*). These activations indicate that covert attention can substantially affect neural responses in the visual system even when attended and ignored stimuli are spatially superimposed.

The crucial test for brain responses to meaningful familiar words compares the activation evoked by words versus consonants within the letter stream. When the letter stream was attended, words minus consonants revealed strong activity in a left-lateralized network of areas, including posterior basal temporal, parietal, and prefrontal cortex (figure 15.2b and table 15.1). This is consistent with previous lesion and functional imaging studies of word processing (*12, 13, 20*). Because words differ from consonant strings in several respects (for example, legal orthography and phonology, lexical status, semantics), the activations may involve all the corresponding word-related processes. Note that word-related activations were found here for attended letter streams, even though our repetition-detection task did not require participants to treat words any differently from nonwords. In this respect, our results agree with previous imaging studies that similarly found word-related activations even in nonlexical tasks (*13*).

Those studies argued on that basis that word processing takes place automatically, as many psychological accounts have proposed (*2, 7, 21*). However, these data argue against fully automatic word processing for the new situation in

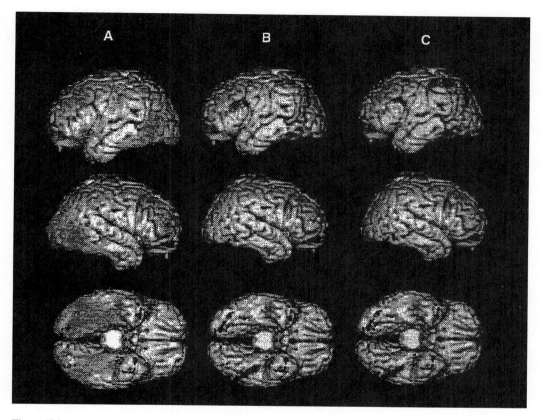

Figure 15.2
(*a*) Effects of attention on fMRI activity. Three views of a T1-weighted anatomical template in Talairach space, on which are superimposed areas where attention to the picture stream produced significant activation compared with all letter streams (green) or vice versa (attend letter streams minus picture stream; red). (*b*) Simple effect of words compared with consonants when attending letters. Three anatomical views, on which are superimposed in red those areas where words minus consonants produced significant activation when attention was directed to the letter stream (see also left half of table 15.1). (*c*) Interaction between attention and word processing. Three anatomical views on which those areas where evoked activity specifically reflected the critical interaction between attention and word identity (where the effect of words minus consonants was greater during attention to the letter streams than during attention to the picture stream) are superimposed in red.

Table 15.1
Coordinates and z scores for activation related to word processing

Cortical region	Attended words minus consonants				Interaction of words and attention			
	Talairach coordinates (mm)			z score	Talairach coordinates (mm)			z score
Left inferior frontal (BA44)	−39	6	27	4.70 ($P = 0.09$)	−39	6	27	4.41
Left posterior temporal (BA37)	−39	−36	−24	4.63	−51	−51	−18	5.71
					−42	−39	−24	4.85
Left posterior parietal (BA7/40)	−33	−33	57	4.59	−33	−33	57	5.36
	−27	−72	33	4.49 ($P = 0.06$)	−24	−75	42	6.50
					−30	−57	39	5.57
Right posterior parietal (BA7)	36	−63	24	4.23 ($P = 0.17$)	36	−60	33	5.32

Note: Shown are loci with higher activity for words versus consonants when attention was directed to the letter stream (left columns) and loci where such word-related activity was greater during attention to the letter stream than during attention to the picture stream (right columns). Coordinates shown are for the maxima within each area of activation ($P < 0.05$; corrected for multiple comparisons except where a different corrected value is specifically indicated).

which the letter streams were unattended, with the pictures being attended instead. The critical interaction between which stream was attended and whether words were presented (that is, testing for a larger effect of words minus consonants when the letter stream was attended) revealed robust left-hemisphere activations virtually identical to those for the simple effect of words when attended (figure 15.2, c and b). Moreover, comparing the same stimuli as before (that is, meaningful words minus consonant strings), but with the letter stream unattended, did not activate a single voxel in these cortical areas, neither in the group analysis (18) nor in further analyses of individual participants at low threshold (22). The time-course data for attended words versus consonants and for unattended words versus consonants are shown in figure 15.3. Note that there is no tendency for a stronger response to words than consonants when the letter stream is unattended (23).

These functional imaging data show that word processing can strongly depend on attention, contrary to previous claims in both psychology

(2, 21) and functional imaging (13) for full automaticity. The data suggest that word processing is not merely modulated but is abolished when attention is fully withdrawn. If unattended words suffered only from inattentional amnesia (14), a differential response to words versus consonant strings should have been found at the time they were presented even when unattended because of automatic processing. By contrast, if ignored words suffer true inattentional blindness, the differential response that is observed for words when attended should be completely eliminated when they are unattended. Our results support the latter prediction. When covert attention was directed to other material for a demanding task, even words presented directly at the fovea produced no detectable differential cortical activity whatsoever (figure 15.3). Differential activation for words compared with consonants was seen neither in classic language areas nor in any area of visual cortex when unattended (18, 22).

The posterior basal temporal activation (see figure 15.2b) found for attended words has been observed in previous imaging studies of word

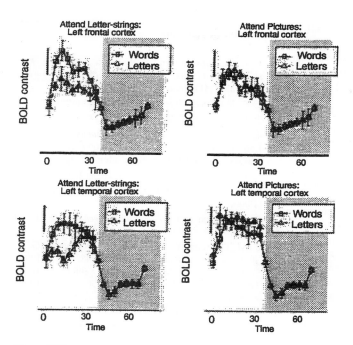

Figure 15.3
Time course of foci of activity in left frontal (upper) and left posterior basal temporal cortex (lower). All four panels use the same plotting conventions. Average BOLD contrast evoked at each locus (see table 15.1 for coordinates) is plotted as a function of time, collapsing across epochs and participants. Note that the areas whose time courses are shown were identified as those areas showing a maximal simple main effect of words under attention to letters. Unshaded areas represent scans acquired in the experimental conditions (see (10) and (11)) and shaded areas represent those acquired during the passive fixation baseline. Error bars indicate interparticipant standard error and dark scale bar represents 0.5% BOLD signal change. Activity evoked when the letter stream contained meaningful words is plotted with black squares and a solid line, and activity when the same stream included only meaningless letter strings is plotted with triangles and a dotted line.

processing (13, 22). Lesions to this area can produce alexia or visual anomia (24). A recent study showed that words activate this area not only in sighted readers but also in blind Braille readers, which suggests that it is an important association area for high-level representation of word identity (20). These data extend previous findings by showing that word-related activation of this area critically depends on attention. Its previous activation during implicit reading tasks, with no lexical response required, was interpreted as showing fully automatic word processing (13).

However, unlike this experiment, those studies presented individual words in total isolation, for up to 1 s, so the lexical properties of the stimulus were unlikely to be ignored. Our study shows that the basal temporal activation for words can be eliminated under conditions of true inattention.

The activations for attended words in left prefrontal cortex (figure 15.2b), close to Broca's area, have also been observed in previous imaging studies of word processing (12), where a role for this area in phonological retrieval and semantics was suggested. We also found activations for attended words in several areas of left parietal cortex and a homologous area on the right. Enhanced activity in left parietal cortex for words has previously been associated with orthographic to phonological conversion and with word meaning in a distributed semantic system (25). Again, our data suggest that such activity may be obliterated under conditions of full inattention.

Our imaging results imply true inattentional blindness for ignored words in the following sense. We do not suggest that our participants were blind to the presence of letters (26) when they were attending the superimposed pictures, but rather they were blind to those properties that distinguish words from random strings of consonants. The phenomenal experience when performing the task is indeed of knowing that both a (red) picture and a (green) letter string are present concurrently in the two rapid streams but being aware of the identity of each item only for the attended stream. The functional imaging data accord with this phenomenology. The success of our method may lie in the taxing demands of the picture task establishing conditions of full inattention for the words (27). Under conditions that do not fully engage attention, incidental processing of linguistic properties may take place even during nonlexical tasks. Indeed, as in previous studies of word processing, which presented letter strings in total isolation (13), words in the attended stream produced lexical activations here despite the nonlexical nature of our repetition task. These activations were eliminated only when the picture stream was being attended instead and the words were ignored. Although unattended words might be processed to a greater extent under conditions that impose a lower load than the present demanding picture task (28) or that use only a single stream of stimuli (29), our results suggest that, under the appropriate conditions of true inattention, words can be directly fixated but not read.

References and Notes

1. W. A. Johnston and V. J. Dark, *Annu. Rev. Psychol.* 37, 43 (1986); H. E. Pashler, *The Psychology of Attention* (MIT Press, Cambridge, MA, 1998).

2. C. MacLeod, *Psychol. Bull.* 109, 163 (1991).

3. D. Holender, *Behav. Brain Sci.* 9, 1 (1996).

4. C. Cherry, *On Human Communication* (Wiley, London, 1957); D. E. Broadbent, *Perception and Communication* (Pergamon, London, 1958).

5. J. Lewis, *J. Exp. Psychol.* 85, 225 (1970).

6. S. P. Tipper and J. Driver, *Mem. Cogn.* 16, 64 (1988).

7. J. Deutsch and D. Deutsch, *Psychol. Rev.* 70, 80 (1963).

8. M. Corbetta, F. M. Miezin, S. Dobmeyer, G. L. Shulman, S. E. Petersen, *Science* 248, 1556 (1990); D. C. Somers, A. M. Dale, A. E. Seiffert, R. B. H. Tootell, *Proc. Natl. Acad. Sci. U.S.A.* 4, 1663 (1999); A. Martinez et al., *Nat. Neurosci.* 2, 364 (1999); S. Treue and C. M. Trujillo, *Nature* 399, 575 (1999).

9. J. Driver and J. D. Mattingley, *Curr. Opin. Neurobiol.* 5, 191 (1995).

10. Six right-handed participants (two male and four female; 23 to 29 years old) gave informed consent to participate. Displays like those in figure 15.1 were presented every 500 ms for 250 ms. All pictures belonged to the Snodgrass-Vanderwart set [J. G. Snodgrass and M. Vanderwart, *J. Exp. Psychol. Hum. Learn. Mem.* 6, 174 (1980)]. Superimposed on the pictures were strings of five letters, comprising either random consonants or high-frequency concrete nouns. Total stimulus size was about 5°, centered at fixation. In different scanning epochs, the letter stream included either letter strings alone or 60% concrete nouns mixed with letter strings. When words were present, they were introduced only after the first eight items, as previous work has shown that people notice distractors more at the beginning of a stream [A. M. Treisman, R. Squire, J. Green, *Mem. Cogn.* 2, 641 (1974)]. Participants performed a single task while they underwent brain imaging (11), detecting immediate repetitions of stimuli within whichever stream (letters or pictures) they attended. This task was performed for epochs of 36.9 s with repetition targets occurring pseudorandomly every six stimuli on average. To ensure that attending pictures was demanding,

pictures had different orientations within any repeated pair, rotated 30° clockwise or counterclockwise from their natural axis (figure 15.1). Repetitions also took place in the unattended stream (requiring no response), uncorrelated in time with repetition in the attended stream. A button press response was required with auditory feedback for hits and misses. Participants were instructed about which stream to attend by an auditory cue in the rest epoch preceding each task epoch. The number of targets per epoch was balanced across conditions. Task order followed a within-participant Latin-square design. During both attention to letter strings and attention to pictures, any words were drawn from one of two different lists balanced for word frequency, concreteness, and imageability and were fully counterbalanced across participants.

11. A Siemens VISION (Siemens, Erlangen) acquired blood oxygenation level–dependent (BOLD) contrast functional images at 2 T. Image volumes were acquired continuously every 4100 ms, each comprising 48 contiguous 3-mm-thick slices to give whole-brain coverage with an in-plane resolution of 3 mm by 3 mm. Functional imaging was performed in four scanning runs comprising 288 volumes in total. In each scanning run, after eight image volumes were discarded to allow for T1 equilibration effects, the experimental conditions were presented for 36.9 s (nine scans) alternating with fixation control (rest) for nine scans. Condition order was counterbalanced across participants.

12. For reviews see C. J. Price [*Trends Cogn. Sci.* 2, 281 (1998)] and J. A. Fiez and S. E. Petersen [*Proc. Natl. Acad. Sci. U.S.A.* 95, 914 (1998)].

13. R. Wise et al., *Brain* 114, 1803 (1991); M. T. Menard, S. M. Kosslyn, W. L. Thompson, N. M. Alpert, S. L. Rauch, *Neuropsychologia* 34, 185 (1996); C. J. Price, R. J. Wise, R. S. J. Frackowiak, *Cereb. Cortex* 6, 62 (1996).

14. J. M. Wolfe, in *Fleeting Memories*, V. Coltheart, Ed. (MIT Press, Cambridge, MA, 1999), pp. 71–94.

15. A. Mack and I. Rock, *Inattentional Blindness* (MIT Press, Cambridge, MA, 1998).

16. After scanning, a surprise recognition memory test was presented. Participants indicated by button press whether each word shown had been presented during the scanning experiment. Three randomly intermingled word lists were tested (attended words, unattended words, and never-seen foils), matched for word frequency, concreteness, and imageability, with list membership counterbalanced across participants. Memory for attended words was better than for unattended words ($t = 5.2$, $P < 0.05$) and the latter did not differ from the chance rate given by false-positive responses to never-seen foils ($t = 0.08$, $P > 0.5$).

17. I. Rock and D. Gutman, *J. Exp. Psychol. Hum. Percept. Perform.* 7, 275 (1981).

18. Statistical parametric mapping software (SPM 99, http://www.fil.ion.ucl.ac.uk/spm) was used. The imaging time series was realigned, spatially normalized to stereotactic Talairach space, and smoothed with a Gaussian kernel of 10 mm full-width at half-maximum. Voxels activated during the experimental conditions were identified by a statistical model containing four delayed boxcar waveforms that represented the mean activity evoked in the experimental conditions. High-pass filtering removed participant-specific low-frequency drifts in signal, and global changes were removed by proportional scaling. Each component of the model served as a regressor in a multiple regression analysis. Masking with the contrast between the four experimental conditions versus baseline fixation was used to restrict our analysis to areas activated by the experimental conditions. A statistical threshold of $P < 0.05$, corrected for multiple comparisons, was used except where specified. Further inspection of any simple effect of unattended words minus consonants lowered the threshold to uncorrected $P < 0.001$ but still found no activation.

19. G. R. Fink et al., *Nature* 382, 626 (1996).

20. C. Buchel, C. Price, K. Friston, *Nature* 394, 274 (1998).

21. M. I. Posner, *Chronometric Explorations of Mind* (Erlbaum, Hillsdale, NJ, 1978); G. C. Van Orden, J. C. Johnston, B. L. Hale, *J. Exp. Psychol. Learn. Mem. Cogn.* 14, 371 (1988).

22. Spatial variability among activations across subjects might obscure an otherwise consistent neural response to ignored words. To test this, we repeated the analysis, but with the voxel of peak activation to attended words selected within individual subjects (for all the cortical areas in table 15.1, within a 10-mm radius of the group activation coordinates) to identify any activation to unattended words. Again, we found no significant differential activation (all $P < 0.05$).

23. The numerically lower activity for unattended words versus unattended consonants in figure 15.3 raises the possibility that inhibitory mechanisms might

suppress responses to unattended words [possibly related to the psychological phenomenon of negative priming (6)]. However, the apparent lowering of activity was not reliable; our data showed neither significant activation nor deactivation for unattended words in these cortical areas. Moreover, psychologically, negative priming is typically eliminated under conditions of high attentional load [N. Lavie and E. Fox, *J. Exp. Psychol. Hum. Percept. Perform.*, in press; A. Treisman and B. DeSchepper, in *Attention & Performance XVI*, T. Inui and J. L. McClelland, Eds. (MIT Press, Cambridge, MA, 1996), pp. 15–46] such as the present demanding picture task.

24. E. DeRenzi, A. Zambolin, G. Crisi, *Brain* 110, 1099 (1987); A. R. Damasio and H. Damasio, *Neurology* 33, 1573 (1983).

25. R. Vandenberghe, C. Price, R. Wise, O. Josephs, R. S. J. Frackowiak, *Nature* 383, 254 (1996).

26. Future work could examine whether activity due to letters depends on attention by comparing ignored consonants with false fonts or other scripts.

27. A. Treisman, *Psychol. Rev.* 76, 282 (1969); N. Lavie, *J. Exp. Psychol. Hum. Percept. Perform.* 21, 451 (1995).

28. G. Rees, C. D. Frith, N. Lavie, *Science* 278, 1616 (1997).

29. S. J. Luck, E. K. Vogel, K. L. Shapiro, *Nature* 383, 616 (1996).

30. Supported by the Wellcome Trust and by an Economic and Social Research Council (U. K.) grant to J. D. We thank F. Crick, R. Frackowiak, C. Koch, and C. Mummery for helpful comments and the late I. Rock for inspiration.

16 Aspects of the Theory of Comprehension, Memory, and Attention

Donald G. MacKay

Introduction

One of the major issues in theories of attention is the level of processing unattended inputs. To what extent do we comprehend unattended sentences? It was probably Wundt (1897) who proposed the first answer to this question, as well as the first systematic theory of comprehension and attention. Wundt held that we process sentences at two distinct levels—one level involving preattentive processes and the other involving attentive processes. The first level of processing provides a preliminary analysis—a superficial or "surface" description of phrases as they appear in the sentence. Attention plays no role in this preliminary or surface analysis, but is essential for the second level of analysis—the level producing perception of the relations among words and phrases of the sentence, relations such as "subject" and "object." According to Wundt (1897, p. 292) "the relations are conceived as coming into existence with the help of attentional processes."

The present paper provides evidence for a modern version of Wundt's theory. In this version the perceptual mechanism P consists of two distinct but interrelated levels or components. The first level involves a limited capacity short-term memory (M1) and the second, a large long-term memory (M2) (after Miller and Chomsky 1963). As in Wundt (1897), we assume that analytic processes at these two levels differ. M1 contains a finite-state device which performs a limited analysis of linguistic input. These M1 computations consist of semantic feature analyses of words (e.g., John—a male person, etc.) and surface syntactic analyses specifying the syntactic categories (noun, noun phrase, verb, verb phrase) and morphophonemic aspects (e.g., THINGS is THING + plural) of words in the sentence. M1 carries out these analyses for both

attended and unattended words transmitting the results of its computations to M2.

Processing in M2 differs in two ways from processing in M1. The first difference is that M2 works out the deep or underlying relations among the symbols computed by M1—relations such as subject, object. An extensive and complex set of rules is required to reconstruct these underlying relations—rules more powerful than the finite-state look-up procedures of M1. The second difference is that M2 only processes attended inputs, whereas M1 handles all inputs, attended and unattended. Partial support for this assumption is found in Norman (1969) who showed that unattended inputs get into short-term memory but not into long-term memory.

This theory generates several empirically testable corollaries, two of which are outlined below. Although the first corollary will not be tested in the present study, it nevertheless serves to illustrate the detailed mechanics of the theory. Corollary one is that M1 will be incapable of detecting or resolving certain types of ambiguity. Only M2 can detect the two meanings in underlying structure ambiguities. To illustrate this point more precisely, suppose that P is analyzing sentence (1) which is ambiguous at the underlying structure level. M1 assigns:

(1) John is quick to please.

(Underlying structure ambiguity)

lexical meaning to each word in (1) (e.g., John—a male person, etc.) along with a preliminary syntactic analysis basically similar to the surface structure in figure 16.1. It is important to note that this M1 analysis fails to capture the fact that we eventually see JOHN as either the object or the subject of "please." And since M1 cannot specify these underlying relations, M1 is therefore incapable of discovering underlying ambiguities such as (1). According to our model, M2 processes are needed for reconstructing the al-

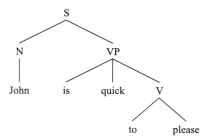

Figure 16.1
Surface structures analysis of the underlying structure ambiguity "John is quick to please" (details omitted after Miller and Chomsky 1963).

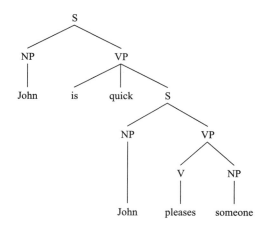

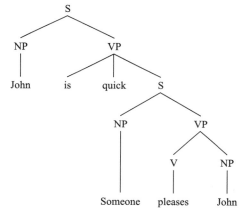

ternative interpretations of underlying structure ambiguities. Specifically, to uncover the underlying relations of (1), M2 must transform the input from M1 (shown in figure 16.1) into structural descriptions similar to (a) and (b) in figure 16.2.

However, M1 can detect lexical ambiguities such as (2), since two lexical readings would be generated when M1 looks up the dictionary meanings for BARK.

(2) The hunters noticed the bark.

(Lexical ambiguity)

M1 can also detect surface structure ambiguities which occur whenever two different form classes (e.g., noun, verb) can be assigned to words in a sentence. For example (3) represents a surface structure ambiguity since *her-dog-biscuits* can be decoded as either *Pronoun-Adjective-Noun* or *Adjective-Noun-Noun*. These surface structure alternatives would be discovered when M1 assigns syntactic categories to words.

(3) The hunters fed her dog biscuits.

(Surface structure ambiguity)

Of the three levels of ambiguity, lexical, surface and deep, the preliminary analyses of M1 will uncover the first two but not the last, a deduction from our theory that has been examined

Figure 16.2
The deep structure analysis of the two interpretations of "John is quick to please" (details omitted after Miller and Chomsky 1963).

in detail in MacKay (in press). But the present paper is concerned with the second corollary outlined below.

Since only M1 analyzes unattended inputs, our theory predicts that unattended words will only be processed at the lexical and surface syntax levels. Deep structure relations will be perceived if and only if the input is attended (i.e., processed by M2). We used Cherry and Taylor's (1954) dichotic listening task to test this deduction. Our subjects had to shadow continuously and without error a sentence rapidly presented to one ear of a stereo headset, ignoring inputs to the other ear. After Moray (1959) we define errorlessly shadowed inputs under these conditions as *attended* and other inputs as *unattended.*

Unknown to subjects, the attended sentences in our studies contained an ambiguity for which the two interpretations were about equally likely (as determined in a pilot study). Our question was whether unattended material would bias the meaning subjects see in processing these attended ambiguities. For example, we presented a lexical ambiguity such as (2) to the attended ear and a "bias word" (DOG) to the unattended ear. If this unattended word biases or makes more likely the DOG bark interpretation of (2), we can conclude that unattended input is processed at the lexical level as predicted in our model. However, an analogous biasing effect for underlying ambiguities is impossible according to our model. Unattended inputs should not bias an underlying ambiguity such as (1) since the transformational rules necessary to reconstruct the deep or underlying relations for this bias effect are only applied to attended inputs. If we find a bias effect at the underlying structure level, our model must be wrong.

Study 1: Initial Determination of Bias

Study 1 was a preliminary test undertaken to determine the initial Bias or likelihood of the meanings of ambiguous sentences used later in our shadowing experiments. We determined Bias in two ways. One formula for Bias was based on the frequency with which subjects see a given interpretation of an ambiguous sentence. Bias in this sense is defined by the percentage of subjects in the sample who see one of the meanings first. Using this measure we determined the Bias of 80 ambiguous sentences recorded in

random order on a Sony TC200 stereo tape recorder by the same female experimenter as in later experiments. Thirty-three UCLA undergraduates listened to the 80 sentences one at a time, turned over a response sheet after each sentence, and indicated which of the meanings he saw first. No subject claimed to see both meanings simultaneously.

Our second method for determining the Bias of our sentences involved subjective likelihood ratings. After indicating on his response sheet which of the two meanings he saw first, the subject estimated the likelihood of these meanings in that particular sentential context. If the subject thought the two meanings were equally likely, he gave both alternatives a rating of 50%. If he thought one meaning was much more probable than the other, he rated that meaning 90% and the other 10%, and so on. The subject was instructed to make these "likelihood ratings" without regard for which meaning he saw first. Using this method, Bias was defined by the average likelihood rating for the two interpretations of an ambiguity.

The results of Study 1 were as follows. Using method 1, Bias ranged from 50% to 100%, mean 74%. Using method 2, Bias ranged from 50% to 83%, mean 63%. But these two methods provided equivalent measures within a certain range of Bias. For sentences with Bias from 30 to 70% the two measures of Bias never differed by more than 5%. But for the range from 70 to 100%, the second method gave consistently less extreme estimates of Bias. In the experiments to follow we discarded sentences with extreme Bias, using only "unbiased ambiguities" (ambiguities with Bias close to 50%). Since the two measures of Bias were equivalent for unbiased ambiguities, and since the second measure was more reliable than the first (each subject contributes more data) and provides a more direct estimate of the salience of the readings of an ambiguous sentence, we propose to use likelihood ratings to measure Bias in this and future studies involving ambiguity.

General Procedures, Instructions, and Analyses: Studies 2–4

For the experiments reported in Studies 2–4 we selected 46 sentences from Study 1, using Bias as our criterion (mean Bias 50%; range from 35 to 65%). Subsets of these 46 sentences made up the materials in the five experiments to follow.

The first three experiments involved lexical ambiguities and are reported as Study 2. The last two experiments included both surface and underlying structure ambiguities, but the results are separately reported for surface ambiguity (Study 3) and underlying structure ambiguity (Study 4). The equipment included a Sony TC200 stereo tape recorder for presenting the stimuli to a low impedence stereo headset worn by the subject. A second, identical machine recorded the subject's responses.

Subjects were instructed to pay close attention to inputs arriving at one ear and to ignore inputs to the other ear. The left ear was attended on one half of the trials and the right on the other half, with ear order counterbalanced across the subjects. Attention was controlled by having the subject vocally shadow the material on the attended ear or write it out on a slip of paper as it was being presented. The subject was instructed to shadow or write out the attended sentence without lag, errors or pauses. The subject was also warned that he later had to recall the sentence in the attended ear.

The attended sentences were all 15 ± 1 syllables long and unknown to the subjects, contained one of the three types of ambiguity discussed above. The series of up to 28 experimental sentences was followed by an equal number of "recognition trials." For example, if the first sentence presented was (4), then on the first recognition trial the subject had to choose between (5) and (6) as to which was closest in meaning to

(4)   They threw stones toward the bank
      yesterday.   (Lexical ambiguity)

(5)   They threw stones toward the side of the river yesterday.
                                    (Recognition alternative A)

(6)   They threw stones toward the savings and loan association yesterday.
                                    (Recognition alternative B)

the sentence he heard originally. In this way we were able to determine which meaning the subject had seen without his knowing that the experiment had anything to do with ambiguity. This procedure therefore precluded the possibility that subjects were searching for ambiguity or were processing the attended sentences in an unnatural manner. The recognition trials proceeded in the same order as the experimental sentences.

The "unattended" or non-shadowed channel contained either one or two words, uttered by the same (female) experimenter at the same rate and loudness as the sentences on the attended or shadowed channel. The experimenter read the sentences at a rapid rate (0.200 s per syllable on the average) in a normal subdued intonation with no pauses between words or phrases. The subject was instructed to ignore all inputs to the "unattended ear." Each experiment was preceded by a practice session in which the subject shadowed or wrote out five unambiguous practice sentences while unrelated words occurred on the unattended channel.

Two main statistical procedures were used in analyzing the data of our experiments. In the first procedure, the sentence was the unit of analysis and the dependent variable was the Bias Shift, defined as:

$$\text{Bias Shift} = \text{BE} - \text{BI}.$$

Thus if meaning A of sentence (4) (i.e., BANK of A RIVER) received an Initial Bias of 45% in Study 1, and an Experimental Bias of 75% when RIVER was the unattended word in Study 2, then the Bias Shift for meaning A is $75 - 45 = 30\%$. Note that the Bias Shift can be either negative or positive, depending on the results of Study 2. But only a significantly positive Bias Shift indicates that the unattended bias words influenced the processing of the sentence in the attended ear. Using this Bias Shift method of data analysis, our null hypothesis held that BE would exceed BI in the predicted direction no more often than chance expectation. A sign test with sentences as the unit of analysis and BI and BE as the variables was used to test this null hypothesis.

The second method of data analysis employed a chi-square test to determine whether the number of subjects seeing the predicted meaning exceeded chance expectation (50%). This test had the advantage of using subjects as the unit of analysis—a standard procedure for statistical tests in psychology. However, the chi-square test is somewhat less sensitive than the sign test discussed above since it fails to take into consideration the variations in BI, the initial Bias of the sentences. But this drawback is perhaps not serious since the average BI for sentences in the experiments to follow was always 50%.

Study 2: Unattended Processing of Lexical Meaning

Hypothesis 1: Unattended Lexical Meaning Can Shift the Bias of Simultaneously Shadowed Sentences Containing Lexical Ambiguities

Twenty-six sentences containing lexical ambiguities were designed to test Hypothesis 1. The ambiguous words usually occurred towards the middle of the sentence, the mean syllabic position of the ambiguities being 5.1 syllables from the beginning. Another word was recorded on the unattended channel. This unattended word was centred relative to the ambiguous word on the attended channel, the relative positioning being determined by ear with the recorder running at one fourth its normal speed. For half the subjects, the unattended word was related to one interpretation of the ambiguity as in hypothetical

example (8), and for the remaining subjects it was related to the other interpretation, as in (9).

(7)   They threw stones toward the bank
      yesterday.   (Lexical ambiguity)

(8)   RIVER
                    (Unattended word)

(9)   MONEY
                    (Unattended word)

The subjects were 16 UCLA undergraduates who had not taken part in Study 1. The subjects were instructed to verbally shadow the attended sentences without errors or pauses longer than 1.0 s.

Results and Discussion

About 7% of the trials involved errors in shadowing, the majority being omissions and unacceptable pauses or onset lags longer than 1.0 s. In no case was the unattended word shadowed by mistake. Only sentences shadowed continuously and without error were considered in the analyses to follow, so as to rule out the hypothesis that subjects had time to switch attention to the unattended ear.

The mean Bias Shift for all 26 sentences in this study was +4.2% (interquartile range 3–25%). Using our first analytic procedure, this Bias Shift was statistically reliable ($P < 0.03$, sign test with sentences as the unit of analysis and BI and BE as variables). Using our second method of analysis, these data were significant at the 0.02 level ($\chi^2 = 6.01$, $df = 1$, subjects as unit of analysis). At first sight, this 4.2% Bias Shift may seem rather small (though reliable). However, the small size of our Bias Shifts may reflect noise inherent in our recognition technique, since some subjects may have forgotten which meaning they saw at the time of test. Hindsight suggests an additional control or comparison condition where the relevant alternatives, say RIVER BANK and SAVINGS INSTITUTION, are presented along with a completely novel alternative, say TREE. False recognitions of the novel word in this condition would give us a signal-to-noise base line against which to compare the Bias Shifts.

However, the significance of our Bias Shift suggests that unattended inputs are processed at the lexical level and can alter the Bias of lexically ambiguous sentences (at least to some extent). That is, the lexical meaning of the unattended word must have been analyzed and integrated with the lexical analyses of the attended sentences. Our data therefore support the hypothesis that unattended words are processed at the meaning level. In this regard our findings contradict Treisman's (1960) hypothesis that "shadowing experiments suggest there is a single channel for analyzing meaning" (p. 246) and Broadbent's (1958) hypothesis that information capacity becomes limited at the meaning stage, so that we can handle only one semantic input at a time, either keeping to one message or switching between the two. Broadbent and others add that switching between channels becomes more likely when new signals arrive suddenly on a hitherto unoccupied channel or when contextually probable signals arrive on an unattended channel. However, this "attention switching" hypothesis seems unlikely for the present experimental paradigm. The subjects in our experiment must have been paying unremittent attention to the sentences in the relevant ear rather than switching attention to the words in the irrelevant ear since we only scored sentences that were shadowed continuously and without error. Moreover, the Bias Shift in this study is probably not dependent on the "sudden arrival" of the bias word on the unattended channel, since Lackner and Garrett, in Garrett (1970), obtained similar results by embedding the bias word in a sentence presented on the unattended channel.

Nor does it seem likely that the meaning of the unattended words was attained by switching to a precategorical acoustic store (PAS) following the end of the attended sentence. This hypothetical switch would occur at least 2.0 s after the unattended words arrived in PAS. But material in PAS decays too rapidly for the unattended words to be grasped in this way (cf. Crowder and Morton 1969).

Hypothesis 2: A Replication of Experiment 1

This experiment had the same purpose, materials and design as the experiment just reported. The only difference was that the subject wrote out the attended sentence as he heard it, instead of shadowing it verbally. The subject had to begin his written transcription within 1.0 s of sentence onset and continue at maximum rate without error, pauses or correction. This procedure had the advantage that feedback from the subject's own voice could not mask the input to the unattended ear. We therefore expected a larger Bias Shift in this experiment since even partial masking of the unattended words in the previous experiment might preclude semantic analysis and thereby rule out an interaction with the ongoing semantic processing of the attended sentence. The subjects were 20 UCLA undergraduates who had not served in our previous experiments.

Results and Discussion

About 5% of the trials involved errors in writing out the sentences, omissions again being most frequent. As before, only errorless trials were scored in the analyses to follow. The unattended words caused a 9.5% Bias Shift in the expected direction (interquartile range 0–20%). This Bias Shift was statistically significant using our first method of analysis ($P < 0.05$ two-tailed sign test with sentences as unit of analysis). These data were also significant using our second method of analysis ($\chi^2 = 4.88$, $df = 1$, $P < 0.05$, subjects as unit of analysis). These findings therefore reinforce the conclusion of the previous experiment: that the meaning of unattended words is analyzed at the lexical level and interacts with the ongoing semantic processing of the attended sentence.

As we expected, the Bias Shift in the present experiment exceeded that in the previous experiment (9.5% vs. 4.2%), although this difference was statistically unreliable ($P < 0.06$, two-tailed sign test with sentences as the unit of analysis and Bias Shift as the variable).

Hypothesis 3: The Awareness Issue

Are our subjects fully aware of the word presented to the unattended channel? And are they more aware of an unattended word if it is related to the attended input than if it is not? To test these hypotheses we included a twenty-seventh ambiguous sentence just prior to the recognition trials in the experiments just discussed. The unattended word on this trial was related to the ambiguity as in (8) for half the subjects and unrelated as in (10) for the remaining subjects. Immediately after presentation of the sentence,

(10)   They threw stones towards the bank
           yesterday   (Lexical ambiguity)
                                    MOTHER
                             (Unattended word)

the experimenter handed the subject a card containing the following instructions: "Stop shadowing (writing). What was the word in your other ear?" _____

Results and Discussion

When the unattended sentence was shadowed or written without error in this condition, only one subject (out of 36) correctly reported the unattended word. This single correct response occurred in the first experiment (verbal shadowing) when the unattended word (MOTHER) bore no relation to the ambiguity. This result indicates that the unattended word usually failed to reach the level of awareness required for verbal report under the conditions of our experiments. This apparent lack of awareness or failure in recall is consistent with the findings of Cherry and Taylor (1954), Broadbent (1958), Treis-

man (1960) and Lewis (1970). But Cherry and Broadbent argued that since subjects can only recall the "general physical characteristics" of unattended messages (pitch, intensity, location), then no further analyses are going on. This conclusion is unwarranted. The fact that subjects are not fully aware of or cannot recall the signal to the unattended ear is not evidence that the signal was not processed. Lack of awareness of failure to recall does not imply absence of analysis.

We suggest that lexical analyses of unattended words occurred in this and previous experiments but that these analyses were no longer available for recall at the time of test. That is, unattended material is processed in short-term memory (M1) and decays so rapidly that analyses of unattended words were obliterated at the time of test in this and previous experiments. However, we suggest that more sensitive tests such as the recognition procedure of Kahnemann (1969) and Norman (1969) should corroborate the occurrence of lexical analyses demonstrated under Hypotheses 1 and 2 of the present study. Using a recognition procedure subjects should choose synonyms of unattended words more often than semantically unrelated words.

However, the present experiment rules out an explanation proposed by Garrett (1970) for the failures to report unattended words. Garrett (1970) argued that "subjects cannot report some of the material in the unattended ear perhaps because they *believe* it was part of the signal to the attended ear" (p. 59). Under this hypothesis one would expect subjects in our experiments to incorporate the unattended words into their shadowing or writing out of the sentences. Since this did not occur, Garrett's hypothesis seems implausible.

Hypothesis 4: The Nature of Interaction Between Attended and Unattended Inputs

The experiments just reported show that semantic analyses of unattended lexical inputs somehow interact with the ongoing semantic processing or interpretation of attended messages. Understanding the nature of this interaction requires a detailed model of the mechanism for lexical analysis. In the model of MacKay (1970), lexical analyses take place in an internal dictionary which receives words as input and generates the semantic features of these words as output. The semantic features of different meanings for ambiguous words have different weightings depending on frequency of occurrence, context and set. The projection rules, which relate the meanings of words in a sentence, contribute to these weightings (thereby eliminating many potential or partial ambiguities). But projection rules are irrelevant to the present study since all of our sentences were fully ambiguous. To illustrate the mechanics of the internal dictionary in our present experiments, consider example (7), lexical ambiguity BANK and unattended word RIVER. The internal dictionary generates two sets of semantic features for BANK which have approximately equal weighting, giving a salience or Bias or 50% in Study 1. In Study 2 these features of BANK are generated while the unattended word RIVER is being analyzed, which further activates the features for the RIVER BANK meaning of BANK. Since more strongly activated features tend to be used in the interpretation of the whole sentence (see MacKay 1970), this unattended input would bias the RIVER BANK interpretation of BANK, thereby explaining the results of Experiments 1 and 2.

But what should happen when two bias words are presented simultaneously on the unattended channel, one denoting one interpretation of the ambiguity, and the other denoting the other interpretation, as in hypothetical examples (11) and (12)? MacKay (1970) predicted:

(11)   They threw stones toward the bank
       yesterday.   (Lexical ambiguity)

(12)   money river
                              (Unattended words)

an interaction between the biasing effects of these unattended words, such that bias from one word would cancel or counteract bias from the other, the end result being 0% Bias Shift.

We used 16 sentences to test this hypothesis, the order of the two unattended words being counterbalanced across subjects. As before, the unattended words were centred relative to the ambiguous word on the attended channel.

Two additional conditions were introduced in this experiment. In one condition, both unattended words were related to the same meaning of the ambiguous sentence as in (13) and (14). In the other condition the same word was simply repeated as in (15) and (16).

(13)   River   Shore   (Unattended words)

(14)   Shore   River   (Unattended words)

(15)   River   River   (Unattended words)

(16)   Shore   Shore   (Unattended words)

We predicted that the RIVER-RIVER condition (same word repeated) would result in a smaller Bias Shift than the RIVER-SHORE condition, since more semantic features of the relevant interpretation of the ambiguous sentence would be activated when different words are presented than when the same word is repeated.

There were two sentences in each of these latter conditions, order of the conditions being counterbalanced across subjects, 20 UCLA students who had not taken part in our earlier experiments.

Results and Discussion
Consider first the RIVER-MONEY condition where the unattended words relate to opposite meanings of the ambiguity (16 sentences). A very slight Bias Shift towards the initial word was found. Bias shifted an average of +1.80% in the direction of the initial word. Using our first method of analysis, this Bias Shift was non-

significant ($P > 0.7$, sign test with sentences as unit of analysis). Using our second method of analysis, these data were non-significant at the 0.5 level ($\chi^2 = 0.78$, $df = 1$, subjects as unit of analysis).

Next consider the RIVER-SHORE condition where the bias words were both related to one of the meanings of the ambiguity. Here the Bias Shift toward the expected meaning was +14.0%. Because of the small number of sentences in this condition, it was impossible to test the reliability of this Bias Shift using a sign test with sentences as unit of analysis. But using our second analytic procedure, this Bias Shift was significant at the 0.01 level ($\chi^2 = 7.54$, $df = 1$, subjects as unit of analysis).

Finally the RIVER-RIVER condition involved a repeated word related to one of the meanings of the ambiguity. Here the Bias Shift was smaller than in the RIVER-SHORE condition but nevertheless highly reliable. The average shift was +10% (statistically significant beyond the 0.02 level, $\chi^2 = 5.48$, $df = 1$, subjects as unit of analysis).

These findings support the predictions of MacKay (1970) and suggest the possibility of two types of interaction between analyzers for lexical input. Results of the RIVER-MONEY condition suggest a negative interaction such that lexical analyses of MONEY cancel or interfere with lexical analyses of RIVER, giving 0% Bias Shift. Other interpretations of this outcome are possible, however.

Results of the RIVER-RIVER and SHORE-RIVER conditions suggest the possibility of a positive interaction between analyzers for lexical input. The same word repeated (RIVER-RIVER) gave a smaller Bias Shift than two different words (RIVER-SHORE), suggesting that more semantic features of the relevant interpretation are activated when different words are presented than when the same word is repeated. However this hypothesis requires further test with sufficient materials for statistical comparisons.

Study 3: Unattended Processing of Surface Structure

Study 3 was similar to Study 2 except for type of ambiguity. In Study 3 subjects attended to surface structure ambiguities and ignored two simultaneously presented words.

Hypothesis 5: The Form Class of Unattended Words Will Shift the Bias of Surface Structure Ambiguities

Hypothesis 5 is based on the theory outlined in the introduction, where M1 analyzes the form class of unattended words. Eight sentences similar to (17) were designed to test Hypothesis 5. The sentences and the two words on the unattended channel were recorded in a syllable-timed monotone so as to eliminate the stress and timing factors which normally bias these ambiguities in conversational speech.

The ambiguities involved virtually every syntactic category: verbs, verb particles, prepositions, adjectives, adverbs, and nouns. The unattended words had the same surface structure as one of the readings of the ambiguity. For example the surface syntax of the bias words in (18) is verb + verb particle, which should bias (17) toward the interpretation "to inspect" according to Hypothesis 5.

(17) When Tom looked over the fence, he didn't like what he saw.

(Surface ambiguity)

(18) phoned up

(Unattended words)

As before, the unattended words overlapped with the ambiguities in time. But the lexical meaning of the unattended words was irrelevant to either interpretation of the ambiguities, thereby ruling out a semantic bias in the manner of Study 2. The subjects were 10 UCLA undergraduates who had not taken part in the earlier experiments.

Results and Discussion

A +13.0% Bias Shift was obtained in this condition. Using our first method of analysis, this Bias Shift was statistically significant ($P < 0.03$, sign test with sentences as the unit of analysis). Using our second method of analysis, these data were reliable at the 0.05 level ($\chi^2 = 4.9$, $df = 1$, subjects as unit of analysis). These findings tend to confirm Hypothesis 5, and within the framework of our model, suggest that M1 must analyze the syntactic categories of unattended words, so as to influence the ongoing syntactic categorization of the attended sentence. In addition, these data suggest that the device for processing unattended inputs (M1) has a span of at least two words, a point of some importance for interpreting the negative results in the experiments to follow.

Hypothesis 6: Lexical Meaning of Unattended Words Will Bias the Interpretation of Surface Structure Ambiguities

To test Hypothesis 6 we presented the eight surface structure ambiguities discussed above to 10 new subjects using the same general procedure as before. Both unattended words in this condition belonged to the same syntactic category (verb, noun, adjective, or adverb) and so could not produce a Bias Shift in the manner of Hypothesis 5. For example, both unattended words in (20) are verbs, which should have no effect on the ongoing syntactic categorization of (19).

(19)   When Tom looked over the fence, he
       didn't like what he saw.
                                (Surface ambiguity)

(20)   examined   inspected
                               (Unattended words)

But the lexical meaning of the unattended words correspond to one of the meanings of the ambiguity. For example, the lexical meaning of the unattended words in (20) corresponds to the "examine" interpretation of (19), which should bias the interpretation of this ambiguity, according to Hypothesis 6.

Results and Discussion

The data did not support Hypothesis 6. The Bias Shift in this condition was -1.5%. Using our first method of analysis, this Bias Shift was statistically unreliable ($P > 0.5$, sign test with sentences as unit of analysis). These data were also nonsignificant using our second method of analysis ($P > 0.8$, $\chi^2 = 0.10$, $df = 1$, subjects as unit of analysis).

The negative results in this experiment must be viewed in conjunction with the positive results in Experiment 1. Since subjects in Experiment 1 processed the lexical meaning of unattended words, subjects in the present experiment probably also carried out lexical analyses, but for some reason, these lexical analyses had no effect on the ongoing syntactic categorization of words in the attended ear. Perhaps then, syntactic categories of words are assigned independently of lexical meaning, semantic features having no effect on form class assignments. This may be because semantic feature analyses follow form class assignments in the processing of sentences. In fact, assignment of syntactic categories before semantic features seems logically necessary in certain instances. For example, the same phonetic input can give rise to the syntactic categorizations THE SAND WHICH IS THERE and THE SANDWICHES THERE, but it seems logically impossible to assign semantic features in such cases before a definite syntactic categorization is achieved. In the present experiment the assignment of syntactic features before semantic features would account for the fact that semantic analyses had no effect on syntactic categorization, an interpretation congruent with, although not necessary for the general model outlined in the introduction.

Study 4: Unattended Processing of Underlying Structure

The procedures in Study 4 were similar to those in Study 3 except that the attended ambiguities were of the deep structure variety.

Hypothesis 7: The Underlying Structure of Unattended Words Can Bias the Interpretation of Underlying Structure Ambiguities

This hypothesis is based on the assumption of Bever, Kirk, and Lackner (1969) that the underlying structure of sentences is processed in short-term memory (M1).

Ten underlying structure ambiguities were designed to test Hypothesis 7.

For instance:

(21)   They knew that flying planes could be dangerous.   (Underlying ambiguity)

(22)   growling lions
                                        (Unattended words)

Flying planes in (21) can take two underlying relations: *planes* (*that*) *are flying* and *for someone to fly planes*. Note that the unattended words in (22) captured the first set of relations but not the second. The input *growling lions* has the underlying structure *lions* (*that*) *are growling*, which should bias (21) toward the interpretation *planes* (*that*) *are flying* according to Hypothesis 7. Note also that the bias words correspond in form class with the ambiguous words. However, as Chomsky (1963) points out, form class is irrelevant to the resolution of underlying structure ambiguities, so that Bias in the manner of Hypothesis 5 is impossible. The subjects in this experiment were the same as for the test of Hypothesis 5.

Results and Discussion

The data did not support Hypothesis 7. Using our first analytic procedure, unattended words in this condition had no significant effect on Bias ($P > 0.5$, sign test). Using our second method of analysis, these data were also non-significant at the 0.5 level ($\chi^2 = 0.72$, $df = 1$, subjects as unit of analysis).

These negative results cannot be considered conclusive support for our theory, since one cannot accept a model on the basis of the null hypothesis holding for the data. But alternative explanations seem difficult indeed. One alter-

native explanation holds that a Bias effect did occur in processing the sentences but the subjects simply forgot which underlying interpretation they saw at the time of test, responding on a chance basis to the recognition alternatives. However, this interpretation seems unlikely. Sachs (1967) has shown that deep structure assignments are *more* resistant to forgetting than lexical assignments. A "forgetting" hypothesis is therefore inconsistent with the positive findings in Study 2.

It is also difficult to explain the negative results in this experiment in terms of a one word limit in immediate memory for unattended inputs: the positive results for Hypothesis 6 indicate a span of at least two words. Identical reasoning rules out the hypothesis that M1 and M2 only reflect different sizes of working space (defined by number of words), that is, that processing of non-shadowed material is quantitatively but not qualitatively different from processing of shadowed material.

Nor can the negative results for Hypothesis 7 be explained by the assumption that underlying ambiguities are just not susceptible to bias effects. Bias effects do occur at the underlying structure level when bias words are attended. For example, Marshall (1965) showed that if subjects attentively process a sentence like (8) just prior to an underlying ambiguity like (9), the subjects are biased towards the underlying interpretation "John pleases someone." This finding (along with controls omitted here) indicates that Bias sentence (8) was processed

(8)   Mary is eager to help.   (Bias sentence)

(9)   John is quick to please.
                              (Underlying ambiguity)

at the deep structure level, and that biasing effects at the underlying structure level do occur when the bias material is attended. Our failure to find a similar bias effect for unattended inputs suggests that subjects may not process unattended inputs at the deep structure level. Within the framework of our model, our data suggest that M1 does not process the underlying relations between words. Attentive processing in M2 is needed for reconstructing the deep structure of linguistic inputs and for biasing an ambiguity at the deep structure level.

Hypothesis 8: The Lexical Meaning of Unattended Words Can Bias the Interpretation of Underlying Structure Ambiguities

Hypothesis 8 was advanced in MacKay (1970) and is directly analogous to Hypothesis 6 discussed above. Ten sentences similar to (23) were designed to test Hypothesis 8. The two "bias words" had the same lexical meaning as one of the interpretations of the ambiguity. For example

(23)   They said that the growing of the flowers was marvellous.   (Underlying ambiguity)

(24)   development growth
                        (Unattended words)

the lexical meaning of both bias words in (24) corresponds to one of the deep structure of (23): i.e. NP (*flowers*) + VP (*were growing*) rather than NP (*someone*) + V (*grew*) + NP (*the flowers*). The subjects were the same as in the test of Hypothesis 6.

Results and Discussion

Hypothesis 8 was not supported. Using our first analytic procedure the unattended words in this condition had no significant effect on Bias ($P > 0.5$, sign test with sentences as unit of analysis). Using our second analytic procedure, these data were non-significant at the 0.1 level ($\chi^2 = 0.20$, $df = 1$, subjects as unit of analysis). Taken in conjunction with the positive results for Hypothesis 1, these negative results suggest that lexical analyses of unattended words have no effect on the ongoing reconstruction of the deep structure of an attended sentence. Within the framework of our model, this means that lexical analyses of unattended words do not influence

or determine which rules are applied in reconstructing the deep structure or underlying relations between words in an attended sentence. However, we must again keep in mind the difficulties of arguing from acceptance of a null hypothesis.

Hypothesis 9: A Replication and Extension of Hypothesis 8

In this experiment both lexical meaning and underlying relations of the unattended words correspond to one of the interpretations of the attended ambiguities, which were again of the underlying type ($N = 10$). For example, the input *sportsmen slain* in (26) has the underlying structure NP (*someone*) + V (*slays*) + NP (*the sportsmen*) which corresponds to the interpretation NP (*someone*) + V (*shoots*) + NP (*the hunters*) in (25). The lexical meaning of *sportsmen slain* also corresponds to the underlying interpretation *someone shoots the hunters*. Hypothesis 9 holds that the combined effect

(25)   They thought the shooting of the hunters was dreadful.   (Underlying ambiguity)

(26)   sportsmen slain
                             (Unattended words)

of lexical meaning and underlying relations will bias these underlying structure ambiguities. The 20 subjects of Hypothesis 7 and 8 also served in this condition.

Results and Discussion

Hypothesis 9 was not supported. A negative Bias Shift of -3.0% was found, which using our first method of analysis was non-significant at the 0.5 level (sign test with sentences as unit of analysis). Using our second method of analysis, these data were non-significant at the 0.2 level ($\chi^2 = 1.20$, $df = 1$, subjects as unit of analysis). Within the framework of our model these negative findings reinforce the hypothesis that we do not process the deep structure of unattended inputs. M1 does not handle the underlying relations between words. Processing of unattended inputs seems to be limited to syntactic categorization (Hypothesis 5) and analyses of lexical meaning (Hypothesis 2).

General Discussion

Our findings fail to support Broadbent's (1958) model of attention, among others. We have shown that the meaning of unattended words must be analyzed to some extent even when the subject cannot recall or report their content, and when switching of attention between channels has been ruled out. Our data therefore suggest that unattended inputs are not filtered at a peripheral level: the "selective processes" in attention must follow the assignment of lexical meanings to words, a conclusion in agreement with Lewis (1970), Kahnemann (1969), and Deutsch and Deutsch (1963). However, our findings are not in complete agreement with the model of Deutsch and Deutsch (1963). We found a limit to the processing of unattended inputs: our data suggested that deep structure relations between words are only processed when the input is attended.

These findings favour a model basically similar to Wundt's (1897). In this model, unattended inputs only receive a preliminary or surface analysis in M1—a short-term memory containing a context-sensitive device for looking up the lexical meaning(s) and form class(es) of words. M1 passes on these limited analyses to M2 but only when the input is attended does M2 apply the transformational rules for deriving the deeper relations between the input symbols of M1.

This adaptation of Wundt's model represents an integration of postulates concerning memory, attention and comprehension, and the theory is consistent with established findings in all three fields.[1] According to the theory, memory for unattended input is limited (in capacity and durability) while memory for attended input is much greater—facts already demonstrated by Norman (1969) and Treisman (1965). According to the theory, material stored in short-term memory differs in form and content from material stored in long-term memory—a fact emphasized by Broadbent (1969) and others: "Long-term memory is not simply short-term memory crystallized into more durable form" (Broadbent, p. 171). According to the model, material stored in long-term memory is highly abstract—a fact underlined by Zangwill (1969) among others: "Long-term memory is highly selective ... and shows a strikingly abstractive character." And according to the model, memory for underlying structure (M2) is more durable than memory for surface structure and lexical items of a sentence (M1)—a fact demonstrated by Sachs (1967) among others.

Finally, the model suggests that processing in short-term memory is limited not just in capacity and durability, but also in scope. Analyses in M1 are carried out by a finite automaton—a device incapable of handling repeated self-embedding (Miller and Chomsky 1963). The model therefore explains (at least in part) why sentences containing repeated self-embeddings (e.g., (27)) are so difficult to store in short-term memory (Miller and Isard 1964).

(27)   The malt the rat the cat ate ate tasted
        good.   (Multiple self-embedding)

In addition, the model predicts that ordinary sequences without the property of repeated self-embedding will not receive full analysis in M1—a prediction which captures the findings of the present studies. Our model is also consistent with a recent study on the search for ambiguity by an amnesic patient (MacKay, in press). As a result of bilateral removal of mesial parts of the temporal lobes and hippocampus, this patient (H. M.) has normla short-term memory, but is almost completely unable to form new long-term traces. Within the framework of our model, H.

M. is unable to transfer information from M1 to M2, or to process new information in M2. Our experiment required H. M. to find the two meanings of various types of ambiguity. Without going into our control procedures, the results showed that H. M. was incapable of finding the two meanings of underlying structure ambiguities, although he was able to resolve surface and lexical ambiguities. These results, in conjunction with control conditions omitted here, strongly support our model. As pointed out in the introduction the model predicts that M1 will be incapable of resolving underlying ambiguities. And since H. M. is only capable of M1 processing, our model explains his inability to resolve the meanings of underlying ambiguities.

Of course M1 must have access to some form of long-term memory in order to look up the form class(es) and semantic features of a word. This, we suggest, hippocampal patients can do: they are able to retrieve long-term lexical traces established before their operation. Access to the internal dictionary for their native language is unimpaired. However, we suggest that hippocampal patients will be unable to learn or fully process the underlying relations of syntactic structures they have not encountered in the past.

Already established parameters are easily introduced in our model of the internal lexicon. The analyzers for specifying semantic features in the internal lexicon may be hierarchically organized and differ in threshold (biologically important analysers having permanently lower thresholds). Thresholds may also fluctuate depending on short-term context, set and instructions. Output activity of the dictionary analyzers may be proportional to importance, importance weightings in the lexicon being determined by past experience (after Deutsch and Deutsch 1963). Other parameters in attention models (e.g., arousal level, rehearsal) are also easy to introduce in our model. But we need not postulate a filter or attenuation mechanism to reduce the strength of input signals. Rather we suggest that attended signals are simply processed at deeper levels, resulting ultimately in awareness and long-term storage in M2.

In addition we assume that the feature analyzers are unique. For example, various related inputs such as *sister, woman, mother, girl* will all boost the activity of a unique analyzer for the semantic feature "female." This "uniqueness" assumption is crucial for explaining our bias effects. According to the uniqueness hypothesis an input such as SHORE boosts the activity of a unique set of feature analyzers, to a large extent the same analyzers as for BANK of a RIVER. We have already noted how this additional boost would bias the interpretation of lexical ambiguities such as BANK even when the bias word SHORE is unattended. This uniqueness postulate may also explain why our RIVER-SHORE condition produced greater bias effects than RIVER-RIVER or SHORE-SHORE. The RIVER-SHORE input boosts the activity of more features for the RIVER BANK interpretation than either of the other input conditions.

We also postulate an "either-or" interaction between the conflicting analyzers for ambiguous words. This "either-or" postulate accounts for the serial nature of perception in experiments on the search for ambiguity: subjects see one meaning then the other, but they virtually never see both meanings at once. For example they see LIKE as *either* a verb *or* a preposition but not both simultaneously, and they see CRANE as *either* non-living (HOIST) *or* living (BIRD) but not both simultaneously (MacKay and Bever 1967). The "either-or" postulate may also account for the disappearance of the bias effect in the RIVER-MONEY condition of Study 2. The bias effect of one word cancelled the bias effect of the other according to our "either-or" postulate.

Areas for Further Research

Our model generates a number of predictions for further research. One prediction concerns the assumption that M1 is modality independent, that is, M1 receives and integrates data from different modalities or input channels. Under this hypothesis, it should be possible to bias the interpretation of BARK in (28) by simultaneously presenting a picture of a barking dog.

(28)   The hunters noticed the bark yesterday.
(Lexical ambiguity)

The sound of a dog's bark on an unattended channel should have a similar biasing effect. Moreover, the finite automaton of M1 should process and integrate lexical meanings of familiar words regardless of language modality. For example, if (28) is the attended sentence for a group of English-German bilinguals, the unattended word GEBELL (German for DOG'S BARK) should bias the ongoing interpretation of the English word BARK.

A second areas for further research concerns the "click" phenomenon. The click phenomenon is observed in tasks where the subject listens to a sentence in one ear while a click is presented to the other ear: when the subject writes out the sentence and marks where he thinks the click occurred, his errors in localization are found to vary with the syntactic structure of the sentence. Even the underlying structure of sentences can influence these localization errors and from this, Bever, Lackner, and Kirk (1969) argued that the underlying structure of sentences must be processed in immediate memory. However, the assumption that click studies only involve short-term memory or perceptual processes seems questionable. For example Ladefoged (1967) obtained the click phenomenon without any click, that is, by instructing subjects to report or guess the locations of "subliminal" (actually nonexistent) clicks. Ladefoged's click phenomenon cannot be explained in terms of perception or even short-term memory for a click, but must reflect a fairly long-term response bias. Under this "response bias" hypothesis, previous click studies may reflect a complete (M2) rather than

superficial (M1) analysis of the sentences. Thus the findings of Bever et al. (1969) may be consistent with our model, even though their interpretation is not.

But note that we might be able to force the subject to respond to the click before his analysis of the sentence is complete, for example, by measuring manual reaction times to the clicks as in Abrams, Bever, and Garrett (1969). Our model suggests that only the surface structure of the sentence will influence an "on line" response such as this whereas underlying constituents will only influence the "post-facto" responses based on the more complete (M2) analyses of the sentence.

Acknowledgments

This research was supported by UCLA Grant 2428 and USPHS Grant 166668-01.

The author thanks K. Achevsky and Dr T. Zelinken for their assistance.

Note

1. The model does not explain why semantic interference is so difficult to find in M1 (see Baddeley and Dale 1966). However this phenomenon does not contradict our model. Explanations of noninterference require a model of interference. Lack of semantic interference does not imply lack of semantic processing in M1, a phenomenon which other studies have already demonstrated (e.g., Henley, Noyes, and Deese 1968).

References

Abrams, K., Bever, T. G. and Garrett, M. (1969). Syntactic structure modulates attention during speech perception. Paper referenced in Bever, Lackner, and Kirk, *Perception and Psychophysics*, 5, (4), 225–34.

Baddeley, A. D. and Dale, H. C. A. (1966). The effect of semantic similarity in retroactive interference in long- and short-term memory. *Journal of Verbal Learning and Verbal Behavior*, 5, 417–20.

Bever, T. G., Lackner, J. R. and Kirk, R. (1969). The underlying structures of sentences are the primary units of immediate speech processing. *Perception and Psychophysics*, 5, (4), 225–34.

Bever, T. G., Kirk, R. and Lackner, J. (1969). An autonomic reflection of syntactic structure. *Neuropsychologia*, 7, 23–8.

Broadbent, D. (1958). *Perception and Communication.* London: Pergamon.

Broadbent, D. E. (1969). Communication models for memory. In Talland, G. A. and Waugh, N. (Eds), *The Pathology of Memory.* Pp. 167–73. New York: Academic Press.

Cherry, C. and Yaylor, W. (1954). Some further experiments on the recognition of speech with one and with two ears. *Journal Acoustical Society of America*, 26, 554–9.

Chomsky, N. (1963). Formal properties of grammars. In Luce, R. D., Bush, R. R. and Galanter, E. (Eds), *Handbook of Mathematical Psychology.* New York: Wiley.

Crowder, R. G. and Morton, J. (1969). Precategorical acoustic storage (PAS). *Perception and Psychophysics*, 5, (6), 365–73.

Deutsch, J. and Deutsch, D. (1963). Attention: some theoretical considerations. *Psychological Review*, 70, 80–90.

Garrett, M. (1970). Does ambiguity complicate the perception of sentences? In Flores D'Arcais, G. B. and Levelt, W. J. M. (Eds), *Advances in Psycholinguistics.* Amsterdam: North Holland.

Henley, N. M., Noyes, H. L. and Deese, J. (1968). Semantic structure in short-term memory. *Journal of Experimental Psychology*, 77, (4), 587–92.

Kahnemann, D. (1969). Paper presented to the XIX International Congress of Psychology, London, July 1969.

Ladefoged, P. (1967). *Three Areas of Experimental Phonetics.* London: Oxford University Press.

17 To See or Not To See: The Need for Attention to Perceive Changes in Scenes

Ronald A. Rensink, J. Kevin O'Regan, and James J. Clark

Although people must look in order to see, looking by itself is not enough. For example, a person who turns his or her eyes toward a bird singing in a tree will often fail to see it right away, "latching onto" it only after some effort. This also holds true for objects in plain view: A driver whose mind wanders can often miss important road signs, even when these are highly visible. In both situations, the information needed for perception is available to the observer. Something, however, prevents the observer from using this information to see the new objects that have entered the field of view.

In this article, we argue that the key factor is attention. In particular, we propose that the visual perception of change in a scene occurs only when focused attention is given to the part being changed. In support of this position, we show that when the low-level cues that draw attention are swamped, large changes in images of real-world scenes become extremely difficult to identify, even if these changes are repeated dozens of times and observers have been told to expect them. Changes are easily identified, however, when a valid verbal cue is given, indicating that stimulus visibility is not reduced. Changes are also easily identified when made to objects considered to be important in the scene. Taken together, these results indicate that—even when sufficient viewing time has been given—an observer does not build up a representation of a scene that allows him or her to perceive change automatically. Rather, perception of change is mediated through a narrow attentional bottleneck, with attention attracted to various parts of a scene based on high-level interest.

The phenomenon of *induced change blindness* has previously been encountered in two rather different experimental paradigms. The first, concerned with visual memory, was used to investigate the detection of change in briefly presented arrays of simple figures or letters (e.g., Pashler 1988, Phillips 1974). An initial display was presented for 100–500 ms, followed by a brief interstimulus interval (ISI), followed by a second display in which one of the items was removed or replaced on half the trials. Responses were forced-choice guesses about whether a change had occurred. Observers were found to be poor at detecting change if old and new displays were separated by an ISI of more than 60–70 ms.

The second type of paradigm, stemming from eye movement studies, was used to examine the ability of observers to detect changes in an image made during a saccade (e.g., Bridgeman, Hendry, and Stark 1975; Grimes 1996; McConkie and Zola 1979). A variety of stimuli were tested, ranging from arrays of letters to images of real-world scenes. In all cases, observers were found to be quite poor at detecting change, with detection good only for a change in the saccade target (Currie, McConkie, Carlson-Radvansky, and Irwin 1995).

Although blindness to saccade-contingent change has been attributed to saccade-specific mechanisms, the blurring of the retinal image during the saccade also masks the transient motion signals that normally accompany an image change. Because transients play a large role in drawing attention (e.g., Klein, Kingstone, and Pontefract 1992; Posner 1980), saccade-contingent change blindness may not be due to saccade-specific mechanisms, but rather may originate from a failure to allocate attention correctly. The blindness to changes in briefly presented displays may have a similar cause: In those experiments, detection was not completely at chance, but instead was at a level corresponding to a monitoring of four to five randomly selected items, a value similar to the number of items that can be attended simultaneously (Pashler 1987; Pylyshyn and Storm 1988; Wolfe, Cave, and Franzel 1989).

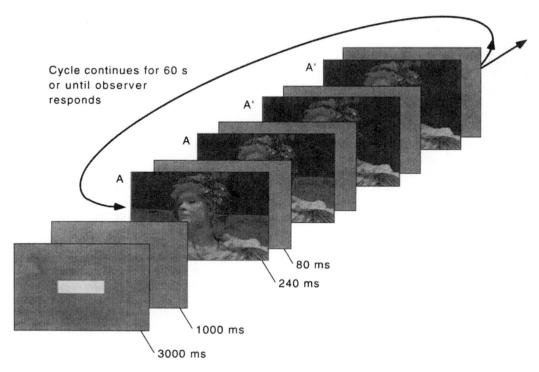

Cycle continues for 60 s
or until observer
responds

A'

A'

A

A

80 ms

240 ms

1000 ms

3000 ms

Figure 17.1
General design of the flicker paradigm. Trials began with a 3-s gray field containing a white rectangle (in which a word appeared when a cue was used). This was followed by a 1-s gray field, followed by a flicker sequence that continued until the observer responded or 60 s had elapsed. In the example here, original image A (statue with background wall) and modified image A' (statue with wall removed) are displayed in the order A, A, A', A', ..., with gray fields between successive images.

In order to examine whether both types of change blindness might be due to the same attentional mechanism, and whether this mechanism might also lead to change blindness under more normal viewing conditions, we developed a *flicker paradigm*. In this paradigm, an original image A repeatedly alternates with a modified image A', with brief blank fields placed between successive images (figure 17.1). Differences between the original and modified images can be of any size and type. (In the experiments presented here, the changes were chosen to be highly

visible.) The observer freely views the flickering display and hits a key when the change is perceived. To prevent guessing, we ask the observer to report the type of change and describe the part of the scene that was changing.

This paradigm allows the ISI manipulations of the brief-display techniques to be combined with the free-viewing conditions and perceptual criteria of the saccade-contingent methods. And because the stimuli are available for long stretches of time and no eye movements are required, the paradigm also provides the best opportunity possible for an observer to build a representation conducive to perceiving changes in a scene. The change blindness found with the brief-display techniques might have been caused by insufficient time to build an adequate representation of the scene; saccade-contingent change blindness might have been caused by disruptions due to eye movements. Both of these factors are eliminated in the flicker paradigm, so that if they were indeed the cause of the difficulties in the other paradigms, perception of change in the flicker paradigm should be easy. But if attention is the key factor, a different outcome would be expected. The flicker caused by the blank fields would swamp the local motion signals due to the image change, preventing attention from being drawn to its location. Observers would then fail to see large changes under conditions of extended free viewing, even when these changes were not synchronized to saccades.

General Method

In the experiments reported here, flicker sequences were usually composed of an original image A and modified version A' displayed in the sequence A, A, A', A',..., with gray blank fields placed between successive images (figure 17.1). Each image was displayed for 240 ms and each blank for 80 ms. Note that each image was presented twice before being switched. This procedure created a degree of temporal uncertainty as to when the change was being made, and also allowed for a wider range of experimental manipulation.

All the experiments used the same set of 48 color images of real-world scenes. Images were 27° wide and 18° high. A single change—in color, location, or presence versus absence—was made to an object or area in each. To test for the influence of higher level factors, we divided changes further according to the degree of interest in the part of the scene being changed. Interest was determined via an independent experiment in which five naive observers provided

a brief verbal description of each scene: *Central interests* (CIs) were defined as objects or areas mentioned by three or more observers; *marginal interests* (MIs) were objects or areas mentioned by none. The average changes in intensity and color were similar for the MIs and the CIs, but the areas of the MI changes (average = 22 sq. deg) were somewhat larger than the areas of the CI changes (average = 18 sq. deg). In all cases, changes were quite large and easy to see once noticed. For example, a prominent object could appear and disappear, switch its color between blue and red, or shift its position by a few degrees (figure 17.2).

Ten naive observers participated in each experiment. They were instructed to press a key when they saw the change, and then to describe it verbally. Before each experiment, observers were told of the types of change possible, and were given six practice trials (two examples of each type) to familiarize themselves with the task. Images were presented in random order for each subject. The dependent variable was the average number of alternations (proportional to the reaction time) needed to see the change. Averages were taken only from correct responses (i.e., responses in which the observer correctly identified both the type of change occurring and the object or area being changed). As might be expected given the large changes, identification error rates were low, averaging only 1.2% across the experiments.

Experiment 1

Experiment 1 examined whether the basic flicker paradigm could indeed induce change blindness. Images were displayed for 240 ms and blanks for 80 ms, with images repeated before being switched (figure 17.1). If insufficient viewing time were the reason for the change blindness found in the brief-display experiments, we expected changes in this experiment to be seen within at most a few seconds of viewing. If saccade-specific mechanisms were responsible for the

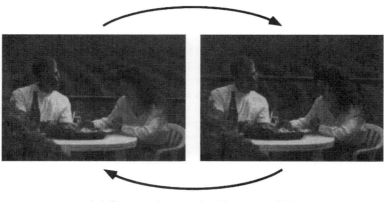

(a) Change in marginal interest (MI)

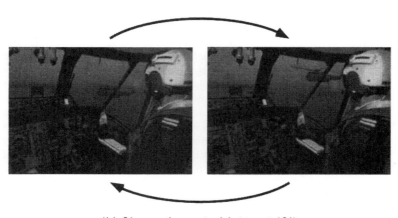

(b) Change in central interest (CI)

Figure 17.2
Examples of changes in scenes. Original and modified images alternated every 640 ms. A change in a marginal in-terest is illustrated by the changed position of the railing behind the people in (a). Although the railing is easily seen, and its location shift is large (3°), and average of 16.2 alternations (10.4 s) was required for identification. A change in a central interest is illustrated by the changed position of the helicopter in (b). Although the change in location is roughly the same as in (a), and the size and contrast of the items changed are comparable, identification of the change in (b) required on average only 4.0 alternations (2.6 s).

change blindness found in the saccade experiments, we expected changes in this experiment to be easy to see simply by keeping the eyes still. But if the failures to detect change in the previous paradigms were due to an attentional mechanism, we expected changes under these flicker conditions to take a long time to see.

The results of Experiment 1 (figure 17.3a) show a striking effect: Under flicker conditions, changes in MIs were extremely difficult to see, requiring an average of 17.1 alternations (10.9 s) before being identified; indeed, for some images, observers required more than 80 alternations (50 s) to identify a change that was obvious once noticed. Changes in CIs were noticed much more quickly, after an average of 7.3 alternations (4.7 s). Because discriminability was not equated for the three different types of change, performance between them cannot be compared. However, within each type of change, perception of MI changes took significantly longer than perception of CI changes ($p < .001$ for presence vs. absence; $p < .05$ for color; $p < .001$ for location), even though MI changes were on average more than 20% larger in area.

To confirm that the changes in the pictures were indeed easy to see when flicker was absent, the experiment was repeated with the blanks in the displays removed. A completely different pattern of results emerged: Identification required only 1.4 alternations (0.9 s) on average, showing that observers noticed the changes quickly. No significant differences were found between MIs and CIs for any type of change, and no significant differences were found between types of change ($p > .3$ for all comparisons).

Experiment 2

One explanation for the poor performance found in Experiment 1 might be that old and new scene descriptions could not be compared because of time limitations. Although the blanks between

images lasted only 80 ms—well within the 300-ms duration of iconic memory (e.g., Irwin 1991, Sperling 1960)—it has been shown that approximately 400 ms are needed to process and consolidate an image in memory (Potter 1976). The images in Experiment 1 were displayed for only 240 ms, which may have interfered with consolidation, and thus with the ability to compare successive images.

In Experiment 2, therefore, the blanks between pairs of identical images were "filled in" by replacing them with an 80-ms presentation of the "surrounding" images. Thus, instead of presenting each image for 240 ms, followed by a blank for 80 ms, and then presenting it again for another 240 ms, we presented images without interruption for 560 ms ($240 + 80 + 240$) at a time. Because the blanks between the original and modified images were kept, original image A and modified image A' were now presented in the sequence A, A', A, A' ..., with changes continuing to be made at the same rate as before. If memory processing were the limiting factor, the longer display of the images in this experiment should have allowed consolidation to take place, and so caused the changes to be much more easily seen.

The results (figure 17.3b), however, show that this did not occur. Although there was a slight speedup for MI changes, this was not large; indeed, response times for MIs and CIs for all three kinds of change were not significantly different from their counterparts in Experiment 1. Note that these results also show that the temporal uncertainty caused by the repeating images in Experiment 1 does not affect performance greatly: Pairs of identical 240-ms images separated by 80 ms have much the same effect as a single image presented for 560 ms.

Experiment 3

Another possible explanation for the occurrence of change blindness under flicker conditions is

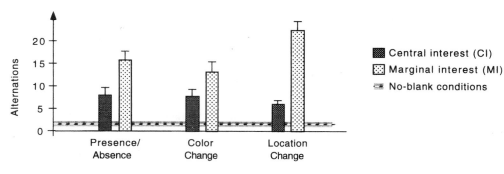

(a) - Standard flicker condition

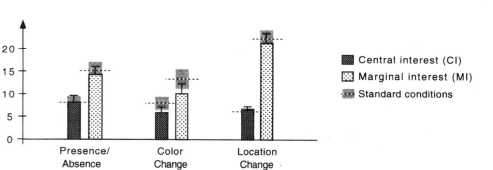

(b) - Extended display duration

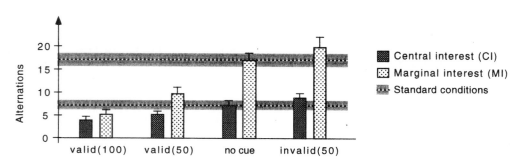

(c) - Effects of cue validity

that the flicker reduces the visibility of the items in the image to the point where they simply become difficult to see. To examine this possibility, in Experiment 3 we repeated Experiment 1, but with a verbal cue (single word or word pair) placed in a white rectangle for 3 s at the beginning of each trial. Two different cuing conditions were used. In the *partially valid* condition, cues were divided equally into valid cues (naming the part of the scene changed) and invalid cues (naming some other part). In the *completely valid* condition, cues were always valid. If visibility is indeed the limiting factor, no large effect of cuing should have occurred—the target would simply remain difficult to find. Otherwise, performance should have been greatly sped up by valid cues, and relatively unaffected (or even slowed down) by invalid ones.

As figure 17.3c shows, valid cues always caused identification of both MI and CI changes to be greatly sped up. This speedup was significant for both the partially valid condition ($p < .001$ for MI; $p < .03$ for CI) and the completely valid condition ($p < .001$ for both MI and CI). Indeed, in the completely valid condition, the difference in response times for MIs and CIs declined to the point where it was no longer significant. Note that this latter result indicates that the faster performance for CIs in Experiment 1 is unlikely to be due to the simple salience of their features: Such a near-equality of search times would hardly be expected if the CIs contained features salient enough to preferentially catch the attention of observers.

In contrast to valid cues, invalid cues caused a slight slowdown in performance (although this was not found to be significant). Taken together, then, these results show that observers could readily locate a cued target under flicker conditions, thereby demonstrating that visibility was not a limiting factor.

General Discussion

The preceding experiments show that under flicker conditions, observers can take a surprisingly long time to perceive large changes in images of real-world scenes. This difficulty is due neither to a disruption of the information received nor to a disruption of its storage. It does, however, depend greatly on the significance of the part of the scene being changed, with identification being faster for structures of central interest than for those of marginal interest.

We therefore make the following proposal:

• Visual perception of change in an object occurs only when that object is given focused attention;

• In the absence of focused attention, the contents of visual memory are simply overwritten (i.e., replaced) by subsequent stimuli, and so cannot be used to make comparisons.

Although it is not yet possible to specify the detailed operation of the attentional mechanisms involved, it is likely that the allocation of atten-

Figure 17.3
Identification of change under flicker conditions. Error bars indicate one standard error; the shaded areas surrounding the dashed lines indicate the standard errors of comparison conditions. Results under the basic conditions of Experiment 1 are shown in (*a*). The dashed line indicates baseline performance when no blanks are present. The effect of longer image duration is shown in (*b*). The dashed lines indicate the results of Experiment 1. The effects of verbal cues are shown in (*c*). Valid cues were presented on 100% and 50% of the trials in the completely and partially valid cue conditions, respectively. These cues are referred to as "valid(100)" and "valid(50)" in the graph. Invalid cues were presented on 50% of the trials in the partially valid condition. These cues are referred to as "invalid(50)" in the graph.

tion causes the relevant structures to form *object files* (Kahneman, Treisman, and Gibbs 1992), or at least lets them be entered into a relatively durable store, such as visual short-term memory (e.g., Coltheart 1980, Irwin 1991, Sperling 1960), so that comparisons can be made.

In this view, all the effects encountered in these experiments can be traced back to the allocation of attention, which is either "pulled" by transient motions or "pushed" by volitional control (e.g., Klein et al. 1992, Posner 1980). Under normal conditions, the motion signals resulting from a change draw attention to its location and so allow the observer to perceive it. When these signals are delocalized by flicker, their influence is effectively removed; attention is then directed entirely by static low-level properties such as feature gradients (Nothdurft 1992) and high-level volition. If there are no distinct low- or high-level cues (true of most stimuli we used), detection of change will require a slow, item-by-item scan of the entire image, giving rise to long identification times. The faster identification of CI than MI changes—despite the smaller area of the CI changes—would result from the attraction of attention via the high-level interest of CI objects.

If this view is correct, it points toward tighter connections between lines of research in four rather different areas of vision: eye movements, visual attention, visual memory, and scene perception. For example, the failure to find representations capable of providing automatic detection of change supports the view of eye movement researchers (e.g., Bridgeman et al. 1975, Irwin 1991, McConkie and Zola 1979) that there simply is no spatiotopic buffer where successive fixations are added, compared, or otherwise combined. Note that although our experiments did not explicitly address the issue of image addition (superposition), the difficulty in detecting positional shifts suggests that such superposition is unlikely; otherwise, observers could simply have looked for instances of doubled structures (i.e., images in which the original and the shifted object were both present side by side). In any event, it appears that much—if not all—of the blindness to saccade-contingent change is simply due to the disruption of the retinal image during a saccade, which causes swamping of the local motion signals that would normally draw attention. A similar explanation can also account for the change blindness encountered in the brief-display studies, suggesting that a common framework may encompass both of these effects.

The results presented here are also related to studies finding (Mack et al. 1992; Neisser and Becklen 1975; Rock, Linnett, Grant, and Mack 1992) that attention is required to explicitly perceive a stimulus in the visual field. In those studies, observers giving their complete attention to particular objects or events in a scene became "blind" to other, irrelevant objects. This effect required that observers not suspect that the irrelevant objects would be tested, for even a small amount of (distributed) attention would cause these objects to be perceived. The present results are more robust, in that blindness occurred even when observers knew that changes would be made, and so could distribute their attention over the entire picture array if it would help. Thus, although distributed attention apparently facilitates the perception of object presence, it does not facilitate the perception of change. Presumably, distributed attention is not sufficient to move a structure from visual memory into the more durable store that would allow the perception of change to take place.

In addition to proposing that attended items are entered into a relatively stable store, we propose that unattended items are overwritten by new stimuli that subsequently appear in their location. This latter point is based on the finding that change blindness occurs even when images are separated by an ISI of only 80 ms, a time well within the 300-ms limit of iconic memory; if no such replacement took place, observers could simply have used the superposed images of original and shifted objects to find positional shifts.

Such a replacement of unattended items has been proposed to explain metacontrast masking (Enns and DiLollo 1997), and it is possible that the same mechanism is involved in the change blindness we observed. In any event, this mechanism implies that two rather different fates await items in visual memory: Attended items are loaded into a durable store and are perceived to undergo transformation whenever they are changed, whereas unattended items are simply replaced by the arrival of new items, with no awareness that replacement has occurred.

Finally, the work presented here also suggests a tighter connection between attention and scene perception. Recall that the valid cues in Experiment 3 caused performance to be greatly sped up. It could be argued that looking for change induces a coding strategy quite different from that of normal viewing; for example, when observers search for a cued object, attention might be more fully engaged and so might "weld" visual representations into a form more suitable for detecting change. But the invalid cues did not help at all, showing that attentional scanning of this kind does not by itself cause any increase in speed.

This result indicates that perception of change is not helped by a person's having attended to an object at some point in its past. Rather, the perception of change can occur only during the time that the object is being attended (or at least during the time it is held in the limited-capacity durable store). After attention is removed, the perception of change vanishes, and any previously attended items again become susceptible to replacement. A similar "evaporation" of attentional effect has been found in visual search, in which feature conjunctions appear to obtain no benefit from having been previously attended (Wolfe 1996). Thus, just as the detailed perception of a scene is mediated by a rapidly shifting fovea of limited area, so is it also mediated by a rapidly shifting attentional mechanism limited in the number of items it can handle at any one time.

The limited capacity of this mechanism requires that it be used effectively if a scene is to be perceived quickly. But how can appropriate guidance be given if the scene has not yet been recognized? Previous work has shown that the gist of a scene can be determined within 100–150 ms (Biederman, Mezzanotte, and Rabinowitz 1982; Intraub 1981; Potter 1976); it may well be that the gist includes a description of the most interesting aspects, which are then used to guide attention. By measuring the relative speed of perceiving changes to various parts of a scene, researchers might be able to determine the order in which attention visits the constituent objects and regions. The resultant "attentional scan path" may prove to be an interesting new tool in the study of scene perception, providing a useful complement to techniques that study eye movements and memory for objects as a function of how well they fit the gist of a scene (e.g., Friedman 1979, Loftus and Mackworth 1978). Furthermore, the correlation we found between reaction time and degree of interest (as derived from written descriptions) opens up another interesting possibility, namely, that the flicker paradigm can be adapted to determine what nonverbal observers (e.g., animals and young children) find interesting in the world.

Why can people look at but not always see objects that come into their field of view? The evidence presented here indicates that the key factor is attention, without which observers are blind to change. The fact that attention can be concurrently allocated to only a few items (e.g., Pashler 1987, Pylyshyn and Storm 1988, Wolfe et al. 1989) implies that only a few changes can be perceived at any time. Although such a low-capacity mechanism might seem to be rather limiting, this need not be the case: If it can switch quickly enough so that objects and events can be analyzed whenever needed, little is gained by the simultaneous representation of all their details (Ballard, Hayhoe, and Whitehead 1992; Dennett 1991; O'Regan 1992; Stroud 1955). Thus, given that attention is normally drawn to any change in a scene and is also attracted to those parts most relevant for the task at hand, the subjective impression of an observer will generally be of a richly detailed environment, with accurate representation of those aspects of greatest importance. It is only when low-level transients are masked or are disregarded because of inappropriate high-level control that the management of this dynamic representation breaks down, causing its relatively sparse nature to become apparent.

Acknowledgments

The authors would like to thank Jack Beusmans, Jody Culham, Andy Liu, Ken Nakayama, Whitman Richards, Nava Rubin, and Jeremy Wolfe for their comments on an earlier draft. Also, thanks to Vlada Aginsky and Monica Strauss for their help in running the experiments.

References

Ballard, D. H., Hayhoe, M. M., and Whitehead, S. D. (1992). Hand-eye coordination during sequential tasks. *Philosophical Transactions of the Royal Society of London B, 337*, 331–339.

Biederman, I., Mezzanotte, R. J., and Rabinowitz, J. C. (1982). Scene perception: Detecting and judging objects undergoing relational violations. *Cognitive Psychology, 14*, 143–177.

Bridgeman, B., Hendry, D., and Stark, L. (1975). Failure to detect displacements of the visual world during saccadic eye movements. *Vision Research, 15*, 719–722.

Coltheart, M. (1980). Iconic memory and visible persistence. *Perception & Psychophysics, 27*, 183–228.

Currie, C., McConkie, G. W., Carlson-Radvansky, L. A., and Irwin, D. E. (1995). *Maintaining visual stability across saccades: Role of the saccade target object* (Technical Report No. UIUC-BI-HPP-95-01). Champaign: Beckman Institute, University of Illinois.

Dennett, D. C. (1991). *Consciousness explained.* Boston: Little, Brown and Co.

Enns, J. T., and DiLollo, V. (1997). Object substitution: A new form of masking in unattended visual locations. *Psychological Science 8*, 135–139.

Friedman, A. (1979). Framing pictures: The role of knowledge in automatized encoding and memory for gist. *Journal of Experimental Psychology: General, 108*, 316–355.

Grimes, J. (1996). On the failure to detect changes in scenes across saccades. In K. Akins (Ed.), *Perception* (Vancouver Studies in Cognitive Science, Vol. 5, pp. 89–109). New York: Oxford University Press.

Intraub, H. (1981). Rapid conceptual identification of sequentially presented pictures. *Journal of Experimental Psychology: Human Perception and Performance, 7*, 604–610.

Irwin, D. E. (1991). Information integration across saccadic eye movements. *Cognitive Psychology, 23*, 420–456.

Kahneman, D., Treisman, A., and Gibbs, B. (1992). The reviewing of object files: Object-specific integration of information. *Cognitive Psychology, 24*, 175–219.

Klein, R., Kingstone, A., and Pontefract, A. (1992). Orienting of visual attention. In K. Rayner (Ed.), *Eye movements and visual cognition: Scene perception and reading* (pp. 46–65). New York: Springer.

Loftus, G. R., and Mackworth, N. H. (1978). Cognitive determinants of fixation location during picture viewing. *Journal of Experimental Psychology: Human Perception and Performance, 4*, 547–552.

Mack, A., Tang, B., Tuma, R., Kahn, S., and Rock, I. (1992). Perceptual organization and attention. *Cognitive Psychology, 24*, 475–501.

McConkie, G. W., and Zola, D. (1979). Is visual information integrated across successive fixations in reading? *Perception & Psychophysics, 25*, 221–224.

Neisser, U., and Becklen, R. (1975). Selective looking: Attending to visually significant events. *Cognitive Psychology, 7*, 480–494.

Nothdurft, H. C. (1992). Feature analysis and the role of similarity in pre-attentive vision. *Perception & Psychophysics, 52*, 355–375.

O'Regan, J. K. (1992). Solving the "real" mysteries of visual perception: The world as an outside memory. *Canadian Journal of Psychology, 46*, 461–488.

Pashler, H. (1987). Detecting conjunctions of color and form: Reassessing the serial search hypothesis. *Perception & Psychophysics, 41*, 191–201.

Pashler, H. (1988) Familiarity and visual change detection. *Perception & Psychophysics*, *44*, 369–378.

Phillips, W. A. (1974). On the distinction between sensory storage and short-term visual memory. *Perception & Psychophysics*, *16*, 283–290.

Posner, M. I. (1980). Orienting of attention. *Quarterly Journal of Experimental Psychology*, *32*, 3–25.

Potter, M. C. (1976). Short-term conceptual memory for pictures. *Journal of Experimental Psychology: Human Learning and Memory*, *2*, 509–522.

Pylyshyn, Z. W., and Storm, R. W. (1988). Tracking multiple independent targets: Evidence for a parallel tracking mechanism. *Spatial Vision*, *3*, 179–197.

Rock, I., Linnett, C., Grant, P., and Mack, A. (1992). Perception without attention: Results of a new method. *Cognitive Psychology*, *24*, 502–534.

Sperling, G. (1960). The information available in brief visual presentations. *Psychological Monographs*, *74*, 1–29.

Stroud, J. M. (1955). The fine structure of psychological time. In H. Quastler (Ed.), *Information theory in psychology: Problems and methods* (pp. 174–207). Glencoe, IL: Free Press.

Wolfe, J. M. (1996). Post-attentive vision. *Investigative Ophthalmology & Visual Science*, *37*, 214.

Wolfe, J. M., Cave, K. R., and Franzel, S. L. (1989). Guided search: An alternative to the feature integration model for visual search. *Journal of Experimental Psychology: Human Perception and Performance*, *15*, 419–433.

18 Function of the Thalamic Reticular Complex: The Searchlight Hypothesis

Francis Crick

This paper presents a set of speculative hypotheses concerning the functions of the thalamus and, in particular, the nucleus reticularis of the thalamus and the related perigeniculate nucleus. For ease of exposition I have drawn my examples mainly from the visual system of primates, but I expect the ideas to apply to all mammals and also to other systems, such as the language system in man.

Visual System

It is now well established that in the early visual system of primates there are at least 10 distinct visual areas in the neocortex. (For a recent summary, see Van Essen and Maunsell (1).) If we include all areas whose main concern is with vision, there may be perhaps twice that number. To a good approximation, the early visual areas can be arranged in a branching hierarchy. Each of these areas has a crude "map" of (part of) the visual world. The first visual area (area 17, also called the striate cortex) on one side of the head maps one-half of the visual world in rather fine detail. Its cells can respond to relatively simple visual "features," such as orientation, spatial frequency, disparity (between the two eyes), and so on. This particular area is a large one so that the connections between different parts of it are relatively local. Each part therefore responds mainly to the properties of a small local part of the visual field (2).

As one proceeds to areas higher in the hierarchy, the "mapping" becomes more diffuse. At the same time the neurons appear to respond to more complex features in the visual field. Different cortical areas specialize, to some extent, in different features, one responding mainly to motion, another more to color, etc. In the higher areas a neuron hardly knows where in the visual field the stimulus (such as a face) is arising, while the feature it responds to may be so complex that individual neurons are often difficult to characterize effectively (3, 4).

Thus, the different areas analyze the visual field in different ways. This is not, however, how we appear to see the world. Our inner visual picture of the external world has a unity. How then does the brain put together all of these different activities to produce a unified picture so that, for example, for any object the right color is associated with the right shape?

The Searchlight

The pioneer work of Treisman and her colleagues (5–8), supported more recently by the elegant experiments of Julesz (9–11), have revealed a remarkable fact. If only a very short space of time is available, especially in the presence of "distractors," the brain is unable to make these conjunctions reliably. For example, a human subject can rapidly spot an "S" mixed in with a randomly arranged set of green Xs and brown Ts—it "pops out" at him. His performance is also rapid for a blue letter mixed in with the same set. However, if he is asked to detect a green T (which requires that he recognize the *conjunction* of a chosen color with a chosen shape), he usually takes much more time. Moreover, the time needed increases linearly with the number of distractors (the green Xs and brown Ts) as if the mind were searching the letters *in series*, as if the brain had an internal attentional searchlight that moved around from one visual object to the next, with steps as fast as 70 ms in favorable cases. In this metaphor the searchlight is not supposed to light up part of a completely dark landscape but, like a searchlight at dusk, it intensifies part of a scene that is already visible to some extent.

If there is indeed a searchlight mechanism in the brain, how does it work and where is located? To approach this problem we must study the general layout of the brain and, in particular, that of the neocortex and the thalamus. The essential facts we need at this stage are as follows.

Thalamus

The thalamus is often divided into two parts: the dorsal thalamus, which is the main bulk of it, and the ventral thalamus. (For a general account of the thalamus, see the review by Jones (12).) For the moment when I speak of the thalamus I shall mean the dorsal thalamus.

Almost all input to the cortex, with the exception of the olfactory input, passes through the thalamus. For this reason it is sometimes called the gateway to the cortex. There are some exceptions—the diffuse projections from the brain-stem, the projections from the claustrum, and also some projections from the amygdala and basal forebrain—that need not concern us here.

This generalization is not true for projections *from* the cortex, which do not need to pass through the thalamus. Nevertheless, for each projection *from* a region of the thalamus there is a corresponding reverse projection from that part of the cortex *to* the corresponding region of the thalamus. In some cases at least this reverse projection has more axons than the forward projection.

Most of the neurons in the thalamus are relay cells—that is, they receive an input from outside the thalamus (for example, the lateral geniculate nucleus of the thalamus gets a major input from the retina) and project directly to the cortex. Their axons form type I synapses and therefore are probably excitatory. There is a minority of small neurons in the thalamus—their exact number is somewhat controversial—that appear to form type II synapses and are therefore probably inhibitory.

While on the face of it the thalamus appears to be a mere relay, this seems highly unlikely. Its size and its strategic position make it very probable that it has some more important function.

Reticular Complex

Much of the rest of the thalamus is often referred to as the ventral thalamus. This includes the reticular complex (part of which is often called the perigeniculate nucleus), the ventral lateral geniculate nucleus, and the zona incerta. In what follows I shall, for ease of exposition, use the term reticular complex to include the perigeniculate nucleus. Again, "thalamus" means the dorsal thalamus. Although much of the following information comes from the cat or the rat, there is no reason to think that it does not also apply to the primate thalamus.

The reticular complex is a thin sheet of neurons, in most places only a few cells thick, which partly surrounds the (dorsal) thalamus (13–32) (see figure 18.1). All axons from the thalamus to the cerebral cortex pass through it, as do all of the reverse projections from the cortex to the thalamus. The intralaminar nuclei of the thalamus, which project very strongly to the striatum,

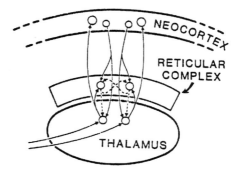

Figure 18.1
The main connections of the reticular complex, highly diagramatic and not at all to scale. Solid lines represent excitatory axons. Dashed lines show GABAergic (inhibitory) axons. Arrows represent synapses.

also send their axons through it, as may some of the axons from the globus pallidus that project back to the thalamus.

It is believed that many of the axons that pass in both directions through the reticular complex give off collaterals that make excitatory synaptic contacts in it (15, 18, 21, 29, 30). If the thalamus is the gateway to the cortex, the reticular complex might be described as the guardian of the gateway. Its exact function is unknown.

Not only is its position remarkable, but its structure is also unusual. It consists largely (if not entirely) of neurons whose dendrites often spread rather extensively in the plane of the nucleus (29). The size of these neurons is somewhat different in different parts of the complex (31). Their axons, which project to the thalamus, give off rather extensive collaterals that ramify, sometimes for long distances, within the sheet of the reticular complex (19, 29). This is in marked contrast with most of the nuclei of the thalamus, the principal cells of which have few, if any, collaterals either within each nucleus or between nuclei. The nuclei of the thalamus (with the exception of the intralaminar nuclei) keep themselves to themselves. The neurons of the reticular complex, on the other hand, appear to communicate extensively with each other. Moreover, it is characteristic of them that they fire in long bursts at a very rapid rate (25).

An even more remarkable property of reticular neurons concerns their output. Whereas all of the output neurons of the thalamus make type I synapses and appear to be excitatory, many (if not all) of the neurons in the reticular complex appear to be GABAergic (GABA = γ-aminobutyric acid) and thus almost certainly inhibitory (26–28). The excitation in the complex must come almost exclusively from the activity of the various axons passing through it.

Both the input and the output of the complex are arranged topographically (16, 29, 30, 32). It seems likely that if a particular group of axons going from the thalamus to the cortex passes through a small region of the reticular complex, the reverse projection probably passes through or near that same region. There may well be a rough map of the whole cortex on the reticular complex, though how precise this map may be is not known. It should be remembered, however, that the spread of the receiving dendrites of the reticular nucleus is quite large.

The projection of the reticular complex to the thalamus is also not random. Though any individual axon may spread fairly widely, there is a very crude topography in the arrangement. The projection from any one part of the reticular complex probably projects to that part of the thalamus from which it receives input as well as other neighboring parts. The exact nature of these various mappings would repay further study.

The neurons of the reticular complex project to the (dorsal) thalamus. The evidence suggests that they mainly contact the principal (relay) cells of the thalamus (22). What effect does the reticular input have on the behavior of the cells in the dorsal thalamus?

Obviously this is a crucial question. Let us consider two oversimplified but contrasting hypotheses. The first is that the main effect of the reticular complex is inhibitory. This would lead to the following general picture. The traffic passing through the reticular complex will produce excitation. Let us assume that one patch of the complex is more excited than the rest because of special activity in the thalamo-cortical pathways. The effect of this will be two-fold. That region will tend to suppress somewhat the other parts of the reticular complex, because of the many inhibitory collaterals. It will also suppress the corresponding thalamic region. These two effects will damp down the thalamus in its most active region and have the opposite effect (since the inhibition from the reticular complex will be reduced there) on the remaining parts. The total effect will be to even out the activity of the thalamus. This is not a very exciting conclusion.

The function of the reticular complex would be to act as an overall thermostat of thalamic activity, making the warm parts cooler and the cool parts warmer.

The second hypothesis is just the opposite. Let us assume that the effect of the reticular complex on the dorsal thalamus is mainly excitation in some form or other. Then we see that, once again, an active patch in the complex will tend to suppress many other parts of the complex. This time, however, the effect will be to heat up the warmer parts of the thalamus and cool down the cooler parts. We shall have positive feedback rather than negative feedback, so that "attention" will be focused on the most active thalamo-cortical regions.

How can GABAergic neurons produce some sort of excitatory effect on the relay cells of the thalamus? One possibility is that they might synapse only onto the local inhibitory neurons in the thalamus. By inhibiting these inhibitory cells they would thereby increase the effect of incoming excitation on the relay cells.

This is certainly possible but the anatomic evidence (22) suggests that in the main the neurons of the reticular complex project directly to the thalamic relay neurons. One would expect that this would inhibit these neurons. We must therefore ask if thalamic neurons show any unusual types of behavior.

Properties of Thalamic Neurons

The recent work of Llinás and Jahnsen (33–35) on thalamic slices from the guinea pig confirms that this is indeed the case. Their papers should be consulted for the detailed results, which are complicated, but, broadly, they show that all thalamic neurons display two relatively distinct modes of behavior. When the cell is near its normal resting potential (say, -60 mV) it responds to an injected current by firing (producing axonal spikes) at a fairly modest rate,

usually between 25 and 100 spikes per second. The rate increases with the value of the current injected.

If, on the other hand, the negative potential of the membrane is increased somewhat (that is, if the cell is hyperpolarized) to, say, -70 mV, then a neuron responds to an injected current, after a short delay, with a spike or a *short fast burst of spikes*, firing briefly at rates nearer *300 spikes per second.* Moreover, the after-effect of this burst is that, even though the injected current is maintained constant, the cell will not produce a further burst for a time of the order of 80–150 ms. Jahnsen and Llinás (34, 35), by means of many elegant controls, have shown that this behavior depends on a number of special ion channels, including a Ca^{2+}-dependent K^+ conductance.

Thus, it is at least possible that the effect of the GABAergic neurons of the reticular complex on the thalamic relay cells is to produce a brief burst of firing in response to incoming excitations, followed by a more prolonged inhibition. Whether this is actually the effect they produce in natural circumstances remains to be seen, since it is not easy to deduce this with certainty from the results of Jahnsen and Llinás on slices.

The Searchlight Hypothesis

What do we require of a searchlight? It should be able to sample the activity in the cortex and/or the thalamus and decide "where the action is." It should then be able to intensify the thalamic input to that region of the cortex, probably by making the active thalamic neurons in that region fire more rapidly than usual. It must then be able to turn off its beam, move to the next place demanding attention, and repeat the process.

It seems remarkable, to say the least, that the nature of the reticular complex and the behavior of the thalamic neurons fit this requirement so neatly. The extensive inhibitory collaterals in the reticular complex may allow it to select a small region that corresponds to the most active part of the thalamo-cortical maps. Its inhibitory output, by making more negative the membrane potential of the relevant thalamic neurons, could allow them to produce a very rapid, short burst and also effectively turns them off for 100 ms or so. This means that the reticular complex will no longer respond at that patch and its activity can thus move to the next most active patch. We are thus led to two plausible hypotheses:

(1)   The searchlight is controlled by the reticular complex of the thalamus.

(2)   The expression of the searchlight is the production of rapid firing in a subset of active thalamic neurons.

So far I have lumped the perigeniculate nucleus (17–24) in with the reticular nucleus proper which adjoins it. It seems probable that the lateral geniculate nucleus (which in primates projects mainly to the first visual area of the cortex) sends collaterals of its output to the perigeniculate nucleus, while the rest of the dorsal thalamus sends collaterals to the reticular nucleus proper (20). This suggests that there may be at least two searchlights: one for the first visual area and another for all of the rest. Indeed, there may be several separate searchlights. Their number will depend in part on the range and strength of the inhibitory collaterals within the reticular complex. Clearly, much more needs to be known about both the neuroanatomy and the neurophysiology of the various parts of the reticular complex.

Malsburg Synapses

We must now ask: what could the searchlight usefully do? Treisman's results (5–8) suggest that what we want it to do is to form *temporary* "conjunctions" of neurons. One possibility is that the conjunction is expressed merely by the relevant neurons firing simultaneously, or at least in a highly correlated manner. In artificial intelligence the problem would be solved by "creating a line" between the units. There is no way that the searchlight can rapidly produce new dendrites, new axons, or even new axon terminals in the brain. The only plausible way to create a line in a short time is to strengthen an existing synapse in some way. This is the essence of the idea put forward in 1981 by von der Malsburg in a little known but very suggestive paper.* After describing the conjunction problem in general terms he proposed that a synapse could alter its synaptic weight (roughly speaking, the weight is the effect a presynaptic spike has on the potential at the axon hillock of the postsynaptic cell) on a fast time scale ("fractions of a second"). He proposed that when there was a strong correlation between presynaptic and postsynaptic activity, the strength of the synapse was temporarily increased—a dynamic version of Hebb's well-known rule (36)—and that with *un*correlated pre- and postsynaptic signals the strength would be temporarily decreased below its normal resting value.

Notice that we are not concerned here with *long-term* alterations in weight, as we would if we were considering learning, but very short-term *transient* alterations that would occur during the act of visual perception. The idea is not, however, limited to the visual system but is supposed to apply to all parts of the neocortex and possibly to other parts of the brain as well.

Most previous theoretical work on neural nets does not use this idea, though there are exceptions (37, 38). The usual convention is that while a net, or set of nets, is *performing*, the synaptic weights are kept constant. They are only allowed to alter when *learning* is being studied. Thus, von

---

*von der Malsburg, C. (1981) Internal Report 81-2 (Department of Neurobiology, Max-Planck-Institute for Biophysical Chemistry, Goettingen, F.R.G.).

der Malsburg's idea represents a rather radical alteration to the usual assumptions. I propose that such (hypothetical) synapses be called Malsburg synapses. Notice that in the cortex the number of synapses exceeds the number of neurons by at least three orders of magnitude.

Let us then accept for the moment that Malsburg synapses are at least plausible. We are still a long way from knowing the exact rules for their behavior—How much can their strength be increased? What exactly determines this increase (or decrease) of strength? How rapidly can this happen? How does this temporary alteration decay?—to say nothing of the molecular mechanisms underlying such changes.

In spite of all of these uncertainties it seems not unreasonable to assume that the effect of the searchlight is to activate Malsburg synapses. We are thus led to a third hypothesis.

(3)   The conjunctions produced by the searchlight are mediated by Malsburg synapses, especially by rapid bursts acting on them.

We still have to explain exactly how activated Malsburg synapses form associations of neurons. This is discussed by von der Malsburg in his paper in some detail but most readers may find his discussion hard to follow. His argument depends on the assumption that the system needs to have more than one such association active at about the same time. He describes at some length how correlations, acting on Malsburg synapses, can link cells into groups and thus form what he calls topological networks. What characterizes one such cell assembly is that the neurons in it fire "simultaneously," an idea that goes back to Hebb (36). von der Malsburg suggests that two kinds of signal patterns can exist in a topological network: waves running through the network or groups of cells switching synchronously between an active and a silent state. He next discusses how a set of cells rather than a single cell might form what he calls a "network element." Finally,

after an elaborate development of this theme he broaches the "bandwidth problem." In simple terms, how can we avoid these various groups of cells interfering with each other?

Cell Assemblies

The cell assembly idea is a powerful one. Since a neuron can usually be made to fire by several different combinations of its inputs, the *significance* of its firing is necessarily ambiguous. It is thus a reasonable deduction that this ambiguity can be removed, at least in part, by the firing pattern of an *assembly* of cells. This arrangement is more economical than having many distinct neurons, each with very high specificity. This type of argument goes back to Young (39) in 1802.

There has been much theoretical work on what we may loosely describe as associative nets. The nets are usually considered to consist of neurons of a similar type, receiving input, in most cases, from similar sources and sending their output mainly to similar places. If we regard neurons (in, say, the visual system) as being arranged in some sort of hierarchy, then we can usefully refer to such an assembly as a *horizontal* assembly.

Von der Malsburg's ideas, however, permit another type of assembly. In his theory a cell at a higher level is associated with one at a lower level (we are here ignoring the direction of the connection), and these, in turn, may be associated with those at a still lower level. (By "associated with" I mean that the cells fire approximately simultaneously.) For example, a cell at a higher level that signified the general idea "face" would be temporarily associated, by Malsburg synapses, with cells that signified the parts of the face, and, in turn, perhaps with their parts. Such an assembly might usefully be called a *vertical* assembly. It is these vertical assemblies that have to be constructed anew for each different visual scene, or for each sentence, etc.

Without them it would be a difficult job to unite the higher level concepts with their low level details in a rather short time. This idea is reminiscent of the K lines of Minsky.[†]

The idea of *transient* vertical assemblies is a very powerful one. It solves in one blow the combinational problem—that is, how the brain can respond to an almost unlimited number of distinct sentences, passages of music, visual scenes, and so on. The solution is to use *temporary* combinations of a subset of a much more limited number of units (the 10^{12} or so neurons in the central nervous system), each new combination being brought into action as the circumstances demand and then largely discarded. Without this device the brain would either require vastly more neurons to do the job or its ability to perceive, think, and act would be very severely restricted. This is the thrust of von der Malsburg's arguments.

A somewhat similar set of ideas about simultaneous firing has been put forward by Abeles. His monograph (40) should be consulted for details. He proposes the concept of "synfire chains"—sets of cells, each set firing synchronously, connected in chains, which fire sequentially. He gives a plausible numerical argument, based mainly on anatomical connectivity, which suggests that to establish a functioning synfire chain only a few (perhaps five or so) synapses would be available at any one neuron. Since this is such a small number he deduces that the individual synapses must be strengthened (if these five synapses by themselves are to fire the cell) perhaps by a factor of 5 or so. However, he gives no indication as to how this strengthening might be done.

Abeles' argument stresses the importance to the system of the *exact time of firing* of each spike, rather than the *average* rate of firing,

which is often taken to be the more relevant variable. This exact timing is also an important aspect of von der Malsburg's ideas. These arguments can also be supported by considering the probable values of the passive cable constants of cortical dendrites. Very rough estimates (for example, $\tau = 8$ ms, $X = \lambda/5$) suggest that inputs will not add satisfactorily unless they arrive within a few milliseconds of each other (see figure 3.18 in ref. 41).

Notice the idea that a cell assembly consists of neurons firing simultaneously (or at least in a highly correlated manner) is a very natural one, since this means that the impact of their joint firing on *other* neurons, elsewhere in the system, will be large. The content of the cell assembly—the "meaning" of all of the neurons so linked together—can in this way be impressed on the rest of the system in a manner that would not be possible if all of the neurons in it fired at random times, unless they were firing very rapidly indeed. Therefore, our fourth hypothesis follows.

(4) Conjunctions are expressed by cell assemblies, especially assemblies of cells in different cortical regions.

It should not be assumed that cell assemblies can only be formed by the searchlight mechanism. Some important ones may well be laid down, or partly laid down, genetically (e.g., faces?) or be formed by prolonged learning (e.g., reading letters or words?).

It is clear that much further theoretical work is needed to develop these ideas and make them more precise. If the members of a vertical assembly fire approximately synchronously, exactly how regular and how close together in time do these firings have to be? Are there special pathways or devices to promote more simultaneous firing? Are dendritic spikes involved? How does one avoid confusion between different cell assemblies? Do neurons in *different* cell assemblies briefly inhibit each other, so that accidental synchrony is made more difficult? And so on.

[†]Minsky, M. (1979) Artificial Intelligence Memo No. 516 (Artificial Intelligence Laboratory, Massachusetts Institute of Technology, Cambridge, MA).

The idea that the dorsal thalamus and the reticular complex are concerned with attention is not novel (19, 42, 43). What is novel (as far as I know) is the suggestion that they control and express the internal attentional searchlight proposed by Treisman (5–8), Julesz (9, 10), Posner (44, 45), and others. For this searchlight at least two features are required. The first is the rapid movement of the searchlight from place to place while the eyes remain in one position, as discussed above. There is, however, another aspect. The brain must know what it is searching *for* (the green *T* in the example given earlier) so that it may know when its hunt is successful. In other words, the brain must know *what* to attend to. That aspect, which may involve other cortical areas such as the frontal cortex, has not been discussed here. The basic searchlight mechanism may depend on several parts of the reticular complex, but these may be influenced by top-down pathways, or by other searchlights in other parts of the reticular complex, which may be partly controlled by which ideas are receiving attention. An important function of the reticular complex may be to limit the number of subjects the thalamus can pay attention to at any one time.

Experimental Tests

These will not be discussed here in detail. It suffices to say that many of the suggestions, such as the behavior of the dorsal thalamus and the reticular complex, are susceptible to fairly direct tests. The exact behavior of reticular neurons and thalamic neurons is difficult to predict with confidence, since they contain a number of very different ion channels. Experiments on slices should therefore be complemented by experiments on animals. Obviously, most of such experiments should be done on alert, behaving animals, if possible with natural stimuli. An animal under an anesthetic can hardly be expected to display all aspects of attention. Various psychophysical tests are also possible.

Other aspects of these ideas, such as the behavior of Malsburg synapses, may be more difficult to test in the immediate future. It seems more than likely that dendritic spines are involved, both the spines themselves and the synapses on them (46, 47).

The existence and the importance of rapid bursts of firing can also be tested. Such bursts, followed by a quiet interval, have been seen in neurons in the visual cortex of a curarized, unanesthetized and artificially respired cat when they respond to an optimal visual signal [see figure 18.1 in Morrell (48)]. It is unlikely that the two systems—the rapid-burst system and the slow-firing system—will be quite as distinct as implied here. In fact, as von der Malsburg has pointed out, one would expect them to interact.

Thus, all of these ideas, plausible though they may be, must be regarded at the moment as speculative until supported by much stronger experimental evidence. In spite of this, they appear as if they might begin to form a useful bridge between certain parts of cognitive psychology, on the one hand, and the world of neuroanatomy and neurophysiology on the other.

Acknowledgments

This work originated as a result of extensive discussions with Dr. Christopher Longuet-Higgins. I thank him and many other colleagues who have commented on the idea, in particular, Drs. Richard Anderson, Max Cowan, Simon LeVay, Don MacLeod, Graeme Mitchison, Tomaso Poggio, V. S. Ramachandran, Terrence Sejnowski, and Christoph von der Malsburg. This work has been supported by the J. W. Kieckhefer Foundation and the System Development Foundation.

Note

Recent unpublished experimental work suggests that the reticular complex may produce bursts of firing in some thalamic neurons but merely an increase of firing rate in others.

References

1. Van Essen, D. C. and Maunsell, J. H. R. (1983) *Trends Neurosci.* 6, 370–375.

2. Hubel, D. H. and Wiesel, T. H. (1977) *Proc. R. Soc. London Ser. B* 198, 1–59.

3. Bruce, C., Desimone, R. and Gross, C. G. (1981) *J. Neurophys.* 46, 369–384.

4. Perrett, D. I., Rolls, E. T. and Caan, W. (1982) *Exp. Brain Res.* 47, 329–342.

5. Treisman, A. (1977) *Percept. Psychophys.* 22, 1–11.

6. Treisman, A. M. and Gelade, G. (1980) *Cognit. Psychol.* 12, 97–136.

7. Treisman, A. and Schmidt, H. (1982) *Cognit. Psychol.* 14, 107–141.

8. Treisman, A. (1983) in *Physical and Biological Processing of Images*, eds. Braddick, O. J. and Sleigh, A. C. (Springer, New York), pp. 316–325.

9. Julesz, B. (1980) *Philos. Trans. R. Soc. London Ser. B.* 290, 83–94.

10. Julesz, B. (1981) *Nature (London)* 290, 91–97.

11. Bergen, J. R. and Julesz, B. (1983) *Nature (London)* 303, 696–698.

12. Jones, E. G. (1983) in *Chemical Neuroanatomy*, ed. Emson, P. C. (Raven, New York), pp. 257–293.

13. Sumitomo, I., Nakamura, M. and Iwama, K. (1976) *Exp. Neurol.* 51, 110–123.

14. Dubin, M. W. and Cleland, B. G. (1977) *J. Neurophys.* 40, 410–427.

15. Montero, V. M., Guillery, R. W. and Woolsey, C. N. (1977) *Brain Res.* 138, 407–421.

16. Montero, V. M. and Scott, G. L. (1981) *Neuroscience* 6, 2561–2577.

17. Ahlsén, G., Lindström, S. and Sybirska, E. (1978) *Brain Res.* 156, 106–109.

18. Ahlsén, G. and Lindström, S. (1982) *Brain Res.* 236, 477–481.

19. Ahlsén, G. and Lindström, S. (1982) *Brain Res.* 236, 482–486.

20. Ahlsén, G., Lindström, S. and Lo, F.-S. (1982) *Exp. Brain Res.* 46, 118–126.

21. Ahlsén, G. and Lindström, S. (1983) *Acta Physiol. Scand.* 118, 181–184.

22. Ohara, P. T., Sefton, A. J. and Lieberman, A. R. (1980) *Brain Res.* 197, 503–506.

23. Hale, P. T., Sefton, A. J., Baur, L. A. and Cottee, L. J. (1982) *Exp. Brain Res.* 45, 217–229.

24. Ide, L. S. (1982) *J. Comp. Neuro.* 210, 317–334.

25. Schlag, J. and Waszak, M. (1971) *Exp. Neurol.* 32, 79–97.

26. Houser, C. R., Vaughn, J. E., Barber, R. P. and Roberts, E. (1980) *Brain Res.* 200, 341–354.

27. Oertel, W. H., Graybiel, A. M., Mugnaini, E., Elde, R. P., Schmechel, D. E. and Kopin, I. J. (1983) *J. Neurosci.* 3, 1322–1332.

28. Ohara, P. T., Lieberman, A. R., Hunt, S. P. and Wu, J.-Y. (1983) *Neuroscience* 8, 189–211.

29. Scheibel, M. E. and Scheibel, A. B. (1966) *Brain Res.* 1, 43–62.

30. Jones, E. G. (1975) *J. Comp. Neurol.* 162, 285–308.

31. Scheibel, M. E. and Scheibel, A. B. (1972) *Exp. Neurol.* 34, 316–322.

32. Minderhoud, J. M. (1971) *Exp. Brain Res.* 12, 435–446.

33. Llinás, R. and Jahnsen, H. (1982) *Nature (London)* 297, 406–408.

34. Jahnsen, H. and Llinás, R. (1984) *J. Physiol.* 349, 205–226.

35. Jahnsen, H. and Llinás, R. (1984) *J. Physiol.* 349, 227–247.

36. Hebb, D. O. (1949) *Organization of Behavior* (Wiley, New York).

37. Little, W. A. and Shaw, G. L. (1975) *Behav. Biol.* 14, 115–133.

38. Edelman, G. M. and Reeke, G. N. (1982) *Proc. Natl. Acad. Sci. USA* 79, 2091–2095.

39. Young, T. (1802) *Philos. Trans.* 12–48.

40. Abeles, M. (1982) *Local Cortical Circuits: Studies of Brain Function* (Springer, New York), Vol. 6.

41. Jack, J. J. B., Noble, D. and Tsien, R. W. (1975) *Electric Current Flow in Excitable Cells* (Clarendon, Oxford).

42. Yingling, C. D. and Skinner, J. E. (1977) in *Attention, Voluntary Contraction and Event-Cerebral Potentials*, ed. Desmedt, J. E. (Karger, Basel, Switzerland), pp. 70–96.

43. Skinner, J. E. and Yingling, C. D. (1977) in *Attention, Voluntary Contraction and Event-Cerebral Potentials*, ed. Desmedt, J. E. (Karger, Basel, Switzerland), pp. 30–69.

44. Posner, M. I. (1982) *Am. Psychol.* 37, 168–179.

45. Posner, M. I., Cohen, Y. and Rafal, R. D. (1982) *Philos. Trans. R. Soc. London Ser. B* 298, 187–198.

46. Perkel, D. H. (1983) *J. Physiol. (Paris)* 78, 695–699.

47. Koch, C. and Poggio, T. (1983) *Proc. R. Soc. London Ser. B.* 218, 455–477.

48. Morrell, F. (1972) in *Brain and Human Behavior*, eds. Karczmar, A. G. and Eccles, J. C. (Springer, New York), pp. 259–289.

19 Selective Attention Gates Visual Processing in the Extrastriate Cortex

Jeffrey Moran and Robert Desimone

Our retinas are constantly stimulated by a welter of shapes, colors, and textures. Since we are aware of only a small amount of this information at any one moment, most of it must be filtered out centrally. This filtering cannot easily be explained by the known properties of the visual system. In primates, the visual recognition of objects depends on the transmission of information from the striate cortex (V1) through prestriate areas into the inferior temporal (IT) cortex (1). At each successive stage along this pathway there is an increase in the size of the receptive fields; that is, neurons respond to stimuli throughout an increasingly large portion of the visual field. Within these large receptive fields will typically fall several different stimuli. Thus, paradoxically, more rather than less information appears to be processed by single neurons at each successive stage. How, then, does the visual system limit processing of unwanted stimuli? The results of our recording experiments on single neurons in the visual cortex of trained monkeys indicate that unwanted information is filtered from the receptive fields of neurons in the extrastriate cortex as a result of selective attention.

The general strategy of the experiment was as follows. After isolating a cell, we first determined its receptive field while the monkey fixated on a small target. On the basis of the cell's response to bars of various colors, orientations, and sizes, we determined which stimuli were effective in driving the cell and which were ineffective. Effective stimuli were then presented at one location in the receptive field concurrently with ineffective stimuli at a second location. The monkey was trained on a task that required it to attend to the stimuli at one location but ignore the stimuli at the other. After a block of 8 or 16 trials, the monkey was cued to switch its attention to the other location. Although the stimuli at the two locations remained the same, the locus of the animal's attention was repeatedly switched between the two locations. Since the identical sensory conditions were maintained in the two types of blocks, any difference in the response of the cell could be attributed to the effects of attention.

The task used to focus the animal's attention on a particular location was a modified version of a "match-to-sample" task. While the monkey held a bar and gazed at the fixation spot, a sample stimulus appeared briefly at one location followed about 500 ms later by a brief test stimulus at the same location. When the test stimulus was identical to the preceding sample, the animal was rewarded with a drop of water if it released the bar immediately, whereas when the test stimulus differed from the sample the animal was rewarded only if it delayed release for 700 ms. Stimuli were presented at the unattended location at the times of presentation of the sample and test stimuli, affording two opportunities to observe the effects of attention on each trial (2).

We recorded from 74 visually responsive cells in prestriate area V4 of two rhesus monkeys and found that the locus of the animal's attention in a cell's receptive field had a dramatic effect on the cell's response (figure 19.1a). When an effective and an ineffective sensory stimulus were present in a cell's receptive field, and the animal attended to the effective stimulus, the cell responded well. When the animal attended to the ineffective stimulus, however, the response was greatly attenuated, even though the effective (but ignored) sensory stimulus was simultaneously present in the receptive field. Thus when there were two stimuli in the receptive field the response of the cell was determined by the properties of the attended stimulus.

To characterize the magnitude of the attenuation, an attenuation index (AI) was derived for each cell by dividing the response (minus baseline) to an effective stimulus when it was being ignored by the response to the same stimulus

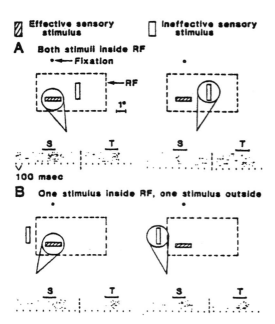

Figure 19.1
Effect of selective attention on the responses of a neuron in prestriate area V4. (*a*) Responses when the monkey attended to one location inside the receptive field (RF) and ignored another. At the attended location (circled), two stimuli (sample and test) were presented sequentially and the monkey responded differently depending on whether they were the same or different. Irrelevant stimuli were presented simultaneously with the sample and test but at a separate location in the receptive field. In the initial mapping of the receptive field, the cell responded well to horizontal and vertical red bars placed anywhere in the receptive field but not at all to green bars of any orientation. Horizontal or vertical red bars (effective sensory stimuli) were then placed at one location in the field and horizontal or vertical green bars (ineffective stimuli) at another. The responses shown are to horizontal red and vertical bars but are representative of the responses to the other stimulus pairings. When the animal attended to the location of the effective stimulus at the time of presentation of either the sample (S) or the test (T), the cell gave a good response (left), but when the animal attended to the location of the ineffective stim-

when it was being attended. For the large majority of cells in V4, the outcome of ignoring an effective sensory stimulus in the receptive field was to reduce the response by more than half (median AI, 0.36 for the sample stimulus and 0.33 for the test) (figure 19.2a).

In the design described, the effective stimuli at one location in the receptive field always differed in some sensory quality, such as color, from the ineffective stimuli at the other location. Thus attenuation of the response to an ignored stimulus could have been based on either its location or its sensory qualities. For example, for the cell described in the legend to figure 19.1, effective horizontal or vertical red bars were presented at one location while ineffective horizontal or vertical green bars were presented at the other. When the monkey attended to the green bars, the cell's response to the irrelevant red bars might have been attenuated because they were red or because they were at the wrong location. To test whether attenuation could be based on spatial location alone, for some cells we randomly intermixed the stimuli at the two locations so that, for example, red or green could appear at either spatial location on any trial.

When the locations of the effective and ineffective sensory stimuli were switched randomly, the responses of cells were still determined by the stimulus at the attended location. Cells responded well when the effective sensory stimu-

ulus, the cell gave almost no response (right), even though the effective stimulus was present in its receptive field. Thus the responses of the cell were determined by the attended stimulus. Because of the random delay between the sample and test stimulus presentations, the rasters were synchronized separately at the onsets of the sample and test stimuli (indicated by the vertical dashed lines). (*b*) Same stimuli as in (*a*), but the ineffective stimulus was placed outside the receptive field. The neuron responded similarly to the effective sensory stimulus, regardless of which location was attended.

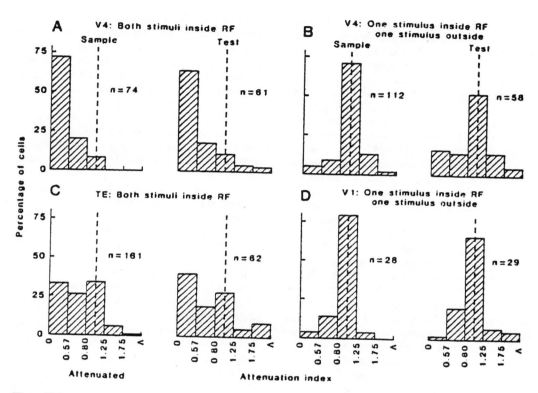

Figure 19.2

Comparison of effect of attention in area V4 (*a* and *b*), the IT cortex (*c*), and the striate cortex (V1) (*d*). An attenuation index (AI) for each cell was calculated by first subtracting its baseline firing rate from the responses to the sample and test stimuli. The responses to stimuli when ignored were then divided by responses to the same stimuli when attended. AI values less than 1 (dashed line) indicate that responses were reduced when a stimulus was ignored. The number of cells is indicated by *n*. For a few cells, irrelevant stimuli were paired only with the sample stimuli.

lus appeared at the attended location and poorly when it appeared at the ignored location (median AI, 0.57 for the sample and test stimuli). Thus attenuation of irrelevant information can be based purely on spatial location.

When attention is directed to one of two stimuli in the receptive field of a V4 cell, the effect of the unattended stimulus is attenuated, almost as if the receptive field has contracted around the attended stimulus. What, then, would be the effect on the receptive field if attention were directed outside it? To answer this, for 112 visually responsive cells (including 51 in the original sample) we placed an effective sensory stimulus inside the receptive field and an ineffective stimulus outside (figure 19.1b). The cells gave a good response regardless of which stimulus was attended (figure 19.2b). Thus, when attention is directed outside a receptive field, the receptive field appears to be unaffected. Furthermore, since the firing rates of cells were the same regardless of whether attention was directed inside or outside the receptive field, we can conclude that attention does not serve to enhance responses to attended stimuli.

To test whether the attenuation of irrelevant information also occurs at the next stage of processing after V4, we recorded from 161 visually responsive neurons in the IT cortex. As in V4, when the animal attended to one stimulus inside the receptive field and ignored another, the response to the ignored stimulus was reduced. Unlike receptive fields in V4, which were typically 2° to 4° wide in the central visual field, those in the IT cortex were so large that the responses of cells could be influenced by attention to stimuli throughout at least the central 12° of both the contralateral and ipsilateral visual fields (the maximum distance that could be tested). The magnitude of the effect was somewhat smaller than in V4 (figure 19.2c), possibly because IT neurons generally gave weaker, more variable responses than neurons in V4.

The results from area V4 and the IT cortex indicate that the filtering of irrelevant information is at least a two-stage process. In V4 only those cells whose receptive fields encompass both attended and unattended stimuli will fail to respond to unattended stimuli. In the IT cortex, where receptive fields may encompass the entire visual field, virtually no cells will respond well to unattended stimuli.

In contrast to area V4 and the IT cortex, there was no effect of attention in V1. When relevant and irrelevant stimuli were in a receptive field (typically 0.5° to 0.9° wide), the animal could not perform the task. When one stimulus was located inside the field and one just outside, the monkey was able to perform the task, but, as in V4 under this condition, attention had little or no effect on the cells (figure 19.2d).

Our results indicate that attention gates visual processing by filtering out irrelevant information from within the receptive fields of single extrastriate neurons. This role of attention is different from that demonstrated previously in the posterior parietal cortex (3), to our knowledge the only other cortical area in which spatially directed attention has been found to influence neural responses. In the posterior parietal cortex, some neurons show enhanced responses when an animal attends to a stimulus inside the neuron's receptive field compared to when the animal attends to a stimulus outside the field.

Since parietal neurons have large receptive fields with little or no selectivity for stimulus quality, these cells may play a role in directing attention to a spatial location (4), but by themselves do not provide information about the qualities of attended stimuli. By contrast, in area V4 and the IT cortex selective attention may allow the animal to identify and remember the properties of a particular stimulus out of the many that may be acting on the retina at any given moment. If so, then the attenuation of response to irrelevant stimuli found in V4 and the IT cortex may underlie the attenuated processing of irrelevant stimuli shown psychophysically in humans (5).

Acknowledgments

We thank M. Mishkin for his support in all phases of the study.

References and Notes

1. C. G. Gross, in *Handbook of Sensory Physiology*, vol. 7, part 3, *Central Processing of Visual Information*, R. Jung, Ed. (Springer, Berlin, 1973), pp. 451–482; L. G. Ungerleider and M. Mishkin, in *Analysis of Visual Behavior*, D. J. Ingle, M. A. Goodale, R. J. W. Mansfield, Eds. (MIT Press, Cambridge, 1984), pp. 549–586; R. Desimone, S. J. Schein, J. Moran, L. G. Ungerleider, *Vision Res.* 25, 441 (1985).

2. Both sample and test stimuli were presented for 200 ms, with a delay between them of 400–600 ms. The sample and test were randomly chosen on each trial from a set of two stimuli, and the irrelevant stimuli were chosen from a different set of two. If the animal attempted to perform the task on the basis of the irrelevant stimuli, its performance would be governed by chance. The performance of the animals was 94 percent correct. The cue to the animal to switch the locus of its attention was to delete the test-time stimulus from the previously relevant location for two trials. On the first of these trials, the animals' performance dropped to 65 percent correct and their reaction time increased by 90 ms, indicating that they had been ignoring the irrelevant stimuli. The neural responses on the two cue trials were not counted. The locus of attention was switched frequently enough to achieve a minimum of ten trials per stimulus configuration. Fixation was monitored by a magnetic search coil, and trials were aborted if the eyes deviated from the fixation target by more than 0.5°.

3. J. C. Lynch, V. B. Mountcastle, W. H. Talbot, T. C. T. Yin, *J. Neurophysiol.* 40, 362 (1977); M. C. Bushnell et al., ibid. 46, 755 (1981).

4. M. I. Posner, J. A. Walker, F. J. Friedrich, R. D. Rafal, *J. Neurosci.* 4, 1863 (1984).

5. D. E. Broadbent, *Acta Psychol.* 50, 253 (1982); D. Kahneman and A. Treisman, in *Varieties of Attention*, R. Parasuraman and D. R. Davies, Eds. (Academic Press, New York, 1984).

20 Attention: The Mechanisms of Consciousness

Michael I. Posner

What is it to be conscious? This has become a central question in many serious scientific circles (1–6). Proposals range from the anatomical, for example, locating consciousness in the thalamus (6) or in thalamic-cortical interactions (2, 6), to the physical, for example, the proposal that consciousness must rest on quantum principles (1, 4). Some proposals combine physical and anatomical reasoning. For example, Beck and Eccles (1) argue that conscious processing acts to increase the probability of quantal discharge at the synapse.

In this paper I propose to discuss the issue of consciousness in light of recent findings about attentional networks of the human brain that lead to selection of sensory information, activate ideas stored in memory, and maintain the alert state. I don't believe that any of these mechanisms are "consciousness" itself, just as DNA is not "life," but I do believe that an understanding of consciousness must rest on an appreciation of the brain networks that subserve attention, in much the same way as a scientific analysis of life without consideration of the structure of DNA would seem vacuous.

Attention

The study of attention has a long history within psychology. William James (7) wrote at the turn of the century, "Everyone knows what attention is. It is the taking possession by the mind in clear and vivid form of one out of what seem several simultaneous objects or trains of thought."

The dominance of behavioral psychology postponed research into the internal mechanisms of selective attention in the first half of this century. The finding that the integrity of the brain stem reticular formation was a necessity to maintain the alert state provided some anatomical reality to the study of an aspect of attention (8). The quest for information-processing mechanisms to support the more selective aspect of attention began after World War II with studies of selective listening. A filter was proposed that was limited for information (in the formal sense of information theory) and located between highly parallel sensory systems and a limited-capacity perceptual system (9).

Selective listening experiments supported a view of attention that suggested early selection of relevant message, with nonselective information being lost to conscious processing. However, on some occasions it was clear that unattended information was processed to a high level because there was evidence that an important message on the unattended channel might interfere with the selected channel.

In the 1970s psychologists began to distinguish between automatic and controlled processes. It was found that words could activate other words similar in meaning (their semantic associates), even when the person had no awareness of the words' presence. These studies indicated that the parallel organization found for sensory information extended to semantic processing. Thus, selecting a word meaning for active attention appeared to suppress the availability of other word meanings. Attention was viewed less as an early sensory bottleneck and more as a system for providing priority for motor acts, consciousness, and memory (10).

Another approach to problems of selectivity arose in work on the orienting reflex (11). The use of slow autonomic systems (e.g., skin conductance as measures of orienting) made it difficult to analyze the cognitive components and neural systems underlying orienting. During the last 15 years there has been a steady advancement in our understanding of the neural systems related to visual orienting from studies using single-cell recording in alert monkeys (12). This work showed a relatively restricted number of areas in which the firing rates of neurons were enhanced selectively when monkeys were trained to attend to a location, at the level of the superior colliculus (i.e., the midbrain), selective enhancement could only be obtained when eye movement was involved, but in the posterior parietal lobe of the cerebral cortex, selective enhancement occurred even when the animal maintained fixation. An area of the thalamus, the lateral pulvinar, was similar to the parietal lobe in containing cells with the property of selective enhancement.

Until recently, there has been a separation between human information processing and neuroscience approaches to attention using non-human animals. The former tended to describe attention, either in terms of a bottleneck that prevented limited-capacity central systems from overload or as a resource that could be allocated to various processing systems in a way analogous to the use of the term in economics. On the other hand, neuroscience views emphasized several separate neural mechanisms that might be involved in orienting and maintaining alertness. Currently, there is an attempt to integrate these two within a cognitive neuroscience of attention. An impressive aspect of current developments in this field is the convergence of evidence from various methods of study. These include performance studies using reaction time, dual-task performance studies, recording from scalp electrodes, and lesions in humans and animals, as well as various methods for imaging and recording from restricted brain areas, including individual cells (13).

Current progress in the anatomy of the attention system rests most heavily on two important methodological developments.

1. The use of microelectrodes with alert animals allowed evidence for the increased activity of cell populations with attention (12).

2. Anatomical (e.g., computerized tomography or magnetic resonance imaging) and physiological [e.g., positron emission tomography (PET) and functional magnetic resonance imagery]

methods of studying parts of the brain allowed more meaningful investigations of localization of cognitive function in normal people (13).

The future should see the use of localizing methods together with methods of tracing the time course of brain activity in the human subject. This combination should provide a convenient way to trace the rapid time-dynamic changes that occur in the course of human information processing.

Three fundamental working hypotheses characterize the current state of efforts to develop a combined cognitive neuroscience of attention.

1. There exists an attentional system of the brain that is anatomically separate from various data-processing systems that can be activated passively by visual and auditory input.

2. Attention is carried out by a network of anatomical areas. It is neither the property of a single brain area nor is it a collective function of the brain working as a whole.

3. The brain areas involved in attention do not carry out the same function, but specific computations are assigned to different areas (13).

It is not possible to specify the complete attentional system of the brain, but something is known about the areas that carry on three major attentional functions: orienting to sensory stimuli, particularly locations in visual space; detecting target events, including ideas stored in memory; and maintaining the alert state. Each of these areas of research provides information that relate to the theories of consciousness discussed in my first paragraph, but as will be apparent from the discussion below, each relates only partially to common definitions of conscious processing.

Visual Orienting

How can one study attention? Crick argues for the selection of a model system that involves

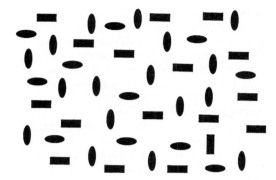

Figure 20.1
Searching this display for a vertical rectangle requires attention to successive locations because the nontargets include both vertical (ellipses) and rectangles (horizontal). Reaction times in this task are linearly related to the number of distracters. (This figure was reproduced with permission from ref. 37 [copyright Elsevier, Cambridge, U.K.].)

consciousness in a limited domain. His choice is awareness during visual search. Visual search has also been a traditional vehicle for the study of attention. For example, if you are asked to report a vertical rectangle in figure 20.1, the time to do so is linearly related to the number of distractors. This situation is thought to occur because one has to orient attention to each location. An individual may do so by making an eye movement, but it is also clear that the eyes can remain fixed and each position examined covertly. We now know quite a lot about the mechanism that performs this covert operation from studies of normal subjects, brain-lesioned patients, and monkeys (13).

When subjects switch attention from location to location, they activate processes in the parietal lobe of the opposite hemisphere (14). These cortical areas are involved in programming the switch of attention in the opposite visual field. The mechanisms of the parietal lobe are not symmetric. PET evidence shows that the right parietal lobe is involved with attention shifts in both visual fields, whereas the left parietal lobe seems restricted to rightward shifts of attention (14). There is a further hemispheric specialization as well. The left hemisphere seems to be more involved when attending to local information that might be important in recognizing objects, whereas the right hemisphere seems more involved when global features are involved, such as in general navigation in an environment (15).

These hemispheric differences are especially important in understanding how brain damage influences our awareness of the visual world. In normal people the two hemispheres operate as a unit in visual search, so that it does not matter if all of the distractors are located in one visual field or if they are distributed across the visual fields. However, if the two hemispheres are separated surgically by cutting the fiber tract that runs between them, this unity no longer applies, and each hemisphere's system operates separately, yielding a search rate that is twice as fast (16). Yet the patient is not really aware that a change has taken place due to the operation. If there is damage to the right parietal lobe, subjects will be very likely to neglect targets in search tasks like those of figure 20.1. In other words, they can be unconscious of information on the side of space opposite the lesion. These same mechanisms are used when these neglect patients recall information from memory, and they neglect the left side of visual images (17).

We know something of the route by which the parietal mechanism influences information about the target identity. The most prominent hypothesis about this route is that it involves the pulvinar nucleus of the thalamus. There is good evidence of activity in this general region when subjects must pull out a target from surrounding clutter (18). Thus the interaction of thalamus and the cortex plays an important role in our consciousness of the target. This finding fits well with the general idea outlined by Crick.

What are the consequences of attending to a visual object? We know from cellular recording studies in monkeys (12) and from neuroimaging studies in people (13) that attention provides a relative increase of neural activity when compared with comparable unattended information. For example, an instruction to attend to the color, form, or motion of visual input increases neural activity in the regions that process this information (19). This finding is certainly consonant with the proposal that mental events work on the rate of transmission of neural impulses that has been suggested by several theories of consciousness (1, 3).

However, the principle of relative amplification by attention is a very general one (13). It is found in all areas of the brain that have been studied. Attention to sensory information amplifies brain areas used to processes that modality; similarly, attention to motor output activates brain areas used to generate the movement. This principle also appears to apply to higher-level cognitive processes (13). For example, creating a visual image from a verbal instruction is now known to produce activation in visually specific areas of the cortex that would be used to process visual input of the same type.

What is still not known is exactly how this amplification is accomplished. There are theories at the neural level (20) and cellular observations that suggest a role for suppression of the unattended processes (21, 22), but the detailed cellular mechanisms remain to be clarified.

Are the thalamic-visual cortex interactions we have been describing "consciousness" as suggested by Crick? One definition of consciousness involves awareness of the outside world, and the interactions of thalamic areas with the visual cortex are certainly important for achieving focal awareness. By focal awareness I mean the type of recognition that one has of the target in figure 20.1. To locate the target one must effortfully engage different locations to be certain that they contain the constellation of features (form and orientation) required. However, it would not be appropriate to say you are unaware of other objects in the field that are not the focus of attention. One is roughly aware of the density of nonattended objects—their extent and basic format. It is possible to distinguish the type of focal awareness needed to locate the target from a more general awareness of the background (23). Damage to the attention network involving the parietal lobe and associated thalamic areas produces a kind of loss of focal awareness on one side of the world. Neglect induced by parietal lesion may leave the patient unconscious of this lack of awareness, just as the split brain person is unaware that search of the visual world has lost integration. However, patients with parietal lesions usually recover awareness of information opposite the lesion but show a permanent loss of the ability of stimuli arising there to produce orienting away from already attended events. This may lead to a failure to see objects on the left side of figure 20.1, but if cued to that location, they become conscious of them. In addition, normal subjects can attend to aspects of visual stimuli, such as their color or form, without activation of the parietal mechanisms we have been describing. These facts seem to argue that the parietal-thalamic system represents an important pathway by which conscious processing is achieved, rather than consciousness itself. Nonetheless, the clarification of neglect that has arisen from recent studies has helped us grasp some important elements of achieving focal awareness.

Attending to Ideas

Suppose you are asked to locate the vertical rectangle in figure 20.1. Must you search all the target locations or can you confine your search to the vertical objects only? There is considerable evidence that search can be guided by information about the color or orientation or other nonlocational features of the target (24). How is this implemented in the brain? It seems that the recruitment and control of posterior brain areas, in this case, is supervised by an anatomi-

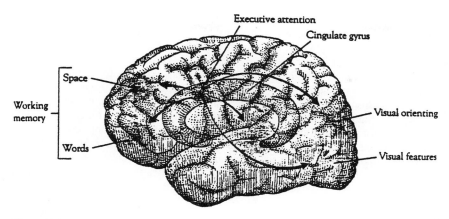

Figure 20.2

The executive attentional system involves frontal structures, including the anterior cingulate, and acts upon many different brain areas (reproduced with permission from ref. 13 [copyright Freeman, New York]).

cally distinct system that involves more anterior structures that have sometimes been called an executive network (ref. 13, pp. 168–174) (figure 20.2). In the study of attentional amplification of color, form, or motion mentioned above there was evidence for activation of a frontal attentional system, but no parietal activation was found (19). It thus appears that two different attentional systems serve as sources of activation for color or form (frontal areas) and for location (parietal), although both may enter via the thalamus to amplify activity within the visual system at the same site (e.g., V4).

In guided search, selection by location and selection by color or form occur simultaneously with relatively little interference (24), unlike the situation for location when the corpus collosum is intact, in which attention cannot be shared between the two fields (16). One speculative possibility would be that time sharing is possible when two anatomically distinct attentional sources are involved.

The frontal areas that serve to guide search appear to involve a network that includes at least portions of the basal ganglia and of the anterior cingulate gyrus (ref. 13, pp. 168–174). The anterior portion of the cingulate gyrus appears to be involved in a wide range of activities that have been termed collectively "executive function" (25). In PET language studies, when subjects were required to name the use of familiar nouns (e.g., pound to hammer) activation of the anterior cingulate along with left lateral cortex language areas was most prominent. When subjects were required to respond to the ink color in which a conflicting color name was presented (Stroop effect), there was strong activation of the anterior cingulate along with prestriate color areas (13). The detection of multiple color form or motion targets in comparison with passive viewing of the same stimuli also activated the anterior cingulate (19). All of these situations involve selection of targets from competing inputs, which is considered a traditional role of attention. In the case of this executive attentional network, the nature of the target does not seem to matter very much.

The term "executive" suggests two important overall functions. An executive is informed about the processes taking place within the organization. A system that would be related to our subjective experience of focal attention would clearly play this function for a subset of current (sensory) and stored (memory) information. There are reasons for relating anterior cingulate function to focal awareness of the target (13). For example, the intensity of cingulate activity tends to increase with number of targets in a set of stimuli and decreases with practice on any single stimulus set. These findings correspond to cognitive theories linking focal attention to number and difficulty of target detection.

A second function of an executive is to exercise some control over the system. The anatomy of the anterior cingulate provides pathways for connecting it to both the posterior parietal area and to anterior areas active during language tasks (26). Working memory is generally thought to involve both a representation of past events and an executive system involved in sustaining and transforming this representation (27). Recent PET (28, 29) and neurophysiological (30, 31) studies show that lateral areas of the prefrontal cortex play a key role in holding on-line a representation of past events. Cellular recordings in the awake monkey indicate that cells within the dorsolateral prefrontal cortex maintain a representation of the spatial environment when monkeys have to hold in mind a location to which to move their eyes after the stimulus disappears (30). Other cells within the inferior convexity hold a representation of the identity of past stimuli (31). Lateral areas of the left frontal and posterior cortex are also active in studies when people must obtain a quick association to word stimuli (13). While specialized areas of the lateral prefrontal cortex appear to hold the relevant information on-line, the anterior cingulate would be playing a role in the executive functions of awareness and control discussed in cognitive studies and often found impaired in subjects with frontal damage. Previously, the empirical results that support the important role of the anterior cingulate as a part of this network were summarized as follows (32):

1. The anterior attention network seems to be much more directly related to awareness than the posterior network, as has been indicated by the PET studies cited previously. The use of subjective experience as evidence for a brain process related to consciousness has been criticized by many authors. However, we note that the evidence for the activation of the anterior cingulate is entirely objective; it does not rest upon any subjective report. Nevertheless, if one defines consciousness in terms of awareness, it is necessary to show evidence that the anterior attention network is related to phenomenal reports in a systematic way. In this section, we note *five points*, each of which appears to relate *subjective experience* to activation of the anterior attention system. First, the degree of activation of this network increases with the number of targets presented in a semantic monitoring task and decreases with the amount of practice in the task. At first one might suppose that target detection is confounded with task difficulty. But in our semantic monitoring task the same semantic decision must be made irrespective of the number of actual targets. In our tasks no storage or counting of targets was needed. Thus, we effectively dissociated target detection from task difficulty. Nonetheless, anterior cingulate activation was related to number of targets present. The increase in activation with number of targets and reduction in such activation with practice corresponds to the common finding in cognitive studies that conscious attention is involved in target detection and is required to a greater degree early in practice. As practice proceeds, feelings of effort and continuous attention diminish, and details of performance drop out of subjective experience.

2. Second, the anterior system appears to be active during tasks requiring the subject to detect visual stimuli, when the targets involve color form, motion, or word semantics.

3. Third, the anterior attention system is activated when listening passively to words, but

not when watching those words. This finding appears to correspond subjectively to the intrusive nature of auditory words to consciousness when they are presented in a quiet background. They seem to capture awareness. Reading does not have this intrusive character. For a visual word to dominate awareness, an act of visual orienting is needed to boost its signal strength.

4. Fourth, the anterior attention system is more active during conflict blocks of the Stroop test than during nonconflict blocks. This is consistent with the commonly held idea that conflict between word name and ink color produces a strong conscious effort to inhibit saying the written word. Finally, there is a relation between the vigilance system and awareness. When one attends to a source of sensory input in order to detect an infrequent target, the subjective feeling is of emptying the head of thoughts or feelings. This subjective "clearing of consciousness" appears to be accompanied by an increase in activation of the right frontal lobe vigilance network and a reduction in the anterior cingulate. Just as feelings of effort associated with target detection or inhibiting prepotent responses are accompanied by evidence of cingulate activation, so the clearing of thought is accompanied by evidence of cingulate inhibition.

Dennett (33) provided a strong philosophical critique of those who implicitly cling to a view that there is an arena of consciousness or what he calls the Cartesian Theater of the Mind. Nonetheless, the specific points made above seemed to identify cingulate activation with aspects of awareness in so much tighter a way than previous efforts that it seems reasonable to set them down with as much clarity as possible. A somewhat similar view of the role of the cingulate in conjunction with the hippocampus has been discussed by Edelman (3). Edelman views these two brain structures as involved in the integration of interoceptive and exteroceptive information needed for conscious processing. In his work he distinguishes what he calls attention (which is

the increase in neural activity within brain areas currently of the organism's concern) from consciousness, which is the source of these activations in the cingulate-hippocampal system. There is a semantic difference in that I have called the former, the site at which attention works, and the latter, attentional networks, but the distinction appears minor.

One new development is an increased understanding of how the brain actually executes a voluntary instruction to attend to something (ref. 13, pp. 141–148). Studies employing PET have revealed important anatomical aspects of word reading. Two major areas of activation appear within the visual system. A right posterior temporal parietal area is activated passively by visual features, whether in consonant strings or words. In PET studies, areas of the left frontal area are active when subjects deal with the meaning of a word. When the process is extended by requiring association of several words to a given input or by slowing the rate of presentation, this left frontal area is joined by a posterior activation in Wernecke's area.

To study semantic and feature activation together, we used tasks that clearly involved both. We measured electrical activity from scalp electrodes. One task was looking for a visual feature; the semantic task required the subject to determine if the word referred to a natural or a manufactured item. Our reasoning was that in the visual task, subjects would be attending to the feature level, and in the semantic task attention would be directed to the meaning of the word. If, as has been described in the PET work, attention serves to amplify computations, it should be possible to see amplifications of the voltages in the waveforms in the right posterior area in feature analysis and in the left frontal area in semantics, depending upon the task used. We used exactly the same stimuli in the two tasks.

Results showed that electrical activity from the left frontal area was more positive at ≈ 200–300 ms when the task was semantic, whereas the right posterior area showed more positivity when the task was feature search. These effects were not confined to single electrode sites. For the posterior area, it was possible to compare the electrode sites first showing the greater right hemisphere activation at 100 ms associated with the processing of visual attributes automatically with those showing the amplification due to voluntary attribute search at ≈250 ms. Our comparison supported the idea that roughly the same areas that first carried out the visual-attribute computations on the letter string were reactivated 100 ms later when subjects were looking for the thick letter. This fit with the idea that subjects can voluntarily reactivate areas of the brain that performed the task automatically when they are instructed to deal with that computation voluntarily. The semantic effect was found at several frontal sites bilaterally. This result differs from the PET data, which were strictly left lateralized, although there was some evidence that the left frontal area showed the effect more strongly than the right.

A popular idea in modern physiology is called reentrant processing. Basically, this is the idea that higher-level associations are made by fibers that reenter the brain areas which processed the initial input (3, 34). Reentrant processing may be contrasted with more traditional notions that higher functions are confined to higher-associational areas of the brain. In our studies, the visual computation occurs at 100 ms, followed by a semantic computation that begins at ≈200 ms. When the instruction is to search the string for a visual feature, the electrodes around the area originally performing the visual computation are reactivated. Similarly, when asked to make a semantic computation, the area thought to perform such computations was amplified in electrical activity.

If the brain operates in this way, we might then be able to instruct the subject to compute the same functions in different orders and thus reprogram the order of the underlying computations. To investigate this, we defined what we call a conjunction task by asking subjects either to respond to targets that had thick letters and were animate or were animate and had thick letters. Both tasks were identical except for the order of the computations.

We did not expect the subjects to actually compute the functions in a serial fashion. The reaction times for targets suggested that the subjects were able to reorder the priority of the underlying computations in the conjunction task. The electrical activity also reflected the instructed priority. The results provide us with a basis for understanding how the brain can carry out so many different tasks upon visual input. Some aspects of the underlying computations are not affected by instructions. The visual attribute area of the right posterior brain seems to carry out the computation on the input string at 100 ms, irrespective of whether the person is concerned with visual features as a part of the task or not. However, when the task is identified as looking for a thick letter, these same brain areas are reactivated and presumably carry out the additional computations necessary to make sure that one of the letters has just enough thickening to constitute a target. Attention thus can amplify computations within particular areas but often does so by reentering the area, not by amplifying its initial activation. The order of these underlying computations can be reprogrammed by attending at different times, just as the order of attended locations in visual search can be changed at will.

The data on computing conjunctions implies two important ideas related to the attentional control of information processing.

1. The results of attentional control are widely distributed, resulting in amplification of activity in the anatomical areas that originally computed that information.

2. The source of this attentional control need not involve a system that has access to the information being amplified but can be a system that has connections to places where the computations occur.

As the result of activity within the attention network, the relevant brain areas will be amplified and/or irrelevant ones will be inhibited, leaving the brain to be dominated by the selected computations. If this were the correct theory of attentional control, one would expect to find the source of attention to lie in systems widely connected to other brain areas, but not otherwise unique in structure. As pointed out by Goldman-Rakic (26), this appears to be the basic organization of frontal midline networks. Anterior cingulate connections to limbic, thalamic, and basal ganglia pathways would distribute its activity to the widely dispersed connections we have seen to be involved in cognitive computations.

Maintaining the Alert State

The earliest studies of the anatomy of attention involved maintenance of the alert state. Cognitive psychologists have studied changes in alerting, by warning signals to prepare for the task. There is evidence that an increase in alertness improves the speed of processing events. The trade-off between improved speed and reduced accuracy with warning signals has led to a view that alerting does not act to improve the buildup of information concerning the nature of the target but, instead, acts on the attentional system to enhance the speed of actions taken toward the target (ref. 13, pp. 174–176).

There has been some improvement in our understanding of the neural systems related to alerting over the last few years. Patients with lesions of the right frontal area have difficulty in maintaining the alert state. In addition, experimental studies of blood flow in normal people during tasks that require maintaining alertness show right frontal activation.

The neurotransmitter norepinephrine appears to be involved in maintaining the alert state. This norepinephrine pathway arises in the midbrain, but the right frontal area appears to have a special role in its cortical distribution. Among posterior visual areas in the monkey, norepinephrine pathways are selective for areas involved in visual spatial attention. Recent studies (35) using drugs to reduce norepinephrine in alert monkeys show that this reduction blocks the increased processing speed usually found with warning signals, thus supporting the role of norepinephrine in achieving alertness.

Applications and Future Directions

We have a start on understanding the circuitry that underlies orienting of attention. However, more detailed cellular studies in monkeys are necessary to test these hypotheses and to understand more completely the time course and the control structures involved in covert orienting of attention. Even more fascinating is the possibility that the microstructure of areas involved in attention will be different somehow in organization from those areas carrying out passive data processing. Such differences could give us a clue as to the way in which brain tissue might relate to subjective experience.

Much remains unknown concerning the more anterior executive system. Studies of blood flow and metabolism in normal people should be adequate to provide candidate areas involved in aspects of attention. It will then be possible to test further the general proposal that these constitute a unified system and that constituent computations are localized.

The idea of attention as a network of anatomical areas makes relevant study of both the comparative anatomy of these areas and their development in infancy (ref. 13, pp. 181–192). In the first few months of life, infants develop nearly adult abilities to orient to external events, but the cognitive control produced by the executive attention network requires many months or years of development. Studies of orienting and motor control are beginning to lead to an understanding of this developmental process. As more about the maturational processes of brain and transmitter system is understood, it could be possible to match developing attentional abilities with changing biological mechanisms. The neural mechanisms of attention must support not only common development among infants in their regulatory abilities, but also the obvious differences among infants in their rates and success of attentional control.

There are many disorders that are often supposed to involve attention—including neglect, depression, schizophrenia, and attention-deficit disorder. The specification of attention in terms of anatomy and function has already proven useful in clarifying some of the underlying bases for these disorders (ref. 13, pp. 217–222). The development of theories of deficits might also foster the integration of psychiatric and higher-level neurological disorders, both of which might affect the brain's attentional system.

Consciousness

The issues of selection and control central to the study of attention are also important aspects of most theories of consciousness. Sperry (36), in particular, has argued that cognitive control over earlier evolving neural systems represents an emergent property of complex networks.

The study of visual attention has implicated a cortical-thalamic network used for orienting that has many similarities to the visual awareness system favored by Crick (2) as a model for the study of consciousness. Although there may be doubts about whether it is a complete model, the importance of studies of this system as a way of integrating human and monkey research is clear. Study of higher forms of attentional selectivity has focused on frontal structures that have something in common with the analysis of consciousness proposed by Edelman (3) and others. The role of the cingulate and other frontal areas in the development of volition remains of critical importance. Neuroimaging

studies have tended to confirm the role of attention in providing a relative amplification of neural activity within specific sensory or motor sites at which computations take place. This is a view favored by Beck and Eccles (1), as well as many others, as a critical aspect of consciousness. Whether the progress in studies of attention and brain mechanisms will provide a complete analysis of consciousness or whether fundamentally new mechanisms such as those that might come from quantum physics (1, 4) will be needed is, of course, a matter of opinion, but what seems clear is that there has been very considerable recent progress toward understanding brain networks relevant to the production of conscious experience, and the tools are present for considerable future development.

Acknowledgments

This research was supported by grants from the Office of Naval Research and by the J. S. McDonnell Foundation and Pew Memorial Trusts through a grant to the University of Oregon.

References

1. Beck, F. and Eccles, J. C. (1992) *Proc. Natl. Acad. Sci. USA* 89, 11357–11361.

2. Crick, F. (1994) *The Astonishing Hypothesis* (Scribner's, New York).

3. Edelman, G. M. (1989) *The Remembered Present* (Basic, New York).

4. Penrose, R. (1989) *The Emperor's New Mind* (Oxford Univ. Press, Oxford).

5. Zeki, S. (1993) *A Vision of the Brain* (Blackwell, Oxford).

6. Baars, B. (1988) *A Cognitive Theory of Consciousness* (Cambridge Univ. Press, Cambridge, U.K.).

7. James, W. (1907) *Psychology* (Holt, Rinehart & Winston, New York).

8. Moruzzi, G. and Magoun, H. V. (1949) *Electroencephalogr. Clin. Neurophysiol.* 1, 445–473.

9. Broadbent, D. E. (1958) *Perception and Communication* (Pergamon, London).

10. Allport, D. A. (1989) in *Foundations of Cognitive Science*, ed. Posner, M. I. (Bradford Books/MIT Press, Cambridge, MA), pp. 636–682.

11. Sokolov, Y. N. (1963) *Perception and the Conditioned Reflex* (Pergamon, London).

12. Wurtz, R. H., Goldberg, M. E. and Robinson, D. L. (1980) *Prog. Psychobiol. Physiol. Psychol.* 9, 43–83.

13. Posner, M. I. and Raichle, M. E. (1994) *Images of Mind* (Sci. Am. Library, New York).

14. Corbetta, M., Miezin, F. M., Shulman, G. L. and Petersen, S. E. (1993) *J. Neurosci.* 13, 1202–1226.

15. Robertson, L. C., Lamb, M. R. and Knight, R. T. (1988) *J. Neurosci.* 8, 3757–3769.

16. Luck, S. J., Hillyard, S. A., Mangun, G. R. and Gazzaniga, M. S. (1989) *Nature* (*London*) 342, 543–545.

17. Bisiach, E. (1992) in *The Neuropsychology of Conscious*, eds. Milner, A. D. and Rugg, M. (Academic, London), pp. 113–137.

18. LaBerge, D. and Buchsbaum, M. S. (1990) *J. Neurosci.* 10, 613–619.

19. Corbetta, M., Miezin, F. M., Dobmeyer, S., Shulman, G. L. and Petersen, S. E. (1991) *J. Neurosci.* 11, 2388–2402.

20. Van Essen, D. C., Anderson, C. H. and Olshausen, B. A. (1994) in *Large Scale Neuronal Theories of the Brain*, eds. Koch, C. and Davis, J. (MIT Press, Cambridge, MA), pp. 271–300.

21. Moran, J. and Desimone, R. (1985) *Science* 229, 782–784.

22. Chelazzi, L., Miller, E. K., Duncan, J. and Desimone, R. (1993) *Nature* (*London*) 363, 345–347.

23. Iwasaki, S. (1993) *Cognition* 49, 211–233.

24. Wolfe, J. K. M., Cave, K. R. and Franzel, S. L. (1989) *J. Exp. Psychol. Hum. Perception Performance* 15, 419–433.

25. Vogt, B. A., Finch, D. M. and Olson, C. R. (1992) *Cereb. Cortex* 2/6, 435–443.

26. Goldman-Rakic, P. S. (1988) *Annu. Rev. Neurosci.* 11, 137–156.

27. Baddeley, A. D. (1990) *Working Memory* (Oxford Univ. Press, Oxford).

28. Jonides, J., Smith, E. E., Koeppe, R. A., Awh, E., Minoshima, S. and Mintun, M. A. (1993) *Nature* (*London*) 363, 623–635.

29. Paulesu, E., Frith, C. D. and Frackowiak, R. S. (1993) *Nature* (*London*) 363, 342–345.

30. Funahashi, S., Chafee, M. V. and Goldman-Rakic, P. (1993) *Nature* (*London*) 365, 753–756.

31. Wilson, F. A. W., Scalaidhe, S. P. O. and Goldman-Rakic, P. (1993) *Science* 260, 1955–1958.

32. Posner, M. I. and Rothbart, M. K. (1992) in *The Neuropsychology of Conscious*, eds. Milner, A. D. and Rugg, M. (Academic, London), pp. 91–112.

33. Dennett, D. (1991) *Consciousness Explained* (Little Brown, Boston).

34. Edelman, G. and Mountcastle, V. (1978) *The Mindful Brain* (MIT Press, Cambridge, MA).

35. Witte, E. A. (1993) Doctoral dissertation (Univ. of Oregon, Eugene).

36. Sperry, R. W. (1988) *Am. Psychol.* 43, 607–613.

37. Posner, M. I. and Dehaene, S. (1994) *Trends Neurosci.* 17, 75–79.

21 Attention, Awareness, and the Triangular Circuit

David LaBerge

Introduction

The operations of attention are crucial to the successful performance of our everyday tasks. A large amount of research by experimental psychologists has shown that the attentional process helps us to select a target item from distractors in a cluttered visual scene (e.g., Treisman and Gelade 1980, Yantis 1993), it helps us to prepare in advance for an expected stimulus so that we may respond more quickly and correctly to it (e.g., Posner 1980, Eriksen and Yeh 1985, Downing 1988), and it helps us to maintain particular cognitive activities for their own sake (LaBerge 1995b). But these ubiquitous pragmatic, or instrumental, benefits of attention should not overshadow the importance of the attentional process to our ongoing awareness of the worlds outside and inside our bodies. William James expressed the broad scope of attention in a clear and concise form more than 100 years ago (James 1890, p. 402) when he wrote "My experience is what I agree to attend to."

This statement contains assertions concerning both attention and awareness. Two aspects of attention are implied in James's claim. The first aspect concerns what is being attended, and the second concerns the action of personal choice. Stated otherwise, the first aspect is the "what," which is the object of attending, and the second aspect is the control of what is attended by the act of agreement. This paper proposes that the attention event is characterized by simultaneous activity in brain sites corresponding to the object and to the controlling action and that these sites are interconnected within a triangular circuit that also includes a third structure that amplifies the activity at the object site.

James' statement also includes the pronouns "my" and "I," which refer to the self. In particular, the expression "my experience" implies a close relationship between the self and the experience of attending to an object. This paper proposes that the experience of attending to an object becomes an experience of being aware of that object when it is conjoined with attending to a representation of the self. In other words, as an event of attending to some object, experience becomes awareness when the self becomes involved, that is, when "an experience" becomes "my experience." The present paper attempts to justify these claims concerning the triangular circuit of attention and the conditions for awareness on the basis of reasonable conjecture, using mainly the findings from studies of brain structures and their interconnections, and from studies of their activities while subjects are engaged in cognitive tasks.

The heavy emphasis on brain locations and their interconnections in the present paper stems from the guiding assumption that if you know *where* something happens you are closer to discovering *how* it happens. In the past two decades, several new anatomical and physiological measures have become available that have enabled researchers to determine the specialized functions of neurons at particular locations in the brain when cognitive tasks are being performed and to determine the patterns in which these locations are interconnected. This new information about how brain structure and function relate to specific cognitive tasks is now of sufficient detail to generate new notions for constructing testable theories of how cognitive processes are carried out. In particular, these developments in neuroscience measures hold the promise of untangling traditionally intractable problems relating to awareness or consciousness (Banks 1993). The purpose of the present essay is to use the available knowledge bridging the fields of cognition and neuroscience to describe a structure whose operations are crucial for the processes of attention and awareness. This notion is the triangular circuit (LaBerge 1995a,b) that joins widely separated regions of the brain in the process of attention.

The "object" of attention, whether an object of sense or an object of thought, is generally believed to be coded in some form within specific areas or modules of the cerebral cortex. Visual shapes are coded in clusters of neurons within the inferotemporal cortex (IT), and visual locations are coded in clusters of neurons within the posterior parietal cortex (PPC), while plans of action and semantic attributes of objects involve codes that appear to be distributed across specific modules of the frontal cortex. When one of these cortical codes becomes the object of attention, we presume that the corresponding module increases its activity relative to its surrounding sites. The resulting profile of activity across the target object and its immediately surrounding sites may be called the *expression* aspect of attention (LaBerge 1995a,b). The controlling "agent" of attention is presumed to be coded within specific areas of the prefrontal cortex (PFC), and modules within these areas also become active when a specific object is voluntarily chosen for attentional activation (Smith et al. 1995, Liotti et al., unpublished). Thus, these PFC modules are said to serve the *control* aspect of attention (LaBerge 1995a,b).

But a controlling PFC module cannot be regarded as a homunculus, in which "first causes" of attentional choice originate. When William James wrote about the close connection between attention and experience (quoted a few paragraphs back), he went on to explain at length that the particular things we agree to attend to depend on their *interest* to us. It turns out that activities in the controlling modules of the PFC are themselves influenced by the basal ganglia, which is a subcortical structure that is closely connected with the motivation-related hypothalamus. While our main concern in this paper is with the relationship between the cortical areas in which attention is expressed and controlled, it is important to keep in mind that these attentional events occur within the contextual influences of the habitual and momentary interests of the person, which appear to involve brain structures other than the ones being considered here (e.g., the basal ganglia and hypothalamus).

The Expression of Attention

Attentional operations exert their effects on ongoing cognitive-related events by modulating the activity levels of neurons in the cerebral cortex. This claim is based on the results of a large number of attention studies that employ a variety of physiological measures, including single-cell recordings, ERPs, MFGs, PET, and fMRI (for examples, see Gazzaniga 1995, LaBerge 1995b), which identified the cortical sites where neurons change their activity levels when subjects vary their attention to the several aspects of a typical behavioral task.

The foregoing physiological indicators measure cortical activity at different spatial (and temporal) scales, ranging from the small spatial scale for the single neuron to the scale of millions of neurons that activate the ERP, MEG, PET, and fMRI measures. Between the extremes of this range lies the scale size of the functional unit of the cortex, which presumably corresponds to the functional unit of cognition. It is the mean activity within this functional unit that is assumed here to be modulated by attentional operations.

The functional unit of the cerebral cortex is widely assumed to be not the individual neuron but ensembles of neurons (e.g., Lansner and Fransen 1994, Rose and Siebler 1995). For some time, physiologists have assumed that the functional unit is the group of neural circuits contained in vertical, cylinder-like structures of the cortical sheet called cortical columns (Mountcastle 1978, Freeman 1975, Goldman-Rakic 1990, Tanaka 1992) or minicolumns (Mountcastle 1957, Peters and Sethares 1991, Purves et al. 1992, Szentagothai 1983). A cortical column corresponds to the mass of neural tissue lying under a 1 mm × 1 mm square area along the surface of the cortex and spanning the 1.5- to 2.0-mm thickness of the cortical sheet. The number of neurons contained within the typical cortical column is said to be on the order of 100,000 (e.g., Amit 1995), while a typical column in area V1 contains nearer to 180,000 neurons (O'Kusky and Colonnier 1982). The cortical column is sometimes subdivided into mini-columns of varying sizes, for example, in V1 the ocular dominance, color, and orientation-specific minicolumns have widths of about 400, 200, and 30 μm wide, respectively, containing about 23,000, 5500, and 140 neurons, respectively (Peters and Sethares 1991). Vertical groups of neurons are centered around the long vertical dendrites of layer 5 neurons, forming a cylinder-like volume having a diameter of approximately 30 μm. This minicolumn, which contains about 140 neurons, has also been proposed as the functional unit of the cortex (Peters and Sethares 1991, Peters 1994), as have minicolumns of approximately the same size, containing 100–200 neurons (Mountcastle 1957, Purves et al. 1992, Szentagothai 1983). According to Peters (1994), a given minicolumn may simultaneously serve eye preference, orientation, and color. The suggested organization of the minicolumn around layer 5 neurons is of significance to the present paper, because (as it will be shown later in this paper) axons of layer 5 neurons provide the major source of inputs to thalamic relay neurons in the triangular circuit. However, since it is highly likely that minicolumns function in groups, it seems appropriate to use the term columns to refer to these groups.

Recently, columns having circular or elliptic shapes with diameters of approximately 0.5 mm have been directly observed by optical imaging of the cortical surface of the anterior infer-otemporal area (Wang, Tanaka, and Tanifuji 1996), which is a region crucial for object identification. Single-cell recordings of individual neurons inside one of these columns responded to a particular class of geometric shapes, while neurons in the immediate neighborhood of the column did not respond to that class of stimuli. Thus, anatomical evidence continues to favor the proposal, made over 30 years ago, that the functional unit of the cerebral cortex is a columnar cluster of neuronal circuits, and the width of the quasi-circular shape of the surface area under which the column lies, according to available estimates, appears to vary between 0.5 and 1.0 mm, so that a column contains on the order of 50,000 to 100,000 neurons.

Therefore, the appropriate level of description of the events taking place within a column would appear to be not the individual neuron, nor a local circuit of several neurons, but rather a large bundle of circuits, whose organization is tailored to the particular function of that column. This level of description for the functional unit of cortex is of considerable importance to the cognitive scientist, because the organizational complexity existing at the level of the circuit bundle has the potential to exhibit the enormous variety of activity patterns (electrical or electromagnetic) necessary to produce the innumerable variety of cognitive events that take place within the human brain. In somewhat the same manner, the organizational complexity of molecules, as combinations of relatively few types of atoms, can exhibit the countless variety of existing chemical substances. However, this informal comparison between chemical substances and cognitive events does not imply that a given cognitive event corresponds to one cortical column. It seems more likely that combinations of cortical columns within and between cortical regions constitute the cognitive unit (see Lansner and Fransen 1994), so that the individual column could be regarded as a cognitive miniunit, in much the same way that an orientation column is divided into minicolumns whose cells have a preference for a particular orientation. Furthermore, several columns are involved for cases of coarse coding, for example, location coding in the posterior parietal cortex (e.g., Andersen et al.

1985). Later in this paper, it will be proposed that simultaneous activity in columns of two separated cortical regions define the attentional event, so that, regarded as a unit of cognition, the attentional event involves not one but two functional units of the cerebral cortex.

The present description of the cortical column as a functional unit does not imply that the relationship between a given column of neurons and a particular function is fixed, either at birth or after learning. A considerable amount of research has shown that the columns can change their functions (e.g., their sensitivities to oriented visual bars and to tactual stimulation of the fingers) over time periods during which certain kinds of sensory stimulation occurred (O'Leary, Schlaggar, and Tuttle 1994; Merzenich, Gilbert, and Wiesel 1992).

Clusters of cortical columns are activated when a subject begins to engage in a cognitive task, and since the typical cognitive task is presumed to involve several different columns or column clusters, columns in many areas of cortex typically will become active during the first seconds of task performance. These increases in column activities are the events that brain imaging techniques measure, albeit indirectly. The ERP and EEG measure electrical fields, and the MEG measures magnetic fields, both fields being produced by millions of neurons, while fMRI measures blood flow, and PET measures either blood flow or glucose uptake, both substances being drawn, in some manner, to the columns by their increased neural activity. When tasks are varied in appropriate ways and the resulting brain images compared, the column clusters corresponding to specific task components can be located in three-dimensional brain maps of a brain atlas (e.g., Talairach and Tournoux 1988).

Expression of Attention in a Cortical Area

Given the foregoing description of cortical column activity as the brain correlate of a component of a cognitive event, the expression aspect of attention can be defined relatively clearly. Viewed cognitively, the expression of attention is the *emphasis* of a particular component of a cognitive event, and viewed cortically, the expression of attention corresponds to a difference in activity levels between the column clusters corresponding to the attended (target) component and its neighboring (distractor) components (or the surround, if the attended component is presented in isolation). For example, consider the task of identifying the letter shape that is located in the fourth position from the left end of the letter string EMPHASIS (see figure 21.1). The left side of figures 21.1b–d shows the activation contours across columns (presumably in V4 and/or IT) after the expression of attention has reached its asymptote. The variations in thickness of the lines used in constructing the letters is intended only to illustrate the several ways by which one could emphasize the letter H if one actually modified the stimulus display; here, the stimulus display for all four examples is the printed word shown in figure 21.1a). The development over time of the attentional expression to the target letter H is shown in the right half of figure 21.1 for these cases. When the familiar word is displayed to the subject, activities in V4/IT columns corresponding to the locations of the coded letter shapes increase to some level, and then a difference in activity begins to develop between the target columns and the neighboring columns. This difference in columnar activity constitutes the expression of attention.

Figure 21.1 depicts three different ways to produce an activity difference between the attended columns and the distractor columns. Figure 21.1b shows the development of attentional expression by operations that enhance activities in columns corresponding to the location of the letter H; figure 21.1c shows the development of attentional expression by operations that suppress activities in columns corresponding to the location of letters in the surrounding neighborhood of the letter H; and figure 21.1d shows the development of atten-

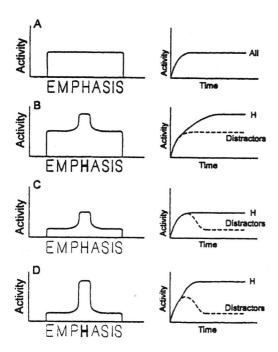

Figure 21.1

Schematic diagrams of three operations by which the location of a part of a stimulus array is selected by attentional expressions (shown in *b*, *c*, and *d*). The stimulus-induced activity of the entire stimulus array prior to selective emphasis is represented in (*a*). The time course of the activities in cortical columns corresponding to locations of the target and surrounding distracters of the stimulus array are shown on the right side of the figure. The brain site for this example is V4 and/or IT.

tional expression by both the enhancement of columns corresponding to the letter H and the suppression of the columns corresponding to the neighboring letters.

Thus, the expression of attention in this kind of task could be based on one of three types of operations: enhancement of the target columns, suppression of surrounding distractor columns, or a combination of these two operations. In the research literature, the target-enhancement operation has been implicitly assumed in the use of the metaphors spotlight, zoom lens, resource allocation, and gain; the distractor-suppression operation has been implicit in the use of the terms filter, gate, and channel. In the present context involving descriptions of cortical column activities, an appropriate metaphor might benefit our understanding of how a cortical column operates, not only when column activity is at high levels that characterize attention, but also at low levels which characterize automatic processing. However, for purposes of the present paper, it seems appropriate simply to use the general descriptive term "column activity level" to describe cortical correlates of attention, keeping in mind that the term "column" represents bundles of neural circuits that exhibit particular activity patterns when triggered by appropriate external or internal signals.

One particular contrasting property of the suppression and enhancement operations is the upper limit on the size of the difference between the target and the distractor activity. The range of suppressions in the distractor columns lies between the initial level and zero (see figure 21.1), while the range of enhancements in the target column lies between the initial level and the upper limit of column activity. Given that the upper limit of neuron firing rates is 1000 Hz and that firing rates of neurons modulated by attention in single-cell studies are on the order of 20–100 Hz (Chelazzi et al. 1993, Motter 1993), the range of suppression effects would appear to be much smaller than the range of potential enhancement effects.

Which of the three types of selective emphasis is evoked in studies of visual spatial attention, using the generic display shown in figure 21.1 as an example? The total activity across the participating columns is above baseline for all three types of selective operations; hence for each type of operation, brain images (e.g., PET and fMRI) would be expected to show higher levels of activation for the cortical region containing these columns, compared to a condition in which attention is not directed to the task. In order to distinguish the three operations effectively, it would be desirable to use a more fine-grained measure that reveals activity levels at the scale of columns, since measures such as PET and fMRI do not satisfactorily resolve activities separated by less than 3 or 4 mm.

At the scale of the single neuron, activities in separate but closely positioned cortical columns can be resolved, and single-cell recordings in monkeys have provided data that appear to favor one or another of the three operations of attentional selection shown in figures 21.1b–d. Chelazzi et al. (1993) displayed two shapes in different quadrants of the visual field and recorded from neurons whose receptive fields contained the shapes. When the monkey attended to one of the two shapes, the trajectories of neural firing rates evoked by the attended (target) shape and by the unattended (distractor) shape showed a pattern that was very similar to the pair of trajectories shown in figure 21.1c. If one assumes that these particular neurons reflect the net effect of the neurons operating within the circuits of their respective columns, the Chelazzi et al. (1993) data indicate that selective attention operates by *suppression* of column activity in columns corresponding to the locations of the distractors. Other studies of single-cell activity (e.g., Moran and Desimone 1985, Schall and Hanes 1993) also support the suppression type of attentional expression in visual spatial attention tasks.

An earlier study by Spitzer, Moran, and Desimone (1988) found that increased attention during a color discrimination task enhanced firing rates in V4 neurons. More recent single-cell recordings of neuronal activity during spatial attention tasks (Motter 1993, Buracas and Albright 1995, Treue and Maunsell 1995) revealed neurons whose firing rates are increased when attention is directed to a stimulus that falls within their receptive fields, following the general pattern of the pair of trajectories shown in figure

21.1b. Assuming that these neurons reflect the net activity of their respective columns, one could conclude that these data indicate that selective attention operates by the enhancement of activity in columns corresponding to the target item's location.

At first glance, these two sets of data obtained from single-cell recordings during spatial attention tasks would seem to be contradictory. However, if the cortical column is assumed to be the functional unit, then it is conceivable that some of the approximately 100,000 individual neurons within that column could exhibit a suppressive pattern and others exhibit the enhancement pattern while the net activity level of the column exhibits either suppression or enhancement. Thus, if the column is regarded as the functional unit of cortical processing instead of the neuron, then data from a small sample of single neurons become less persuasive as a means of determining whether attentional expression arises from enhancement of the target site or suppression of the distractor site(s).

Another approach to distinguishing the three operations of attentional expression depicted in figure 21.1 considers the properties of the anatomical fibers arriving from outside a particular column that trigger activity in that column. What controls which columns will become enhanced and/or suppressed, or by how much, when attention is directed to a specific target location? Clearly, instructions to a subject can determine which item is to be attended to (e.g., name the last letter of the word EMPHASIS), and the saliency of a particular item can attract attention to itself (e.g., a red letter among black letters). In the present example, shown in figure 21.1, the letters in the stimulus display are presumed to be equally salient, so that the choice of the target item is determined by instructions or training procedures. Therefore, the signals that control which columns are chosen for modulated activity come from within the brain.

When signals arrive at columns of cortex from long-range distances (i.e., outside the immediate cortical area), they are, without known exception, exclusively of the excitatory type when the origin of the signals is another cortical area (Jones 1985, Salin and Bullier 1995). Also, when the origin of the signals arriving at a cortical column is the thalamus, the signals are, without known exception, of the excitatory type (Jones 1985). Inhibitory fibers in the cortex extend over very small distances (up to 1–2 mm), and thus their direct effects are virtually always local. Approximately 80% of cortical neurons are excitatory, and approximately 85% of the synapses in cortex are excitatory (Braitenberg and Schuz 1991). Hence, it would appear that the input fibers to a column that arrive from distant cortical or subcortical areas are likely to have an overall excitatory effect and not an inhibitory general effect on the receiving column neurons.

Given that voluntary influences on the expression of attention arrive by means of excitatory fibers over long-distance connections, a crucial question concerns how these excitatory signals result in either an enhancement or a suppression of activities in a cortical column corresponding to the location of a target or a distractor. Three examples of the relationship of attentional expression to an outside controlling influence are illustrated in figure 21.2, corresponding to three theories of selective attention that are at least 20 years old. The diagram in figure 21.2a represents complete filtering of sensory input (Broadbent 1958), the diagram in figure 21.2b represents attenuated filtering of sensory input (Treisman 1960), and the diagram in figure 21.2c represents the enhancement of sensory input (LaBerge 1975, LaBerge and Samuels 1974). In these diagrams, sensory information corresponding to the locations of the target and four distractors (e.g., the task is to identify the fourth letter from the left in the word EARTH) trigger an initial level of energy that is approximately equal across the columns that express attention, as illustrated in figure 21.1a. After attentional operations have selected the target columns, the activation from the target columns exceeds that of neighboring

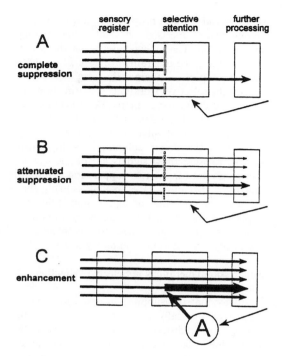

Figure 21.2
Schematic diagrams of selective attention operations according to some theories of attention in the psychological literature. (*a*) Complete suppression or filtering of distractor codes (Broadbend 1958); (*b*) attenuated suppression or filtering of distractor codes (Treisman 1960); (*c*) enhancement of the target code (Laberge and Samuels 1974).

columns, and the featural information from the target item then dominates the information sent on to other areas for further processing (e.g., for identification in IT or for storage in the hippocampus), as illustrated in figures 21.1b–d.

Clearly, the selection of the target column requires top-down signals, particularly when the target-distractor similarity is high and there is no appreciable preattentive "popout" (Treisman and Gelade 1980, Julesz and Bergen 1983) of one item from the others, owing to its having some special featural property (e.g., a red object among black objects, or a slanted line among vertical lines). The arrows inserted at the lower right of the three diagrams in figure 21.2 represent the top-down signals that are needed to control the selective operations performed on the target and distractor columns. For the enhancement diagram illustrated in figure 21.2c, the selective operation of enhancement can be directly applied to the target column(s) by top-down signals, because these signals are of the excitatory type. But for the two suppression diagrams illustrated in figures 21.2a–b it is unlikely that the selective operation of suppression is directly applied to the distractor columns by top-down excitatory signals, since these signals travel over excitatory fibers and not inhibitory fibers.

Suppression Operations in Selective Attention

One way that the suppressive operations (illustrated schematically in figure 21.1c) could be applied to the distractor columns is locally, by lateral inhibitory fibers arising from the target column. Local suppression operations would seem particularly appropriate when the distractor is in the same receptive field as the target and are consistent with the descriptive account given by Desimone (1992) that attention shrinks the size of the receptive field. Another way of accounting for the reduction in activation in distractor columns is by assuming that activation simply decays in the absence of supporting signals from top-down sources. Decay of distractor site activation, following initial sensory excitation, would seem appropriate when the distractor lies outside the receptive field of the target. However, for both accounts of suppression-like results, the level of activation exhibited by the target columns is presumed to be largely determined by retinal neurons, which respond to the intensity characteristics of the stimulus. Thus, retina-driven signals in the target columns, under the regulatory influences of top-down sig-

nals, subsequently inhibit the activities in neighboring distractor columns, or else these activities simply decay.

Enhancement Operations in Selective Attention

In the case of the enhancement operation, the energy used for target column activity during attentional expression arises from a top-down source. The signals controlling which columns will be enhanced act on those columns in an enhancement manner to increase their levels of activation (as shown in figure 21.1b). Distractor columns do not require suppression from initial activity levels, but some suppression of distractor columns could accompany target column enhancement (as shown in figure 21.1d).

Candidates for the top-down, extraretinal sources of energy for the activation levels of a target column are within the visual cortex itself, the prefrontal cortex, the thalamus, and the neuromodulatory centers in the brain stem. Neuromodulatory centers are necessary for the state of wakefulness and states of alertness, which themselves are preconditions for states of attention and awareness (e.g., Steriade, McCormick, and Sejnowski 1993). Although fibers from the brainstem neuromodulatory nuclei project richly to thalamic nuclei as well as directly to cortical areas, the distribution of these fibers is too diffuse to account for more localized patterns of activity believed to underlie selective attention (see figure 21.1).

Within a single column of the visual cortex there exist a sufficient number of feedback connections to produce significant self-amplification (Douglas et al. 1995). Hence, it is possible that cortical self-amplifying circuits could be triggered and/or regulated by signals from external sources, such as the prefrontal cortex or thalamus.

Another nonretinal source of column-activity amplification is another cortical area, for example, the posterior parietal area, where locations of objects are known to be coded (e.g., Andersen, Essick, and Siegel 1985), or the prefrontal cortex, where neuronal activity is known to increase at the time when shapes and locations, currently held in working memory, are selected for an overt response (Wilson, O'Scalaidhe, and Goldman-Rakic 1993). Signals from the prefrontal voluntary regions, operating indirectly through the posterior parietal area or possibly directly to V4/IT, could select which columns in V4/IT express attention.

In view of the foregoing considerations, and in view of the considerations yet to be described concerning the triangular circuit, the prefrontal area emerges as a promising candidate for the source of attentional control. Prefrontal areas lie in the anterior cortex, the cortical region in which actions appear to be represented, so that controls on attentional expressions in posterior areas of perception clearly imply that an *action* of some kind is taken by the system.

However, the combination of the two brain sites corresponding to attentional expression and attentional control is not regarded here as sufficient for the attentional event to exist. While fibers arising from the prefrontal areas (sometimes operating indirectly through another cortical area such as the posterior parietal area when the location of the object is being controlled) presumably carry the signals needed to choose the columns in V4/IT (that are appropriate to the location and shape of the selected target item) it is questionable whether or not fibers from these other cortical areas also carry the range of firing rates needed to induce directly the higher levels of activity in the columns that correspond to the attended item. High rates of firing can obscure the temporal properties of a signal train that is precisely tuned to choose the appropriate columns for attentional expression. To keep separate the informational and modulatory properties of prefrontal control, a supplemental route from the prefrontal (and/or parietal) areas is needed to carry the modulatory signals that

are needed to intensify the activity levels in the target columns.

The principal pathways of fibers connecting the control areas of the prefrontal cortex to cortical columns where attention is expressed are prefrontal to IT (Webster et al. 1994) for shape, and prefrontal to PPC (Goldman-Rakic, Chafee, and Friedman 1993) for location, but another pathway of fibers connects these prefrontal areas with their posterior cortical target columns. This other pathway passes through the thalamus, and the thalamic circuitry has the modulatory ability to enhance the rate of neural signals passing through it, according to a simulation analysis (LaBerge, Carter, and Brown 1992). Thus, the two pathways by which a prefrontal area connects to another cortical area form a triangle, in which the direct link is mainly concerned with choosing precisely which columns shall be activated, and the indirect link (which passes through the thalamus) is mainly concerned with how much the chosen column shall be intensified. In order to clarify the way in which the triangular circuit separates the informational and modulatory aspects of signaling between cortical areas, the structure of the circuit will be described with some detail in the following section.

The Triangular Circuit

Since most of the knowledge we have of cortical and thalamic circuitry has been obtained from studies of the primary visual cortex and its adjacent areas, the description given here of the triangular circuit is based on a schematic diagram of the triangular circuit involving areas V1 and V2. In figure 21.3, the direct (forward) connecting fibers between a V1 column and a V2 column arise from layer 2 of the V1 column and terminate in the middle layers of the V2 column. The indirect connecting fibers between a V1 column and a V2 column arise from Layer 5 of the V1 column, and terminate on a thalamic relay neu-

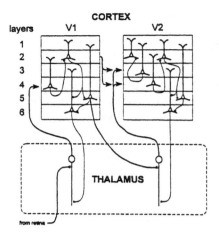

Figure 21.3
Schematic diagrams of excitatory neurons within a pair of cortical columns and within a thalamic nucleus, along with their main interconnections. The forward connection from the first column (e.g., in area V1) to the second column (e.g., in area V2) occurs both directly and indirectly by means of a synapse in a thalamic nucleus, forming a triangular circuit.

ron, which in turn projects to the middle layers of a V2 column. The effect of a Layer 5 neuron of V1 on a V2 column is somewhat analogous to the effect of an optic nerve cell on a V1 column.

Evidence from neural tracing studies (e.g., Ungerleider, Galkin, and Mishkin 1983) indicate that V1 fibers synapse in the pulvinar nucleus of the thalamus (which projects directly to V2) and that these fibers arise from Layer 5 of V1 (Conley and Razkowski 1990). Relay neurons in the pulvinar project directly to area V2 (Jones 1985), as well to the other visual areas in the posterior cortex (including V1). Thus, the triangular circuit depicted in figure 21.3 begins with neurons in a V1 column that connect with a V2 column by a direct connection and by an indirect connection by way of the thalamus.

The route between V1 and V2 that enlists thalamic neurons, shown in figure 21.3, appears to have characteristics that enhance firing rates. Layer 5 neurons fire in bursts of a few spikes at rates at least as high as 250 Hz, with intraburst firing rates on the order of 15 Hz (Connors and Gutnick 1990, Gray and McCormick 1996), and therefore these neurons have the ability to drive their target neurons to high rates of firing. The intrinsically spiking Layer 5 neurons synapse near the cell bodies of thalamic neurons and are therefore in a privileged position to drive the spike outputs of the cell body (synapses on relay cell bodies are virtually always inhibitory). Layer 6 neurons, whose fibers have smaller diameters and thus can be distinguished from those of Layer 5, synapse well away from the cell body, mostly at remote locations on the dendrite (Sherman 1990). The function of Layer 6 axons is believed to be mainly that of lowering the threshold of the thalamic neuron, so that signals arriving at synapses near the cell body will have a greater probability of inducing the cell body to fire (McCormick and Von Krosigk 1992). Thus, the feedback loop involving Layer 6 neurons and the thalamic relay neuron appear to facilitate synaptic transmission of Layer 5 neurons contacting that relay neuron and thereby potentiate the already strong effects of the bursting Layer 5 neurons on the receiving relay neuron.

It is therefore conjectured that the thalamocortical loop, involving the ascending thalamic relay fibers together with the feedback fibers from Layer 6 neurons, has the ability to enhance firing rates of input fibers arriving from Layer 5 cells of another column. This conjecture was supported by a study in which the thalamocortical circuit was modeled as a neural network so that simulations of its operations could be carried out for a selective attention task (LaBerge, Carter, and Brown 1992). The neural network was based on the known interconnections of all the types of thalamic neurons, including the local inhibitory cells and the reticular nucleus inhibitory cells, which are located between the relay cells and the cortical columns to which they project.

In that study, the corticothalamic neurons (in Layer 6) were assumed to contribute to the activity of the relay cell in the usual manner, that is, by adding their effects to the effects contributed by the Layer 5 inputs. The results of the simulations in that study showed firing-rate trajectories of the thalamic relay neurons and the receiving cortical neurons that resemble closely the pattern of trajectories for target and distractor location columns shown in figures 21.1b and 21.1d. Small initial differences between inputs to the relay cells serving target and distractor columns (i.e., inputs from Layer 5 cells in cortical areas of attentional control) were strongly magnified (e.g., by a factor of 25 or more) by the thalamocortical circuit. When the network parameters were changed to incorporate the assumption that corticothalamic neurons contribute to the activity of the relay cell only by varying the synaptic weights of the Layer 5 input fibers, the simulation results (unpublished) showed trajectory patterns for the target and distractor columns that were similar in all major respects to the patterns obtained in the published simulation study.

Thus, the part of the triangular circuit that flows through thalamic neurons contains characteristics that can greatly enhance the firing rates of the Layer 5 output neurons from the column of origin, while this output is being transmitted to the middle layers of the destination column.

Supporting evidence for the existence of the triangular circuit in other regions of the cortex is provided by the confirmation of large Layer 5 fibers that synapse near the relay cell body and small Layer 6 fibers that synapse at the distal regions of the relay dendrites for the auditory cortex (Ojima 1994) and for the prefrontal cortex (Schwartz, Dekker, and Goldman-Rakic 1991). Since all regions of the cortex are connected with the thalamus (it has been said in a personal communication by a noted neurophysiologist that thalamic cells constitute the seventh layer of cortex), it seems highly probable that the trian-

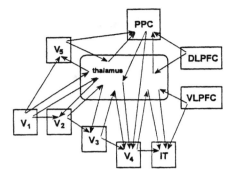

Figure 21.4
Schematic diagrams of some of the triangular circuits in the visual system. The triangular circuits serving visual attention are believed to originate in the dorsolateral prefrontal cortex (DLPFC) for location and in the ventrolateral prefrontal cortex (VLPFC) for shape. Effects in the posterior parietal cortex (PPC) of DLPFC activations may be relayed to V4 via an attentional triangular circuit to select the location of a part of a stimulus array (e.g., as shown in figure 21.1)

gular circuit exists wherever cortical columns in one area communicate with columns in another area. Figure 21.4 shows the diagram of several proposed triangular circuits (LaBerge 1995a,b) that are particularly relevant to attentional processing in the brain.

The proposed triangular circuits of figure 21.4 function to amplify corticocortical connections in both bottom-up and top-down directions (by adding activity to the cortical neuron or by lowering its threshold, or by both operations). Triangular circuits confined to the posterior cortical regions presumably enhance bottom-up sources of cortical column activation. The set of triangular circuits of most interest in this paper are those that project activation in the top-down direction to posterior cortical columns in which attention is expressed. For example, data from both single-cell recordings (e.g., Wilson, O'Scalaidhe, and Goldman-Rakic 1993) and PET (e.g., Smith et al. 1995; Liotti et al., unpublished) show that the DLPFC area is crucially involved in voluntary control of attention for locations, while the VLPFC area is crucially involved in voluntary control of attention for shape and color (see Rajkowska and Goldman-Rakic 1995 for a mapping of the human DLPFC). It is conjectured here that the enhancement operations provided by the thalamic part of the triangular circuit are stronger and of longer duration when the circuit involves top-down sources of activation than when it involves only bottom-up sources of activation.

It seems likely that voluntary control of attention from frontal areas may be relayed through intermediate cortical areas before it reaches a region of interest to the investigator. A noteworthy example is the route of voluntary control of selective attention to a target surrounded by distractors (see figure 21.1). Anatomical tracing studies have not confirmed to date a direct connection between the DLPFC and area V4 in the monkey (Felleman and Van Essen 1991), and therefore voluntary choice of a particular target location to be attended may produce its first attentional expression in PPC location codes, and then the outputs from these activated codes project to V4, where the corresponding target location receives enhanced activation (see figure 21.4).

Physiological Measures of Thalamic Involvement in Attention

If triangular circuits provide the modulatory enhancements necessary for attentional expressions in cortical columns, then physiological measures should show increased activity in the thalamus while a subject is attending to a task. Studies using single-cell recordings showed that pulvinar neurons increased their firing rates to a visual stimulus when that stimulus was a target of an impending eye movement or when the animal simply attended to it without a subsequent eye movement (Peterson, Robinson, and Keys

1985). Patients with lesion of the posterior thalamus on one side were slower to respond to visual stimuli in the contralateral visual field (Rafal and Posner 1987). Chemical deactivation of the pulvinar on one side impairs disengagement of visual attention toward one side (Petersen, Robinson, and Morris 1987) and interferes with performance when a target is displayed with a distractor but not when the target is presented alone (Desimone, Wessinger, Thomas, and Schneider 1990).

Several PET experiments with humans have shown activation of the pulvinar during visual attention. When subjects attended to the shape of many objects in a multidimensional visual display in order to detect small changes in their size, activations were found in a region containing the right pulvinar (Corbetta et al. 1991). Activations were located in the right pulvinar when subjects concentrated attention to a single target shape in a known location to the right or left of center fixation (LaBerge and Buchsbaum 1990). Using the same concentrated-attention task of the LaBerge and Buchsbaum (1990) experiment, Liotti et al. (1994; unpublished) compared hard and easy levels of attentional difficulty with a control condition and examined changes throughout most of the brain. The right pulvinar effect was strongly confirmed for the hard task (when the hard task condition was compared with the easy task condition as well as with the control task).

Two other thalamic regions showed activations when the hard condition was compared with the easy and control conditions. One activated thalamic region contained the mediodorsal nucleus, which connects strongly with the prefrontal cortex and also with the PPC; this region was also activated in the Corbetta et al. (1991) study with shapes and in the Heinze et al. (1994) study in which subjects sustained focal attention on locations in the right visual field. The other region activated by the hard task in the Liotti et al. study was the ventrolateral nucleus, which connects with both the frontal areas and the basal ganglia. Corbetta et al. (1991) found activations at or near this region when subjects discriminated shape sizes or changes in the velocity of shape movements, and Corbetta et al. (1993) found activations in this region when subjects shifted attention toward the right in the right visual field. Thus, three regions of the thalamus have been shown to be selectively active when humans are attending to visual shapes and their locations.

At the same time that thalamic nuclei are active in these visual attention tasks, cortical regions that are directly connected with these thalamic nuclei are also active. Occipital-temporal areas and posterior parietal areas, which are closely connected with the pulvinar nucleus, showed activations in the Corbetta et al. (1991) and Liotti et al. (1994) studies. These areas are presumed to exhibit the expressions of attention to location and shapes. Prefrontal areas in the dorsal (the DLPFC) region and ventral (the VLPFC) region were also activated in the Liotti et al. study. These areas of the prefrontal cortex are strongly implicated in the voluntary control of location and shape, respectively (e.g., Wilson, O'Scalaidhe, and Goldman-Rakic 1993, Frith, Friston, Liddle, and Frackowiak 1991). Thus, taken together, these PET studies show activations both in thalamic nuclei and in the cortical areas of attentional expression and attentional control that are reciprocally connected with these thalamic nuclei.

The Control of Attentional Expressions

According to the view of the present paper, the brain area that is crucial for attentional control (particularly the temporal integration of activity within the triangular circuit) lies in the prefrontal cortex. However, there are opposing views. Posner and Petersen (1990) proposed that the site of executive control is located in the anterior cingulate cortex. Studies of human patients with

bilateral frontal lesions (Brickner 1952, Hebb and Penfield 1940) did not show the degree of deficit in everyday cognitive functioning that would be expected if all attentional control were lost. However, specific tests of attention (e.g., spatial cuing, selection, preparation) were yet to be developed, so that the more challenging aspects of attention such as its higher intensities and longer durations could not be estimated. It is known that lesions of varying sizes and locations in the frontal cortex (e.g., Warren and Akert 1964) commonly report heightened distractablity in the delayed response task and a general inability to shift responses appropriately to meet changing demands of a task, both indicators implying some degree of deficit in attentional control. Thus, on the available evidence, one cannot rule out the possibility that the frontal (in particular, the prefrontal) area normally functions to control attention, and if the frontal area is not available some other area or areas can carry out some of the operations of attentional control, presumably by means of a triangular circuit involving the thalamus.

Enhanced activity in cortical regions of attentional expression, shown consistently by PET and ERP studies of selective attention, is what would be expected if attentional selection operates by enhancement of the target columns. Compared to cortical regions of expression, the amount by which activity is increased in regions concerned with the control of attention is conjectured to be considerably lower. Analogously, the voltage levels in circuits of the control panels of power stations are typically much lower than the high voltage levels at the generators and transformers in the field that are regulated by the control panels. It is presumed that the services performed by attention, such as selecting and priming columns (e.g., columns that code locations and shapes of objects), require relatively high activation contrasts, owing to the relatively high activations that can exist in sensory pathways of the posterior cortex. In comparison, columns in the control regions of the prefrontal cortex would seem to need relatively low activations to consider what sensory columns will be chosen as the target of activation and to consider how strongly and for how long the activation will be projected to the target columns. Furthermore, rapid shifting of attentional control is of great advantage to the organism, and changes in activation patterns in the cortical domains of control would seem to be accomplished more quickly if the constituent activation levels are low rather than high.

If one assumes that cortical regions of attentional control operate at lower levels of column activation than cortical regions of attentional expression, then some means of amplification must be inserted between the areas of control and the areas of expression. A core conjecture of this paper is that the thalamus serves as the mechanism that amplifies signals sent (top-down) from regions of attentional control to regions of attentional expression located in posterior and anterior cortical areas. The thalamic amplifier of neuronal signaling is located on one of the two pathways that make up the triangular circuit connecting the control areas with the expression areas.

The triangular circuits involved in bottom-up pathways also provide the benefits of thalamic enhancements for corticocortical connections (see figure 21.4), but it is conjectured that these enhancements are typically of shorter durations and lower intensities than the enhancements produced by top-down pathways of voluntary control. It is rare that external stimuli are strong enough to prevent voluntary attention from overriding their effects. For example, when a pulsating sound and/or light from an emergency vehicle or a smoke alarm begins, our attention may be momentarily disoriented, but we are able to direct our attention successfully to other objects in the scene while the alarm stimuli persist. When the configuration of an ambulance vehicle and flashing red lights are located close together in our visual field, we manage successfully to attend to the shape of the vehicle and identify it, because the intensity of the top-down

control is raised to a higher level than the intensity of the bottom-up sensory input. Thus, it is conjectured that columns of attentional expression can almost always reach higher levels of activation when they are controlled by top-down sources than when they are driven by bottom-up sources.

The Compact Disc Player Metaphor of Attentional Expression, Intensification, and Control in the Triangular Circuit

The overall operation of the triangular circuit during attentional processing (as illustrated schematically in figure 21.5) may be seem too complex to grasp at first, owing to the different sets of operations involved in each of the attentional aspects residing at the three nodes of the

ATTENTION, AWARENESS, AND THE TRIANGULAR CIRCUIT

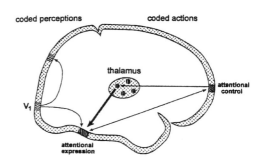

Figure 21.5
Schematic diagram of the three major (human) brain sites connected in an attentional triangular circuit that results in attentional intensification of activity in a cortical column cluster. The presumed control site in prefrontal cortex directly selects the site of attentional expression in the occipitotemporal cortex, and this control site also regulates the intensity of the cortical expression in the occipitotemporal cortex by means of the indirect connection through a thalamic nucleus. The posterior cortical areas serve mainly perceptions, while the anterior cortical areas serve mainly actions, and sites of attention expression may exist in both areas.

triangular circuit. A well-chosen metaphor can sometimes promote the understanding of complex systems of operations, providing that it is made clear exactly what properties of the metaphor are intended to be mapped onto the system at hand and what properties of the metaphor are not so intended.

The metaphor of attentional operations within the triangular circuit being proposed here is the compact disc player (CD player), which is assumed to contain a bank of thousands of discs. Each disc corresponds to a column, or column cluster, in the cerebral cortex. Each CD corresponds to a cortical column that codes a memory of some cognitive event, some events being brief and others more prolonged. Although special columns in the prefrontal cortex serve as the control centers of the brain, the control center of the CD player is presumed to the human hand that voluntarily selects a particular CD of interest. It could be said that the control center can "dial" a CD and that this action corresponds to the voluntary choice of what the system will be attending to in the next few moments.

In the operation of a CD player, the dialing or selection of a particular CD is not sufficient to hear it. The volume knob of the CD player must also be adjusted to increase the intensity of output from the chosen CD to an audible level. Analogously, the selection by the prefrontal control center of a particular cortical patch does not also activate the columns in that patch to a level that qualifies as an expression of attention without appropriate amplification from the thalamus (see figure 21.5). It is assumed that the present CD player contains a separate volume knob for each CD, corresponding to the existence in the thalamus of separate sectors for each column cluster in the cortex. Thus the controlling hand in the CD-player metaphor does two things: it dials the particular CD and adjusts the volume knob associated with it.

The role of stimulus-evoked attention is represented in the CD-player metaphor by the external triggering of a particular CD or group of CDs (assume that the CD player is connected to the Internet, whose incoming signals select CDs). For example, visual stimuli trigger into activity particular columns of neurons in V1 corresponding to oriented bars and color, and when stimuli appear as abrupt onsets (e.g., Yantis 1993), columns corresponding to their locations are particularly strongly activated. These V1 columns in turn trigger into activity columns of V2, V3, V5, and so on. In like manner, when CDs are triggered externally, they subsequently trigger automatically other CDs to which they are connected within the CD-player circuitry.

The CDs triggered from external sources typically register very brief peaks of activity, and these events are communicated to the control center. The control center then voluntarily chooses whether or not to sustain the activities of these CDs by returning activation to the CDs directly and by turning up their volume knobs. If the control center does not return the activation, the stimulus-induced CD activity decays quickly.

Some cortical columns, such as V1, appear to be inaccessible to control from the prefrontal cortex, and it has been conjectured that attention is not expressed in these columns (e.g., Crick and Koch 1995). One might reason that there is adaptive value in having the initial registration of visual stimuli be as faithful as possible to the features of the physical stimulus and that changing the patterns of column activation from within could seriously distort the initial registration patterns. The fact that subjects can attend strongly to cued locations and to cued attributes of objects (both cases involving columns beyond those of V1) is known to put the subjects at a disadvantage when they expect objects in other locations (e.g., Posner 1980) or expect the object to have other attributes (e.g., LaBerge 1973). In the CD-player metaphor, it is assumed that some CDs are not accessible by the control center, but when those CDs are externally activated they subsequently activate other CDs that are accessible to the control center.

At this point, one might be concerned that the typical state of affairs involves the simultaneous playing of many CDs, which results in a chaotic cacophony of sounds. Yet our everyday perception of the world seems one of harmony, not cacophony. It would seem, therefore, that the CD player must have a means of constraining which CDs are sustained simultaneously, at least over some minimum time necessary for the control center to participate in the activity. This issue has been termed the "binding problem." Columns corresponding to the several attributes of a typical visual shape lie in cortical locations separated by centimeters, but these columns are somehow joined by an intrinsic "harmony" by the ways in which their constituent neurons respond. The harmony in this case has been proposed as having the form of synchronous firing (e.g., Gray et al. 1989).

Another way to constrain which columns are bound simultaneously is by means of common activations from an "extrinsic control" source, similar to an "object file" (Kahneman, Treisman, and Gibbs 1992). When a particular object is accessed within the control center, its relevant attributes are also accessed, and each of these in turn simultaneously accesses its corresponding patches of columns in the posterior cortex. On this correlated-intensity account of binding, the role of the control center is crucial, which contrasts with the typical synchronous-firing account of binding for which no extrinsic control source is necessary. Although it is not yet clear how the event of binding occurs in the brain, or whether all cases of binding take place by the same process, it would appear that widely separated columns corresponding to attributes of an object express their attentional enhancements in a correlated manner.

Attention and the Detection of Signals in Noise

Attention to a specific location can increase speed and accuracy in the detection of signals occurring at that location (e.g., Bashinski and Bacharach 1980, Hawkins et al. 1990, Posner, Nissen, and Ogden 1978). A considerable amount of research has been devoted to deciding whether these performance benefits result from the operation of attention during the early perceptual stages of processing (e.g., Hillyard and Mangun 1987, Eimer 1994) or only at later decision stages (e.g., Palmer 1993, Shaw 1978), where the appropriate response is selected. The CD-player metaphor will be employed here to clarify how selective attention could operate early in the brain, after a brief review of the issues and some preliminary assumptions.

Resolution of the controversy concerning the existence vs nonexistence of early attentional selection has met several obstacles. Response-time data from behavioral experiments are often regarded as being compromised by the error data (for a review, see Luce 1986). The response times of even a small proportion of errors can be construed to indicate the use of a particular speed–accuracy trade-off strategy on the part of the subject. For example, the obtained pattern of correct mean-response times can be interpreted as mixtures of stimulus-driven responses, fast guesses, and slow guesses. Whether or not a guess is made on a trial typically requires a decision, and that decision depends upon the payoffs associated with the possible outcomes of the decision. Since some guesses are included among the correct responses, the average value of the correct response times will be influenced by the decision-driven guesses.

Another approach to revealing the effects of early attention in detection of signals involves measures of ERPs (event-related potentials). Data from these experiments have identified enhancements of waveform components that begin as early as 80–110 ms following stimulus onset (e.g., Hillyard and Mangun 1987, 1995, Mangun and Hillyard 1991). One kind of account of these data given by a late-selection viewpoint assumes that decision biases can shift the entire waveform in a negative or positive direction and thereby give the false impression that an enhancement of an early wave reflects a process that operates at an early perceptual stage.

While many response-time and ERP experiments (e.g., Hawkins et al. 1990, Woldorff et al. 1993) continue to address these and other problems voiced by proponents of the late-selection view, a basic issue lies in the background of the early selection question. The issue is: how can a sensory signal in an inherently noisy channel of the brain be enhanced without at the same time enhancing the noise as well? Put otherwise, how can the sensory signal-to-noise ratio be increased by any conceivable attentional operation? Of course, if the signal and the noise are distributed differently across several channels, then one can concentrate the selective sampling of information at those channels that have the strongest signal-to-noise ratio (see Luce and Green 1978, Bonnel and Miller 1994). But enhancing the selective weight of a given channel enhances the noise as well as the signal in that channel.

The problem of enhancing noise along with the signal is inherent in the notion of a channel along which information flows (Shannon and Weaver 1949), an idea that has long served as a root metaphor for much of the information-processing type of theorizing in cognitive psychology. However, some neurophysiologists (e.g., Freeman 1995) have questioned the paradigmatic assumption that signals arising at the sensory surface undergo various transformations as they flow along "channels" or "streams" within the brain toward regions that generate responses. Instead of assuming that sensory events initiate a streamlike flow of information-bearing signals along major pathways of the cortex, it is suggested that a sensory event (e.g., an oriented bar) triggers column clusters of neurons into activities whose patterns are dominated by the characteristic structure of the bundles of circuits within the columns, and not by the particular characteristics of the pulse train carried by the sensory input fibers to the columns. Thus columns pass activation onto other columns by acts of triggering, so that the effect of transmission of activation along a major brain "pathway" resembles more the way a wave of

excitation progresses down a row of dominoes than the way an electromagnetic wave entering the antenna of a radio undergoes a series of electronic transformations as it flows toward the sound-generating magnet in the speaker. The important distinction here lies in the choice of words such as "activates," "triggers," or "excites" rather than the words "is transformed by" or "is processed by" to describe the relation of a neural signal to the cortical column it contacts.

How does the assumption that neural signals "activate" rather than "are transformed by" cortical columns provide another perspective on the question of how attention can increase the signal-to-noise ratio of sensory stimulation? A signal of a particular kind, for example, a brief flash of a light or a brief tone, is detected when the appropriate posterior cortical columns are activated to a level that in turn projects activity to prefrontal columns of control. The prefrontal columns return excitation to the posterior columns, so that their activity levels are sustained (and perhaps increased further) for the minimum time required to qualify as an attended detection event. This activation of the expression-control loop in the brain is analogous to events in the CD-player metaphor that begin with an external selection of a particular CD, which in turn is communicated to the controlling hand, which then may either ignore that CD or adjust the selector dial along with the volume dial to that CD, in order to sustain that CD's activity at an appropriate sound level.

How could attention operate at early stages of sensory processing to increase the effect of the input signal without also increasing the effect of the noise? First, it is assumed that a sensory signal of a particular type begins the series of events leading to a successful detection by activating its corresponding set of cortical columns. If the signal is too weak (relative to background noise) to activate its column cluster, then no perceptual detection event occurs. However, if the particular sensory columns are already in an active state, then the weak signal can raise that activity to the level required to begin the events leading to a detection.

The active state of the particular set of sensory columns prior to the onset of the weak sensory signal is assumed to be produced by preparatory attention, controlled from voluntary regions of the prefrontal cortex in anticipation of the particular kind of sensory stimulus that will soon occur. The prior state of activity of the sensory columns could also conceivably be produced by the residual activations of recent presentations of the same, or a similar, stimulus. In the typical case, however, it is assumed that preparatory attention for the upcoming stimulus, and/or its location, activates the corresponding cortical columns to a level which allows an otherwise ineffective signal to trigger those columns to respond in the manner that begins the events culminating in a detection. In the research literature, the terms "cuing" (LaBerge, Van Gelder, and Yellott 1970) and "priming" (Posner and Snyder 1975) have been used to describe the operations that preactivate mechanisms of sensory detection.

Preactivation in the CD-player metaphor may be produced when the controlling hand sets the particular CD in motion, but does not engage the laser readout mechanism. An external signal (e.g., from the Internet) has the capability of selecting a particular CD by briefly engaging its laser readout and disc rotation. If the external signal is too weak (the signal-to-noise ratio is too small) to activate that CD when that CD is in the inactive state, it still may be able to excite the CD into action if that CD has been preactivated, that is, if that CD's disc rotation has already been engaged. In effect, preactivation of a particular CD raises the probability that a given signal-to-noise ratio produced by an external input will trigger that CD into action. Thus, for the typical detection of a signal in noise, preactivation of the receiving column produces the same result as raising the signal-to-noise ratio of the external input.

The present preactivation account, which has appeared before in the psychological literature (LaBerge, Van Gelder, and Yellott 1970, Posner and Snyder 1975), is not without problems that need resolving. One problem is to distinguish the column activity produced by the effective sensory input and the column activity produced by top-down attention. It is likely that mean intensity of column activity alone cannot satisfactorily separate the two ways of activating the columns. One reason is that it is assumed here that top-down attention can, on occasion, induce higher levels of activity than bottom-up sensory inputs, so that some false detections should almost always occur when preparatory attention for the stimulus event is high. Another reason is that if imaging an object involves the same columns as perceiving the object (Farah 1985, Kosslyn et al. 1993), some properties of the column activity presumably must differentiate between the real and the imagined.

One approach to this problem may be to consider how the patterns of circuit activity (which includes inactive as well as active circuits) within a column can differ according to whether the column is activated by bottom-up sensory inputs or top-down attentional inputs. In the CD-player metaphor, it is assumed that each CD has two kinds of (simultaneously) active states, corresponding to the rotation motion of the disc and the action of the laser readout mechanism, and that each active state is assumed to allow variations in intensity.

Conceivably, the rotation mechanism could represent a component of the CD that is mainly modulatory, while the readout mechanism could represent a component that is mainly informational. By analogy, the neurons in Layers 5 and 6 of a cortical column appear to function mainly in the modulatory mode, while the neurons in Layers 2 and 3 appear to function mainly in the informational mode. Since circuits within a column tend to be vertically organized (around the long dendrites of Layer 5 neurons (Peters 1994)), it would appear that a typical circuit will exhibit the interactions between these two types of neurons. While any detailed description of column circuit operations is highly speculative at the present time, there are known properties of cortical columns (including which layers send signals to and receive signals from other cortical and subcortical areas) that suggest that the typical column has sufficient complexity to support the notion of separable activity levels for informational and modulatory operations. For relevant descriptions of cortical column structure and function the reader is referred to Douglas and Martin 1990.

Thus, top-down preparatory attentional control is assumed to activate modulatory components of a cortical column corresponding to some sensory event to be detected. The increased activity within that column increases the probability that an otherwise ineffective sensory input (i.e., having a low signal-to-noise ratio) will raise the column activity to a level leading to a detection event. In this way preactivated columns in early stages of perception can increase the accuracy and speed of detection.

The hypothesis that the typical cortical column can allow some degree of independence in informational and modulatory activities suggests a way to solve the "problem of the inverse," which arises in considerations of how top-down control operates in the brain. Top-down activation of a column cluster that codes a letter, for example, does not produce the same pattern of activity as bottom-up activation of the same column cluster (imagining the letter H does not produce the same cognitive experience as perceiving the letter H). If it is assumed that a cortical column does not respond with exactly the same pattern to bottom-up and top-down inputs while allowing some degree of overlap, then the column event of imagining a letter (from top-down control) can be different from perceiving the same letter (from bottom-up stimulation). In the CD-player metaphor, the informational aspect of column activity is represented by the laser readout mechanism and the modulatory aspect

of column activity by the disc rotation. Bottom-up evocation of the particular CD (from external sources) engages mainly the laser readout mechanism, and top-down selection of a particular CD involves mainly setting its disc in motion. Thus, the two directions of activations to a given column cluster produce different activity patterns within the column cluster, and this is conjectured to account for the different experiences of perceiving and imagining a stimulus object.

How the Brain Attends: A Synopsis

Many of the ideas presented thus far can be summarized under the question of how the brain attends to some object, plan of action, sensory sensation, or feeling. Attention is assumed here to be an event in the brain having three aspects that are connected by the triangular circuit. The three aspects are the expression of attention in cortical columns, the mechanism that directly activates the columns, and the control over which columns will express attention and how intense the expression will be (see figure 21.5). The brain sites corresponding to each of these aspects are, respectively: (a) for *expression*, columns in the posterior and anterior cortex that serve cognitive functions, such as perceptions of objects and attributes, and the organizing and the executing of action plans, such as greeting a friend or rehearsing a telephone number; (b) for the *mechanism*, column-like sectors of thalamic nuclei, whose excitatory neurons activate neurons in the corresponding cortical columns; and (c) for the *control*, cortical columns of the prefrontal regions of the anterior cortex. Neurons in these three brain sites are interconnected by a triangular circuit, and when the three sites corresponding to all three of these attentional aspects are simultaneously active, it is said that an attentional event occurs.

The triad of sites connected by the triangular circuit is initially activated by two different classes of sources, one within the system and one outside the system. Internal sources normally activate the triangular circuit at the prefrontal control node of the circuit. These sources are connected with motivational sites of the brain and may operate through momentary considerations of the person's interests or may operate relatively automatically by habitual interests, all presumably involving the basal ganglia. External sources are sensory stimuli that activate the cortical column site where attention is eventually expressed. However, it is assumed here that activating these cortical sites of attentional expression from sources outside the system does not itself constitute an attentional event, owing to its brevity and rapidly decaying intensity (e.g., Fruhstorfer et al. 1970). In order to achieve a sufficiently intense and long-lasting activation in a column cluster, the appropriate prefrontal area must be signaled to return activation through the thalamic route of the triangular circuit (see figure 21.5).

It is conjectured that the durations of activity in the brain sites at the three nodes of the triangular circuit are relatively short when a person is engaged in tasks that require rapid object identification and rapid selection of actions, particularly when the objects and actions are familiar. If the tasks are highly routinized, then much of the object identification and action selection occur automatically, that is, without the need for prefrontal control operating through the triangular circuit. For example, many of the perceptual and comprehension components of reading are routinized for the skilled reader, so that cortical areas can carry out their parts of the task at relatively low activity levels. In general, then, automatic column activations triggered during well-learned sensorimotor tasks are presumed to be of relatively short duration and of relatively low intensity.

In contrast to everyday tasks that involve, and often require, rapid perceptions and actions, there are situations that invite us to savor the activities in particular cortical columns that serve sensations and feelings. When we stare at con-volutions in the petals of a red rose, or listen to the slow resolution of a Bach cadence, or let a line of verse echo for a moment, or roll a fine Burgundy wine across the tongue, our attentional system enhances and sustains these sensations. In these cases, where it is desirable to intensify and prolong experiences, the triangular attention circuit is presumed to be relatively highly active, because it is the source of the amplification of activities in the corresponding cortical columns.

Attention and Awareness

The conditions necessary for the existence of an awareness event in the brain have historically resisted clear definitions that are accepted by a broad sector of the research community. Part of the problem may be that "awareness" has been used synonymously with "consciousness," which has been called a "mongrel" concept, owing to the variety of its definitions (Block 1995). Another part of the problem may be that during an alert state of wakefulness, the boundary between awareness and nonawareness of an event is not a sharp one, and that when awareness of an event does occur it may be expressed cognitively and neurally in more than one way and with more than one level of intensity. The treatment here of the difficult topic of awareness will consist largely of a few conjectures that are directed to the matters of the boundary between awareness and nonawareness and the varieties of expressions of awareness.

The reason that awareness is being considered in this paper is that it appears that a case can be made that one of the necessary conditions for an awareness event is the existence of an attentional event, where the attentional event is defined by the activity of a triangular circuit of attention, which includes controlling columns located in the prefrontal cortex. The assumption of prefrontal involvement in awareness has been made by Crick and Koch (1995), together with the assumption that there are also groups of active neurons somewhere in cortex that correspond to the feature of a visual scene that is the object of awareness. If one adds to these two kinds of active regions the activity of a thalamic nucleus and links the three regions in a triangular circuit, then the result involves the structure of attention described in the present paper.

Baars (1995) has stated that activity in both thalamic and cortical structures (as well as in brainstem reticular nuclei) is a necessary and sufficient condition for a state of waking consciousness to exist. Bogen (1995) has implicated the intralaminar nuclei of the thalamus in awareness, owing in part to their widespread connections across the cortex, their direct efferents to the basal ganglia, and their sensitivity to very small lesions. As viewed here, and briefly discussed earlier, the broad cortical distribution of brainstem neuromodulatory fibers, together with that of the intralaminar thalamic fibers, serves to modulate general states of waking and alertness, which are preconditions for the more local activation patterns required for attention and awareness. Therefore, this paper emphasizes the distinction between the brain state of wakefulness and the state of attending to one of the many available cognitive aspects of wakefulness (e.g., a sensory, ideational, or feeling aspect). Thus, to produce the cognitive state needed to give an appropriate answer to the question of "what it is like" to the phenomenally conscious requires that the brain attend to some aspect or aspects of waking (phenomenal) experience.

The awareness event, as proposed here, has a property that distinguishes it from the simple act of attending to some aspect of waking experience. Awareness introduces the agent or actor that is involved when attention is voluntarily directed to some event (object, feeling, or thought). Simply attending to an event requires action on the part of the cortical areas of control, but the representation of the responsible "actor" may be absent. For example, one may attend strongly to a bird that is struggling against the window without attentively processing one's own participation in the action of attending to it. Another example is given by Sartre (1957), in which I am running down the street to catch a bus and attending to "the bus having to be caught" but without attending to "myself having to catch it" (I may include myself in the attended events after I catch the bus). Thus, additional brain areas are active when attention is directed to the actor along with the external event.

Specifically, it is proposed that the awareness event requires that the event of attending to some object (e.g., of perception, idea, or plan of action) be accompanied by an event of attention directed to a representation of the self. Being "aware" of something is a predicate that appears to call for a subject, and the subject is supplied by activation of the cortical areas in which the concept of selfhood is represented, presumably frontal cortical areas (Gazzaniga 1985). The role of references to the self in states of awareness has been treated at length elsewhere (e.g., Harth 1995, Russell 1996). When objects give rise to perceptions, or sensations, these events may be followed by statements such as "I am perceiving X," or "I am sensing X," or "my experience is X" (as in the James quote at the beginning of this paper), which reflect the additional processing of some representation of the self. Thus, it is assumed here that the event of awareness requires that attention be directed to the regions where the subject is expressed at the same time that attention is directed to the cortical regions where the object is expressed (noting that, on occasion, subject and object may be the same). Simultaneous activation of the two triangular circuits is assured if they were both activated from a common brain area in the frontal cortex, that is, the two triangular circuits would be joined at their common control center. To distinguish the two kinds of triangular attention circuits, they will be labeled object-attended and self-attended circuits.

The action of activating both the object-attended and the self-attended triangular circuits produces more than the simultaneous (or near-simultaneous) increase in activity at the object- and self-attended cortical sites of attentional expression. Within each triangular circuit the feedback from the expression site to the prefrontal area of control is synchronized with the activations flowing from the common control site to the expression site. As a result of the temporal coincidence between the two triangular circuits, not only is attention being directed to the self along with attention to an object, but attention is being directed to "the self doing the control" of attention to the object.

For some readers it may be difficult to accept the present definition of awareness, particularly if they have used the term synonymously with consciousness. The commonly received impression is that what it is like to be aware is the same as what it is like to be conscious. To help clarify the present definition of awareness, one might consider a case in which the person is "conscious" (in the sense of being in wakeful cortical state), but awareness is lost while attention is retained. When falling asleep, one sometimes experiences a stage in which images of events unfold under their own control. If one recognizes this state as a mark of going to sleep ("I am falling asleep"), the act of realizing one's drowsy state often returns one to the former alert state. Apparently, one can attend to the spontaneous drama of images during drowsiness without impeding further progress toward sleep, but if the self-representation is suddenly activated by attending to "myself in the process of falling asleep," then the resultant state of self-awareness may restore the alert state of wakefulness by its increased cortical activity. It could be said that during the drowsy state, one attends to the spontaneous dance of images without awareness, but when attention to the self is added, awareness appears.

The properties coded by the representation of selfhood accessed by the self-attended triangular circuit undoubtedly vary greatly across individuals, but there may be a common com-ponent of the representations, one that perhaps provides a means of locating the object-attended event in space and time. The location marker is almost always associated with the body, and the body surface is richly represented within the cortex (Damasio 1994). The location of the body with respect to a changing environmental scene is updated continually within the self-representation. Thus, for example, I can realize that I perceived a windy day yesterday or that I am now perceiving a windy day, where "I" is associated with my body being in a particular place relative to the windy-day event.

But the self conceivably may be referenced on occasion without attending to one's bodily land-scape. Verbal representations linked strongly to one's personal history are readily accessed from memory and serve as the self-attended event. One would expect that, on many occasions, the verbal representation will automatically activate bodily landscape codes, and vice versa, so that attention to the self would typically involve both sets of representations. Thus, the way in which one involves the self-representation while attending to some other object can vary from person to person, and from one time to another time for the same person.

Attention to self-representation is assumed to involve the triangular circuit in a manner similar to attention to objects of perception, cognition, and action. Bodily landscapes and verbal categories are represented by sets of corresponding cortical columns whose activity is controlled by voluntary prefrontal columns acting through the thalamus in triangular circuits. While activity in the columns of self-expression may be automatically induced in particular situations, it does not count as an awareness event unless the prefrontal area amplifies that activity to a particular level and sustains it there for some minimum duration.

In the pathological condition of depersonalization, the self-representation is dissociated from the perceptions of the body, so that perceptions and actions by the body are believed to be happening to someone other than the self (e.g., Jacobs and Bovasso 1992, Simeon and Hollander 1993). In the present context, the system dysfunction could occur in the prefrontal areas where the controls of attention to the self-representations and to the object representations (and action representations) are closely related. The prefrontal area is believed to have a crucial role in the temporal integration of operations that control the actions of monkeys and humans (Fuster 1991). If defects occur in the temporal coordination of the actions controlling activities in the self-attended and object-attended triangular circuits, then the person's experience of self as an agency of control could be compromised, resulting in the observed disorder of depersonalization, which disrupts the sense of awareness.

Relatively brief durations of combined object-attended and subject-attended events suffice for a *realization* event of awareness, for example, when we give an answer to the question, "Are you aware that the sky is bright blue today?" Of course, such questions could have easily translated into the form "Do you perceive that the sky is bright blue today?" and therefore it is difficult to know whether or not the self-attended event occurred or not. But the point being made here is that when the self-attended event occurs in such situations, the event is typically a brief one of realization.

In contrast to the brief duration of attention in events of realization, attention is prolonged during a *sensation*, which may accompany perceptual realizations. An example is a reaction to the statement "Look at that bright blue sky!" The longer durations of object-attending during sensations may give rise to parallel durations of self-attending, with the consequence that bodily landscape sensations are evoked. Sensations of the bodily landscape kind are typically described as "feelings" (Damasio 1994). Sensations and feelings vary in intensity, and it is assumed that the activities in the prefrontal cortex, acting through the attentional triangular circuit, are able not only to prolong sensations and feelings but also to modulate their levels of intensity.

When events of realization and sensation are separately considered in this manner, one can describe how a person who is eating a fantastic meal could devote a series of brief attentional events to realizing (and verbally labeling) the kinds of seasonings, textures, and tastes without directing prolonged attention to particular taste sensations to enjoy them for their own sake. Cognitive styles can be characterized by the relative dominance of realizations or sensations. Realizations are useful for purposes of communication to others or for remembering the realized events for oneself, both being activities that are of central value in the academic world. Prolonged and intense sensations not only serve one's immediate pleasures, but, if one is a cook or an artist, can inspire creations that bring like pleasures to others.

It is sometimes said that individuals sometimes "forget themselves" when they are writing, or engaged in vigorous conversation, or enraptured by music. The interpretation of this subjective observation in terms of the present notion is that at such moments attention is not being directed to one of the self-representations.

The term "heightened awareness" as typically used in the literature appears to refer to object-attended events whose corresponding column expressions are at a high level of activity, while some lesser degree of attentional activity exists in the columns representing the self. When self-attending is intensified, with or without some degree of object-attending, the corresponding term in the literature appears to be "heightened self-awareness." Under relatively intense and prolonged attention to the self, it is more likely that the attended representation is the bodily landscape than verbal representations, owing to the relatively brief durations of verbal realizations. Hence, during prolonged attention to bodily sensations, heightened awareness typically involves attention to feelings, whereas brief attention to a verbal self-description does not.

General Summary

The two main points being made in this paper are that attention to an object requires the simultaneous activity of three brain regions that are connected by a triangular circuit and that awareness of an object requires an additional component, which is attention to some representation of the self. For both kinds of attention, object-attention and self-attention, the three types of brain regions connected by the triangular circuit are cortical columns of attentional expression, a group of thalamic neurons that enhance activities in these columns, and a set of prefrontal cortical columns that control the choice of columns and control the level and duration of enhanced activity. The thalamic component of the attentional triangular circuit operates by modulating firing rates in a column without changing the informational signaling existing in that column. The expression of attention in a set of cortical columns may involve widely separated columns, such as attending both to a particular object's shape and to its direction of movement. The expression of attention to self-representations also may involve widely separated cortical columns corresponding to the bodily landscape and/or cortical columns corresponding to verbal-based memories of autobiographical events. An event of awareness may be relatively brief, as when we realize the coincident occurrences of the self and the perception of an object; and an event of awareness may be relatively prolonged, as when the sheer sensation of the object's attributes, and/or the sheer feeling of the self's bodily landscape, is allowed to intensify and be sustained for a time. Thus, according to the definition of awareness given by the present paper, an attention event is a necessary but not sufficient condition for an awareness event, so that there can be attention without awareness, but no awareness without attention.

References

Amit, D. J. (1995). The Hebbian paradigm reintegrated: Local reverberations as internal representations. *Behavioral and Brain Sciences*, 18, 617–657.

Andersen, R. A., Essick, G. K., and Siegel, R. M. (1985). Encoding of spatial location by posterior parietal neurons. *Science*, 230, 456–458.

Baars, B. J. (1995). Tutorial commentary: Surprisingly small subcortical structures are needed for the state of waking consciousness, while cortical projection areas seem to provide perceptual contents of consciousness. *Consciousness and Cognition: An International Journal*, 4, 159–162.

Banks, W. P. (1993). Problems in the scientific pursuit of consciousness. *Consciousness and Cognition: An International Journal*, 2, 255–263.

Bashinski, H. S., and Bachrach, V. R. (1980). Enhancement of perceptual sensitivity as the result of selectively attending to spatial locations. *Perception and Psychophysics*, 28, 241–248.

Block, N. (1995). On a confusion about a function of consciousness. *Behavior and Brain Sciences*, 18, 227–320.

Bogen, J. E. (1995). On the neurophysiology of consciousness. I. An overview. *Consciousness and Cognition: An International Journal*, 4, 52–62.

Bolz, J., Gilbert, C. D., and Wiesel, T. N. (1989). Pharmacological analysis of cortical circuitry. *Trends in Neuroscience*, 12, 292–296.

Bonnel, A.-M., and Miller, J. (1994). Attentional effects on concurrent psychophysical discriminations: Investigations of a sample-size model. *Perception and Psychophysics*, 55, 162–179.

Braitenberg, V., and Schulz, A. (1991). *Anatomy of the cortex*. Berlin: Springer-Verlag.

Brickner, R. M. (1952). Brain of patient "A" after bilateral frontal lobectomy: Status of the frontal lobe problem. *Archives of Neurological Psychiatry*, 68, 293–313.

Broadbent, D. E. (1958). *Perception and communication*. London: Pergamon.

Buracas, G. T., and Albright, T. D. (1995). Neural correlates of target detection during visual search in area MT. *Society for Neuroscience Abstracts*, 21, 1759.

Chelazzi, L., Miller, E. K., Duncan, J., and Desimone, R. (1993). A neural basis for visual search in inferior temporal cortex. *Nature*, 363, 345–347.

Conley, M., and Raczkowski, D. (1990). Sublaminar organization within layer VI of the striate cortex in Galago. *Journal of Comparative Neurology*, 302, 425–436.

Connors, B. W., and Gutnick, M. J. (1990). Intrinsic firing patterns of diverse neocortical neurons. *Trends in Neuroscience*, 13, 99–104.

Corbetta, M., Miezin, F. M., Dobmeyer, S., Shulman, G. L., and Petersen, S. E. (1991). Selective and divided attention during visual discrimination of shape, color, and speed: Functional anatomy by positron emission tomography. *Journal of Neuroscience*, 11, 2382–2402.

Corbetta, M., Miezin, F. M., Shulman, G. L., and Petersen, S. E. (1993). A PET study of visuospatial attention. *Journal of Neuroscience*, 13, 1202–1226.

Crick, F., and Koch, C. (1995). Are we aware of neural activity in primary visual cortex. *Nature*, 375, 121–123.

Crick, F., and Koch, C. (1990). Towards a neuro-biological theory of consciousness. *Seminars in the Neurosciences*, 2, 263–275.

Damasio, A. R. (1994). *Descartes' error: Emotion, reason, and the human brain*. New York: Avon.

Desimone, R. (1992). Neural circuits for visual attention in the primate brain. In G. A. Carpenter and S. Grossberg (Eds.). *Neural networks for vision and image processing* (pp. 343–364). Cambridge, MA: MIT Press.

Desimone, R., Wessinger, M., Thomas, L., and Schneider, W. (1990). Attentional control of visual perception: Cortical and subcortical mechanisms. *Cold Spring Harbor Symposia on Quantitative Biology*, 55, 963–971.

Douglas, R. J., Koch, C., Mahowald, M., Martin, K. A. C., and Suarez, H. H. (1995). Recurrent excitation in neocortical circuits. *Science*, 269, 981–985.

Douglas, R. J., and Martin, K. A. C. (1990). In G. M. Shepherd (Ed.), *The synaptic organization of the brain*. New York: Oxford Univ. Press.

Douglas, R. J., Martin, K. A. C., and Whitteridge, D. (1989). A canonical microcircuit for neocortex. *Neural Computation*, 1, 480–488.

Downing, C. J. (1988). Expectancy and visual-spatial attention: Effects on perceptual quality. *Journal of Experimental Psychology: Human Perception and Performance*, 1, 188–202.

Eimer, M. (1994). "Sensory gating" as a mechanism for visuospatial orienting: Electrophysiological evidence from trial-by-trial cuing experiments. *Perception and Psychophysics*, 55, 667–675.

Eriksen, C. W., and Yeh, Y. Y. (1985). Allocation of attention in the visual field. *Journal of Experimental Psychology: Human Perception and Performance*, 11, 583–597.

Farah, M. J. (1985). Psychophysical evidence for a shared representational medium for mental images and percepts. *Journal of Experimental Psychology: General*, 114, 91–103.

Felleman, D. J., and Van Essen, D. C. (1991). Distributed hierarachical processing in the primate cerebral cortex. *Cerebral Cortex*, 1, 1–47.

Freeman, W. J. (1975). *Mass action in the nervous system*. New York: Academic Press.

Freeman, W. J. (1995). *Societies of brains*. Hillsdale, NJ: Erlbaum.

Frith, C. D., Friston, K., Liddle, P. F., and Frackowiak, R. S. J. (1991). Willed action and the prefrontal cortex in man: A study with PET. *Proceedings of the Royal Society of London (Biology)*, 244, 241–246.

Frukhstorfer, H., Soveri, P., and Jarvilehto, T. (1970). Short-term habituation of the auditory evoked response in man. *Electroencephalography and Clinical Neurophysiology*, 28, 153–161.

Fuster, J. M. (1991). The prefrontal cortex and its relation to behavior. *Progress in Brain Research*, 87, 201–211.

Gazzaniga, M. S. (1985). *The social brain: Discovering the networks of the mind*. New York: Basic Books.

Gazzaniga, M. S. (1995). *The cognitive neurosciences*, Cambridge, MA: MIT Press.

Goldman-Rakic, P. S. (1990). Cellular and circuit basis of working memory in prefrontal cortex of nonhuman primates. *Progress in Brain Research*, 85, 325–336.

Goldman-Rakic, P. S., Chafee, M., and Friedman, H. (1993). Allocation of function in distributed circuits. In T. Ono, L. R. Squire, M. E. Raichle, D. I. Perrett, and M. Fukuda (Eds.), *Brain mechanisms of perception and memory: From neuron to behavior.* (pp. 445–456). New York: Oxford Univ. Press.

Gray, C. M., Konig, P., Engel, A. K., and Singer, W. (1989). Oscillatory responses in cat visual cortex exhibit inter-columnar synchronization which reflects global stimulus properties. *Nature*, 338, 334–337.

Gray, C. M., and McCormick, D. A. (1996). Chattering cells: Superficial pyramidal neurons contributing to the generation of synchronous oscillations in the visual cortex. *Science*, 274, 109–115.

Harth, E. (1995). The sketchpad model. *Consciousness and Cognition: An International Journal*, 4, 346–368.

Hawkins, H. L., Hillyard, S. A., Luck, S. J., Mouloua, M., Downing, C. J., and Woodward, D. P. (1990). Visual attention modulates signal detectability. *Journal of Experimental Psychology: Human Perception and Performance*, 16, 802–811.

Hebb, D. O., and Penfield, W. (1940). Human behavior after extensive bilateral removals from the frontal lobes. *Archives of Neurological Psychiatry*, 44, 421–438.

Heinze, H. J., Mangun, G. R., Burchert, W., Hinrichs, H. I., Scholz, M. N., Munte, T. F., Gos, A., Johannes, S., Scherg, M., Hundeshagen, H., Gazzaniga, M. S., and Hillyard, S. A. (1994). Combined spatial and temporal imaging of brain activity during visual selective attention in humans. *Nature*, 392, 543–546.

Hillyard, S. A., and Mangun, G. R. (1987). Sensory gating as a physiological mechanism for visual selective attention. In R. Johnson, Jr., R. Parasuraman, and J. W. Rohrbaugh (Eds.), *Current trends in event-related potential research* (pp. 61–67). New York: Elsevier.

Hillyard, S. A., and Mangun, G. R. (1995). Neural systems mediating selective attention. In M. Gazzaniga (Ed.), *The cognitive neurosciences*. Cambridge, MA: MIT Press.

Jacobs, J. R., and Bovasso, G. B. (1992). Toward the clarification of the construct of depersonalization and its association with affective and cognitive dysfunctions. *Journal of Personality Assessment*, 59, 352–365.

James, W. (1890). *Principles of psychology* (Vol. 1). New York: Holt.

Jones, E. G. (1985). *The thalamus*. New York: Plenum.

Julesz, R., and Bergen, J. R. (1983). Textons, the fundamental elements in preattentive vision and perception of textures. *Bell Systems Technical Journal*, 62, 1619–1645.

Kahneman, D., Treisman, A., and Gibbs, B. J. (1992). The reviewing of object files: Object-specific integration of information. *Cognitive Psychology*, 24, 175–219.

Kosslyn, S. M. (1994). *Image and brain*. Cambridge MA: MIT Press.

Kosslyn, S. M., Alpert, N. M., Thompson, W. L., and Maljkovic, V. (1993). Visual mental imagery activates topographically organized visual cortex: PET investigations. *Journal of Cognitive Neuroscience*, 5, 263–287.

LaBerge, D. (1973). Identification of the time to switch attention: A test of a serial and a parallel model of attention. In S. Kornblum (Ed.), *Attention and performance IV*. New York: Academic Press.

LaBerge, D. (1975). Acquisition of automatic processing of perceptual and associative learning. In P. M. A. Rabbitt and S. Dornic (Eds.), *Attention and performance V*. New York: Academic Press.

LaBerge, D. (1995a). *Attentional processing: The brain's art of mindfulness*. Cambridge, MA: Harvard Univ. Press.

LaBerge, D. (1995b). Computational and anatomical models of selective attention in object identification. In M. Gazzaniga (Ed.), *The cognitive neurosciences*. Cambridge, MA: MIT Press.

LaBerge, D., and Buchsbaum, M. S. (1990). Positron emission tomographic measurements of pulvinar activity during an attention task. *Journal of Neuroscience*, 10, 613–619.

LaBerge, D., Carter, M., and Brown, V. (1992). A network simulation of thalamic circuit operations in selective attention. *Neural Computation*, 4, 318–331.

LaBerge, D., and Samuels, S. J. (1974). Toward a theory of automatic information processing in reading. *Cognitive Psychology*, 6, 293–323.

LaBerge, D., Van Gelder, P., and Yellott, J. I. (1970). A cueing technique in choice reaction time. *Perception and Psychophysics*, 7, 57–62.

Lansner, A., and Fransen, E. (1994). Improving the realism of attractor models by using cortical columns as functional units. In J. M. Bower (Ed.), *The neurobiology of computation: Proceedings of the Annual Computational Neuroscience Meeting*. Dordrecht: Kluwer.

Liotti, M., Fox, P. T., and LaBerge, D. (1994). PET measurements of attention to closely spaced visual shapes. *Society for Neurosciences Abstracts*, 20, 354.

Liotti, M., Fox, P. T., and LaBerge, D. (unpublished). Brain activations during high and low levels of concentrated attention to visual shape and location.

Luce, R. D. (1986). *Response times*. New York: Oxford Univ. Press.

Luce, R. D., and Green, D. M. (1978). Two tests of a neural attention hypothesis for auditory psychophysics. *Perception and Psychophysics*, 23, 363–371.

Mangun, G. R., and Hillyard, S. A. (1987). The spatial allocation of visual attention as indexed by event-related brain potentials. *Human Factors*, 29, 195–212.

McCormick, D. A., and Von Krosigk, M. (1992). Corticothalamic activation modulates thalamic firing through glutamate "metabotropic" receptors. *Proceedings of the National Academy of Sciences USA*, 89, 2774–2778.

Merzenich, M. M., Nelson, R. J., Stryker, M. P., Cynader, M. S., Schoppmann, A., and Zook, J. M. (1984). Somatosensory cortical map changes following digit amputation in adult monkeys. *Journal of Comparative Neurology*, 224, 591–605.

Moran, J., and Desimone, R. (1985). Selective attention gates visual processing in the extrastriate cortex. *Science*, 229, 782–784.

Motter, B. C. (1993). Focal attention produces spatially selective processing in visual cortical areas V1, V2, and V4 in the presence of competing stimuli. *Journal of Neurophysiology*, 70, 909–919.

Mountcastle, V. B. (1957). Modality and topographic properties of single neurons of cat's sensory cortex. *Journal of Neurophysiology*, 20, 408–434.

Mountcastle, V. B. (1978). *The mindful brain*. Cambridge, MA: MIT Press.

Ojima, H. (1994). Terminal morphology and distribution of corticothalamic fibers originating from layers 5 and 6 of cat primary auditory cortex. *Cerebral Cortex*, 6, 646–663.

O'Kusky, J., and Colonnier, M. (1982). A laminar analysis of the number of neurons, glia and synapses in the visual cortex (area 17) of adult macaque monkeys. *Journal of Comparative Neurology*, 210, 278–290.

O'Leary, D. D. M., Schlaggar, B. L., and Tuttle, R. (1994). Specification of neocortical areas and thalamocortical connections. *Annual Review of Neuroscience*, 17, 419–439.

Palmer, J. (1994). Set-size effects in visual search: The effect of attention is independent of the stimulus for simple tasks. *Vision Research*, 34, 1703–1721.

Peters, A. (1994). The organization of the primary visual cortex in the macaque. In A. Peters and K. S. Rockland (Eds.), *Cerebral cortex* (pp. 1–35). New York: Plenum.

Peters, A., and Sethares, C. (1991). Organization of pyramidal neurons in area 17 of monkey visual cortex. *Journal of Comparative Neurology*, 306, 1–23.

Petersen, S. E., Robinson, D. L., and Keys, W. (1985). Pulvinar nuclei of the behaving rhesus monkey: Visual responses and their modulation. *Journal of Neurophysiology*, 54, 867–886.

Petersen, S. E., Robinson, D. L., and Morris, J. D. (1987). Contributions of the pulvinar to visual spatial attention. *Neuropsychologia*, 25, 97–105.

Posner, M. I. (1980). Orienting of attention. *Quarterly Journal of Experimental Psychology*, 32, 3–25.

Posner, M. I., Nissen, M. J., and Ogden, W. C. (1978). Attended and unattended processing modes: The role of set for spatial location. In H. L. Pick and I. J. Saltzman (Eds.), *Modes of perceiving and processing information*. Hillsdale, NJ: Erlbaum.

Posner, M. I., and Petersen, S. E. (1990). The attention system of the human brain. *Annual Review of Neuroscience*, 13, 25–41.

Posner, M. I., and Snyder, C. R. R. (1975). Facilitation and inhibition in the processing of signals. In P. M. A. Rabbitt and S. Dornic (Eds.), *Attention and performance V* (pp. 669–681). New York: Academic Press.

Purves, D., Riddle, D. R., and LaMantia, A. S. (1992). Iterated patterns of brain circuitry (or how the cortex gets spots). *Trends in Neuroscience*, 15, 362–368.

Rafal, R. D., and Posner, M. I. (1987). Deficits in human visual spatial attention following thalamic lesions. *Proceedings of the National Academy of Sciences USA*, 84, 7349–7353.

Rajkowska, G., and Goldman-Rakic, P. S. (1995). Cytoarchitectonic definition of prefrontal areas in the normal human cortex: II. Variability in location of areas 9 and 46 and relationship to the Talairach coordinate system. *Cerebral Cortex*, 5, 323–337.

Rose, G., and Siebler, M. (1995). Cooperative effects of neuronal ensembles. *Experimental Brain Research*, 106, 106–110.

Russell, J. (1996). *Agency: Its role in mental development*. Hove, England: Taylor and Francis.

Salin, P.-A., and Bullier, J. (1995). Corticocortical connections in the visual system: Structure and function. *Physiological Reviews*, 75, 107–154.

Sartre, J.-P. (1957). *The transcendence of the ego: An existentialist theory of consciousness*. New York: Noonday Press.

Schwartz, M. L., Dekker, J. J., and Goldman-Rakic, P. S. (1991). Dual mode of corticothalamic synaptic termination in the mediodorsal nucleus of the rhesus monkey. *Journal of Comparative Neurology*, 309, 289–304.

Shall, J. D., and Hanes, D. P. (1993). Neural basis of saccade target selection in frontal eye field during visual search. *Nature*, 366, 467–469.

Shannon, C. E., and Weaver, W. (1949). *The mathematical theory of communication*. Urbana: Univ. of Illinois Press.

Shaw, M. L. (1978). A capacity allocation model for reaction time. *Journal of Experimental Psychology: Human Perception and Performance*, 4, 596–598.

Sherman, S. M. (1990). Thalamus. In G. M. Shepherd (Ed.), *The synaptic organization of the brain*. New York: Oxford Univ. Press.

Simeon, D., and Hollander, E. (1993). Depersonalization disorder. *Psychiatric Annals*, 23, 382–388.

Smith, E. E., Jonides, J., Koeppe, R. A., Awh, E., Schumacher, E. H., and Minoshima, S. (1995). Spatial versus object working memory: PET investigations. *Journal of Cognitive Neuroscience*, 7, 337–356.

Spitzer, H., Desimone, R., and Moran, J. (1988). Increased attention enhances both behavioral and neuronal performance. *Science*, 240, 338–340.

Steriade, M., McCormick, D. A., and Sejnowski, T. J. (1993). Thalamocortical oscillations in the sleeping and aroused brain. *Science*, 262, 679–685.

Szentagothai, J. (1975). The "module-concept" in cerebral cortex architecture. *Brain Research*, 95, 475–496.

Talairach, J., and Tournoux, P. (1988). *Co-planar stereotaxic atlas of the human brain*. New York: Thieme Verlag.

Tanaka, K. (1992). Inferotemporal cortex and higher visual functions. *Current Opinion in Neurobiology*, 2, 502–505.

Treisman, A., and Gelade, G. (1980). A feature integration theory of attention. *Cognitive Psychology*, 12, 97–136.

Treisman, A. (1960). Contextual cues in selective listening. *Quarterly Journal of Experimental Psychology*, 12, 242–248.

Treue, S., and Maunsell, J. H. (1996). Attentional modulation of visual motion processing in cortical areas MT and MST. *Nature*, 382, 539–541.

Ungerleider, L. G., Galkin, T. W., and Mishkin, M. (1983). Visuotopic organization of projections from striate cortex to inferior and lateral pulvinar in rhesus monkey. *Journal of Comparative Neurology*, 217, 137–157.

Wang, G., Tanaka, K., and Tanifuji, M. (1996). Optical imaging of functional organization in the monkey inferotemporal cortex. *Science*, 272, 1665–1668.

Warren, J. M., and Ekert, K. (1965). *The frontal granular cortex and behavior*. New York: McGraw-Hill.

Webster, M. J., Bachevalier, J., and Ungerleider, L. G. (1994). Connections of inferior temporal areas TEO and TE with parietal and frontal cortex in macaque monkeys. *Cerebral Cortex*, 5, 470–483.

Wilson, F. A., O'Scalaidhe, S. P., and Goldman-Rakic, P. S. (1993). Dissociation of object and spatial processing domains in primate prefrontal cortex. *Science*, 260, 1955–1958.

Woldorff, M. G., Gallen, C. C., Hampson, S. A., Hillyard, S. A., Pantev, C., Sobel, D., and Bloom, F. E. (1993). Modulation of early sensory processing in human auditory cortex during auditory selective attention. *Proceedings of the National Academy of Sciences USA*, 90, 8722–8726.

Yantis, S. (1993). Stimulus-driven attentional capture and attentional control settings. *Journal of Experimental Psychology: Human Perception and Performance*, 19, 676–681.

IV IMMEDIATE MEMORY: THE FLEETING CONSCIOUS PRESENT

Immediate memory is closely associated with consciousness. In immediate memory we can compare a currently conscious item to one that faded a few seconds ago. But faded items can be retrieved intact for about ten seconds, and the argument can be made therfore that items must exist unconsciously even after they have faded. It seems therefore that conscious information does not degrade immediately, even when it is no longer conscious. Thus immediate memory allows us to treat consciousness as an experimental variable. (See Introduction.)

Brains have a basic need for rapid, short-term memories. Events that arrive a few seconds apart need to be related to each other. In reading this sentence, the reader must understand the first few words in relation to the last ones, even though they were read at different moments in time. Likewise, in order to speak a sentence, earlier and later words must be related to each other even before the vocal tract begins to move. And when things in the world must be anticipated, expectations and responses must be prepared in time to outrun that predator or to catch that prey. It therefore makes sense to have a number of holding bins, short-term buffer memories, in which earlier events can be held until later ones can catch up. All adaptive computational systems have such buffer memories. And in the brain, all the immediate memories we know about are closely associated with the "fleeting present" of consciousness.

Sensory Memory

Immediate memory may be divided into two kinds: sensory memories, which typically last on the order of seconds, and working memory, which may be defined as the rehearsable component of immediate memory and may last for tens of seconds. An example of sensory memory in vision (termed iconic memory) is the "double-take," which takes place when one looks back at something briefly glimpsed. Such a double-take

results from information taken in, stored briefly in literal form, and processed after a very brief delay. The equivalent in auditory memory (echoic memory) would be hearing a word not at first understood, then an instant later realizing what was said. In contrast, working memory involves rehearsable elements, like the digits of a telephone number or the steps of a rating scale. These can be mentally rehearsed to make sure they remain available for some time. Baddeley (1993; chap. 25, this volume) has proposed an influential model suggesting that working memory may have both a verbal and a visual-spatial component.

Much effort has been expended to make these ideas testable and precise. A classic study by Sperling (1960; chap. 22, this volume) is often taken to reflect a visual buffer memory. It is particularly important for the study of consciousness because Sperling discovered a way to obtain information from brief visual exposures even when it was impossible for subjects to recall all of the material. In this "partial report procedure," subjects are shown a 3×4 grid of letters or numbers for a fraction of a second. Observers typically claim that they can see all the letters, but they can only recall three or four of them. Thus they pass the "consciousness report" operational criterion suggested in the Introduction, but they fail by the accuracy criterion. Objectively, it seems difficult to verify the claim that observers truly have momentary conscious access to the entire display. Yet people continue to insist that they are momentarily conscious of all the elements in the array.

Sperling brilliantly found a way for observers to reveal their knowledge objectively, by asking them *after* the exposure to report *any* arbitrarily cued letter. Under these circumstances people can accurately report any letter, which suggests that they do indeed have fleeting access to all of them. Given that the response cue is only given after the array has disappeared, it is clear that the correct information must have come from memory, not from the physical input. Now we can be confident that subjects in the Sperling experiment have momentary conscious access to momentary memory for all the elements in the visual display. Both the accuracy and the "consciousness report" criterion are satisfied.

The Sperling experiment serves as a reminder that conscious events may decay in a few hundred milliseconds, so that immediate report is often essential. Sometimes even very recent events can be hard to recall—very fleeting ones, for example, or novel stimuli that cannot be organized into a single experience, or stimuli that are followed by a distracting event. Indeed, the very act of retrieving and reporting recent material may interfere with accurate recall.

Sperling's classic experiment has been interpreted as evidence for a rapid sensory memory, and similar evidence has been found for buffer memories for hearing and touch.

Rehearsable Working Memory

The part of immediate memory that can be rehearsed is now usually called working memory (WM). The best-studied aspect is the verbal component of WM—the domain in which we rehearse new words and telephone numbers. There is a remarkably small limit to the number of unrelated words, numbers, objects, or rating categories that can be kept in WM (Miller 1956; chap. 23, this volume). With rehearsal, we can recall about 7 ± 2 items, and without rehearsal, between 3 and 4 items. This is a fantastically small number for a system as large and sophisticated as the human brain; an inexpensive calculator can store many times more. WM is limited in duration as well, to perhaps 10 s, if items are not rehearsed.

WM is a most peculiar memory because although it is limited in size, the "size" of each item can be indefinitely large. For example, one can keep the following unrelated items in WM: "consciousness, quantum physics, mother, Europe, modern art, love, self." Each of these stands for a world of knowledge—but it is highly organized knowledge. The relationship between two properties of "mother" are likely to be interconnected, because they are part of an organized body of beliefs. This is one aspect of *chunking*, the fact that information that can be coherently organized can be treated as a single element in WM. Consider the series: 67712491009166010002. It far exceeds our WM capacity, being 20 units long. But we need only read each series of four numbers backwards to discover that there are only five "chunks" or organized units: the well-known years 1776, 1492, 1900, 1066, and 2000. Chunking greatly expands the capacity of WM. It serves to emphasize that WM is always assessed by way of a *novel, unintegrated* series of items. As soon as items become permanently memorized, or when we discover a single principle that can simplify a whole input string, many items begin to behave as one. This is the single most important point of G. A. Miller's classic paper that begins this section.

Atkinson and Shiffrin (1971; chap. 24, this volume) provide a classic statement of the relationships between immediate memory, sensory input, and long-term memory. The evidence for chunking itself implies that WM depends fundamentally on long-term memory (LTM)—the great storehouse of information that can be recalled or recognized (see Section 5). The fact that 1066 is known as the year of the Norman invasion of England is stored in LTM, and this must somehow become available to tell us that 1066 can be treated as a single, integrated chunk. Not surprisingly, several authors have argued that working memory may be nothing but the currently activated, separate components of long-term memory.

Working memory is not the same as consciousness, but conscious experience and WM are closely related. We are only conscious of currently rehearsed items, not of the ones that are in the background. Yet the unconscious items in WM are readily available to focal consciousness.

It is useful to treat consciousness as a kind of momentary working memory in some respects (Baars 1988, 1997). WM then becomes a slightly larger current memory store, one that holds information a bit longer than consciousness does.

The Brain Basis of Working Memory

Baddeley (1993; chap. 25, this volume) presents a more integrated conception of working memory. First, his proposal for WM is not limited to verbal material (the phonological loop) but includes a visual component, the visual-spatial sketchpad. Next, there is an executive aspect of WM functioning: We can voluntary decide to rehearse material, to transform visual images, and to talk about what is in our WM. Perhaps most dramatically, Baddeley cites brain-imaging evidence that appears to support several decades of psychological studies. Inner rehearsal of WM items appears to activate both Broca's and Wernicke's areas in the left hemisphere, regions that have been known to be involved with the production and perception of speech since the nineteenth century. Thus it seems that inner speech activates the same parts of the brain that produce and perceive outer speech. Similar results have been found in visual imagery, which activates normal visual cortex (see Section 5).

Goldman-Rakic (1992; chap. 26, this volume) presents discoveries about nerve cells that may underlie working memory, using a delayed-matching task as a way to operationalize the concept in monkeys. Pyramidal neurons in prefrontal cortex appear to be involved in such WM functions, an interesting point in light of similar prefrontal functions in humans. In support of these discoveries, Gabrieli et al. (1998) show that semantic working memory processes activate large portions of prefrontal cortex, using fMRI. The emphasis in their article is on the meaning component of WM, which appears to activate more anterior neurons. It may be that conscious access to meaning has a right prefrontal locus,

though word meaning is often associated with sensory images as well, which are presumably more posterior.

Working memory is classically conceived as being controlled by an "executive component" to reflect the fact that people are typically asked to mentally rehearse items in WM "at will." They can stop and start mental rehearsal, they can select some items and avoid others, they can transform items in certain ways, and they generally exercise a great deal of control when asked to do so. But not much has been said about this executive component until recently, though it obviously relates closely to William James's "self as agent" and to Freud's conception of the ego as a controlling agency in mental life. Here again, brain-imaging studies are helping to fill in some of the blank spots in theory and evidence. E. E. Smith and J. Jonides (1999; chap. 27, this volume) provide a summary of current knowledge, with particular emphasis on the role of prefrontal cortex in memory storage and executive control.

The Widely Distributed Ramifications of Working Memory

Working memory affects more than a few areas of the brain. Using EEG, E. Roy John, Paul Easton, and Robert Isenhart (1997; chap. 28, this volume) show widespread brain processing of stimuli presented in a working memory task. This surprisingly simple, brain-wide pattern occurs during the first few hundred milliseconds after stimulus presentation and may involve a widespread comparison process between the expected and actual stimulus. The time domain is the same one in which conscious visual events are established, and the results may have significant implications for what Francis Crick and others have called the "binding problem"—how the various aspects of a stimulus combine to create a single, coherent conscious percept (e.g., Crick and Koch 1990).

It is worth remarking that the electrical activity of the waking brain is vastly complicated, so that many scientists have viewed the problem of finding meaningful simplicity in EEG as hopeless. That judgment has changed somewhat with the development of powerful computational tools and the study of event-related potentials (ERPs). By studying stimulus-locked brain voltages averaged over trials, some very clear patterns have emerged. ERPs are clearly sensitive to cognitive processes, both conscious and unconscious. Nevertheless, their interpretation has proved difficult.

Classical ERPs typically average voltages across the time domain, and in recent years ERPs have been collected at many points across the scalp, adding a spatial component. One of the distinctive contributions of the chapter by John, Easton, and Isenhart is a novel factor analytic technique, Spatial Principal Components Analysis (SPCA), to extract the major spatial components of activity across the brain. The largest single component accounts for fully half of the data: It is a wave of activity emerging from occipital cortex and diminishing toward the front of the brain, seen in all five subjects and across tasks. It is tempting to suppose that this component shows visual activity sweeping from visual to frontal cortex. The second component accounts for a fifth of the variance in the data and appears to be a concentric waveform, centered approximately in the area of the thalamus. Structures in this area, such as the intralaminar and mediodorsal thalamic nuclei and the anterior cingulate cortex, have also been associated with consciousness and effortful atttention (Posner 1994, Bogen 1995). The third component, accounting for another 14% of the data, appears as a left-to-right wave of activity, perhaps corresponding to left-hemisphere verbal and executive functions. Together these three components account for 84% of the variance.

These findings raise many questions, of course. If the results appear to be robust on further testing, they may significantly increase our understanding of those crucial first few hundred milliseconds during which widely distributed populations of neurons cooperate and compete to establish coherent conscious contents, further triggering widespread unconscious activity, and perhaps reemerging in consciousness, in the ceaseless interplay that Sherrington classically called the "enchanted loom" of the brain. Finding pattern and simplicity in that interplay is a step toward understanding.

References

Baars, B. J. (1997) *In the Theater of Consciousness: The Workspace of the Mind.* New York: Oxford University Press.

Baars, B. J. (1988) *A Cognitive Theory of Consciousness.* New York: Cambridge University Press.

Bogen, J. E. (1995) On the neurophysiology of consciousness: I. An overview. *Conscious Cogn* 4: 52–62.

Crick, F. H. C., and C. Koch (1990) Towards a neurobiological theory of consciousness. *Seminars in Neurosciences* 2: 263–275.

Gabrieli, J. D., J. B. Brewer, and R. A. Poldrack (1998) Images of medial temporal lobe functions in human learning and memory. *Neurobiol Learn Mem* 70: 275–283.

Rosner, M. I. (1994) Attention: The mechanisms of consciousness. *Proc Natl Acad Sci USA* 91: 7398–7403.

22 The Information Available in Brief Visual Presentations

George Sperling

How much can be seen in a single brief exposure? This is an important problem because our normal mode of seeing greatly resembles a sequence of brief exposures. Erdmann and Dodge (1898) showed that in reading, for example, the eye assimilates information only in the brief pauses between its quick saccadic movements. The problem of what can be seen in one brief exposure, however, remains unsolved. The difficulty is that the simple expedient of instructing the observer of a single brief exposure to report what he has just seen is inadequate. When complex stimuli consisting of a number of letters are tachistoscopically presented, observers enigmatically insist that they have seen more than they can remember afterwards, that is, report afterwards.[1] The apparently simple question "What did you see?" requires the observer to report both what he remembers and what he has forgotten.

The statement that *more is seen than can be remembered* implies two things. First, it implies a memory limit, that is, a limit on the (memory) report. Such a limit on the number of items which can be given in the report following any brief stimulation has, in fact, been generally observed; it is called the span of attention, apprehension, or immediate memory (see Miller 1956b). Second, *to see more than is remembered* implies that more information is available during, and perhaps for a short time after, the stimulus than can be reported. The considerations about available information are quite similar, whether the information is available for an hour (as it is in a book that is borrowed for an hour), or whether the information is available for only a fraction of a second (as in a stimulus which is exposed for only a fraction of a second). In either case it is quite probable that for a limited period of time more information will be available than can be reported. It is also true that initially, in both examples, the information is available to vision.

In order to circumvent the memory limitation in determining the information that becomes available following a brief exposure, it is obvious that the observer must not be required to give a report which exceeds his memory span. If the number of letters in the stimulus exceeds his memory span, then he cannot give a whole report of all the letters. Therefore, the observer must be required to give only a partial report of the stimulus contents. Partial reporting of available information is, of course, just what is required by ordinary schoolroom examinations and by other methods of sampling available information.

An examiner can determine, even in a short test, approximately how much the student knows. The length of the test is not so important as that the student not be told the test questions too far in advance. Similarly, an observer may be "tested" on what he has seen in a brief exposure of a complex visual stimulus. Such a test requires only a partial report. The specific instruction which indicates which part of the stimulus is to be reported is then given only after termination of the stimulus. On each trial the instruction, which calls for a specified part of the stimulus, is randomly chosen from a set of possible instructions which cover the whole stimulus. By repeating the interrogation (sampling) procedure many times, many different random samples can be obtained of an observer's performance on each of the various parts of the stimulus. The data obtained thereby make feasible the estimate of the total information that was available to the observer from which to draw his report on the average trial.

The time at which the instruction is given determines the time at which available information is sampled. By suitable coding, the instruction may be given at any time: before, during, or after the stimulus presentation. Not only the available information immediately following the termination of the stimulus, but a continuous function relating the amount of information available to the time of instruction may be obtained by such a procedure.

Many studies have been conducted in which observers were required to give partial reports, that is, to report only on one aspect or one location of the stimulus. In prior experiments, however, the instructions were often not randomly chosen, and the set of possible instructions did not systematically cover the stimulus. The notions of testing or sampling were not applied.[2] It is not surprising, therefore, that estimates have not been made of the total information available to the observer following a brief exposure of a complex stimulus. Furthermore, instructions have generally not been coded in such a way as to make it possible to control the precise time at which they were presented. Consequently, the temporal course of available information could not have been quantitatively studied. In the absence of precise data, experimenters have all too frequently assumed that the time for which information is available to the observer corresponds exactly to the physical stimulus duration. Wundt (1899) understood this problem and convincingly argued that, for extremely short stimulus durations, the assumption that stimulus duration corresponded to the duration for which stimulus information was available was blatantly false, but he made no measurements of available information.

The following experiments were conducted to study quantitatively the information that becomes available to an observer following a brief exposure. Lettered stimuli were chosen because these contain a relatively large amount of information per item and because these are the kind of stimuli that have been used by most previous investigators. The first two experiments are essentially control experiments; they attempt to confirm that immediate memory for letters is independent of the parameters of stimulation, that it is an individual characteristic. In the third experiment the number of letters available immediately after the extinction of the stimulus

is determined by means of the sampling (partial report) procedure described above. The fourth experiment explores decay of available information with time. The fifth experiment examines some exposure parameters. In the sixth experiment a technique which fails to demonstrate a large amount of available information is investigated. The seventh experiment deals with the role of the historically important variable: order of report.

General Method

Apparatus

The experiments utilized a Gerbrands tachistoscope.[3] This is a two-field, mirror tachistoscope (Dodge 1907b), with a mechanical timer. Viewing is binocular, at a distance of about 24 inches. Throughout the experiment, a dimly illuminated fixation field was always present.

The light source in the Gerbrands tachistoscope is a 4-watt fluorescent (daylight) bulb. Two such lamps operated in parallel light each field. The operation of the lamps is controlled by the microswitches, the steady-state light output of the lamp being directly proportional to the current. However, the phosphors used in coating the lamp continue to emit light for some time after the cessation of the current. This afterglow in the lamp follows an exponential decay function consisting of two parts: the first, a blue component, which accounts for about 40% of the energy, decays with a time constant which is a small fraction of a millisecond; the decay constant of the second, yellow, component was about 15 ms in the lamp tested. Figure 22.1 illustrates a 50-ms light impulse on a linear intensity scale. The exposure time of 50 ms was used in all experiments unless exposure time was itself a parameter. Preliminary experiments indicated that , with the presentations used, exposure duration was an unimportant parameter. Fifty millisecond was sufficiently short so that eye movements during the exposure were rare, and it could conveniently be set with accuracy.

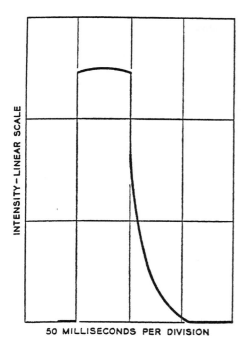

50 MILLISECONDS PER DIVISION

Figure 22.1
A 50-ms light flash, such as was used in most of the experiments. (Redrawn from a photograph of an oscilloscope trace)

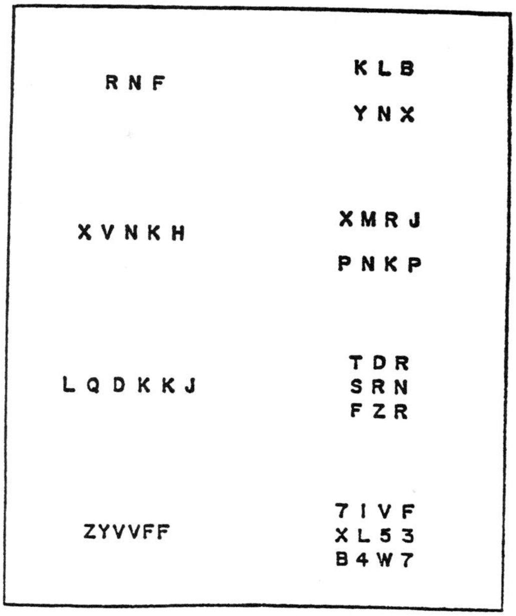

Figure 22.2
Typical stimulus materials. Col. 1: 3, 5, 6, 6-massed. Col. 2: 3/3, 4/4, 3/3/3, 4/4/4 L&N.

Stimulus Materials

The stimuli used in this experiment were lettered 5 × 8 cards viewed at a distance of 22 inches. The lettering was done with a Leroy No. 5 pen, producing capital letters about 0.45 inch high. Only the 21 consonants were used, to minimize the possibility of Ss interpreting the arrays as words. In a few sets of cards the letter Y was also omitted. In all, over 500 different stimulus cards were used.

There was very little learning of the stimulus materials either by the Ss or by the E. The only learning that was readily apparent was on several stimuli that had especially striking letter combinations. Except for the stimuli used for training, no S ever was required to report the same part of any stimulus more than two or three times, and never in the same session.

Figure 22.2 illustrates some typical arrays of letters. These arrays may be divided into several categories: (a) stimuli with three, four, five, six, or seven letters normally spaced on a single line; (b) stimuli with six letters closely spaced on a single line (6-massed); (c) stimuli having two rows of letters with three letters in each row (3/3), or two rows of four letters each (4/4); (d) stimuli having three rows of letters with three letters in each row (3/3/3). The stimulus information, calculated in bits, for some of the more complex stimuli is 26.4 bits (6-letters, 6-massed, 3/3), 35.1 bits (4/4), and 39.5 bits (3/3/3).

In addition to stimuli that contained only letters, some stimuli that contained both letters and numbers were used. These had eight (4/4 L&N,

35.7 bits) and twelve symbols (4/4/4 L&N, 53.6 bits), respectively, four in each row. Each row had two letters and two numbers—the positions being randomly chosen. The S was always given a sample stimulus before L&N stimuli were used and told of the constraint above. He was also told that O when it occurred was the number "zero" and was not considered a letter. Calculated with these constraints, the information in each row of four letters and numbers (17.9 bits) on such a card is nearly equal to the information in a row of four randomly chosen consonants (17.6 bits), even though there are different kinds of alternatives in each case.

Subjects

The nature of the experiments made it more economical to use small numbers of trained Ss rather than several large groups of untrained Ss. Four of the five Ss in the experiment were obtained through the student employment service. The fifth S (RNS) was a member of the faculty who was interested in the research. Twelve sessions were regularly scheduled for each S, three times weekly.

Instructions and Trial Procedures

S was instructed to look at the fixation cross until it was clearly in focus; then he pressed a button which initiated the presentation after a 0.5-s delay. This procedure constituted an approximate behavioral criterion of the degree of dark adaptation prior to the exposure, namely, the ability to focus on the dimly illuminated fixation cross.

Responses were recorded on a specially prepared response grid. A response grid appropriate to each stimulus was supplied. The response grid was placed on the table immediately below the tachistoscope, the room illumination being sufficient to write by. The Ss were instructed to fill in all the required squares on the response grid and to guess when they were not certain. The Ss were not permitted to fill in consecutive X's, but were required to guess "different letters." After a re-

sponse, S slid the paper forward under a cover which covered his last response, leaving the next part of the response grid fully in view.

Series of 5–20 trials were grouped together without a change in conditions. Whenever conditions or stimulus types were changed, S was given two or three sample presentations with the new conditions or stimuli. Within a sequence of trials, S set his own rate of responding. The Ss (except ND) preferred rapid rates. In some conditions, the limiting rate was set by the E's limitations in changing stimuli and instruction tones. This was about three to four stimuli per minute.

Each of the first four and last two sessions began with and/or ended with a simple task: the reporting of all the letters in stimuli of three, four, five, and six letters. This procedure was undertaken in addition to the usual runs with these stimuli to determine if there were appreciable learning effects in these tasks during the course of the experiment and if there was an accuracy decrement (fatigue) within individual sessions. Very little improvement was noted after the second session. This observation agrees with previous reports (Whipple 1914). There was little difference between the beginning and end of sessions.

Scoring and Tabulation of Results

Every report of all Ss was scored both for total number of letters in the report which agreed with letters in the stimulus and for the number of letters reported in their correct positions. Since none of the procedures of the experiments had an effect on either of these scores independently of the other, only the second of these, *letters in the correct position*, is tabulated in the results. This score, which takes position into account, is less subject to guessing error,[4] and in some cases it is more readily interpreted than a score which does not take position into account. As the maximum correction for guessing would be about 0.4 letter for the 4/4/4 (12-letter) material—and considerably less for all other materials—no such correction is made in the treatment of the data. In general, data were not tabulated more accurately than 0.1 letter.

Data from the first and second sessions were not used if they fell below an S's average performance on these tasks in subsequent sessions. This occurred for reports of five and of eight (4/4) letters for some Ss. A similar criterion applied in later sessions for tasks that were initiated later. In this case, the results of the first "training" session(s) are not incorporated in the total tabulation if they lie more than 0.5 letter from S's average in subsequent sessions.

Experiment 1: Immediate Memory

When an S is required to give a complete (whole) report of all the letters on a briefly exposed stimulus, he will generally not report all the letters correctly. The average number of letters which he does report correctly is usually called his *immediate memory span* or *span of apprehension for that particular stimulus material under the stated observation conditions.* An expression such as immediate-memory span (Miller 1956a) implies that the number of items reported by S remains invariant with changes in stimulating conditions. The present experiment seeks to determine to what extent the span of immediate memory is independent of the number and spatial arrangement of letters, and of letters and numbers on stimulus cards. If this independence is demonstrated, then the qualification "for that particular stimulus material" may be dropped from the term immediate-memory span when it is used in these experiments.

Procedure

Ss were instructed to write all the letters in the stimulus, guessing when they were not certain. All 12 types of stimulus materials were used. At least 15 trials were conducted with each kind of stimulus with each S. Each S was given at least 50 trials with the 3/3 (6-letter) stimuli which had yielded the highest memory span in preliminary experiments. The final run made with any

kind of stimulus was always a test of immediate-memory. This procedure insured that Ss were tested for memory when they were maximally experienced with a stimulus.

Results

The lower curves in figure 22.3 represent the average number of letters correctly reported by each S for each material.[5] The most striking re-

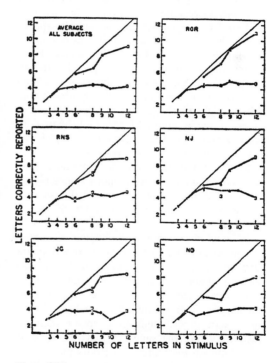

Figure 22.3
"Channel capacity curves." Immediate memory and letters available (output information) as functions of the number of stimulus letters (input information). Lower curves = immediate memory (experiment 1); upper curves = letters available immediately after termination of the stimulus; diagonal lines = maximum possible score (i.e., input = output). Code: × = letters on one line; + = 6-massed; O = 3/3, 4/4, 5/5; △ = 3/3/3; □ = 4/4 L&N, 4/4/4 L&N.

sult is that immediate memory is constant for each *S*, being nearly independent of the kind of stimulus used. The immediate-memory span for individual *S*s ranges from approximately 3.8 for JC to approximately 5.2 for NJ with an average immediate-memory span for all *S*s of about 4.3 letters. (The upper curves are discussed later.)

The constancy which is characteristic of individual immediate-memory curves of figure 22.3 also appears in the average curve for all *S*s. For example, three kinds of stimuli were used that had six letters each: six letters normally spaced on one line, 6-massed, and 3/3-letters (see figure 22.2). When the data for all *S*s are pooled, the scores for each of these three types of materials are practically the same: the range is 4.1–4.3 letters. The same constancy holds for stimuli containing eight symbols. The average number of letters correctly reported for each of the two different kinds of eight letter stimuli, 4/4, 4/4 L&N, is nearly the same: 4.4, 4.3, respectively.

Most *S*s felt that stimuli containing both letters and numbers were more difficult than those containing letters only. Nevertheless, only NJ showed an objective deficit for the mixed material.

In conclusion, the average number of correct letters contained in an *S*'s whole report of the stimulus is approximately equal to the smaller of (a) the number of letters in the stimulus or (b) a numerical constant—the span of immediate memory—which is different for each *S*. The use of the term immediate-memory span is therefore justified within the range of materials studied. This limit on the number of letters that can be correctly reported is an individual characteristic, but it is relatively similar for each of the five *S*s of the study.

Experiment 2: Exposure Duration

The results of experiment 1 showed that, regardless of material, *S*s could not report more than an average of about 4.5 items per stimulus exposure. In order to determine whether this limi-

tation was a peculiar characteristic of the short exposure duration (0.05 s), it was necessary to vary the exposure duration.

Procedure

As in the previous experiment, *S*s were instructed to report all the letters in the stimulus. The stimuli were six letter cards (3/3). NJ, who was able to report more than five correct letters in experiment 1, was given 4/4 stimuli in order to make a possible increment in his accuracy of responding detectable. The *S*s were given 10 trials in each of the four conditions, .015-, .050-, .150- (.200-), .500-s exposure duration, in the order above. In a later session, additional trials were conducted at .015-s exposure as a control for experiment 5. These trials are averaged with the above data.

Results and Discussion

Figure 22.4 illustrates the number of letters correctly reported as a function of the duration of exposure. The main result is that exposure duration, even over a wide range, is not an important parameter in determining the number of letters

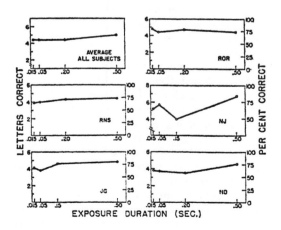

Figure 22.4

Letters correctly reported as a function of exposure duration.

an S can recall correctly. Both individually and as a group, Ss show no systematic changes in the number of letters correctly reported as the exposure duration was varied from 0.015 to 0.500 s. The invariance of the number of letters reported as a function of exposure durations up to about 0.25 s for the kind of presentation used (dark pre- and postexposure fields) has long been known (Schumann 1904).

Experiment 3: Partial Report

Experiments 1 and 2 have demonstrated the span of immediate memory as an invariant characteristic of each S. In experiment 3 the principles of testing in a perceptual situation that were advanced in the introduction are applied in order to determine whether S has more information available than he can indicate in his limited immediate-memory report.

The S is presented with the stimulus as before, but he is required only to make a partial report. The length of this report is four letters or less, so as to lie within S's immediate-memory span. The instruction that indicates which row of the stimulus is to be reported is coded in the form of a tone. The instruction tone is given after the visual presentation. The S does not know until he hears the tone which row is called for. This is therefore a procedure which samples the information that S has available after the termination of the visual stimulus.

Procedure

Initially, stimulus materials having only two lines were used, that is, 3/3 and 4/4. The S was told that a tone would be sounded, that this tone would come approximately simultaneously with the exposure, and that it would be either a high tone (2500 cps) or a low tone (250 cps). If it were a high tone, he was to write only the upper row of the stimulus; if a low tone, only the lower row. He was then shown a sample card of 3/3 letters and given several high and low tones. It was suggested that he keep his eyes fixated on the fixation point and be equally prepared for either tone. It would not be possible to outguess the E who would be using a random sequence of tones.

The tone duration was approximately o.5 s. The onset of the tone was controlled through the same microswitch that controlled the off-go of the light, with the completion of a connection from an audio-oscillator to the speaker. Intensity of the tone was adjusted so that the high (louder) tone was "loud but not uncomfortable."

In each of the first two sessions, each S received 30 training trials with each of the materials 3/3, 4/4. In subsequent sessions Ss were given series of 10 or more "test" trials. Later, a third, middle (650 cps) tone was introduced to correspond to the middle row of the 3/3/3 and 4/4/4 stimuli. The instructions and procedure were essentially the same as before.

In any given session, each tone might not occur with equal frequency for each type of stimulus. Over several sessions, usually two, this unequal frequency was balanced out so that an S had an exactly equal number of high, medium, and low tones for each material. If an S "misinterpreted" the tone and wrote the wrong row, he was asked to write what he could remember of the correct row. Only those letters which corresponded to the row indicated by the tone were considered.

Treatment of the Data

In the experiments considered in this section, S is never required to report the whole stimulus but only one line of a possible two or three lines. The simplest treatment is to plot the percentage of letters correct. This, in fact, will be done for all later comparisons. The present problem is to find a reasonable measure to enable comparison between the partial report and the immediate-memory data for the same stimuli. The measure, *percent correct*, does not describe the results of the immediate-memory experiments parsimoniously. In experiment 1 it was shown that Ss report a constant number of letters, rather than a constant percentage of letters in the stimulus.

The measure, *number of letters correct*, is inappropriate to the partial report data because the number of letters which *S* reports is limited by the *E* to at most three or four. The most reasonable procedure is to treat the partial report as a random sample of the letters which the *S* has available. Each partial report represents a typical sample of the number of letters *S* has available for report. For example, if an *S* is correct about 90% of the time when he is reporting three out of nine letters, then he is said to have 90% of the nine letters—about eight letters—available for partial report at the time the instruction tone is given.

In order to calculate the number of available letters, the average number of letters correct in the partial report is multiplied by the number of equiprobable (nonoverlapping), partial reports. If there are two tones and two rows, multiplication is by 2.0; if three, by 3.0. As before, only the number of correct letters in the correct position is considered.

Results

The development of the final, stable form of the behavior is relatively rapid for *S*s giving partial reports. The average for all *S*s after 30 trials (first session) with the 3/3 stimuli was 4.5; on the second day the average of 30 more trials was 5.1. On the third day *S*s averaged 5.6 out of a possible six letters. Most of the improvement was due to just one *S*: ND who improved from 2.9 to 5.8 letters available. In the 3/3/3 stimulus training, all *S*s reached their final value after the initial 40 trials on the first day of training. The considerable experience *S*s had acquired with the partial reporting procedure at this time may account for the quick stabilization. NJ, whose score was 7.7 letters available on the first 20 trials, was given almost 150 additional trials in an unsuccessful attempt to raise this initial score.

In figure 22.3 the number of letters available as a function of the number of letters in the stimulus are graphed as the upper curves. For all stimuli and for all *S*s, the available information calculated from the partial report is greater than that contained in the immediate-memory report. Moreover, from the divergence of the two curves it seems certain that, if still more complex stimuli were available, the amount of available information would continue to increase.

The estimate above is only a lower bound on the number of letters that *S*s have available for report after the termination of the stimulus. An upper bound cannot be obtained from experiments utilizing partial reports, since it may always be argued that, with slightly changed conditions, an improved performance might result. Even the lower-bound measurement of the average available information, however, is twice as great as the immediate-memory span. The immediate-memory span for the 4/4/4 (12-letters and numbers) stimuli ranges from 3.9 to 4.7 symbols for the *S*s, with an average of 4.3. Immediately after an exposure of the 4/4/4 stimulus material, the number of letters available to the *S*s ranged from 8.1 (ND) to 11.0 (ROR), with an average of 9.1 letters available. This number of letters may be transformed into the bits of information represented by so many letters. For the 4/4/4 (12-letters and numbers) material, the average number of bits available, then, is 40.6, with a range from 36.2 to 49.1 (out of a possible 53.6 bits). These figures are considerably higher than the usual estimates. For example, in a recent review article Quastler (1956) writes: "All experimental studies agree that man can ... assimilate less than 25 bits per glance" (p. 32). The data obtained in experiment 3 not only exceed this maximum, but they contain no evidence that the information that became available to the *S*s following the exposure represented a limit of "man" rather than a maximum determined by the limited information contained in the stimuli which were used.

Experiment 4: Decay of Available Information

Part 1: Development of Strategies of Observing

It was established in experiment 3 that more information is available to the *S*s immediately after termination of the stimulus than they could report. It remains to determine the fate of this surplus information, that is, the "forgetting curve." The partial report technique makes possible the sampling of the available information at the time the instruction signal is given. By delaying the instruction, therefore, decay of the available information as a function of time will be reflected as a corresponding decrease in the accuracy of the report.

Procedure

The principal modification from the preceding experiment is that the signal tone, which indicates to the S which row is to be reported, is given at various other times than merely "zero delay" following the stimulus off-go. The following times of indicator tone onset relative to the stimulus were explored: 0.05 s before stimulus onset (−0.10 s), ±0.0-, +0.15-, +0.30-, +0.50-, +1.0-s delays after stimulus off-go. The stimuli used were 3/3, 4/4.

The Ss were given five or more consecutive trials in each of the above conditions. These trials were always preceded by at least two samples in order to familiarize S with the exact time of onset. The particular delay of the instruction tone on any trial was thus fixed rather than chosen randomly. The advantages of this procedure are (a) optimal performance is most likely in each delay condition, if S is prepared for that precise condition (cf. Klemmer 1957), (b) minimizing delay changes makes possible a higher rate of stimulus presentations. On the other hand, a random sequence of instruction tone delays would make it more likely that S was "doing the same thing" in each of the different delay conditions.

The sequence in which the different delay conditions followed each other was chosen either as that given above (ascending series of delay conditions) or in the reverse order (descending series). Within a session, a descending series always followed an ascending series and vice versa, irrespective of the stimulus materials used. At least two ascending and two descending series of

delay conditions were run with each S and with each material after the initial training (Experiment 3) with that material. This number of trials insures that for each S there are at least 20 trials at each delay of the indicator tone.

Results and Discussion

The development of the typical behavior is illustrated by the S, ROR, in figure 22.5a–c. Figure 22.5a shows ROR's performance in a single session, the first posttraining session. The upper and lower curves represent the ascending and descending series of tone instruction delays, respectively. The arrows indicate the order. Although each point is based upon only five trials, the curves are remarkably similar and regular. Clearly, most of the letters in excess of ROR's memory span are forgotten within about 0.25 s. The rapid forgetting of these letters justifies calling this a short-term memory and accounts for the fact that it may easily be overlooked under less than optimal conditions. In the following session (figure 22.5b) the descending series was given first. Here orderly behavior disintegrates. In the third session (figure 22.5c) two modifications were introduced: (a) the number of trials in each delay condition was increased to eight and (b) a new delay condition was given—namely, a signal tone coming 0.05 s before the stimulus

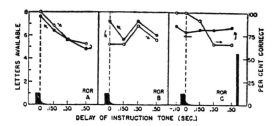

Figure 22.5
Partial report of eight (4/4) letters, three consecutive sessions. Arrows indicate the sequence in which conditions followed within a session. The light flash is shown on same time scale at lower left of each figure. Bar at right indicates immediate memory for this material. One subject (ROR).

onset. The curves are again regular, but they are obviously different for the ascending and descending series. For the session indicated in figure 22.5c an analysis of the errors by position shows that in the ascending series the errors are evenly split between the top and bottom rows of the stimulus; in the descending series, the top row is favored 3:1.

ROR's performance is analyzable in terms of two kinds of observing behavior (strategies) which the situation suggests. He may follow the instruction, given by E prior to training, that he pay equal attention to each row. In this case, errors are evenly distributed between rows. Or, he may try to anticipate the signal by guessing which instruction tone will be presented. In this case, S is differentially prepared to report one row. If the signal and S's guess coincide, S reports accurately; if not, poorly. Such a guessing procedure would lead to the variability observed in figure 22.5b. On the other hand, S may prefer always to anticipate the same row—in the case of ROR (figure 22.5c, descending series), the top row. This would again allow reliable scores, provided only that there are an equal number of instruction signals calling for the top and bottom rows. Concomitantly, a differential accuracy of report for the two rows is observed. (ROR's preference for the top row is again prominent in experiment 7, figures 22.10, 22.11.)

Equal attention responding is initially reinstated on the third day. The obvious change in procedure which is responsible is the introduction of a tone 0.05 s before the stimulus onset (−0.10 s "after" its termination). This signal is sufficiently in advance of the stimulus so that perfect responding is possible by looking at only the row indicated by the signal tone. ROR scores 100%, both in this condition and in the succeeding zero delay. The whole (ascending series) decay curve of figure 22.5c is highly similar to that of figure 22.5a. A run with 3/3 stimuli was interposed between the ascending and descending series shown in figure 22.5c. Since the guessing procedures were easily sufficient for a nearly

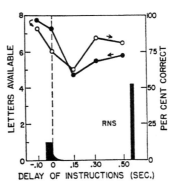

Figure 22.6
Partial report of eight (4/4) letters, last of three sessions. Arrows indicate the sequence in which conditions followed within session. The light flash is shown on same time scale at lower left. Bar at right indicates immediate memory for this material. (RNS)

perfect score with 3/3 materials, when the descending series of delay conditions was run, ROR continued guessing. While guessing was advantageous at the long delays, at the short delays it was a decided disadvantage.

Figure 22.6 illustrates the performances of RNS, a sophisticated observer. RNS described the two strategies (equal attention, guessing) to E. In accordance with the instructions to do as well as he could, RNS said that he switched from the first to the second strategy at delays longer than 0.15 s. Thus in the three short delay conditions, RNS divided his errors almost evenly (19:21) between the favored (top) and the unfavored rows; in the two longer delays, errors were split 4:26. The dip in the curve indicates that RNS did not switch strategies quite as soon as he could have, for optimal performance. Such a dip is characteristically seen in experiments of this kind.

The other Ss exhibit similar curves.[6] These are not presented, as the main features have already been demonstrated by ROR and RNS. In summary, the method of delaying the instruction tone is a feasible one for determining the decay of the short-term memory contents, but experience with the difficult, long delays causes a considerable increase in the variability of Ss' performance which is carried over even to the short delay conditions. This has been attributed to Ss' change from an equal attention to a guessing strategy in observing the stimulus.[7]

Part 2: Final Level of Performance

The analysis of the preceding experiment has indicated that two distinct kinds of observing behavior develop when the instruction to report is delayed. The accuracy of report resulting from the first of these behaviors (equal attention) is correlated with the delay of the instruction tone; it is associated with the Ss initially giving equal attention to all parts of the stimulus. The accuracy of the other kind of report (guessing) is uncorrelated with the delay of the instruction; it is characterized by Ss' differential preparedness for some part of the stimulus (guessing). Equal attention observing is selected for further study here. The preceding experiment suggests three modifications that would tend to make equal attention observing more likely to occur, with a corresponding exclusion of guessing.

1. The use of stimuli with a larger number of letters, that is, 3/3/3 and 4/4/4. Differential attention to a constant small part of the stimulus is less likely to be reinforced, the larger the stimulus. The use of three tones instead of two diminishes the probability of guessing the correct tone.

2. Training with instruction tones that begin slightly before the onset of the stimulus. It is not necessary for S to guess in this situation since he can succeed by depending upon the instruction tone alone. This situation not only makes equal attention likely to occur, but differentially reinforces it when it does occur.

When delays of longer length are tested, priority should be given to an ascending series of delays so that S will, at the beginning of a particular delay sequence, have a high probability of entering with the desired observing behavior. This probability might be nearly 1.0 by interposing a series of trials on which the instruction is given in advance of, or immediately upon, termination of the stimulus and requiring that S perform perfectly on this task before he can continue to the particular delay being tested.[8] This tedious procedure was tried; but, as it did not have an appreciable effect upon the results, it was discontinued. The problem is that Ss learn to switch between the two modes of behavior in a small number of trials.

3. The E may be able to gain *verbal* control over Ss' modes of responding. Initially, however, even S cannot control his own behavior exactly. This suggests a limit to what E can do. For example, frequently Ss reported that, although they had tried to be equally prepared for each row, after some tones they realized that they had been selectively prepared for a particular row. This comment was made both when the tone and the row coincided and (more frequently) when they differed.

Some verbal control is, of course, possible. An instruction that was well understood was:

You will see letters illuminated by a flash that quickly fades out. This is a visual test of your ability to read letters under these conditions, not a test of your memory. You will hear a tone during the flash or while it is fading which will indicate which letters you are to attempt to read. Do not read the card until you hear the tone, [etc.].

The instruction was changed at the midway point in the experiment. The S was no longer to do as well as he could by any means, but was limited to the procedure described above. Part 2 of this experiment, utilizing 9- and 12-letter stimuli, was carried out with the three modifications suggested above.

Results

The results for 3/3/3 and 4/4/4 letters and numbers are shown for each individual S in figures

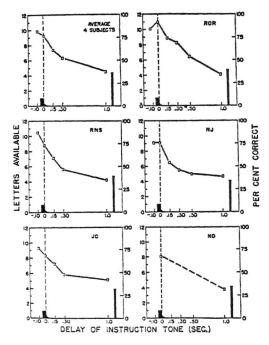

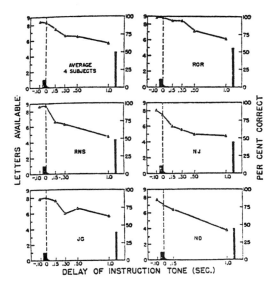

Figure 22.7
Decay of available information: nine (3/3/3) letters. Light flash is shown on same time scale at lower left. Bar at right indicates immediate memory for this material.

Figure 22.8
Decay of available information: twelve (4/4/4) letters and numbers. Light flash is shown on same time scale at lower left. Bar at right indicates immediate memory for this material.

22.7 and 22.8. The two ordinates are linearly related by the equation:

$$\frac{\text{percent correct}}{100} \times \text{no. letters in stimulus}$$

$$= \text{letters available}$$

Each point is based on all the test trials in the delay condition. The points at zero delay of instructions for NJ and JC also include the training trials, as these Ss showed no subsequent improvement.

The data indicate that, for all Ss, the period of about 1 s is a critical one for the presentation of

the instruction to report. If Ss receive the instruction 0.05 s before the exposure, then they give accurate reports: 91% and 82% of the letters given in the report are correct for the 9- and 12-letter materials, respectively. These partial reports may be interpreted to indicate that the Ss have, on the average, 8.2 of 9 and 9.8 of 12 letters available. However, if the instruction is delayed until one sec. after the exposure, then the accuracy of the report drops 32% (to 69%) for the 9-letter stimuli, and 44% (to 38%) for the 12-letter stimuli. This substantial decline in accuracy brings the number of *letters available* very near to the number of letters that Ss give in immediate-memory (whole) reports.

The decay curves are similar and regular for each S and for the average of all Ss. Although individual differences are readily apparent, they are small relative to the effects of the delay of the

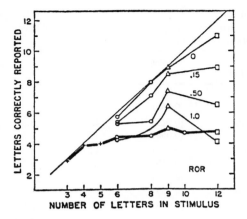

Figure 22.9
Immediate-memory and available information. The parameter is the time at which available information is sampled (delay of instruction). Heavy line indicates immediate memory for the same materials. One subject (ROR).

instruction. For example, when an instruction was given with zero delay after the termination of the stimulus, the *least* accurate reports by any Ss are given by ND, who has 8.1 letters available immediately after the termination of the stimulus. With a 1-s delay of instructions, the *most* accurate reports were given by JC, who has only 5.1 letters available at this time.

In figure 22.3, in which whole reports and partial reports were compared, only that particular partial report was considered in which the instruction tone followed the stimulus with zero delay. It is evident from this experiment that the zero delay instruction is unique only in that it is the earliest possible "after" instruction, but not because of any functional difference.

In figure 22.9, therefore, the 0.15-, 0.50-, and 1.00-s instruction delays are also plotted for one S, ROR. Data for the six- (3/3) and eight- (4/4) letter stimuli are taken from the two ascending delay series with each material that yielded monotonic results. Figure 22.9 clearly highlights

the significance of a precisely controlled coded instruction, given within a second of the stimulus off-go, for the comparison of partial and immediate-memory reports. One second after termination of the stimulus, the accuracy of ROR's partial reports is no longer very different from the accuracy of his whole reports.

Experiment 5: Some Exposure Parameters

In experiment 3 it was shown that the number of letters reported correctly is almost independent of the exposure duration over a range from 15 to 500 ms. It is well known, however, that the relation between the accuracy of report and the exposure duration depends upon the pre- and postexposure fields (Wundt, 1899).

In a technique developed in Helmholtz's laboratory (Baxt 1871) the informational (stimulus) field is followed, after a variable delay, by a noninformational, homogeneous, bright postexposure field. Using this method, Baxt showed that the number of reportable letters was a nearly linear function of the delay of the bright post-exposure field.[9]

Other combinations of pre- and postexposure fields have also been tried (Dodge 1907a). The usual tachistoscopic presentation utilizes gray pre- and postexposure fields (Woodworth 1938). Baxt's procedure, however, is the most disadvantageous for the observer. A similar procedure was therefore selected, in order to study whole and partial reports in a vastly different visual presentation from that of the previous experiments.

Procedure

1. Ss were instructed to write all the letters of the stimulus; 3/3 stimuli were used. After several sample presentations of a stimulus card followed by a light postexposure field, Ss were given a random sequence of normal (pre- and postexposure fields dark) and Baxt (preexposure dark, postexposure field light) trials. The Baxt

trials do not correspond exactly to the presentation that Baxt used. In this experiment, the post-exposure field is the same intensity as the stimulus (informational) field, whereas Baxt usually used more intense postexposure fields; also, the stimulus field always remains *on* until the onset of the postexposure field, whereas Baxt used a fixed 5-ms duration for the stimulus field. The postexposure field itself remains on for about 1 s. The preexposure field is always dark, as in all the previous experiments. Two exposure durations, 0.015 and 0.050 s, were tested.

2. Three Ss were tested with the Baxt presentation of a 3/3/3 stimulus at an exposure duration of 0.015 s. The partial report procedure was used to determine the effects of the postexposure field on the number of letters available.

3. The same three Ss were run as their own controls. The procedure was exactly the same as in paragraph 2 above except that the postexposure field was normal (dark).

Results

The complete results are given in tables 22.1 and 22.2. In all tests, the Baxt procedure reduces

Table 22.1

A comparison of response accuracy with two different post-exposure fields

Subject	Exposure (sec.)	Normal	Baxt
RNS	(0.015)	3.9	2.5
	(0.050)	4.0	2.2
ROR	(0.015)	4.8	3.5
	(0.050)	4.4	2.8
ND	(0.015)	3.8	1.9
	(0.050)	3.7	2.3
NJ	(0.015)	5.1	2.4
	(0.050)	5.4	3.4
JC	(0.015)	4.1	2.7
	(0.050)	3.8	3.4
Mean	(0.015)	4.3	2.6
	(0.050)	4.3	2.8

Note: Number of letters correctly reported. Whole report of six (3/3) letter stimuli. Normal = pre- and post-exposure fields dark; Baxt = pre-exposure field dark, post-exposure field white.

Table 22.2

A comparison of response accuracy with two different post-exposure fields

Delay of Instruction (sec.):	0.0		0.15	
Exposure Duration (sec.): Subject	0.015	0.05	0.015	0.05
RNS (N)	8.0	8.7	5.4	6.6
(B)	2.0		2.2	
ROR (N)	8.6	8.9	8.3	8.5
(B)	6.3		5.4	
ND (N)	7.3	7.0	5.8	6.4
(B)	2.2		1.7	
Mean (N)	8.0	8.2	6.5	7.2
(B)	3.5		3.1	

Note: Number of letters available (fraction of letters correct in partial report × number of letters in stimulus). Stimuli: nine (3/3/3) letters. (N) = normal (pre- and post-exposure fields dark), (B) = Baxt (pre-exposure field dark, post-exposure field white).

the response accuracy of all *S*s to about one-half of their normal score. This finding confirms the earlier studies. However, a linear relation between exposure duration and the number of letters reported was not observed. The failure to find a linear relation may be due to the previously mentioned differences between the presentations.

For RNS and ND, the number of letters available is nearly the same (about two) in the partial report of 9-letter stimuli as the whole report of 6-letter stimuli. The fact that in both procedures the number of letters given by *S*s is the same suggests that a Baxt presentation reduces the number, or the length of time that letters are available, and that it does not directly affect the immediate-memory span.

ROR's partial reports of Baxt presentations are considerably more accurate than those of the other *S*s, although they are not as accurate as his reports in control presentations. ROR seemed to show improvement on successive Baxt trials. JC, another *S* who seemed to show improvement, was given additional Baxt trials on which he continued to improve slowly. Unfortunately, it was unfeasible to determine the asymptotic performance of these two *S*s. Whether the difference in performance between ROR, and RNS and ND is attributable to some overt response, such as squinting or blinking, was not determined.

Table 22.2 also enables the comparison of 0.015- and 0.050-s exposures of 3/3/3 stimuli. A decrease in exposure duration has only a slight effect on the number of letters available. This suggests, as in the immediate-memory experiments, that the duration of a tachistoscopic exposure is not as important a determinant of the number of letters available as the fields which follow the exposure.

Experiment 6: Letters and Numbers

In experiment 3 partial reports were found to be uniformly more accurate than whole reports. In one case, stimuli of eight letters were used and only one row of four letters was reported. Designating the letters to be reported by their location is only one of a number of possible ways. In the following experiment, a quite similar set of stimuli is used; each stimulus has two letters and two numbers in each of the two rows. The partial report again consists of only four symbols, but these are designated either as letters or as numbers rather than by row. In addition, a number of controls which are also relevant to experiment 3 are conducted.

Procedure

1. Training: The *S*s were given practice trials with the instruction: "Write down only the numbers if you hear a short pip (tone 0.05-s duration) and only the letters if you hear the long tone (0.50-s duration)." The tones were then given with zero delay following the stimulus off-go. The stimuli were 4/4 L&N.

2. In the following session, tests were conducted with five different instructions:

a. Letters only—Instructions given well in advance of stimulus to write only the letters in the following card(s). (8 trials)
b. Numbers only—Write only the numbers in the following card(s). (8 trials)
c. Top only—Write only the top row in the following card(s). (4 trials)
d. Bottom only—Write only the bottom row in the following card(s). (4 trials)
e. Instruction tone—Write either letters or numbers as indicated by tone. Tone onset 0.05 s before stimulus onset. (16 trials) ROR was also given additional trials at longer delay times.

Results

The results are illustrated in table 22.3. For purposes of comparison, the number of correct letters is multiplied by two when an instruction was used which required *S* to report only four of the eight symbols of the stimulus. This includes instructions given well in advance of the stimu-

Table 22.3
Comparison of five procedures

Subject	Letters only	Numbers only	Average L&N	Instr. tone −0.10	Immediate- memory	One row only
RNS	5.0	4.5	4.8	4.3	4.6	7.3
ROR	6.5	6.5	6.5	6.3	4.5	7.3
ND	3.5	3.8	3.6	4.1	4.1	7.5
NJ	4.0	5.0	4.5	4.6	4.3	—
JC	3.3	4.0	3.6	3.4	4.1	8.0
Mean	4.5	4.8	4.6	4.5	4.3	—

Note: Average letters and/or numbers available (fraction of letters—numbers—correct in partial report × number of symbols in stimulus). Stimuli: eight (4/4) letters and numbers.

lus. All measures, then, have 8.0 as the top score and are thus equivalent within a scale factor to percent correct measures. The range is 0–8 instead of 0–100. Scores which are based on partial reports are therefore directly comparable to the partial report scores (letters available) obtained in experiments 3, 4, and 5.

When stimuli consist of letters and numbers, but Ss report only the letters or only the numbers, then the Ss' partial reports are only negligibly more accurate than their whole reports of the same stimuli. The average number of letters available (calculated from the partial report) is just 0.2 letter above the immediate-memory span for the same material. For practical purposes, the partial report score is the same score that Ss would obtain if they wrote all the letters and numbers they could (that is, gave a whole report) but were scored only for letters or only for numbers, independently by the experimenter. The partial report of letters only (or of numbers only) does not improve even when the instruction is given long in advance verbally instead of immediately before the exposure by a coded signal tone.

The estimate of the number of available letters and numbers which is obtained from the partial report of letters (or numbers) only is also the same as the estimate that would be obtained if,

on each trial, Ss wrote only one row—either the top or the bottom—according to their whim. Reporting only one row of four letters and numbers is a task at which the Ss succeed with over 90% accuracy. Even if they are scored for the whole stimulus, by arbitrarily reporting only one row they would still achieve a score of almost 50% correct or almost four letters available. This is why no delay series were conducted. If Ss had ignored the instruction to write only the letters (or numbers) and had written only a single row on each trial, they would have shown less than a 0.5 letter decrement, no matter what the delay of the instruction.

Only ROR showed a substantial improvement when reporting only the numbers (or letters). He was the only S with whom it made sense to conduct a systematic delay series, although checks with other Ss confirmed this conclusion. Table 22.4 indicates that two extra symbols are available to ROR for report only when the tone is given before the stimulus, but not if it is given immediately after. It should be noted that the information in the instruction tone comes only after it has been on for 0.05 s. At this time it either continues or is terminated. The actual "instruction" is thus given 0.05 s after the tone onset. ROR therefore requires that the *instruction* be given within 0.05 s of the stimulus ter-

Table 22.4
Partial reports or letters or numbers

Subj.	Prior Verbal Instr.	Delay of Instr.		Tone (sec.) +0.25	Immediate Memory
		−0.10	0.0		
ROR	6.5	6.3	4.7	4.4	4.5

Note: Average of symbols available (fraction of letters—numbers—correct in partial report × number of symbols in stimulus). Stimuli: eight (4/4) letters and numbers.

mination if any benefit of the partial report procedure is to be retained.

Whether the *S*s would have shown improvement with a large amount of additional training in the partial report of letters or numbers cannot be stated. Table 22.3 shows that, when *S*s are required in advance to report only one row, this task is trivial. The substantial advantage of partial reports of rows (report by position) over partial reports of numbers or letters (report by category) when the instruction is given verbally long in advance of the exposure is retained even when the instruction is coded and given shortly after the exposure.

The failure in experiment 6 to detect a substantial difference in accuracy between partial reports of only letters (or only numbers) and whole reports clearly illustrates that partial reports by position are more effective for studying the capacity of short-term information storage than partial reports by category.

Experiment 7: Order of Report

Interpretations of the effects of instructions upon the report following a single brief visual exposure have often been concerned with either the perceptual sensitizing effects of an instruction given before the exposure or with the importance of forgetting between the exposure and a postexposure instruction to report. The decay curves of experiment 4 include both of these effects.

Previous studies, however, have usually assumed the order in which the various parts (aspects, dimensions, etc.) of the stimulus are reported to be the significant correlate of postexposure forgetting. The possibility that information might be well retained even though not immediately reported has been mentioned (Broadbent 1958), but experimental investigations of such an effect by an independent variation of the order of report by Wilcocks (1925), Lawrence and Laberge (1956), and Broadbent (1957a) have apparently shown otherwise. Broadbent (1957a) has also shown a case in which independent variation of the order of report did not reduce overall response accuracy.

In the present experiment, order of report is introduced as a purely "nuisance" variable for the *S*. The *S* is instructed to get as many letters correct as possible, but the *E* randomly manipulates the order in which they are to be reported. The experiment is a survey of how *S*s adapt to this kind of interference with the normal order of their report.

Procedure

The *S*s were instructed to write the row indicated by the tone (high, low) first, then to write the other row. They were to try to get as many *total* letters correct as possible, it being of no importance in which particular row the correct letters might be. The instruction tone was given with 0.0-, .30- (or .50-), and 1.0-s delay after the termination of the stimulus.

Controls

In addition to the trials with a high or low tone, two sets of 8 (or 10) trials were given with a neutral, middle tone. The instruction was: "Write all the letters in any order you wish, but do not begin writing until you hear the tone." The tone was sounded with 0.0-s delay following termination of the stimulus and also with 1.0-s delay. It bears repeating here that *S*s were not permitted just to mark X's but were required to guess various letters.

Results

Controls: The instruction which required *S*s to wait for 1.0 s before beginning to write their answer was ignored by the *S*s, since it was almost physically impossible to begin writing sooner. Consequently the two different controls—trials on which *S* was required to "wait" for 1.0 sec. and trials on which *S* could begin his report immediately—are grouped together. These data, which are almost exactly the same as the memory span data (experiment 1), are presented on the far right in figure 22.10.

The *S*s' responses on the control trials are analyzed in terms of the correlation between the location of letters on the stimulus and the accuracy of the report of these letters in the response. The symbols T and B above IM in figure 22.10 represent the percentage of the letters of the top and of the bottom rows that *S*s report correctly. The middle point is the average percentage of the letters of the top and bottom rows that were correctly reported by *S*s. The middle point is therefore also the average percentage correct of all the letters that were reported. Figure 22.10 shows that all *S*s report the top row of the stimulus more accurately than the bottom row, if they are not instructed with regard to the order in which they must report the rows.

The average accuracy with which *S*s report the top and the bottom rows, when instructions

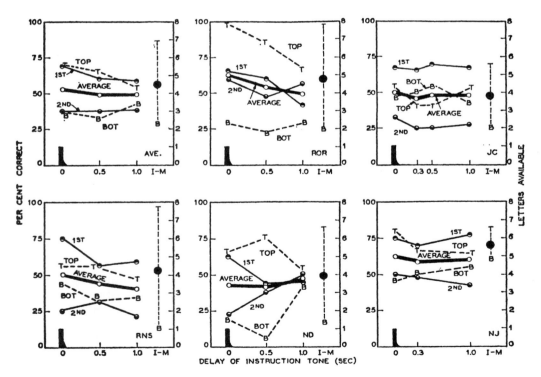

Figure 22.10
Accuracy of the first (second) row reported and of the top (bottom) row as a function of the delay of the instruction to report one row first. Light flash is indicated at lower left; immediate memory (IM) at right.

to report one or the other of these rows are given with various delays after the exposure, is also illustrated in figure 22.10. The accuracy of reports of the top row decreases slightly as the delay of the instructions increases. In other respects, however, the data show no systematic changes in accuracy with changes in the delay of instructions. The data clearly indicate that the top row is generally reported more accurately than the bottom row although the instruction to report each row is given with equal frequency.

The same data may also be analyzed with regard to the accuracy of the row that must be reported first and the row that is reported last. All *S*s except ROR are more accurate when they report the first row (the row called for by the instruction tone) than the second row. For most *S*s, therefore, the order of report is correlated with the accuracy of report.

There is a slight tendency for the accuracy of report of the row which is reported first to decrease as the delay of the instructions increases. On the whole, however, the overall accuracy of report decreases slightly with the delay of the instruction to report one row first. The experimental interference with the normal order of report does not change the overall number of letters reported correctly by any *S* by more than about 0.5 letter.

In this task, unlike the preceding ones, individual differences are more striking than the similarities. The pooled data are highly untypical of three of the five *S*s. Figure 22.11 was devised as a two-dimensional, graphical analysis of variance to compress the details of figure 22.10 into one figure.[10] Each coordinate represents the accuracy of one row of the report relative to the whole report. Thus the ordinate represents the number of letters that an individual *S* reports correctly in the top row of the stimulus (independently of order) divided by the total number of letters (both rows) that he reports correctly. Similarly, the abscissa represents the percentage of the total correct letters reported by *S* that are contained in his report of the first row. Since

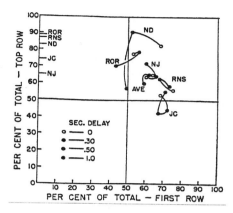

Figure 22.11
Graphical analysis of position on stimulus versus order of report as contributors to response accuracy. Each point represents the average of all trials of an S at a particular delay of instruction. The order in which the points are connected corresponds to the magnitude of the delays. (Upper left) Position preference in control (immediate memory) report.

each coordinate is relative to *S*'s own accuracy, no point of the graph is inaccessible to *S* provided that, if necessary, he is willing to sacrifice some accuracy. Since the interference with *S*'s order of report in this experiment had only slight effects on the overall accuracy of *S*'s report, this method of presenting the data is justifiable.

From figure 22.11 it is immediately evident that, for example, 50% of the correct letters that JC reports are from the top row and, by implication, 50% are from the bottom row of the stimulus. More than 70% of the correct letters that JC reports are in the first row reported by him. ROR represents the converse, preferring to report the top row accurately, remaining indifferent to whether it is called for first or last. Other *S*s lie between these extremes, each *S* maintaining approximately the same relative accuracy for the top and the first rows throughout the various delay conditions. Each *S*, therefore, operates within a characteristic, limited area of the graph. ND is an exception. At zero delay of the instruction tone, both position and order account heavily for the correct letters reported by ND. At 0.5-s delay, ND ignored the order (preferring to concentrate on the top row), and at 1.0-s delay she lost her position (top row) preference as well. In these three conditions, the total number of letters correctly reported by ND remained approximately the same, within 0.5 letter of the control condition. At 1.0-s delay *neither position nor the order contribute to ND's accuracy of report*.

All *S*s operate in the upper right quadrant of figure 22.11. This illustrates the finding that no *S* consistently reported the bottom row more accurately than the top, nor the last row better than the row first called for by the instruction tone. It does not, of course, indicate that *S*s could not report the bottom row or the last row more accurately under other conditions. While *S*s normally behave quite consistently, the data of ND show that they may try a number of different procedures. The instructions given the *S*s prior to the experiment were not restrictive. No specific procedure for making a report was suggested to the *S*s, because the purpose of the experiment was to find out how *S*s respond when they are not given detailed instructions. With suitable instructions, training, and reinforcements, *S*s could probably be induced to make most of the possible kinds of reports that can be diagrammed by figure 22.11. This remains an empirical problem.

The results obtained in this experiment support the conclusions that both a position preference and the order of report ordinarily correlate with the accuracy of response, but that probably *neither are necessary* conditions for response accuracy. Some *S*s can relinquish the position preference and a favorable order of report with no appreciable decrement in accuracy. This finding is in opposition to Lawrence and Laberge's (1956) contention that accuracy is accounted for by the order of report. Accuracy and order are often correlated, but if a favorable order

of report is not *necessary* for accuracy, then it cannot be the cause of accuracy.

When *S* is given a signal indicating which row is to be reported first (experiment 7), the accuracy of report of the row indicated by the signal (the first row reported) may be compared to the accuracy of the partial report (experiment 3). The overt procedure on each trial is quite similar in experiments 3 and 7. The only difference is that in the order of report experiment, after the *S*s have finished writing the row indicated by the signal, they must also write down the other row. In the partial report procedure they do not have to write the second row. The partial report and the order of report experiments also share a common dependent variable: the accuracy of report of the row indicated by the instruction signal.

In view of the similarity in procedure, it is surprising that the accuracy of this common datum should be so different in the two experiments. For example, when *S*s give only the partial reports (the instruction signal being given immediately after termination of the stimulus), then they report 90% of the letters correctly in one row of 4/4 stimuli. When they are required to write the other row also, then they report only 69% of the first four letters correctly. Every *S*, individually, gives a more accurate partial report (experiment 3) than a report of the first row—of two rows to be reported (experiment 7). The consistent superiority of the partial report over the first half of a whole report prevails even when the instruction to report is delayed for 0.5 (or 0.3) s. In all cases where data are available, each *S* reports a row of four letters more accurately when he does not have to write another row of four letters afterwards. That what *S*s must write later should affect the accuracy of what they write first must be explained—if we disregard teleological explanation—by the effect of prior instructions on the accuracy of the report. In other words, if order of report is effective in determining the accuracy of report, then this effect must be a function of instructions given prior to any report at all. For some Ss, no effect of order of report upon response accuracy was observed.

The two findings, that partial reports are uniformly more accurate than whole reports and that order of report may be uncorrelated with accuracy, contradict Lawrence and Laberge's conclusion that "partial" reports are essentially similar to "first" reports. In fact, the second finding (that in some circumstances order of report and accuracy of report are not correlated) provides a direct counterexample to their conclusion. Their different results may be in part due to the vastly different stimuli which they used. Lawrence and Laberge's entire stimuli each contained less information than two randomly chosen letters.

Discussion

In all seven experiments, Ss were required to report the letters of briefly exposed lettered stimuli. Two kinds of reports were explored: *partial reports*, which required the Ss to report only a specified part of the stimulus, and *whole reports*, which required the Ss to report all the letters of the stimulus. Experiment 3 demonstrated that the accuracy of partial reports was consistently greater than the accuracy of whole reports. Another important difference between partial and whole reports is the correlation of accuracy with the delay of the instruction to report. This was shown in experiment 4 in which the time delay of the instruction signal, which indicated the row of the stimulus to be reported, was varied. The accuracy of the partial report was found to be a sharply decreasing function of the time at which the instruction was given. If the instruction signal was delayed for 1 s after the exposure, the accuracy of the partial report was no longer very different from that of the whole report. In experiment 7 it was shown that the accuracy of the whole report does not change as the time of the signal to report is varied—over the same range of time—up to 1 s after the exposure.

The two kinds of report can also be considered in terms of the information (in these experiments, letters) which they indicate the S has available for report. In the whole report, the S reports all the information that he can. When he gives a partial report, the S may have additional available information that is not required for the report. A calculation of the information available to the Ss for their partial reports indicates that between two and three times more information is available for partial reports than for the whole reports. This discrepancy between the two kinds of report is short-lived. Information in excess of that indicated by the whole report was available to the Ss for only a fraction of a second following the exposure. At the end of this time, the accuracy of partial reports is no longer very different from that of whole reports.

The whole report has already been extensively studied by psychologists. The maximum number of items an individual can give in such a report is called his *span of immediate memory*; whole reports are usually called *immediate-memory reports*. Experiments 1 and 2 extend the well-known conclusions that the span of immediate memory is an individual characteristic and that it is constant over a wide range of stimuli and exposure conditions. Although, in immediate-memory experiments, items are conventionally presented sequentially, experiments 1 and 2 illustrate that this is not necessary—that a simultaneous presentation may also give results characteristic of immediate-memory experiments.

The main problems to be considered here concern the partial—whole report discrepancy: (a) Why is the partial report more accurate than the whole report? (b) Why does the partial report retain this added accuracy only for a fraction of a second after the exposure?

The answers proposed are a systematic elaboration of an observation that is readily made by most viewers of the actual tachistoscopic presentation. They report that the stimulus field appears to be still readable at the time a tone is heard which follows the termination of the stimulus by 150 ms. In other words, the subjective image or sensation induced by the light flash outlasts the physical stimulus at least until the tone is heard. The stimulus information is thus "stored" for a fraction of a second as a persisting image of the objective stimulus. As the visual image fades, its legibility (information content) decreases, and consequently the accuracy of reports based upon it decreases.

There is other evidence, besides such phenomenological accounts, that suggests that information is available in the form of an image for a short time after extinction of the physical stimulus. In the first place, it is inconceivable that the observers should stop seeing the stimulus at exactly the moment the light is turned off. The rise and fall of sensation may be rapid, but they are not instantaneous. The question is not *whether* the observer continues to see the stimulus after the illumination is turned off, but for *how long* he continues to see the stimulus. A number of different kinds of psychophysical measurements of the rise and fall of sensation have been attempted. These estimates of the persistence of the visual sensation vary from a minimum of 0.05 s (Wundt 1899) to almost 1 s (McDougall 1904). The most representative estimates are in the neighborhood of 1/6 s (cf. Piéron 1934), a figure that is in good agreement with the results.[11]

In experiment 5 it was shown that the postexposure field strongly influences the accuracy of both the partial and the whole report. This experiment indicates that the available information is sensitive to interference by *noninformational visual stimuli* which follow the exposure. The dependence of available information upon noninformational visual stimulation is just the dependence that would be expected of a visual image.

Finally, there are subtle aspects of the sequence of letters reported by an S which characterize the information that is available to him. In sequentially spoken letters, for example, there is a limit—two—on the number of letters that can

be adjacent to any given letter. Different limits apply to a two-dimensional visual display. If information is stored in a form topologically similar to the stimulus, this may be detected by noting the sequential dependencies that limit successive responses to the stimulus.

Probably the kinds of sequential responding that would most clearly distinguish visual from auditory information storage would be (a) the ability of the S to read the rows of the visual stimulus backwards as well as forwards, or to report the columns or the diagonals, and (b) his inability to do an equivalent task when presented with the information sequentially. (All these procedures merely require the report of adjacent letters if the stimulus is two dimensional.) Unfortunately, these particular experiments were not conducted.

The foregoing experiments offer some relevant evidence. In contrast to spoken letters and numbers, which are most accurately recalled if they occur at the beginning or end of a sequence (Pollack 1952),[12] no obvious gradients of accuracy were found in the foregoing experiments. The middle row actually tended to be slightly better reported than the other rows. Therefore, it is unlikely that the *entire* visual stimulus (12-letters and numbers) was transformed into an auditory (sequential) representation for storage. Such an entire transformation is also unlikely, though not impossible, because of the relatively small time between the stimulus exposure and the report.

An analysis of errors reveals numerous cases of errors that may be classified as "misreading" (for example, confusions between E and F, B and R) and as "mishearing" (for example, confusions between B and D, D and T; Miller and Nicely 1955). Still other confusions (for example, C and G) are ambiguous. All of these types of errors occurred whenever errors occurred at all. The ubiquity of misreading and mishearing errors, taken at face value, suggests that both visual and auditory storage of information are always involved in both whole and partial reports. A nonquantitative error analysis is therefore not likely to shed much light on the question of visual imagery. The frequent mishearing errors suggest that the storage of letters, just prior to a written report, may share some of the characteristics of audition. Like the preceding analysis of the constraints upon successive responses, error analysis requires considerable research before it can be quantitatively applied to problems of imagery.

This then is the evidence—phenomenological reports, the effects of the postexposure fields, the known facts of the persistence of sensation, and the detailed characteristics of the responses— that is consistent with the hypothesis that information is initially stored as a visual image and that the Ss can effectively utilize this information in their partial reports. In the present context, the term, visual image, is taken to mean that (a) the observer behaves as though the physical stimulus were still present when it is not (that is, after it has been removed) and that (b) his behavior in the absence of the stimulus remains a function of the same variables of visual stimulation as it is in its presence. The units of a visual image so defined are always those of an equivalent "objective image," the physical stimulus. It is as logical or illogical to compute the information contained in a visual image (as was done in experiments 3 and 4) as it is to compute the information in a visual stimulus.

"Visual image" and "persistence of sensation" are terms suggested by the asynchrony between the time during which a stimulus is present and the time during which the observer behaves as though it were present. Although asynchrony is inevitable for short exposure durations, there is, of course, no need to use the term "visual image" in a description of this situation. One might, for example, refer simply to an "information storage" with the characteristics that were experimentally observed. This form of psychological isolationism does injustice to the vast amount of relevant researches.

Imagery that reputedly occurs long after the original stimulation (memory images, eidetic images, etc.) is of interest as well as imagery that occurs for only a few tenths of a second following stimulation. Whether the term "imagery," as it has been used here to describe the immediate effects of brief stimulation, is an appropriate term for the description of the lasting effects of stimulation is an empirical problem. It is hoped, however, that the principles and methods developed here will not be without relevance to these traditional problems.

Persistence of Vision and Afterimages

Between the short persistence of vision and the remembrance of a long-passed event, there is an intermediate situation, the afterimage, which requires consideration. In discussing afterimages, it will be useful to distinguish some phases of vision that normally follow an intense or prolonged stimulus. First, there is the "initial" (or primary, or original) "image" (or sensation, or impression, or perception, or response). Any combination of a term from the first and from the second of these groups may be used. The initial image is followed by a latent period during which nothing is seen and which may in turn be followed by a complex sequence of afterimages. Afterimages may be either positive or negative; almost any sequence is possible, but the initial image is almost always positive.[13] Some authors distinguish the initial image from a positive afterimage (for example, McDougall 1904); others do not (for example, von Helmholtz 1924–25). It is often implicit in such distinctions that the persistence of the initial image is due to a continued excitatory process, whereas afterimages arise from receptor fatigue. If there is no repeated waxing and waning of sensation, but merely a single rise and fall, one cannot distinguish two phases in the primary image, one corresponding to the "initial image" and the other to an identical "positive afterimage" of it.

Although it is difficult to prove that visual information is stored in the initial image, there can be no gainsaying that an afterimage may be a rich store of information. Positive or negative afterimages may carry many fine details, including details that were not visible at the time of stimulation (von Helmholtz 1924–25). Afterimages generally last for at least several seconds, and following high energy stimulation they normally last for several minutes (Berry and Imus 1935). The clarity of the details, of course, deteriorates with the passage of time. Since afterimages appear to move when the eye is moved, they usually have been considered retinal phenomena. Taken together, these facts imply that *there is a considerable capacity for visual information storage in the retina*. If the illumination of the stimulus cards used in the foregoing experiments had been sufficiently intense to blaze the letters upon the retina and thereby take maximum advantage of its information storage capacity, there would have been little doubt afterwards as to the nature or location of most of the available information. The stimulus presentations actually used, however, rarely elicited reports of afterimages; Ss usually reported seeing simply a single brief flash. The problem is therefore to determine the persistence of the image of the brief flash, or equivalently, the duration of seeing (the stimulus) or the persistence of vision (of the stimulus), rather than the duration of an afterimage. These terms are used to suggest that the S feels he is responding directly to the stimulus rather than to aftereffects of stimulation.

Psychologists have often carelessly assumed that the absence of discernible afterimages following a visual presentation was sufficient to insure that the duration of sensation will correspond to the duration of the physical stimulus, that is, that there is no persistence of vision at all. Wundt (1899) was one of the first to take vigorous exception to this naive view. Wundt's most compelling example was drawn from Weyer (1899). Weyer had found that two 40-μs light flashes had to be separated by 40 to 50 ms

in order for them to be seen as two distinct flashes; at smaller separations they were seen as a single flash. In the dark adapted eye, the minimum separable interval that consistently yielded reports of "two flashes" was 80–100 ms.

Wundt argued that the two flashes could not be seen as distinct until the sensation occasioned by the first flash had ceased. Thus, under optimum conditions, the minimum duration of the sensation of a short flash was at least 40 ms which, in this case, was 1,000 times the stimulus duration. Wundt thought that, in order to determine the duration of a longer flash, one must merely add the 40 ms of fade-out time to the actual physical light duration. While these details of Wundt's reasoning may be questioned, his main point, based on the example of the short flash, is indisputable: one does not directly control the time for which information is visually available simply by manipulating exposure duration. The experiments reported here provide a direct proof of this assertion.

An Application of the Results to "Before and After" Experiments

The previous experiments showed that more information is available to Ss for a few tenths of a second after the exposure than they can give in a complete report of what they have seen. It was suggested that the limit on the number of items in the memory report is a very general one, the span of immediate-memory, which is relatively independent of the nature of the stimulus. Evidence was offered that information in excess of the immediate-memory span is available to the S as a rapidly fading visual image of the stimulus. If more information is available to him than he can remember, the S must "choose" a part of it to remember. In doing so, he has chosen the part to forget. In experiments 3 and 4, Ss exercised only locational choices, that is, portions of the stimulus were remembered only on the basis of their location. Locational choices are probably not the only effective choices that the S can make. During the short time that information is available to him, the S may process it in any way in which he normally handles information. Usually, what he does, or attempts to do, is determined by the instructions. The S's (unobservable) response to the stimulus is probably the same whether the instruction to make this response is given before the stimulus presentation or after it; the difference between the two cases lies in the information that the response can draw upon. If the stimulus contains more information than the S's immediate-memory span, and if the postexposure instruction is delayed until the S has little of this extra information available, then a difference in the accuracy of the responses with prior- and postexposure instructions will be observed. If the stimulus does not contain more information than can be coded for immediate memory, or if the postexposure instruction is given soon enough so that the S can utilize the still available information effectively, then only minor differences in the accuracy of responses with prior- and postexposure instructions will be observed. If the stimulus is destitute of information (for example, a single, mutilated, dimly illuminated letter of the alphabet) then a host of other factors which are normally insignificant may become crucial. In this case, the "stimulus" itself may well be irrelevant (Goldiamond 1957), and the effects of instructions given before or after the exposure must be predicted on some other basis.

There are some simple experiments in which it is known a priori that the effects of instructions given either before or after the exposure will be exactly the same. This degenerate situation can be illustrated by a stimulus which is exposed for 1 μs and with sufficient energy to be clearly visible. By suitable coding, the preexposure and postexposure instructions can be separated by only 2 μs. The example serves to emphasize that what is implicitly referred to by "before and after" is not the exposure but something else: traditionally, the sensitization and/or forgetting that presumably occur in conjunction with the exposure. Thus, the theory that has been presented here merely gives an explicit statement of assumptions that have long been implicit.

Unobservable Responses and the Order of Report

The subjective response to the high signal tone is "looking up." Since eye movements cannot occur in time to change the retinal image with any of the presentations used (Diefendorf and Dodge 1908) a successful looking-up must be described in terms of a shift in "attention." Nonetheless, such a shift in attention can be quantitatively studied by means of a stabilized retinal image (Pritchard 1958) although Wundt (1912), who did not use this modern, technically difficult technique, was able to give many essential details. The reaction time for the attentional response, like the reaction time for more observable responses, is greater than zero. Therefore, if the S is given an instruction before the presentation, he can prepare for, or sensitize himself to, the correct row of the stimulus even though there is not time enough for a useful eye movement. The response to an instruction which is given 0.05 s before the stimulus is probably the same as the response to a similar instruction that is given 0.1 s later, immediately after the exposure. The short time difference, 0.1 s, accounts for the similar accuracy of responding in these two conditions.

Once his attention is directed to the appropriate row, the S still has to read the letters. This, too, takes time. Baxt's (1871) data indicate that the time required to read a letter is about 10 ms. Baxt's experiment, with some modifications, was repeated by the author, and similar results were obtained.[14]

How is all this relevant to the order of report? The order in which the letters are finally reported can be an important variable because of (a) purely temporal factors (letters that are reported first will be more accurately reported only because they are reported sooner after the exposure, the actual order of reporting the letters per se being relatively unimportant) or (b) interaction effects (the report of some letters is detrimental to the report of the remaining letters, that is, letters reported later suffer from proactive interference by the letters reported earlier).

That purely temporal factors cannot be very important can be seen from the slope of the curves describing available information as a function of time. In the foregoing experiments, the amount of available information approached the immediate-memory span at about 0.5–1.0 s after the exposure; further decrements in available information as a function of time are slight. The report of the letters usually does not begin until 1.0–1.5 s after the exposure. The passage of time during the actual time that letters are being reported, therefore, cannot account for appreciable accuracy changes as a function of the order of report.

The second possible effect of order of report—the interfering effect of the letters reported first upon unreported letters—cannot be so readily discounted. Proactive interference would imply that partial reports are more accurate than whole reports by an amount dependent upon their relative lengths. The results of experiment 4 tend to support this view. At delays of the instruction signal greater than 0.3 s, partial reports of three letters (from stimuli of nine letters) indicate more available letters than do partial reports of 4 letters (from stimuli of 12 letters). On the other hand, in experiment 7 one S, ROR, does not show decreased accuracy as a function of the length of his report. ROR is able to report eight letters as accurately when he begins his report with three or four incorrect letters as when he ends his report with three or four incorrect letters. Other Ss did not systematically attempt to report incorrect letters first. Had they been required to report incorrect letters first, they might well have been able to do so.

The choice of what part of the stimulus to attend to or of which letters to read is the choice of what fraction of the stimulus information to utilize. This choice can be made successfully only while the information is still available. The Ss prefer to report what they remember first, but this does not imply that they remember it because they report it first. It is difficult to disentangle the many factors that determine precisely what stimulus letters will appear in the response, but important choices of what information is to be recalled must occur while there is still something to choose from. Since the actual report begins only when there are available but a few letters in excess of the immediate-memory span, the order of report can at most play only the minor role of determining which of the few "excess" letters will be forgotten.[15]

The Questions of Generality and Repeatability

To what extent are the results obtained limited to the particular conditions of the foregoing experiments? The possibility that the actual physical fading of the light source is important to the availability of information can be rejected not only on prior grounds (see Apparatus) but also by the empirical findings. For example, in figure 22.9, the curve representing the number of letters available 0.15 s after exposure is quite similar to the 0.0-s delay curve. There is no visible energy emitted by the light source 0.15 s after its termination.

In the present case, the answer to the problem of repeatability of the results is made less speculative by three separate investigations that have since been conducted with similar techniques to those reported here.

The experiments have been repeated by the author[16] with a different tachistoscope, timer, and a light source that has only a negligible afterglow. All the main findings were reproducible.

Klemmer and Loftus (1958) confirmed the existence of a short-term, high information storage. They used a display consisting of four discrete line patterns, the S being required to report only one of these. The instruction was coded either as a signal light or verbally. Decay curves obtained when the instruction is delayed are similar to those reported above. A similar experiment has also been conducted by Averbach,[17] who used a television tachistoscope to present stimuli containing up to 16 letters. A pointer appeared above the letter to be reported. Initially, Ss had about twelve letters available for report, but the number decreased rapidly when the visual instruction was delayed.

It is usually technically more difficult to code instructions visually than acoustically. Although the principle of sampling in order to determine available information is common to both kinds of instructions, visually coded instructions differ in some interesting ways from acoustically coded instructions. For example, the time taken to "interpret"—or even to find—a visual instruction may well depend on its location relative to the fixation point. Moreover, there may be spatial interactions between the visual "instruction" and the symbols to be reported. On the other hand, prior to training, the task of interpreting a visual marker is easier for Ss than the equivalent task with an acoustically coded instruction. Ultimately, such differences are probably only of secondary importance since the two kinds of experiments agree quite well.

Three main findings emerge from the experiments reported here: a large amount of information becomes available to observers of a brief visual presentation, this information decays rapidly, the final level is approximately equal to the span of immediate memory. Although the exact, quantitative aspects of information that becomes available following a brief exposure unquestionably depend upon the precise conditions of presentation, it seems fair to conclude that the main results can be duplicated even under vastly different circumstances in different laboratories.

Summary and Conclusions

When stimuli consisting of a number of items are shown briefly to an observer, only a limited number of the items can be correctly reported.

This number defines the so-called span of immediate memory. The fact that observers commonly assert that they can *see* more than they can *report* suggests that memory sets a limit on a process that is otherwise rich in available information. In the present studies, a sampling procedure (partial report) was used to circumvent the limitation imposed by immediate memory and thereby to show that at the time of exposure, and for a few tenths of a second thereafter, observers have two or three times as much information available as they can later report. The availability of this information declines rapidly, and within one second after the exposure the available information no longer exceeds the memory span.

Short-term information storage has been tentatively identified with the persistence of sensation that generally follows any brief, intense stimulation. In this case, the persistence is that of a rapidly fading, visual image of the stimulus. Evidence in support of this hypothesis of visual information storage was found in introspective accounts, in the type of dependence of the accuracy of partial reports upon the visual stimulation, and in an analysis of certain response characteristics. These and related problems were explored in a series of seven experiments.

An attempt was first made to show that the span of immediate memory remains relatively invariant under a wide range of conditions. Five practiced observers were shown stimuli consisting of arrays of symbols that varied in number, arrangement, and composition (letters alone, or letters and numbers together). It was found (experiments 1 and 2) that each observer was able to report only a limited number of symbols (for example, letters) correctly. For exposure durations from 15 to 500 ms, the average was slightly over four letters; stimuli having four or fewer letters were reported correctly nearly 100% of the time.

In order to circumvent the immediate-memory limit on the (whole) report of what has been seen, observers were required to report only a part—designated by location—of stimuli exposed for 50 ms (partial report). The part to be reported, usually one out of three rows of letters, was small enough (three to four letters) to lie within the memory span. A tonal signal (high, middle, or low frequency) was used to indicate which of the rows was to be reported. The S did not know which signal to expect, and the indicator signal was not given until after the visual stimulus had been turned off. In this manner, the information available to the S was sampled immediately after termination of the stimulus.

Each observer, for each material tested (6, 8, 9, 12 symbols), gave partial reports that were more accurate than whole reports for the same material. For example, following the exposure of stimuli consisting of 12 symbols, 76% of the letters called for in the partial report were given correctly by the observers. This accuracy indicates that the total information available from which an observer can draw his partial report is about 9.1 letters (76% of 12 letters). This number of randomly chosen letters is equivalent to 40.6 bits of information, which is considerably more information than previous experimental estimates have suggested can become available in a brief exposure. Furthermore, it seems probable that the 40-bit information capacity observed in these experiments was limited by the small amount of information in the stimuli rather than by a capacity of the observers.

In order to determine how the available information decreases with time, the instruction signal, which indicated the row of the stimulus to be reported, was delayed by various amounts, up to 1.0 s (experiment 4). The accuracy of the partial report was shown to be a sharply decreasing function of the delay in the instruction signal. Since, at a delay of 1.0 s, the accuracy of the partial reports approached that of the whole reports, it follows that the information in excess of the immediate-memory span is available for less than a second. In contrast to the partial report, the accuracy of the whole report is not a function of the time at which the signal to report is given (experiment 7).

The large amount of information in excess of the immediate-memory span, and the short time during which this information is available, suggests that it may be stored as a persistence of the sensation resulting from the visual stimulus. In order to explore further this possibility of visual information storage, some parameters of visual stimulation were studied. A decrease of the exposure duration from 50 to 15 ms did not substantially affect the accuracy of partial reports (experiment 5). On the other hand, the substitution of a white post-exposure field for the dark field ordinarily used greatly reduced the accuracy of both partial and whole reports. The ability of a homogeneous visual stimulus to affect the available information is evidence that the process depends on a persisting visual image of the stimulus.

Whether other kinds of partial reports give similar estimates of the amount of available information was examined by asking observers to report by category rather than by location. The observer reported numbers only (or the letters only) from stimuli consisting of both letters and numbers (experiment 6). These partial reports were no more accurate than (whole) reports of all the letters and numbers. The ability of observers to give highly accurate partial reports of letters designated by location (experiment 3), and their inability to give partial reports of comparable accuracy when the symbols to be reported are designated as either letters or numbers, clearly indicates that all kinds of partial reports are not equally suitable for demonstrating the ability of observers to retain large amounts of information for short time periods.

In the final study (experiment 7), the order of report was systematically varied. Observers were instructed to get as many letters correct as possible, but the order in which they were to report the letters was not indicated until after the exposure. An instruction tone, following the exposure, indicated which of the two rows of letters on the stimulus was to be reported first. This interference with the normal order of report reduced only slightly the total number of letters that were reported correctly. As might be expected, the first row—the row indicated by the instruction tone—was reported more accurately than the second row (order effect). There was, however, a strong tendency for the top row to be reported more accurately than the bottom row (position effect). Although, as a group, the observers showed both effects, some failed to show either the order or the position effect, or both. The fact that, for some observers, order and position are not correlated with response accuracy suggests that order of report, and position, are not the major *causes* of, nor the necessary conditions for, response accuracy. The high accuracy of partial report observed in the experiments does not depend on the order of report or on the position of letters on the stimulus, but rather it is shown to depend on the ability of the observer to read a visual image that persists for a fraction of a second after the stimulus has been turned off.

Acknowledgments

This paper is a condensation of a doctoral thesis (Sperling 1959). For further details, especially on methodology, and for individual data, the reader is referred to the original thesis. It is a pleasure to acknowledge my gratitude to George A. Miller and Roger N. Shepard whose support made this research possible and to E. B. Newman, J. Schwartzbaum and S. S. Stevens for their many helpful suggestions. Thanks are also due to Jerome S. Bruner for the use of his laboratory and his tachistoscope during his absence in the summer of 1957. This research was carried out under Contract AF 33(038)-14343 between Harvard University and the Operational Applications Laboratory, Air Force Cambridge Research Center, Air Research Development Command.

Notes

1. Some representative examples are Bridgin 1933, Cattell 1883, Chapman 1930, Dallenbach 1920, Erdmann and Dodge 1898, Glanville and Dallenbach 1929, Külpe 1904, Schumann 1922, Wagner 1918, Whipple 1914, Wilcocks 1925, and Woodworth 1938.

2. The experiments referred to are (cf. Sperling 1959) Külpe 1904; Wilcocks 1925; Chapman 1932; Long, Henneman, and Reid 1953; Long and Lee 1953a; Long and Lee 1953b; Long, Reid, and Garvey 1954; Lawrence and Coles 1954; Adams 1955; Lawrence and Laberge 1956; and Broadbent 1957a.

3. Ralph Gerbrands Company, 96 Ronald Road, Arlington 74, Massachusetts.

4. If there are a large number of letters in the stimulus, the probability that these same letters will appear somewhere on the response grid, irrespective of position, becomes very high whether or not S has much information about the stimulus. In the limit, the correspondence approaches 100% provided only that the relative frequency of each letter in the response matches its relative frequency of occurrence in the stimulus pack. If the response is scored for both letter *and* position, then the percent guessing correction is independent of changes in stimulus size.

5. See Sperling (1959) for tables giving the numerical values of all points appearing in this and in all other figures.

6. See Sperling (1959) for tables containing individual averages of all trials for each S at each delay of instruction tone: 3/3, 4/4.

7. Increase in variability (with consequent decrement in accuracy and/or speed) is not unusual after difficult conditions. For example, Cohen and Thomas (1957) in a clinically oriented study have reported an exactly analogous "hysteresis" phenomenon in a study of discriminative reaction time. Hysteresis refers to the fact that, when the difficulty of an experimental task is changed, the corresponding change in accuracy of response lags behind the change in task.

8. It takes, on the average, a very large number of trials for S to get 10 consecutive perfect trials even if he has 6 or 7 of 9 letters available or knows with 2/3 probability what the tone will be. Success in this task within a reasonable time limit demands a level of excellence reached only with "equal attention" observing, as judged by the other criteria.

9. This important method was described by Ladd (1899) and James (1890) in their textbooks, but it is no longer well known. Consequently it has been "rediscovered," most recently, by Lindsley and Emmons (1958). Baxt (1871) intended that the bright second

field would interfere with the lingering image of the first (informational) field. Unfortunately, the effect depends in a complex way upon the intensity of the two fields. Derived time values must be used with caution. In some cases the Baxt technique may actually result in no loss of legibility, the second field producing a negative "afterimage" instead of merely interfering with the positive image (cf. footnote 13).

10. Figure 22.11 is based upon a suggestion by E. B. Newman. A statistical analysis of variance was not attempted since it would have had to be carried out separately on each S. There was not enough data to make this worthwhile, and figure 22.11 serves the same purpose.

11. Measurements of the persistence of sensation have almost invariably used techniques which have at most questionable validity. Wundt's method depends upon masking, the effect of the persisting stimulus upon another stimulus. The masking power of a stimulus may be quite different from its visibility. McDougall's measurements, as well as those cited by Piéron, depend upon motion of a stimulus across the retina. Such measurements are undoubtedly influenced by the strong temporal and spatial interactions of the eye (Alpern 1953). Schumann's ingenious application of the method of Baxt to the determination of persistence is probably the only experiment that utilizes pattern stimulation. The other methods have not been tried with pattern stimuli although there is, a priori, no good reason why they have not been. The possibility that the persistence of pattern information is quite different from persistence of "brightness" has not been investigated.

12. Summarized in Luce 1956.

13. Bidwell (1897) and Sperling (1960) describe conditions for seeing a negative "afterimage without prior positive image." The method involves a presentation quite similar to that of Baxt (1871).

14. Sperling, G. Unpublished experiments conducted at the Bell Telephone Laboratories, 1958.

15. There are many ways in which proactive interference might occur. For example, if letters are stored "sequentially" prior to report (see Broadbent 1957b), then the importance of order of report may lie in the agreement of the two sequences: storage and report.

16. Sperling, G. Unpublished experiments conducted at the Bell Telephone Laboratories, 1958.

17. Averbach, E. Unpublished experiments conducted at the Bell Telephone Laboratories, 1959.

References

Adams, J. S. The relative effectiveness of pre- and poststimulus setting as a function of stimulus uncertainty. Unpublished master's dissertation, Department of Psychology, University of North Carolina, 1955.

Alpern, M. Metacontrast. *J. Opt. Soc. Amer.*, 1953, 43, 648–657.

Baxt, N. Über die Zeit welche nötig ist damit ein Gesichtseindruck zum Bewusstsein kommt und über die Grösse (Extension) der bewussten Wahrnehmung bei einem Gesichtseindrucke von gegebener Dauer. *Pflüger's Arch. ges. Physiol.*, 1871, 4, 325–336.

Berry, W., and Imus, H. Quantitative aspects of the flight of colors. *Amer. J. Psychol.*, 1935, 47, 449–457.

Bidwell, S. On the negative after-images following brief retinal excitation. *Proc. Roy. Soc. Lond.*, 1897, 61, 268–271.

Bridgin, R. L. A tachistoscopic study of the differentiation of perception. *Psychol. Monogr.*, 1933, 44 (1, Whole No. 197), 153–166.

Broadbent, D. E. Immediate memory and simultaneous stimuli. *Quart. J. exp. Psychol.*, 1957, 9, 1–11. (a)

Broadbent, D. E. A mechanical model for human attention and memory. *Psychol. Rev.*, 1957, 64, 205–215. (b)

Broadbent, D. E. *Perception and communication.* New York: Pergamon, 1958.

Cattell, J. M. Über die Trägheit der Netzhaut und des Sehcentrums. *Phil. Stud.*, 1883, 3, 94–127.

Chapman, D. W. The comparative effects of determinate and indeterminate aufgaben. Unpublished doctor's dissertation, Harvard University, 1930.

Chapman, D. W. Relative effects of determinate and indeterminate "Aufgaben." *Amer. J. Psychol.*, 1932, 44, 163–174.

Cohen, L. D., and Thomas, D. R. Decision and motor components of reaction time as a function of anxiety level and task complexity. *Amer. Psychologist*, 1957, 12, 420. (Abstract).

Dallenbach, K. M. Attributive vs. cognitive clearness. *J. exp. Psychol.*, 1920, 3, 183–230.

Diefendorf, A. R., and Dodge, R. An experimental study of the ocular reactions of the insane from photographic records. *Brain*, 1908, 31, 451–489.

Dodge, R. An experimental study of visual fixation. *Psychol. Monogr.*, 1907, 8 (4, Whole No. 35). (a)

Dodge, R. An improved exposure apparatus. *Psychol. Bull.*, 1907, 4, 10–13. (b)

Erdmann, B., and Dodge, R. *Psychologische Untersuchungen über das Lesen auf experimenteller Grundlage.* Halle: Niemeyer, 1898.

Glanville, A. D., and Dallenbach, K. M. The range of attention. *Amer. J. Psychol.*, 1929, 41, 207–236.

Goldiamond, I. Operant analysis of perceptual behavior. Paper read at Symposium on Experimental Analysis of Behavior, APA Annual Convention, 1957.

James, W. *The principles of psychology.* New York: Holt, 1890.

Klemmer, E. T. Simple reaction time as a function of time uncertainty. *J. exp. Psychol.*, 1957, 54, 195–200.

Klemmer, E. T., and Loftus, J. P. *Numerals, nonsense forms, and information.* USAF Cambridge Research Center, Operational Applications Laboratory, Bolling Air Force Base, 1958. (Astia Doc. No. AD110063)

Külpe, O. Versuche über Abstraktion. In, *Bericht über den erste Kongress für experimentelle Psychologie.* Leipzig: Barth, 1904. Pp. 56–68.

Ladd, G. T. *Elements of physiological psychology: A treatise of the activities and nature of the mind.* New York: Scribner, 1889.

Lawrence, D. H., and Coles, G. R. Accuracy of recognition with alternatives before and after the stimulus. *J. exp. Psychol.*, 1954, 47, 208–214.

Lawrence, D. H., and Laberge, D. L. Relationship between accuracy and order of reporting stimulus dimensions. *J. exp. Psychol.*, 1956, 51, 12–18.

Lindsley, D. B., and Emmons, W. H. Perception time and evoked potentials. *Science*, 1958, 127, 1061.

Long, E. R., Henneman, R. H., and Reid, L. S. Theoretical considerations and exploratory investigation of "set" as response restriction: The first of a series of reports on "set" as a determiner of perceptual responses. *USAF WADC tech. Rep.*, 1953, No. 53–311.

Long, E. R., and Lee, W. A. The influence of specific stimulus cuing on location responses: The third of a series of reports on "set" as a determiner of perceptual responses. *USAF WADC tech. Rep.*, 1953, No. 53–314. (a)

Long, E. R., and Lee, W. A. The role of spatial cuing as a response-limiter for location responses: The second of a series of reports on "set" as a determiner of perceptual responses. *USAF WADC tech. Rep.*, 1953, No. 53–312. (b)

Long, E. R., Reid, L. D., and Garvey, W. D. The role of stimulus ambiguity and degree of response restriction in the recognition of distorted letter patterns: The fourth of a series of reports on "set" as a determiner of perceptual responses. *USAF WADC tech. Rep.*, 1954, No. 54–147.

Luce, D. R. *A survey of the theory of selective information and some of its behavioral applications.* New York: Bureau of Applied Social Research, 1956.

McDougall, W. The sensations excited by a single momentary stimulation of the eye. *Brit. J. Psychol.*, 1904, 1, 78–113.

Miller, G. A. Human memory and the storage of information. *IRE Trans. Information Theory*, 1956, IT-2, No. 3, 129–137. (a)

Miller, G. A. The magic number seven, plus or minus two: Some limits on our capacity for processing information. *Psychol. Rev.*, 1956, 63, 81–97. (b)

Miller, G. A., and Nicely, P. E. An analysis of perceptual confusions among some English consonants. *J. Acoust. Soc. Amer.*, 1955, 27, 338–352.

Piéron, H. L'évanouissement de la sensation lumineuse: Persistance indifferenciable et persistance totale. *Ann. psychol.*, 1934, 35, 1–49.

Pollack, I. The assimilation of sequentially encoded information. *Hum. Resources Res. Lab. memo Rep.*, 1952, No. 25.

Pritchard, R. M. Visual illusions viewed as stabilized retinal images. *Quart. J. exp. Psychol.*, 1958, 10, 77–81.

Quastler, H. Studies of human channel capacity. In H. Quastler, *Three survey papers.* Urbana, Ill.: Control Systems Laboratory, Univer. Illinois, 1956. Pp. 13–33.

Schumann, F. Die Erkennung von Buchstaben und Worten bei momentaner Beleuchtigung. In, *Bericht über den erste Kongress für experimentelle Psychologie.* Leipzig: Barth, 1904. Pp. 34–40.

Schumann, F. The Erkennungsurteil. *Z. Psychol.*, 1922, 88, 205–224.

Sperling, G. Information available in a brief visual presentation. Unpublished doctor's dissertation, Department of Psychology, Harvard University, 1959.

Sperling, G. Afterimage without prior image. *Science*, 1960, 131, 1613–1614.

von Helmholtz, H. *Treatise on physiological optics.* Vol. II. *The sensations of vision.* (Transl. from 3rd German ed.) Rochester, New York: Optical Society of America, 1924–25.

Wagner, J. Experimentelle Beitrage zur Psychologie des Lesens. *Z. Psychol.*, 1918, 80, 1–75.

Weyer, E. M. The Zeitschwellen gleichartiger und disparater Sinneseindrucke. *Phil. Stud.*, 1899, 15, 68–138.

Whipple, G. M. *Manual of physical and mental tests.* Vol. I. *Simpler processes.* Baltimore: Warwick & York, 1914.

Wilcocks, R. W. An examination of Külpe's experiments on abstraction. *Amer. J. Psychol.*, 1925, 36, 324–340.

Woodworth, R. S. *Experimental psychology.* New York: Holt, 1938.

Wundt, W. Zur Kritik tachistosckopischer Versuche. *Phil. Stud.* 1899, 15, 287–317.

Wundt, W. *An introduction to psychology.* London: Allen & Unwin, 1912.

The Magical Number Seven, Plus or Minus Two: Some Limits on Our Capacity for Processing Information

George A. Miller

My problem is that I have been persecuted by an integer. For seven years this number has followed me around, has intruded in my most private data, and has assaulted me from the pages of our most public journals. This number assumes a variety of disguises, being sometimes a little larger and sometimes a little smaller than usual, but never changing so much as to be unrecognizable. The persistence with which this number plagues me is far more than a random accident. There is, to quote a famous senator, a design behind it, some pattern governing its appearances. Either there really is something unusual about the number or else I am suffering from delusions of persecution.

I shall begin my case history by telling you about some experiments that tested how accurately people can assign numbers to the magnitudes of various aspects of a stimulus. In the traditional language of psychology these would be called experiments in absolute judgment. Historical accident, however, has decreed that they should have another name. We now call them experiments on the capacity of people to transmit information. Since these experiments would not have been done without the appearance of information theory on the psychological scene, and since the results are analyzed in terms of the concepts of information theory, I shall have to preface my discussion with a few remarks about this theory.

Information Measurement

The "amount of information" is exactly the same concept that we have talked about for years under the name of "variance." The equations are different, but if we hold tight to the idea that anything that increases the variance also increases the amount of information we cannot go far astray.

The advantages of this new way of talking about variance are simple enough. Variance is always stated in terms of the unit of measurement—inches, pounds, volts, and so on—whereas the amount of information is a dimensionless quantity. Since the information in a discrete statistical distribution does not depend upon the unit of measurement, we can extend the concept to situations where we have no metric and we would not ordinarily think of using the variance. And it also enables us to compare results obtained in quite different experimental situations where it would be meaningless to compare variances based on different metrics. So there are some good reasons for adopting the newer concept.

The similarity of variance and amount of information might be explained this way: When we have a large variance, we are very ignorant about what is going to happen. If we are very ignorant, then when we make the observation it gives us a lot of information. On the other hand, if the variance is very small, we know in advance how our observation must come out, so we get little information from making the observation.

If you will now imagine a communication system, you will realize that there is a great deal of variability about what goes into the system and also a great deal of variability about what comes out. The input and the output can therefore be described in terms of their variance (or their information). If it is a good communication system, however, there must be some systematic relation between what goes in and what comes out. That is to say, the output will depend upon the input, or will be correlated with the input. If we measure this correlation, then we can say how much of the output variance is attributable to the input and how much is due to random fluctuations or "noise" introduced by the system during transmission. So we see that the measure of transmitted information is simply a measure of the input-output correlation.

There are two simple rules to follow. Whenever I refer to "amount of information," you will understand "variance." And whenever I refer to "amount of transmitted information," you will understand "covariance" or "correlation."

The situation can be described graphically by two partially overlapping circles. Then the left circle can be taken to represent the variance of the input, the right circle the variance of the output, and the overlap the covariance of input and output. I shall speak of the left circle as the amount of input information, the right circle as the amount of output information, and the overlap as the amount of transmitted information.

In the experiments on absolute judgment, the observer is considered to be a communication channel. Then the left circle would represent the amount of information in the stimuli, the right circle the amount of information in his responses, and the overlap the stimulus-response correlation as measured by the amount of transmitted information. The experimental problem is to increase the amount of input information and to measure the amount of transmitted information. If the observer's absolute judgments are quite accurate, then nearly all of the input information will be transmitted and will be recoverable from his responses. If he makes errors, then the transmitted information may be considerably less than the input. We expect that, as we increase the amount of input information, the observer will begin to make more and more errors; we can test the limits of accuracy of his absolute judgments. If the human observer is a reasonable kind of communication system, then when we increase the amount of input information the transmitted information will increase at first and will eventually level off at some asymptotic value. This asymptotic value we take to be the *channel capacity* of the observer: it represents the greatest amount of information that he can give us about the stimulus on the basis of an absolute judgment. The channel capacity is the upper limit on the extent to which the observer can match his responses to the stimuli we give him.

Now just a brief word about the *bit* and we can begin to look at some data. One bit of information is the amount of information that we need to make a decision between two equally likely alternatives. If we must decide whether a man is less than six feet tall or more than six feet tall and if we know that the chances are 50–50, then we need one bit of information. Notice that this unit of information does not refer in any way to the unit of length that we use—feet, inches, centimeters, and so on. However you measure the man's height, we still need just one bit of information.

Two bits of information enable us to decide among four equally likely alternatives. Three bits of information enable us to decide among eight equally likely alternatives. Four bits of information decide among 16 alternatives, five among 32, and so on. That is to say, if there are 32 equally likely alternatives, we must make five successive binary decisions, worth one bit each, before we know which alternative is correct. So the general rule is simple: every time the number of alternatives is increased by a factor of two, one bit of information is added.

There are two ways we might increase the amount of input information. We could increase the rate at which we give information to the observer, so that the amount of information per unit time would increase. Or we could ignore the time variable completely and increase the amount of input information by increasing the number of alternative stimuli. In the absolute judgment experiment we are interested in the second alternative. We give the observer as much time as he wants to make his response; we simply increase the number of alternative stimuli among which he must discriminate and look to see where confusions begin to occur. Confusions will appear near the point that we are calling his "channel capacity."

Absolute Judgments of Unidimensional Stimuli

Now let us consider what happens when we make absolute judgments of tones. Pollack (17) asked listeners to identify tones by assigning numerals to them. The tones were different with respect to frequency, and covered the range from 100 to 8000 cps in equal logarithmic steps. A tone was sounded and the listener responded by giving a numeral. After the listener had made his response he was told the correct identification of the tone.

When only two or three tones were used the listeners never confused them. With four different tones confusions were quite rare, but with five or more tones confusions were frequent. With fourteen different tones the listeners made many mistakes.

These data are plotted in figure 23.1. Along the bottom is the amount of input information in bits per stimulus. As the number of alternative tones was increased from 2 to 14, the input in-formation increased from 1 to 3.8 bits. On the ordinate is plotted the amount of transmitted information. The amount of transmitted information behaves in much the way we would expect a communication channel to behave; the transmitted information increases linearly up to about 2 bits and then bends off toward an asymptote at about 2.5 bits. This value, 2.5 bits, therefore, is what we are calling the channel capacity of the listener for absolute judgments of pitch.

So now we have the number 2.5 bits. What does it mean? First, note that 2.5 bits corresponds to about six equally likely alternatives. The result means that we cannot pick more than six different pitches that the listener will never confuse. Or, stated slightly differently, no matter how many alternative tones we ask him to judge, the best we can expect him to do is to assign them to about six different classes without error. Or, again, if we know that there were N alternative stimuli, then his judgment enables us to narrow down the particular stimulus to one out of $N/6$.

Most people are surprised that the number is as small as six. Of course, there is evidence that a musically sophisticated person with absolute pitch can identify accurately any one of 50 or 60 different pitches. Fortunately, I do not have time to discuss these remarkable exceptions. I say it is fortunate because I do not know how to explain their superior performance. So I shall stick to the more pedestrian fact that most of us can identify about one out of only five or six pitches before we begin to get confused.

It is interesting to consider that psychologists have been using seven-point rating scales for a long time, on the intuitive basis that trying to rate into finer categories does not really add much to the usefulness of the ratings. Pollack's results indicate that, at least for pitches, this intuition is fairly sound.

Next you can ask how reproducible this result is. Does it depend on the spacing of the tones or the various conditions of judgment? Pollack varied these conditions in a number of ways. The

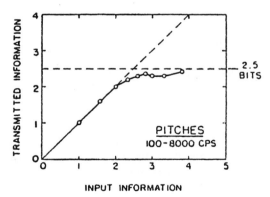

Figure 23.1
Data from Pollack (17, 18) on the amount of information that is transmitted by listeners who make absolute judgments of auditory pitch. As the amount of input information is increased by increasing from 2 to 14 the number of different pitches to be judged, the amount of transmitted information approaches as its upper limit a channel capacity of about 2.5 bits per judgment.

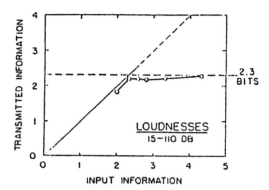

Figure 23.2
Data from Garner (7) on the channel capacity for absolute judgments of auditory loudness.

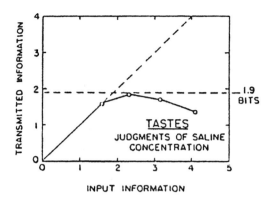

Figure 23.3
Data from Beebe-Center, Rogers, and O'Connell (1) on the channel capacity for absolute judgments of saltiness.

range of frequencies can be changed by a factor of about 20 without changing the amount of information transmitted more than a small percentage. Different groupings of the pitches decreased the transmission, but the loss was small. For example, if you can discriminate five high-pitched tones in one series and five low-pitched tones in another series, it is reasonable to expect that you could combine all ten into a single series and still tell them all apart without error. When you try it, however, it does not work. The channel capacity for pitch seems to be about six and that is the best you can do.

While we are on tones, let us look next at Garner's (7) work on loudness. Garner's data for loudness are summarized in figure 23.2. Garner went to some trouble to get the best possible spacing of his tones over the intensity range from 15 to 110 db. He used 4, 5, 6, 7, 10, and 20 different stimulus intensities. The results shown in figure 23.2 take into account the differences among subjects and the sequential influence of the immediately preceding judgment. Again we find that there seems to be a limit. The channel capacity for absolute judgments of loudness is 2.3 bits, or about five perfectly discriminable alternatives.

Since these two studies were done in different laboratories with slightly different techniques and methods of analysis, we are not in a good position to argue whether five loudnesses is significantly different from six pitches. Probably the difference is in the right direction, and absolute judgments of pitch are slightly more accurate than absolute judgments of loudness. The important point, however, is that the two answers are of the same order of magnitude.

The experiment has also been done for taste intensities. In figure 23.3 are the results obtained by Beebe-Center, Rogers, and O'Connell (1) for absolute judgments of the concentration of salt solutions. The concentrations ranged from 0.3 to 34.7 gm. NaCl per 100 cc. tap water in equal subjective steps. They used 3, 5, 9, and 17 different concentrations. The channel capacity is 1.9 bits, which is about four distinct concentrations. Thus taste intensities seem a little less distinctive than auditory stimuli, but again the order of magnitude is not far off.

On the other hand, the channel capacity for judgments of visual position seems to be significantly larger. Hake and Garner (8) asked observers to interpolate visually between two scale

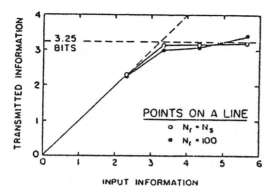

Figure 23.4
Data from Hake and Garner (8) on the channel capacity for absolute judgments of the position of a pointer in a linear interval.

markers. Their results are shown in figure 23.4. They did the experiment in two ways. In one version they let the observer use any number between zero and 100 to describe the position, although they presented stimuli at only 5, 10, 20, or 50 different positions. The results with this unlimited response technique are shown by the filled circles on the graph. In the other version the observers were limited in their responses to reporting just those stimulus values that were possible. That is to say, in the second version the number of different responses that the observer could make was exactly the same as the number of different stimuli that the experimenter might present. The results with this limited response technique are shown by the open circles on the graph. The two functions are so similar that it seems fair to conclude that the number of responses available to the observer had nothing to do with the channel capacity of 3.25 bits.

The Hake-Garner experiment has been repeated by Coonan and Klemmer. Although they have not yet published their results, they have given me permission to say that they obtained channel capacities ranging from 3.2 bits for very short exposures of the pointer position to 3.9 bits

for longer exposures. These values are slightly higher than Hake and Garner's, so we must conclude that there are between 10 and 15 distinct positions along a linear interval. This is the largest channel capacity that has been measured for any unidimensional variable.

At the present time these four experiments on absolute judgments of simple, unidimensional stimuli are all that have appeared in the psychological journals. However, a great deal of work on other stimulus variables has not yet appeared in the journals. For example, Eriksen and Hake (6) have found that the channel capacity for judging the sizes of squares is 2.2 bits, or about five categories, under a wide range of experimental conditions. In a separate experiment Eriksen (5) found 2.8 bits for size, 3.1 bits for hue, and 2.3 bits for brightness. Geldard has measured the channel capacity for the skin by placing vibrators on the chest region. A good observer can identify about four intensities, about five durations, and about seven locations.

One of the most active groups in this area has been the Air Force Operational Applications Laboratory. Pollack has been kind enough to furnish me with the results of their measurements for several aspects of visual displays. They made measurements for area and for the curvature, length, and direction of lines. In one set of experiments they used a very short exposure of the stimulus—1/40 s—and then they repeated the measurements with a 5-s exposure. For area they got 2.6 bits with the short exposure and 2.7 bits with the long exposure. For the length of a line they got about 2.6 bits with the short exposure and about 3.0 bits with the long exposure. Direction, or angle of inclination, gave 2.8 bits for the short exposure and 3.3 bits for the long exposure. Curvature was apparently harder to judge. When the length of the arc was constant, the result at the short exposure duration was 2.2 bits, but when the length of the chord was constant, the result was only 1.6 bits. This last value is the lowest that anyone has measured to date. I should add, however, that these values are apt to be slightly too low because the data from all subjects were pooled before the transmitted information was computed.

Now let us see where we are. First, the channel capacity does seem to be a valid notion for describing human observers. Second, the channel capacities measured for these unidimensional variables range from 1.6 bits for curvature to 3.9 bits for positions in an interval. Although there is no question that the differences among the variables are real and meaningful, the more impressive fact to me is their considerable similarity. If I take the best estimates I can get of the channel capacities for all the stimulus variables I have mentioned, the mean is 2.6 bits and the standard deviation is only 0.6 bit. In terms of distinguishable alternatives, this mean corresponds to about 6.5 categories, one standard deviation includes from 4 to 10 categories, and the total range is from 3 to 15 categories. Considering the wide variety of different variables that have been studied, I find this to be a remarkably narrow range.

There seems to be some limitation built into us either by learning or by the design of our nervous systems, a limit that keeps our channel capacities in this general range. On the basis of the present evidence it seems safe to say that we possess a finite and rather small capacity for making such unidimensional judgments and that this capacity does not vary a great deal from one simple sensory attribute to another.

Absolute Judgments of Multidimensional Stimuli

You may have noticed that I have been careful to say that this magical number seven applies to one-dimensional judgments. Everyday experience teaches us that we can identify accurately any one of several hundred faces, any one of several thousand words, any one of several thousand objects, and so forth. The story certainly would not be complete if we stopped at this point. We must have some understanding of

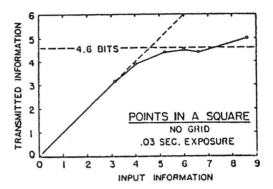

Figure 23.5
Data from Klemmer and Frick (13) on the channel capacity for absolute judgments of the position of a dot in a square.

why the one-dimensional variables we judge in the laboratory give results so far out of line with what we do constantly in our behavior outside the laboratory. A possible explanation lies in the number of independently variable attributes of the stimuli that are being judged. Objects, faces, words, and the like differ from one another in many ways, whereas the simple stimuli we have considered thus far differ from one another in only one respect.

Fortunately, there are a few data on what happens when we make absolute judgments of stimuli that differ from one another in several ways. Let us look first at the results Klemmer and Frick (13) have reported for the absolute judgment of the position of a dot in a square. In figure 23.5 we see their results. Now the channel capacity seems to have increased to 4.6 bits, which means that people can identify accurately any one of 24 positions in the square.

The position of a dot in a square is clearly a two-dimensional proposition. Both its horizontal and its vertical position must be identified. Thus it seems natural to compare the 4.6-bit capacity for a square with the 3.25-bit capacity for the position of a point in an interval. The point in the square requires two judgments of the interval type. If we have a capacity of 3.25 bits for estimating intervals and we do this twice, we should get 6.5 bits as our capacity for locating points in a square. Adding the second independent dimension gives us an increase from 3.25 to 4.6, but it falls short of the perfect addition that would give 6.5 bits.

Another example is provided by Beebe-Center, Rogers, and O'Connell. When they asked people to identify both the saltiness and the sweetness of solutions containing various concentrations of salt and sucrose, they found that the channel capacity was 2.3 bits. Since the capacity for salt alone was 1.9, we might expect about 3.8 bits if the two aspects of the compound stimuli were judged independently. As with spatial locations, the second dimension adds a little to the capacity but not as much as it conceivably might.

A third example is provided by Pollack (18), who asked listeners to judge both the loudness and the pitch of pure tones. Since pitch gives 2.5 bits and loudness gives 2.3 bits, we might hope to get as much as 4.8 bits for pitch and loudness together. Pollack obtained 3.1 bits, which again indicates that the second dimension augments the channel capacity but not so much as it might.

A fourth example can be drawn from the work of Halsey and Chapanis (9) on confusions among colors of equal luminance. Although they did not analyze their results in informational terms, they estimate that there are about 11–15 identifiable colors, or, in our terms, about 3.6 bits. Since these colors varied in both hue and saturation, it is probably correct to regard this as a two-dimensional judgment. If we compare this with Eriksen's 3.1 bits for hue (which is a questionable comparison to draw), we again have something less than perfect addition when a second dimension is added.

It is still a long way, however, from these two-dimensional examples to the multidimensional stimuli provided by faces, words, and so forth. To fill this gap we have only one experiment, an

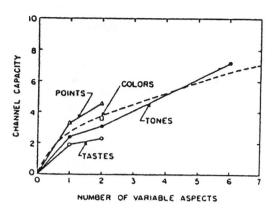

Figure 23.6
The general form of the relation between channel capacity and the number of independently variable attributes of the stimuli.

auditory study done by Pollack and Ficks (19). They managed to get six different acoustic variables that they could change: frequency, intensity, rate of interruption, on-time fraction, total duration, and spatial location. Each one of these six variables could assume any one of five different values, so altogether there were 5^6, or 15,625 different tones that they could present. The listeners made a separate rating for each one of these six dimensions. Under these conditions the transmitted information was 7.2 bits, which corresponds to about 150 different categories that could be absolutely identified without error. Now we are beginning to get up into the range that ordinary experience would lead us to expect.

Suppose that we plot these data, fragmentary as they are, and make a guess about how the channel capacity changes with the dimensionality of the stimuli. The result is given in figure 23.6. In a moment of considerable daring I sketched the dotted line to indicate roughly the trend that the data seemed to be taking.

Clearly, the addition of independently variable attributes to the stimulus increases the channel capacity, but at a decreasing rate. It is interesting to note that the channel capacity is increased even when the several variables are not independent. Eriksen (5) reports that, when size, brightness, and hue all vary together in perfect correlation, the transmitted information is 4.1 bits as compared with an average of about 2.7 bits when these attributes are varied one at a time. By confounding three attributes, Eriksen increased the dimensionality of the input without increasing the amount of input information; the result was an increase in channel capacity of about the amount that the dotted function in figure 23.6 would lead us to expect.

The point seems to be that, as we add more variables to the display, we increase the total capacity, but we decrease the accuracy for any particular variable. In other words, we can make relatively crude judgments of several things simultaneously.

We might argue that in the course of evolution those organisms were most successful that were responsive to the widest range of stimulus energies in their environment. In order to survive in a constantly fluctuating world, it was better to have a little information about a lot of things than to have a lot of information about a small segment of the environment. If a compromise was necessary, the one we seem to have made is clearly the more adaptive.

Pollack and Ficks's results are very strongly suggestive of an argument that linguists and phoneticians have been making for some time (11). According to the linguistic analysis of the sounds of human speech, there are about eight or ten dimensions—the linguists call them *distinctive features*—that distinguish one phoneme from another. These distinctive features are usually binary, or at most ternary, in nature. For example, a binary distinction is made between vowels and consonants, a binary decision is made between oral and nasal consonants, a ternary decision is made among front, middle, and back phonemes, and so on. This approach gives us quite a different picture of speech perception than we might otherwise obtain from our studies of the speech spectrum and of the ear's ability to discriminate relative differences among pure tones. I am personally much interested in this new approach (15), and I regret that there is not time to discuss it here.

It was probably with this linguistic theory in mind that Pollack and Ficks conducted a test on a set of tonal stimuli that varied in eight dimensions, but required only a binary decision on each dimension. With these tones they measured the transmitted information at 6.9 bits, or about 120 recognizable kinds of sounds. It is an intriguing question, as yet unexplored, whether one can go on adding dimensions indefinitely in this way.

In human speech there is clearly a limit to the number of dimensions that we use. In this instance, however, it is not known whether the limit is imposed by the nature of the perceptual machinery that must recognize the sounds or by the nature of the speech machinery that must produce them. Somebody will have to do the experiment to find out. There is a limit, however, at about eight or nine distinctive features in every language that has been studied, and so when we talk we must resort to still another trick for increasing our channel capacity. Language uses sequences of phonemes, so we make several judgments successively when we listen to words and sentences. That is to say, we use both simultaneous and successive discriminations in order to expand the rather rigid limits imposed by the inaccuracy of our absolute judgments of simple magnitudes.

These multidimensional judgments are strongly reminiscent of the abstraction experiment of Külpe (14). As you may remember, Külpe showed that observers report more accurately on an attribute for which they are set than on attributes for which they are not set. For example, Chapman (4) used three different attributes and compared the results obtained when the observers were instructed before the tachistoscopic presentation with the results obtained when they were not told until after the presentation which one of the three attributes was to be reported. When the instruction was given in advance, the judgments were more accurate. When the instruction was given afterwards, the subjects presumably had to judge all three attributes in order to report on any one of them and the accuracy was correspondingly lower. This is in complete accord with the results we have just been considering, where the accuracy of judgment on each attribute decreased as more dimensions were added. The point is probably obvious, but I shall make it anyhow, that the abstraction experiments did *not* demonstrate that people can judge only one attribute at a time. They merely showed what seems quite reasonable, that people are less accurate if they must judge more than one attribute simultaneously.

Subitizing

I cannot leave this general area without mentioning, however briefly, the experiments conducted at Mount Holyoke College on the discrimination of number (12). In experiments by Kaufman, Lord, Reese, and Volkmann random patterns of dots were flashed on a screen for 1/5 of a second. Anywhere from 1 to more than 200 dots could appear in the pattern. The subject's task was to report how many dots there were.

The first point to note is that on patterns containing up to five or six dots the subjects simply did not make errors. The performance on these small numbers of dots was so different from the performance with more dots that it was given a special name. Below seven the subjects were said to *subitize*; above seven they were said to *estimate*. This is, as you will recognize, what we once optimistically called "the span of attention."

This discontinuity at seven is, of course, suggestive. Is this the same basic process that limits our unidimensional judgments to about seven categories? The generalization is tempting, but not sound in my opinion. The data on number

estimates have not been analyzed in informational terms; but on the basis of the published data I would guess that the subjects transmitted something more than four bits of information about the number of dots. Using the same arguments as before, we would conclude that there are about 20 or 30 distinguishable categories of numerousness. This is considerably more information than we would expect to get from a unidimensional display. It is, as a matter of fact, very much like a two-dimensional display. Although the dimensionality of the random dot patterns is not entirely clear, these results are in the same range as Klemmer and Frick's for their two-dimensional display of dots in a square. Perhaps the two dimensions of numerousness are area and density. When the subject can subitize, area and density may not be the significant variables, but when the subject must estimate perhaps they are significant. In any event, the comparison is not so simple as it might seem at first thought.

This is one of the ways in which the magical number seven has persecuted me. Here we have two closely related kinds of experiments, both of which point to the significance of the number seven as a limit on our capacities. And yet when we examine the matter more closely, there seems to be a reasonable suspicion that it is nothing more than a coincidence.

The Span of Immediate Memory

Let me summarize the situation in this way. There is a clear and definite limit to the accuracy with which we can identify absolutely the magnitude of a unidimensional stimulus variable. I would propose to call this limit the *span of absolute judgment*, and I maintain that for unidimensional judgments this span is usually somewhere in the neighborhood of seven. We are not completely at the mercy of this limited span, however, because we have a variety of techniques for getting around it and increasing the accuracy of our judgments. The three most important of these devices are (a) to make relative rather than absolute judgments; or, if that is not possible, (b) to increase the number of dimensions along which the stimuli can differ; or (c) to arrange the task in such a way that we make a sequence of several absolute judgments in a row.

The study of relative judgments is one of the oldest topics in experimental psychology, and I will not pause to review it now. The second device, increasing the dimensionality, we have just considered. It seems that by adding more dimensions and requiring crude, binary, yes-no judgments on each attribute we can extend the span of absolute judgment from 7 to at least 150. Judging from our everyday behavior, the limit is probably in the thousands, if indeed there is a limit. In my opinion, we cannot go on compounding dimensions indefinitely. I suspect that there is also a *span of perceptual dimensionality* and that this span is somewhere in the neighborhood of ten, but I must add at once that there is no objective evidence to support this suspicion. This is a question sadly needing experimental exploration.

Concerning the third device, the use of successive judgments, I have quite a bit to say because this device introduces memory as the handmaiden of discrimination. And, since mnemonic processes are at least as complex as are perceptual processes, we can anticipate that their interactions will not be easily disentangled.

Suppose that we start by simply extending slightly the experimental procedure that we have been using. Up to this point we have presented a single stimulus and asked the observer to name it immediately thereafter. We can extend this procedure by requiring the observer to withhold his response until we have given him several stimuli in succession. At the end of the sequence of stimuli he then makes his response. We still have the same sort of input-output situation that is required for the measurement of transmitted information. But now we have passed from an experiment on absolute judgment to what is traditionally called an experiment on immediate memory.

Before we look at any data on this topic I feel I must give you a word of warning to help you avoid some obvious associations that can be confusing. Everybody knows that there is a finite span of immediate memory and that for a lot of different kinds of test materials this span is about seven items in length. I have just shown you that there is a span of absolute judgment that can distinguish about seven categories and that there is a span of attention that will encompass about six objects at a glance. What is more natural than to think that all three of these spans are different aspects of a single underlying process? And that is a fundamental mistake, as I shall be at some pains to demonstrate. This mistake is one of the malicious persecutions that the magical number seven has subjected me to.

My mistake went something like this. We have seen that the invariant feature in the span of absolute judgment is the amount of information that the observer can transmit. There is a real operational similarity between the absolute judgment experiment and the immediate memory experiment. If immediate memory is like absolute judgment, then it should follow that the invariant feature in the span of immediate memory is also the amount of information that an observer can retain. If the amount of information in the span of immediate memory is a constant, then the span should be short when the individual items contain a lot of information and the span should be long when the items contain little information. For example, decimal digits are worth 3.3 bits apiece. We can recall about seven of them, for a total of 23 bits of information. Isolated English words are worth about 10 bits apiece. If the total amount of information is to remain constant at 23 bits, then we should be able to remember only two or three words chosen at random. In this way I generated a theory about how the span of immediate memory should vary as a function of the amount of information per item in the test materials.

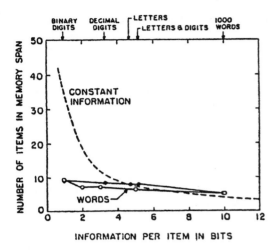

Figure 23.7
Data from Hayes (10) on the span of immediate memory plotted as a function of the amount of information per item in the test materials.

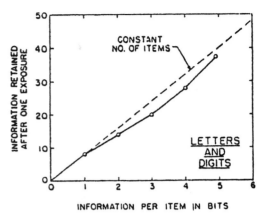

Figure 23.8
Data from Pollack (16) on the amount of information retained after one presentation plotted as a function of the amount of information per item in the test materials.

The measurements of memory span in the literature are suggestive on this question, but not definitive. And so it was necessary to do the experiment to see. Hayes (10) tried it out with five different kinds of test materials: binary digits, decimal digits, letters of the alphabet, letters plus decimal digits, and with 1,000 monosyllabic words. The lists were read aloud at the rate of one item per second and the subjects had as much time as they needed to give their responses. A procedure described by Woodworth (20) was used to score the responses.

The results are shown by the filled circles in figure 23.7. Here the dotted line indicates what the span should have been if the amount of information in the span were constant. The solid curves represent the data. Hayes repeated the experiment using test vocabularies of different sizes but all containing only English monosyllables (open circles in figure 23.7). This more homogeneous test material did not change the picture significantly. With binary items the span

is about nine and, although it drops to about five with monosyllabic English words, the difference is far less than the hypothesis of constant information would require.

There is nothing wrong with Hayes's experiment, because Pollack (16) repeated it much more elaborately and got essentially the same result. Pollack took pains to measure the amount of information transmitted and did not rely on the traditional procedure for scoring the responses. His results are plotted in figure 23.8. Here it is clear that the amount of information transmitted is not a constant, but increases almost linearly as the amount of information per item in the input is increased.

And so the outcome is perfectly clear. In spite of the coincidence that the magical number seven appears in both places, the span of absolute judgment and the span of immediate memory are quite different kinds of limitations that are imposed on our ability to process information. Absolute judgment is limited by the amount of information. Immediate memory is limited by the number of items. In order to capture this distinction in somewhat picturesque terms, I have fallen into the custom of distinguishing between *bits* of information and *chunks* of information. Then I can say that the number of bits of information is constant for absolute judgment and the number of chunks of information is constant for immediate memory. The span of immediate memory seems to be almost independent of the number of bits per chunk, at least over the range that has been examined to date.

The contrast of the terms *bit* and *chunk* also serves to highlight the fact that we are not very definite about what constitutes a chunk of information. For example, the memory span of five words that Hayes obtained when each word was drawn at random from a set of 1000 English monosyllables might just as appropriately have been called a memory span of 15 phonemes, since each word had about three phonemes in it. Intuitively, it is clear that the subjects were recalling five words, not 15 phonemes, but the logical distinction is not immediately apparent. We are dealing here with a process of organizing or grouping the input into familiar units or chunks, and a great deal of learning has gone into the formation of these familiar units.

Recoding

In order to speak more precisely, therefore, we must recognize the importance of grouping or organizing the input sequence into units or chunks. Since the memory span is a fixed number of chunks, we can increase the number of bits of information that it contains simply by building larger and larger chunks, each chunk containing more information than before.

A man just beginning to learn radiotelegraphic code hears each *dit* and *dah* as a separate chunk. Soon he is able to organize these sounds into letters and then he can deal with the letters as chunks. Then the letters organize themselves as words, which are still larges chunks, and he

begins to hear whole phrases. I do not mean that each step is a discrete process, or that plateaus must appear in his learning curve, for surely the levels of organization are achieved at different rates and overlap each other during the learning process. I am simply pointing to the obvious fact that the dits and dahs are organized by learning into patterns and that as these larger chunks emerge the amount of message that the operator can remember increases correspondingly. In the terms I am proposing to use, the operator learns to increase the bits per chunk.

In the jargon of communication theory, this process would be called *recoding*. The input is given in a code that contains many chunks with few bits per chunk. The operator recodes the input into another code that contains fewer chunks with more bits per chunk. There are many ways to do this recoding, but probably the simplest is to group the input events, apply a new name to the group, and then remember the new name rather than the original input events.

Since I am convinced that this process is a very general and important one for psychology, I want to tell you about a demonstration experiment that should make perfectly explicit what I am talking about. This experiment was conducted by Sidney Smith and was reported by him before the Eastern Psychological Association in 1954.

Begin with the observed fact that people can repeat back eight decimal digits, but only nine binary digits. Since there is a large discrepancy in the amount of information recalled in these two cases, we suspect at once that a recoding procedure could be used to increase the span of immediate memory for binary digits. In table 23.1 a method for grouping and renaming is illustrated. Along the top is a sequence of 18 binary digits, far more than any subject was able to recall after a single presentation. In the next line these same binary digits are grouped by pairs. Four possible pairs can occur: 00 is renamed 0, 01 is renamed 1, 10 is renamed 2, and 11 is renamed 3. That is to say, we recode from a base-two arithmetic to

Table 23.1

Ways of recoding sequences of binary digits

Binary Digits (Bits)		1	0	1	0	0	0	1	0	0	1	1	1	0	0	1	1	1	0
2:1	Chunks	10		10		00		10		01		11		00		11		10	
	Recoding	2		2		0		2		1		3		0		3		2	
3:1	Chunks	101			000			100			111			001			110		
	Recoding	5			0			4			7			1			6		
4:1	Chunks	1010				0010				0111				0011				10		
	Recoding	10				2				7				3						
5:1	Chunks	10100					01001					11001					110			
	Recoding	20					9					25								

a basefour arithmetic. In the recoded sequence there are now just nine digits to remember, and this is almost within the span of immediate memory. In the next line the same sequence of binary digits is regrouped into chunks of three. There are eight possible sequences of three, so we give each sequence a new name between 0 and 7. Now we have recoded from a sequence of 18 binary digits into a sequence of 6 octal digits, and this is well within the span of immediate memory. In the last two lines the binary digits are grouped by fours and by fives and are given decimal-digit names from 0 to 15 and from 0 to 31.

It is reasonably obvious that this kind of recoding increases the bits per chunk, and packages the binary sequence into a form that can be retained within the span of immediate memory. So Smith assembled 20 subjects and measured their spans for binary and octal digits. The spans were 9 for binaries and 7 for octals. Then he gave each recoding scheme to five of the subjects. They studied the recoding until they said they understood it—for about 5 or 10 minutes. Then he tested their span for binary digits again while they tried to use the recoding schemes they had studied.

The recoding schemes increased their span for binary digits in every case. But the increase was not as large as we had expected on the basis of their span for octal digits. Since the discrepancy increased as the recoding ratio increased, we reasoned that the few minutes the subjects had spent learning the recoding schemes had not been sufficient. Apparently the translation from one code to the other must be almost automatic or the subject will lose part of the next group while he is trying to remember the translation of the last group.

Since the 4:1 and 5:1 ratios require considerable study, Smith decided to imitate Ebbinghaus and do the experiment on himself. With Germanic patience he drilled himself on each recoding successively, and obtained the results shown in figure 23.9. Here the data follow along rather nicely with the results you would predict on the basis of his span for octal digits. He could remember 12 octal digits. With the 2:1 recoding, these 12 chunks were worth 24 binary digits. With the 3:1 recoding they were worth 36 binary digits. With the 4:1 and 5:1 recodings, they were worth about 40 binary digits.

It is a little dramatic to watch a person get 40 binary digits in a row and then repeat them back without error. However, if you think of this merely as a mnemonic trick for extending the memory span, you will miss the more important point that is implicit in nearly all such mnemonic devices. The point is that recoding is an extremely powerful weapon for increasing the

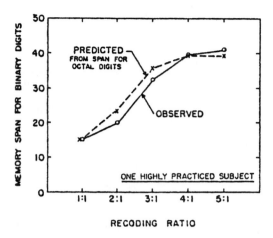

Figure 23.9
The span of immediate memory for binary digits is plotted as a function of the recoding procedure used. The predicted function is obtained by multiplying the span for octals by 2, 3, and 3.3 for recoding into base 4, base 8, and base 10, respectively.

amount of information that we can deal with. In one form or another we use recoding constantly in our daily behavior.

In my opinion the most customary kind of recoding that we do all the time is to translate into a verbal code. When there is a story or an argument or an idea that we want to remember, we usually try to rephrase it "in our own words." When we witness some event we want to remember, we make a verbal description of the event and then remember our verbalization. Upon recall we recreate by secondary elaboration the details that seem consistent with the particular verbal recoding we happen to have made. The well-known experiment by Carmichael, Hogan, and Walter (3) on the influence that names have on the recall of visual figures is one demonstration of the process.

The inaccuracy of the testimony of eyewitnesses is well known in legal psychology, but the distortions of testimony are not random—they follow naturally from the particular recoding that the witness used, and the particular recoding he used depends upon his whole life history. Our language is tremendously useful for repackaging material into a few chunks rich in information. I suspect that imagery is a form of recoding, too, but images seem much harder to get at operationally and to study experimentally than the more symbolic kinds of recoding.

It seems probable that even memorization can be studied in these terms. The process of memorizing may be simply the formation of chunks, or groups of items that go together, until there are few enough chunks so that we can recall all the items. The work by Bousfield and Cohen (2) on the occurrence of clustering in the recall of words is especially interesting in this respect.

Summary

I have come to the end of the data that I wanted to present, so I would like now to make some summarizing remarks.

First, the span of absolute judgment and the span of immediate memory impose severe limitations on the amount of information that we are able to receive, process, and remember. By organizing the stimulus input simultaneously into several dimensions and successively into a sequence of chunks, we manage to break (or at least stretch) this informational bottleneck.

Second, the process of recoding is a very important one in human psychology and deserves much more explicit attention than it has received. In particular, the kind of linguistic recoding that people do seems to me to be the very lifeblood of the thought processes. Recoding procedures are a constant concern to clinicians, social psychologists, linguists, and anthropologists and yet, probably because recoding is less accessible to experimental manipulation than nonsense syllables or T mazes, the traditional experimental psychologist has contributed little or nothing to their analysis. Nevertheless, experimental techniques can be used, methods of recoding can be specified, behavioral indicants can be found. And I anticipate that we will find a very orderly set of relations describing what now seems an uncharted wilderness of individual differences.

Third, the concepts and measures provided by the theory of information provide a quantitative way of getting at some of these questions. The theory provides us with a yardstick for calibrating our stimulus materials and for measuring the performance of our subjects. In the interests of communication I have suppressed the technical details of information measurement and have tried to express the ideas in more familiar terms; I hope this paraphrase will not lead you to think they are not useful in research. Informational concepts have already proved valuable in the study of discrimination and of language; they promise a great deal in the study of learning and memory; and it has even been proposed that they can be useful in the study of concept formation. A lot of questions that seemed fruitless twenty or thirty years ago may now be worth another look. In fact, I feel that my story here must stop just as it begins to get really interesting.

And finally, what about the magical number seven? What about the seven wonders of the world, the seven seas, the seven deadly sins, the seven daughters of Atlas in the Pleiades, the seven ages of man, the seven levels of hell, the seven primary colors, the seven notes of the musical scale, and the seven days of the week? What about the seven-point rating scale, the seven categories for absolute judgment, the seven objects in the span of attention, and the seven digits in the span of immediate memory? For the present I propose to withhold judgment. Perhaps there is something deep and profound behind all these sevens, something just calling out for us to discover it. But I suspect that it is only a pernicious, Pythagorean coincidence.

Acknowledgments

This paper was first read as an Invited Address before the Eastern Psychological Association in Philadelphia on April 15, 1955. Preparation of the paper was supported by the Harvard Psycho-Acoustic Laboratory under Contract N5ori-76 between Harvard University and the Office of Naval Research, U. S. Navy (Project NR142-201, Report PRN-174). Reproduction for any purpose of the U. S. Government is permitted.

References

1. Beebe-Center, J. G., Rogers, M. S., and O'Connell, D. N. Transmission of information about sucrose and saline solutions through the sense of taste. *J. Psychol.*, 1955, 39, 157–160.

2. Bousfield, W. A., and Cohen, B. H. The occurrence of clustering in the recall of randomly arranged words of different frequencies-of-usage. *J. gen. Psychol.*, 1955, 52, 83–95.

3. Carmichael, L., Hogan, H. P., and Walter, A. A. An experimental study of the effect of language on the reproduction of visually perceived form. *J. exp. Psychol.*, 1932, 15, 73–86.

4. Chapman, D. W. Relative effects of determinate and indeterminate *Aufgaben, Amer. J. Psychol.*, 1932, 44, 163–174.

5. Eriksen, C. W. Multidimensional stimulus differences and accuracy of discrimination. *USAF, WADC Tech, Rep.*, 1954, No. 54–165.

6. Eriksen, C. W., and Hake, H. W. Absolute judgments as a function of the stimulus range and the number of stimulus and response categories. *J. exp. Psychol.*, 1955, 49, 323–332.

7. Garner, W. R. An informational analysis of absolute judgments of loudness. *J. exp. Psychol.*, 1953, 46, 373–380.

8. Hake, H. W., and Garner, W. R. The effect of presenting various numbers of discrete steps on scale reading accuracy. *J. exp. Psychol.*, 1951, 42, 358–366.

9. Halsey, R. M., and Chapanis, A. Chromaticity-confusion contours in a complex viewing situation. *J. Opt. Soc. Amer.*, 1954, 44, 442–454.

10. Hayes, J. R. M. Memory span for several vocabularies as a function of vocabulary size. In *Quarterly Progress Report*, Cambridge, Mass: Acoustics Laboratory, Massachusetts Institute of Technology, Jan.–June, 1952.

11. Jakobson, R., Fant, C. G. M., and Halle, M. *Preliminaries to speech analysis.* Cambridge, Mass.: Acoustics Laboratory, Massachusetts Institute of Technology, 1952. (Tech. Rep. No. 13.)

12. Kaufman, E. L., Lord, M. W., Reese, T. W., and Volkmann, J. The discrimination of visual number. *Amer. J. Psychol.*, 1949, 62, 498–525.

13. Klemmer, E. T., and Frick, F. C. Assimilation of information from dot and matrix patterns. *J. exp. Psychol.*, 1953, 45, 15–19.

14. Külpe, O. Versuche über Abstraktion. *Ber. ü. d. I Kongr. f. exper. Psychol.*, 1904, 56–68.

15. Miller, G. A., and Nicely, P. E. An analysis of perceptual confusions among some English consonants. *J. Acoust. Soc. Amer.*, 1955, 27, 338–352.

16. Pollack, I. The assimilation of sequentially encoded information. *Amer. J. Psychol.*, 1953, 66, 421–435.

17. Pollack, I. The information of elementary auditory displays. *J. Acoust. Soc. Amer.*, 1952, 24, 745–749.

18. Pollack, I. The information of elementary auditory displays. II. *J. Acoust. Soc. Amer.*, 1953, 25, 765–769.

19. Pollack, I., and Ficks, L. Information of elementary multi-dimensional auditory displays. *J. Acoust. Soc. Amer.*, 1954, 26, 155–158.

20. Woodworth, R. S. *Experimental psychology.* New York: Holt, 1938.

24 The Control of Short-Term Memory

Richard C. Atkinson and Richard M. Shiffrin

The notion that the system by which information is stored in memory and retrieved from it can be divided into two components dates back to the nineteenth century. Theories distinguishing between two different kinds of memory were proposed by the English associationists James Mill and John Stuart Mill and by such early experimental psychologists as Wilhelm Wundt and Ernst Meumann in Germany and William James in the United States. Reflecting on their own mental processes, they discerned a clear difference between thoughts currently in consciousness and thoughts that could be brought to consciousness only after a search of memory that was often laborious. (For example, the sentence you are reading is in your current awareness; the name of the baseball team that won the 1968 World Series may be in your memory, but to retrieve it takes some effort, and you may not be able to retrieve it at all.)

The two-component concept of memory was intuitively attractive, and yet it was largely discarded when psychology turned to behaviorism, which emphasized research on animals rather than humans. The distinction between short-term memory and long-term memory received little further consideration until the 1950s, when such psychologists as Donald E. Broadbent in England, D. O. Hebb in Canada, and George A. Miller in the United States reintroduced it (see "Information and Memory," by George A. Miller; *Scientific American*, August, 1956). The concurrent development of computer models of behavior and of mathematical psychology accelerated the growth of interest in the two-process viewpoint, which is now undergoing considerable theoretical development and is the subject of a large research effort. In particular, the short-term memory system, or short-term store (STS), has been given a position of pivotal importance. That is because the processes carried out in the short-term store are under the immediate control of the subject and govern the flow of information in the memory system; they can be called into play at the subject's discretion, with enormous consequences for performance.

Some control processes are used in many situations by everyone and others are used only in special circumstances. "Rehearsal" is an overt or covert repetition of information—as in remembering a telephone number until it can be written down, remembering the names of a group of people to whom one has just been introduced or copying a passage from a book. "Coding" refers to a class of control processes in which the information to be remembered is put in a context of additional, easily retrievable information, such as a mnemonic phrase or sentence. "Imaging" is a control process in which verbal information is remembered through visual images; for example, Cicero suggested learning long lists (or speeches) by placing each member of the list in a visual representation of successive rooms of a well-known building. There are other control processes, including decision rules, organizational schemes, retrieval strategies, and problem-solving techniques; some of them will be encountered in this article. The point to keep in mind is the optional nature of control processes. In contrast to permanent structural components of the memory system, the control processes are selected at the subject's discretion; they may vary not only with different tasks but also from one encounter with the same task to the next.

We believe that the overall memory system is best described in terms of the flow of information into and out of short-term storage and the subject's control of that flow, and this conception has been central to our experimental and theoretical investigation of memory. All phases of memory are assumed to consist of small units of information that are associatively related. A set of closely interrelated information units is

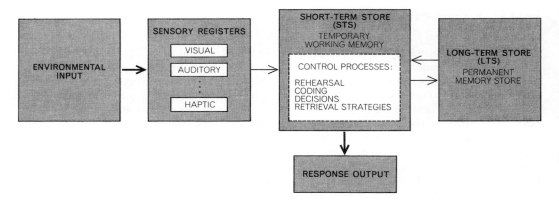

Figure 24.1
Information flow through the memory system is conceived of as beginning with the processing of environmental inputs in sensory registers (receptors plus internal elements) and entry into the short-term store (STS). While it remains there the information may be copied into the long-term store (LTS), and associated information that is in the long-term store may be activated and entered into the short-term store. If a triangle is seen, for example, the name "triangle" may be called up. Control processes in the short-term store affect these transfers into and out of the long-term store and govern learning, retrieval of information, and forgetting.

termed an image or a trace. Note that "image" does not necessarily imply a visual representation; if the letter-number pair *TKM*–4 is presented for memory, the image that is stored might include the size of the card on which the pair is printed, the type of print, the sound of the various symbols, the semantic codes and numerous other units of information.

Information from the environment is accepted and processed by the various sensory systems and is entered into the short-term store, where it remains for a period of time that is usually under the control of the subject. By rehearsing one or more items the subject can keep them in the short-term store, but the number that can be maintained in this way is strictly limited; most people can maintain seven to nine digits, for example. Once an image is lost from the short-term store it cannot thereafter be recovered from it. While information resides in short-term storage it may be copied into the long-term store (LTS), which is assumed to be a relatively permanent memory from which information is not lost.

While an image is in short-term storage, closely related information in the long-term store is activated and entered in the short-term store too. Information entering the short-term store from the sensory systems comes from a specific modality—visual, auditory, or whatever—but associations from the long-term store in all modalities are activated to join it. For instance, an item may be presented visually, but immediately after input its verbal "name" and associated meanings will be activated from the long-term store and placed in the short-term one (figure. 24.1).

Our account of short-term and long-term storage does not require that the two stores necessarily be in different parts of the brain or involve different physiological structures. One might consider the short-term store simply as being a temporary activation of some portion of the long-term store. In our thinking we tend to equate the short-term store with "consciousness," that is, the thoughts and information of which we are currently aware can be considered part of the contents of the short-term store. (Such a statement lies in the realm of phenomenology and cannot be verified scientifically, but thinking of the short-term store in this way may help the reader to conceptualize the system.) Because consciousness is equated with the short-term store and because control processes are centered in and act through it, the short-term store is considered a working memory: a system in which decisions are made, problems are solved and information flow is directed. Retrieval of information from short-term storage is quite fast and accurate. Experiments by Saul Sternberg of the Bell Telephone Laboratories and by others have shown that the retrieval time for information in short-term storage such as letters and numbers ranges from 10 to 30 ms per character.

The retrieval of information from long-term storage is considerably more complicated. So much information is contained in the long-term store that the major problem is finding access to some small subset of the information that contains the desired image, just as one must find a particular book in a library before it can be scanned for the desired information. We propose that the subject activates a likely subset of information, places it in the short-term store and then scans that store for the desired image. The image may not be present in the current subset, and so the retrieval process becomes a search in which various subsets are successively activated and scanned (figure 24.2). On the basis of the information presented to him the subject selects the appropriate "probe information" and places it in the short-term store. A "search set," or subset of information in the long-term store closely associated with the probe, is then activated and put in the short-term store. The subject selects from the search set some image, which is then examined. The information extracted from the selected image is utilized for a decision: has the desired information been found? If so, the search is terminated.

If the information has not been found, the subject may decide that continuation is unlikely

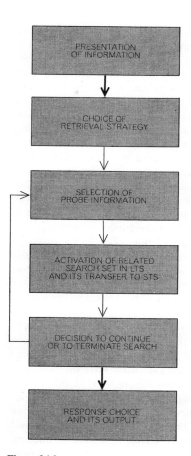

Figure 24.2
Retrieval from the long-term store requires a choice of strategy and selection of certain information as a "probe" that is placed in the short-term store. The probe activates a "search set" of information in the long-term store. The search set is placed in the short-term store and is examined for the desired information. If it is not found, search is halted or recycled with new probe.

to be productive or he may decide to continue. If he does, he begins the next cycle of the search by again selecting a probe, which may or may not be the same probe used in the preceding cycle depending on the subject's strategy. For example, a subject asked to search for states of the United States starting with the letter M may do so by generating states at random and checking their first letter (in which case the same probe information can be used in each search cycle), or he may generate successive states in a regular geographic order (in which case the probe information is systematically changed from one cycle to the next). It can be shown that strategies in which the probe information is systematically changed will result more often in successful retrieval but will take longer than alternative "random" strategies. (Note that the Freudian concept of repressed memories can be considered as being an inability of the subject to generate an appropriate probe.)

This portrayal of the memory system almost entirely in terms of the operations of the short-term store is quite intentional. In our view information storage and retrieval are best described in terms of the flow of information through the short-term store and in terms of the subject's control of the flow. One of the most important of these control processes is rehearsal. Through overt or covert repetition of information, rehearsal either increases the momentary strength of information in the short-term store or otherwise delays its loss. Rehearsal can be shown not only to maintain information in short-term storage but also to control transfer from the short-term store to the long-term one. We shall present several experiments concerned with an analysis of the rehearsal process.

The research in question involves a memory paradigm known as "free recall," which is similar to the task you face when you are asked to name the people present at the last large party you went to. In the typical experimental procedure a list of random items, usually common English words, is presented to the subject one at a time. Later the subject attempts to recall as many words as possible in any order. Many psychologists have worked on free recall, with major research efforts carried out by Bennet Murdock of the University of Toronto, Endel Tulving of Yale University and Murray Glanzer of New York University. The result of principal interest is the probability of recalling each item in a list as a function of its place in the list, or "serial-presentation position." Plotting this function yields a U-shaped curve (figure 24.3a). The increased probability of recall for the first few words in the list is called the primacy effect; the large increase for the last eight to 12 words is called the recency effect. There is considerable evidence that the recency effect is due to retrieval from short-term storage and that the earlier portions of the serial-position curve reflect retrieval from long-term storage only. In one experimental procedure the subject is required to carry out a difficult arithmetic task for 30 s immediately following presentation of the list and then is asked to recall. One can assume that the arithmetic task causes the loss of all the words in short-term storage, so that recall reflects retrieval from long-term storage only. The recency effect is eliminated when this experiment is performed; the earlier portions of the serial-position curve are unaffected (figure 24.3b). If variables that influence the long-term store but not the short-term one are manipulated, the recency portion of

Figure 24.3
Probability of recall in free-recall experiments varies in a characteristic way with an item's serial position in a list: a "primacy effect" and a "recency effect" are apparent (a). If an arithmetic task is interpolated between presentation and recall, the recency effect disappears (b). Words in long lists are recalled less well than words in short lists (c). Slower presentation also results in better recall (d). The curves are idealized ones based on experiments by James W. Dees, Bennet Murdock, Leo Postman, and Murray Glanzer.

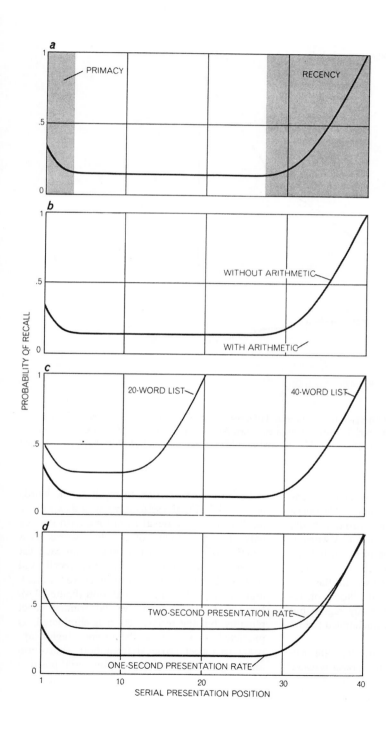

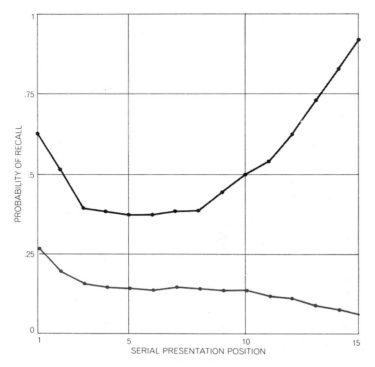

Figure 24.4
Effect of delay is tested by asking subjects to recall at the end of a session all words from the entire session, and then plotting probability of recall against serial position within each list. An experiment by Fergus Craik compares immediate recall (black) with delayed recall (gray). The delayed-recall curve emphasizes transitory nature of recency effect.

the serial-position curve should be relatively unaffected, whereas the earlier portions of the curve should show changes. One such variable is the number of words in the presented list. A word in a longer list is less likely to be recalled, but the recency effect is quite unaffected by list length (figure 24.3c). Similarly, increases in the rate of presentation decrease the likelihood of recalling words preceding the recency region but leave the recency effect largely unchanged (figure 24.3d).

In free recall experiments many lists are usually presented in a session. If the subject is asked

at the end of the session to recall all the words presented during the session, we would expect his recall to reflect retrieval from long-term storage only. The probability of recalling words as a function of their serial position within each list can be plotted for end-of-session recall and compared with the serial-position curve for recall immediately following presentation (figure 24.4). For the delayed-recall curve the primacy effect remains, but the recency effect is eliminated, as predicted. In summary, the recency region appears to reflect retrieval from both short-term and long-term storage whereas the serial-position

ITEM PRESENTED	ITEMS REHEARSED (REHEARSAL SET)
1 REACTION	REACTION, REACTION, REACTION, REACTION
2 HOOF	HOOF, REACTION, HOOF, REACTION
3 BLESSING	BLESSING, HOOF, REACTION
4 RESEARCH	RESEARCH, REACTION, HOOF, RESEARCH
5 CANDY	CANDY, HOOF, RESEARCH, REACTION
6 HARDSHIP	HARDSHIP, HOOF, HARDSHIP, HOOF
7 KINDNESS	KINDNESS, CANDY, HARDSHIP, HOOF
8 NONSENSE	NONSENSE, KINDNESS, CANDY, HARDSHIP
⋮	⋮
20 CELLAR	CELLAR, ALCOHOL, MISERY, CELLAR

Figure 24.5
Overt-rehearsal experiment by Dewey Rundus shows the effect of rehearsal on transfer into long-term storage. The subject rehearses aloud. A partial listing of items rehearsed in one instance shows typical result: early items receive more rehearsals than later items.

curve preceding the recency region reflects retrieval from long-term storage only.

In 1965, at a conference sponsored by the New York Academy of Sciences, we put forward a mathematical model explaining these and other effects in terms of a rehearsal process. The model assumed that in a free-recall task the subject sets up a rehearsal buffer in the short-term store that can hold only a fixed number of items. At the start of the presentation of a list the buffer is empty; successive items are entered until the buffer is filled. Thereafter, as each new item enters the rehearsal buffer it replaces one of the items already there. (Which item is replaced depends on a number of psychological factors, but in the model the decision is approximated by a random process.) The items that are still being rehearsed in the short-term store when the last item is presented are the ones that are immediately recalled by the subject, giving rise to the recency effect. The transfer of information from the short-term to the long-term store is postulated to be a function of the length of time an item resides in the rehearsal buffer; the longer the time period, the more rehearsal the item receives and therefore the greater the transfer of information to long-term storage. Since items presented first in a list enter an empty or partly

empty rehearsal buffer, they remain longer than later items and consequently receive additional rehearsal. This extra rehearsal causes more transfer of information to long-term storage for the first items, giving rise to the primacy effect.

This rehearsal model was given a formal mathematical statement and was fitted to a wide array of experiments, and it provided an excellent quantitative account of a great many results in free recall, including those discussed in this article. A more direct confirmation of the model has recently been provided by Dewey Rundus of Stanford University. He carried out free-recall experiments in which subjects rehearsed aloud during list presentation. This overt rehearsal was tape-recorded and was compared with the recall results. The number of different words contained in the "rehearsal set" (the items overtly rehearsed between successive presentations) was one after the first word was presented and then rose until the fourth word; from the fourth word on the number of different words in the rehearsal set remained fairly constant (averaging about 3.3) until the end of the list. The subjects almost always reported the members of the most recent rehearsal set when the list ended and recall began. A close correspondence is evident between the number of rehearsals and the

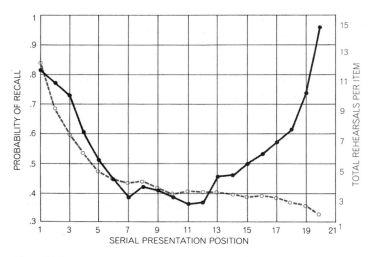

Figure 24.6
Effect of rehearsal is demonstrated by comparison of an item's probability of recall (solid black line) with the total number of rehearsals item receives (broken gray line). The two are related in regions reflecting retrieval from long-term storage (preceding recency region). That is, long-term storage efficacy depends on number of rehearsals and is reflected in retrieval.

recall probability for words preceding the recency effect; in the recency region, however, a sharp disparity occurs (figures 24.5 and 24.6). The hypothesis that long-term storage is a function of the number of rehearsals can be checked in other ways. The recall probability for a word preceding the recency region was plotted as a function of the number of rehearsals received by that word; the result was an almost linear, sharply increasing function. And words presented in the middle of the list given the same number of rehearsals as the first item presented had the same recall probability as that first item.

With efficacy of rehearsal established both for storing information in the long-term store and for maintaining information in the short-term store, we did an experiment in which the subjects' rehearsal was manipulated directly. Our subjects were trained to engage in one of two types of rehearsal. In the first (a one-item rehearsal set) the most recently presented item was

rehearsed exactly three times before presentation of the next item; no other items were rehearsed. In the second (a three-item rehearsal set) the subject rehearsed the three most recently presented items once each before presentation of the next item, so that the first rehearsal set contained three rehearsals of the first word, the second rehearsal set contained two rehearsals of the second word and one rehearsal of the first word, and all subsequent sets contained one rehearsal of each of the three most recent items (figures 24.7 and 24.8).

When only one item is rehearsed at a time, each item receives an identical number of rehearsals and the primacy effect disappears, as predicted. Note that the recency effect appears for items preceding the last item even though the last item is the only one in the last rehearsal set. This indicates that even when items are dropped from rehearsal, it takes an additional period of time for them to be completely lost from short-

ONE-ITEM REHEARSAL SCHEME

SERIAL POSITION	ITEM PRESENTED	ITEMS REHEARSED	TOTAL REHEARSALS PER ITEM
1	A	AAA	3
2	B	BBB	3
3	C	CCC	3
4	D	DDD	3
5	E	EEE	3
6	F	FFF	3
.	.	.	.
.	.	.	.
.	.	.	.
14	N	NNN	3
15	O	OOO	3
16	P	PPP	3

THREE-ITEM REHEARSAL SCHEME

SERIAL POSITION	ITEM PRESENTED	ITEMS REHEARSED	TOTAL REHEARSALS PER ITEM
1	A	AAA	5
2	B	BBA	4
3	C	CBA	3
4	D	DCB	3
5	E	EDC	3
6	F	FED	3
.	.	.	.
.	.	.	.
.	.	.	.
14	N	NML	3
15	O	ONM	2
16	P	PON	1

Figure 24.7
Number of rehearsals is controlled with two schemes. In one (top) only the current item is rehearsed and all items have three rehearsals. In the other (bottom) the latest three items are rehearsed; early ones have extra rehearsals. (Letters represent words.)

term storage. The curve for the three-item rehearsal condition shows the effect also. The last rehearsal set contains the last three items presented and these are recalled perfectly, but a recency effect is still seen for items preceding these three. It should also be noted that a primacy effect occurs in the three-rehearsal condition. This was predicted because the first item received a total of five rehearsals rather than three. A delayed-recall test for all words was given at the end of the experimental session. The data confirmed that long-term-store retrieval closely par-

allels the number of rehearsals given an item during presentation, for both rehearsal schemes.

These results strongly implicate rehearsal in the maintenance of information in the short-term store and the transfer of that information to the long-term system. The question then arises: What are the forgetting and transfer characteristics of the short-term store in the absence of rehearsal? One can control rehearsal experimentally by blocking it with a difficult verbal task such as arithmetic. For example, Lloyd R. Peterson and Margaret Peterson of Indiana

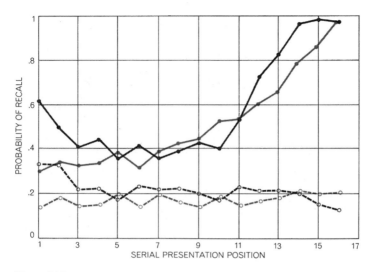

Figure 24.8
Primacy effect disappears with one-item rehearsal (gray), in which all items have equal rehearsal, but remains with three-item rehearsal (black). Recency effect is pronounced for both schemes in immediate recall (solid lines). Curves for delayed recall (broken lines), which reflect only retrieval from long-term storage, parallel the number of rehearsals.

University [see "Short-Term Memory," by Lloyd R. Peterson; *Scientific American*, July, 1966] presented a set of three letters (a trigram) to be remembered; the subject next engaged in a period of arithmetic and then was asked to recall as many letters of the trigram as possible. When the probability of recall is plotted as a function of the duration of the arithmetic task, the loss observed over time is similar to that of the recency effect in free recall (figure 24.9). Short-term-store loss caused by an arithmetic task, then, is similar to loss from short-term storage caused by a series of intervening words to be remembered. The flat portion of the curve reflects the retrieval of the trigram from long-term storage alone and the earlier portions of the curve represent retrieval from both short-term and long-term storage; the loss of the trigram from short-term storage is represented by the decreasing probability of recall prior to the asymptote.

Does the forgetting observed during arithmetic reflect an automatic decay of short-term storage that occurs inevitably in the absence of rehearsal or is the intervening activity the cause of the loss? There is evidence that the amount of new material introduced between presentation and test is a much more important determinant of loss from short-term storage than simply the elapsed time between presentation and test. This finding is subject to at least two explanations. The first holds that the activity intervening between presentation and test is the *direct* cause of an item's loss from short-term storage. The second explanation proposes that the rate of intervening activity merely affects the number of rehearsals that can be given the item to be remembered and thus *indirectly* determines the rate of loss.

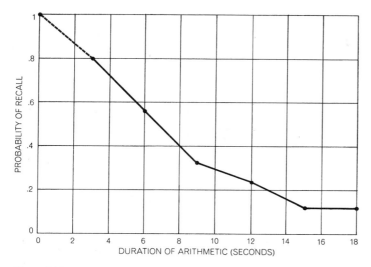

Figure 24.9
Arithmetic task before recall reduces the probability of recall. Lloyd R. Peterson and Margaret Peterson charted recall probability against duration of arithmetic. The probability falls off with duration until it levels off when recall reflects retrieval from long-term storage alone. Does curve reflect only lack of rehearsal or also nature of intervening task?

It has recently become possible to choose between these two explanations of loss from the short-term store. Judith Reitman of the University of Michigan substituted a signal-detection task for the arithmetic task in the Petersons' procedure. The task consisted in responding whenever a weak tone was heard against a continuous background of "white" noise. Surprisingly, no loss from short-term storage was observed after 15 s of the task, even though subjects reported no rehearsal during the signal detection. This suggests that loss from the short-term store is due to the type of interference during the intervening interval: signal detection does not cause loss but verbal arithmetic does. Another important issue that could potentially be resolved with the Reitman procedure concerns the transfer of information from the short-term to the long-term store: Does transfer occur only at initial presentation and at subsequent re-

hearsals, or does it occur throughout the period during which the information resides in the short-term store, regardless of rehearsals?

To answer these questions, the following experiment was carried out. A consonant pentagram (a set of five consonants, such as *QJXFK*) was presented for 2.5 s for the subject to memorize. This was followed by a signal-detection task in which pure tones were presented at random intervals against a continuous background of white noise. The subjects pressed a key whenever they thought they detected a tone. (The task proved to be difficult; only about three-fourths of the tones presented were correctly detected.) The signal-detection period lasted for either 1 s, 8 s, or 40 s, with tones sounded on the average every 2.5 s. In conditions 1, 2, and 3 the subjects were tested on the consonant pentagram immediately after the signal detection; in conditions 4, 5, and 6, however, they were required to carry out 30 s

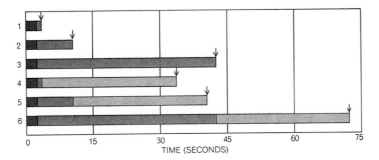

Figure 24.10
Two tasks were combined in an experiment with these six conditions. Five consonants were presented for 2.5 s (dark gray) followed by a signal-detection task for 1 s, 8 s, or 40 s (medium gray), followed in three cases by arithmetic (light gray). Then came the test (arrows). Rehearsal during detection was included in a control version.

of difficult arithmetic following the signal detection before being tested (figure 24.10). In order to increase the likelihood that rehearsal would not occur, we paid the subjects for performing well on signal detection and for doing their arithmetic accurately but not for their success in remembering letters. In addition they were instructed not to rehearse letters during signal detection or arithmetic. They reported afterward that they were not consciously aware of rehearsing. Because the question of rehearsal is quite important, we nevertheless went on to do an additional control experiment in which all the same conditions applied but the subjects were told to rehearse the pentagram aloud following each detection of a tone.

The results indicate that arithmetic causes the pentagram information to be lost from the short-term store but that in the absence of the arithmetic the signal-detection task alone causes no loss (figure 24.11). What then does produce forgetting from the short-term store? It is not just the analysis of any information input, since signal detection is a difficult information-processing task but causes no forgetting. And time alone causes no noticeable forgetting. Yet verbal information (arithmetic) does cause a large loss. Mrs. Reitman's conclusion appears to be correct:

forgetting is caused by the entry into the short-term store of other, similar information.

What about the effect of rehearsal? In the arithmetic situation performance improves if subjects rehearse overtly during the signal-detection period. Presumably the rehearsal transfers information about the pentagram to the long-term store; the additional transfer during the long signal-detection period is reflected in the retrieval scores, and the rehearsal curve rises. The no-rehearsal curve is horizontal over the last 32 s of signal detection, however, confirming that no rehearsal was occurring during that period. The fact that the lowest curve is flat over the last 32 s has important implications for transfer from the short-term store to the long-term. It indicates that essentially no transfer occurred during this period even though, as the results in the absence of arithmetic show, the trace remained in the short-term store. Hence the presence of a trace in the short-term store is alone not enough to result in transfer to the long-term store. Apparently transfer to the long-term system occurs primarily during or shortly after rehearsals. (The rise in the lowest curve over the first 8 s may indicate that the transfer effects of a presentation or rehearsal take at least a few seconds to reach completion.)

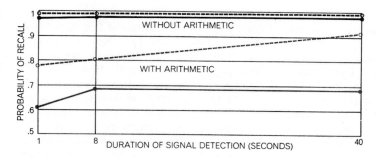

Figure 24.11
Nature of tasks is seen to have an effect. In the absence of arithmetic, signal detection leaves the short-term store virtually unaffected, with rehearsal (broken black curve) or without (solid black). Arithmetic, however, causes loss from the short-term store (gray); decreased recall shown reflects retrieval from long-term store only. Retrieval improves with duration of signal detection if there is rehearsal, which increases transfer to the long-term store (broken gray curve) but not in the absence of rehearsal (solid gray).

The emphasis we have given to rote rehearsal should not imply that other control processes are of lesser importance. Although much evidence indicates that transfer from short-term storage to long-term is strongly dependent on rehearsals, effective later retrieval from long-term storage can be shown to be highly dependent on the type of information rehearsed. Coding is really the choosing of particular information to be rehearsed in the short-term store. In general, coding strategies consist in adding appropriately chosen information from long-term storage to a trace to be remembered and then rehearsing the entire complex in the short-term store. Suppose you are given (as is typical in memory experiments) the stimulus-response pair *HRM*–4; later *HRM* will be presented alone and you will be expected to respond "4." If you simply rehearse *HRM*–4 several times, your ability to respond correctly later will probably not be high. Suppose, however, *HRM* reminds you of "homeroom" and you think of various aspects of your fourth-grade classroom. Your retrieval performance will be greatly enhanced. Why? First of all, the amount and range of information stored appears to be greater with coding than with rote

rehearsal. Moreover, the coding operation provides a straightforward means by which you can gain access to an appropriate and small region of memory during retrieval. In the above example, when *HRM* is presented at the moment of test, you are likely to notice, just as during the initial presentation, that *HRM* is similar to "homeroom." You can then use "homeroom" (and the current temporal context) as a further probe and would almost certainly access "fourth grade" and so generate the correct response.

As the discussion of coding suggests, the key to retrieval is the selection of probe information that will activate an appropriate search set from the long-term store. Since in our view the long-term store is a relatively permanent repository, forgetting is assumed to result from an inadequate selection of probe information and a consequent failure of the retrieval process. There are two basic ways in which the probe selection may prove inadequate. First, the wrong probe may be selected. For instance, you might be asked to name the star of a particular motion picture. The name actually begins with *T* but you decide that it begins with *A* and include *A* in the probe information used to access the long-term store. As a result the correct name may not be included in the search set that is drawn into the short-term store and retrieval will not succeed.

Second, if the probe is such that an extremely large region of memory is accessed, then retrieval may fail even though the desired trace is included in the search set. For example, if you are asked to name a fruit that sounds like a word meaning "to look at," you might say "pear." If you are asked to name a living thing that sounds like a word meaning "to look at," the probability of your coming up with "pear" will be greatly reduced. Again, you are more likely to remember a "John Smith" if you met him at a party with five other people than if there had been 20 people at the party. This effect can be explained on grounds other than a failure of memory search, however. It could be argued that more attention was given to "John Smith" at the smaller party. Or if the permanence of long-term storage is not accepted, it could be argued that the names of the many other people met at the larger party erode or destroy the memory trace for "John Smith." Are these objections reasonable? The John Smith example is analogous to the situation in free recall where words in long lists are less well recalled from long-term storage than words in short lists.

The problem, then, is to show that the list-length effect in free recall is dependent on the choice of probe information rather than on either the number of words intervening between presentation and recall or the differential storage given words in lists of different size. The second issue is disposed of rather easily: in many free-recall experiments that vary list length, the subjects do not know at the beginning of the list what the length of the list will be. It is therefore unlikely that they store different amounts of information for the first several words in lists of differing length. Nevertheless, as we pointed out, the first several words are recalled at different levels.

To dispose of the "interference" explanation, which implicates the number of words between presentation and recall, is more difficult. Until fairly recently, as a matter of fact, interference theories of forgetting have been predominant [see "Forgetting," by Benton J. Underwood, *Scientific American*, March, 1964, and "The Interference Theory of Forgetting," by John Ceraso, October, 1967]. In these theories forgetting has often been seen as a matter of erosion of the memory trace, usually by items presented following the item to be remembered but also by items preceding the item to be remembered. (The list-length effect might be explained in these terms, since the average item in a long list is preceded and followed by more items than the average item in a short list.) On the other hand, the retrieval model presented in this article assumes long-term storage to be permanent; it maintains that the strength of long-term traces is independent of list length and that forgetting results from the fact that the temporal-contextual probe cues used to access any given list tend to elicit a larger search set for longer lists, thereby producing less efficient retrieval.

In order to distinguish between the retrieval and the interference explanations, we presented lists of varying lengths and had the subject attempt to recall not the list just studied (as in the typical free-recall procedure) but the list before the last. This procedure makes it possible to separate the effect of the size of the list being recalled from the effect of the number of words intervening between presentation and recall. A large or a small list to be recalled can be followed by either a large or a small intervening list. The retrieval model predicts that recall probability will be dependent on the size of the list being recalled. The interference model predicts that performance will be largely determined by the number of words in the intervening list.

We used lists of five and of 20 words and presented them in four combinations: 5–5, 5–20, 20–5, 20–20; the first number gives the size of the list being recalled and the second number the size of the intervening list. One result is that there is no recency effect (figure 24.12). This

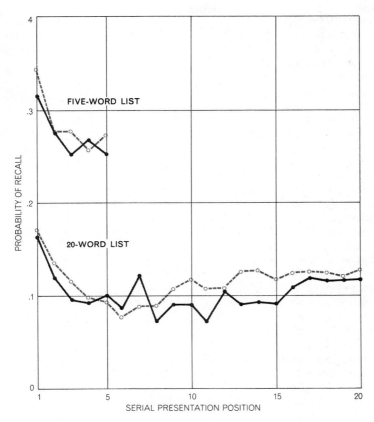

Figure 24.12
Length of list rather than amount of "interference" governs recall probability. Subjects were asked to recall the list before the one just studied. Five-word lists (top) were recalled better than 20-word lists (bottom) whether they were followed by intervening lists of five words (black) or of 20 words (broken gray). The data are averages from three experiments.

would be expected since there is another list and another recall intervening between presentation and recall; the intervening activity causes the words in the tested list to be lost from short-term storage and so the curves represent retrieval from long-term storage only. The significant finding is that words in lists five words long are recalled much better than words in lists 20 words long, and the length of the intervening list has little, if any, effect. The retrieval model can predict these results only if a probe is available to access the requested list. It seems likely in this experiment that the subject has available at test appropriate cues (probably temporal in nature) to enable him to select probe information pertaining to the desired list. If the experimental procedure were changed so that the subject was asked to recall the tenth preceding list, then selection of an adequate probe would no longer be possible. The results demonstrate the importance of probe selection, a control process of the short-term store.

The model of memory we have described, which integrates the system around the operations of the short-term store, is not in any sense a final theory. As experimental techniques and mathematical models have become increasingly sophisticated, memory theory has undergone progressive changes, and there is no doubt that this trend will continue. We nevertheless think it is likely that the short-term store and its control processes will be found to be central.

25 Verbal and Visual Subsystems of Working Memory

Alan D. Baddeley

The term "working memory" refers to the system responsible for the temporary maintenance of information necessary for performing such cognitive tasks as reasoning, understanding, and learning. Evidence from a range of studies based on the functioning of working memory in normal and brain-damaged patients, led myself and G. Hitch to propose a model for working memory that assumes it has three components. The first is an attentional controller, a "central executive" that is responsible for strategy selection and cognitive control. This central system is aided by two subsidiary slave systems, the "phonological loop" that is responsible for maintaining and manipulating speech-based information, and the "visuo-spatial sketchpad" that is responsible for holding and manipulating visual images [1, 2].

The Phonological Loop

The phonological loop is thought to be a system with two components: a brief memory store able to hold acoustic or phonological information, coupled with an articulatory control system capable of maintaining information by subvocal rehearsal and also of entering new information into the memory store by means of subvocal naming. Evidence for the phonological memory store comes from the acoustic similarity effect, whereby sequences of items that are similar in sound, such as the words MAN, CAD, MAT, MAP, CAN, are harder to remember and repeat back than dissimilar words such as PIT, DAY, HOT, COW, PEN, while similarity of meaning between the words has little or no effect [3]. The articulatory control process is reflected in the presence of the word-length effect, whereby the capacity for immediate memory is inversely related to the time it takes to say the relevant words [4].

A recent study by Longoni, Richardson, and Aiello [5] has combined these two variables in a single experiment and demonstrated that they appear to operate independently. This study, which involved experiments in both Italian and English, provides further evidence for the presence of separate storage and articulatory-rehearsal components of the phonological loop. Previous evidence obtained from patients with impaired phonological working memories suggested the involvement of the perisylvian region of the left hemisphere, but left unanswered the question of whether the two subsystems are anatomically separable [6].

A recent study by Paulesu, Frith, and Frackowiak [7] used positron emission tomography (PET) scanning to investigate the anatomical localization of the phonological component of working memory in normal subjects. PET scanning measures changes in regional cerebral blood flow, which are assumed to reflect changes in the activation levels of different regions of the brain. The study of Paulesu et al. involved the immediate recall of sequences of visually presented consonants—a standard phonological memory task. Such a task, however, is likely to involve visual and motor components, in addition to the two hypothetical memory components. Paulesu et al. tackled this problem by the subtraction method, where the experimental condition involving verbal memory was contrasted with a condition involving immediate visual memory, and a task involving subvocalization without memory was compared with an equivalent visual task (figure 25.1).

The PET scanning experiments showed that when subjects are required to perform a task involving phonological subvocalization, but not demanding memory, neuronal activation occurs in Broca's area. In an experimental condition involving immediate memory, a process that is assumed to involve both subvocalization and

Cognitive components of the tasks	Experiment 1		Experiment 2	
Phonological store				
Subvocal rehearsal system				
Grapheme/phoneme transcoding				
Visual analysis/store				
	Phonological memory	Visual memory	Rhyming task	Shape similarity
	Tasks			

Figure 25.1

Schematic layout illustrating the cognitive components (pink squares) involved in the two studies carried out by Paulesu et al. The first experiment contrasted memory for consonants with memory for Korean letters, which had previously been shown to rely on purely visual coding. Experiment 2 compared a rhyme judgment task, involving phonological processing but not memory, with a task involving shape judgments. (Adapted from (7)).

storage, activation also occurs in the left supra-marginal gyrus, suggesting that this is the location of the short-term phonological memory store (figure 25.2). The evidence for separable storage and articulatory rehearsal subsystems is consistent with the previously described behavioural data from normal subjects, and also the suggested location of the memory store is consistent with evidence gained from the study of lesions in patients with phonological memory deficits.

The Visuo-spatial Sketchpad

The visual-spatial sketchpad is thought to be responsible for the maintenance of visuo-spatial images [1, 2]. It has been suggested that it may have at least two components, one that is principally associated with the storage of visual information such as pattern and colour, and a second component that is responsible for representing spatial information. Although experiments on normal subjects are generally consistent with such a visuo-spatial separation, they do not provide unequivocal evidence. Stronger evidence for a separation comes from studies of neuropsychological patients, with the suggestion that the visual aspects of the system occur in the occipital lobes, and that spatial coding appears to have a more parietal localization [8]. Work by Goldman-Rakic [9] using single cell recording during a visual memory task performed by awake monkeys suggests a further involvement of the frontal lobes.

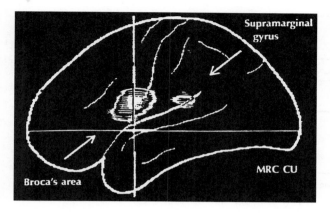

Figure 25.2
The cortical areas involved respectively in phonological memory and subvocal rehearsal. (Data kindly provided by Paulesu et al.).

A recent study by Jonides et al. [10] has investigated this question using PET scanning. Their task is illustrated in figure 25.3. In the memory test condition, subjects are briefly shown a pattern of dots. Their memory is then tested by presenting a circle and asking the subject to decide whether the dot would have fallen within the circle, had they been presented simultaneously. It was found that the subjects can perform this task but make errors, in contrast to the control condition in which the dot pattern is presented at the same time as the circle, which requires a perceptual rather than a memory judgement. Subtracting the level of brain activation present during the perceptual condition from that involved when memory is required indicates the location of the additional processing demanded by immediate visual memory and, by implication, the anatomical basis of the visuo-spatial sketchpad.

As figure 25.4* demonstrates, visual memory led to significantly greater neuronal activation in four areas, all in the right hemisphere. Activation of two of these, the occipital and parietal lobes, is consistent with earlier lesion studies, whereas the frontal lobe activation is broadly consistent with the single cell-recording work of Goldman-Rakic. Jonides et al. speculate that the occipital lobe activation may reflect the initial creation of the image, whereas determination of its spatial coordinates may depend on parietal lobe processing. Following the work by Goldman-Rakic, they suggest a frontal lobe involvement in image maintenance. The observation of premotor activation, however, remains a problem as both the memory and the perceptual control condition involved an equivalent motor response.

To the best of my knowledge, Paulesu et al. and Jonides et al. [10] are the first two studies in which PET scanning is used to analyse the characteristics of working memory. The fact that they produce results that are consistent with the model based on behavioural data from normal subjects and neuropsychological patients is gratifying, but raises the question of whether the PET scans are telling us anything we did

---

*Figure 25.4 deleted because it could not be reproduced accurately.

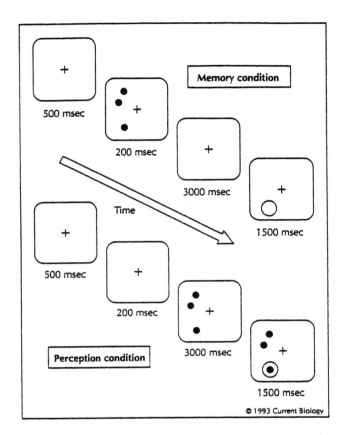

Figure 25.3
The experimental procedure used by Jonides et al. to study visuo-spatial working memory. The upper part of the figure illustrates the events in the memory condition of the experiment in which subjects attempt to retain dots and subsequently decide whether any of them fell within the location specified by the circle. The lower part shows the control condition involving visual judgment without memory. (Adapted from (10)).

not already know. I think they do—in part, because existing evidence bearing on the issues raised, though strong, is far from overwhelming. There is, furthermore, one question to which the PET scan-derived anatomical data speak much more cogently than the behavioural evidence. This is the issue of whether a particular pattern of behavioural results should be interpreted as reflecting separate subsystems, or whether it is better explained in terms of differential processes within a single system. Purely behavioural data are typically ambiguous on this point, whereas PET scanning studies, such as those discussed, provide powerful evidence for separable subsystems.

Finally, the fact that both of these studies have produced results that are coherent and consistent with a substantial body of existing data provides useful and necessary evidence for the validity and theoretical potential of PET scanning. Although it is clearly necessary for these results to be replicated by other groups using a wider range of materials, they appear to open the way to further studies asking more detailed questions about the structure and functioning of working memory.

References

1. Baddeley AD, Hitch G: Working memory. In *The Psychology of Learning and Motivation, vol 8*. Edited by Bowers GA. New York: Academic Press; 1974:47–89.

2. Baddeley AD: Working memory. *Science* 1992, 255:556–559.

3. Baddeley AD: Short-term memory for word sequences as a function of acoustic, semantic and formal similarity. *Q J Exp Psychol* 1966, 18:362–365.

4. Baddeley AD, Thomson N, Buchanan M: Word length and the structure of short-term memory. *J Verbal Learning and Verbal Behav* 1975, 14:575–589.

5. Longoni AM, Richardson JT, Aiello A: Articulatory rehearsal and phonological storage in working memory. *Memory Cogn* 1993, 21:11–22.

6. Vallar G, Shallice T: *Neuropsychological Impairments of Short-term Memory*. Cambridge: Cambridge University Press; 1990.

7. Paulesu E, Frith CD, Frackowiak RSJ: The neural correlates of the verbal component of working memory. *Nature* 1993, 362:342–345.

8. Farah MJ: Is visual memory really visual? Overlooked evidence from neuropsychology. *Psychol Rev* 1988, 95:307–317.

9. Goldman-Rakic PW: Topography of cognition: parallel distributed networks in primate association cortex. *Annu Rev Neurosci* 1988, 11:137–156.

10. Jonides J, Smith EE, Koeppe RA, Awh E, Minoshima S, Mintun MA: Spatial working memory in humans as revealed by PET. *Nature* 1993, 363:623–625.

26 The Prefrontal Landscape: Implications of Functional Architecture for Understanding Human Mentation and the Central Executive

P. S. Goldman-Rakic

Introduction

The prefrontal cortex is the area of the brain most often associated with executive processes in humans. Concerning this venerated organ of mind, two points are rarely contested: first, that this large expanse of neocortex has a compartment organization based on its cytoarchitectonic subdivisions; and second, that injury to this cortex in humans and animals results in a diversity of behavioural abnormalities. One of the major questions confronted by our field is that of how function maps onto structure in association cortex. Do the different regions carry out distinctive functions, for example, inhibitory control, motor planning, and spatial memory, as argued at different times by numerous contributors to the prefrontal literature (e.g., Fulton 1950, Mishkin 1964, Brutkowski 1965, Fuster 1980, Pribram 1987)? Is there a hierarchical relationship between superior and inferior dorsolateral cortex as recently proposed by Owen et al. (1996)? Or is the prefrontal cortex organized into subregions according to informational domain with the different domains sharing a common specialization that can uniquely be identified with prefrontal cortex (Goldman-Rakic 1987)? According to this latter view, content, not function, is mapped onto major cytoarchitectonic fields. It would be premature to draw strong conclusions and firm answers to the questions that will be raised here. However, a field advances when discrete hypotheses can be generated, compared and eventually some of them falsified. Furthermore, an understanding of the "functional map" in prefrontal cortex has direct implications for the nature and existence of a general purpose central executive (Baddeley and Hitch 1974, Baddeley 1986) and/or a supervisory attentional system (Shallice 1982), as well as for defining the concept of polymodal cortex, the nature of consciousness and the organization of mind. This essay addresses the landscape of prefrontal cortex anatomically and functionally, based on the premise that structure and function are inextricably related. And I would argue further, that every theory of cortical function should be integrated with knowledge of regional circuitry and physiology. This meeting has provided an opportunity to review different organizational schemes and suggest ways they may be harmonized and/or tested in future research.

Tradition of Functional Duality

A major organizing principle of prefrontal function since mid-century has been that of a duality between the dorsolateral and orbital cortices. An early example of this partition can be found in the Salmon Lecture delivered by John Fulton (1950). Fulton subdivided the prefrontal cortex into mesopallium—posterior areas 13 and 14 of Walker—and neopallium—Walker's areas 9, 10, 11 and 12, 46, and 8. The mesopallium was part of the visceral brain involved in emotion and affect while the neopallium was considered important for intellectual functions. The trend for orbital lesions, particularly posterior or mesopallial areas to produce selective impairments on tasks which evoke emotional or appetitive responses and for lateral lesions of the convexity to produce impairments on tests requiring integration of information has persisted in one form or another to the present day. The caudal regions of the orbital cortex have long been associated with the interceptive and palpable senses (Fulton 1950) and anatomical evidence is accumulating to show that the orbital areas subserving these functions are definable in terms of the relevant afferent inputs (e.g., Baylis et al. 1995, Carmichael and Price 1995). Dias et al. (1996) have shown deficits in reversing stimulus-reward associations following orbital lesions in the marmoset presumably attributable to connections with limbic areas. Finally, clinical studies reveal an autonomic pattern of deficits associated with orbital lesions (Damasio et al. 1991), although cognitive deficits have also been observed (Eslinger and Damasio 1985, Freedman and Oscar-Berman 1986).

The neopallium or dorsolateral convexity in turn can also be further differentiated into functional territories. In an influential 1964 essay, Mishkin introduced a division of labour between dorsal and ventral portions of the neopallium according to which the dorsolateral convexity represented by the principal sulcus was concerned with spatial function, while the ventral part, or the inferior prefrontal convexity (including the cortex of the lateral orbital cortex) was associated with the maintenance of what was termed 'central sets' (Mishkin 1964). Although then, as now, impairment on delayed-response tasks defined the dorsolateral contribution, emphasis was placed more on its spatial nature and less in terms of the immediate memory process. The tradition of functional diversity was further elaborated by Fuster (1989) who expanded duality of function into the functional trinity of preparatory set, retrospective provisional memory and suppression of external and internal influences. In Fuster's system, the first two functions were associated with the dorsal prefrontal convexity; the last mentioned with the orbital prefrontal cortex. Importantly, however, these three functions were considered subordinate to the synthetic role of prefrontal cortex in 'the formation of temporal structures of behaviour with a unifying purpose or goal' (Fuster 1980, p. 126). With respect to memory, Fuster and Alexander (1971), Pribram and Tubbs (1967), and Goldman and Rosvold (1970) all placed emphasis on the temporal structuring of delayed-response tasks, considering their spatial properties as subsidiary. Further, Fuster considered the memory function of prefrontal cortex to be highly localized to one subarea of cortex

which subserved both non-spatial as well as spatial processing. Depression of activity in the principal sulcus region by cooling produced both non-spatial and spatial impairments (Bauer and Fuster 1976). On the other hand, surgical removals of the dorsolateral and inferior convexity portions of the dorsolateral cortex have yielded evidence of dissociation between the spatial and non-spatial memory systems of the prefrontal cortex. Passingham, for one, found deficits on delayed colour matching task following inferior convexity lesions; delayed alternation was unimpaired by the same lesion. Conversely, lesions of the principal sulcus produce impairments on spatial delayed-response tasks and rarely on non-spatial tasks (for review, see Goldman-Rakic 1987). Nevertheless, the interpretation often given to this dissociation is that the inferior convexity plays a role in inhibiting or overcoming incorrect or prepotent response tendencies while the dorsolateral prefrontal cortex, exemplified by the salient delayed-response deficits, is central to the memorial programming of appropriate motor programmes.

More recent studies have offered additional views of prefrontal functional architecture. Petrides has advanced the idea of a two-stage hierarchical organization of prefrontal cortex according to which the midfrontal areas 9 and 46 carry out sequential processing and self-monitoring functions while the inferior convexity areas 45 and 47 (in humans) are engaged in a lower level function entailing "comparison between stimuli in short-term memory as well as the active organization of sequences of responses based on conscious explicit retrieval of information from posterior cortical association systems." In the Petrides model, each level can operate on either spatial or nonspatial information.

This brief review of the literature is intended to make one point—how widespread and deeply rooted is the view that the prefrontal cortex is a composite of functionally distinct or hierarchically arranged areas engaged respectively with the cardinal psychological processes of attention, affect, emotion, memory and motor aspects of behaviour. In this paper I will expand on another view that (1) the dorsolateral prefrontal cortex as a whole has a generic function—"on-line" processing of information or working memory in the service of a wide range of cognitive functions; (2) that this process is iteratively represented throughout several and possibly many subdivisions of the prefrontal neopallium; and (3) that each autonomous subdivision integrates attentional, memorial, motor and possibly affective dimensions of behaviour by virtue of network connectivity with relevant sensory, motor, and limbic areas of brain. This view is compatible with the diversity of behavioural deficits described for frontal lobe patients and animals with experimental lesions, and differs mainly with interpretations of data rather than with the data itself, which, in my view, is remarkably consistent (reviewed in Goldman-Rakic 1987).

Working Memory and "On-line" Processing

The tissue surrounding the caudal half of the principal sulcus (Walker's area 46; Brodmann's area 9) including portions of the frontal eye field (area 8) in the rhesus monkey qualifies as a mental sketch pad and central processor of visuo-spatial information. Lesions restricted to this region have been shown repeatedly to impair performance on spatial delayed-response tasks which tax an animal's working memory ability, that is, to hold an item of information "in mind" for a short period of time and to update information from moment to moment. The impairments are selective in two critical respects; performance on tasks which engage memory for objects such as visual discrimination object reversal, learning set, match-to-sample is not affected by the same lesions nor do these lesions impair performance which relies on associative memory (e.g., Jacobsen 1936, Goldman et al. 1971, Passingham 1975, Mishkin and Manning 1978) or sensory-guided responses (e.g., Funa-

hashi et al. 1993a, Sawaguchi and Goldman-Rakic 1993, Chafee and Goldman-Rakic 1994). In general, neither the consistent rules of a task nor its sensorimotor requirements cause a problem for the prefrontally lesioned animal. The monkey's difficulty lies in recalling information and using it to guide a correct response. Thus, on the basis of neuropsychological evidence, I have suggested that the brain obeys the distinction between working and associative memory, and that prefrontal cortex is pre-eminently involved in the former while other areas of the neopallium and hippocampus are likely the necessary critical substrates of memory consolidation and long-term storage (Goldman-Rakic 1987).

Single neuron recording has been used extensively to dissect the neuronal elements involved in working memory processes. This approach also can provide fresh insights into issues of functional allocation as well as deliver convergent validation of their essential nature. In the oculomotor delayed response paradigm utilized for this purpose, briefly presented visuo-spatial stimuli are remembered in order to provide guidance *from memory* for subsequent saccadic eye movements (figure 26.1a). The essential feature of this task is that the item to be recalled (in this case, the location of an object) has to be updated on every trial as in the moment-to-moment process of human mentation. The prefrontal cortex contains classes of neurons engaged respectively in registering the sensory cue, in holding the cued information "on line," and in releasing the motor responses in the course of task performance whether the task is conducted in the manual (Fuster and Alexander 1971) or oculomotor (Goldman-Rakic et al. 1991) mode. In aggregate, dorsolateral prefrontal cortex contains a local circuit that encompasses the entire range of subfunctions necessary to carry out an integrated response: sensory input, through retention in short-term memory, to motor response. Thus, attentional, memorial and response control mechanisms exist within this one area of prefrontal cortex and need not be allo-

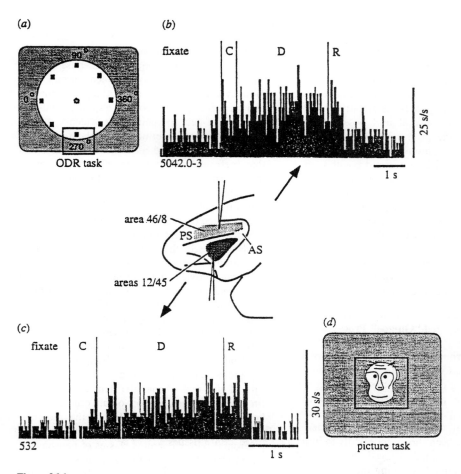

Figure 26.1
Multiple memory domains are illustrated in this diagram of the monkey prefrontal cortex. The dorsolateral area around the principal sulcus and anterior arcuate is important for spatial working memory; that for features or attributes of objects, in the inferior convexity of the prefrontal cortex. (*a*) Diagram of ODR task; (*b*) activity of a neuron recorded from area 46 during the ODR task. The neuron shown was activated in the delay whenever the monkey had to recall the target presented at the 270° location and at no other location; (*c*) a neuron activated in the delay whenever the stimulus to be recalled was a picture of a particular face during a picture working memory task; the same neuron was unresponsive to other memoranda or in relation to direction of response. (*d*) Diagram of picture working memory task. These results illustrate that prefrontal neurons can code selective aspects of or selected images in working memory. (Modified from Funahashi et al. 1989 and Wilson et al. 1993.)

cated to separate architectonic regions. Much remains to be learned about a dedicated area like the principal sulcus, including whether it has further functional subspecializations that have yet to be delineated.

Prefrontal neurons that express "memory fields" are particularly relevant to this discussion (see figure 26.1b). The concept of a "memory field" is based on the finding that the same neuron appears to always code the same location and different neurons code different locations. Consequently, individual neurons capable of holding specific visuo-spatial coordinates "on line" appear to be aggregated into a working memory system within an area of the prefrontal cortex. These aggregates likely form modular or columnar units defined by common visual-spatial coordinates but with the specialized subfunctions of cue registration, maintenance of the mnemonic trace and response preparedness allocated to different neurons within a column (Goldman-Rakic 1984). Again, much remains to be learned about these modules but, even at a microarchitectural level of cortical function, sensory, memorial and motor subfunctions are represented in the circuitry of the module. We have demonstrated that temporary inactivation of one or a few modules results in loss of "online" memory for particular target locations (Sawaguchi and Goldman-Rakic 1991). Further, in instances where the memory field of a neuron is not maintained throughout the delay and the activity falters, the animal is highly likely to make an error (Funahashi et al. 1989). The finding that neuronal firing is content-specific and directly associated with accurate recall provides a dramatic example of a compartmentalized and constrained architecture for memory processing equivalent to that observed in sensory systems. Additionally, it has been shown that prefrontal neurons can code the direction of an impending response iconically, that is, without reference to the direction of the response (Funahashi et al. 1993b). These and other results provide strong evidence at a cellular level for the theorized role of prefrontal neurons in working memory, that is, maintenance of representational information in the *absence* of the stimulus that was initially present. Knowledge of these neuronal properties helps to provide an explanation for the observation that monkeys and humans with prefrontal lesions have little difficulty in moving their eyes to a visible target or reaching for a desired object; rather their problem is organizing and directing these same motor responses to *remembered* targets and objects. In the same vein, damage to the prefrontal cortex does not impair knowledge about the world or long-term memory; it impairs only the ability to bring this knowledge to mind and utilize it to guide behaviour.

Working Memory, Mental Processing, and Perseveration

Two issues have dominated thinking in the area of prefrontal localization. One already mentioned is the degree of dissociation between areas subserving motor control, disinhibition and perseveration on the one hand and memory processes on the other. Another related issue is the separate location of a temporary storage component and a processing component of working memory (Just and Carpenter 1985, Baddeley 1986). Both issues can be addressed in non-human primates to some degree with an antisaccade task in which monkeys are trained to suppress the automatic or prepotent tendency to respond in the direction of a remembered cue and instead respond in the opposite direction, a transformation that is not particularly easy for human subjects (Guitton et al. 1985). The antisaccade task could be viewed as a member of a class of tasks like the Stroop test, which require prepotent response tendencies to be overridden by opponent or unlike responses. In our experiment with monkeys (Funahasi et al. 1993), we implemented a compound delayed-response paradigm, in which, on some trials, the monkey learned to make deferred eye movements to the same direction signalled by a brief visual cue (standard oculomotor delayed-response (ODR) task), and on other trials, cued by a change in the colour of the fixation spot, to suppress that response and direct its gaze to the opposite direction (delayed anti-saccade task, DAS). The monkeys succeeded in learning this difficult task at high (85% and above) levels of accuracy, in itself an indication that monkeys are capable of holding "in mind" two sequentially presented items of information—the colour of the fixation point and the location of a spatial cue and transforming the direction of response from left to right (or the reverse) based on a mental synthesis of that information. Approximately one-third of the task-related population coded the direction of the impending response, showing a pattern of activation in the delay period that presaged rightward or leftward responses. However, the majority (approximately 60%) of prefrontal neurons were iconic, that is, their activity in the delay period reflected the location of the cue, whether the intended movement was toward or away from the designated target. These results, together with numerous other single unit studies of prefrontal neurons, establish the following two major points: (1) the same area of cortex harbours sensory, mnemonic and response coding mechanisms, thus supporting an integral localization of the functions of attention, memory and motor response; and (2) the very same neuron involved in commanding an oculomotor response is also engaged when opposing responses are suppressed and/or redirected. Thus prefrontal neurons engaged in directing a response from memory are at the same time part of the mechanism engaged to inhibit the immediate or prepotent tendency to respond. Based on these findings, we would interpret the common association of verbal fluency and Stroop-like deficits discussed in the recent study by Burgess and Shallice (1996) as a failure to suppress a prepotent response (naming the word) due to an

inability to use working memory to initiate the correct response (naming the colour of the word based on recent instruction). Perseveration and disinhibition may be the inevitable result of a loss of the neural substrate necessary to generate the correct response.

Multiple Working Memory Domains

According to the working memory analysis of prefrontal function, a working memory function should be demonstrable in more than one area of the prefrontal cortex and in more than one knowledge domain. Thus, different areas within prefrontal cortex will share in a common process—working memory; however, each will process different types of information. Thus, informational domain, not process, will be mapped across prefrontal cortex. Evidence on this point has recently been obtained in our laboratory from studies of non-spatial memory systems in areas on the inferior convexity of the prefrontal cortex (O Scalaidhe et al. 1992, Wilson et al. 1992, Wilson et al. 1993). In particular, we explored the hypothesis that the inferior convexity of the prefrontal cortex comprising Walker's areas 12 and 45 may contain specialized circuits for recalling the attributes of stimuli and holding them in short-term memory—thus processing non-spatial information in a manner analogous to the mechanism by which the principal sulcus mediates memory of visuo-spatial information. The inferior convexity cortex lying below and adjacent to the principal sulcus is a likely candidate for processing non-spatial—colour and form—information, in that lesions of this area produce deficits on tasks requiring memory for the colour or patterns of stimuli (e.g., Passingham 1975, Mishkin and Manning 1978) and the receptive fields of the neurons in this area, unlike those in area 46 on the dorsolateral cortex above, represent the fovea (Mikami et al. 1982, Suzuki and Azuma 1983), the region of the retina specialized for the analysis of fine detail and colour—stimulus attributes important for the recognition of objects.

We recorded from the inferior convexity region in monkeys trained to perform delayed-response tasks in which spatial or feature *memoranda* had to be recalled on independent, randomly interwoven trials. For the spatial delayed-response trials (SDR), stimuli were presented 13° to the left or right of fixation while the monkeys gazed at a fixation point on a video monitor. After a delay of 2500 ms, the fixation point disappeared, instructing the animal to direct its gaze to the location where the stimulus appeared before the delay. For the picture delayed-response (PDR) trials, various patterns were presented in the centre of the screen (figure 26.1d); one stimulus indicated that a left-directed and the other a right-directed response would be rewarded at the end of the delay. Thus, both spatial and feature trials required exactly the same eye movements at the end of the delay; but differed in the nature of the mnemonic representation that guided those responses.

We found that neurons were responsive to events in both delayed response tasks. However, a given neuron was generally responsive to the spatial aspects or the feature aspects and not both (Wilson et al. 1993). Thus, the majority of the neurons examined in both tasks were active in the delay period when the monkey was recalling a stimulus pattern which required a 13° response to the right *or* left. The same neurons did not respond above baseline during the delay preceding an identical rightward or leftward response on the PDR trials. Neurons exhibiting selective neuronal activity for patterned memoranda were almost exclusively found in or around area 12 on the inferior convexity of the prefrontal cortex, beneath the principal sulcus, while neurons that responded selectively in the SDR were rarely observed in this region, appearing instead in the dorsolateral cortical regions where spatial processing has been localized in our previous studies. In addition, we discovered that the neurons in the inferior convexity

were highly responsive to complex stimuli, such as pictures of faces or specific objects. We subsequently used pictures of monkey or human faces as memoranda in a working memory task and demonstrated that such stimuli could indeed serve as memoranda in memory tasks (figure 26.1a, c). The same cells are unresponsive on trials when the monkey has to remember a different face or pattern nor do they code the direction of an impending response (Wilson et al. 1993). Finally, we have shown that the areas from which face or object selective neurons are recorded are connected directly with area TE in the inferiotemporal cortex which is a major relay of the ventral pathway for object vision (Mishkin et al. 1982) and an area rich in cells that respond to the features of visual stimuli, including faces (e.g., Rolls and Baylis 1986, Tanaka et al. 1991). Together with the evidence for dissociation of inferior prefrontal and dorsolateral prefrontal lesions vis-à-vis object processing (reviewed in Goldman-Rakic 1987), these several results establish that non-spatial attributes of an object or stimulus may be processed separately from those dedicated to the analysis of spatial location and vice versa. Furthermore, within inferior prefrontal cortex, different features appear to be encoded by different neurons (Wilson et al. 1993, in preparation). Thus, feature and spatial memory—what and where an object is—are dissociable not only at the areal level but at the cellular level as well. Altogether these findings support the prediction that different prefrontal subdivisions represent different informational domains rather than different processes and thus, more than one working memory domain exists in the prefrontal cortex—one in and around the caudal principal sulcus concerned with spatial information and another on the caudal inferior convexity concerned with object information. If the inferior prefrontal cortex carries out temporal integration of information analogous to the spatial processing of the dorsolateral region, as we have proposed, then it will surely be engaged in "comparison between stimuli in short-term memory as well as the active organization of sequences of responses based on conscious explicit retrieval of information from posterior cortical association systems" as formulated by Petrides an colleagues (Owen et al. 1996). The question to be decided in future research is whether this function is at a lower level of a hierarchical processing than the "monitoring" function proposed by the same authors for superior prefrontal cortical areas. To decide this, the performance of monkeys with cortical lesions in superior areas will have to be directly compared to that of monkeys with inferior convexity lesions on the same set of tasks.

The functional architecture suggested by physiological and lesion studies in monkeys appear to be supported by findings from positron emission tomography and magnetic resonance imaging in humans. Thus, the middle frontal gyrus where area 46 is located is consistently activated as human subjects access visuo-spatial information from long-term storage and/or immediate experience through representation-based action (e.g., McCarthy et al. 1994, Nichelli et al. 1994, Baker et al. 1996, Gold et al. 1996, Goldberg et al. 1996, Owen et al. 1996, Smith et al. 1996, Sweeney et al. 1996). In contrast, working memory for the features of objects or faces engages anatomically more lateral and inferior prefrontal regions (Adcock et al. 1996, Cohen et al. 1994, Courtney et al. 1996, McCarthy et al. 1996) and semantic encoding and retrieval as well as other verbal processes engages still more inferior, insular, and/or anterior prefrontal regions (Paulesu et al. 1993, Raichle et al. 1994, Demb et al. 1995, Fiez et al. 1996, Price et al. 1996). The superior to inferior localization of spatial, object and linguistic processing in imaging studies of human cognition support a multiple domain hypothesis of prefrontal functional architecture and indicate that there may be a common bauplan for their network organization.

As to the remaining expanse of prefrontal areas, less is known. The evidence from recent studies of the orbital surface indicate that this general region of the frontal lobe may be similarly compartmentalized as to informational domain, though it is not yet clear that these regions have domain-specific "on-line" memory functions. However, Rolls in this meeting has mapped a taste area in the caudolateral orbitofrontal cortex near an area concerned with olfaction (Tanabe et al. 1974), together providing sensory definition to the mesopallial map. Certainly, the studies of Rolls and others (Tanabe et al. 1974, Baylis et al. 1995, Carmichael and Price 1995) clearly define gustatory and olfactory regions in the mesopallial areas. What lies in between these and the dorsolateral regions—in the ventromedial and ventrolateral expanse of the orbital cortex—remains to be explored as do the dorsomedial and medial areas of the prefrontal cortex. Studies of orbital lesions in humans have revealed an autonomic pattern of deficits (Damasio et al. 1991) as well as subtle executive deficits in real world social contexts (Grattan et al. 1994, Eslinger et al. 1995).

Levels of Processing: Distributed Networks Subserve Sensory, Motor, Limbic, and Mnemonic Components Constrained by Informational Domain

Although the prefrontal cortex has a pre-eminent role in working memory functions, it does so as part of an integrated network of areas, each dedicated to carrying out specialized functions. Each working memory domain is embedded in and supported by a distinct and essentially independent network of cortical areas; thus networks are functionally integrated by domain. For example, the prefrontal areas engaged in spatial working memory are interconnected with portions of posterior parietal cortex (Cavada and Goldman-Rakic 1989), while the feature working memory areas of the inferior prefrontal cortex are interconnected with area TE in the temporal lobe (Barbas 1988, 1993; Bates et al. 1994, Rodman 1994, Webster et al. 1994, Carmichael and Price 1995). A network is comprised of sensory association (temporal and parietal), premotor (cingulate motor areas, pre-SMA) and limbic (retrosplenial cingulate, parahippocampal or perirhinal) areas at a minimum and virtually all of the connections within a network are reciprocal (Selemon and Goldman-Rakic 1985). Thus, this model of prefrontal network organization contrasts with other theories of prefrontal organization which distribute attention, affect,

memory and motor action among the different cytoarchitectonic regions of the prefrontal cortex. The multiple domain model distributes these functions among the cortical areas within networks defined by informational domain.

Allocation of function within a widespread cortical network is a subject currently under examination by a number of laboratories. Here I give two examples from our own work with respect to the spatial cognition network (Selemon

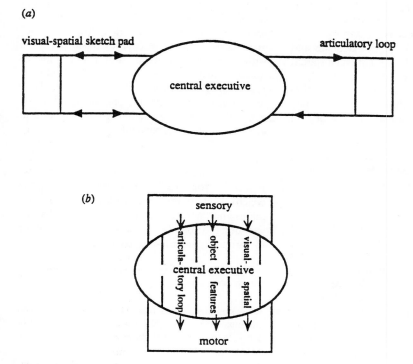

Figure 26.2

(*a*) Diagram of the central executive (psychologically based; Baddeley 1989). The model consists of a central executive and two slave systems—the phonological loop and the visuo-spatial sketchpad. The slave systems and central processor are presumed to be localized in separated regions of the cortex. (*b*) Model of the "central executive" based on functional architecture elucidated in studies of non-human primates (Goldman-Rakic 1996). According to this neurologically based model, the central executive may be considered an emergent property of coactivated multiple domain-specific processors located in prefrontal cortex but interconnected both with the domain-relevant long-term storage sites in posterior regions of the cortex (sensory) and with appropriate motor pathways.

and Goldman-Rakic 1988). Posterior parietal regions carry directionally specific information in all phases of the delayed response task (cue, delay, and response) and thus, neurons in posterior parietal cortex mirror those in prefrontal cortex (Chafee et al. 1989, Chafee and Goldman-Rakic 1994). In contrast to the parietal cortex, neuronal activity in posterior cingulate cortex is, in general, not directionally tuned but rather posterior cingulate neurons appear to be engaged in a non-specific form of activation related to response anticipation (figure 26.2; Carlson et al. 1993). Both the single unit studies described here and a series of 2-deoxyglucose metabolic imaging studies in the literature (e.g., Friedman and Goldman-Rakic 1994) indicate that when spatial memories are activated, parietal, cingulate and prefrontal components of the spatial cognition network are coactivated, though each area may be essential for different aspects of the task in question.

The Supervisory Attentional System, the Central Executive, and the Domain-Specific Slave Systems

One of the most powerful and influential ideas in cognitive psychology is Baddeley's working memory model (Baddeley 1986). This tripartite model of cognitive architecture invokes a supervisory controlling system called the "central executive" and two slave systems, the "articulatory loop" and the "visuo-spatial scratch pad" or "sketch pad," specialized for language and spatial material, respectively (figure 26.2). The model recognizes the separation of informational domains for lower level tasks handled by the "slave" systems but retains the traditional notion of a general purpose, panmodal processor in the central executive that manages control and selection processes, similar to the supervisory attentional system of Shallice (1982). The findings reviewed above provide an alternative model in which the expression of central executive processing is a result of the interaction of multiple independent information processing modules each with its own sensory, mnemonic and motor control features. This multiple domain model reduces but does not necessarily eliminate "the residual area of ignorance" called the central executive but it does open the question of how these independent systems cooperate to result in an integrated behavioural script.

Our view is that the central executive may be composed of multiple segregated special purpose processing domains rather than one central processor served by slave systems converging to a central processor; and that each specialized domain consists of local and extrinsic networks with sensory, mnemonic, motor and motivational control elements (figure 26.2; Goldman-Rakic 1987). This process-oriented view explains the dysexecutive syndrome—disorganization, perseveration and distractibility—as a default in one or more independent working memory domains. The working memory specialization of the prefrontal cortex is especially suited to retrieve information from long-term memory and process it "on line." It is possible to view the coactivation of multiple working memory domains and their associated cortical networks as a well designed parallel processing architecture for the brain's highest level cognition.

References

Adcock, R. A., Constable, R. T., Gore, J. C. and Goldman-Rakic, P. 1996 Functional magnetic resonance imaging of frontal cortex during performance of non-spatial memory tasks. *Neuroimage* 3, S526.

Baddeley, A. 1986 *Working memory.* Oxford University Press.

Baddeley, A. D. and Hitch, G. 1974 Working memory. In *The psychology of learning and motivation. Advances in research and theory* (ed. G. H. Bower), pp. 47–89. New York: Academic Press.

Baker, S. C., Frith, C. D., Frackowiak, R. S. J. and Dolan, R. J. 1996 Active representation of shape and spatial location in man. *Cereb. Cortex.* 6, 612–619.

Barbas, H. 1988 Anatomic organization of basoventral and mediodorsal visual recipient prefrontal regions in the rhesus monkey. *J. Comp. Neurol.* 276, 313–342.

Bates, J. F., Wilson, F. A. W., O Scalaidhe, S. P. and Goldman-Rakic, P. S. 1994 Area TE connections with inferior prefrontal regions responsive to complex objects and faces. *Soc. Neurosci. Abstr.* 20, 434.10.

Bauer, R. H. and Fuster, J. M. 1976 Delayed matching and delayed-response deficit from cooling dorsolateral prefrontal cortex in monkeys. *J. Comp. Physiol. Psychol.* 90, 293–302.

Baylis, L. L., Rolls, E. T. and Baylis, G. C. 1995 Afferent connections of the caudolateral orbitofrontal cortex taste area of the primate. *Neurosci.* 64, 801–812.

Brutkowski, S. 1965 Functions of prefrontal cortex in animals. *Physiol. Rev.* 45, 721–746.

Burgess, P. W. and Shallice, T. 1996 Response suppression, initiation and strategy use following frontal lobe lesions. *Neuropsychologia* 34, 263–273.

Carlson, S., Mikami, A. and Goldman-Rakic, P. S. 1993 Omnidirectional delay activity in the monkey posterior cingulate cortex during the performance of an oculomotor delayed response task. *Soc. Neurosci. Abstr.* 19, 800.

Carmichael, S. T. and Price, J. L. 1995 Sensory and premotor connections of the orbital and medial prefrontal cortex of macaque monkeys. *J. Comp. Neurol.* 363, 642–664.

Cavada, C. and Goldman-Rakic, P. S. 1989 Posterior parietal cortex in rhesus monkey: II. Evidence for segretated corticocortical networks linking sensory and limbic areas with the frontal lobe. *J. Comp. Neurol.* 287, 422–445.

Chafee, M. and Goldman-Rakic, P. S. 1994 Prefrontal cooling dissociates memory- and sensory-guided oculomotor delayed response functions. *Soc. Neurosci. Abstr.* 20, 335.1.

Chafee, M., Funahashi, S. and Goldman-Rakic, P. S. 1989 Unit activity in the primate posterior parietal cortex during delayed response performance. *Soc. Neurosci. Abstr.* 15, 786.

Cohen, J. D., Forman, S. D., Braver, T. S., Casey, B. J., Servan-Schreiber, D. and Noll, D. C. 1994 Activation of the prefrontal cortex in a nonspatial working memory task with functional MRI. *Hum. Brain Map* 1, 293–304.

Courtney, S. M., Ungerleider, L. G., Keil, K. and Haxby, J. V. 1996 Object and spatial visual working memory activate separate neural systems in human cortex. *Cereb. Cortex* 6, 39–49.

Damasio, A. R., Tranel, D. and Damasio, H. C. 1991 Somatic markers and the guidance of behavior: Theory and preliminary testing. In *Frontal lobe function and dysfunction* (ed. H. S. Levin, H. M. Eisenberg, and A. L. Benton), pp. 217–229. New York: Oxford University Press.

Demb, J. B., Desmond, J. E., Wagner, A. D., Vaidya, C. J., Glover, G. H. and Gabrieli, J. D. E. 1995 Semantic encoding and retrieval in the left inferior prefrontal cortex: A functional MRI study of task difficult and process specificity. *J. Neurosci.* 15, 5870–5878.

Dias, R., Robbins, T. W. and Roberts, A. C. 1996 Dissociation in prefrontal cortex of affective and attentional shifts. *Nature* 380, 69–72.

Eslinger, P. J. and Damasio, A. R. 1985 Severe disturbance of higher cognition after bilateral frontal lobe ablation: Patient EVR. *Neurology* 35, 1731–1741.

Eslinger, P. J., Grattan, L. M. and Geder, L. 1995 Impact of frontal lobe lesions on rehabilitation and recovery from acute brain injury. *NeuroRehabilitation* 5, 161–182.

Fiez, J. A., Raife, E. A., Balota, D. A., Schwarz, J. P., Raichle, M. E. and Petersen, S. E. 1996 A positron emission tomography study of the short-term maintenance of verbal information. *J. Neurosci.* 16, 808–822.

Freedman, M. and Oscar-Berman, M. 1986 Bilateral frontal lobe disease and selective delayed response deficits in humans. *Behav. Neurosci.* 100, 337–342.

Fulton, J. F. 1950 *Frontal lobotomy and affective behavior.* New York: Norton.

Funahashi, S., Bruce, C. J. and Goldman-Rakic, P. S. 1989 Mnemonic coding of visual space in the monkey's dorsolateral prefrontal cortex. *J. Neurophysiol.* 61, 1–19.

Funahashi, S., Bruce, C. J. and Goldman-Rakic, P. S. 1993a Dorsolateral prefrontal lesions and oculomotor delayed-response performance: Evidence for mnemonic scotomas. *J. Neurosci.* 13, 1479–1497.

Funahashi, S., Chafee, M. V. and Goldman-Rakic, P. S. 1993b Prefrontal neuronal activity in rhesus monkeys performing a delayed anti-saccade task. *Nature* 365, 753–756.

Fuster, J. M. 1980 *The prefrontal cortex.* New York: Raven Press.

Fuster, J. M. 1989 *The prefrontal cortex*, 2nd edn. New York: Raven Press.

Fuster, J. M. and Alexander, G. E. 1971 Neuron activity related to short-term memory. *Science* 173, 652–654.

Gold, J. M., Berman, K. F., Randolph, C., Goldberg, T. E. and Weinberger, D. R. 1966 PET validation and clinical application of a novel prefrontal task. *Neuropsychology* 10, 3–10.

Goldberg, T. E., Berman, K. F., Randolph, C., Gold, J. M. and Weinberger, D. R. 1996 Isolating the mnemonic component in spatial delayed response: A controlled PET 0–15 water regional cerebral blood flow study in normal humans. *NeuroImage.* 3, 69–78.

Goldman, P. S. and Rosvold, H. E. 1970 Localization of function within the dorsolateral prefrontal cortex of the rhesus monkey. *Experimental Neurology* 27, 291–304.

Goldman, P. S., Rosvold, H. E., Vest, B. and Galkin, T. W. 1971 Analysis of the delayed-alternation deficit produced by dorsolateral prefrontal lesions in the rhesus monkey. *J. Comp. Physiol. Psychol.* 77, 212–220.

Goldman-Rakic, P. S. 1984 The frontal lobes: Uncharted provinces of the brain. *TINS* 7, 425–429.

Goldman-Rakic, P. S. 1987 Circuitry of primate prefrontal cortex and regulation of behavior by representational memory. In *Handbook of physiology, the nervous system, higher functions of the brain* (ed. F. Plum), sect. I, vol, V, pp. 373–417. Bethesda, MD: American Physiological Society.

Goldman-Rakic, P. S., Funahashi, S. and Bruce, C. J. 1991 Neocortical memory circuits. *Q. J. Quantitative Biology* 55, 1025–1038.

Grattan, L. M., Bloomer, R. H., Archambault, F. X. and Eslinger, P. J. 1994 Cognitive flexibility and empathy after frontal lobe lesion. *Neuropsychiat. Neuropsychol. Behav. Neurol.* 7, 251–259.

Guitton, D., Buchtel, H. A. and Douglas, R. M. 1985 Frontal lobe lesions in man cause difficulties in suppressing reflexive glances and in generating goal-directed saccades. *Exp. Brain Res.* 58, 455–472.

Jacobsen, C. F. 1936 Studies of cerebral function in primates. *Comp. Psychol. Monogr.* 13, 1–8.

Just, M. A. and Carpenter, P. A. 1985 Cognitive coordinate systems: Accounts of mental rotation and individual differences in spatial ability. *Psych. Rev.* 92, 137–172.

McCarthy, G., Blamire, A. M., Puce, A. et al. 1994 Functional magnetic resonance imaging of human prefrontal cortex activation during a spatial working memory task. *Proc. natn. Acad. Sci. U.S.A.* 91, 8690–8694.

McCarthy, G., Puce, A., Constable, R. T., Krystal, J. H., Gore, J. C. and Goldman-Rakic, P. S. 1996 Activation of human prefrontal cortex during spatial and nonspatial working memory tasks measured by functional MRI. *Cereb. Cortex.* 6, 600–610.

Mikami, A., Ito, S. and Kubota, K. 1982 Visual response properties of dorsolateral prefrontal neurons during a visual fixation task. *J. Neurophysiol.* 47, 593–605.

Mishkin, M. 1964 Perseveration of central sets after frontal lesions in monkeys. In *The frontal granular cortex and behavior* (ed. J. M. Warren and K. Akert), pp. 219–241. New York: McGraw-Hill.

Mishkin, M. and Manning, F. J. 1978 Non-spatial memory after selective prefrontal lesions in monkeys. *Brain Res.* 143, 313–323.

Mishkin, M., Ungerleider, L. G. and Macko, K. A. 1982 Object vision and spatial vision: Two cortical pathways. *TINS* 6, 414–417.

Nichelli, P., Grafman, J., Pietrini, P., Alway, D., Carton, J. C. and Miletich, R. 1994 Brain activity in chess playing. *Nature* 369, 191.

O Scalaidhe, S. P., Wilson, F. A. W. and Goldman-Rakic, P. S. 1992 Neurons in the prefrontal cortex of the macaque selective for faces. *Soc. Neurosci. Abstr.* 18, 705.

Owen, A. M., Evans, A. C. and Petrides, M. 1996 Evidence for a two-stage model of spatial working memory processing with the lateral frontal cortex: A positron emission tomography study. *Cereb. Cortex* 6, 31–38.

Passingham, R. E. 1975 Delayed matching after selective prefrontal lesions in monkeys (*Macac mulatta*). *Brain Res.* 92, 89–102.

Paulescu, E., Frith, C. D. and Frackowiak, R. S. J. 1993 Localization of a human system for sustained attention by positron emission tomography. *Nature* 362, 342–345.

Pribram, K. H. 1987 The subdivisions of the frontal cortex revisited. In *The frontal lobes revisited* (ed. E. Perecman), pp. 11–39. New York: The IRBN Press.

Pribram, K. H. and Tubbs, W. E. 1967 Short-term memory, parsing and the primate frontal cortex. *Science* 156, 1765–1767.

Price, C. J., Wise, R. J. S. and Frackowiak, R. S. J. 1996 Demonstrating the implicit processing of visually presented words and pseudowords. *Cereb. Cortex* 6, 62–70.

Raichle, M. E., Fiez, J. A., Videen, T. O. et al. 1994 Practice-related changes in human brain functional anatomy during non-motor learning. *Cereb. Cortex* 4, 8–26.

Rodman, H. R. 1994 Development of inferior temporal cortex in the monkey. *Cereb. Cortex* 4, 484–498.

Rolls, E. T. and Baylis, G. C. 1986 Size and contrast have only small effects on the responses to faces of neurons in the cortex of the superior temporal sulcus of the monkey. *Exp. Brain Res.* 65, 38–48.

Sawaguchi, T. and Goldman-Rakic, P. S. 1991 D1 dopamine receptors in prefrontal cortex: involvement in working memory. *Science* 251, 947–950.

Sawaguchi, T. and Goldman-Rakic, P. S. 1993 The role of D1-dopamine receptor in working memory: Local injections of dopamine antagonists into the prefrontal cortex of rhesus monkeys performing an oculomotor delayed-response task. *J. Neurophysiol.* 71, 515–528.

Selemon, L. D. and Goldman-Rakic, P. S. 1985 Longitudinal topography and interdigitation of corticostriatal projections in the rhesus monkey. *J. Neuroscience*, 5, 776–794.

Selemon, L. D. and Goldman-Rakic, P. S. 1988 Common cortical and subcortical target areas of the dorsolateral prefrontal and posterior parietal cortices in the rhesus monkey: Evidence for a distributed neural network subserving spatially guided behavior. *J. Neuroscience* 8, 4049–4068.

Shallice, T. 1982 Specific impairments in planning. *Proc. Roy. Soc.* 298, 199–209.

Smith, E. E., Jonides, J. and Koeppe, R. A. 1996 Dissociating verbal and spatial working memory using PET. *Cereb. Cortex* 6, 11–20.

Suzuki, H. and Azuma, M. 1983 Topographic studies on visual neurons in the dorsolateral prefrontal cortex of the monkey. *Exp. Brain Res.* 53, 47–58.

Sweeney, J. A., Mintun, M. A., Kwee, M. B. et al. 1996 Positron emission tomography study of voluntary saccadic eye movements and spatial working memory. *J. Neurophysiol.* 75, 454–468.

Tanabe, T., Ooshima, Y. and Takagi, S. F. 1974 An olfactory area in the prefrontal lobe. *Brain Res.* 80, 127–130.

Tanaka, K., Saito, H., Fukada, Y. and Moriya, M. 1991 Coding visual images of objects in the inferotemporal cortex of the macaque monkey. *J. Neurophysiol.* 66, 170–189.

Webster, M. J., Bachevalier, J. and Ungerleider, L. G. 1994 Connections of inferior temporal areas TEO and TE with parietal and frontal cortex in macaque monkeys. *Cereb. Cortex* 4, 470–483.

Wilson, F. A. W., O Scalaidhe, S. P. and Goldman-Rakic, P. S. 1992 Areal and cellular segregation of spatial and of feature processing by prefrontal neurons. *Soc. Neurosci. Abstr.* 18, 705.

Wilson, F. A. W., O Scalaidhe, S. P. and Goldman-Rakic, P. S. 1993 Dissociation of object and spatial processing domains in primate prefrontal cortex. *Science* 260, 1955–1958.

Storage and Executive Processes in the Frontal Lobes

Edward E. Smith and John Jonides

The frontal cortex comprises a third of the human brain; it is the structure that enables us to engage in higher cognitive functions such as planning and problem solving (1). What are the processes that serve as the building blocks of these higher cognitive functions, and how are these implemented in frontal cortex?

Recent discussions of this issue have focused on working memory, a system used for temporary storage and manipulation of information. The system is divided into two general components: short-term storage and a set of "executive processes." Short-term storage involves active maintenance of a limited amount of information for a matter of seconds; it is a necessary component of many higher cognitive functions (2) and is mediated in part by the prefrontal cortex (PFC) (3). Executive processes are implemented by PFC as well (4). Although executive processes often operate on the contents of short-term storage, the two components of working memory can be dissociated: there are neurological patients who have intact short-term storage but defective executive processes and vice versa (5).

We review here neuroimaging studies of these two components of working memory. We consider experiments that have used positron emission tomography (PET) or functional magnetic resonance imaging (fMRI) to image participants while they engage in cognitive tasks that are designed to reveal processes of interest, such as tasks that isolate short-term storage of verbal material. We concentrate on studies in which participants performed an experimental and a control task while being scanned and in which the control task has typically been chosen so that it differs from the experimental task only in a process of interest; a comparison of the experimental and control tasks thus reveals activations due to the process of interest (6). These paradigms contrast with standard neuropsychological tasks that may have diagnostic value for patients with frontal cortical lesions but that do not reveal individual cognitive processes.

Storage Processes and the Frontal Lobes

Many neuroimaging studies are founded on Baddeley's (7) model of working memory. In part, it posits separate storage buffers for verbal and visual-spatial information. Baddeley further argued that verbal storage can be decomposed into a phonological buffer for short-term maintenance of phonological information and a subvocal rehearsal process that refreshes the contents of the buffer. We examine evidence about each aspect of this model as it relates to frontal cortex.

Verbal Storage

Some evidence about storage mechanisms comes from experiments with the item-recognition task (8) (figure 27.1a). In most of these studies, a small set of target letters was presented simultaneously, followed by an unfilled delay interval of several seconds, followed by a single-letter probe; the participant's task was to decide whether the probe matched any of the target letters. Compared with a control task, the item-recognition task results in activations in left posterior parietal cortex (Brodmann's area (BA) 40) and three frontal sites (Broca's area (BA 44) and left supplementary motor and premotor areas (BA 6)). (The latter three areas, along with other important frontal areas and divisions, are presented schematically in figure 27.2). Given that these frontal areas are known to be involved in the preparation of speech (9) and that participants rehearse the targets silently during the delay, the frontal speech areas likely mediate subvocal rehearsal of the targets. As evidence for

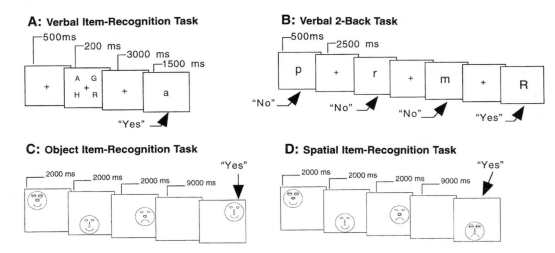

Figure 27.1
Schematic representation of four tasks used to study working memory. (*a*) Verbal item-recognition task, which taps mainly short-term storage for verbal information. A trial includes (i) fixation point, (ii) four uppercase letters, (iii) blank delay interval, and (iv) a lowercase probe letter. The participant's task is to decide whether the probe names one of four target letters. (*b*) Verbal 2-back task, which presumably involves executive processes (temporal coding) as well as storage of verbal material. Each letter is followed by a blank delay interval, and the participant's task is to decide whether each letter has the same name as the one that occurred two back in the sequence. (*c*) Object item-recognition task, which taps short-term storage for object information. A trial includes (i) a sequence of three target faces, (ii) a blank delay interval, and (iii) a probe face. The participant's task is to decide whether the probe face is the same as any of the target faces. (*d*) Spatial item-recognition task, which taps short-term storage for spatial information. A trial includes the same events as in the object task, but the participant's task is to decide whether the probe face is in the same location as any of the target faces.

this claim, the activation in Broca's area closely matches that obtained in an explicitly phonological task, rhyme judgments (10). (Evidence from neurological patients suggests that the posterior parietal region mediates a storage buffer (11, 12).)

Further evidence for localizing rehearsal in the frontal speech areas comes from a PET study that used a "2-back" task (13) (see figure 27.1b). Participants viewed a sequence of single letters separated by 2.5 s each; for each letter they had to decide whether it was identical in name to the letter that appeared two items back in the sequence. The experiment used two different controls. In one, participants saw a sequence of letters but simply had to decide whether each

letter matched a single target letter. Subtracting this control from the 2-back condition yielded many of the areas of activation that have been obtained in item-recognition tasks, including the left frontal speech regions and the parietal area. The second control required participants to rehearse each letter silently. Subtracting this rehearsal control from the 2-back task should have removed much of the rehearsal circuitry since rehearsal is needed in both tasks; indeed, in this subtraction, neither Broca's area nor the premotor area remained active. Hence, this experiment isolated a frontal rehearsal circuit.

Several other PET and fMRI studies have used 2-back and 3-back tasks. All have found

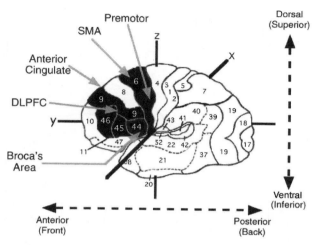

Figure 27.2

Schematic of the left lateral cortex, displaying major prefrontal areas (numbers correspond to Brodmann areas). The areas of greatest interest are shaded, and they include Broca's area, DLPFC, the anterior cingulate (not visible in the schematic, as it lies on the medial side of the cortex), SMA, and premotor. Also shown are the x, y, and z dimensions, which are used to report the coordinates of activations (where the three dimensions intersect, all coordinates are zero). In addition, anterior-posterior and dorsal-ventral directions, which are used in anatomical descriptions, are indicated.

activation in Broca's area and the premotor cortex (14, 15). In addition, two studies have used a free-recall paradigm to study short-term storage, and they also found activation in frontal speech regions (16). Thus, frontal regions that no doubt evolved for the purpose of spoken language appear to be recruited to keep verbal information active in working memory.

Figure 27.3 summarizes the relevant results; figure 27.3a shows data from item-recognition tasks, which require mainly storage, whereas figure 27.3b shows data from n-back tasks and free-recall tasks, which presumably require executive processes as well as storage. In figure 27.3a, in the sagittal view, the activations cluster posteriorly in the frontal lobes—running from the premotor and supplementary motor area (SMA) ventrally to Broca's area; this is the rehearsal circuit. In the coronal and axial views of figure

27.3a, the activation foci show a left lateral tendency; indeed, the mean x coordinate is significantly less than zero ($t(31) = -2.9$; $P < 0.01$), indicating a center of mass in the left hemisphere. The lateralization pattern changes when nonstorage processes are added to the task. In the axial and coronal projections of figure 27.3b, the activation foci were bilateral, not left-lateralized. Furthermore, in addition to the clusters in premotor and SMA, Broca's, and posterior parietal lobe, these tasks also produce a cluster in dorsolateral prefrontal cortex (DLPFC), as shown in the sagittal view of figure 27.3b. In fact, the mean y coordinate of frontal activations ($y > 0.25$) in figure 27.3b is significantly anterior to that in figure 27.3a ($t(79, 52) = 4.18$; $P < 0.001$). These activations therefore reflect the distinction between tasks requiring mainly storage and those requiring additional processing.

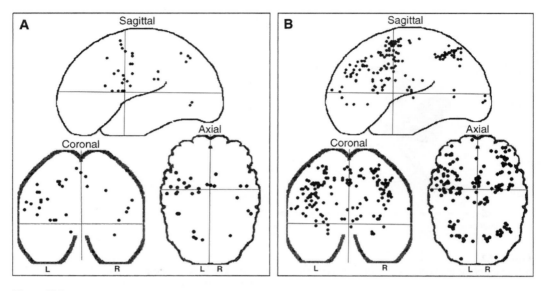

Figure 27.3
Neuroimaging results for verbal working memory are summarized by sets of three projections, with each containing points and axes conforming to standard Talairach space (40). Each projection collapses one plane of view for each activation focus—that is, the sagittal view collapses across the x plane as though one were looking through the brain from the side; the coronal view collapses across the y plane as though one were looking through the brain from the front or back; and the axial view collapses across the z plane as though one were looking through the brain from the top. Included in the summary are published ^{15}O PET or fMRI studies of verbal working memory that reported coordinates of activation and had a memory load of six or fewer items. (Cerebellar activation foci, not shown, were predominantly in the right hemisphere, which is consistent with the crossed connections of cerebellum and cerebrum.) (*a*) Activation foci from studies that involve mainly storage. Awh et al. (13), item recognition; Jonides et al. (15), 0- and 1-back; Jonides et al. (33), item recognition; Paulesu et al. (10), item recognition. (*b*) Activation foci from studies that require executive processing as well as storage. Awh et al. (13), 2-back; Braver et al. (15), 2- and 3-back; Cohen et al. (14), 2-back; Cohen et al. (15), 2- and 3-back; D'Esposito et al. (28), 2-back; Fiez et al. (16), free recall; Jonides et al. (15), 2- and 3-back; Jonides et al. (16), free recall; Schumacher et al. (15), 3-back; Smith et al. (15), 3-back.

Spatial and Object Storage

Research on nonverbal working memory has been influenced by physiological work with nonhuman primates (3). Single-cell recordings made while monkeys engage in spatial-storage tasks have found "spatial memory" cells in DLPFC (which is usually taken to include BA 46 and 9). These cells selectively fire during a delay period and are position specific. Recordings made while monkeys engage in object-storage tasks have found delay-sensitive "object memory" cells in a more ventral region of PFC that are object specific (17). The implications of these findings are that (i) spatial and object working memory have different neural bases, and (ii) at least part of the circuitry for these two types of memory is in PFC, with spatial information being represented more dorsally than object information (18).

Neuroimaging evidence supports a distinction between human spatial and object working memory as well (19–21). In one paradigm used to demonstrate the distinction, three target faces were presented sequentially in three different locations, followed by a probe face in a variable location. In the object working-memory task (see figure 27.1c), participants decided whether the probe matched any of the three targets in identity; in the spatial task (see figure 27.1d), they decided whether the probe matched any of the targets in position. The object task activated regions in the right DLPFC whereas the spatial task activated a region in the right premotor cortex. Follow-up studies have shown that the region in DLPFC remains active during a delay period in the object task, whereas the premotor area remains active during a delay in the spatial task, thus strengthening the case that the two areas mediate separate kinds of storage (22, 23).

Figure 27.4 summarizes the relevant results. The sagittal and coronal projections reveal a dorsal-ventral difference between spatial and object working-memory tasks, respectively, particularly in posterior cortex. For posterior cortex ($y > -25$), the average z coordinate of the spatial-memory activation foci was significantly greater (more dorsal) than that of object-memory activation foci ($t(41, 45) = 9.87$; $P < 0.001$). The anterior cortex ($y > -25$) also shows a significant dorsal-ventral difference ($t(37, 47) = 3.24$; $P < 0.004$). Specifically, spatial working-memory activations seem to cluster primarily in the premotor area, whereas object working-memory activations spread from premotor to DLPFC.

Although the dorsal-ventral difference is in line with the results from monkeys, there are two findings from spatial tasks that differ from the results obtained with monkeys: the presence of activation in premotor cortex and the failure to consistently find activation in DLPFC. The first finding has considerable support, as spatial tasks routinely activate the right premotor area (24). Perhaps the true functional homologue of DLPFC in monkeys is the premotor region in humans (25), or perhaps the major site of spatial working-memory in monkeys is more posterior than was originally believed (18). The issue remains unresolved.

Can the activations obtained in the spatial tasks be divided into storage and rehearsal functions, parallel to verbal working memory? One possibility is that the right premotor activation is a reflection of spatial rehearsal. By this account, spatial rehearsal involves covertly shifting attention from location to location, and doing so requires recruitment of an attentional circuit, including premotor cortex (26). Support for this account comes from the fact that neuroimaging results from studies of spatial working memory and spatial attention show overlap in activation in a right premotor site (27).

Implications

The research reviewed and the meta-analyses presented in figures 27.3 and 27.4 are relevant to two major proposals about the organization of PFC. One is that PFC is organized by the modality of the information stored; for example,

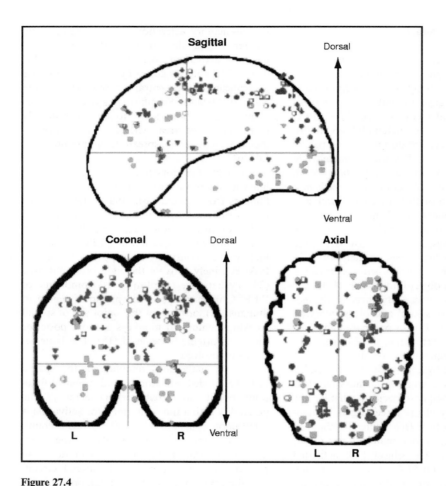

Figure 27.4
Neuroimaging results for spatial (blue) and object (red) working memory are summarized on three projections, with each containing points and axes conforming to standard Talairach space (40) (see figure 27.3 legend). Included in the summary are published ^{15}O PET or fMRI studies of spatial or object working memory that reported coordinates of activation. Courtney et al. (19) (●): item recognition (faces), item recognition (locations); Courtney et al. (22) (■): item recognition (faces); Courtney et al. (23) (▲): item recognition (faces), item recognition (locations); D'Esposito et al. (28) (◗): 2-back (locations); Faillenot et al. (21) (▼): item recognition (objects), item recognition (orientation); Jonides et al. (24) (▮): item recognition (locations); McCarthy et al. (19) (✳): item recognition (locations); Owen et al. (20) (◆): item recognition (locations), spatial span; Owen et al. (21) (✚): n-back (locations), n-back (objects); Smith et al. (19) (❑): item recognition (locations), item recognition (objects); Smith et al. (15) (○): 2-back (locations); Sweeney et al. (41) (◖): memory guided saccades (locations).

spatial information is represented more dorsally than object information (17). The second proposal is that PFC is organized by process, with ventrolateral regions (BA 45 and 47) mediating operations needed to sustain storage and dorsolateral regions (BA 46 and 9) implementing the active manipulation of information held in storage (see references in (28)). Our review provides support for both organizational principles. Relevant to the first, we have noted that verbal storage tasks activate left-hemisphere speech areas, spatial storage activates the right premotor cortex, and object storage activates more ventral regions of PFC (as shown in figure 27.4). Relevant to the second, verbal tasks that require only storage lead primarily to activations that typically do not extend into DLPFC, whereas verbal tasks that require executive processes as well as storage lead to activations that include DLPFC (figure 27.3) (28).

Executive Processes and Frontal Cortex

Most researchers concur that executive processes are mediated by PFC and are involved in the regulation of processes operating on the contents of working memory. Although there is lack of consensus about a taxonomy of executive processes, there is some agreement that they include (i) focusing attention on relevant information and processes and inhibiting irrelevant ones ("attention and inhibition"); (ii) scheduling processes in complex tasks, which requires the switching of focused attention between tasks ("task management"); (iii) planning a sequence of subtasks to accomplish some goal ("planning"); (iv) updating and checking the contents of working memory to determine the next step in a sequential task ("monitoring"); and (v) coding representations in working memory for time and place of appearance ("coding"). Tasks manifesting each of these executive processes are known to be selectively impaired in patients with prefrontal damage (4). Of the five executive pro-

cesses noted, the first two appear to be the most elementary and the most interrelated; for these reasons, we focus on attention and inhibition and task management.

Attention and Inhibition

A paradigmatic case of attention and inhibition is the Stroop test (29). Participants are presented a set of color names printed in different colors and asked to report the print colors; performance is poorer when the print color differs from the color name than when it is the same (it takes longer to say blue to the word red printed in blue than to the word blue printed in blue). The effect arises because two processes are in conflict: a prepotent one that automatically names the word and a weaker but task-relevant process that names the print color. Successful performance requires focusing attention on the task-relevant process and inhibiting the task-irrelevant one (30). More generally, the executive process of attention and inhibition is recruited whenever two processes are in conflict.

PET studies of the Stroop test show substantial variation in regions of activation, although one broad region is the anterior one-third of cingulate cortex (31). Activations in the anterior cingulate have been obtained in other experiments that induce a conflict between processes or response tendencies as well (32). These studies suggest that the anterior cingulate may be involved in the resolution of cognitive conflict.

If executive processes are indeed distinct from short-term storage, it should be possible to add attention and inhibition to a short-term storage task. Two recent studies have attempted to do this by introducing conflict into the verbal item-recognition task (again, see figure 27.1a) (33, 34). These studies included trials in which distractor probes—probes that were not in the memory set—were familiar, thereby putting into competition a decision based on familiarity and one based on the target items being coded as "current targets." Conflict led to activation in the left lateral prefrontal cortex, however, not the anterior cingulate.

Why are different areas of activation found in studies of attention and inhibition? One possibility is that the anterior-cingulate region mediates the inhibition of preprogrammed responses. Incorrect responses may often be preprogrammed in tasks such as Stroop's but not in the item-recognition task; hence, only the former would recruit the cingulate region. By contrast, the frontal site activated in studies of item-recognition may reflect operation of attention and inhibition earlier in the processing sequence. This interpretation is consistent with an fMRI study in which participants were led to prepare a response to an expected probe but on occasional trials had to respond differently to an unexpected probe and hence had to inhibit the prepared response (35). Statistical techniques were used to isolate trials that should have involved response inhibition; analyses of these trials revealed activations in the anterior cingulate, not in prefrontal cortex (36, 37).

Task Management

A canonical case of task management arises when participants are presented with dual tasks. For example, they might be presented a series of numbers and have to add three to the first number, subtract three from the second, and so on through successive trials (38). Both tasks require some nonautomatic or "controlled" processes, and a critical aspect of task management is switching from one controlled process to another.

An fMRI study has examined dual-task performance (39). In one task, participants had to decide whether each word presented in a series named an instance of the category Vegetable; in the other task, participants had to decide whether two visual displays differed only by a matter of rotation; in the dual-task condition, participants performed the categorization and rotation tasks concurrently. Only the dual-task condition activated frontal areas, including DLPFC (BA 46) and the anterior cingulate. The frontal areas overlap those found in attention and inhibition tasks, but in this case the anterior cingulate does not dominate the picture. The communality of results should be expected if a critical component of scheduling is management of the same attentional process that is involved in attention and inhibition tasks.

Concluding Remarks

Neuroimaging studies of humans show that storage and executive processes are major functions of the frontal cortex. The distinction between short-term storage and executive processes appears to be a major organizational principle of PFC. With regard to storage, the PFC areas most consistently activated show modality specificity (verbal versus spatial versus object information), and generally they appear to mediate rehearsal processes, at least for verbal and spatial information. Neuroimaging analyses of executive processes are quite recent, and they have yet to lead to clear dissociations between processes. Perhaps the highest priority, then, is to turn further attention to executive processes and their implementation in frontal cortex.

Acknowledgments

Supported by grants from the National Institute on Aging and the Office of Naval Research. We are indebted to the members of our laboratory for discussion of these issues and to D. Badre for his substantial contributions to the preparation of this manuscript.

References and Notes

1. A. R. Luria, *Higher Cortical Functions in Man* (Basic Books, New York, 1966).

2. P. A. Carpenter, M. A. Just, P. Shell, *Psychol. Rev.* 97, 404 (1990).

3. J. M. Fuster, *The Prefrontal Cortex: Anatomy, Physiology, and Neuropsychology of the Frontal Lobe* (Lippincott-Raven, New York, 1997); P. S. Goldman-Rakic, in *Handbook of Physiology. Nervous System*, vol. 5, Higher Functions of the Brain, F. Plum, Ed. (American Physiological Society, Bethesda, MD, 1987), pp. 373–417.

4. D. T. Stuss and D. F. Benson, *The Frontal Lobes* (Raven, New York, 1986).

5. M. D'Esposito and B. R. Postle, *Attention and Performance XVIII* (Academic Press, New York, 2000).

6. M. I. Posner, S. E. Petersen, P. T. Fox, M. E. Raichle, *Science* 240, 1627 (1988).

7. A. Baddeley, *Working Memory* (Clarendon Press/Oxford Univ. Press, Oxford, 1986).

8. E. E. Smith, J. Jonides, C. Marshuetz, R. A. Koeppe, *Proc. Natl. Acad. Sci. U.S.A.* 95, 876 (1998).

9. J. M. Fuster, *Memory in the Cerebral Cortex: An Empirical Approach to Neural Networks in the Human and Nonhuman Primate* (MIT Press, Cambridge, MA, 1995).

10. E. Paulesu, C. D. Frith, R. S. Frackowiak, *Nature* 362, 342 (1993).

11. T. Shallice, *From Neuropsychology to Mental Structure* (MIT Press, Cambridge, MA, 1988).

12. None of the cited item-recognition studies found activation in DLPFC. However, a recent item-recognition experiment found DLPFC activation with a memory load of six items compared with three items, which suggests a role for DLPFC with larger memory loads (B. Rypma, V. Prabhakaran, J. E. Desmond, *NeuRoimage* 9, 2 (1999). Follow-up work suggests that the role of DLPFC in this task is to mediate executive processes during encoding of the larger loads (M. D'Esposito, personal communication).

13. E. Awh et al., *Psychol. Sci.* 7, 125 (1996).

14. J. D. Cohen et al., *Hum. Brain Mapp.* 1, 293 (1994).

15. E. H. Schumacher et al., *Neuroimage* 3, 79 (1996); E. E. Smith, J. Jonides, R. A. Koeppe, *Cereb. Cortex* 6, 11 (1996); T. S. Braver, J. D. Cohen, J. Jonides, E. E. Smith, D. C. Noll, *Neuroimage* 5, 49 (1997); J. D. Cohen et al., *Nature* 386, 604 (1997); J. Jonides et al., *J. Cognit. Neurosci.* 9, 462 (1997).

16. J. A. Fiez et al., *J. Neurosci.* 16, 808 (1996); J. Jonides et al., ibid. 18, 5026 (1998).

17. F. A. Wilson, S. P. Scalaidhe, P. S. Goldman-Rakic, *Science* 260, 1955 (1993).

18. There is currently some controversy about the degree of separation of object and spatial regions in PFC in nonhuman primates. Recent findings indicate that dorsal or ventral regions can contain neurons that process either spatial or object information or both (S. C. Rao, G. Rainer, E. K. Miller, *Science* 276, 821 (1997); G. Rainer, W. F. Asaad, E. K. Miller, *Proc. Natl. Acad. Sci. U.S.A.* 95, 15008 (1998)). However, even these studies find some neural segregation—a sizable proportion of neurons tested by Rainer et al. are selective only for location, and these neurons predominate in posterior locations.

19. E. E. Smith et al., *J. Cogn. Neurosci.* 7, 337 (1995); G. B. McCarthy et al., *Proc. Natl. Acad. Sci. U.S.A.* 91, 8690 (1994); S. M. Courtney, L. G. Ungerleider, K. Keil, *Cereb. Cortex* 6, 39 (1996).

20. A. M. Owen, A. C. Evans, M. Petrides, *Cereb. Cortex.* 6, 31 (1996).

21. I. Faillenot, H. Sakata, N. Costes, *Neuroreport* 8, 859 (1997); A. M. Owen et al., *Proc. Natl. Acad. Sci. U.S.A.* 95, 7721 (1998).

22. M. Courtney, L. G. Ungerleider, K. Keil, J. V. Haxby, *Nature* 386, 608 (1997).

23. S. M. Courtney, L. Petit, J. M. Maisog, L. G. Ungerleider, J. V. Haxby, *Science* 279, 1347 (1998).

24. J. Jonides et al., *Nature* 363, 623 (1993); P. A. Reuter-Lorenz, J. Jonides, E. E. Smith, A. Hartley, A. Miller, C. Marshuetz, R. A. Koeppe, *J. Cogn. Neurosci.* 12, 174–187 (2000).

25. L. G. Ungerleider, S. M. Courtney, J. V. Haxby, *Proc. Natl. Acad. Sci. U.S.A.* 95, 883 (1998).

26. E. Awh, J. Jonides, P. A. Reuter-Lorenz, *J. Exp. Psychol. Hum. Percept. Perform.* 24, 780 (1998).

27. E. Awh and J. Jonides, in *The Attentive Brain*, R. Parasurama, Ed. (MIT Press, Cambridge, MA, 1997), pp. 353–380.

28. Two other recent meta-analyses of neuroimaging studies of working memory also found evidence that PFC is organized by storage versus executive processes (M. D'Esposito et al., *Cogn. Brain Res.* 7, 1 (1998); A. M. Owen, *Eur. J. Neurosci.* 9, 1329 (1997)). However, neither of these meta-analyses found evidence that PFC was organized by modality. There are at least two reasons for this discrepancy from the present analyses. Neither of the previous meta-analyses focused on ver-

bal storage or included recent fMRI studies that isolate delay-period activity and that provide relatively strong evidence for a difference between spatial and object storage (22, 23).

29. J. R. Stroop, J. Exp. Psychol. 18, 643 (1935).

30. F. N. Dyer, Mem. Cogn. 1, 106 (1973); J. D. Cohen, K. Dunbar, J. L. McClelland, Psychol. Rev. 97, 332 (1990); C. M. Macleod, Psychol. Bull. 109, 163 (1991).

31. J. V. Pardo, P. J. Pardo, K. W. Janer, Proc. Natl. Acad. Sci. U.S.A. 87, 256 (1990); C. J. Bench et al., Neuropsychologia 31, 907 (1993); C. S. Carter, M. Mintun, J. D. Cohen, Neuroimage 2, 264 (1995); M. S. George et al., J. Neuropsychol. Clin. Neurosci. 9, 55 (1997); S. F. Taylor, S. Kornblum, E. J. Lauber, Neuroimage 6, 81 (1997); S. W. Derbyshire, B. A. Vogt, A. K. Jones, Exp. Brain Res. 118, 52 (1998).

32. S. F. Taylor, S. Kormblum, S. Minoshima, Neuropsychologia 32, 249 (1994); M. Iacoboni, R. P. Woods, J. C. Mazziotta, J. Neurophysiol. 76, 321 (1996); G. Bush, P. J. Whalen, B. R. Rosen, Hum. Brain Mapp. 6, 270 (1998).

33. J. Jonides, E. E. Smith, C. Marshuetz, R. A. Koeppe, P. A. Reuter-Lorenz, Proc. Natl. Acad. Sci. U.S.A. 95, 8410 (1998).

34. M. D'Esposito et al., paper presented at Cognitive Neuroscience Society Meeting, San Francisco (1998).

35. C. S. Carter et al., Science 280, 74 (1998).

36. The anterior cingulate is also activated in tasks that do not involve response inhibition, indicating that the cingulate serves multiple functions. (R. D. Badgaiyan and M. I. Posner, Neuroimage 7, 255 (1998); P. J. Whalen et al., Biol. Psychiatry 44, 1219 (1998)).

37. Attention and inhibition may also be involved in self-ordering tasks, such as the following: on each series of trials, a set of forms is presented in random positions, and participants must point to a form they have not selected on a previous trial in that series. This task activates the anterior cingulate and DLPFC, similar to tasks that involve attention and inhibition (M. Petrides, B. Alivisatos, A. C. Evans, Proc. Natl. Acad. Sci. U.S.A. 90, 873 (1993)). Some researchers have proposed that self-ordering tasks reflect the executive process of monitoring, but alternatively they may involve an appreciable working memory load and some inhibition, either of which may cause the frontal activations.

38. A. Spector and I. Biederman, Am. J. Psychol. 89, 669 (1976).

39. M. D'Esposito et al., Nature 378, 279 (1995).

40. J. Talairach and P. Tournoux, A Co-Planar Stereotaxic Atlas of the Human Brain: An Approach to Medical Cerebral Imaging (Thieme, New York, 1988).

41. J. A. Sweeney et al., J. Neurophysiol. 75, 454 (1996).

28 Consciousness and Cognition May Be Mediated by Multiple Independent Coherent Ensembles

E. Roy John, Paul Easton, and Robert Isenhart

Introduction

In order for human beings to adapt reliably to their experiences, an integrated representation of the recent past must be readily accessible and must interact with current input in essentially an automatic way. This function is indispensable for continuity of subjective experience to exist from one moment to the next and to facilitate immediate identification of those environmental features which have changed. Rapid recognition of recent antecedents which might have noteworthy consequences, possibly requiring energetic action or meriting permanent storage, must depend upon essentially automatic brain mechanisms which perhaps act as filters. A large body of research, initially from clinical and neurophysiological experiments and more recently from brain imaging studies, has investigated the mediation of behaviors requiring incoming information to be evaluated in the context of recent experience. An extensive, steadily proliferating set of brain regions has been identified as somehow taking part in this process. Such studies have usually evaluated the mediating processes as if they were discrete elements of one single system, functioning in a holistic but sequentially organized manner. However, such adaptive behaviors may be the product of multiple parallel functional subsystems, which engage different fractions of the neuronal populations within many of the anatomical regions and whose activity may overlap in time as well as in space. Failure to recognize dynamic partition of these populations and spatiotemporal patterns of covariance may obscure insights into how memory is utilized and information processing organized, limiting our understanding to a mere catalog of participating structures.

Further, it is becoming increasingly clear that perception, memory formation, and cognitive processes are mediated by neuronal ensembles, not by individual neurons. Informational significance appears to be attributed by the brain to temporal coherence or synchronization in spatially distributed sets of neurons. It is important to understand how such self-selected representational populations are organized and interact dynamically. Neuronal networks appear to oscillate in a synchronized way. It has been pointed out (Lopes da Silva 1996) that such oscillatory behavior may not be an epiphenomenon merely reflecting the functional organization of neuronal networks. Rather, it may reflect switching mechanisms gating the flow and facilitating the transfer of information between neural subsystems, binding together dispersed assemblies of neurons in a common functional state to subserve perception or the formation of memory traces and to mediate integrated consciousness of input. Abundant evidence indicates that multiple neuronal networks are simultaneously active in parallel during the processing of neural information, at both the subcortical and cortical levels. The coherent firing of neurons in such functional assemblies tends to oscillate with zero phase shift between distant regions, perhaps resulting from multilevel feedback and feedforward.

In view of the foregoing considerations, it seems highly desirable to develop methods for the separation of the hypothesized independent but parallel networks of coherent ensembles, overlapping in time as well as in space. Coherence, or normalized covariance, of voltage fluctuations in different brain regions can serve as an indication of significant coupling and cooperation among the underlying neuronal populations. Accordingly, we studied the *spatial* covariance matrices of fluctuating time series in different locations across a voltage surface, as well as the *temporal* covariance matrices across voltage time series in different spatial locations. Two kinds of coupling can be distinguished: spatial coupling, in which similar time series activity is shown in different brain regions across an interval of time, and temporal coupling, in which similar spatial patterns among a set of brain regions are shown in different moments of time. The topographical organization of locations which are temporally coherent can be quantified by spatial principal component analysis, or SPCA (Skrandies and Lehmann 1982, Gasser et al. 1983a,b; Hjorth and Rodin 1988, Skrandies 1989).

For example, consider the simple example below, illustrating four regions from which an ERP was recorded to a particular stimulus: In region 1, the ERP contains a large early component "A" and no later component. In region 2, the ERP contains no early component but a large later component "B". In region 3, the ERP contains a large early component "A" and no later component. In region 4, the ERP contains no early component but a large later component "B". Thus:

	Component	
	Early	Late
Region 1	A	o
Region 2	o	B
Region 3	A	o
Region 4	o	B

Spatial Principal Component Analysis would identify two spatial principle components: SPC1, loading upon regions 1 and 3; SPC2, loading upon regions 2 and 4. Temporal Principal Component Analysis would identify two temporal principal components: TPC 1, accounting for the variance of early component A in regions 1 and 3; TPC 2, accounting for the variance of the late component B in regions 2 and 4.

The high temporal resolution available by electrophysiological analyses, combined with spatial principal component analysis, may illuminate the sequential engagement of overlapping patterns of spatial covariance in coactive sys-

tems of coherently discharging neurons, thereby clarifying the interaction between input, motivational process, and memory retrieval in adaptive behavior. In previous work, we have shown that the sequences of coherent activation of neuronal ensembles within brain regions could be segmented analytically into a limited set of independent processes with high temporal covariance. These same processes, but with different weighting coefficients in each region, contributed to the evolution of voltages in the time domain at every place across the scalp (John et al. 1993). This observation leads naturally to the suggestion that the patterns of spatial covariance of the weighting coefficients of these independent temporal processes might be similarly segmented. The decomposition of the fluctuations among spatial relationships during stimulus evoked temporal fluctuations of voltages might provide a quantitative description of dynamic aspects of brain organization in space and time. This article presents the results obtained in studies with this goal, during the evoked potential analysis epochs following presentation of meaningful and meaningless stimuli during tasks requiring delayed matching to samples.

Anatomical Dispersion of Memory

It has long been proposed that short-term memory "traces" may depend upon reverberatory activity in specific cell assemblies (de No 1938, Hilgard and Marquis 1940, Hebb 1949), with recurrent patterns of discharge arising from circulation around an initially responsive neuronal network (Burns 1954, Burns and Mogenson 1958, Verzeano and Negishi 1960, Buzsaki et al. 1994). However, life events are actually comprised multiple contemporaneous stimuli, with multidimensional attributes. Each separate attribute is segregated by highly specific neuronal analyzers and dispersed to localized receptortopic sensory receiving areas. Extensive anatomical dispersion of brain processes mediating the temporary storage of information in the brain for subsequent evaluation (working memory, or WM) has been consistently reported by investigators using a wide variety of experimental techniques.

Multidisciplinary Confirmation
Distinct cell assemblies must store different information, since specific categories of information even within the same modality can be lost after brain injury (Swartz et al. 1994, Zola-Morgan and Squire 1993). This suggests parallel processing by multiple representational systems, each with possibly independent mnemonic modules (Mesulam 1990, Goldman-Rakic 1988). Convergent evidence from studies of single neuron activity (Fuster 1989, Funahashi et al. 1990), sensory evoked potentials (Neville et al. 1986; Kutas 1988; Barrett and Rugg 1989; Friedman 1990; Fuel et al. 1990; Ruchkin et al. 1990, 1992; Dupont et al. 1993; Begleiter et al. 1993; Petrides et al. 1993; Heinze et al. 1994; Nielsen-Boheman and Knight 1994; Rugg and Doyle 1994; Zatore et al. 1994), event-related desynchronization of the brain (Pfurtscheller and Berghold 1989, Pfurtscheller and Klimesch 1990), regional cerebral blood flow (Grasby et al. 1993, Haxby et al. 1993), positron emission tomography (Corbetta et al. 1991, Paulescu et al. 1991, Becker et al. 1993, Frackowiak 1994, Raichle 1994, Swartz et al. 1994), magnetoencephalography (Starr et al. 1991, Sosaki et al. 1994), functional activation magnetic resonance (McCarthy et al. 1993, Cohen et al. 1994), and neuropsychological studies of deficits and sparing after brain lesions in animals and humans (Mesulam 1990, Zola-Morgan and Squire 1993, Levine et al. 1994) has established the involvement of extensive distinct brain regions in mediation of WM. Each kind of memory is probably mediated by a different anatomically extensive and distributed system, demonstrated for basic sensory and motor functions, language, and thinking as well as for memory, using a variety of imaging modalities (Roland and Friberg 1985, Papanicolau et al. 1987, Fox et al. 1988, Sergent et al. 1992,

Petsche et al. 1992). Functional connectivity analysis has substantiated the existence of different system organizations engaged by these tasks (Worsley et al. 1992, Friston et al. 1993, McLaughlin et al. 1992, Moller and Strother 1991).

Anatomical Regions Implicated
Depending upon the sensory modality of the stimulus and whether the task requires mediation by a verbal-articulatory loop (Baddeley 1986) or a visual sketchpad (Barrett and Rugg 1989, Friedman 1990), the numerous regions which have been implicated by these diverse methods in short-term or WM have included prefrontal cortex (PFC) (Shallice 1982; Goldman-Rakic 1987; Ruchkin et al. 1990, 1992; Paulescu et al. 1991; Sergent et al. 1992; Becker et al. 1993; Dupont et al. 1993; Cohen et al. 1994), basal forebrain (Dokker et al. 1991), left and right temporal lobe including the superior, middle, and inferior gyri (Milner 1990, Sugishita et al. 1990), medial temporal lobe (Zola-Morgan and Squire 1993, Squire et al. 1992), mesial-temporal cortex (Vallor and Baddeley 1984; Zatore et al. 1992; Abeles et al. 1993; Haxby et al. 1993, 1995; Petrides et al. 1993; Wilson et al. 1993; Cohen et al. 1994; O'Sullivan et al. 1994; Rugg and Doyle 1994; Sosaki et al. 1994; Swartz et al. 1994; Zatore et al. 1994), inferotemporal cortex (Baylis and Rolls 1993), hippocampus (Roland and Friberg 1985, Goldman-Rakic 1987, Grasby et al. 1993, Petrides et al. 1993, Squire et al. 1992, Habib and Houle 1994, Shallice et al. 1994), cingulate gyrus (Dupont et al. 1993, Petrides et al. 1993, Zatore et al. 1994), parieto-occipital cortex (Barrett and Rugg 1989, Fuel et al. 1990, Begleiter et al. 1993), the diencephalon (Markowitsch 1988), and the brainstem (Doty and Ringo 1994, Levine et al. 1994).

Many of these regions have been shown to be involved bilaterally as well as unilaterally (Risberg 1987, Luck et al. 1989, Ingvar 1991, Starr et al. 1991, Haxby et al. 1993, Doty and Ringo 1994, Zatore et al. 1994). A variety of WM tasks have been found to activate the same brain areas, while multiple areas were engaged in parallel by the same task (Wilson et al. 1993, Cohen et al. 1994, Swartz et al. 1994, O'Sullivan et al. 1994, Goldman-Rakic 1994, Raichle 1994, McCarthy 1995). The principal sulcus region of prefrontal cortex and multiple regions of the parietal cortex have been shown, by the use of 2DG autoradiography, to be concurrently activated in rhesus monkeys performing working memory tasks, suggesting that these regions represent two nodes in a neural network mediating spatial working memory (Friedman and Goldman-Rakic 1994). Using $H_2 O^{15}$ to obtain repeated PET scans, many different brain regions, including parts of association cortex, frontal cortex, inferior frontal cortex, thalamus, and cerebellum, were shown to be concurrently activated while subjects accessed two different kinds of memory, focused episodic memory (recollections of specific personal experiences) or random episodic memory (face association). Some portions of this widespread memory network were common to both types of memory (Andreasen et al. 1995).

These facts make it unlikely that WM storage is highly localized or organized topographically by information type. It seems inescapable that ensembles encoding information in a representational system widely dispersed throughout multiple brain regions, each responsive to distinctive elements within a complex set of stimulus attributes, must be integrated and activated holistically to accomplish almost instantaneous recognition of the recurrence of the stored event. This poses the "binding problem."

Spatio Temporal Coherence

When an environmental stimulus occurs, neurons lying within a number of brain regions are coherently activated. Phase-locked firing and resonant oscillations among cell assemblies which display coherent firing within a region in response to afferent input have been observed in multiple single unit or multiunit recordings (Singer 1990,

Abeles et al. 1993, Singer 1994, Buzsaki et al. 1994, Nicolelis et al. 1995) and in computer simulations (Abeles et al. 1994). Behavioral significance causes synchronized discharge to occur across extensive neuronal regions (John 1972, Ramos et al. 1976, Merzenich 1995). *The representational assembly is organized ad hoc, with simultaneous temporal patterns across distant spatial locations constituting the signature of membership* (John 1968, Singer 1990, Abeles et al. 1993, Buzsaki et al. 1994, Singer 1994, Merzenich 1995).

A recently reported study used principal components analysis to represent the time-integrated activity of large sets of single neurons, simultaneously recorded in multiple cortical, thalamic, and brainstem regions in the trigeminal system of freely moving rats (Nicolelis et al. 1995). The first principal component (PC1) received loadings from simultaneous unit firings in many regions and correlated better with tactile inputs from facial whiskers than did the activity of single neurons, indicating sensory encoding by spatiotemporal coherence. Similar conclusions have been proposed by others on the basis of distributed multiunit or macropotential recordings in behaving animals (John 1972, Ramos et al. 1976). More recently, spatially coherent neuronal activity and coherent oscillations have been described by other workers, in response to visual, auditory, somatosensory, or olfactory discriminanda. Concluding that macropotentials provided the best experimental access to spatiotemporal patterns of cortical activity, these workers subjected sets of macropotential traces of time series from cortical spatial arrays to principal component analysis. Factor loadings of the first principal components (PC1) provided quantitative descriptors of the spatial patterns of voltage fields. Highly accurate classifications of the positive and negative stimuli in each sensory modality were achieved by correlating the voltage field of cortical responses evoked by the stimulus presentation with the first spatial principal components, which account for the highest proportion of the total variance (Freeman and Barrie 1994).

Event-Related Potential Evidence of Parallel Processing

Quantitative electroencephalographic (QEEG) changes may represent generalized changes in background activity related to cognitive performance (Jasper and Penfield 1949, Legewie et al. 1969, Gevins et al. 1981, Tucker et al. 1985, Sergent et al. 1987, Ojemann et al. 1989, Pfurtscheller and Klimesch 1990), whereas event-related potentials (ERPs) more closely represent chronometry of mental activity (Posner 1978). The ERP N200 component has been associated with early memory activation during selective attention, omitted stimuli, lexical decision, and word matching cognitive tasks. Its amplitude varies with magnitude of stimulus mismatch (Kramer and Donchin 1987). The frontal/central distribution of N200 increases with degree of semantic association, greater over the left hemisphere (Boddy 1986). N200 varies with difficulty of discrimination, related to response latency (Ritter et al. 1983). A second negative component, N400, varies with degree of semantic relatedness between prime and target stimuli (Munte et al. 1989), in visual, auditory, and sign language presentation, and is sensitive to familiarity of faces, first presentation of a word, and mental rotation of abstract forms. N400 may reflect retrieval of current episodic context, independent from long-term memory activation (Rugg and Nagy 1987), reflecting working memory of task relevant context, whether of semantic or other representation (Stuss et al. 1983).

The most studied endogenous ERP components are the P300 or late positive components (LPC) (Sutton et al. 1965). Multiple LPCs exist, differentially sensitive to cognitive variables (Friedman et al. 1978), associated with matching of expectations, selective attention processes, and with the amount of controlled processing (Schneider and Shiffrin 1977). LPCs reflect stimulus evaluation, independent of response selec-

tion and execution (Magliero et al. 1984), and vary with stimulus familiarity, especially during semantic encoding (Sanquist et al. 1980). LPCs reflect an update of an internal WM template after stimulus evaluation (McCarthy and Donchin 1983) and decrease in amplitude but increase in latency with memory set size and load (Kramer et al. 1986) in both recall and recognition tasks. Ruchkin et al. (1992) used ERPs to study WM, reporting evidence for specialized systems for short-term storage of phonological and visuospatial information, with marked differences between the topography and morphology of ERPs elicited by these types of WM. They found some common aspects of timing and topography in two tasks, which were consistent with features expected were a central executive process to exist. Begleiter et al. (1993) have reported identification of a visual memory potential (VMP), usually maximal at about 240 ms in temporal regions, reflecting WM during DMS. Most recently, in studies using large numbers of electrodes chronically implanted in patients awaiting neurosurgery (Halgren et al. 1994a,b, 1995a,b), ERP evidence was obtained indicating parallel as well as sequential engagement of many brain regions during cognitive tasks.

ERP waveshapes from functionally interacting regions have been correlated and transmission delays measured by the lagged covariance (Gevins 1990). Statistical signal analysis, based upon the assumption that brain regions which are functionally related have similar waveshapes, has been used to study memory requiring graphic, phonemic, semantic, and grammatical judgments in a delayed match from sample language task, revealing somewhat different topography among these conditions (Gevins 1990). Gevins and Cutillo (1993) suggested that distinct Event Related Convenience (ERC) patterns associated with WM only occur during intervals in which the information in an active state is being utilized for task performance. More recently, Gevins et al. (1996) have commented on the striking amount of similarity of topography in EPs obtained during spatial versus verbal WM tasks. They suggested that functional networks established during specific WM tasks might interact with a system common to all attention-demanding tasks.

The overview above suggests that information encoding multiple attributes of complex sensory stimuli is distributed and stored in multiple anatomical regions, which represent and retrieve these dispersed fragments of experience by parallel processes. Many disparate techniques have been used to scrutinize the engagement of particular brain regions in cognition, working memory storage, and retrieval of its component elements. The purpose of the studies reported here was to obtain insights into the spatio temporal coherence and operational principles of the functional brain subsystems which cooperatively integrate these elements for real time holistic utilization, rather than to focus further upon the participation of any unique region in some specific task.

Materials and Methods

Subjects

The subjects in this study were nine normally functioning members of the laboratory staff (six male and three female). All subjects were right handed.

Recording Method

Silver–silver chloride disk electrodes were affixed to the scalp with electrode paste at the 19 positions of the 10/20 System plus Fpz and Oz.[1] EOG electrodes were placed diagonally above and below the right eye and an EKG electrode was placed on the left shoulder. The linked earlobes served as reference electrode and the average reference was constructed. Data were collected using a Lexicor Corp. Lexigraph, with a bandwidth from 0.15 to 30 Hz, amplified 32 K, and sampled with 16 bits at a rate of 128 Hz.

Stimulus Presentation

Subjects were seated comfortably in a darkened room, 0.5 m in front of a computer screen serving as a stimulus generator, with a two-button mouse at their right hand. Using the right index finger, the subject pressed the left button on the ("same") mouse if *every* item in the *matching set S2* had been present in the initial or *priming set S1* (or their sums were equal), but the right button ("different") if *any* item in S2 had not been in S1 (or their sums were unequal).

All stimuli were generated by computer and presented sequentially on the monitor screen of an Amiga Model 4000 personal computer. In the studies reported here, the stimuli consisted of black "probes" (fixation crosses), presented in Intervals 1 and 3, or information items of approximately equal contrast, presented in Interval 2 (Priming Sample) and Interval 4 (Matching Sample). Four tasks were administered, differing only in the content of six information items in the priming and matching sets (see "Tracer stimuli"): *Faces* (monochrome photos from a high school yearbook); *Letters* (single block letters); and single digit numbers to be retained (*Digits*) or added (*Sums*). *Faces* stimuli could not be matched for contrast but were of approximately equal area and brightness. Probes, letters, and numerical stimuli were comprised of solid black contours about 4 mm in the thickness and a vertical extent of about 44 mm (about 5° visual angle), centered within a white field about 11 cm wide by 8 cm high (about 13° visual angle) in a black border. Stimuli were presented on the monitor screen as a flash with a rise time of about 16 ms (the refresh rate of the video monitor) and a duration of 333 ms. There was an interval of 667 ms between the *onsets* of successive stimuli (1.5 stimuli per second). This standard trial format is illustrated in figure 28.1.

CONSCIOUSNESS, COGNITION, AND COHERENT ENSEMBLES

```
┌─────────────────────────────────────────────────────────────────────┐
│ INTERVAL:                                                           │
│    1              2              3              4                    │
│ 6 Probes = P1   6  Priming = S1   6  Probes = P2   6 Matching = S2   │
│                                                                     │
│ + + + + +      + + + + + +    + + + + + +    + + + + + +             │
│                                                                     │
│ ←— 4 secs —→    ←— 4 secs —→   ←— 4 secs —→   ←— 4 secs —→          │
└─────────────────────────────────────────────────────────────────────┘
```

Si = Individual Digits, Sums, Letters, or Faces
Pj = Non-contingent probes (Fixation Points)

Figure 28.1
Schematic of the standard structure of stimulus presentation in intervals 1–4 of each trial of every DMS task.

Data Acquisition and Analysis

The strategy adopted for this study incorporated several features into Data Acquisition which were considered critical.

"Tracer" Stimuli

In early studies of brain mechanisms of learning and memory, using chronically indwelling electrodes to study the EEG, ERPs, and multiple unit activity as animals acquired and performed a variety of conditioned responses (John and Killam 1959, 1960; John 1968, 1972, 1976; John and Morgades 1969), tracer stimuli were utilized. Visual and auditory stimuli, which were to serve as cues for discriminative behaviors, were presented at differential tracer repetition rates for each behavior response. "Labeled activity," mediating the processing of this information by different neuroanatomical structures, was identified by searching the EEG power spectrum or unit discharges for enhanced activity at the tracer frequency or by ERP waveshape changes triggered by each tracer cycle. This method provided a criterion, which was sufficient, albeit not necessary, to establish the participation of any brain region in processing cue-relevant informa-tion. The present study examined the engage-ment of brain regions in human subjects during the performance of delayed matching from sam-ple (DMS) tasks, identifying labeled activity by very narrow band (VNB) spectral analysis of the EEG and by ERPs elicited by repetitive sets of six successive fixation points in the center of the visual field serving as "probes," *preceding and following priming sets S1 and matching sets S2*, each containing six information items presented sequentially at a tracer frequency of 1.5 Hz.

Noncontingent Probes The waveshape or am-plitude of the response evoked by an irrelevant environmental stimulus, presented before and during performance of some task in no way contingent upon that probe, will change in those brain regions where substantial proportions of neurons which otherwise would respond to the probe are presumably engaged by the task demands. Such a decrement in probe amplitude might reflect engagement by the task, habitua-tion or "distraction." These alternative explora-tions appear unlikely in the present study, since ERPs to the Matching Set stimuli do not show a consistent decrement relative to the previous Priming Set and are larger than responses to P2.

The methods of the "noncontingent probe," or NCP, have been discussed elsewhere in detail (Papanicolau et al. 1984, 1987). Reports cited previously have shown that substantial proportions of cells in the prefrontal cortex respond to a stimulus, while nearby neurons discharge persistently during a subsequent delay in a matching task (Goldman-Rakic 1987, Fuster 1989, Funahashi et al. 1990). Other evidence cited above indicates that, while WM is engaged by a DMS task, significant levels of residual activity persist sufficiently in many brain regions to affect relatively global indicators such as cerebral blood flow and glucose metabolism. *If memory traces require reverberation or sustained activity within some subset of neurons activated as a consequence of stimulus input, then participating assemblies in extensive anatomical areas should be unresponsive to challenges by subsequent probes.* The spatial distribution of this inhibitory representation should be distinctive for different memory content.

Intervals Accordingly, the DMS tasks used in this study were each designed to consist of six intervals, each of 4 s duration: *Interval 1*—Control Set (P1) of six information-free probes, *Interval 2*—a Priming Set (S1) of six information items, *Interval 3*—a second Delay Set (P2) of six information-free probes, *Interval 4*—a Matching Set (S2) of six information items, *Interval 5*—six probes presented while the subject pressed the appropriate mouse button, and *Interval 6*—six probes which were green if response was correct but red if incorrect. The presentation of six items in each 4-s interval thus established a tracer frequency of 1.5 Hz. It was anticipated that there would be a significant difference between the NCPs elicited by the probes before (P1) and after (P2) presentation of the Priming Set, reflecting the sustained engagement of substantial proportions of neuronal populations in different brain regions by the retention of a representation of the Priming Series in working memory. Twenty or 30 trials were presented in

each task session. Several task sessions were presented each day, with *Digits* and *Sums* always in successive sessions on the same day. Accuracy ranged from 80 to 100% and only data from correct trials were included in results discussed in this paper. This paper will only examine data from the first four intervals of this sequence, obtained using the structure which was illustrated in figure 28.1.

Functional Landscapes

In recent studies (Lehmann et al. 1987, Strik and Lehmann 1993, Pascual-Marqui et al. 1995), methods have been presented for the quantitative evaluation of momentary scalp EEG or ERP voltage distributions, or "landscapes." These methods include the computation of Global Field Power, or GFP, which quantifies the spatial variance of temporal sequences of voltage across the set of electrodes. Points where GFP peaks occur can be identified in the time series of voltage across these spatial arrays. The *centroids* of positive and negative regions of the voltage surface are calculated for every GFP peak. Specific locations for the positive and negative centroids are used to identify a particular corresponding "microstate."

A "brain microstate" has been defined (Lehmann et al. 1987) as a functional state during which specific neural computations are performed. Each microstate is uniquely characterized by a fixed spatial distribution of active neuronal generators with synchronized time-varying intensity. The voltages arising from these multiple generators are summated at the scalp, resulting in a field "landscape." While no unique set of neuronal generators can be inferred to underlie a particular landscape, *changes in the scalp field imply changes in the source distribution.* GFP peaks are often observed to wax and wane while centroid positions remain unchanged and the landscape appears stable, especially during cognitive tasks. The persistence and frequent recurrence of similar landscapes during GFP peaks at particular latencies, in our view, lends plausibility to the suggestion that a unique distribution of neuronal generators may, in fact, underlie each distinctive landscape.

Multiple functional neuroanatomical subsystems are activated, in parallel and in series, as information is encoded, stored, retrieved, and compared to satisfy the requirements of the delayed matching tasks used in these studies. Sequences of landscapes observed during performance of cognitive tasks may arise from temporally non-overlapping sequential or overlapping parallel activation of subsystems. The identification of these underlying subsystems is a major aim of these studies. It is assumed that the available set of subsystems will be largely genetically determined, very much the same in any human being. Different individuals may allocate these information processing resources differently, and different cognitive tasks or stages of processing may utilize them in different dynamic combinations. Different levels of activation of a relatively limited number of functional subsystems may underlie the vast variety of field landscapes observable on the scalp. Persistence of a landscape implies a prolonged microstate, reflecting sustained activation of a subsystem dominant during that interval.

Landscape analysis was considered advantageous for the present studies because it provided an initial approach to quantification of systems which might be engaged during DMS task performance. Particular attention was paid to *differences* between landscape sequences elicited by the noncontingent probes before and after presentation of the Priming Set, because such differences might reflect sustained engagement of an extensive neuronal population mediating retention of information in working memory during the delay period. Our observation of prolonged periods during cognitive tasks in which centroid locations remained stable, although absolute voltage values might change at surface locations, confirmed previous reports (Lehmann et al. 1987, Strik and Lehmann 1993, Pascual-Marqui et al. 1995). This observation

was particularly frequent about 200 ms after stimulus presentation, at the time when subjective perception of the stimulus has been shown to occur (Libet 1973, Hassler 1979). Correlational analyses among probe difference landscapes and information stimulus landscapes were examined. Such correlation studies evaluated the possibility that "feed forward" of sustained activity in the neuronal population engaged by the working memory, possibly mediated by long-term potentiation, inhibition, or reverberatory oscillations among multiple coherent ensembles, was utilized by the brain for coincidence detection. Subsequent stimulus complexes might thereby be recognized by a present–past comparator, supporting a recently proposed filter model which incorporates such a process (Harth 1995).

Spatial and Temporal Principal Component Analysis

Surface voltage landscapes presumably arise from the time-varying levels of activation or inhibition coherently engaging large proportions of the neurons in each of several functional neuroanatomical subsystems contemporaneously active in parallel during cognition. The voltage fields generated by these coactive subsystems must overlap in space and time. The same set of genetically determined brain resources is presumed to be available to every human being. The allocation of these resources might vary from individual to individual, as a function of cognitive style, and from task to task, as a function of the specific information processing requirements. Some subsystems in the set might also account for a relatively constant amount of voltage variance because those subsystems are engaged by non-information-specific tasks, such as maintenance of alertness, motivation, and vegetative or motor functions.

Factor Loadings Spatial Principal Component Analysis (SPCA), with or without Varimax rotation (SPCVA), was therefore applied to the sequences of voltage landscapes across the scalp

(Skrandies and Lehmann 1982, Gasser et al. 1982). Temporal Principal Component Analysis with Varimax rotation (TPCVA) was also applied to decompose the set of surface voltage time series into temporally independent sequential components (John et al. 1964, 1965, 1993, 1994; John 1972). These methods were intended to seek evidence that a finite set of functional neuroanatomical systems, common to all subjects in these studies, might account for the great preponderance of variance displayed during performance of any one of a variety of cognitive tasks. The factor loadings of this set of SPCs would be essentially the same in every individual, possibly reflecting the common underlying neuroanatomy. Variations were expected in the percentage of variance accounted for by each of those SPCs, from person to person and task to task. It must be acknowledged that the SPCs may simply constitute a precise multivariate statistical description of surface topography. Such parsimonious statistical descriptors would be useful and important as such. This problem is further addressed in the Discussion.

Factor Scores The momentary factor scores of each separate SPC would quantify the time-varying engagement of each of these functional neuroanatomical systems by the cognitive and representational demands, fluctuating throughout the task performance intervals. Particular SPCs might plausibly be expected to mediate registration and encoding of sensory information, while others might be more engaged by retrieval from WM and recognition or identification of subsequent events. Factor score differences for particular SPCs between intervals P2 versus P1 might identify subsystems mediating WM and between S1 versus P1 might identify subsystems mediating encoding of information.

The methods and results presented in this article, thus, are hoped to demonstrate the feasibility as well as the desirability of a paradigm shift, departing from the analysis of attribute processing in any specific region to refocus upon the global integration of such activity, dispersed across many regions, into one holistic brain organization of systems mediating conscious experiential evaluation and cognition.

Results obtained from these studies and focused upon VNB EEG, labeled activity, and ERP activity in specific brain regions during particular tasks have been previously reported (John and Easton 1995, John et al. 1996). This article presents the results obtained with analytical methods directed at global system features.

Data Analysis Methods

Stimulus-Response Categories Trials in four stimulus-response categories were segregated: Trials in which sets S1 and S2 matched and were identified correctly (Class 1) or incorrectly (Class 2); trials in which sets S1 and S2 did not match, which the subject perceived accurately (Class 3) or failed to detect (Class 4). Data in these four classes were processed separately. Performance by the different subjects on these tasks ranged from 80 to 100% correct, with small differences in response latency across tasks. This suggested that the task difficulty was comparable and modest.

Averages Two kinds of averages were constructed: (1) *Interval averages*, in which corresponding four second long intervals (control probes P1, priming set S1, delay probes P2, matching set S2) from trials in the same stimulus-response category were averaged together. Interval averages thus contained sequential evoked potential epochs from six successive events; (2) *Event averages*, in which the six items within each task interval were averaged together from trials in the same category. Event analysis thus combined six times more analysis epochs than interval averages, yielding a better signal to noise ratio but obscuring possible effects of serial position of an item.

"Landscapes" or Field Maps Topographic maps of the voltage fields on the scalp were constructed using interpolation of the set of simultaneous voltages from 19 electrodes of the 10/20 system, digitized at each sampling time point.

Global Field Power At each time point, the GFP was computed, defined as the total variance of voltage across the set of nineteen electrodes. The sequence of mean GFP values was constructed for every event average and interval average across the 20 trials within each task session. The latency of GFP peaks was identified (Lehmann et al. 1987).

Centroid Computation At 8-ms intervals across the analysis epoch of the event or interval average, the centroids of the positive and negative voltage regions on the scalp were computed and their locations identified on the corresponding landscapes (Lehmann et al. 1987).

Interlandscape Recognition—"Correlograms" Inspection of absolute voltage landscapes (relative to the average reference), GFP peaks, and centroids at successive 8-ms increments revealed the recurrence of more or less similar, recognizable voltage fields, persisting across extended periods. In order to quantify this apparent similarity objectively, the Pearson product moment correlation coefficient, r_{ij}, was computed between the voltage values at the 19 electrodes at any time, t_i, and the sequence of values, at all times t_j, within the interval and event average analysis epochs for all intervals across all the trials in any category. The resulting temporal sequence of values was displayed as the *correlogram*, $r_{ij}(t)$. The probability of the observed values of r was assessed by the Fischer Z-transform (Wilkins 1962).

Difference Landscapes The differences of voltage at each electrode were calculated at corresponding latency points, across the entire analysis epochs of interval and event averages, between the task intervals P1, S1, P2, and S2 to construct the *difference landscapes* P2-P1, S1-P1, and S2-S1.

Matrices Covariance, cross-covariance, and coherence matrices were computed in order to quantify (1) the *similarity between the time series of voltage* values among each electrode versus every other electrode, across the epoch of the interval or event averages, and (2) the *similarity between the instantaneous set of voltages* (voltage landscape) among the 19 electrodes for any time point versus the voltage landscape at every other time point across the interval or event averages.

SPCA Spatial Principal Component Analysis was performed on the matrices defined in section H above, which quantified the spatial coupling in somewhat different matrices. The *factor loadings* of the spatial principal components decompose the landscape into "subscenes" which are independent modes of voltage coherence across the cortex. (No matter how the coupling matrix was quantified, the resulting SPCs were found to display highly similar loadings; see Gasser et al. 1983.)

Spatial Factors

The spatial factors presented here, represented as interpolated head maps, were obtained by taking the cross-covariance matrix for the 21 derivations, averaged over the first four intervals of each trial. From such matrices, we obtained a set of five principal components (usually accounting for about 90% of the total variance across all deviations). The Varimax factors were then obtained from these principal components. The factors (or factor loadings) are 21 point vectors, 1 point for each derivation, and are pictured as *interpolated* head maps.

Each factor was regressed against the averages of each of the first four intervals (over the interval average values of the 21 channels, for each time point) to get the factor scores for each interval. From these, we obtained the total fractional variance accounted for by each factor. The *factor scores* were normalized by the average variance in each of the four intervals and were depicted as *graphs of amplitude against time.*

We also reaveraged the averaged evoked potentials (AEPs) over time segments of one-sixth the duration of the interval, to obtain the average response to a single stimulus (event average) in any particular interval, and performed the same regressions as described above.

Varimax Rotation Varimax rotation was applied to the Spatial Principal Components. For any SPC set, the Varimax rotation redistributes the identical amount of variance into loadings which maximize the variance contributed from particular regions of the space while minimizing the variance from the remaining regions.

Spatial Principal Component or Varimax loadings depict the extent to which proportions of the neuron population in any region display activity (reflected as integrated postsynaptic potentials across that cell assembly) not only coherent within the population in that anatomical region but also coherent with neuronal groups in other regions. It should be clear that *other subsets of neurons in the same region may display quite a different pattern of coherence with each other and with other regions, and thus participate in a different factor loading.*

TPCVA If the coupling matrices (covariance, cross-covariance, coherence) are computed not for temporal coherence across space (SPCA) but for spatial patterns across time, analytical temporal segmentation can be achieved (John et al. 1993, 1994).

In this case we took the temporal cross-covariance for segments of 67 time points, corresponding to a time interval of two-thirds of a second. Each time segment began with a stimulus in any one of the first four intervals. The matrices were averaged over all derivations. The

factors (or factor loadings) were depicted as *67 point graphs of amplitude against time.*

The largest factors were then regressed against the AEPs of each of the four intervals to obtain the factor scores. These were 21 point vectors which showed how the weighting of the factor was distributed over the head. The *factor scores were* depicted as *head maps,* either one for every stimulus item within each interval or, by averaging across the six events, a single head map for each factor in each interval.

Also, in both methods, scores for differences between selected conditions were calculated by subtracting one set of scores from the other. This is mathematically equivalent to constructing a difference AEP between conditions and calculating the scores from that.

TPCVA segments the time series of the interval or event average analysis epochs across all leads to identify the extent to which sequential sets of time points covary with each other. Each set of covarying time points, or *factor loading,* can be considered to arise from a hypothetical generator or functional neuroanatomical system, which can describe a portion of the morphology of the waveshapes in all leads during some temporal subepoch. It should be clear that contributions of different factor loadings can overlap in time at the same electrode(s).

Results

Landscape Topographies

Interpolated topographic maps of the average voltage fields ("landscapes") were computed for both interval average and event averages, at 8-ms intervals. GFP peaks occurred at approximately 100–120, 160–176, 200–216, and 304–320 ms in the various tasks performed by each of our subjects.

Figure 28.2 shows sequential landscapes every 8 ms from 120 to 312 ms, during performance of *Digits* and *Letters* by one subject. Note the close

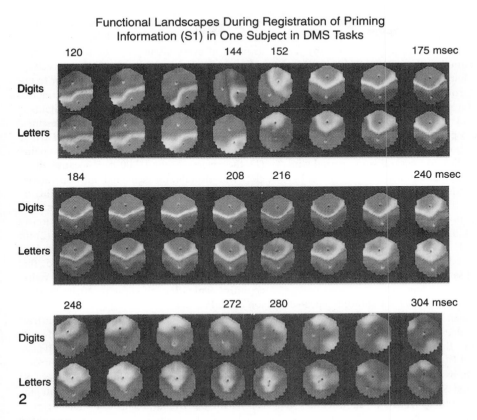

Figure 28.2
Functional landscapes recorded during performances by one subject of two different DMS tasks. The subject was required to decide whether every one of six items in a matching set, S2, had been among the six items contained in the previous priming set, S1, independent of order within the set. These landscapes, relative to the average references, were computed after averaging together the six information items in set S1 across 30 trials of each task. Since accuracy was 100%, each event average was based upon a sample of 180 stimuli which were accurately perceived and stored in WM. These topographic maps display the voltages interpolated from the values at 21 electrodes, sampled every 8 ms from 120 to 304 ms of latency after the onset of the stimuli. Each map depicts the landscape seen from above with the face upward. Red hues depict positive and blue hues negative voltages. The blue dot on each map indicates the centroid of the positive domain, while the red dot indicates the negative centroid. Nuances of shading within these domains have been obscured in some instances by saturation of color scale reproduction, which does not affect the position of the centroids. Full scale on this color palette was ± 5.0 µV.

similarity of landscapes between *Digits* and *Letters* at 120 ms (peak of P1) and the subsequent differences between the responses evoked by the two sets of stimuli although they were equated for field size, luminance, and contrast. As the EP swings first through the negative peak in posterior regions (at about 160 ms) and then toward a positive peak in posterior regions (at about 240 ms), the topography across the surface persists and the position of the centroids remains quite stable, followed by a transition period with rapid change beyond 300 ms.

Different landscapes appeared within different intervals of a task. Landscapes during corresponding intervals across tasks also differed. This was strikingly seen when *Digits* and *Sums* were compared, indicating that the observed field changes reflected endogenous processes such as cognition and set, not simply stages in automatic processing of visual input.

The region around 200 ms showed repeated instants in which the landscapes during P2 but not P1 resembled that during S1. If the differences between the pre- and post-information probes, P2 and P1, reflected the WM of different mental operations performed on identical stimuli in the *Digits* and *Sums* tasks, then the "difference landscapes" resulting from the subtraction of P1 from P2 should differ between the two tasks. Such differences reflect the distribution of neurons in extensive populations initially responsive to the visual stimulation during P1, but not activated by stimulation during P2. These differences may reflect nonspecific differences in functional systems engaged by the two tasks or in the actual content of the mental operation. It is unlikely that these differences reflect habituation to repeated visual stimulation, since ERPs elicited by the matching set during S2 closely resemble those elicited by the priming set during S1.

Landscapes of Working Memory

In order to estimate whether neuronal ensembles engaged by WM constituted an actual facsimile of S1, used subsequently for comparison with S2, the topographic similarity of P2-P1 and S2 was assessed at every latency by computing correlations across the electrode array between voltage values at consecutive time points. In order to test the stability of the postulated facsimile across successive presentations of the six serial items of information during S1 and S2, this assessment was performed on the interval averages. Particular attention was paid to two latency domains: (1) the region around 200 ms, because direct electrical stimulation delivered intraoperatively to thalamic or cortical brain regions at this interval after a stimulus is presented has been demonstrated to block subjective perception of the event (Hassler 1979, Libet 1973), and (2) the region around 300 ms, because ample psychophysiological research has demonstrated that late positive components around P300 reflect cognitive evaluations of stimulus attributes (Sutton et al. 1965).

The correlograms in figure 28.3 demonstrate highly significant, recurrent statistical similarities between the *difference landscape* (P2-P1), at about 200 ms, presumably reflecting a neuronal population engaged by holding the traces of S1 in WM, and the six serial items of the matching set S2, for the *Digits* task in one subject (upper panel) and the *Sums* tasks in a second subject (lower panel). The figure also illustrates that correlograms between the *landscape* at 216 ms of the probe P1 (top panel) or the *difference landscape* (P2-P1) at the longer latency 400 ms (bottom panel) were not statistically significant.

Figure 28.4 shows the matrix of cross-correlation coefficients evaluating similarities between *every* difference landscape during the 4-s *interval difference*, P2-P1 (top to bottom) and the 4-s *Interval 4* containing the six items of the matching set, S2 (left to right). The color scale goes from a correlation coefficient of +1.0 (red) to −1.0 (blue). This matrix demonstrates the recurrence of high positive or inverse similarity between the sequence of difference landscapes attributed to the retention of a "trace" in WM

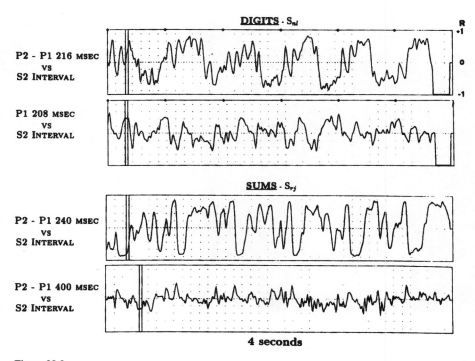

Figure 28.3

These graphs illustrate the similarity between the landscape of working memory and those elicited by subsequent presentation of the matching set. Landscape cross-correlation functions, obtained by calculating the Pearson correlation coefficient, r, between the WM landscapes (P2-P1) at about 200 ms and the succession of landscapes of the matching set of information (S2) in 8-ms steps across the 4 s of Interval 4, are shown for *Digits*, subject S_{nl} (graph 1) and *Sums*, subject S_{rj} (graph 3). Control data from the same subjects show lower correlations between S2 and the pre-information probe P1 at 208 ms (graph 2) and between S2 and P2-P1 landscapes at longer latencies (graph 4). Note that r must exceed 0.575 to achieve $p < .01$ for these data.

and the sequence of items S2 which must be matched to the contents of WM.

Decomposition of Landscape Sequences by SPCA

Inspection of instantaneous landscape sequences in many subjects performing the four delayed matching tasks used in this study revealed certain common features. Persistent topographies were consistently observed, and difference land-

scapes repeatedly obtained, which were highly correlated with the landscapes evoked by the stimuli presented in the different tasks. Within a subject, distinctive difference landscapes emerged in every task. *Momentary* landscapes with similar topography could be briefly discerned in different tasks and different subjects, in agreement with the observations commented upon by others (Gevins et al. 1996). However, the sequence of landscapes across event averages for different subjects performing the same tasks were

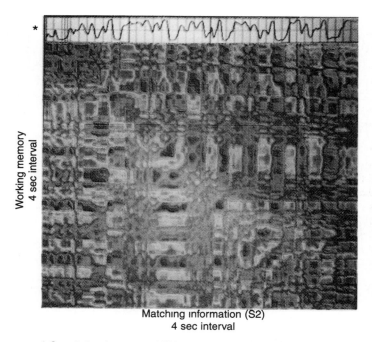

Matching information (S2)
4 sec interval

* Correlation between a WM landscape at 240 msec and match-
4   ing information landscapes throughout Interval 4 (0-4 sec).

Figure 28.4
Matrix of cross-correlations of every landscape of working memory (P2-P1) versus every landscape of matching information (S2) across the 4-s intervals of *Sums* for one subject. Each point in this matrix represents the Pearson correlation coefficient, *r*, between the WM and S2 landscapes at the corresponding latencies on the two axes. Red, maximum positive $r \approx 1.0$; blue, maximum negative $r \approx -1.0$.

very different. This lack of consistency among sequential average landscapes across subjects was concordant with the high variability across subjects, previously noted in our analyses of average ERPs and of very narrow band spectral composition of EEGs obtained from these same data using "tracer" stimulus technique (John et al. 1996).

Ideally, parsimony suggests that one be able to represent all landscapes, generated during the performance of any task by every subject, by a limited set of global descriptors which will reveal

fundamental similarities in the underlying functional neuroanatomical subsystems. Differences in electrophysiological patterns of activation between tasks and among individuals must be expected, because of idiosyncratic allocation of available information processing resources. Nonetheless, all human brains must contain the same neuroanatomical structures which can become available for incorporation into dynamic functional subsystems, functioning in parallel to mediate different brain operations. The relative contribution of these different operators to the

Table 28.1

	Component	
	Early	Late
Region 1	A	o
Region 2	o	B
Region 3	A	o
Region 4	o	B

total instantaneous variance of voltage at the surface should depend upon the extent of their momentary engagement in the corresponding operations. Momentary similarity of landscapes across individuals or between tasks may indicate momentary dominance of total system voltage variance due to salience of a particular non-specific *operator*, rather than the specific information *content* of the mental operation at that instant.

Spatial Principal Component and Varimax Factor Loadings (SPCA)

Accordingly, we subjected the voltage time-series observed at each electrode, while all eight subjects were engaged in a total of 55 sessions at rest or during performance of one of the four matching tasks, to SPCA. Five Spatial Principal Components accounted for 89.7% of the total variance of voltages recorded across the surface of the scalp in all of these sets of data (table 28.1).

The five major spatial principal components might be characterized as: (1) A contrast between occipital/parietal/posterior temporal versus frontal (*anterior versus posterior*); (2) central regions versus surround, especially frontal (*center versus surround*); (3) left anterior–posterior temporal versus right (*L versus R temporal*); (4) right posterior temporal versus central (*right temporal versus central*); (5) left anterior temporal versus all other regions (*left frontal temporal*), closely resembling loadings reported by others

(Skrandies and Lehmann 1982, Gasser et al. 1988, Hjorth and Rodin 1988).

While the Varimax rotated factors reallocated the *amount* of variance accounted for by the SPCs, the Varimax and Principal Component *loadings* were remarkably similar. This similarity provides support for the proposition that the observed loadings reflect the "natural" structure of functional subsystems of anatomically extensive coherent populations of neurons, activated independently but overlapping in space and time, rather than resulting merely from the forced mathematical constraints of principal component analysis.

Figure 28.5a depicts the factor loadings for the first five SPCAs for five subjects performing the *Sums* tasks. This figure illustrates the basic correspondence of these loadings across subjects performing the same task. Figure 28.5b shows the factor loadings for the first five SPCAs for a sixth subject at rest and performing four different tasks. This figure illustrates the engagement of the same basic resources in different cognitive activities. The factor *scores* shown above each loading in figures 28.5a,b quantify the variable allocation of these resources among individuals or across tasks.

These *factor loadings* correspond to the surface projection of voltages arising from the coherent but independent activation of varying proportions of large neuronal population, distributed in different neuroanatomical structures. This coherent activation results in covarying shifts of integrated postsynaptic membrane potentials, detectable at the scalp surface above extensive cortical regions. These spatially distributed, coherently active but independent populations constitute different *functional neuro-anatomical subsystems*. Note that the *percentage* of the total variance accounted for by a given SPC varies somewhat across individuals and among some tasks, although the loading remains basically similar. This reflects the fluctuation in the fraction of neurons locally recruited into the coherent assembly.

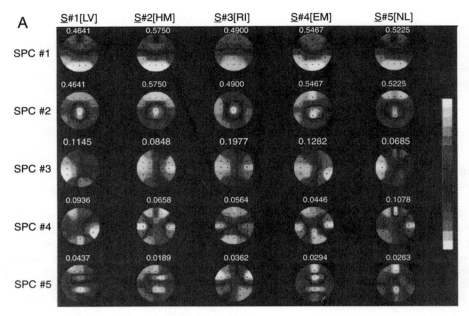

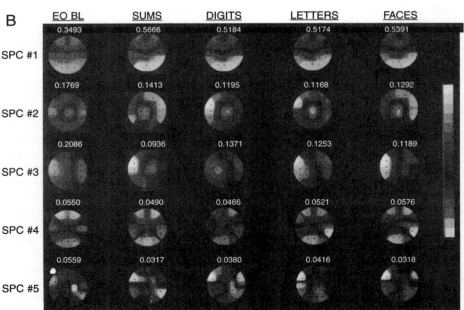

It must be pointed out that the same neuron may be engaged by two (or more) different subsystems at different times or in different tasks. In an information processing system, where multiple parallel processors contribute to the serial stages in information registration, encoding, storage, retrieval, and interpretation, it is to be expected that multiple functional subsystems may be simultaneously engaged. Such shifting engagement may be reflected in the changes in local participation in a particular SPC loading from task to task seen in figure 28.5b and from moment to moment (see figure 28.6).

Factor Score Curves

The proportion of neurons in any particular neuroanatomical structure, coherently engaged by one of these subsystems together with subsets of neurons in other brain regions, fluctuates from moment to moment reflecting the varying contribution of that subsystem to the successive stages of information processing in a specific task. Accordingly, the *factor scores*, which correspond to the momentary contribution of each such subsystem to the total voltage variance at each instant, wax and wane. Multiple factor score curves quantify the extent to which engagement of portions of the neuronal population in each brain region fluctuates in time with other coherent but independent, anatomically distributed functional subsystems and describe the coexisting, overlapping spatial modes of coherence.

The neurons coherently activated by the information-free noncontingent probes during the control interval P1 reflect the population of visually responsive cells globally distributed among different brain regions. The fluctuations of surface voltage landscapes during the analysis epoch of the P1 events accordingly can be considered analogous to a *baseline surface*.

The presentation of the information items S1 produces a different sequence of landscapes, which might be considered as analogous to *modulation* of the baseline surface by the priming set. Subtraction of P1 from S1 should remove the baseline contribution, leaving a "difference surface" (S1-P1) revealing the modulation by information, analogous to *demodulation*.[2] Similarly, subtraction of the baseline surface landscapes from the landscapes elicited by the delay probes should reveal modulated surface, P2-P1, hypothesized to reflect the working memory trace. Finally, subtraction of the landscapes elicited by the priming set, reflecting registration, encoding, and storage of the S1 information items, from the landscapes elicited by the matching set (S2-S1), reflecting registration and encoding of the S2 information as well as retrieval and comparison of those items with the working memory S1, should be sensitive to the retrieval and matching comparators.

Figure 28.6 depicts the factor scores quantifying the time course of engagement of the subsystems represented by SPC1 and SPC2 in (figure 28.6a) the registration and encoding of information about the priming set (S1-P1), (figure 28.6b)

Figure 28.5
Factor *loadings* of the first five Spatial Principal Components (SPC), which accounted for an average of 89.7% of the total voltage across the head in 55 sessions by eight subjects. The loadings depict the coherent *excitation* (red-orange hues) or *inhibition* (blue-green hues) of neuronal populations in extensive anatomical brain regions, relative to the average reference. These temporally synchronous patterns of spatially coherent networks accounted for the indicated percentages of the global voltage variance (shown above each loading) of the landscapes, which occurred across all four intervals of the 20–30 correct trials during each task. In each topographic SPC map, the landscape is viewed from the top with the face toward the top. (*a*) Loadings for the first five SPCs from each of five subjects performing the same DMS task (*Sums*). (*b*) Loadings for the first five SPCs from a sixth subject at rest (EO) and during *Sums*, *Digits*, *Letters*, and *Faces*.

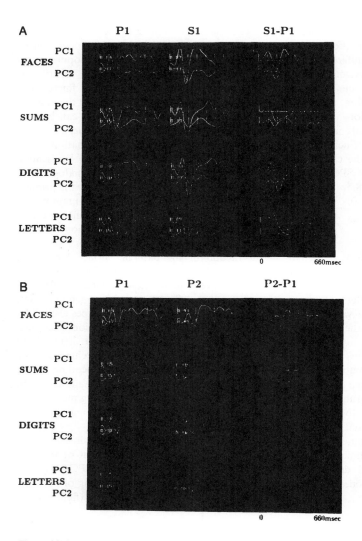

Figure 28.6

Factor *scores* (curves) of the first two Spatial Principal Components (PC1 [*top*] and PC2 [*bottom*]) showing differing temporal fluctuations in the allocation of these brain resources by one subject, during *event averages* within the four intervals of four different tasks. (*a*) Factor score curves throughout the event averages of (first column) the probes *P1* during Control Interval 1, (second column) the information items *S1* during Priming Interval 2, (third column) the demodulated "information" obtained by calculating the *difference wave, S1-P1.* Four sets of paired factor scores curves (for PC1 and PC2) are shown for the different DMS tasks *Faces, Sums, Digits, and Letters.* Note the very marked similarities between the PC1 curves for the probes *P1* during the baseline Control Interval 1 in the four different tasks (column 1). Minor differences in PC2 may reflect differences in expectation or "set." Columns 2 (S1)

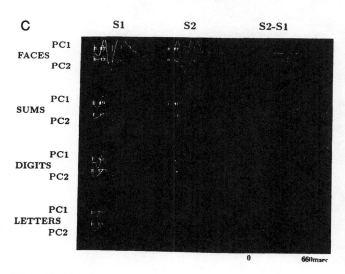

Figure 28.6 (continued)
and 3 (S1-P1) show marked differences in the information waves encoding these four classes of information, presented using size, luminance, and contrast equated screens (except faces). The analysis epochs of each event average were 667 ms, with vertical time marks every 100 ms. (*b*) Factor score curves as explained above, but showing fluctuations of PC1 and PC2 during the event averages of (column 1) the probes *P1* during Control Interval 1, (column 2) the probes (P2) during the Delay Interval 2, and (column 3) the working memory estimate, *P2-P1*. Note the clear differences in the WM curves, among all four tasks, in the allocation of both PC1 and PC2. (*c*) Factor score curves as above, showing fluctuations during the *event averages* of (column 1) the information in the Priming Set, *S1*, (column 2) the information in the Matching Set, *S2*, and (column 3) the differences reflecting the retrieval and matching process required to compare S2 to S1, *S2-S1*. Note the clear differences in PC1 across all four tasks.

the working memory of the priming set (P2-P1), and (figure 28.6c) the retrieval and matching comparator (S2-S1), in one subject.

The differences between resource allocation curves of SPC1 and SPC2 during the presentation of the control probes P1 and the priming set S1 represent the demodulation of the information from the postulated baseline surface. The allocation difference curves (S1-P1) for this "energy-free" encoding of the information are shown in figure 28.6a, for the information items in the *Faces* (F), *Sums* (S), *Digits* (D), and *Letters* (L) tasks. Note the close similarity of the SPC1 curve for the P1 event averages (column 1) in each of the four tasks, indicating comparable and stable baselines. Minor differences in PC2

may reflect "set." SPC1 and SPC2 together accounted for 72–76% of the total variance in each of these examples. In contrast, very marked differences between temporal variations reflecting the engagement in the four tasks of the coherent functional neuroanatomical subsystems corresponding to the loading of SPC1 can be clearly seen in columns 2 (S1) and 3 (S1-P1). The major differences begin at about 150 ms in all four tasks, most marked for SPC1. The differences in the allocation of SPC1 between 100 and 400 ms are especially remarkable in the case of D and S. Since the physical stimuli were identical, these differences seem reasonable to attribute to the difference in cognitive operations performed upon them in those two tasks. Differ-

Digits

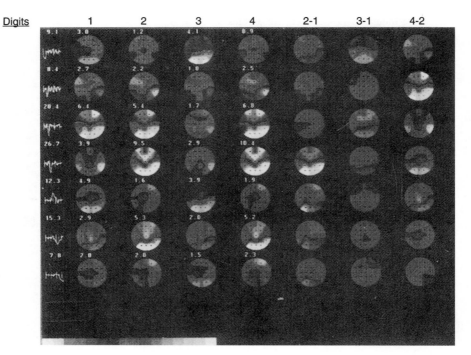

Sums

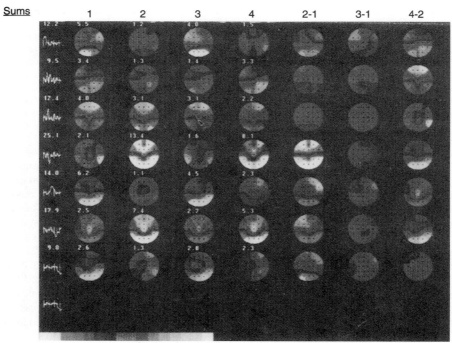

ences can also be seen between F and L, most marked in SPC1 between 200 and 300 ms and in SPC2 between 100 and 200 ms. These differences may reflect the fact that letters but not novel faces can be verbally tagged, but it should be pointed out that the contrast in the half tone photos used as stimuli in F was unavoidably impossible to match with the letter items in L.

Figure 28.6b shows differences in the allocation curves between the control probes P1 and the physically identical delay probes P2, which are somewhat diminished between 100 and 300 ms, presumably reflecting sustained engagement of some neural assemblies in maintaining the "trace" of S1. These diminutions cannot reasonably be attributed to habituation or fatigue of the visual system due to the repeated flashing stimuli in the visual field, since vigorous engagement of both SPC1 and SPC2 is seen during presentation of the subsequent matching set, S2. Note that engagement, especially of SPC1, is markedly and consistently greater when information items rather than probes of equal luminance and contrast were in the visual field.

Clear differences in the postulated demodulated working memory trace, P2-P1, are shown in figure 28.6b, for F, L, D, and S. These estimates of the engagement of the two functional subsystems indicate maximum and differential participation by SPC1 in visual working memory. Note that this process is maximal between 150 and 300 ms. Since the loading of SPC1 is maximally positive in posterior temporal and occipital regions, *while frontal regions are coher-*

ently out of phase, this finding appears to implicate reciprocal interactions between frontal cortex and primary and secondary visual cortices. A clear differential but secondary involvement of SPC2 is also evident, involving similar reciprocal transactions between right frontotemporal regions, possibly evaluating spatial attributes of the visual information and linking them to a left temporal-central verbal encoding process.

Inspection of figure 28.6c, illustrating the difference between S2 vs S1, suggests that the processes of retrieval of visual information from working memory and matching it to present visual input are accomplished by a comparator primarily engaging the subsystem represented by SPC1. This retrieval and matching process thus appears to bear a marked similarity to stimulus encoding and WM, involving reciprocal, out of phase transactions between coherent frontal cortical regions and the receiving areas of the visual system.

Temporal Principal Component Varimax Analysis

In previous work (John et al. 1993, 1994), we have used Temporal Principal Component Varimax Analysis for quantitative description of ERP morphology. In this method, each Varimax factor loading constitutes a set of *time* points across which voltages covary. Essentially, by treating each electrode as a subject, this method enables the time variance of voltage on the head

Figure 28.7
Results of TPCVA of *Digits* (top) and *Sums* (bottom) in one subject. Along the left margin the *factor loadings* of the first six temporal factors are arrayed as wave shapes from top to bottom, rank ordered according to the latency at which the maximum global variance was contributed across the set of 21 event averaged ERPs. The topographic maps in the different columns depict the *factor scores* quantifying the percentage of variance in the time series of the voltages at each electrode, contributed by the corresponding factor: (column 1) control probes, *P1*; (column 2) information in the Priming Set, *S1*; (column 3) delay interval probes, *P2*, (column 4) items in the Matching Set, *S2*; (column 5) the information waves, *S1-P1*; (column 6) the Working Memory estimate, *P2-P1*; (column 7) the difference reflecting the retrieval and matching process, *S2-S1*. Note the marked similarity between these temporal factor score maps and the maps of SPC loadings shown in figure 28.5.

to be objectively segmented into sequentially covarying ERP voltage segments which can be considered as independent components, although temporal overlap may occur.

A small set of TPCVA, about five or six factors, will usually account for about 94% of the temporal variance of voltages across the head during an ERP analysis epoch (John et al. 1993). In figure 28.7 are depicted the results of TPCVA of *Digits* and *Sums* in one subject (the same data are decomposed into SPC loadings in figure 28.5b and described by the SPC factor score curves in figure 28.6). For each temporal *factor loading* (component), shown at the left (from top to bottom), in increasing order of the latency at which maximum contribution to ERP variance occurs (from top to bottom), the average *factor scores* during the interval (cross product of factor loading X ERP) across every electrode are depicted as a color-coded interpolated topographic map. On these maps, hues of red through orange indicate increasing *positive* factor scores and blue through white indicate increasing *negative* factor scores.

In the figure, average factor scores are depicted for the *Digits* (top panel) and *Sums* (bottom panel) tasks as follows: (column 1) during control probe set, P1; (column 2) during priming set, S1; (column 3) during delay interval probes, P2; (column 4) during matching set, S2; (column 5) the difference between S1 and P1; (column 6) the difference between P2 and P1; and (column 7) the difference between S2 and S1. Note the occasional similarity between the topographic maps for *factor scores* for particular Temporal Varimax Components in figure 28.7 and the Spatial Principal Component *loadings* shown in figure 28.5.

Discussion

An extensive, multidisciplinary body of EEG, ERP, neurophysiological, and multimodal imaging evidence, summarized in the introduction, indicates that widespread brain regions participate in the storage of information in WM and its retrieval to identify subsequent events. Analyses of data from these delayed matching tasks reported elsewhere, using tracer stimuli, very narrow band EEG power spectra, event-related desynchronization (ERD) and synchronization (ERS), and ERPs, reported elsewhere, similarly showed widespread brain involvement in the representation, storage, and retrieval of a variety of types of information presented visually. While each method of analysis revealed marked changes in brain activity during cognitive activity, differing within an individual from task to task, little correspondence in such correlates of cognition was found among individuals. Further, each analytic method implicated different brain regions in mediation of the task, apparently sensitive o different aspects of the neuronal activation (John et al. 1997). *The task-related changes which were observed depended upon the method of analysis which was used.* Yet, within a task and any particular type of analysis such changes were highly significant. Which method correctly revealed the true relevant brain activation?

"Baseline Surfaces" and Modulation

Using topographic mapping of interval averages or event averages during DMS, widespread voltage shifts appeared across the scalp. Topographic "landscapes" with centroids in stable locations were observed to persist, sometimes for tens or even hundreds of milliseconds. One can consider that the preinformation probes, P1, activate the total population of visually responsive neurons, evoking a global integrated postsynaptic potential fluctuation which may be considered a *baseline surface*. This distributed coherent activity generates a corresponding sequence of landscapes. The information items in the priming set, S1, activate this population in a more differentiated way, significantly altering the state of varying proportions of the neurons in different brain regions containing specialized feature extractors sensitive to particular attributes of the afferent information. A "representational cell assembly" is thereby organized, consisting of the subset of visually responsive neurons which has been self-selected by its coherent activation, modulating the baseline surface as the postsynaptic potentials elicited by S1 are generated. The sequence of landscapes is thereby altered. It is plausible to argue that persistent engagement of that cell assembly perhaps mediates WM, since only those neurons registered input. Those neurons in widespread regions, preempted either by reverberatory or inhibitory maintenance of a "memory trace" (de No 1938, Hilgard and Marquis 1940, Hebb 1949), are no longer available to participate in the global population of visually responsive cells activated by the probes in the delay period, P2. This might be expected to constitute a *negative modulation* of the baseline surface previously evoked by the information free probes, P1, with a consequent change of landscape sequences.

Removal of the baseline surface, by subtraction of P1 from S1, can be considered analogous to *demodulation* and should leave the surface projection of the representational cell assembly, unmasked from the nonspecific global response to visual stimulation. Subtraction of P1 from P2 should leave the "negative modulation" defined by the set of neurons activated by the probe stimuli *before but not after* loading the priming information S1 into the working memory, potentially the "negative image" of the cell assembly initially engaged by S1. If so, these differences should display marked topographic similarities both to S2 as well as S1. The fact that the landscape topography of S2 at GFP peaks is almost identical with that of S1, while that of P2 is so markedly different from that of P1, offers assurance that the changes seen in response to P2 are neither due to nonspecific effects of stimulus repetition nor habituation.

Correlational analysis across landscapes at successive timepoints reveals that the sequential topography of the difference landscapes P2-P1

across the interval average *recurrently* displays high similarity to the landscape sequences during S1-P1 and S2-P1, about six times during the duration of the 4-s interval average. These correlograms attain highest values during a sustained period around 200 ms after each of the six stimuli, the latency at which subjective perception of prior information input appears to occur (Hassler 1979, Libet 1973) This high correlation value showing similarity among landscape topographies alternates in polarity, suggesting that stimulus input itself produces a positive excitation followed by a phase in which the previously stimulated cells are briefly inhibited.

Although these effects were regularly observed, in contrast the specific details of local VNB activation, ERD or ERS, ERP waveshape, or landscape topography were relatively variable, with a disappointing poverty of replicable features across different subjects performing similar tasks (John et al. 1997), although strong effects in multiple regions were found within every subject. There was an inconsistent relationship between localized findings and expectations derived from current beliefs about localization of function. This paucity of intersubject replicability may reflect differences in allocation of brain resources to these cognitive tasks, which may be idiosyncratic to each subject and reflect "cognitive style." However, the anatomical brain resources available must be genetically determined and available to all subjects. This reasoning leads to the expectation that there should exist a common, qualitatively invariant set of functional neuroanatomical subsystems which are engaged in parallel processing of information in qualitative modes, which may vary quantitatively according to individual cognitive styles.

SPC analysis revealed a limited set of such qualitative modes. The *loading* of an SPC is determined by the spatial pattern of covariance of subsets of neurons within extensive populations, which are engaged in coherent activity although dispersed in many anatomical regions. Difference in stimulus attributes, among items of information and in cognitive operations to be performed on these items of information, may alter the proportion of neurons in any region entering a particular coherent mode at any instant. Neurons in a given region may also switch rapidly by recruitment, from coherent participation in one mode into a different mode. A small set of five SPCs or their Varimax rotated transforms accounted for about 90% of the total voltage variance in all of the tasks and subjects studied thus far. This could probably be increased to about 95% by using a total of eight principal components.

SPC1 was characterized by a loading which contrasted a posterior positivity, maximum in bilateral posterior temporal, parietal, and occipital regions, with a generalized negativity in more anterior regions. One might speculate that this loading reflected the registration ot visual information on primary receiving and secondary processing cortical regions of the visual system. This spatial principal component accounted for the largest proportion of voltage variance, about 50% across all sessions with all tasks.

SPC2 was characterized by a loading which contrasted positivity in medial and lateral prefrontal, mesial frontal, anterior and posterior temporal, bilateral parietal, and occipital regions with negativity in bilateral central and frontal regions. One might speculate that this loading integrates the focusing of attention involving the anterior cingulate cortex reflected by the mesial frontal positivity, incorporation of the representation of recent (WM) attributes of the visual priming stimuli reflected by the posterior temporal, parietal, and occipital positivity, subvocal verbalization about the stimuli held in WM reflected in the positivity of the anterior temporal regions, and consciousness awareness and evaluation of the information represented by SPC 1 relative to the prior priming set reflected by the positivity in the medial and frontal prefrontal cortex. SPC 2 accounted for an average of about 17% of the total variance across all tasks.

SPC3 contrasted left anterior/posterior temporal regions to right. This loading suggested dichotomous or alternating processing of the verbal attributes of incoming stimuli in temporal regions of one hemisphere while nonverbal or spatial attributes were processed in corresponding regions on the other side. This speculation is concordant with the conceptual model proposed by Baddeley (1986).

It must be considered possible that this result may essentially be a mathematical artifact of the Principal Component method, which reliably produces statistical descriptors to account parsimoniously for the variance in a system. Such quantitative descriptors of scalp fields would nonetheless have utility. Further, the topography of the spatial factor loadings suspiciously resembles the sequence of spherical harmonics. Reassurance that these results reflect subsystem neurophysiology comes from four lines of evidence: (1) There is strong resemblance between the Spatial Principal Component and Varimax loadings, suggesting that these loadings reveal a "natural" structure rather than merely reflecting the arbitrary mathematical constraints of PCA; (2) observation of *instantaneous landscape* sequences reveals repeated appearance of topographies similar to these Spatial Principal Component or Varimax *loadings*, as illustrated above; (3) the temporal segmentation by Temporal Principal Component Varimax analysis described above yields *factor scores* across regions within various task intervals which, when displayed as factor score topographic maps, are similar to the Spatial Principal Component *loadings*; and (4) the use of a different mathematical approach to accomplish adaptive segmentation of landscape sequences yields a set of basic landscape topographies basically similar to the Spatial Principal Component loadings reported here (Pascual-Marqui et al. 1995).

It is undesirable that no unique set of generators can be presumed to underlie a particular surface voltage landscape. Similarly, a particular SPCA or TPCVA factor loading cannot be assumed to reflect the activity of a specific functional neuroanatomical distribution of neuronal activity. Ultimately, multimodal correlations of fMRI or PET images with SPC loadings during the same behavioral performance will be required to establish such correspondence. Yet, the consistent emergence of a highly similar set of factor loadings in different subjects and tasks and the prolonged persistence and frequent recurrence of landscapes closely resembling particular loadings lend plausibility to the proposal that they do reflect subsystem neurophysiology. The orderly fluctuations of the factor scores of Spatial Principal Components 1 and 2, in particular, and the similarity between factor score curves and familiar event related potential morphology suggests that more positive identification of their origins may be elucidated by judicious behavioral, psychophysiological, and pharmacological analysis.

These findings suggest that a high proportion of the neurons engaged in the processing of visual information and the maintenance of the capabilities required to perform adaptive cognitive behavior are engaged by five functional organizations, or "subsystems," dispersed within the brain. The proportion of neurons in any neuroanatomical region engaged by a particular one of these functional subsystems may vary from moment to moment. Individual neurons may be recruited into or depart from the coherent activity within such a subsystem, as the work load requires. These multiple subsystems, comprised of coactive neuronal populations which share different and independent temporal patterns of coherent activity, coexist in time within the same brain regions. Analyses of momentary allocation of these resources in different intervals of various cognitive tasks show dynamic temporal changes in their engagement. The nature of these changes suggests the primary role of a dynamic, reciprocally out-of-phase subsystem which mediates transactions between frontal cortex and posterior cortical areas. This subsystem (SPC1) seems to be engaged heavily during encoding, storage, and retrieval of visual information.

The loading of a Spatial Principal Component reflects the proportion of neurons across the cortical surface whose coherent activation produces the scalp voltages, reflecting their integrated postsynaptic membrane potentials. Further assessment of this interpretation will await the confirmation or contradiction of the proposed basic subsystem structure or coherence modes by methods such as LORETA (Low Resolution Electrophysiological Tomography Analysis) (Pascual-Marqui 1994) and functional MRI (Cohen et al. 1994). We are currently carrying out pilot studies using both methods for this purpose. The extraction of a particular SPC from the covariance matrix computed across a sequence of landscapes indicates that the underlying coherent neuronal assembly is oscillating in a common mode. Whether that common mode is rhythmic, as in the spontaneous EEG, or fluctuations of local field potentials, as in the event-related potential or ERP, it has been suggested that it may serve a number of possible functions (Lopes da Silva 1996):

1. Binding together single neurons dispersed within and among diverse anatomical regions such that they can form a unit of information processing

2. Rerouting information flow among brain systems by gating channels

3. Matching information transfer between assemblies in distinct areas

4. Modulating synaptic transmission and plasticity in specific synaptic systems

Evaluation of these different functional roles will be explored by studying the effects of alterations produced by pharmacological interventions or pathological states. Changes in SPC loadings and factor scores in a variety of cognitive tasks which are believed to require different allocation of brain resources should also be observed, as the functional relevance of these loadings is further examined.

Notes

1. It is unfortunate that only 21 electrodes were used in these studies but funds for a larger set of EEG amplifiers were not available. While studies using more electrodes reveal fine structure in scalp voltage fields not evident from only 21 locations (Gevins and Cutillo 1993, Gevins et al. 1996), we consider the present study a valid illustration of an approach and the results as a qualitative first approximation to the identification of basic resources in the brain. Preliminary exploration of the EEG dimensionality using 128 electrodes (P. Valdes-Sosa et al., personal communication) suggest that 90% of the surface voltage variance can be accounted for by 9–10 spatial principal components. The first four SPCs have loadings very similar to those shown below.

2. The use of these terms (baseline, modulation, demodulation) is intended merely as a conceptual aid and in no way is to be interpreted as suggestion of a model to be considered literally.

References

Abeles, M., Bergman, H., Mongalit, E., and Vaadia, E. (1993). Spatio-temporal firing patterns in the frontal cortex of behaving monkeys. *Journal of Neurophysiology*, 70, 1629–1638.

Abeles, M., Purt, Y., Bergman, H., and Vaadia, E. (1994). Synchronization in neuronal transmission and its importance for information. In Buzsaki, G., Llinas, R., & Singer, W. (Eds.), *Temporal coding in the brain* (pp. 39–50). Berlin: Springer-Verlag.

Andreasen, N. C., O'Leary, D. S., Cizaldo, T., Arndt, S., Rezai, K., Watkins, G. L., Boles Pinto, L. L., and Hichwa, R. D. (1995). Remembering the past: Two facts of episodic memory explored with positron emission tomography. *American Journal of Psychiatry*, 152, 1576–1585.

Baddeley, A. D. (1986). Working memory. In *Oxford psychology, series II* (pp. 1–289). Oxford: Clarendon.

Barrett, S. E., and Rugg, M. D. (1989). ERPs and the semantic matching. *Neuropsychology*, 27, 913–922.

Baylis, G. C., and Rolls, E. T. (1993). Responses of neurons in the inferior temporal cortex in short-term and serial recognition memory tasks. *Experimental Brain Research*, 65, 614–622.

Becker, J. T., Mintum, M. A., Diehl, D., DeKosky, S. T., and Dolkin, J. (1993). Functional neuroanatomy of verbal memory as revealed by word list recall during PET scanning. *Society of Neuroscience Abstracts*, 19, 1079.

Begleiter, H., Projesz, B., and Wang, W. (1993). A neurophysiologic correlate of visual short-term memory in humans. *Electroencephalography and Clinical Neurophysiology*, 87, 46–53

Boddy, J. (1986). Event-related potentials in chronometric analysis of primed word recognition with different stimulus onset asynchronies. *Psychophysiology*, 23(2), 232–245.

Burns, B. D. (1954). The production of afterbursts in isolated cerebral cortex. *Journal of Physiology*, 125, 427–446.

Burns, B. D., and Mogenson, G. (1958). Effects of cortical stimulation on habit acquisition. *Canadian Journal of Psychology*, 12, 77–82.

Buzsaki, G., Bragin, A., Chrobak, J. J., Nadasdy, Z., Sik, S., Hsu, M., and Ylinen, A. (1994). Oscillatory and intermittent synchrony in the hippocampus: Relevance to memory trace. In Buzsaki, G., Llinas, R., and Singer, W. (Eds.), *Temporal coding in the brain* (pp. 145–172). Berlin: Springer-Verlag.

Cohen, J., Forman, S., Braver, T., Casey, B., Servan-Schrelber, D., and Noll, D. (1994). Activation of the prefrontal cortex in a nonspatial WM task with FMRI. *Human Brain Mapping*, 1(4), 293–404.

Corbetta, M., Miezin, F. M., Dobmeyer, S., Sbuhman, G. L., and Petersen, S. F. (1991). Selective and divided attention during visual discriminations of shape, color and speed: Functional anatomy by positron emission topography. *Journal of Neuroscience*, 1, 2383–2402.

de No, R. L. (1938). Analysis of the activity of the chains of internuncial neurons. *Journal of Neurophysiology*, 1.

Dokker, A. J., Conner, D. J., and Thal, L. J. (1991). The role of cholinergic projections from the nucleus basalis in memory. *Neuroscience and Biobehavioral Reviews*, 15, 299–317.

Doty, R. W., and Ringo, J. L. (1994). Hemispheric distribution of memory traces. In Delacour, J. (Ed.),

The memory system of the brain (pp. 636–656). Singapore: World Scientific.

Dupont, P., Orban, G. A., and Vogels, R. (1993). Different perceptual tasks performed with the same visual stimulus attribute activate different regions of the brain. *Proceedings of the National Academy of Science USA*, 90, 10927–10931.

Fox, P. T., Mintum, M. A., Reiman, E. M., and Raichle, M. E. (1988). Enhanced detection of focal brain responses. *Journal of Cerebral Blood Flow and Metabolism*, 8, 642–653.

Frackowiak, R. (1994). Functional maps of verbal memory and language. *Trends in Neuroscience*, 17, 109–115.

Freeman, W. J., and Barrie, J. M. (1994). Chaotic oscillations and the genesis of meaning in cerebral cortex. In Buzsaki, G. L., Llinas, R., Singer, W., Bertroz, A., and Y., C. (Eds.), *Temporal coding in the brain* (pp. 13–38). Berlin: Springer-Verlag.

Friedman, D. (1990). Cognitive event-related potential (ERP) components during continuous recognition memory for pictures. *Psychophysiology*, 27, 136–148.

Friedman, D., Vaughan, H., and Erlenmeyer-Kimling, L. (1978). Stimulus and response related components of the late positive complex in a visual discrimination task. *Electroencephalogy and Clinical Neurophysiology*, 45, 319–330.

Friedman, H. R., and Goldman-Rakic, P. S. (1994). Coactivation of prefrontal cortex and inferior parietal cortex in working memory tasks revealed by 2DG functional mapping in the rhesus monkey. *Journal of Neuroscience*, 14(5), 2775–2788.

Friston, K. J., Frith, C. D., Liddle, P. F., and Frackowiak, R. (1993). Functional connectivity: The principal component analysis of large PET data sets. *Journal of Cerebral Blood Flow and Metabolism*, 13, 5–15.

Fuel, G., Goldenberg, W., Lang, G., Lindmger, M., Steiner, L., and Deeke, L. (1990). Cerebral correlates of imaging colors, faces and a map. II Negative cortical d. c. potentials. *Neuropsychologia*, 28, 81–93.

Funahashi, S., Bruce, C. J., and Goldman-Rakic, P. S. (1990). Visuospatial coding of primate prefrontal neurons revealed by oculomotor paradigms. *Journal of Neurophysiology*, 63(4), 814–831.

Fuster, J. M. (1989). *The prefrontal cortex* (2nd ed.). New York: Raven Press.

Gasser, T., Jennen-Steinmetz, C., Sroka, L., Verleger, R., and Möcks, J. (1983a). Development of the EEG of

school-age children and adolescents. II. Topography. *EEG Clin. Neurophysiol.*, 69, 100–109.

Gasser, T., Mocks, J., and Bacher, P. (1983b). Topographic factor analysis of the EEG with applications to development and to mental retardation. *EEG Clin. Neurophysiol.*, 55, 445–463.

Gevins, A. (1990). Distributed neuroelectric patterns of human neocortex during simple cognitive tasks. *Progress in Brain Research*, 85, 337–354.

Gevins, A., and Cutillo, B. (1993). Spatio-temporal dynamics of component processes in human working memory. *Electroencephalography and Clinical Neurophysiology*, 87, 128–143.

Gevins, A., Smith, M. E., Le, J., Leong, H., Bennett, J., Martin, N., L, M., Du, R., and Whitfield, S. (1996). High resolution evoked potential imaging of the cortical dynamics of human working memory. *Electroencephalography and Clinical Neurophysiology*, 98, 327–348.

Gevins, A. S., Doyle, J. C., Cutillo, B. A., Schaffer, R. F., Tannehill, R. L. et al. (1981). Electrical potentials in human brain during cognition. *Science*, 213, 918–922.

Goldman-Rakic, P. S. (1987). Circuitry of primate prefrontal cortex and regulation of behavior by representational knowledge. In F. Plum and V. B. Mountcastle (Eds.), *Handbook of physiology*, (5th ed., pp. 373–407). Bethesda: Am. Physiol. Soc.

Goldman-Rakic, P. S. (1988). Changing concepts of cortical connectivity: Parallel distributed cortical networks. In P. Rakic and W. Singer (Eds.), *Neurobiology of neocortex, dahlem konferenzen* (pp. 177–202). New York: Wiley.

Goldman-Rakic, P. S. (1994). The issue of memory in the study of prefrontal function. In *Motor and cognitive functions of the prefrontal cortex* (pp. 112–121). Berlin: Springer-Verlag.

Grasby, P., Frith, C., Friston, J., Frackowiak. R. J., and Dolan, R. (1993). Activation of the human hippocampal formation during auditory-verbal LTM function. *Neuroscience Letter*, 163, 185–188.

Habib, R., and Houle, S. (1994). Neuroanatomic correlates of retrieval in episodic memory: Auditory sentence recognition. *Proceedings of the National Academy of Science USA*, 91, 2012–2015.

Halgren, E., Baudena, P., Clarke, J. M., Heit, G., Liegeois, C. et al. (1995a). Intracerebral potentials to rare target and distractor auditory and visual stimuli.

Electroencephalography and Clinical Neurophysiology, 94, 191–220.

Halgren. E., Baudena, P., Clarke, J. M., Heit. G., Marinkovic, K., Devaux, B., Vignal, J., and Biraben, A. (1995b). Intracerebral potentials to rare target and distractor auditory and visual stimuli. II. Medial, lateral and posterior temporal lobe. *Electroencephalography and Clinical Neurophysiology*, 94, 299–250.

Halgren, E., Baudena, P., Heit, G., Clarke, M., and Marinkovic, K. (1994a). Spatio-temporal stages in face and word processing. *Journal of Physiology*, 88, 1–50.

Halgren, E., Baudena, P., Heit, G., Clarke, M., Marinkovic, K., and Chauvel, P. (1994b). Spatio-temporal stages in face and word processing. *Journal of Physiology*, 88, 51–80.

Harth, E. (1995). The Sketchpad Model. *Consciousness and Cognition*, 4, 346–368.

Hassler, R. (1979). Striatal regulation of adverting and attention directing induced by pallidal stimulation. *Applied Neurophysiology*, 42, 98–102.

Haxby, J. V., Horwitz, B., Ungerleider, L. C., Masiog, J., Allen, D. C. et al. (1993). Lateralization of frontal lobe activity associated with working memory for faces changes with retention interval: A parametric PET r-CBF study. *Society of Neuroscience Abstracts*, 19, 1284.

Haxby, J. V., Ungerleider, L. G., Horwitz, B., Rapport, S. I., and Grady, C. L. (1995). Hemispheric difference in neural systems for face working memory: A PET-rCBF study. *Human Brain Mapping*, 3, 68–82.

Hebb, D. O. (1949). *The organization of behavior*. New York: Wiley.

Heinze, H. J., Minute, T. F., and Mangum, G. R. (1994). *Cognitive Electrophysiology*. Birkhauser, Boston.

Hilgard, E. R., and Marquis, D. G. (1940). *Conditioning and learning*. New York: Appleton.

Hjorth, B., and Rodin, E. (1988). An eigenfunction approach to the inverse problem of EEG. *Brain Topography*, 1(2), 79–86.

Ingvar, D. H. (1991). Ideography: Mapping ideas in the brain. In *Brain work and mental activity* (pp. 346–359). Copenhagen: Munksgaard.

Jasper, H. H., and Penfield, W. (1949). Electrocorticograms in man: Effect of voluntary movement upon the electrical activity of the precentral gyrus. *Archiv fur Psychiatrie und Nervenkrankheitem*, 262, 163–174.

John, E. R. (1968). *Mechanisms of memory*. New York: Academic Press.

John, E. R. (1972). Switchboard versus statistical theories of learning and memory. *Science*, 177, 850–864.

John, E. R. (1976). Neurometric analysis of brain function. *Triangle*, 15, 77–88.

John, E. R., and Easton, P. (1995). Quantitative electrophysiological studies of mental tasks. *Biological Psychology*, 40(1–2), 101–113.

John, E. R., Easton, P., and Isenhart, R. (1997). Consciousness and cognition may be mediated by multiple independent coherent ensembles. *Consciousness and Cognition*, 6(1).

John. E. R., Easton, P., Isenhart, R., and Gulyashar, A. (1996). Electrophysiological analysis of the registration, storage and retrieval of information in DMS. *International Journal of Psychophysiology*, 24, 127–144.

John, E. R., Easton, P., Prichep, L. S., and Friedman, J. (1993). Standardized Varimax descriptors of ERPs. I. Basic considerations. *Brain Topography*, 6(2), 143–162.

John, E. R., Easton, P., Prichep, L. S., and Friedman, J. (1994). Standardized Varimax descriptors of ERPs. II. Evaluation of psychiatric patients. *Psychiatric Research*, 55, 13–40.

John, E. R., and Killam, K. F. (1959). Electrophysiological correlates of avoidance conditioning in the cat. *Journal of Pharmacology and Experimental Therapeutics*, 125, 252–274.

John, E. R., and Killam, K. F. (1960). Studies of electrical activity of brain during differential conditioning in cats. In *Recent advances in biological psychiatry* (pp. 138–148). Philadelphia: Grune & Stratton.

John, E. R., and Morgades, P. P. (1969). Neural correlates of conditioned responses studied with multiple chronically implanted moving microelectrodes. *Experimental Neurology*, 23, 412–425.

John, E. R., Ruchkin, D. S., Leiman, A., Sachs, E., and Ahn, H. (1965). Electrophysiological studies of generalization using both peripheral and central conditioned stimuli. In *Proc. XXIII international congress of physiological sciences* (Vol. 87, pp. 618–627).

John. E. R., Ruchkin, D. S., and Villegas, J. (1964). Signal analysis and behavioral correlates of evoked potential configurations in cats. In W. C. Corning and

M. Balaban (Eds.), *The mind: Biological approaches to its functions* (Chap. 5, pp. 101–175). New York: Wiley.

Kramer. A. F., and Donchin, E. (1987). Brain potentials as indices of orthographic and phonological interaction during word matching. *Journal of Experimental Psychology*, 13(1), 76–86.

Kramer, A. F., and Schneider, W., Fisk, A., and Donchin, E. (1986). The effects of practice and task structure on components of the event-related brain potential. *Psychophysiology*, 23, 33–47.

Kutas, M. (1988). Review of event-related potential studies of memory. In M. Gazzaniga (Ed.), *Perspective in memory research* (pp. 181–218). Cambridge: MIT Press.

Legewie, H., Simonova, O., and Cruetzfeldt, O. D. (1969). EEG changes during performance of various tasks under open- and closed-eyed conditions. *Electroencephalography and Clinical Neurophysiology*, 27, 470–479.

Lehmann, D., Ozaki, H., and Pal, I. (1987). EEG alpha map series: Brain micro-states by space-oriented adaptive segmentation. *Electroencephalography and Clinical Neurophysiology*, 67, 271–288.

Levine, J. D., Doty, R. W., Astur, R. A., and Provencal, S. L. (1994). Role of the forebrain commisures in Bihemispheric Memonic Integration in Macques. *Journal of Neuroscience*, 14(5), 2575–2530.

Libet, B. (1973). Electrical stimulation of cortex in human subjects, and conscious sensory aspects. In A. Iggo (Ed.), *Handbook of sensory physiology* (Vol. II, Chap. 19, pp. 743–790). Berlin: Springer-Verlag.

Lopes da Silva, F. H. (1996). The generation of electric and magnetic signals of the brain by local networks. In R. Greger and U. Windhorst (Eds.), *Comparative Human Physiology* (pp. 509–531). Berlin: Springer-Verlag.

Luck, S., Hillyard, S., Mangum, G., and Gazzaniga, M. (1989). Independent hemispheric attentional systems mediate visual search in split-brain patients. *Nature*, 342, 543–545.

Magliero, A., Bashore, T. R., Coles, M. G. H., and Donchin, E. (1984). On the dependence of P300 latency on stimulus evaluation processes. *Psychophysiology*, 21, 171–186.

Markowitsch, H. J. (1988). Diencephalic amnesia: A reorientation. *Brain Research Review*, 13, 351–370.

McCarthy, G. (1995). Functional neuroimaging of memory. *The Neuroscientist*, 1(3), 155–163.

McCarthy, G., and Donchin, E. (1983). Chronometric analysis of human information processing. In A Gaillard and W. Ritter (Eds.), *Tutorials in event-related potential research: Endogenous components. Advances in psychology* (Vol. 10, pp. 251–268). Amsterdam: Elsevier.

McCarthy, G., Pruce, A., Rothman, D. L., Goldman-Rakic, P. S., and Shuhman, R. G. (1993). FMRI during a spatial working memory task in humans. *Society of Neuroscience Abstracts*, 19, 190.

McLaughlin, T., Steinberg, B., Christensen, B., Law, I., Parving, A., and Friberg, L. (1992). Potential language and attentional networks revealed through factor analysis of rCBF data measure with SPECT. *Journal of Cerebral Blood Flow and Metabolism*, 12(4), 535–545.

Merzenich, M. (1995). Distributed cortical representations of learned stimuli and behaviors. In *Symposium, Center for Neuroscience, New York University*.

Mesulam, M. (1990). Large scale neurocognitive networks and distributed processing for attention, language and memory. *Annals of Neurology*, 28, 597–611.

Milner, B. (1990). Right temporal lobe contribution to visual perception and visual memory. In E. Iwai and M. Mishkin (Eds.), *Vision, memory and the temporal lobe* (pp. 43–53). New York: Elsevier.

Moller, J. R., and Strother, S. C. (1991). A regional covariance approach to the analysis of functional patterns in positron emission tomographic data. *Journal of Cerebral Blood Flow and Metabolism*, 11, 121–135.

Munte, T. F., Kunkel, H., and Heinze, H. J. (1989). Semantic distance and the electro-physiological priming effect. In E. Basar and T. H. Bullock (Eds.), *Brain dynamics: Progress and perspectives* (pp. 436–448). Berlin: Springer-Verlag.

Neville, H. J., Kutas, M., Chesney, G., and Schmidt A. C. (1986). Event related brain potentials during encoding and recognition memory of congruous and incongruous words. *Journal of Memory and Language*, 25, 75–92.

Nicolelis, M. A. L., Baccala, L. A., Lin, R. C. S., and Chopin, J. K. (1995). Sensorimotor encoding by synchronous neural ensemble activity at multiple levels of the somatosensory system. *Science*, 268, 1353–1358.

Nielsen-Bohlman, L. and Knight, R. (1994). ERPs dissociate immediate and delayed memory. In H. J. Heinze, T. F. Minute, and G. R. Mangum (Eds.),

Cognitive electrophysiology (pp. 169–182). Basel: Birkhauser.

Ojemann, G. A., Fried, I., and Lettich, E. (1989). ECoG correlates of language. I. desynchronization in temporal language cortex during object naming. Electroencephalography and Clinical Neurophysiology, 73, 453–463.

O'Sullivan, B. T., Roland, P. E., and Kawashina, R. (1994). A PET study of somatosensory discrimination in man. Microgeometry is macrogeometry. European Journal of Neuroscience, 6, 137–148.

Papanicolau, A., Deutsch, C., Bourbon, W., Will, K., Loring, D., and Eisenberg, H. (1987). Convergent EP and rCBF evidence of task-specific hemispheric differences. Electroencephalography and Clinical Neurophysiology, 66, 515–520.

Papanicolau, A. C., Levin, H. S., and Eisenberg, H. M. (1984). Evoked potential correlates of recovery from aphasia after focal left hemisphere injury in adults. Neurosurgery, 14(4).

Pascual-Marqui, R., Michel, C., and Lehmann, D. (1995). Segmentation of brain electrical activity into microstates. IEEE Transactions on Biomedical Engineering, 42(7), 658–665.

Pascual-Marqui, R. D. (1994). Low resolution brain electromagnetic tomography. Abstract of paper presented at the International 7th Swiss Brain Mapping Meeting, March 11–12, 1994 in Zurich.

Paulescu, E., Frith, C., and Frackowiak, R. (1991). The neural correlates of the verbal component of WM. Nature, 362, 342–343.

Petrides, M., Alisavotos, B., Evans, A. C., and Meyer, E. (1993). Dissociation of human mid dorsolateral from posterior dorsolateral frontal cortex in memory processing. Proceedings of the National Academy of Science USA, 90, 873–877.

Petsche, H., Lacroix, D., Lincher, K., Rappelsberger, P., and Schmidt-Henrick, E. (1992). Thinking with images or thinking with language: A pilot EEG probability mapping study. International Journal of Psychology, 12, 31–39.

Pfurtscheller, G., and Berghold, A. (1989). Patterns of cortical activation during planning of voluntary movement. EEG Clinical Neurophysiology, 72, 250–258.

Pfurtscheller, G., and Klimesch, W. (1990). Topographical display and interpretation of event-related desynchronization during a visual-verbal task. Brain Topography, 3, 85–93.

Posner, M. I. (1978). Chronometric explorations of the mind. Hillsdale, NJ: Erlbaum.

Raichle, M. E. (1994). Visualizing the mind. Scientific American, 270, 36–43.

Ramos, A., Schwartz, E. L., and John, E. R. (1976). Stable and plastic unit discharge patterns during behavioral generalization. Science, 192, 393–396.

Risberg, J. (1987). Hemispheric functions evaluated by measurements of the regional cerebral blood flow. In D. Ottoson (Ed.), Duality and unity of the brain (pp. 442–453). New York: Plenum.

Ritter, W., Vaughan, H., and Macht, M. (1983). On relating ERP components and stages of information processing. In A. Gaillard and W. Ritter (Eds.), Tutorials in ERP research: Endogenous components. Advances in Psychology (Vol. 10, pp. 143–158). Amsterdam: Elsevier.

Roland, P. E., and Friberg, L. (1985). Localization of cortical areas activated by thinking. Journal of Neurophysiology, 53, 1219–1243.

Ruchkin, D. S., Johnson, R., Jr., Canorme, H., and Ritter, W. (1990). Short term memory storage and retention: An event-related potential study. Electroencephalography and Clinical Neurophysiology, 76, 419–439

Ruchkin, D. S., Jr., R. J., Grafman, J., Conoune H., and Ritter, W. (1992). Distinctions and similarities among working memory processes: An ERP study. Cognitive Brain Research, 1, 53–66.

Rugg, M. D., and Doyle, M. C. (1994). ERPs and stimulus repetition. In H. J. Heinze, T. F. Minute and G. R. Mangum (Eds.), Cognitive electrophysiology. Basel: Birkhauser.

Rugg, M. D., and Nagy, M. E. (1987). Lexical contribution to non-word-repetition effects: Evidence from event-related potentials. Memory and Cognition, 6, 473–481.

Sanquist, T. F., Rohrbaugh, J. W., Syndulko, K., and Lindsley, D. B. (1980). Electro-cortical signs of levels of processing: perceptual analysis and recognition memory. Psychophysiology, 17, 568–576.

Schneider, W., and Shiffrin, R. M. (1977). Controlled and automatic human information processing. I. Detection, search and attention. Psychology Review, 84, 1–66.

Sergent, J., Geuze, R., and vanWinsum, W. (1987). ERD and P300. Psychophysiology, 24(3), 272–277.

Sergent, J., Zuck, E., Levesque, M., and MacDonald, B. (1992). PET study of letter and object processing. *Cortex*, 2(1), 68–80.

Shallice, T. (1982). Specific impairments in planning. *Philosophical Transactions of the Royal Society of London*, 298.

Shallice, T., Fletcher, P., Frith, C. D., Grasby, P., Frakowiak, R. S. J., and Dolan, R. J. (1994). Brain regions associated with acquisition and retrieval of verbal episodic memory. *Nature*, 368, 633–635.

Singer, W. (1990). Search for coherence: A basic principle of cortical self-organization. *Concepts in Neuroscience*, 1(1), 1–26.

Singer, W. (1994). Time as coding space in neocortical processing. In G. Buzsáki, R. Llinás, W. Singer, A Berthoz and Y. Christen (Eds.), *Temporal coding in the brain* (pp. 51–80). Berlin: Springer-Verlag.

Skrandies, W. (1989). Data reduction of multichannel fields: Global field power and principal components. *Brain Topography*, 2, 73–80.

Skrandies, W., and Lehmann, D. (1982). Spatial principal components of multichannel maps evoked by lateral visual half-field stimuli. *EEG Clin. Neurophysiol.*, 54, 662–667.

Sosaki, K., Gemba, H., Mambu, A., and Matauzaki, R. (1994). Activity of the prefrontal cortex on no-go decision and motor suppression. In *Motor and cognitive functions of the prefrontal cortex* (pp. 139–159). Berlin: Springer Verlag.

Squire, L. R., Ojemann, J. G., Meizni, S. M., Petersen, S. E., Videen, T. O., and Raichle, M. E. (1992). Activation of the hippocampus in normal humans: A functional anatomical study of human memory. *Proceedings of the National Academy of Sciences USA* 89, 1837–1841.

Starr, A., Kristeva, R., Cheyne, D., Lindmger, D., and Deeke, L. (1991). Localization of brain activity during auditory verbal short-term memory derived from magnetic recordings. *Brain Research*, 558, 181–190.

Strik, W. K., and Lehmann, D. (1993). Data-determined window size and space-oriented segmentation of spontaneous EEG map series. *Electroencephalography and Clinical Neurophysiology*, 87, 169–174.

Stuss, D., Sarazin, E., Leech, E., and Picton, T. (1983). Event-related potentials during naming and mental rotation. *Electroencephalography and Clinical Neurophysiology*, 56, 133–146.

Sugishita, M., Koike, A., Shimigu, H., and Ishijima, B. (1990). Paired associate learning deficit after dominant (left) temporal lobectomy. In E. Iwai and M. Mishkin (Eds.), *Vision, memory and the temporal lobe* (pp. 55–61). New York: Elsevier.

Sutton, S., Braren, M., John, E. R., and Zubin, J. (1965). Evoked potential correlates of stimulus uncertainty. *Science*, 150, 1187–1188.

Swartz, B. E., Halgren, E., Fuster, J., and Mandelkern, M. (1994). An [18]FDG-PET study of cortical activation during a short-term visual memory task in humans. *NeuroReport*, 5, 925–928.

Tucker, D. M., Dawson, S. L., and Roth, D. L. (1985). Regional changes in EEG power and coherence during cognition: Intensive study of two individuals. *Behavioral Neuroscience*, 99.

Vallor, G., and Baddeley, A. D. (1984). Activation of working memory: Neuropsychological evidence for a phonological short-term store. *Journal of Verbal Learning and Verbal Behavior*, 23, 151–161.

Verzeano, M., and Negishi, K. (1960). Neuronal activity in cortical thalamic networks. *Journal of General Physiology*, 43.

Wilkins, S. (1962). Testing parametric statistical hypotheses. In *Mathematical statistics* (Chap. 13, pp. 394–427, Problem 13.4). New York: Wiley.

Wilson, F. A. W., O'Scalaidke, S. P., and Goldman-Rakic, P. S. (1993). Dissociation of object and spatial processing domains in primate prefrontal cortex. *Science*, 260, 1955–1958.

Worsley, K. J., Evans, A. C., Marrett, S., and Neelin, P. (1992). A three-dimensional statistical analysis for CBF activation studies in human brain. *Journal of Cerebral Blood Flow*, 12, 900–918.

Zatore, R. J., Evans, A. C., and Mayer, E. (1994). Neural mechanisms underlying modal perception and memory for pitch. *International Journal of Neuroscience*, 14, 1908–1919.

Zatore, R. J., Evans, A. C., Meyer, E., and Gjeche, A. (1992). Lateralization of phonetic and pitch discrimination in speech processing. *Science*, 256, 846–849.

Zola-Morgan, S., and Squire, L. (1993). Neuroanatomy of memory. *Annual Review of Neuroscience*, 16, 547–563.

V INTERNAL SOURCES: VISUAL IMAGES AND INNER SPEECH

We can be conscious of internal images in all
sensory modalities, especially vision; in inner
speech; and body-referred feelings associated
with emotion, anticipatory pleasure, and anticipatory pain. All these internally generated
experiences seem to resemble external, stimulus-
driven events. There are now a number of techniques for assessing imagined events that can
meet the widespread operational definition of
conscious experience (see Introduction), though
the imagery literature has been more concerned
with verifying imagery reports than with asking
whether or not the image was conscious. For
example, a famous series of experiments by
Cooper and Shepard (1973) shows that people
can rotate mental images and that the time
needed for rotation is a linear function of the
number of degrees of rotation. This very precise
result has been taken as evidence for the accuracy and reliability of mental images. But it is
not obvious that subjects in this task are necessarily conscious of the image. It is possible for
example that in mentally rotating an image of a
chair, we are conscious of the chair at 0, 90, 180,
and 270 degrees, and less conscious at other
points along the circle.

Visual Imagery in the Brain

Stephen Kosslyn is one of the early pioneers
in the scientific exploration of visual imagery.
The chapter in this section by Kosslyn (1988)
describes major progress in understanding the
brain basis of visualization. In particular, there is
good evidence that visual experiences of internal
origin involve many of the same parts of visual
cortex that are needed to identify external visual
events. Along similar lines, Farah (1989) provides a summary of current knowledge of the
brain basis of visual imagery. These chapters
provide a different perspective on the visual
aspects of working memory (see section IV).

Thinking and Inner Speech—Central Modalities of Human Experience

Most humans go around the world talking to
themselves, though we may be reluctant to do so
out loud. Indeed, we may be so accustomed to
the inner voice that we are no longer aware of its
existence "metacognitively," which leads to the
paradox of people asking themselves, "What
inner voice?" But experiments on inner speech
show its existence quite objectively and reliably.
For several decades Singer and his colleagues
have studied inner speech simply by asking people to talk out loud, which they are surprisingly
willing to do (Singer 1993; chap. 31, this volume). There is good evidence from this work that
the inner voice maintains a running commentary
about our experiences, feelings, and relationships with others; it comments on past events
and helps to make plans for the future. Clinical
researchers have trained children to talk to
themselves in order to control impulsive behavior, and there are many hundreds of experiments
in the cognitive literature on verbal working
memory, which is roughly the domain in which
we rehearse telephone numbers, consider different ideas, and talk to ourselves generally (e.g.,
Baddeley 1990; chap. 25, this volume). Thus we
actually know a great deal about inner speech,
even though it is not always referred to by that
name.

Thinking involves more than just inner speech,
of course. Much thinking appears to be nonverbal, much of it involves abstract ideas which
are not necessarily expressible in speech, some of
it involves visual images and metaphors, and so
on.

Ericsson and Simon (1987; chap. 32, this volume) report on efforts to study thinking in the
laboratory and summarize the extensive body
of research on verbal reports of thinking (for
a much more comprehensive account, consult
Ericsson and Simon 1984/1993). In contrast to

the chapter by Singer, theirs is not a study of spontaneous thinking, but the goal-directed thinking necessary to learn concepts, recall and memorize information, and solve problems. Most of our knowledge of expert and exceptional performance derives from such reports (Ericsson 1996, Ericsson and Lehmann 1996). These findings have led to the development of new theories of skilled performance and the acquisition of extended working memory (Ericsson and Kintsch 1995) that contrasts with the traditional theories with a small, central working memory interacting with a large long-term memory with automatic problem-action rules, or semantic networks (e.g., Newell 1990, Anderson 1983; see Baars 1998; chap. 65, this volume). Obviously, the working memories in cognitive architectures are allied to consciousness.

References

Anderson, J. R. (1983) *The architecture of cognition.* Cambridge, MA: Harvard University Press.

Cooper, L. A., and Shepard, R. N. (1973) Chronometric studies of the rotation of mental images. In W. G. Chase (ed.), *Visual information processing.* New York: Academic Press.

Ericsson, K. A. (1996) The acquisition of expert performance: An introduction to some of the issues. In K. A. Ericsson (ed.), *The road to excellence: The acquisition of expert performance in the arts and sciences, sports, and games.* (pp. 1–50). Hillsdale, NJ: Erlbaum.

Ericsson, K. A., and Kintsch, W. (1995) Long-term working memory. *Psychological Review,* 102, 211–245.

Ericsson, K. A., and Lehmann, A. C. (1996) Expert and exceptional performance: Evidence of maximal adaptations to task constraints. *Annual Review of Psychology,* 47, 273–305.

Ericsson, K. A., and Simon, H. A. (1984/1993) *Protocol analysis: Verbal reports as data.* Cambridge, MA: MIT Press.

Newell, A. (1990) *Unified theories of cognition.* Cambridge, MA: Harvard University Press.

29 Aspects of a Cognitive Neuroscience of Mental Imagery

S. M. Kosslyn

Perhaps the most fundamental insight of contemporary cognitive science is the discovery that mental faculties can be decomposed into multicomponent information-processing systems. Although mental faculties such as "memory," "thinking," "imagery," and so on intuitively may seem to be single abilities, they are not. How visual mental imagery is being analyzed into distinct processing components and how these functionally characterized components are coming to be identified with brain structures is the subject of this article. Only one facet of imagery is considered here, namely the way visual mental images are generated from stored information.

Mental imagery has played a key role in many theories of mental function, both historically and currently (1–3). Imagery consists of brain states like those that arise during perception but occurs in the absence of the appropriate immediate sensory input; such events are usually accompanied by the conscious experience of "seeing with the mind's eye," "hearing with the mind's ear," and so on. Visual imagery is a particularly useful place to begin in that it clearly draws on some of the mechanisms also used in visual perception (2–5), and the anatomy and physiology of vision is becoming relatively well understood (6, 7). Evidence for the use of common mechanisms in imagery and like-modality perception abounds. For example, visual perception is more difficult than auditory perception when one is simultaneously holding a visual mental image, and vice versa when one is holding an auditory mental image (8). In addition, some visual illusions also appear in visual imagery (4). Indeed, there is emerging evidence that visual areas of the brain are selectively activated during visual mental imagery (5).

Generating hypotheses about the processing that underlies imagery is aided by consideration of three kinds of factors. First, it is necessary to begin by characterizing the behavior of imagery mechanisms. Without such information, there is nothing to explain. Second, because a theory of human information processing is in fact a theory about how the brain functions, it is useful to have some knowledge of the underlying neural substrate. Given that imagery shares some modality-specific perceptual mechanisms, facts about the anatomy and physiology of the visual system can be used in generating hypotheses about the processing underlying imagery. Third, it is useful to perform an analysis of what would be required to build a system that would produce the observed behavior. The use of these three kinds of factors is illustrated in the following section.

Generating Visual Mental Images

Probably the most obvious behavioral property of the imagery system is that images are not present all the time, but only occur in specific circumstances. For example, if one is asked to decide whether the uppercase letters of the alphabet have only straight lines or contain any curved lines, images of the letters are likely to be used. These images come to mind only when one begins to perform the task. The question to be considered here is, what is the nature of the processing that produces mental images?

Behavioral Characterization

When asked, most people report that images of simple objects, such as letters or line patterns, seem to pop into mind all at once. However, when the time course of image formation is charted, such introspections are revealed to be incorrect: imaged patterns are built up a part at a time. Consider the following task. First, observe the letter in the grid at the upper left of figure

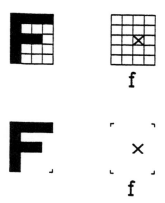

Figure 29.1
(*Top left*) A letter formed by selectively filling in cells of a matrix. (*Top right*) Subjects were shown a lowercase cue and asked whether the corresponding uppercase block letter would occupy the cells containing one or two × marks. Because only 500 ms were allowed between presentation of the lowercase cue and the probe marks, which is not enough time to read the cue and finish forming the image, the decision times in part reflect the time to form the image in the matrix. (*Bottom*) An alternative way of presenting the stimuli, which was expected to induce a different method of arranging parts in the image.

29.1. If that letter were present in the grid at the upper right, would it cover the × mark? In these experiments, subjects first memorized a set of such block letters, which varied from two (L) to five segments (G). The subjects later were shown a blank grid with a lowercase letter beneath it, and were asked to decide whether the corresponding uppercase version of the letter—if drawn in the grid as previously seen—would fill the cells occupied by two such × marks. On half the trials the letter would have covered both × marks, whereas on the other half it would have covered only one (the other was in a cell that would have been adjacent to the letter). Subjects were told to respond as quickly as possible while being as accurate as possible; response time and accuracy were measured.

The key to this method is that the two probe marks appeared in the grid only 500 ms after the lowercase cue letter was presented. Given that up to 250 ms are necessary to read a letter cue (9), and about 250 ms are required to move one's eyes up from the cue, there was not enough time to finish forming the image before the probes appeared. Hence the time to respond should in part reflect the time to form the image (10).

The first result of interest was that the response times increased with the visual complexity (number of segments) of the queried letter (mean slope, 133 ms per segment; SE, 28 ms; $P < 0.0005$). Although this result suggests that more complex forms require more time to image, it could instead reflect the time to search for the probe marks. Thus, it is important that complexity had greatly reduced effects when these subjects evaluated probe marks with the figure actually present (mean slope, 10 ms; SE, 4 ms; $P < 0.05$); the results in the imagery task do not reflect only search and evaluation time. In addition, in another condition the probe marks were eliminated, and subjects now were asked simply to read the lowercase cue and form an image of the corresponding uppercase version in the grid; as soon as the image was fully formed, the subjects were to press a key. These times also increased for letters with more segments, and did so to a similar degree in this task and the image evaluation task (mean slope, 100 ms per segment; SE, 19 ms; $P < 0.0005$; $P > 0.1$ for the comparison of the two slopes). Thus, there is reason to infer that differences in response times in the experimental task reflect differences in image formation time (11).

In addition to varying the complexity of the stimuli, the positions of the probe marks were varied along the individual letters. If the image is being constructed a segment at a time, then some probes ought to require more time to reach than others. A separate group of 25 subjects was asked to copy the block letters into empty grids, and the order in which the segments were drawn

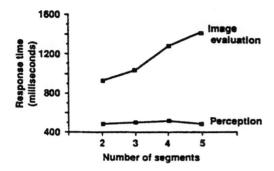

Figure 29.2
The mean time to evaluate probe marks in the image evaluation and perception tasks when the farthest probe mark was on the first, second, third, or fourth segment typically drawn. The image evaluation task required deciding whether probes would have fallen on a letter, and the perception task required deciding whether probes actually did fall on a letter.

was covertly observed; the order was highly consistent, with five of the letters being drawn in the same way by 100% of the subjects, and the remainder being drawn in the same way by at least 75% (when these letters were drawn differently it was always in the order of a single segment). As is illustrated in figure 29.2, more time was required in the image evaluation task when the "farthest" probe mark fell on a segment typically drawn later in the sequence (mean slope, 178 ms per segment; SE = 35 ms; $P < 0.0005$). This effect of probe position did not occur in the perception control task (mean slope, 2 ms per segment; SE, 7 ms; $P > 0.25$). Similar results were found for novel two-dimensional patterns (11) and three-dimensional shapes (12).

Thus, it appears that patterns in images are built up by activating parts individually and that parts are imaged in roughly the order in which they are typically drawn. These inferences were supported by a host of additional experiments controlling for various alternative accounts. For example, it was possible that the effect of probe

position was due to scanning an imaged pattern in search of the probes (which might be different than inspecting a figure that is actually present). If so, then farther probes should require more time to evaluate than nearer ones, even when one has formed the image in advance of the probe; this did not occur. It was also possible that the effects reflect patterns of eye movements; nevertheless, they persisted even when subjects fixated on the center of the screen while performing the task (11, 12).

Additional research has been conducted to discover what factors determine the nature of the parts, and has shown that principles of perceptual organization also determine the part structure of images (13). That is, it has been known since the early part of this century that we see lines and regions as being organized into "perceptual units." For example, the pattern "------" is seen as a line (grouped by the "law of good continuation"), not six isolated dashes; "XXX XXX" is seen as two units (grouped by the "law of proximity"), not six solitary X's; and XXXooo is seen as two units (grouped by the "law of similarity"), not simply three X's and three o's. Similarly, lines that form a symmetrical pattern or that form enclosed areas tend to be grouped as units (14). In the block letter stimuli used in the image generation experiments, adjacent filled cells will form a unit (a bar) as per the law of good continuation. There is good evidence that these sorts of units are not only perceived, but also are stored in memory (13).

Thus, given that visual mental images are formed by activating previously stored perceptual information, it is easy to formulate a hypothesis about why images are constructed a part at a time: namely, when originally viewed the parts were stored individually and hence they are later activated into an image individually. But even so, the data suggest that parts are activated sequentially. Why are they not simply activated all at once to reconstruct the entire object in the image?

Neurological Constraints

One possible reason why parts are imaged sequentially hinges on the way parts and spatial relations among them might be stored in memory. Ungerleider and Mishkin (7) summarize evidence for "two cortical visual systems" in primates (figure 29.3). The ventral system runs from area OC (primary visual cortex) through area TEO down to the inferior temporal lobe. This system has been identified with the analysis of shape ("what"). The dorsal system runs almost directly from circumstriate area OB to OA and then to PG (in the parietal lobe). This system has been identified with the analysis of location ("where").

Three sorts of data have been marshalled to support Ungerleider and Mishkin's claims. First, neuroanatomical investigations have documented the existence of the separate pathways. Indeed, each pathway has now been decomposed into connections among numerous distinct areas (6, 7).

Second, neurophysiological investigations of monkey brains have revealed that cells in both systems are sensitive to visual input, but have different functional properties. For example, cells in the inferior temporal lobe are sensitive to

shape (often being highly tuned for specific shape properties), color, and have very large receptive fields that almost always include the fovea (15, 16). In contrast, cells in the parietal lobe are not particularly sensitive to shape or color, rarely include the fovea in their receptive fields, are sensitive to direction of motion, and some cells in this region respond selectively to an object's location (as gated by eye position) (17).

Third, behavioral data provide dramatic evidence of the distinct visual functions of the two systems. When the temporal lobes are ablated but the parietal lobes are spared, animals are severely impaired in learning to discriminate among patterns, but are relatively unimpaired in learning to discriminate among locations. In contrast, when the parietal lobes are ablated and the temporal lobes are spared, the animals are severely impaired in learning to discriminate locations, but are relatively unimpaired in learning to discriminate among patterns; corresponding results have also been reported in humans after stroke (18).

Information-Processing Analyses

The observation that "what" and "where" are processed separately during perception leads to an explanation of why parts are imaged sequentially if the shape of each part is stored separately, and a part's location is specified relative to another part. If so, then one needs to have the reference part already activated before one can know where a subsequent part belongs in an image. When generating an image of a block letter F, for example, one might have encoded that there is a vertical line on the left, a horizontal line connected at its left side to the top of the vertical line, and another horizontal line connected at its left side to the vertical line midway down (94% of the subjects we have observed print the segments in this order). When forming the image, then, the vertical line on the left is a prerequisite for the other two lines; the locations of the horizontal lines are specified relative to the

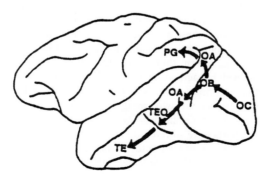

Figure 29.3
The dorsal and ventral systems of the primate brain. (Adapted from (32).)

vertical line. Thus, some parts should be imaged before others. Finally, because one needs to attend to a specific place on the reference part in order to place a new part, and focal attention is restricted to only a single region of space at a time (19), only one part can be imaged at a time.

Consider first the assumption that individual parts of shapes are stored separately. When is this likely to occur? An important fact about the visual system is that it operates at multiple scales of analysis; it is sensitive to coarse overall features and to fine-grained features, and one can attend to a given scale. However, there appears to be a trade-off between scope and resolution (20, 21). For example, one can take in an entire human form, but not see much in the way of details about the face, or one can attend to individual features of the face at high resolution but lose the overall pattern. When one attends to details, the laws of perceptual organization serve to parse objects into parts, as was noted earlier (13). Attending to details is necessary to distinguish among similar objects that have different parts, such as letters; thus, parts should be encoded separately for such objects.

Consider next the assumption that part locations are stored relative to other parts. This assumption follows from an analysis of what would be required to build a machine that recognizes shape: for purposes of perceptual recognition, it is of limited use to store a single pattern to be matched against input as a template. Many objects (such as a dog, scissors, or a person) can assume a very large number of distinct shapes (as, for example, when a dog is scratching, sleeping, running, jumping, and so on). Similarly, many objects assume multiple variants on a shape, such as a letter of the alphabet (which comes in many fonts). In such cases, there are so many distinct shapes, and new ones occur all the time, that shapes may often arise that do not correspond to one previously seen and stored in memory. Thus, encoding a shape as a single pattern may not lead to a match with a previously stored shape.

A more effective way to represent such shapes is to extract specific properties that will not change when the object assumes a new configuration or a shape-variant appears. One such invariant is the type of spatial relation between parts. For example, no matter how a dog is contorted, the parts remain connected in the same way. I refer to this type of representation as categorical because equivalence classes of relations are specified. "Connected to" (or "above," "below," "inside," "next to," and so on) does not correspond to a particular topographic configuration, but rather specifies a large category of such configurations (for example, the foreleg remains "connected to" the upper leg no matter how the leg is bent or stretched. With such categorical representations, part locations are specified relative to other parts (20). If the appropriate categorical relations are used, a description of the arrangement of an object's parts will be the same across its various contortions and variations and, hence, will be useful for recognition.

Neuropsychological Hypothesis Testing

Images thus appear to be formed a part at a time because (i) shapes of individual parts of objects are stored separately, (ii) spatial relations among parts are stored separately from shapes, (iii) spatial relations specify location relative to other parts, (iv) stored parts and relations are used to form mental images, and (v) only a single reference point on a prior part can be located at a time. Hence, because parts can only be added when the reference part is present and the reference location on it has been found, parts will be imaged sequentially.

The separation of the storage of parts and spatial relations suggests a possible distinction between two classes of processes—ones that activate stored visual shapes and ones that gain access to and use stored spatial relations to arrange those shapes correctly. One way to garner evidence for this initial, rather coarse decomposition of the processing underlying image generation is to show that the two kinds of processing can be dissociated during image formation. Farah et al. and Kosslyn et al. have done just this in a series of experiments examining image generation in commissurotomy patients (22, 23).

One task we used required subjects to make judgments about letters. Letters were the initial stimuli of choice in part because of the evidence that they are imaged a segment at a time. The task was to decide from memory whether specific uppercase letters are composed only of straight lines (for example, A and H) or include at least one curved line (for example, B and D) (24); unless one has performed the task many times or intentionally memorized the responses, imagery is used to make this judgment (23). There were two critical assumptions in our experiments. First, we assumed that the shapes of letters are stored as segments and categorical spatial relations among them. Letters come in many different fonts, and one wants to recognize new instances; thus it is efficient to store categorical representations of the spatial relations among parts, which will apply to a wide range of different topographic positions. Second, we assumed that categorical relations are language-like (indeed, they almost always can be labeled by a word or two). This assumption was critical for our experiments because one uncontroversial fact about the functional specialization of the cerebral hemispheres is that for right-handed people the left hemisphere is superior to the right at producing and using language (18).

Therefore, we expected that the left cerebral hemisphere would be better at generating images of letters, assuming that multiple parts would be composed by use of categorical spatial relations. In contrast, we expected no difference between the hemispheres in the ability to form images of single shapes, when separate representations of spatial relations would not be used; visual memories of shape should be equally available in both hemispheres. If we could document such a dis-sociation and implicate image generation differences as its cause, we would have evidence for a distinction between a mechanism that activates stored shapes and one that uses stored spatial relations to arrange them.

Documenting an Image-Generation Deficit

We tested these hypotheses by lateralizing lowercase letter cues. The lateralization procedure consisted of asking subjects to focus on a fixation point, and then to view stimuli presented 1.5° to the left or right of fixation. Because the cues were only presented for 150 ms, the subjects could not move their eyes to examine them, ensuring that the letter was projected onto only one half of the retina. Because the left half of each retina sends input only to the left cerebral hemisphere, and the right half of each retina sends input only to the right cerebral hemisphere, lateralizing stimuli in this way allowed us to provide input to the separate hemispheres (25).

The most detailed examination, which was conducted with patient J. W., will be summarized here (23). This patient had undergone surgery about 3 years before testing (for the treatment of otherwise intractable epilepsy), and magnetic resonance scanning revealed that his corpus callosum was fully sectioned. Because his corpus callosum was transected, information presented to one hemisphere was not available to the other hemisphere.

We began by lateralizing lowercase letters, and asking J. W. to judge whether the corresponding uppercase version had any curved lines. He pressed one key when he decided that the uppercase letter had at least one curved line and another if it had only straight lines. The results were striking: J. W.'s left hemisphere responded perfectly, whereas his right hemisphere was correct only 70% of the time; in a replication experiment, the left hemisphere again was perfect, whereas the right was correct only 65% of the time (26).

This finding is not enough to document an image generation deficit per se. A rather lengthy series of control experiments was required to eliminate various alternative accounts. The most simple control consisted of presenting J. W. with the uppercase letters themselves, and asking him to judge them as they appeared on the screen. Both hemispheres responded correctly on at least 97.5% of the trials. This result indicates that the right hemisphere deficit in the imagery task was not due to its being unable to perform the judgment, to encode letters, or produce appropriate key presses. In other control experiments we showed that both hemispheres could understand the correspondence between the lowercase cues and the uppercase letters, could retain images long enough to interpret their shapes, and could perform multipart tasks.

A Selective Deficit

We expected the right hemisphere to have difficulty generating images of letters if parts are activated sequentially and categorical representations of spatial relations are used to arrange the parts into the image. However, to argue that the difficulty lies in one class of processes and not others, it must be demonstrated that the right hemisphere can perform some imagery tasks, but not those in which the parts must be arranged with the use of categorical relations.

We reasoned that images should be constructed from parts whenever the task requires evaluation or comparison of parts; in these cases, high-resolution images of parts are necessary, and these representations were encoded and stored individually. In contrast, arranging parts should not be necessary to perform a task requiring imaging the overall shape of an object, if such a shape was encoded as a single perceptual unit. That is, even though such a template has little use in perceptual recognition for generalizing over variations in an object's shape, we expected relatively low-resolution patterns of overall shape to be encoded because they provide

information about how an object is oriented in space, which is useful for navigation. If so, then we expected both hemispheres to be able to image such a pattern representing a single object. Although such a pattern would have a relatively low resolution, we reasoned that it should be sufficient to perform tasks that do not require comparing or evaluating parts (and hence high-resolution images of individual parts are not necessary).

In one task, J. W. was asked to decide which of two similar-sized animals (for example, a goat or a hog) was the larger, as seen from the side at the same distance; this task previously had been shown to require imagery (27). The name of one of the animals was lateralized, and hence only one hemisphere had the opportunity to perform the task. Only one error occurred during the entire testing session. This high level of performance is worrisome, however, in that it may reflect a "ceiling effect." The task may be so easy that it is insensitive to differences in hemispheric processing. Thus, we devised a second imagery task that did not require assembling parts, but which was considerably more difficult. J. W. was asked to decide whether named objects (book, nose, and buckle, for example) are taller than they are wide. This was a difficult task, given the stimuli we used, and resulted in overall worse performance. Nevertheless, both hemispheres could perform the task at better than chance levels of performance (50%), and did so equally well (70.8% versus 66.7% correct for the left and right hemispheres, respectively).

One could argue that all that has been shown is a difference for letters versus words. Thus, we conducted another task with the animal names presented in the size judgment experiment, but this task required comparing locations of parts, which we assumed required relatively high-resolution images of the parts—entailing the use of individually stored parts and spatial relations. We now asked J. W. to decide whether the named animal's ears protrude above the top of its skull (for example, an ape and a sheep versus a cat and a mouse). The left hemisphere performed correctly on 87.5% of the trials, whereas the right hemisphere performed correctly on only 45% of the trials. In short, the problem was not limited to letters, but apparently to tasks that involve juxtaposing parts.

Convergent evidence for the distinction between processes that activate images and that arrange parts is also available in the clinical literature. For example, Deleval et al. (28) describe a patient who experienced impaired imagery following left hemisphere damage. This patient claimed, "When I try to image a plant, an animal, an object, I can recall but one part, my inner vision is fleeting, fragmented; if I'm asked to imagine the head of a cow, I know that it has ears and horns, but I can't revisualize their respective places. In the same way, I cannot determine how many fingers a frog paw has, even though I have manipulated this animal each day in the laboratory...."

Contrasting Left and Right Hemisphere Abilities

A second split-brain patient also provided evidence for a functional dissociation between processes that activate images and processes that arrange parts in images, with the left hemisphere being superior when the latter processes were required. However, only two subjects were tested, and these patients may have atypical cerebral organization due to years of severe epilepsy and the disconnection of the cerebral hemispheres at the time of testing. Thus it is important to show that the inferences about component processes and their neural realization generalize to normal people.

To obtain such converging evidence, a group of normal right-handed Harvard University students was tested in a variation of the grids imagery task described above (see the top panels of figure 29.1). After subjects memorized the block letters, they saw lateralized grids with a lowercase cue beneath them (64 trials, half presented

in each visual field). The letters were presented in mixed order, with a letter not repeated in fewer than four trials. The grids now contained only a single "×" probe, as is illustrated in figure 29.1. Because the corpus callosa of these subjects is intact, information presented to one hemisphere will be transmitted to the other; thus, the primary measure of interest here was the time to respond: response times should be fastest when the hemisphere that receives the initial input is more effective in processing (25).

Consistent with the findings from the split-brain patients, these subjects evaluated the probes more quickly when the grid was presented to the right visual field (and hence was projected onto the left side of each retina and was seen first in the left cerebral hemisphere). However, it was possible that this result only reflected the left hemisphere's greater facility at reading the lowercase cues. Hence, as a control, an additional group of students was tested in a modified version of the task. The lowercase cue was now presented in the center (replacing the fixation point), not beneath the grid; after this, an empty grid with one probe mark was lateralized eight times (four in the left field, and four in the right, with no more than three trials appearing in the same field in a row and with the probe mark in a different location on each trial). Each new series of trials began with a different lowercase cue appearing in the center. As is evident in figure 29.4, although these subjects responded faster overall in this blocked design, a left hemisphere advantage was nevertheless obtained. Thus, the left hemisphere was shown to be better than the right hemisphere even in normal subjects at performing this multipart image generation task (29).

These experiments with normal subjects pushed the information-processing analyses one step further. The tests done with the split-brain patients hinged on the assumptions that categorical relations are used to arrange segments of letters and relative positions of animal parts in images, and that such relations are processed

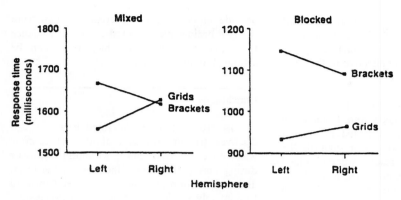

Figure 29.4
The mean time required by normal right-handed people to evaluate single probe marks in lateralized grids. The grids were complete (grids) or reduced to four brackets at the corners (brackets) (see figure 29.1). (*Left*) Results when each letter was imaged only once before a new letter was presented (mixed trials). (*Right*) Results when the letter was imaged eight times in succession after the cue was presented (blocked trials). In mixed trials a lowercase cue was presented beneath the grid; in blocked trials the cue was presented at the central fixation point at the beginning of the trials.

better in the left hemisphere. However, categorical representations cannot be the only method used by the brain to store spatial relations: what is a virtue for recognizing semirigid objects is a drawback for distinguishing among subtly different multipart shapes or for reaching or navigating. For these tasks, one needs to know the actual metric spatial relations among parts or objects. Knowing only that an object is "next to" the wall will not help one very much to find it and pick it up. For these sorts of tasks, the coordinates of an object must be internally represented. In short, information-processing considerations lead to the hypothesis that the brain can store spatial relations in two ways, either in terms of a category or in terms of more precise coordinates (30).

If this is so, then there should be two ways of forming images of a multipart object—by using either categorical or coordinate stored spatial relations to arrange parts. Given the evidence that the right hemisphere is more efficient at representing and processing metric spatial rela-

tions (18), the right hemisphere therefore should be better than the left when parts must be arranged in precise positions in an image. To test this idea, an additional group of students was tested in a modified version of the grids task; this task was the same as the grids task except that the internal lines were removed and only brackets at the four corners were depicted (as is illustrated in the bottom panels of figure 29.1). After subjects memorized the block letters as they appeared within the brackets, probe marks within the brackets were lateralized (lower right corner of figure 29.1), and the subjects were asked to decide whether the probe would fall on the letter were it within the brackets as previously shown. When grid lines are present, a categorical representation of how segments are connected is adequate; the grid lines are a crutch for placing segments properly in accordance with a description. In contrast, when only four corner brackets are present, more precise representations of segment location are necessary to determine whether an imaged letter would cover the

X mark. Thus, it was expected that a process that uses coordinate representations to arrange parts would be recruited in this task, and that this process would be more effective in the right hemisphere.

The results from both the "grids" and "brackets" conditions are illustrated in figure 29.4. As expected, the subjects were faster when the brackets stimuli were presented to the left visual field, and hence were seen first in the right hemisphere. These results were obtained when lowercase cues were presented beneath the brackets ("mixed" presentation) or when an additional group saw them in the center before eight consecutive trials with that letter ("blocked" presentation); in both cases, these results are in sharp contrast to those obtained with grids, when categorical relations were presumably adequate.

In order to consider whether the results with the brackets were due to a right-hemisphere superiority at localizing the probe marks, and not due to image generation per se, a separate group of subjects was given an analog of the task that did not require image generation but did require encoding the probe location and comparing it to an uppercase letter. A probe X was lateralized within brackets (for 150 ms) and then replaced by an uppercase letter (as illustrated at the lower left of figure 29.1, for 100 ms). The task was to judge whether the X mark would have fallen on the letter, had they been superimposed. The letter served to mask the X, requiring subjects to encode its location into memory to be compared to the locations of the letter segments. As expected, the right hemisphere was superior when the metric location of the X had to be stored. However, this right hemisphere advantage was 3.2 times too small to account for the right hemisphere advantage for the brackets imagery task.

In short, both hemispheres can form images of the components, but the hemispheres apparently differ in the preferred way of arranging them. These results from normal subjects not only provide support for the inferences drawn from the split-brain subjects, but also provide evidence for a second means by which parts can be arranged in images (31).

Conclusions

In this article, I have illustrated how one can discover structure in mental abilities where none was obvious. After first examining behavior during task performance, facts about the brain and information-processing analyses can lead to relatively subtle hypotheses about processing. These hypotheses are testable in part by examining selective impairments in neuropathological populations. With this approach, it was found that the act of generating a visual mental image involves at least two classes of processes—ones that activate stored shapes and ones that use stored spatial relations to arrange shapes into an image. The discovery that the left hemisphere is better at arranging shapes when categorical information is appropriate, whereas the right hemisphere is better when coordinate information is necessary, suggests that the processes that arrange parts can be further decomposed into two classes that operate on different sorts of information.

The findings that under some circumstances the left cerebral hemisphere is better at mental imagery is counterintuitive to many. The left hemisphere has traditionally been identified with language, and the right with imagery (22, 23, 28–30). However, neither hemisphere can be said to be the seat of mental imagery: imagery is carried out by multiple processes, not all of which are implemented equally effectively in the same part of the brain.

Acknowledgments

Supported by NIMH grant MH 39478, ONR contract N00014-85-K-0291, and AFOSR contract 88-0012. I thank J. Gabrieli, O. Koenig, and V. Maljkovic for critical readings, S. Hamilton and C. Moheban for technical assistance, and my collaborators and students cited herein for stimulating discussions and critical reviews of earlier works.

References and Notes

1. A. Paivio, *Imagery and Verbal Processes* (Holt, Rinehart, & Winston, New York, 1971).

2. S. M. Kosslyn, *Image and Mind* (Harvard Univ. Press, Cambridge, 1980).

3. R. N. Shepard and L. A. Cooper, *Mental Images and Their Transformations* (MIT Press, Cambridge, 1982).

4. R. A. Finke and R. N. Shepard, in *Handbook of Perception and Human Performance*, K. R. Boff, L. Kaufman, J. P. Thomas, Eds. (Wiley, New York, 1986), vol. 37, p. 1.

5. M. J. Farah, *Psychol. Rev.*, 95; 301–317.

6. D. C. Van Essen, in *Cerebral Cortex*, A. Peters and E. G. Jones, Eds. (Plenum, New York, 1985), vol. 3, p. 259.

7. L. G. Ungerleider and M. Mishkin, in *Analysis of Visual Behavior*, D. J. Ingle, M. A. Goodale, R. J. W. Mansfield, Eds. (MIT Press, Cambridge, 1982), p. 549.

8. S. J. Segal and V. Fusella, *J. Exp. Psychol.* 83, 458 (1970).

9. C. W. Eriksen and B. A. Eriksen, *ibid.* 89, 306 (1971).

10. This method was adapted from one developed to compare imagery and perception by P. Podgorny and R. N. Shepard, *J. Exp. Psychol.: Hum. Percept. Performance* 4, 21 (1978).

11. S. M. Kosslyn, C. B. Cave, D. A. Provost, S. M. Von Gierke, *Cog. Psychol.*, 20, 319–343 (1988).

12. J. D. Roth and S. M. Kosslyn, *Cog. Psychol.*, 20, 344 (1988).

13. S. M. Kosslyn, B. J. Reiser, M. J. Farah, S. J. Fliegel, *J. Exp. Psychol. Gen.* 112, 278 (1983); S. K. Reed and J. A. Johnsen, *Mem. Cog.* 3, 569 (1975).

14. J. E. Hochberg, *Perception* (Prentice-Hall, New York, 1964); L. D. Kaufman, *Sight and Mind* (Oxford Univ. Press, New York, 1974); I. Biederman, *Psychol. Rev.* 94, 115 (1987).

15. C. G. Gross, C. J. Bruce, R. Desimone, J. Fleming, R. Gattass, in *Cortical Sensory Organization II: Multiple Visual Areas*, C. N. Woolsey, Ed. (Humana, Clinton, NJ, 1984), p. 187.

16. R. Desimone, T. D. Albright, C. G. Gross, C. J. Bruce, *J. Neurosci.* 4, 2051 (1984).

17. R. A. Andersen, G. K. Essick, R. M. Siegel, *Science* 230, 456 (1985).

18. E. DeRenzi, *Disorders of Space Exploration and Cognition* (Wiley, New York, 1982); H. Hecaen and M. L. Albert, *Human Neuropsychology* (Wiley, New York, 1978).

19. C. J. Downing and S. Pinker, in *Attention and Performance XI*, M. I. Posner and O. S. I. Marin, Eds. (Erlbaum, Hillsdale, NJ, 1985), p. 177; D. LaBerge, *J. Exp. Psychol.: Hum. Percept. Performance* 9, 371 (1983); M. I. Posner, C. R. R. Snyder, B. J. Davidson, *J. Exp. Psychol.: Gen.* 109, 160 (1980); A. M. Treisman and G. Gelade, *Cog. Psychol.* 12, 97 (1980).

20. D. Marr, *Vision* (Freeman, San Francisco, 1982).

21. H. Egeth in *The Psychology of Learning and Motivation*, G. H. Bower, Ed. (Academic Press, New York, 1977), p. 277; C. W. Eriksen and J. D. St. James, *Percept. Psychophys.* 40, 225 (1986); J. Jonides, *Bull. Psychonomics Soc.* 21, 247 (1983); G. L. Shulman and J. Wilson, *Perception* 16, 89 (1987).

22. M. J. Farah, M. S. Gazzaniga, J. D. Holtzman, S. M. Kosslyn, *Neuropsychologia* 23, 115 (1985).

23. S. M. Kosslyn, J. D. Holtzman, M. J. Farah, M. S. Gazzaniga, *J. Exp. Psychol. Gen.* 114, 311 (1985).

24. This task is a variant of one developed by R. J. Weber and J. Castleman, *Percept. Psychophys.* 8, 165 (1970).

25. J. G. Beaumont, Ed., *Divided Visual Field Studies of Cerebral Organization* (Academic Press, New York, 1982).

26. Both response time and accuracy were always measured in all of these experiments to ensure that errors were not made because of hurried decisions. Such possible speed-accuracy tradeoffs do not undermine the inferences drawn from any of the response time or accuracy results described here.

27. S. M. Kosslyn, G. L. Murphy, M. E. Bemesderfer, K. J. Feinstein, *J. Exp. Psychol.: Gen.* 106, 341 (1977).

28. J. Deleval, J. De Mol, J. Noterman, *Acta Neurol. Belg.* 83, 61 (1983) (M. J. Farah and O. Koenig,

translators). See also M. J. Farah, D. N. Levine, R. Calvanio, *Brain Cog.*, 20, 439 (1988). M. J. Farah, *Cognition* 18, 245 (1984).

29. For additional converging results, see M. J. Farah, *Neuropsychologia* 24, 541 (1986).

30. See S. M. Kosslyn (*Psychol. Rev.* 94, 148 (1987)) for additional explication of, and evidence for, this distinction.

31. Only the results from the first set of trials are summarized here; additional trials were administered to assess possible changes in strategy with practice, as is describe by S. M. Kosslyn, J. R. Feldman, V. Maljkovic, S. Hamilton, unpublished manuscript.

32. M. Mishkin, L. G. Ungerleider, K. A. Macko, *Trends Neurosci.* 6, 414 (1983).

30 The Neural Basis of Mental Imagery

Martha J. Farah

What color are the stars on the American flag? To answer, you probably formed a mental image of the flag, and "saw" that the stars are white. The question to which this article is addressed is, what neural events underlie this ability to form and use mental images? More specifically, what is the relation between the neural bases of mental imagery and visual perception? Are mental imagery processes lateralized to one hemisphere? And, finally, what are the implications of neuroscientific data for our understanding of mental imagery at the functional, or 'information-processing' level of description used in cognitive science?

What the Mind's Eye Tells the Brain's Visual Cortex

The subjective similarity of seeing and imagining suggests that common internal representations might underlie these two experiences. In support of this hypothesis, cognitive psychologists such as Finke,[1] Kosslyn,[2] Paivio,[3] and Shepard[4] have used a variety of ingenious experimental paradigms to gather evidence that imagery and perception have similar behavioral consequences, and that imagery and verbal thought have different behavioral consequences. However, for reasons to be discussed in the last section of this article, not all cognitive psychologists have found these behavioral demonstrations persuasive. It is therefore of interest to turn to neuropsychological and physiological evidence on these issues.

With respect to the relation between imagery and perception, the relevant evidence can be divided into two categories: brain imaging data that implicate activity in cortical visual processing areas during imagery; and studies of brain-damaged patients showing selective deficits in imagery ability that parallel the patients' perceptual deficits. In the first category are electrophysiological and regional blood flow studies of normal subjects during imagery.

One approach has been to record event-related potentials (ERPs) to visual stimuli while subjects hold mental images.[5] If imagery has a systematic effect on the ERP, then there must be some common brain locus at which imagery and perceptual processing interact. More important, if the interaction between imagery and perception is content-specific—for example, if imaging an H affects the ERP to visually presented Hs more than the ERP to visually presented Ts, and imaging a T affects the ERP to Ts more than the ERP to Hs—then the interaction must be taking place in neural structures where information about the differences between Hs and Ts is preserved, that is, in common neural representations. Imagery was found to have a content-specific effect on the ERP within the first 200 ms of stimulus processing, and this effect was localized at the occipital and posterior temporal recording sites, as shown in figure 30.1. Furthermore, the inference that the image-percept interaction was occurring in modality-specific visual cortex is strengthened by the fact that the time course of the effect of imagery on the ERP was the same as that of the first negative peak of the visual ERP waveform, which is believed to originate in extrastriate visual cortex.[6]

The act of generating a mental image from memory also has discernible effects on the ERP.[7] ERPs were recorded to words under two instructional conditions: to encode the word (baseline condition), and to encode the word and form an image of its referent (image condition). The difference between the ERPs to the words in these two conditions should reflect the brain electrical activity synchronized with the generation of mental images. This difference measure, represented in figure 30.2, was also maximal over the occipital and posterior temporal regions of

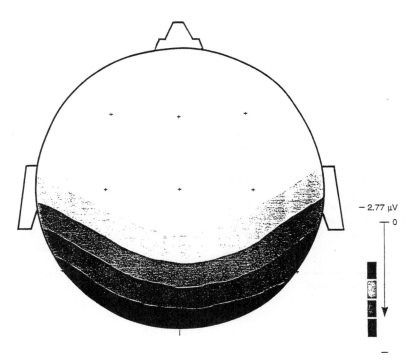

Figure 30.1
Topographic representation of the distribution of the effect of imagery on the visual ERP, obtained by subtracting the ERP to the stimulus when the image and stimulus do not match from the ERP to the stimulus when the image and stimulus match, at 173 ms after stimulus presentation (the latency of the first negative peak of the visual ERP).

the scalp, whether words were visually or auditorily presented.

Regional cerebral blood flow provides another method of localizing brain activity accompanying mental imagery. Roland and Friberg[8] measured regional cerebral blood flow while subjects rested and during a series of different cognitive tasks, one of which involved visual imagery: visualizing a walk through one's neighborhood making alternating right and left turns starting at one's front door. This task caused massive blood flow to the posterior regions of the brain, including the occipital, posterior parietal and posterior inferior temporal areas important

for higher visual processing. Goldenberg et al.[9] devised a simpler imagery task, along with a control task differing from the imagery task only in the absence of imagery. They gave groups of normal subjects the same auditorily presented lists of concrete words to learn under different instructional conditions: one group was told just to listen to the words and try to remember them; and the other group was told to visualize the referents of the words as a mnemonic strategy. Imagery was associated with more blood flow to the occipital lobes, particularly the left inferior occipital region, and with high co-variation of blood flow (which provides another index of re-

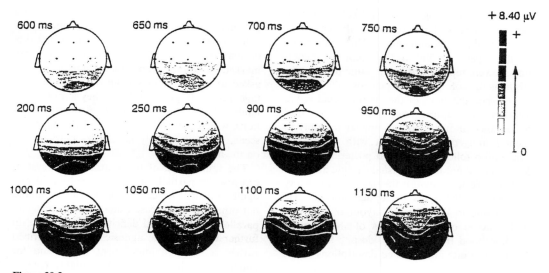

Figure 30.2
Topographic representation of the distribution of the effect of generating an image from memory, obtained by subtracting the ERP to auditorily presented words when subjects passively listen to the words from the ERP to the same stimuli when subjects generate mental images of the words' referents. The effect is shown at 50-ms intervals beginning 600 ms after word onset (upper left diagram) and continuing left to right, and top row to bottom row, through 1150 ms after word onset.

gional brain activity), bilaterally, in the occipital and posterior temporal areas of the brain. Comparable results were obtained when subjects tried to answer questions that require visual imagery (e.g., "is the green of pine trees darker than the green of grass?") compared with those that do not (e.g.,"is the categorical imperative an ancient grammatical form?").[10]

The results of the brain imaging studies implicate occipital, temporal and parietal cortex in mental imagery, the same areas that subserve visual perception. Although it is difficult to distinguish activity in primary visual cortex from that in visual association areas on the basis of these techniques, the ERP results suggest that primary visual cortex is probably not involved: imagery has its earliest effect on the visual ERP at the latency of the first negative component, a component with a presumed extrastriate origin.

This is consistent with the results of single-unit recordings in conscious monkeys, showing cognitive effects on neuronal activity in secondary, but not primary, visual cortex.[11]

If mental imagery does consist of endogenously generated activity in cortical visual areas, then patients with damage to those areas should have imagery deficits that parallel their perceptual deficits. Studies of the effects of focal brain damage on imagery are generally consistent with this prediction. For example, color vision may be impaired after brain damage with relative preservation of other visual capacities, and in these cases, the ability to imagine color is often compromised as well.[12] De Renzi and Spinnler[13] investigated various color-related abilities in a large group study of unilaterally brain-damaged patients, and found an association between impairment on color vision tasks, such as the Ishihara test of color blindness, and color imagery tasks, such as verbally reporting the colors of common objects from memory. This is what one would expect to find if the color of mental images were represented in the same neural substrate as the color of visual percepts.

The specializations of the "two cortical visual systems" for representing visual location and appearance information also appear to apply to mental imagery.[14] A patient with visual disorientation following bilateral posterior parietal lesions could not localize visual stimuli, although he was able to recognize them, and his imagery abilities paralleled his perceptual abilities. He was unable to describe the layout of furniture in his home or the locations of shops in his neighborhood from memory, despite his ability to give accurate and detailed descriptions of the appearances of objects from memory. A patient with visual agnosia following bilateral inferior temporal lesions showed the opposite pattern of perceptual and imagery abilities. He was impaired at recognizing objects, but not localizing them, and he was unable to draw or describe the appearances of objects from memory, despite his ability to give accurate descriptions of the spatial locations of objects and landmarks from memory. In a review of the literature for similar cases, we found that in most published reports of patients with selective "what" or "where" deficits in visual perception for whom imagery was tested, parallel imagery impairments were found.

More selective impairments of perceptual functioning within each of the two cortical visual systems also exist, and have correlates in imagery. For example, the neglect syndrome, characterized by a failure to detect visual stimuli in the side of space opposite a parietal lesion, has been shown by Bisiach and his colleagues to manifest itself in imagery. In one study,[15] two right parietal-damaged patients were asked to form an image of the famous Piazza del Duomo in Milan, with which the patients had been familiar before their brain damage. When asked to imagine viewing it from the position marked

"A" in figure 30.3, and to describe the view, both patients omitted from their descriptions the landmarks that would have fallen on the left side of that scene and named only the landmarks marked "a" on the map. When the patients were asked to repeat the task from the opposite vantage point, at position "B," they omitted the landmarks previously included in their descriptions, which now fell on the left of the imagined scene, and named only landmarks marked "b" on the map.

The functioning of the ventral visual system can also be partially impaired, resulting in recognition deficits for certain classes of stimuli and not others. In these cases, imagery deficits again parallel the perceptual deficits. For example, in further testing of the agnosic patient described earlier, a selective impairment was found for imaging stimuli that could be roughly categorized as "living things," paralleling his greater recognition impairment for those stimuli.[16] Shuttleworth, Syring and Allen[17] reviewed the literature on cases of prosopagnosia (agnosia for faces) and found that impaired imagery for faces was common. Of their own prosopagnosic patient, they report that she had "no voluntary visual recall (revisualization) of faces but was able to revisualize more general items such as buildings and places."

In sum, several lines of evidence converge in implicating cortical visual processing areas in mental imagery. Electrophysiological and regional blood flow measures demonstrate activity in visual areas while normal subjects form mental images. In addition, localized damage to these areas results in selective imagery deficits that parallel the more evident visual perceptual deficits.

Hemispheric Specialization for Mental Imagery

Many higher perceptual and cognitive functions are carried out more proficiently or even exclusively by one hemisphere, and the question

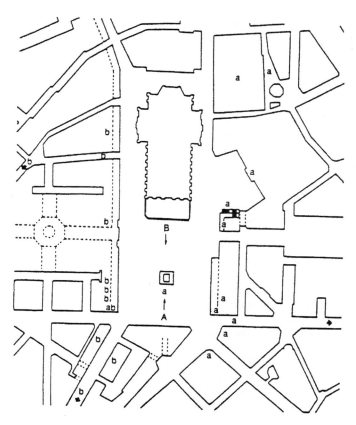

Figure 30.3
Map of the Piazza del Duomo in Milan, showing the two positions "A" and "B" from which patients were asked to imagine viewing the Piazza, and the landmarks that they recalled from each imagined position, labeled "a" and "b," respectively.

therefore arises whether there is any cerebral asymmetry for mental imagery. Ehrlichmann and Barrett[18] pointed out the existence of a widespread assumption that imagery is a specialized function of the right hemisphere, but found little support for this assumption in their critical review of the literature. Farah[19] suggested that different components of mental imagery ability might have different neuroanatomic loci, and identified a subset of cases of loss of

imagery whose profile of abilities and deficits indicated a loss of the image generation process—the ability to form a visual mental image from stored long-term visual memory information. In this subset of cases, the predominant site of damage was the posterior left hemisphere. Subsequent cases have been consistent with this localization[20] and have suggested a relation between the inability to recognize multiple forms that sometimes follows left posterior brain damage[21] and the inability to generate a normally detailed image from memory, which is believed to require the synthesis of separately stored parts of the image.[2] Language and verbal memory need not be impaired in such cases, despite the laterality of the lesion, indicating that imagery and verbal thought depend upon at least partially distinct neural processes.[19]

The results of research with split-brain patients are also consistent with left hemisphere specialization for generating images. In one experiment, carried out with patient J. W.,[22] a single hemisphere was presented with an upper case letter and asked to classify the corresponding lower case letter as ascending (e.g., "f"), descending (e.g., "g") or neither, a judgement that requires generating a mental image. Only the left hemisphere of this patient could perform the task. In contrast, both hemispheres could correctly classify the lower case letters when viewing them, and both could associate the upper case letters with the corresponding lower case forms in free vision, implicating image generation per se as the cause of the right hemisphere's failure in the imagery task. With a different imagery task that did not require visualizing details, judging whether a named animal was larger or smaller than a goat, both of J. W.'s hemispheres performed well, consistent with the idea that the left hemisphere is specialized for synthesizing images that have distinct parts.[23] Two other split-brain patients have been tested on image-generation tasks so far. Like J. W., L. B. showed left hemisphere superiority for the generation of detailed visual images, although his right hemisphere was above chance in at least one image-generation task.[24] Results from patient VP are less clear: she showed initial left hemisphere superiority, but her right hemisphere eventually attained comparable levels of performance.[23] It should be noted that the right hemisphere of this patient is also capable of speech.

Research with normal subjects has also, on the whole, supported the hypothesis of left hemisphere specialization for image generation. For example, imagery has a larger effect on perception in the right than in the left hemifield,[25,26] generating images interferes more with right- than with left-hand motor performance,[27,28] and causes greater suppression of EEG α-rhythm over the left than over the right hemisphere.[29] The results of the brain imaging studies with normal subjects mentioned earlier, in which images were formed while brain activity was monitored, are also relevant: all showed left-sided foci of activity.[7-10] Nevertheless, some studies have shown the opposite trend, for greater right than left hemisphere involvement in image-generation tasks[30,31] and these exceptions may indicate that factors such as practice, individual differences and task requirements modulate the roles of the hemispheres in image generation.[32]

In addition to recalling from memory the appearances of stimuli that are absent, we can also use mental imagery to decide how a stimulus currently in view would look if it were spatially transformed.[33] For example, in deciding whether the pairs of objects depicted in figure 30.4 are identical or mirror images of one another, you probably mentally rotated them. The process of mental image rotation can be dissociated by brain damage from mental image generation,[34] implying that different neural systems are involved, and the available evidence suggests some degree of right hemisphere superiority for mental rotation. For example, Ratcliff[35] assessed the ability of patients with penetrating head wounds to carry out a mental rotation task, and found that the right posteriorly damaged patients were most impaired at this task. Papanicolaou et al.[36] measured regional cerebral blood flow and evoked potentials to task-irrelevant visual probe flashes while normal subjects performed the mental rotation task shown in figure 30.4. They found greater blood flow to the right than to the left hemisphere (especially the right parietal region), and greater suppression of probe-evoked potentials over the right than over the left hemisphere, when sub-

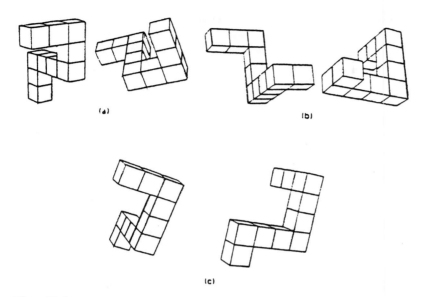

Figure 30.4
Are the objects in each of these pairs identical or is one a mirror image of the other? Response time data from normal subjects indicate that most people answer this question by mentally rotating the objects.[33]

jects performed mental rotation than when they passively viewed the same stimuli. Using a lateralized stimulus-presentation technique, Cohen[25] found evidence that normal subjects rotate mental images with their right hemispheres, and Corballis and Sergent[24] used a similar task to document normal mental rotation ability in the right but not the left hemisphere of split-brain patient L. B.

The Functional Architecture of Mental Imagery: Constraints from Neuropsychology

It has proved difficult for cognitive psychologists to gather decisive evidence on certain issues concerning mental imagery. Data that seem to support the visual nature of images, and the map-like or pictorial format of images, can also be explained in terms of non-visual and prop-

ositional (i.e., language-like) representations. Anderson[37] has argued that this is an inherent limitation of the kinds of data used by cognitive psychologists. If one can control and measure only the inputs and outputs to a "black box," then there will always be alternative theories of the internal processing stages that can account for any set of input-output data. For example, the finding that people take longer to "scan" mentally across subjectively larger mental images appears to support a spatial format for mental images.[2] However, Pylyshyn[38] has suggested that the underlying representations are propositional, and that the scanning times reflect subjects' interpretation of imagery instructions as instructions to *simulate* the scanning of a visual percept.

The neuroscientific data reviewed earlier provide a new source of evidence on these questions. The dissociability of imagery impairments from impairments in verbal thought suggests that thinking in images is distinct from thinking in language. The existence of common neural substrates for imagery and perception demonstrates rather directly that imagery is a function of the visual system and, insofar as occipital representations are retinotopically mapped, carries the further implication that images also have this format. Finally, in addition to addressing questions about imagery that cognitive scientists have already asked, this new source of data suggests new insights about the functional architecture of mental imagery: the dissociability of imagery impairments after dorsal and ventral damage, for example, implies that the normal visual imagery system includes separate subsystems for representing visual appearance and spatial location information.[39]

Acknowledgments

The writing of this article was supported by ONR contract N0014-86-0094, NIH grant NS23458, the Alfred P. Sloan Foundation, and NIH program project grant NS06209 to the Aphasia Research Center of the Boston University School of Medicine. The author thanks Frank Peronnet and his colleagues at INSERM, Unit 280, for their collaboration on the ERP studies, and the anonymous reviewers of this paper for many helpful suggestions.

Selected References

1. Finke, R. A. (1980) *Psychol. Rev.* 87, 113–132

2. Kosslyn, S. M. (1980) *Image and Mind* Harvard University Press

3. Paivio, A. (1971) *Imagery and Verbal Processes* Holt, Rinehart and Winston

4. Shepard, R. N. (1978) *Am. Psychol.* 33, 125–137

5. Farah, M. J., Peronnet, F., Gonon, M. A. and Giard, M. H. (1988) *J. Exp. Psychol. (Gen.)* 117, 248–257

6. Lesevre, N. and Joseph, J. P. (1980) in *Evoked Potentials* (Barber, C., ed.), MIT Press

7. Farah, M. J., Peronnet, F., Weisberg, L. and Monheit, M. A. *J. Cog. Neurosci.* (in press)

8. Roland, P. E. and Friberg, L. (1985) *J. Neurophysiol.* 53, 1219–1243

9. Goldenberg, G., Podreka, I., Steiner, M. and Willmes, K. (1987) *Neuropsychologia* 25, 473–486

10. Goldenberg, G., Podreka, I., Steiner, M., Deecke, L. and Willmes, K. (1988) in *Cognitive and Neuropsychological Approaches to Mental Imagery* (Denis, M., Englekamp, J. and Richardson, J. T. E., eds), pp. 363–373, Martinus Nijhoff

11. Moran, J. and Desimone, R. (1985) *Science* 229, 782

12. Beauvois, M. F. and Saillant, B. (1985) *Cog. Neuropsychol.* 2, 1–48

13. DeRenzi, E. and Spinnler, H. (1967) *Cortex* 3, 194–217

14. Levine, D. N., Warach, J. and Farah, M. J. (1985) *Neurology* 35, 1010–1018

15. Bisiach, E. and Luzzatti, C. (1978) *Cortex* 14, 129–133

16. Farah, M. J., Hammond, K. M., Mehta, Z. and Ratcliff, G. (1989) *Neuropsychologia* 27, 193–200

17. Shuttleworth, E. C., Syring, V. and Allen, N. (1982) *Brain Cog.* 1, 302–332

18. Ehrlichman, H. and Barrett, J. (1983) *Brain Cog.* 2, 39–52

19. Farah, M. J. (1984) *Cognition* 18, 245–272

20. Farah, M. J., Levine, D. N. and Calvanio, R. (1988) *Brain Cog.* 8, 147–164

21. Kinsbourne, M. and Warrington, E. K. (1962) *J. Neurol. Neurosurg. Psychiatry* 25, 339–344

22. Farah, M. J., Gazzaniga, M. S., Holtzman, J. D. and Kosslyn, S. M. (1985) *Neuropsychologia* 23, 115–118

23. Kosslyn, S. M., Holtzman, J. D., Farah, M. J. and Gazzaniga, M. S. (1985) *J. Exp. Psychol. (Gen.)* 114, 311–341

24. Corballis, M. C. and Sergent, J. (1988) *Neuropsychologia* 26, 13–26

25. Cohen, G. (1975) in *Attention and Performance (Vol. 5)* (Rabbit, P. M. A. and Dornic, S., eds), pp. 20–32, Academic Press

26. Farah, M. J. (1986) *Neuropsychologia* 24, 541–551

27. Lempert, H. (1987) *Neuropsychologia* 25, 835–839

28. Lempert, H. (1989) *Neuropsychologia* 27, 575–579

29. Rugg, M. D. and Venables, P. H. (1980) *Neurosci. Lett.* 16, 67–70

30. Kosslyn, S. M. (1988) *Science* 240, 1621–1626

31. Sergent, J. (1989) *J. Exp. Psychol. (Hum. Percept. Perform.)* 15, 170–178

32. Farah, M. J. (1989) *J. Exp. Psychol. (Hum. Percept. Perform.)* 15, 203–211

33. Shepard, R. N. and Cooper, L. A. (1982) *Mental Images and Their Transformations* MIT Press

34. Farah, M. J. and Hammond, K. M. (1988) *Cognition* 29, 29–46

35. Ratcliff, G. (1979) *Neuropsychologia* 17, 49–54

36. Papanicolaou, A. C. et al. (1987) *Electroencephalogr. Clin. Neurophysiol.* 66, 515–520

37. Anderson, J. R. (1978) *Psychol. Rev.* 85, 249–277

38. Pylyshyn, Z. W. (1981) *Psychol. Rev.* 88, 16–45

39. Farah, M. J., Hammond, K. L., Levine, D. N. and Calvanio, R. (1988) *Cog. Psychol.* 20, 439–462

31 Experimental Studies of Ongoing Conscious Experience

Jerome L. Singer

William James's (1890) introduction of the concept of a stream of consciousness, so stimulating to several generations of writers, from his own student Gertrude Stein to James Joyce, Virginia Woolf, William Faulkner, and Saul Bellow, was largely ignored by psychologists for almost 60 years of the twentieth century. More recently, however, as personality researchers and specialists in social cognition attempt to examine the major characteristics of the individual that account for beliefs about self or others and for attitudes that may govern overt behaviour, they find increasing renewed interest in introspection and reports of consciousness (Sabini and Silver 1981, Singer and Kolligian 1987). Brain researchers, students of artificial intelligence, psychophysiologists and investigators of the neural and autonomic concomitants of sleep are intrigued by the opportunity for studying personal "scripts," ongoing images, fantasies and interior monologues (Ellmann and Antrobus 1991, Kreitler and Kreitler 1976, McGuire 1984, Schank and Abelson 1977, Singer and Bonanno 1990, Sperry 1976).

Although one must always keep in mind the limitations of using introspective reports for ascertaining causality sequences, the analyses of Natsoulas (1984), Baars (1987), and Singer and Bonanno (1990) all point to the rich range of information about beliefs and attitudes that emerges from introspective accounts, even from relatively less articulate subjects (Hurlburt 1990, Pekala 1991, Pope 1978).

In this paper, I shall focus on the study of ongoing consciousness through a variety of methods and experimental procedures. I propose we need such a basis for understanding at least one phase of the human condition, our "private personality." Experiences of interior monologue, mental glosses on one's social and physical surround, daydreams, fantasies, anticipations, recurring memories, all of which may interrupt or co-occur with our necessary processing of information, form a consensually agreed upon or physically measurable "external world." My personal strategy for "navigating" the stream of consciousness over forty years of research has involved sets of convergent empirical methods with the hope that groups of new operations can yield reliable methods of measurement. These may lead to identification of the relevant phenomena and perhaps to formulation of theories and testable hypotheses about the determinants of ongoing sequences of thought and their implications for emotional reactions, information processing, the formation of interpersonal attitudes, beliefs about self and possibly even the roots of creativity, on the one hand, or to linkages to physical and mental health, on the other.

Psychometric Approaches to the Study of Daydreams and Ongoing Consciousness

Rorschach Inkblots

As a clinical psychologist, I began my effort to study imagination, daydreams and consciousness through some of the first empirical studies of correlates of responses to the Rorschach inkblots. Hermann Rorschach (1942) had proposed that persons who were inclined to "see" human figures as associations to the blots, especially associations involving humans in action, were also more likely to show a rich fantasy life and engage in much daydreaming. Rorschach also reported that the persons who provided more of such human movement responses (the so-called M score) were more susceptible to inhibition in their movements or were more capable of controlling physical activity or behavioural motion. Research attention has focused chiefly upon linking the M response frequency to measures of fantasy, motor control, creativity, self-awareness and "planfulness" (Moise et al. 1988–1989, Singer and Brown 1977). Dozens of individual difference and factor-analytic studies consistently show that persons who give more M associations to inkblots (especially responses that are reasonably congruent with the blot shapes) are also more likely to tell rich and varied stories in response to thematic apperception test pictures, to score more highly on questionnaire measures of daydreaming frequency, and to provide more varied and cognitively complex free associations and person descriptions in other tests and in psychoanalytic sessions. They are also more likely to sit quietly in waiting rooms, to be able to slow down writing speed voluntarily, to resist laughing if so instructed when listening to a "laughing" record, to show fewer impulsive responses in problem-solving tasks, to be more accurate in time estimates and to manifest less open aggression (Singer and Brown 1977). Clinically, percipients with a low M score respond better to support-expressive or direct therapies, whereas those scoring a higher M value do better in more psychoanalytic types of therapy where imaginative productivity and free associations are critical (Blatt 1990).

Questionnaires and Self-Report Procedures

It soon occurred to me that more direct inquiries about people's daydreams and ongoing thought might provide useful normative data on the phenomena of private experience. Singer and Antrobus (1972) developed a series of 22 scales of 12 items, each designed to measure a wide range of patterns of self-reported inner experience and types of daydreams. This imaginal processes inventory (IPI) has been factor-analysed in several studies with subjects of all ages. An extensive new analysis of the IPI with a large sample of college students has led to a shortened version, the SIPI (Huba et al. 1982, Segal et al. 1980). From the varied uses of the IPI, some generalizations about the normative role of daydreams are possible.

Briefly, many studies indicate that most people report being aware of at least some daydreaming every day, and that their daydreams vary from obvious wishful thinking to elaborate and complex visions of frightening or guilty encounters. Cultural differences in frequency and patterning of daydreaming also emerge. Comprehensive factor analysis of the scales of the IPI indicates that the data yield three major factors that characterize ongoing thought: a positive–constructive daydreaming style, a guilty–dysphoric daydreaming style, and a poor attentional control pattern that is generally characterized by fleeting thoughts and an inability to focus on extended fantasy (Singer and Kolligian 1987, Singer and Bonanno 1990). Giambra (1977a,b) found evidence for factor patterns similar to those reported in our studies and tracked these across an extensive age range; in addition, he checked the test–retest reliability of daydreaming reports in response to this set of scales and found it to be surprisingly high.

Even with reliable and psychometrically well-constructed questionnaires, we are still left with the issue of whether individual respondents can really summarize accurately their ongoing experiences, the frequency of particular daydreams, etc. We must turn to other estimates of ongoing thought or other forms of self-report to ascertain the validity of the questionnaire responses. Reviewing such data, one finds that the self-reports of frequent or vivid daydreaming on questionnaires are correlated with:

1. daydream-like thoughts obtained during signal-detection tasks, with imagery so vivid that the participants don't notice that a faint picture has been projected at the point they are fixating while imagining an object;

2. with particular patterns of eye shifts during reflective thought;

3. with particular emphasis on analogy usage when the structure of the language used in transcripts of regularly sampled thought reports is analysed;

4. with particular forms of drug and alcohol use;

5. with reported fantasies during sexual behaviour;

6. with daily records of dreams recalled;

7. with measures of hypnotic susceptibility;

8. with measures of hallucinations of mental patients or flashbacks of traumatized war veterans, etc (Singer and Bonanno 1990).

The evidence from our own and related questionnaires suggests that the psychometric approach has considerable value in identifying individual stylistic variations in awareness of, and assignment of priorities to, processing centrally generated information.

More Direct Thought-Sampling Procedures

Laboratory Studies of Signal Detection

My colleague John Antrobus and I developed a particular paradigm for attempting to estimate some parameters of ongoing thought. An approach that affords maximum "control" over extraneous stimulation (at the cost of some artificiality or possibly reduced 'ecological validity') is the use of prolonged (45–60 minute) signal-detection sessions by participants seated in sound-proof, reduced-stimulation booths. Because the amount of external stimulation can be controlled, it remains to be determined to what extent individuals will shift their attention away from processing external cues (by which they earn money for accurate signal detection) toward the processing of material that is generated by the presumably ongoing activity of their own brains. Can we ascertain the conditions under which participants, even with high motivation for external signal processing, will show that they are experiencing task-unrelated images and thoughts (TUITs)?

Thus, if an individual detecting auditory signals is interrupted every 15 s and questioned about whether any stimulus-independent thoughts occurred, a "Yes" response is scored as a TUIT. The participant and experimenter agree in advance on a common definition of what constitutes a task-unrelated thought, so that the experimenter has some reasonable assurance that reports conform to an established operational definition. A thought such as "Is that tone more highly-pitched than the one before it?" is considered task-related and elicits a "No" response. A thought such as "I've got to pick up the car keys for my Saturday night date" is scored as a TUIT.

In this research paradigm, keeping the subjects in booths for a fairly long time and obtaining reports of the occurrence of task-unrelated thoughts after each 15 s of signal detection (with tones presented at rates of about one per second) have made it possible to accumulate extensive information on the frequency of occurrence of TUITs, as well as their relationship to the speed of signal presentation, the complexity of the task and other characteristics of the subjects' psychological states.

In addition to generalizations about the nature of cognitive processing (Singer 1988), the signal-detection model permits the study of individual differences. Antrobus et al. (1967) showed that participants known by self-report to be frequent daydreamers were more likely as time went on to report TUITs than individuals who had said on a questionnaire that they were little given to daydreaming. Initially, the frequent daydreamers reported a considerable number of TUITs, but the same level of errors as the infrequent daydreamers. As time went on, however, the frequent daydreamers seemed to be preferring to respond to task-unrelated mentation: their error rate increased significantly, compared with the relatively stable rate of errors for the subjects who showed fewer TUITs.

Controlled studies of ongoing thought during signal detection afford a rich opportunity for investigating the determinants of the thought stream. The introduction of unusual or alarming information prior to entry into the detection booth (overhearing a broadcast of war news) can increase the frequency of TUITs, even though accuracy of detection may not be greatly affected (Antrobus et al. 1966). Mardi Horowitz (1978) has demonstrated that intense emotional experiences prior to engaging in signal detection lead to increased ideation, as measured by thought sampling during the detection period. Such findings have suggested a basis for understanding clinical phenomena such as "unbidden images" (Horowitz 1978) or "peremptory ideation."

Studies using auditory and visual signal detection or vigilance models with interruptions for reports have also shown that TUITs occur more than half of the time, even when subjects are achieving very high detection rates, when signals come as frequently as every 0.5 s or when the density (i.e., chords versus single tones) of signal information is increased. Indeed, there was evidence for parallel processing of the TUITs and the external signals. When external signals were visual, the visual content of TUITs was reduced relative to their verbal content and vice versa when the external signals were auditory. This suggests that our daydream processes in particular sensory imagery modalities (visual or auditory) use the same brain pathways as are needed for processing external cues. Studies of continuous talk in these laboratory settings point to the moderately arousing, vigilance-maintaining quality of ongoing thought and also to the dependence of such thought on physical posture, the social setting, and so on. For example, when experimenters and participants are of the opposite sex there is a significant increase in TUIT reports during signal detections (Singer 1988, Singer and Bonanno 1990).

Thought Sampling in More "Natural" Circumstances

Some methods that sacrifice the rigid controls of the signal-detection booth for greater ecological relevance have been increasingly employed in the development of an approach to determining the characteristics and determinants of waking conscious thought. These involve (1) asking participants to talk out loud while in a controlled environment, with such verbalization being scored according to empirically or theoretically derived categories; (2) allowing the respondent to sit, recline, or stand quietly and interrupting them periodically for reports of thought or perceptual activity; or (3) requiring the person to signal by a button press whenever a new chain of thought begins, and then to report verbally in retrospect or to fill out a prepared rating form characterizing various possible features of ongoing thought.

Klinger (1990) has employed thought sampling in the ways described above to test a series of hypotheses about ongoing thought. He has made a useful distinction between "operant" and "respondent" thought processes. The former category includes thoughts that have a conscious instrumental property—the solution of a specific problem, analysis of a particular issue presently confronting one, examination of the implications of a specific situation in which one finds oneself at the moment. Operant thought is active and directed, and has the characteristics of what Freud called "secondary-process" thinking. As Klinger (1978) has noted, it is volitional; it is checked against new information concerning its effectiveness in moving toward a solution or the consequences of a particular attempted solution; and there are continuing efforts to protect such a line of thought from drifting off target or from being distracted by external cues or by extraneous, irrelevant thought. Operant thought seems to involve a greater sense of mental and physical effort; it is a human capacity especially likely to suffer from fatigue or brain damage.

Respondent thought, in Klinger's terminology, involves all other thought processes. These are non-volitional in the sense of conscious direction of a sequence and most are relatively effortless. Most of what we consider daydreams are instances of respondent thought.

The use of thought sampling in a reasonably controlled environment also permits evaluation of a variety of conditions that may influence or characterize ongoing consciousness. One can score the participants' verbalizations on dimensions such as (1) organized, sequential thought versus degenerative, confused thought; (2) use of imagery, related episodes or event memory material versus logical, semantic structures; (3) reference to current concerns and unfulfilled intentions; (4) reminiscence of past events versus orientation toward the future; and (5) realistic versus improbable content. Two studies of my students may be cited here. Pope (1978) demonstrated that longer sequences of thought more remote from the participants' immediate circumstances were obtained when the respondents were reclining rather than walking freely and when they were alone rather than in company. Zachary (1983) evaluated the relative role of positive and negative emotional experiences just before a thought-sampling period. He found that intensity of experience rather than its emotional quality and, to a lesser extent, the relative ambiguity of the material, determined the frequency of recurrence in the thought stream.

Klinger's own research points to the relative importance of current concerns as determinants of the material that emerges in thought sampling. Current concerns are defined as those that occur between the time one becomes committed to pursuing a particular goal and when one either consummates or abandons this objective (Klinger 1990). Such concerns, as measured psychometrically, make up a useful operational definition of the Freudian wish in its early form as an unfulfilled intention or aspiration that is not necessarily libidinal or sexual (Holt 1976). They may range from unfulfilled intentions (e.g., to pick up a container of milk on the way home) to long-standing unresolved desires (e.g., to please a parent). One can evaluate current concerns before the thought-sampling sessions and estimate the relative importance of goals, the person's perception of the reality of goal achievement, and so on. Only after we have explored the range and influence of such current conscious concerns in sampling of the individual's thoughts, emotions and behavioural responses can we move to infer the influence of unconscious wishes or intentions.

In the 1980s there has been a considerable interest in thought-sampling studies outside the laboratory—research now involves accumulation of data over as long as two weeks, from participants who carry paging devices and report on their thoughts, emotions and current activities when signalled several times a day (Csikszentmihalyi and Larson 1984, Hurlburt 1990, Klinger 1990). The results suggest this method is feasible and suitable for hypothesis testing as well as for accumulating basic descriptive data (as in the Csikszentmihalyi and Larson study of teenagers).

In one such study, participants whose prior measured fantasies pointed to greater longing for closer association with others, reported more thoughts of other people and more positive emotional responses in social situations than did other participants, on the basis of a week-long accumulation of eight daily reports (McAdams and Constantian 1983). The relationship between similarly obtained frequent daily reports of thought and the same participants' scores on a daydreaming questionnaire, our IPI (Singer and Antrobus 1972), was evaluated by Hurlburt (1980). He reported significant correlations between the questionnaire scales of frequent daydreaming and acceptance of daydreaming and the accumulated daily reports of daydreaming, based on two days of dozens of interruptions.

The accumulation of thought samples has also proven useful in studies of clinical groups, such as bulimiacs or patients with panic disorder, where the time, locale and contingent circumstances associated with recurrent thoughts have yielded meaningful data (Singer and Bonanno 1990). I have found that samples of ongoing conscious thought of normal individuals include many of the metaphors or symbols that are also reported by them in recounting subsequent night dreams—that is, the ongoing consciousness is already laying the groundwork for what seem to be the strange or creative settings of the night dream (Singer 1988).

Children's Imaginative Play as a Forerunner of the Thought Stream

With Dorothy Singer, I have carried out a series of observational studies and experiments that involve recording the spontaneous play and language of preschool children, especially between the ages of $2\frac{1}{2}$ and 5 years, when make-believe or pretend play is most prevalent (D. Singer and J. Singer 1990). In this work, we rely on pairs of trained observers who independently record samples of children's behaviour during "free play" periods in the day care centre (or, occasionally, at home). These samples can be obtained on several occasions in a week and, in some studies, recurrently over a year. We must, of course, rely on the spontaneous verbalizations of the child in scoring the degree to which play introduces elements of fantasy and transcends the concrete description of objects or the child's motor actions. One can then look at variables such as affective responses, cooperation with others, leadership and aggression, and also examine the kinds of language forms used.

A detailed review of findings from this approach would take us far afield, but one can assert that, as Jean Piaget (1962) suggested, symbolic play emerging by the third year is a key factor in leading towards more advanced cognitive processes. Yet contrary to Piaget, make-believe does not fade once concrete operational thought appears. It never goes away and seems to be a welcome, if concealed, feature of middle childhood. As we have tried to show (D. Singer and J. Singer 1990), pretending and make-believe either as private experiences of daydreaming or in the form of adult play, for example, carnival dressing-up, persist throughout life.

Task-Unrelated Images and Thoughts During Eleven Days of Signal Detection

With John Antrobus, I studied a group of participants who returned to the laboratory on eleven consecutive days for a one-hour session of detecting auditory signals at a frequency of one per second. They were interrupted every 15 s and pressed buttons indicating if they had experienced (1) no TUIT; (2) a TUIT that involved a perceptual response—for example, to an extraneous noise, physical discomfort, or other sensory-derived reaction not specific to the listening to and discriminating of the auditory signals, the task for which they were paid; (3) a TUIT that involved specific thoughts about the experimental situation, for example, "How much longer?"; (4) a TUIT that involved experimentally remote responses, such as "I'm picturing myself canoeing with Sadie this weekend." The participants had been accustomed, before the experiment, to common definitions and we asked them, during training, to verbalize actual thoughts. They were in relatively sound- and light-proof booths and wore earphones through which the signals (randomly presented high or low pure tones, one class of which was the one demanding a button press) were presented.

Figure 31.1 shows the average findings for the group across eleven days of one-hour sessions of reports every 15 s. The subjects sustained an overall accuracy, as in most of our studies, of 80–100%. The percentage of reports other than "No," that is, the task-unrelated thoughts, remains steady across eleven days at 52–58%. On the first few days, either the perceptual or experiment-related responses represent as much as 40% of the TUITs. By the second or third session most of the TUITs are quite remote from the immediate experience of the signal-detection booth. The participants have accustomed themselves to the setting and, while merrily continuing to process signals, almost all of their reported TUITs represent memories, wishes, fantasies, or

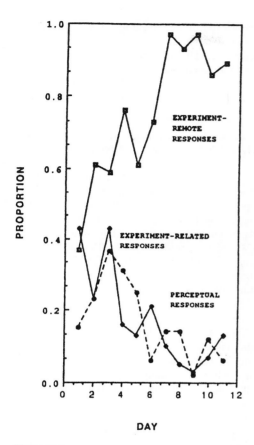

Figure 31.1

The average proportion of the different kinds of task-unrelated images and thoughts (TUITs) in the total TUITs reported during a 45-min. signal-detection period on each of 11 days of participation by five subjects. All types of TUITs reported during each session made up, on average, 55% of the responses obtained after each 15-s period of detecting signals; thus about 45% of the time subjects answered "No" to the query "Were your thoughts unrelated to those specifically about detection of the signals?" Perceptual or experiment-related TUITs drop off sharply as the participants gain more experience in the experimental situation and experimentally remote TUITs become more prominent.

other thoughts far removed from the immediate setting.

We might conclude that even in an environment that makes a continuing demand on us for external signal detection, our brain may be continually active in generating information from long-term memory. We seem to orient ourselves to new settings, then our brain's channel capacity soon allows us to perform accurately our main task of environmental attention while also becoming aware of our centrally generated, long-term memory stimuli.

Determinants of the Content of Ongoing Thought

For a more natural thought-sampling procedure, we set up a hierarchy of possible conditions that might lead to recurrence of material from an experimental situation during later thoughts sampled after experimental intervention from a group of adolescents (Klos and Singer 1981). The thought reports were rated by trained judges for their similarity to the particular experimental scenarios experienced by our subjects. The judges were provided with samples of all the different possible experimental scenarios, but were ignorant of the actual experimental conditions. We could then estimate the probability that the exposure of a participant to a particular experimental condition matched up with its recurrences in the person's later stream of thought.

It was proposed that even for first-year college students, parental involvements were likely to prove especially provocative of further thought. We chose to evaluate the relative recurrence in later thought of (1) generally resolved versus unresolved situations (the old Zeigarnik effect); (2) a mutual non-conflictive parental interaction; (3) a confrontation with a parent that involved a collaborative stance by the adult; and (4) a comparable confrontation in which the parent's attitude was clearly coercive. It was proposed that exposure (through a simulated interaction) to each of these conditions would yield differences in the later recurrence of simulation-relevant thoughts in the participants' consciousness.

More specifically, we predicted that unresolved situations would have a greater impact on later thought than resolved situations, that conflict situations would recur more in later thought than non-conflictive simulated interactions with a parent, and that the confrontation with a coercive parent would cause more later thought than one with a collaborative parent. Finally, we proposed that a history of long-standing stress with one's actual parents would amplify all of these conflict effects. Our experimenters and judges were unfamiliar with participants' scores on the long-standing parent stress measure. In summary, we predicted that while an unresolved, non-conflictive situation might recur more often in later thoughts than a resolved, non-conflictive simulation, more powerful effects on recurrence would emerge for the parent conflict situations and especially for those with a coercive parent, particularly if the subject had a history of parental stress.

The data provided clear support for the major hypotheses. The frequency of thoughts' recurrences occurred in the predicted order (figure 31.2). The effects were clearly amplified by a history of long-standing interpersonal stress with a parent. The "pure incompletion effect" was a modest one, observed mainly in the non-conflictive situation. It was overridden by the increasing coerciveness of the imaginary conflict situations. Of special interest is the fact that, once exposed to a simulated parental conflict, young people with a history of stress reflected this brief, artificial incident in as many as 50% of their later sampled thoughts. If we tentatively generalize from these results, the thought world of adolescents who have had long-standing parental difficulties may be a most unpleasant domain, since many conflictive chance encoun-

ters or even film or television plots may lead to a considerable degree of associative thought recurrence. The implications of a method of this kind (combined with estimates of personality variables or of other current concerns) for studying various groups (e.g., patients after surgery) are intriguing.

Self-Belief Discrepancies in Cocaine Abusers

In some studies recently completed with S. Kelly Avants and Arthur Margolin, we sought to test hypotheses derived from the work of Tory Higgins on the linkage between self-belief discrepancies and specific affective states. Higgins (1987) had proposed that we all formulate, consciously or otherwise, a series of beliefs about ourselves in various manifestations. These can be about our Actual Self, our Ideal Self, our Ought Self (what we think our parents might have wanted us to be), or other representations such as Past, Future, or Dreaded Self. The Actual Self, as reported by a participant's listing of traits or tendencies, reflects how one describes one's self as accurately as possible. One's Ideal Self represents the aspirations one holds for the best one might be, e.g. 'star athlete, popular, deeply respected ...' The Ought Self might reflect more early family or social group expectations, such as "scholarly, obedient, religious ..." A Dreaded Self might yield terms like "sexually impotent, unmarriageable, friendless ...".

Higgins had shown that individuals found to have large measured discrepancies between Actual Self and Ideal Self were also likely to suffer from depression or sadness, while those with discrepancies between Actual Self and Ought Self were more likely to experience agitation, anxiety and fear. Indeed, experimental priming of Actual–Ideal or Actual–Ought Self discrepancies generated sadness or agitated emotional reactions, respectively. Discrepancy scores, which could be calculated by counting non-recurring trait words listed for Actual Self,

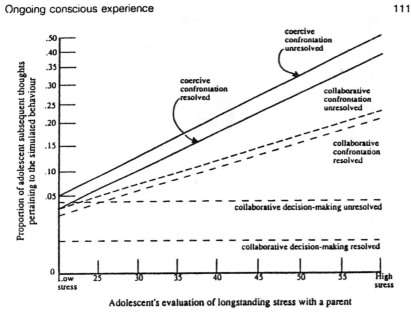

Figure 31.2
Adolescent stress and simulated parental confrontation. Adolescents' thoughts during a 20-min. postexperimental period were rated by judges as bearing a clear similarity to the scenarios of the simulated (1) resolved or unresolved, (2) collaborative or confrontational, or (3) coercive or collaborative conflict situations that subjects had undergone earlier. The abscissa reflects previously obtained measures of the subjects' degree of reported stress with their actual parents. Thus, while unresolved simulations recur in later thought more than resolved ones, and confrontational or conflictual episodes more than collaborative decision-making simulations, the simulated coercive parental conflict is much more likely to recur in later though. All the conflictual effect recurrences are greatly affected by the degree of individauls' experience of long-standing stress with parents. (From Klos and Singer 1981, reproduced with permission of the American Psychological Association.)

Ideal Self, or Ought Self, proved predictive in differentiating depressed (Actual–Ideal) versus socially fearful (Actual–Ought) clinical groups.

We hypothesized, on the premise that cocaine abusers may be self-medicating a depressive mood by using an "up-lifting" drug, that this class of abusers should show more evidence of an Actual Self–Ideal Self discrepancy than either a group of heroin users or a non-abusing control group. Our results clearly support this hypothesis (figure 31.3). We also obtained thought samples of the participants and we could show how cravings for cocaine emerged along with reports of greater Actual–Ideal discrepancies on a day-to-day basis. We then asked these patients to keep logs of their moods and of their thoughts of self (as "Addict," "Ideal," "Craving," etc.), while a cognitive-behavioural therapy intervention sought to help them identify and practise more adaptive self-representations. Follow-up thought samples revealed correlations between each of: less craving, fewer Actual–Ideal discrepancies, more positive Future Selves, and physiologically measured abstinence.

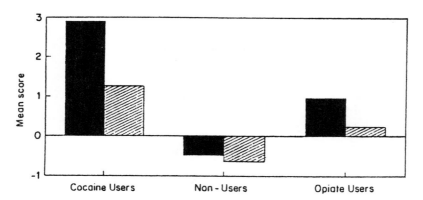

Figure 31.3

Actual Self–Ideal Self and Actual Self–Ought Self discrepancies for cocaine users, opiate users, and nonusers. A high score (arbitrary units) indicates that subjects' descriptions of their Actual Self are considerably different from the way they describe either their Ideal Self or their Ought Self (for definitions, see text). ■, Actual-Ideal; ⊠, Actual-Ought.

We have extended the self-belief discrepancy study to a large sample of normal individuals. We have measured many personality variables, clinical attitudes such as depression, and various manifestations of Self (Actual, Ideal, Ought, Dreaded, Past, Future). Our participants are involved in experiments that seek to prime particular self-discrepancies to determine whether these will increase recurrent thoughts about these concerns. The subjects carry paging devices for a week, which signal them randomly eight times a day so they can report on mood, specific thoughts and contingent events. We hope by this method to ascertain to what extent the conscious thoughts of the respondents show consistency with personality measures and cross-sectionally measured self-schemata, as well as reflecting priming of particular self-belief discrepancies.

A Cognitive-Affective Perspective

I should like to close by summarizing my conclusions from years of applying these methods to the study of ongoing thought. I propose that human beings are best regarded as creatures who are biologically endowed with the necessary capacities and motivated from birth to explore their environments and to move gradually toward labelling and assigning meaning to their experiences. The human information-processing systems are closely tied to the separate, differentiated affective system, so that we are aroused, frightened, angered or depressed by sudden or persistent incongruity between our expectancies (plans, goals or wishes) and the information presented in a given situation. Likewise, we are moved to laughter and joy when incongruities are resolved, or to interest and to exploration when the novelty we confront is at a moderate level rather than an extreme one (Mandler 1984; Singer 1974, 1984; Tomkins 1962). If there is an overarching human motive from this perspective, it is to assign meaning, to make sense of the world. The theorizing and empirical research of the Kreitlers highlights the heuristic value of such an approach for the study of personality (Kreitler and Kreitler 1976).

If we are indeed "wired" to make sense of our environment, to select, to identify, to label, to encode and to schematize new stimulation, what are the sources of this information? For human beings (as far as we can tell), the stimuli derive either from the "objective" world, the consensually measurable physical and social stimuli in our milieu, or from the "subjective" or private world of our memories and ongoing mental processes (Cartwright 1981, Pope and Singer 1978). At any given moment, a human being must assign a priority to responding either to those stimuli that come from external sources (sounds, light patterns, smells, touches, or tastes) or to those that appear to be "internal" (the recollections, associations, images, interior monologues, wishful fantasies, or ruminative worries that characterize consciousness). Bodily sensations or signals of pain or malfunction from our organ systems represent a kind of intermediary source of stimulation, although such experiences often appear to us to have an "objective" quality, despite their inherent embedment within our physical selves. We must generally give greater weight in our instantaneous assignments of priority to externally derived stimuli, or else we are likely to be hit by cars or to bump into poles. But human environments are characterized by sufficient redundancy, and our motor skills and cognitive plans for specific situations generally are so overlearned and well differentiated, that we have ample opportunity to engage in elaborate memories, plans or fantasies, even while driving a car or participating in a business meeting.

Our human condition is such that we are forever in the situation of deciding how much attention to give to self-generated thought and how much to information from the external social or physical environment. This dilemma represents, I believe, a way of formulating the introversion–extroversion dimension of human experience. It may be seen as one manifestation of, or perhaps even as the prototype for, the major existential dilemma of the human being—the persisting dialectical struggle between autonomy and association (Singer and Bonanno 1990). Under the umbrella of the overarching motive for meaning, we humans are always seeking, on the one hand, to feel loved, admired or respected, to feel close to an individual or a group, and, on the other, to sustain a sense of autonomy and individuality, of self-direction, privacy in thought or uniqueness in competence and skill. Although the individual stream of consciousness may be seen as the human's last bastion of privacy and sense of uniqueness, our studies of ongoing consciousness suggest that a great majority of our thoughts are about affiliation and attachment to others!

Acknowledgment

Some of the recent research described herein was supported by a grant from the John D. and Catherine T. MacArthur Foundation to the Program on Conscious and Unconscious Mental Processes, University of California, San Francisco School of Medicine.

References

Antrobus JS, Singer JL, Greenberg S 1966 Studies in the stream of consciousness: experimental enhancement and suppression of spontaneous cognitive processes. Percept Mot Skills 23:399–417

Antrobus JS, Coleman R, Singer JL 1967 Signal detection performance by subjects differing in predisposition to daydreaming. J Consult Psychol 31:487–491

Baars BJ 1987 A cognitive theory of consciousness. Cambridge University Press, Cambridge

Blatt S 1990 Interpersonal relatedness and self definition: two personality configurations and their implications for psychopathology and psychotherapy. In: Singer JL (ed) Repression and dissociation. University of Chicago Press, Chicago, IL, p 299–335

Cartwright RD 1981 The contribution of research on memory and dreaming to a twenty-four-hour model of cognitive behaviour. In: Fishbein W (ed) Sleep, dreams, and memory. (Adv Sleep Res Ser, vol 6) Luce, Manchester, MA

Csikszentmihalyi M, Larson R 1984 Being adolescent. Basic Books, New York

Ellman S, Antrobus JS 1991 The mind in sleep, 2nd edn. Wiley, New York

Giambra LM 1977a Adult male daydreaming across the life span: a replication, further analyses, and tentative norms based upon retrospective reports. Int J Aging Hum Dev 8:197–228

Giambra LM 1977b Daydreaming about the past: the time setting of spontaneous thought intrusions. The Gerontologist 17:35–38

Higgins ET 1987 Self-discrepancy: a theory relating self and affect. Psychol Rev 94:319–340

Holt RR 1976 Drive or wish? A reconsideration of the psychoanalytic theory of motivation. In: Gill MM, Holzman PS (eds) Psychology versus metapsychology: psychoanalytic essays in memory of George S. Klein. (Psychol Issues Monogr 36, vol 9) International University Press, New York, p 158–197

Horowitz MJ 1970 Image formation and cognition. Appleton Century Crofts, New York

Huba GJ, Singer JL, Aneschensel CS, Antrobus JS 1982 The short imaginal processes inventory. Research Psychologists Press, Port Huron, MI

Hurlburt RT 1980 Validation and correlation of thought sampling with retrospective measures. Cognit Ther Res 4:235–238

Hurlburt RT 1990 Sampling normal and schizophrenic inner experience. Plenum Publishing Corporation, New York

James W 1890 The principles of psychology, 2 vols. Republished 1952. Dover Press, New York

Klinger E 1978 Modes of normal conscious flow. In: Pope KS, Singer JL (eds) The stream of consciousness. Plenum Publishing Corporation, New York, p 225–258

Klinger E 1990 Daydreaming. Tarcher, Los Angeles, CA

Klos DS, Singer JL 1981 Determinants of the adolescent's ongoing thought following simulated parental confrontations. J Pers Soc Psychol 41:975–987

Kreitler H, Kreitler S 1976 Cognitive orientation and behavior. Springer-Verlag, New York

Mandler G 1984 Mind and body. Norton, New York

McAdams D, Constantian CA 1983 Intimacy and affiliation motives in daily living: an experience sampling analysis. J Pers Soc Psychol 4:851–861

McGuire WJ 1984 Search for the self: going beyond self-esteem and the reactive self. In: Zucker RZ, Aran-off J, Rabin AI (eds) Personality and the prediction of behavior. Academic Press, New York, p 73–120

Moise F, Yinon Y, Rabinowitz A 1988–1989 Rorschach inkblot movement response as a function of motor activity or inhibition. Imagin Cognit Person 8:39–48

Natsoulas T 1984 The subjective organization of personal consciousness: a concept of conscious personality. J Mind Behav 5:311–336

Pekala R 1991 Quantifying consciousness. Plenum Publishing Corporation, New York

Piaget J 1962 Play, dreams, and imitation. Norton, New York

Pope KS 1978 How gender, solitude and posture influence the stream of consciousness. In: Pope KS, Singer JL (eds) The stream of consciousness. Plenum Publishing Corporation, New York, p 259–289

Pope KS, Singer JL 1978 Regulation of the stream of consciousness: toward a theory of ongoing thought. In: Schwartz GE, Shapiro D (eds) Consciousness and self-regulation. Plenum Publishing Corporation, New York, vol 2:101–135

Rorschach H 1942 Psychodiagnostics. Grune & Stratton, New York

Sabini J, Silver M 1981 Introspection and causal accounts. J Person Soc Psychol 40:171–179

Schank RC, Abelson RP 1977 Scripts, plans, goals, and understanding: an inquiry into human knowledge structures. Erlbaum, Hillsdale, NJ

Segal B, Huba G, Singer JL 1980 Drugs, daydreaming and personality. Erlbaum, Hillsdale, NJ

Singer DG, Singer JL 1990 The house of make-believe: children's play and the developing imagination. Harvard University Press, Cambridge, MA

Singer JL 1974 Imagery and daydream methods in psychotherapy and behavior modification. Academic Press, New York

Singer JL 1984 The human personality. Harcourt Brace Jovanovich, New York

Singer JL 1988 Sampling ongoing consciousness and emotional experience: implications for health. In: Horowitz MJ (ed) Psychodynamics and cognition. University of Chicago Press, Chicago, IL, p 297–346

Singer JL, Antrobus JS 1972 Daydreaming, imaginal processes, and personality: a normative study. In: Sheehan P (ed) The function and nature of imagery. Academic Press, New York, p 175–202

Singer JL, Bonanno GA 1990 Personality and private experience: individual variations in consciousness and in attention to subjective phenomena. In: Pervin L (ed) Handbook of personality: theory and research. Guilford Press, New York, p 419–444

Singer JL, Brown SL 1977 The experience-type: some behavioural correlates and theoretical implications. In: Rickers-Orsiankina MA (ed) Rorschach psychology. Krieger, Huntington, NY, p 325–374

Singer JL, Kolligian J Jr 1987 Personality: developments in the study of private experience. Annu Rev Psychol 38:533–574

Sperry R 1976 A unifying approach to mind and brain: ten year perspective. In: Corner A, Swab DF (eds) Perspectives in brain research. Elsevier Science Publishers, Amsterdam

Tomkins SS 1962 Affect, imagery, consciousness. Springer-Verlag, New York

Zachary R 1983 Cognitive and affective determinants of ongoing thought. PhD thesis, Yale University, New Haven, CT

32 Verbal Reports on Thinking

K. Anders Ericsson and Herbert A. Simon

Introduction

After a long period of studying human performance and abilities, research in psychology is now seeking to understand the underlying cognitive processes. Researchers are looking for observations on thinking that would allow tracing the intermediate steps of the thought processes. Subjects' verbal reports on their thinking would appear to be a major source of information about detailed steps of thought processes. However, investigators have been reluctant to rely on such reports on thinking for historical reasons. After an early period in which psychologists made heavy use of verbal reports (introspection), they fell into disrepute during the era of behaviourism; but they have been revived since the 1970s as a major source of data for cognitive research.

In the course of this history, verbal reports have been used for widely varying purposes and have been gathered and interpreted according to quite different methodologies. In the earlier period, they were a mainstay of classical introspection (Titchener 1912), the analysis of problem solving by Würzburg and Gestalt psychologists (Duncker 1945; Selz 1913, 1922; Wertheimer 1945), clinical analyses of thought (Freud 1914), and analyses of the development of children's thinking (Inhelder and Piaget 1958). In the recent resurgence of their use (Newell, Shaw, and Simon 1958; Newell and Simon 1972), they have been employed within an information-processing framework, chiefly in the study of problem solving.

With the growing use of verbal reports in psychology, it has become important to improve the methodology for collecting and interpreting verbal reports and to provide protocol analysis with a firm theoretical foundation. The early investigators uncritically regarded the verbal reports by trained subjects of their cognitive processes as immediate and direct observations of those processes, veridical and uncontroversial. Given the assumed immediacy of the observations, investigators asked subjects to report specific types of information without any regard for how cognitive processes generating such reports were feasible. When, as a result of these deficiencies, verbal reports collected in different laboratories were found to be mutually inconsistent, opponents of the introspective method, like Watson, argued that the method was unscientific and should be discarded.

The goal of this chapter is to outline a framework for studying thinking that is consistent with the current experimental methodology. Within this framework, verbal reports of subjects are seen as one of many types of observations that provide data on subjects' cognitive processes. This chapter will show how the information processing theory of human cognition can guide us in selecting tasks, recording observations and interpreting verbal reports as evidence or data on underlying cognitive processes. Let us first briefly describe the theory and our theoretical framework.

Theoretical Framework

The most general and weakest hypothesis we require is that human cognition is information processing: that a cognitive process can be seen as a sequence of internal states successively transformed by a series of information processes. An important, and more specific, assumption is that information is stored in several memories having different capacities and accessing characteristics: several sensory stores of very short duration, a short-term memory (STM) with limited capacity and/or intermediate duration, and a long-term memory (LTM) with very large capacity and relatively permanent storage, but with relatively slow fixation and access times compared with the other memories.

Within the framework of this information processing model, it is assumed that information recently acquired (attended to or heeded) by the central processor is kept in STM, and is directly accessible for further processing (e.g., for producing verbal reports), whereas information from LTM must first be retrieved (transferred to STM) before it can be reported.

Subjects' thought processes can therefore be described as a sequence of states of heeded information. A subset of this heeded information is stored in LTM and is retrievable after the thought processes are completed at the end of a task. It is important to note that any observable behaviour used as data for a thought process requires an explicit account of its relation to the states of the thought processes and any mediating additional cognitive processes.

Within the framework of information processing an account of thought processes used in tasks involves a model, often specified in the form of a computer program, which can take the tasks as input and generate the corresponding answers as responses. From an analysis of the relevant tasks (task analysis) it is often possible to enumerate a wide range of a priori acceptable models that generate desired answers as a result of sequences of processing steps. From the acceptable models, the best model is selected by collecting additional observations on the thought processes, like reaction times, eye movements, verbal reports, and so on. The best model is the one that can *regenerate* these additional observations in addition to the desired answers. In the following section we will demonstrate how this framework of regeneration allows us to treat verbal report observations in the same way as more traditional data. The concept of regeneration of observations provides an important criterion for judging how informative the observations are. The amount of information associated with observations is related to their ability to discriminate between many a priori accept-

able models. A more detailed description of information-processing theory is given by Newell and Simon (1972).

Let us now discuss the implications of our theoretical framework for the study of thought processes. The first set of issues concerns how tasks should be selected to best allow us to study thinking. We will show how tasks can be selected to assure thinking and how a task analysis provides a priori expectations regarding the possible thought processes available for generating the answer to the task. The second set of issues concerns how observations relevant to the thought processes should be collected in order to provide valid evidence about the thought processes. This presentation follows a more extensive discussion by Ericsson and Oliver (1988).

Selection of Tasks

Let us first look at the earliest studies of thinking and, using the concept of regeneration, critically evaluate some of the tasks used. Considerable research was done on the free-association task, in which subjects are instructed to say the first word that comes to mind after hearing or seeing a particular word like "needle" or "father" (Jung 1910). This task was thought to involve a single associative step (from the stimulus word to the response word) and hence correspond to the simplest form of thinking that could be studied using introspective reports. Other tasks were designed by Karl Bühler (1951) to get at processes of comprehension by having subjects respond as quickly as possible if they did or did not understand sentences, such as: "We depreciate everything that can be explained." Other types of question testing general knowledge were also used, such as: "Do you know where our other stop-watch is now?"

When one attempts to propose a model for the thought processes involved in free-association and sentence comprehension, it becomes clear how uninformative such responses are in the regeneration sense. In both cases one could conceive of models in which the response was selected prior to the presentation of the task or by some task-irrelevant procedure. Any response in the free-association task is acceptable even though it may be unusual. The early investigators used this methodology because they felt they could trust their subjects to follow the instructions. However, a methodology can be devised where subjects need not be trusted by making their responses to a task more informative.

More modern methodology avoids these problems by determining a priori what is the correct answer. For example, the question "Is Stockholm the capital of Sweden?" has only one correct answer, that is, "Yes." However, in all tasks that require choosing among a few alternative answers, the possibility exists that subjects might simply guess and hence give correct answers by chance. If the two possible responses are "Yes" and "No," correct answers would be obtained about half of the time purely by chance. In studies of thinking it is not uncommon that only correct responses are analysed and the data from subjects with high error rates (more than 10–20%) are completely discarded. A different approach is to request a more informative answer or response: for the instruction "Name the capital of Sweden," the correct answer "Stockholm" would be unlikely to occur as a result of guessing.

Recent studies of thinking have primarily used tasks in logic (Guyotte and Sternberg 1981, Johnson-Laird and Steedman 1978), mathematics (Ginsberg 1983), probability (Estes 1976), and so on, where a given task has a single correct answer. Using tasks in a formalized domain has many advantages. It is easy to generate a large number of different problems among which only the surface elements differ. In addition, the investigator can make a careful analysis of the task, which may suggest what kinds of theory may be reasonable before observations of people performing the task are gathered.

Analysis of Tasks and Strategies

For those tasks for which we know the correct answers or responses, we also know a fair amount about the procedures, methods and knowledge available for producing the answers. A systematic analysis of such information for a certain task or domain of tasks is called a task analysis with a specification of possible strategies.

It is important to realize that a task analysis should be made prior to the collection and analysis of observations. Although the term task analysis is relatively new, experimental psychologists have always been concerned with how subjects generate their responses. The emphasis was on eliminating the possibility that the subject may rely on information that is not associated with the experimental variables. A well-known example is the use of nonsense syllables, like *qub* or *teg*, in memory experiments to eliminate the possibility that subjects could rely on previous knowledge when committing the syllables to memory (Ebbinghaus 1885). As it turned out, subjects actually do draw on their knowledge of words and common spelling patterns when they memorize this material (Montague 1972). Thus, empirical evidence showed that the initial task analysis was inadequate in that subjects used information not considered in advance to be important. This example shows that task analyses are always provisional and should be modified in the light of new findings.

It is particularly important to explicate the knowledge necessary to generate successful solutions when we study tasks that cannot be easily performed with simple strategies, like guessing. In such task domains as mathematics, logic, statistics, and so forth, clearly defined procedures exist for generating correct solutions. These procedures can be described as a sequence of steps, which in turn can be described with flow charts or even computer programs.

Tasks like translation of a particular sentence to a different language can be subjected to a similar task analysis, although the number of different acceptable translations will complicate the analysis. If one can assume that the sentence is translated in strict left-to-right order, the analysis will be considerably simplified. Of particular interest is the availability of linguistic rules as opposed to exceptions and idiomatic constructions. A description of the similarity of the two languages with respect to particular grammatical rules and specific lexical items is likely to be of major importance for assessing plausible cognitive representations and processes. Words with multiple lexical meanings are also likely to be particularly revealing with respect to the translation processes.

An a priori analysis of the possible thought sequences generating an answer to a task is essential. Such a task analysis often reveals that an answer can be generated by several alternative processing sequences. In many cases slight changes in the task or the specific problem can dramatically reduce the number of alternative accounts and provide more informative observations. The task analysis has another important function. It specifies a number of sequences of processing steps with specifications of the information processed at each step. These sequential accounts of possible thought processes are necessary for analysing a wide range of observations of behaviour observed during the thought processes, like sequences of eye-fixations and "think-aloud" reports.

Selecting Types of Observations to be Recorded

Once a task is selected for study, we may ask what observations can be recorded to provide information on the cognitive processes used in that task. The central issue is how these observations reflect underlying cognitive processes. Within the framework of information processing theory we can interpret a wide range of observa-

tions as providing information about the order and duration of processing steps. Figure 32.1 illustrates schematically the temporal sequence of thought processes in generating a solution to a task.

The reaction time, which is the duration measured from the presentation of the problem to the production of the answer, will then consist of the sum of the durations of individual processing steps. If the generated answer is correct, it is likely that one of the sequences of processes specified by our task analysis was used. If the generated answer is incorrect, the subject either lacked some crucial knowledge or made an error in executing one or more of the processing steps. We will call observations that bear on the total performance of a task, that is, reaction time and accuracy of the response, *performance observations*.

There are also several types of observations that give information about the individual processing steps, such as spontaneous verbalizations and eye-movement sequences during the solution of the task. By instructing subjects to think aloud, that is, verbalize their thoughts, during the solution of the task, one can get a sequence of verbalizations corresponding to the sequence of generated thoughts. We will call this type of observation *process observations*.

In addition, we can collect data after a task is completed, such as memory for thought-processes during the task, memory for presented information, and recollections of the strategies used. We will call this final type of observation *post-process observations*. Investigators have traditionally been reluctant to collect process data and post-process observations since they were concerned that procedures used to collect such data might change the subject's thought processes and, indirectly, the performance data.

We have indicated above how different types of observations can be interpreted as reflecting the underlying cognitive processes or processing steps. Next, we will discuss how changes in procedures and experimental situations can allow

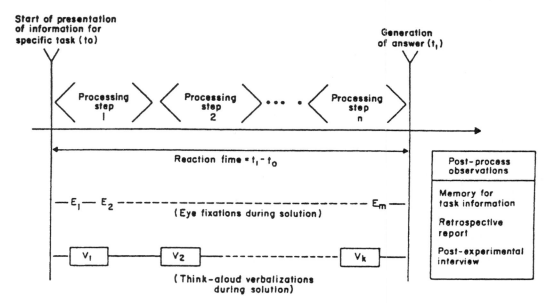

Figure 32.1
Overview of different types of observations that are potentially available for a thinking process for a given task (From Ericsson and Oliver 1989.)

us to make observations that more accurately reflect the important properties of the cognitive processes. Although we are of course most interested in various types of verbal report procedures, we will first discuss the traditional performance measures (i.e., reaction time and response accuracy) to demonstrate that very similar considerations apply to collection of any type of data. We will then turn to a discussion of process data (i.e., various types of concurrent verbal reports) and then finally to post-process data (i.e., retrospective verbal reports and post-experimental questioning).

Performance Observations

It is important to realize that, in a normal context, reaction times can be recorded relatively unobtrusively. But in most studies measuring reaction time as an indicator of underlying processes, several additional steps are taken to obtain a pure estimate of the necessary cognitive processes for that type of task.

It is easy to imagine a subject having a longer reaction time than necessary due to lapses of attention or additional checking on the correctness of a generated answer. In that case, the observed reaction time will not be a pure estimate of the durations of necessary processing steps but will reflect the durations of these extraneous cognitive activities as well. Hence, in studies measuring reaction time, subjects are usually instructed to respond as rapidly as possible without being inaccurate. Under these conditions experimenters should obtain a reasonably accurate reaction time of the necessary processing steps with any extraneous processing eliminated, or at least reduced.

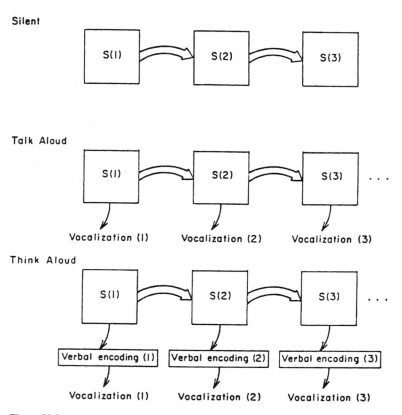

Figure 32.2
The states of heeded information in a cognitive process and their relation to verbalizations under three different conditions.

The correct answers for some types of tasks can be generated by quite different methods and strategies. In most research using reaction-time measures, subjects are given some initial practice (warm-up) on the types of tasks used in the experiment. It is often assumed that the subjects use this warm-up time to come up with the strategy that is most efficient for them. Practice also gives them a chance to decide how careful they must be in order to be both accurate and fast. It is assumed that reaction times at the end of the warm-up phase give reasonably consistent estimates of the time necessary to perform particular sequences of cognitive processes.

The responses in the form of answers given by subjects can also be viewed as summary observations of sequences of cognitive processes in a given task. From a correct answer we can infer correct processing of all of the individual steps, and from an error we can infer incorrect processing of at least one of those steps. These inferences apply to an entire sequence of steps and leave unspecified what might be going on during the individual steps. We will now discuss observations on elements or individual steps of these processing sequences.

Concurrent Verbal Reports

A wide range of procedures may be used to elicit verbal reports on ongoing cognitive processes. We will first outline some theoretical considerations on various characteristics of such procedures and then discuss how some of the desirable procedures can and have been implemented. We will then discuss a broader range of concurrent verbal report procedures with reference to the recommended procedures.

Theoretical Considerations

According to our information processing model described earlier, we can define a cognitive process as a sequence of states in which each state corresponds to information (thoughts) in attention and STM, that is, heeded information (thoughts). To obtain verbal reports, as new information (thoughts) enters attention, the subjects should verbalize the corresponding thought or thoughts. According to this verbal report procedure the new incoming information is *maintained* in attention until the corresponding verbalization of it is completed. The crucial aspect of this procedure is that the sequence of states (i.e., the information contained in attention and STM) remains the same with the verbal report procedure as it would be without the reporting procedure, that is, when the cognitive processes proceed silently. The top panel of figure 32.2 shows a normal (silent) cognitive process with its associated states of heeded information. The middle panel illustrates a "talk-aloud" report in which the subject simply vocalizes "silent speech." The bottom panel illustrates a "think-aloud" report in which subjects must convert the heeded information into a verbalizable form to vocalize it. In each of these

Table 32.1
A transcript of a thinking-aloud protocol from a subject mentally multiplying 36 times 24. On the right side, the same multiplication is performed using the traditional paper and pencil method

OK	36
36 times 24	24
um	144
4 times 6 is 24	720
4	864
carry the 2	
4 times 3 is 12	
14	
144	
0	
2 times 6 is 12	
2	
carry the 1	
2 times 3 is 6	
7	
720	
720	
144 plus 72	
so it would be 4	
6	
864	

three examples the *same* sequence of states is retained.

Before proceeding to some of the complications of our model let us illustrate the types of verbal reports observed. In table 32.1 the observed verbalizations of a subject mentally multiplying 36 × 24 are given.

The observations in this case consist of a sequence of verbalizations each of which can be segmented on the basis of brief pauses and intonation patterns. These verbalizations are relevant to our task analysis that predicts a wide range of intermediate steps depending on the solution process. By matching these logically

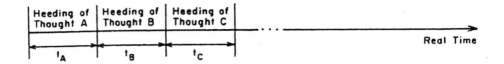

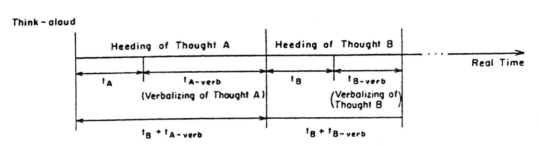

Figure 32.3
The temporal characteristics of heeding of thoughts for silent thought and "think-aloud."

possible intermediate states against the verbalizations we can identify the specific solution process used for this particular task.

The verbal report procedures preserve the sequences of states, and hence the cognitive processes should not change as a result of the additional instruction to verbalize. Ericsson and Simon (1984) made an exhaustive review of studies comparing silent subjects' performance with the performance of "talk-aloud" and "think-aloud" subjects. They found no consistent differences in the generated responses (accuracy). However, several studies indicated that subjects with "think-aloud" instructions required more time to complete their solutions. Let us therefore consider in more detail the temporal relation between thinking and verbalization.

The rate of heeding ("silent speech") has been found to be quite similar to the rate of overt speech (Landauer 1962, Weber and Bach 1969), and hence we can assume that overt vocalization occurs in parallel to the internal heeding without any requirement for additional time.

The situation is rather different for thinking aloud, where an additional verbal encoding of the heeded information is necessary. For that case we need to assume that the time required for vocalization of the corresponding verbalization is considerably greater than the time required for heeding in the silent case. The silent case is illustrated in the upper panel of figure 32.3. In a recent study, Deffner and Ericsson (1985) proposed that the additional time required for full vocalization in "think-aloud" corresponded to maintained attention to the information verbalized. "Think-aloud" would then correspond to initial heeding, as in the silent case, and then maintained heeding during the verbalization, as illustrated in the lower panel of figure 32.3. Hence, to produce the verbalization, the corresponding thought would have to remain heeded and subsequent states would not emerge until the verbalization was completed. An empirical test of this hypothesis could be made by estimating the actual time subjects vocalize, and then subtracting this time from their total solution time. Deffner and Ericsson (1985) found that verbalizations occurred in relatively short speech bursts, and by subtracting this vocalization time they eliminated previously found differences in solution time between thinking-aloud subjects and silent control subjects.

If the additional time required for verbalization in thinking aloud corresponds to maintenance of attention to the information being verbalized, it means that the attention cannot be diverted without interrupting the verbalization. Thinking aloud is, therefore, not well suited to the study of cognitive processes with real-time attentional demands involving motor skills, and tasks requiring intermittent rehearsal of information. In such cases "talk-aloud" or post-process observations like retrospective reports should be preferred. A more complete discussion is given in Ericsson and Simon (1984, chapter 5).

Methodology to Elicit "Talk-Aloud" and "Think-Aloud"

The above theoretical considerations have led us to a verbal report procedure which should provide optimal information about the thought sequence with minimal interference. In this section we will discuss a methodology for eliciting such behaviour in subjects. We will first discuss the initial instruction to subjects, then we will discuss a warm-up procedure, and then, finally, something about how one should remind subjects about the verbal report instructions.

Instructions

We will begin by examining the instructions given by the two psychologists, Duncker and Claparède, who are usually credited with introducing the method of thinking aloud.

The main part of the instruction to think aloud is usually very short, making reference to a procedure that is presumed to be already familiar to the subjects.

"Try to think aloud. I guess you often do so when you are alone and working on a problem." (Duncker 1926; underlined in original)

"Think, reason in a loud voice, tell me everything that passes through your head during your work searching for the solution to the problem." (Claparède 1934)

Thus, in Duncker's instructions, although the word "think" is used, the subjects are asked just to vocalize their thoughts, which are apparently presumed to have the form of inner speech. If the presumption is correct, it is not surprising that such short instructions could elicit the desired behaviour. Verbalizing, under this assumption, would be quite simple, because of the oral code and sequential structure of the internal speech.

In Claparède's instructions, however, the subject is asked to verbalize "everything that passes through [his] head," whether encoded orally or not. In order to comply with such an instruction, the subject would in many cases have to label and encode the content of attention, thus requiring the kinds of recoding process that are postulated in think-aloud verbalization.

Although subjects appear to understand what "thinking aloud" means, they sometimes tend to fall into other forms of verbal communication with which they are more familiar. In a school situation with mathematics tasks, where the students were accustomed to explaining their solutions aloud, Krutetskii (1976) took special pains to warn his subjects against confusing the instruction to think aloud with that of explaining the solution:

"Do not try to explain anything to anyone else. Pretend there is no one here but yourself. Do not tell about the solution but solve it." (Krutetskii 1976)

Ericsson and Simon (1984) have developed complete instructions for "thinking aloud" which have been successfully used by many investigators with occasional changes and adaptations to the particular tasks.

Warm-up

In many TA experiments, the subject is given initial warm-up problems to acquaint him with the experimental situation and accustom him to the microphones and tape recorders. Another important reason for a standardized procedure with warm-up is that we need some means to establish that all subjects are using the same verbal report procedure. Investigators using eye-movement equipment ask subjects to look at objects in different locations in the display to assure agreement between subjects' fixation points and the output of recording devices. Analogously, Ericsson and Simon (1984) recommend that subjects be asked to solve a series of standardized problems while thinking aloud. On the basis of the think-aloud reports on these problems an investigator can assess whether the subjects verbalize in a manner consistent with the instructions. If not, the subject can be reinstructed and given additional warm-up problems. Performance on such selected problems provides a means to distinguish differences in method of verbalization from differences in thought sequences, which cannot be easily separated in protocols on new problems.

Reminders

The experimenter is generally, though not always, present during TA experiments. In the earlier studies, the experimenter had to be present, since there was no other means for recording the subject's verbalizations. Although tape recorders are now used almost universally, the experimenter is still usually present, primarily to monitor the verbalizations by reminding the subject to speak, when he lapses into silence. These reminders, given after 15 s to 1 min pauses (the interval being different in different

studies), are generally standardized, taking the form of "keep talking" or "what are you thinking about?"

Reminders to verbalize of the "keep talking" variety should have a very small, if any, effect on the subject's processing. In fact, according to our theoretical model, subjects will invariably verbalize their thoughts when talking is initiated. However, a reminder of the type, "what are you thinking about?" is more likely to elicit a self-observation process or produce an other-oriented description as a response.

Other Types of Concurrent Verbal Reports

For "talk-aloud" and "think-aloud" reports we have attempted to identify a theoretical foundation by explicating the corresponding verbalization processes and their relation to the heeded information. In this section we will try to extend these considerations to the larger class of concurrent verbal report procedures.

In order to understand better the motivation for the other forms of concurrent report it is better to take on a more "naive" view. When concurrent verbal reports are collected it is desirable to gain as much information as possible about the subjects' cognitive processes. In addition to instructing subjects to think aloud, investigators often ask subjects to describe what they are doing physically or what they are perceiving visually. Another kind of complementary instruction is a request for *explanation*. In order to get as full an understanding as possible of the subjects' processes, they are asked to explain their thinking:

"In order to follow your thoughts we ask you to think aloud, explaining each step as thoroughly as you can." (Smith 1971)

These explanations allow the investigator to get an explicit description of general rules and methods used in the generation of the process. These requests for additional information may appear completely legitimate until we ask what

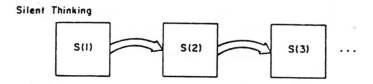

Silent Thinking

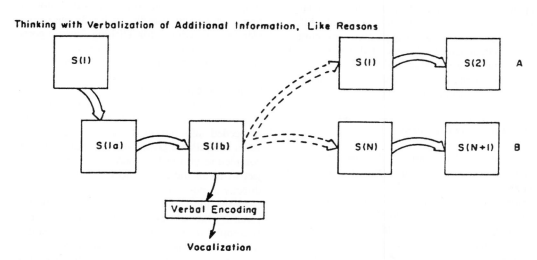

Thinking with Verbalization of Additional Information, Like Reasons

Figure 32.4
A comparison of the states of heeded information for silent thought (*upper panel*) and for thinking with instruction to verbalize reasons for every step (*lower panel*).

kind of cognitive processes would be required to produce this additional information.

If the requested information would be produced with normal "think-aloud" instructions (and the associated cognitive processes) then these additional instructions would be unnecessary. However, if the instructions force subjects to report information not normally heeded, it means that the sequences of heeded states must be changed to bring the additional information into attention for subsequent verbalization. Such changes in the sequence of states are illustrated

in figure 32.4. The sequence of states for silent thinking is given in the upper panel, while the sequence of states associated with an instruction to verbalize additional information is shown in the lower panel. To simplify the comparison we assume that the first state of both sequences, S(1), is identical. After the extra states necessary for the additional verbalization of description or explanation have been generated, it is conceivable that the subject could reinstate the original state, S(1), and proceed with the next steps in the cognitive process (marked as alternative A), especially when a familiar procedure is followed. It is more likely that in tasks requiring productive thinking the state following the additional verbalizing will differ from the state encountered during silent thought (marked as alternative B). In a review of research comparing silent subjects' performance to the performance of subjects with a requirement to verbalize additional information (especially explanations and reasons) (Ericsson and Simon 1984, chapter 2), a large proportion of the studies showed reliable differences between the two groups even in accuracy and characteristics of generated solutions. A requirement to verbalize additional information leads to changes in the sequence of thoughts compared to silent control subjects.

Post-Process Observations

Once subjects have performed a task, one might think that no further information about their cognitive processes could be recorded. However, testing subjects' memory can provide three additional types of observation. In experiments on thinking, the same information may not always be continuously available to subjects. For instance, instructions may be given only once to subjects who must then rely on their memory of the instructions to perform the task. The subjects can therefore be tested after an experiment for their memory of the instructions or for their memory of other types of task information (memory for task information). Another type of observation is obtained by instructing subjects to remember the specific thoughts they had while generating the response (retrospective reports). And a final category of observations is obtained by questioning subjects, after the experiments are completed, about strategies and representations used (postexperimental questioning).

As the focus of this chapter is on verbal reports on thought processes, retrospective reports will first be considered from our theoretical framework and then we will proceed to discuss

the more complex forms of verbal reports associated with postexperimental questioning.

Retrospective Reports

From our theoretical analysis of the cognitive process it follows what kinds of information we would like the subject to report retrospectively. The first section attempts to specify how the subject would be able to retrieve such information, and we will also discuss briefly the recommended procedures for eliciting such reports. Finally, we will discuss the broader range of verbal report and interviewing procedures.

Theoretical Considerations

Within our theoretical framework the cognitive processes are represented as sequences of states of heeded information (thoughts). Hence, even when subjects are giving verbal reports after the completion of a task or tasks, we want the subject to recall these sequences as accurately and directly as possible.

In the ideal case the retrospective report is given by the subject immediately after the task is completed, while much information is still in STM or otherwise directly accessible, and can be directly reported or used as a retrieval cue. It is clear that some additional cognitive processing is required to make certain that the particular memory structures of interest are heeded. Our model predicts that retrospective reports on the immediately preceding cognitive activity can be accessed and specified without the experimenter having to provide the subject with specific information about what to retrieve. In this particular case, the subject will have the necessary retrieval cues in STM after a general instruction is given "to report everything you can remember about your thoughts during the last problem." This form of retrospective verbal report should give us the closest approximation to the actual memory structures.

Even in this favourable case, some problems arise that are common to all kinds of verbal reports from LTM. First, the retrieval operation is fallible, in that other similar memory structures may be accessed instead of those created by the just-finished cognitive process. The probability of this occurring increases markedly if the subjects have just solved a series of similar problems. However, since most accessed memory structures contain redundant information beyond the cues used for retrieval, subjects may use this additional information to validate the retrieval as well as to increase their confidence in the veridicality of the retrieved information. In a subsequent section we will discuss this type of evaluation further and examine the relevant theoretical and empirical literature.

A second general problem when retrieving cognitive structures is to separate information that was heeded at the time of a specific episode, from information acquired previously or subsequently that is associated with it (Müller 1911). For example, if a picture reminds one of an old friend, it may be tempting to use the stored information about that friend to *infer* what the person in the picture looked like. It may be possible to eliminate this artifact by instructing subjects only to report details that they can remember heeding at the time of the original episode (Müller 1911). By imposing a requirement of determinable memory as a basis for reporting, we can avoid many subjects' tendency to fill in information that they can't remember but "must" have thought. It is possible to distinguish such inferred information from the remembered information by showing that such inferences would not be part of the possible sequences of thoughts. Hence, an analysis of the content and temporal characteristics of the generated retrospective reports allows us to assess that the instructions are followed, and we need not rely on simply trusting the subjects.

In analogy with the procedures for instructing subjects to "think-aloud," it appears to be essential to provide warm-up tasks which are particularly suited for retrospective reports. It is easy to monitor the instruction to report specific thoughts. The subject is instructed to think aloud during the solution of the warm-up problems; then the subject's retrospective report is compared to his think-aloud report.

From our theoretical perspective the retrospective reports will contain a sequence of heeded thoughts quite similar to that elicited with "think-aloud" instructions. When the studied cognitive process is of long duration, it is likely that many steps of the cognitive process will not be recalled at the end of the task and will be omitted from the retrospective report.

There are several methods available to reduce the level of omissions. A commonly used procedure is to break down the original task into smaller components with a retrospective report following each. For example, in studies of text comprehension, several investigators have divided the text into sentences. The subject reads the sentences one-by-one and gives a retrospective report after each. This procedure has been found to provide rich information, which allows monitoring concurrent expectations and comprehension, uncontaminated by subsequent events and information contained in the text (Olson, Mack, and Duffy 1981; Waern 1979). Another possibility discussed in Ericsson and Simon 1984 (chapter 5) is to disrupt the cognitive processes at particular points in the solution of the task and ask for an immediate retrospective report. This last method is obviously quite intensive and should only be used on small proportions of randomly selected trials to ensure that the subject maintains normal task performance.

A rather different method attempts to increase subjects' recall by providing better retrieval cues at the time of giving retrospective reports. Asking subjects to recall thoughts of specified kinds is not recommended, unless the experimenter has previously established that thoughts of such kinds occur with all subjects. Otherwise it might bias subjects toward accepting low-confidence memories or even toward fabricating such thoughts. Furthermore, on trials following such probing, subjects might change their cognitive processes in order to effectively monitor further occurrences of such thoughts.

In the absence of a detailed description of a subject's thoughts it is hard to provide helpful and non-biasing retrieval cues. However, many investigators have collected concurrent eye-movements of subjects during the solution of tasks. Several studies (Deffner 1984, Winikoff 1967) have shown that concurrent verbal reports referring to perceptually available objects and information is reliably related to eye-fixations of the areas containing the corresponding information. Hence, displaying the sequence of eye-fixations recorded during the solution should provide effective cues for the subject's recall of the concurrent thoughts. Such aided recall has been used by several investigators, and retrospective verbal reports under these conditions have been found to be longer (measured by a word count) than normal retrospective reports. However, such aided recall raises an important methodological problem. Do the subjects actually recall their thoughts *or* do the subjects infer what they might have, or must have, thought given the displayed sequences of eye-fixations? We are not aware of any studies that have systematically explored this question. It would be possible to test whether subjects could reliably recognize parts of their sequences of eye-fixations from other subjects' for the same task, as well as subjects' ability to predict directly subsequent thoughts and corresponding eye-fixations. Let us now discuss other types of retrospective questioning and interviewing techniques, where the issue of memory versus inference becomes critical.

Other Types of Retrospective Questioning and Interviewing

According to our theoretical assumptions, even a complete retrospective report will only contain a sequence of states of heeded information, as is illustrated in figure 32.5. Many investigators

of human thought have tried to probe subjects for additional information. At the turn of the century, Titchener and other analytic introspectionists sought to describe the individual thoughts as completely as possible. Each thought should be described in terms of its smallest element, that is, its sensory components, as is illustrated in the middle panel of figure 32.5. A different type of information often sought are the relations or connections of states of heeded information. This additional information corresponds to asking why a given heeded thought emerged or why some heeded thought followed another heeded thought, as is illustrated in the lower panel of figure 32.5.

Analysis of Individual Thoughts

The method of introspection, or observing the contents of one's mind, has been used frequently to gain information about thinking and the structure of thought. According to the theoretical assumptions of the analytic introspectionists, each thought could be described by enumerating its sensory elements. Hence, an analysis of a sequence of thoughts during a task should be made through a careful description of the elements of each thought. William James criticized such descriptions because the sensory elements were not immediately available—only the object of thought—and, hence, the sensory component could only be extracted through additional analysis. Later, this view became generally recognized, as concurrent analysis of thought into elements was found to disrupt and change the thought process (Lindworsky 1931).

The problem of disruption was avoided by postponing the analysis of the thoughts until the cognitive processes were completed, that is, retrospective analysis of thought. Within our framework such analysis would correspond to recall of each of the heeded thoughts, but in addition all recalled thoughts need to be processed further to extract their components, preferably their sensory elements. This subsequent analysis of a recalled thought will require additional

Silent Thought

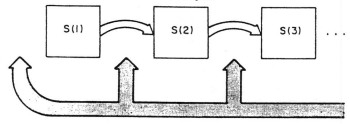

Analytic Introspection

Concurrently Active
Sensory Element

Verbal Reports of Causes of Heeded Thoughts

Figure 32.5
A contrast between the information contained in a retrospective report after silent thought (*upper panel*) and the information requested by analytic introspection (*middle panel*) or by studies requesting causes or reasons for thoughts and actions (*lower panel*).

retrievals, which may or may not yield information related to the originally heeded thought. Even long after the demise of analytic introspection, investigators have asked subjects questions about image characteristics of their thoughts, which would require a similar retrospective analysis for their answers. Although the current research on such issues is quite active, no clear account of the relationship between imagery reports and thinking/memory has emerged (Sheikh 1983). For our present purposes the important conclusion is that the subsequently retrieved elements of a thought were not heeded initially and, therefore, not part of the information heeded originally.

Establishing Reasons and Causes of Thoughts and Actions

It has been traditional in many experiments to ask subjects *why* they did something, or why they preferred some alternatives over others. In a very important review, Nisbett and Wilson (1977) showed that subjects' reasons frequently were inaccurate in accounting for the experimental variables that actually influence their behaviour. The article raised a number of methodological issues that have been discussed in detail elsewhere (Ericsson and Simon 1980, Nisbett and Ross 1980, Smith and Miller 1978, White 1980). For our current purposes it is sufficient to note that giving a reason for one's thought or thought sequence (ideally, a cause relating to external stimuli) is quite different from reporting the thought sequence as remembered. Let us illustrate this point with an example.

When asked to generate a word starting with the letter "A" most undergraduates respond with "apple." If asked for a retrospective report they say that it simply "popped up" or "came," and are unable to report any intermediate thoughts. When asked why they thought of "apple" rather than any of thousands of words, they are quite willing to speculate, "I had an apple for lunch," "In grade school I learned 'A as in apple'," and so on. One likely strategy for arriving at these inferred reasons is to use the response word (i.e.,

"apple"), as a retrieval cue to find any pertinent episodes or associative relations to the given cue (i.e., starting with the letter "A"). These generated characteristics have to be judged for plausibility and can be readily used for inferring "reasons" for other people's behaviour.

Even for cognitive processes involving several intermediate states or thoughts, similar problems exist. Subjects solving mental multiplication problems correctly are essentially unable to tell us why they did, or didn't, use a familiar short cut in a calculation procedure. In recognition of perceptually available objects, or during memory retrieval, there is considerable evidence for processes without intermediate heeded steps where the subject is only aware of the results of the processes. In sum, asking subjects to give more information than they can recall, as part of their retrospective report, is likely to lead to additional inferential processing with no obvious relation to a particular observed cognitive process.

Determining General Strategies and Procedures of Subjects

Most investigators seek to identify the general strategies or procedures used by subjects in performing the experimental tasks. Hence, it has been a long-standing tradition in psychology to interview subjects after the experiment, where questioning cannot possibly bias the earlier recorded performance data. Subjects are often asked to describe how they solved the tasks, and so on. The implicit assumption is that the subjects relied on a single strategy throughout the experiment and that they are able to recall this general strategy. However, there is considerable evidence that subjects' cognitive processes change during the experiment as a function of practice, and different cognitive processes and methods are used for problems in the same task domain. In cases of such diversity of cognitive processes, how do subjects describe their procedures? This question has not been seriously considered by investigators using postexperimental questioning.

Ericsson and Simon (1980) argued that this procedure is questionable if one wants to gain access to subjects' specific memory of their cognitive processes. After a large number of trials, subjects' memory for cognitive processes on individual tasks is quite poor due to interference from many similar solutions and the relatively long delay. Ericsson and Simon (1984) proposed that subjects might rely on their memory for a few, possibly unrepresentative, trials and attempt to abstract some general characteristics. Another possibility is that subjects would recall some of the tasks and retrieve or generate methods for solving these tasks. Regardless of the cognitive processes proposed for generating these verbal descriptions of strategies, it is clear that they would not be a veridical summary of all cognitive processes used in the experiments. Hence, the fact that some investigators have found inconsistencies between postexperimental interview data and actual performance data during the experiments is not surprising.

Summary

In analogy with our discussion of concurrent reports, we have argued for collecting retrospective reports consisting of memory for sequences of heeded thoughts. These reports constitute observations on the cognitive processes on a par with other types of data. After a comprehensive task analysis has been completed, these retrospective reports can then be encoded to supply data on the sequence of cognitive processes employed in a given solution. Analysis of reliable connections between states of heeded information and use of general strategies can be converted into empirically testable hypotheses regarding sequences of heeded information and we need not ask the subject to provide such information. It should be stressed that these other reporting instructions are not judged to be scientifically invalid. With a better understanding of the cognitive processes used to access this additional information, and of the relation between this additional information and the information

heeded during the solutions, such reports should provide converging information on thinking.

Protocol Analysis

Up to this point we have been primarily concerned with task analysis and methodology for collecting verbal reports. The analysis and encoding of reports can be quite straightforward within our theoretical framework. In the most favourable case the task analysis has provided a large number of possible *unique* states with heeded information. In the encoding phase the verbal reports are segmented into verbalizations of heeded thoughts and the corresponding unique state from the task analysis is identified. However, in most actual studies using protocol analysis the mapping between verbal reports and states in the task analysis is not unambiguous and unique, due to the similarity of the heeded information in different states and lack of specificity of the verbal reports. Ericsson and Simon (1984) discuss many methods to deal with such situations. One very general method is to encode selectively a small number of unique and distinct states corresponding to alternative processing models, among which the investigator wants to determine the best one. Further discussion of such methods is not possible within the scope of this chapter. Instead, two examples of encoding and analysis of verbal reports will be presented. The first example demonstrates encoding of think-aloud protocols for a case in which the number of possible thoughts is too large and explicit enumeration is not feasible. The second discusses an analysis of cognitive processes using retrospective reports.

Think-Aloud Protocols from Anagram Problem Solving

In the anagram task, subjects are presented with a scrambled sequence of letters and asked to generate an English word using all the letters.

From previous published work reporting think-ing-aloud protocols collected for the anagram-solving task (Mayzner, Tresselt, and Helbock 1964; Sargent 1940), we know that subjects heed several different kinds of information while solving these problems. Two types of information are especially prominent in protocols.

First, subjects select likely combinations of letters (sequences that occur frequently in English) and use these as constraints for generating longer strings or as probes to LTM to evoke words that contain those combinations. We encode mentions of such combinations in the protocols as C: L1–L2–...–L3 (Position), where C signifies Constraint, L1, L2, L3 are letters, and Position refers to the beginning, middle, or end part of the word.

Second, subjects generate alternative possible solution words. These can derive from attempts to sound out letter combinations or can be related words evoked from LTM. These possible solutions are encoded as A: (spelling of word or combination of syllables), where A signifies Alternative. In table 32.2 we give several short protocols of subjects solving the anagram "NPEHPA." (The first two of these protocols are reproduced from Sargent 1940.)

These protocols depend heavily upon recognition processes and evocation of information from LTM. A computer model could be programmed to produce qualitatively similar protocols, but it is impossible, in the absence of detailed knowledge of how subjects have information stored and indexed in LTM, to predict the sequence of events in any particular subjects' thinking-aloud protocol. In spite of the use of common processes, different subjects arrive at the anagram solution along different routes.

Retrospective Reports

Ericsson and Simon (1984) reviewed the relatively extensive evidence showing that subjects' retrospective verbal reports provide reliable in-

Table 32.2

Transcript of three thinking-aloud protocols from subjects solving the anagram 'NPEHPA'

Protocol 1	
N–P, neph, neph	
Probably PH goes together	C:PH
Phan	A:phan
Phanny	A:phanny
I get phan-ep	A:phan-ep
no. Nap-	A:nap
Phep-an, no	A:phep-an
E is at the end	C:E(end)
Phap-en	A:phap-en
People, I think of	A:people
Try PH after the other letters	C:PH(end)
Naph, no	A:naph
I thought of paper again	A:paper
E and A sound alike couldn't go together without a consonant	
Try double P	C:PP
happy	A:happy
Happen	A:happen
Protocol 2	
Start with P	C:P(beginning)
No, it doesn't the two P's go together	C:PP
Happen	A:happen
Protocol 3	
All right	
Let's see	
NPEHPA	
Let's try what letters go together	
Do you want to tell me when I miss, okay	
PH go together	C:PH
but they're not very likely so how about APP	C:APP
Oh, happen	A:happen
Got it	

Note: The first two protocols were recorded by Sargent (1940). On the right side encodings of the verbalized thoughts are given. (From Ericsson and Simon, 1985.)

formation to predict the latencies for a variety of task domains. The validity of retrospective verbal reports extended to tasks with average latencies of less than two seconds. Systematic attempts to derive a processing model to predict the observed reaction times, on the basis of retrospective reports, are much rarer. Two English investigators, Hamilton and Sanford (1978), studied subjects who made simple judgements of whether two presented letters, like "RP" or "MO," were in alphabetical order or not. In accord with previous investigators, they found that the reaction times were longer when the two presented letters occurred close together in the alphabet than when they were far apart. From the reaction time data alone, one would infer a uniform retrieval process, where factors internal to the retrieval process required more time for order decisions for letters occurring close together in the alphabet. Retrospective verbal reports, for subjects doing individual decisions, indicated two types of cognitive processes. For some of the trials, subjects reported no mediation or direct access of their order judgment. For other trials, subjects reported they ran through brief segments of the alphabet before making a decision of order. For example, when the letter-pair "MO" was presented, a subject reported retrieving "LMNO" before the subject reached the decision that the letters were in alphabetical order. In another case, a subject reported retrieving "RSTUV" before rejecting the letter-pair "RP" as not being in alphabetical order. In a subsequent analysis of the reaction times, Hamilton and Sanford (1978) found very different relations for trials with direct access, versus trials with retrieval of segments of the alphabet. For trials with retrieval, the observed reaction time was a linear function of the number of retrieved letters. The estimated rate of retrieval corresponded closely to rates obtained in studying simple recital of the alphabet. For trials with reports of direct access, no relation of reaction time to the amount of separation of the two letters was found. Hamilton and Sanford (1978)

concluded that the original effect was due to a mixture of two quite different processes, and that closeness of the letters influenced the probability that recall of letters would be necessary before an order decision could be made.

Summary and Conclusions

The goal of this chapter was to analyse verbal reports on cognitive processes and explicate their relation to those processes. The information-processing theory was used as a theoretical framework for describing thinking. Within this framework, thinking can be represented as a sequence of states of heeded information (thoughts). From a task analysis it is possible to specify a number of a priori plausible thought sequences, which are sufficient to generate the correct answer. By collecting observations on the thought processes and by specifying how these observations reflect the sequence and durations of processing steps, many alternative accounts of the thought processes can be eliminated.

Procedures for collecting concurrent and retrospective verbal reports were described, where the verbal reports consist of verbalizations of the sequence of heeded thoughts. These verbalizing procedures allow the thought processes to proceed along their normal course and, with only one exception, at their normal rate. When subjects "think aloud" the rate of thinking has to be slowed down to allow for the additional time required for verbalization of the heeded thought. Concurrent and retrospective verbal reports contain sequences of verbalized thoughts, which can be matched against the a priori plausible thought sequences given by the task analysis.

Other procedures for eliciting concurrent verbal reports were analysed and changes in the thought processes could be identified as a function of complying with the instructions. The problems with other types of retrospective report procedures concerned requests for information beyond memory for heeded thoughts. Attempts were made to specify the information retrieved by these other types of reporting procedures.

Within the framework of information processing we have been able to describe the thought process as a sequence of thoughts and show how a wide range of observations reflect its characteristics. It is important to note that observations in the form of verbal reports are analysed in a manner analogous to other observations, like eye-movements and reaction times. In fact, a considerable number of studies have used the redundancy between observations, like eye-movements and verbal reports, to provide convergent validation of the description of the thought processes.

To build an adequate theory of a dynamic system, like the human brain solving problems, observations must be made on that system at a temporal density commensurate with the speed of its processes. Although they are not fully adequate for catching the fine grain of thought processes, verbal protocols and recordings of eye movements have provided data at the highest densities we have as yet attained. For this reason, they have been, and remain, indispensable experimental tools in contemporary cognitive science.

Note

This chapter is, for the most part, a summary of ideas developed in more detail in Ericsson and Simon (1984, 1985) and Ericsson and Oliver (1988). We would like to sincerely thank Victor Schoenberg for his helpful comments and suggestions on earlier drafts of this chapter.

References

Bühler, K. 1951, On thought connections. In D. Rapaport (ed.), *Organization and Pathology of Thought*. New York: Columbia University Press.

Claparède, E. 1934, Genese de l'hypothèses. *Archives de Psychologie 24*, 1–155.

Deffner, G. 1984, Lautes Denken-Untersuchung zur Qualität eines Datenerhebungsverfahrens. Frankfurt: Lang.

Deffner, G. and Ericsson, K. A. 1985, *Sprechtempo und Pausen bei lautem Denken*. Paper presented at Tagung experimentell arbeitender Psychologen. Wuppertal, West Germany.

Duncker, K. 1926, A qualitative (experimental and theoretical) study of productive thinking (solving of comprehensible problems). *Pedagogical Seminary 33*, 642–708.

Duncker, K. 1945, On problem solving (Entire issue). *Psychology Monographs*, 58:5.

Ebbinghaus, H. 1964, *Memory: A Contribution to Experimental Psychology*. H. A. Ruger and C. E. Bussenius, trans. New York: Dover Publications, Inc. (Originally published 1885).

Ericsson, K. A. and Oliver, W. 1988, Methodology for laboratory research on thinking: Task selection, collection of observations and data analysis. Invited chapter in R. J. Sternberg and E. E. Smith (eds), *The Psychology of Human Thought*. New York: Cambridge University Press.

Ericsson, K. A. and Simon, H. A. 1980, Verbal reports as data. *Psychological Review 87*, 215–51.

Ericsson, K. A. and Simon, H. A. 1984, *Protocol Analysis*. Cambridge, Mass.: MIT Press/Bradford.

Ericsson, K. A. and Simon, H. A. 1985, Protocol analysis. In T. A. van Dijk (ed.), *Handbook of Discourse Analysis*, Vol. 2. New York: Academic Press, 259–68.

Estes, W. K. 1976, The cognitive side of probability learning. *Psychological Review 83*, 37–64.

Freud, S. 1914, *Psychopathology of Everyday Life*. New York: Macmillan.

Ginsberg, H. (ed.) 1983, *The Development of Mathematical Learning*. New York: Academic Press.

Guyotte, M. J. and Sternberg, R. J. 1981, A transitive-chain theory of syllogistic reasoning. *Cognitive Psychology 13*, 461–525.

Hamilton, J. M. E. and Sanford, A. J. 1978, The symbolic distance effect for alphabetic order judgments: A subjective report and reaction time analysis. *Quarterly Journal of Experimental Psychology 30*, 33–43.

Inhelder, B. and Piaget, J. 1958, *The Growth of Logical Thinking from Childhood to Adolescence*. New York: Basic Books.

Johnson-Laird, P. N. and Steedman, M. 1978, The psychology of syllogisms. *Cognitive Psychology 10*, 64–99.

Jung, C. G. 1910, The association method. *American Journal of Psychology* 21, 219–69.

Krutetskii, V. A. 1976, *The Psychology of Mathematical Problem Solving*. Chicago, Ill.: University of Chicago Press.

Landauer, T. K. 1962, Rate of implicit speech. *Perceptual and Motor Skills* 15, 646.

Lindworsky, J. 1931, *Experimental Methodology*. New York: Macmillan.

Mayzner, M. S., Tresselt, M. E. and Helbock, H. 1964, An exploratory study of mediational responses in anagram problem solving. *Journal of General Psychology* 57, 263–74.

Montague, W. E. 1972, Elaborative strategies in verbal learning and memory. In G. H. Bower (ed.), *The Psychology of Learning and Motivation* (Vol. 6). New York: Academic Press.

Müller, G. E. 1911, Zur Analyse der Gedächtnistätigkeit und des Vorstellungsverlaufes: Teil I. *Zeitschrift für Psychologie, Ergänzungsband* 5.

Newell, A., Shaw, J. C. and Simon, H. A. 1958, Elements of a theory of human problem solving. *Psychological Review* 65, 151–66.

Newell, A. and Simon, H. A. 1972, *Human Problem Solving*. Englewood Cliffs, N.J.: Prentice-Hall.

Nisbett, R. E. and Ross, L. 1980, *Human Inference: Strategies and Shortcomings of Social Judgment*. Englewood Cliffs, N.J.: Prentice-Hall.

Nisbett, R. E. and Wilson, T. D. 1977, Telling more than we can know: Verbal reports on mental processes. *Psychological Review* 84, 231–59.

Olson, G. M., Mack, R. L. and Duffy, S. A. 1981, Cognitive aspects of genre. *Poetics* 10, 283–315.

Sargent, S. S. 1940, Thinking processes at various levels of difficulty. *Archives of Psychology* 249, 5–58.

Selz, O. 1913, *Über die Gesetze des geordneten Denkverlaufs*. Stuttgart: Spemann.

Selz, O. 1922, *Zur Psychologie des produktiven Denkens und des Irrtums*. Bonn: Friedrich Cohen.

Sheikh, A. A. (ed.) 1983, *Imagery: Current Theory, Research, and Application*. New York: Wiley.

Smith, C. O. 1971, *The Structure of Intellect Processes Analyses System. A Technique for the Investigation and Quantification of Problem Solving Processes*. Unpublished doctoral dissertation, University of Houston.

Smith, E. R. and Miller, F. S. 1978, Limits on the perception of cognitive processes: A reply to Nisbett & Wilson. *Psychological Review* 85, 355–62.

Titchener, E. B. 1912, The schema of introspection. *American Journal of Psychology* 23, 485–508.

Waern, Y. 1979, *Thinking Aloud during Reading: A Descriptive Model and Its Application* (Report No. 546). Stockholm: Department of Psychology, University of Stockholm.

Weber, R. J. and Bach, M. 1969, Visual and speech imagery. *British Journal of Psychology* 60, 199–202.

Wertheimer, M. 1945, *Productive Thinking*. New York: Harper & Row.

White, P. 1980, Limitations on verbal reports of internal events: A refutation of Nisbett and Wilson and of Gem. *Psychological Review* 87, 105–12.

Winikoff, A. 1967, *Eye Movements as an Aid to Protocol Analysis of Problem Solving Behavior*. Unpublished doctoral dissertation, Carnegie-Mellon University.

VI BELOW THE THRESHOLD OF SENSORY CONSCIOUSNESS

Perhaps the single largest literature today involves subliminal stimulus presentations. These are studies of unconscious processes, but they have relevance to consciousness as well. Controversy has existed about the reality of subliminally provided information since the "New Look in psychology" of the 1950s (Erdelyi 1974). Much of that debate was resolved when Marcel (1983) and others showed that subliminal visual words could reliably "prime" semantically related tasks. Thus a subliminal word like "cat" would influence the response time for deciding whether a supraliminally presented word like "dog" was a real word or not. These reliable findings led to an explosion of research studies on subliminal tasks.

Cheesman and Merikle (1986; chap. 33, this volume) proposed an influential distinction between the "objective threshold," which involves detection of any kind, and the "subjective threshold," the threshold of experienced sensory report. The objective threshold is lower than the subjective threshold. Subliminal processes therefore can be defined as those that take place below the subjective threshold but above the objective one.

Shevrin and Dickman (1980; chap. 34, this volume) represent a long-term research program aimed at testing psychoanalytic ideas about the unconscious by way of subliminally presented stimuli. Their article appeared at a time when the notion of a complex unconscious was itself out of favor. Even today there is controversy over the complexity of subliminal processing, as mentioned above, though there are clearly many complex, intelligent, and abstract processes that are unconscious owing to automaticity and being stored in memory. There is also good evidence for active processing of unattended input, though it may be limited in dealing with novelty. There is additional evidence for dissociation from consciousness in hypnosis, absorption and neurological conditions (see section 8). All of that still adds up to a rather boring unconscious from a psychodynamic point of view, an unconscious that is not rich in impulsive motives, inner conflict, ego defenses, and profound symbolism. There is no consensus today regarding such dynamic unconscious mechanisms, but our methods for studying unconscious processes are still quite primitive. Ignorance is not an argument either for or against any given hypothesis.

Benjamin Libet has carried on an influential research program using subliminal stimulation, both in the somatosensory projection areas of the brain and at the skin receptor sites. His 1982 article (chap. 35, this volume) states some basic claims emerging from the research, including the observations that it may take as long as 0.5 s for a stimulus to come to consciousness, and that cortical stimulation can modify the perception of skin stimuli a half second before. There are a number of "backward referring" phenomena in auditory and visual perception, but it is not clear whether such phenomena occur routinely or as an artifact of experimental conditions. It is difficult to replicate Libet's remarkable studies, given that they often involve patients during neurosurgery. Nevertheless, these are pioneering experiments with great impact on the field.

Subliminal processes appear to be severely limited. There is no evidence, for example, that novel combinations of subliminal words can be combined into coherent wholes (Greenwald 1992; see also MacKay 1973; chap. 16, this volume). Thus subliminally presented words like "mountain" and "goat" may each prime related conscious words, but the combination "mountain goat" may not be integrated subliminally into a meaningful single idea. This is interesting in that it suggests that consciousness may be needed for novel integration of known elements. There are very complex unconscious processes of course, such as the automatic analysis of syntax and meaning in sentence comprehension. But subliminal input processes may be so severely limited that they may not be as revealing as other ways of investigating unconscious processes. Thus the subliminal controversy persists in new ways.

References

Erdelyi, M. H. (1974) A new look at the New Look: Perceptual defense and vigilance. *Psychological Review*, 81, 186–190.

Marcel, A. J. (1983) Conscious and unconscious perception: Experiments on visual masking and word recognition. *Cognitive Psychology*, 15, 197–237.

Greenwald, A. (1992) New Look 3, Unconscious cognition reclaimed. *American Psychologist*, 47, 766–779.

33   Distinguishing Conscious from Unconscious Perceptual Processes

Jim Cheesman and Philip M. Merikle

The relationship between perceptual processing and awareness has been the subject of considerable debate for over 30 years. Over this period of time, a pivotal question has concerned whether or not the meaning of visual stimuli is perceived in the absence of awareness or, in other words, in the absence of conscious perceptual processing. Unfortunately, in spite of an extensive number of investigations directed at answering this question (see Dixon 1971, 1981; Holender 1986, for reviews), there is still no general agreement concerning whether conscious perceptual processing is necessary for the perception of meaning.

The present studies reflect our attempt to resolve some of the issues that have continually plagued research investigating the relationship between perceptual processing and awareness. Our proposed resolution is based on a distinction between subjective and objective recognition thresholds (Cheesman and Merikle 1984), and it follows from our previous suggestion that the boundary between conscious and unconscious perceptual processes should be defined in terms of subjective rather than objective thresholds (Cheesman and Merikle 1985, Merikle and Cheesman 1986). A *subjective threshold* is the level of discriminative responding at which observers claim not to be able to detect or recognize perceptual information at a better than chance level of performance, whereas an *objective threshold* is the level of discriminative responding corresponding to chance level performance. Given that perceptual awareness or consciousness is a subjective state, we propose that the subjective threshold, or the threshold for *claimed* awareness, better captures the phenomenological distinction between conscious and unconscious perceptual experiences and that the subjective threshold, therefore, provides a better definition of the boundary between conscious and unconscious processes than is provided by the objective threshold.

In many of the recent studies directed at distinguishing conscious from unconscious perceptual processes, the masked-prime paradigm, originally reported by Marcel (1974, 1983a), has been used, and the boundary between conscious and unconscious processes has been defined in terms of an objective threshold for forced-choice recognition or detection (Balota 1983; Cheesman and Merikle 1984; Fowler, Wolford, Slade, and Tassinary 1981; Marcel 1980, 1983a; McCauley, Parmelee, Sperber, and Carr 1980; Purcell, Stewart, and Stanovich 1983). In this type of study, the presentation of a target stimulus is preceded by the presentation of a priming stimulus which is either clearly visible or centrally masked so as to preclude it from awareness, as indicated by chance level performance on a forced-choice recognition or detection task. By defining the boundary between conscious and unconscious processes in terms of an objective threshold, conscious perceptual processing in these studies was equated with an ability to make discriminative responses, and, conversely, unconscious perceptual processing was equated with an inability to make such responses. Although this approach for distinguishing conscious from unconscious perceptual processes has considerable theoretical and empirical appeal (cf. Eriksen 1960), the recent masked-prime studies in which this approach has been adopted have provided discrepant empirical findings.

In general, two different patterns of results have emerged from these studies involving masked priming stimuli. The results from one group of studies suggest that the meaning of primes is perceived even when it is impossible to decide if these stimuli have been presented (Balota 1983; Fowler et al. 1981; Marcel 1980, 1983a; McCauley et al. 1980). This conclusion is based on observations indicating that masked primes, presented below an observer's objective threshold, nevertheless affect decision times to target stimuli. On the other hand, the results from other studies suggest that the meaning of primes is perceived only when they can be recognized or detected at a better than chance level of accuracy (Cheesman and Merikle 1984, Purcell et al. 1983). These latter studies raise serious questions concerning whether it is possible to perceive the meaning of stimuli presented at or below an observer's objective threshold, and the results of these studies suggest that the masked-prime studies presumed to demonstrate unconscious perceptual processing may contain serious methodological flaws.

The proposed distinction between objective and subjective thresholds provides a possible basis for resolving this apparent discrepancy between the results obtained in these different masked-prime studies. If it is assumed that subjective rather than objective thresholds were inadvertently established in the masked-primed studies which appear to indicate that priming occurs in the absence of discriminative responding (Balota 1983; Fowler et al. 1981; Marcel 1980, 1983a; McCauley et al. 1980), then the apparently contradictory patterns of results may not be contradictory at all. Our previous research indicates that somewhat higher stimulus energy levels are associated with subjective than with objective thresholds and that considerable perceptual processing, as indicated by discriminative reports, occurs when information is presented at energy levels between the ones defined by these two thresholds (Cheesman and Merikle 1984). Furthermore, the methods used to establish objective thresholds in the masked-prime studies presumed to demonstrate unconscious perceptual processing are not capable of distinguishing between objective and subjective thresholds (cf. Merikle 1982); thus, it is entirely possible that subjective rather than objective thresholds were established in these studies. If this did occur, then the apparently contradictory results found in different masked-prime studies may actually be consistent; all masked-prime studies may actually demonstrate

that considerable perceptual processing occurs when observers *claim* that they are not aware of a stimulus or, in other words, when stimuli are presented below an observer's subjective threshold.

One implication of defining the boundary between conscious and unconscious perceptual processes in terms of an observer's subjective threshold is that discriminative responding, per se, may provide a completely adequate index of all perceptual processing, both conscious and unconscious. Given that the subjective threshold is associated with a higher stimulus energy level than the objective threshold, the transition from unconscious to conscious perceptual processing, as indicated by the subjective threshold, must necessarily occur at a stimulus energy level associated with above chance discriminative responding. According to the proposed view, stimuli presented above the subjective threshold are consciously processed, whereas stimuli presented at energy levels between the objective and subjective thresholds are unconsciously processed. On the other hand, when discriminative responding indicates a complete absence of perceptual processing, then it may be impossible to demonstrate either conscious or unconscious perceptual processes. This view of the relationship between discriminative responding and perceptual processing is entirely consistent with our previously reported findings indicating that priming and forced-choice recognition are equally sensitive measures of perceptual processing (Cheesman and Merikle 1984). This view is also consistent with Eriksen's (1960) earlier conclusion that discriminative responding provides as sensitive an indicator of perceptual processing as any other response.

Unfortunately the empirical problem of distinguishing conscious from unconscious processes is not solved by simply changing the definition of awareness. Many criticisms can be directed at any approach that equates awareness solely with a subjective threshold. The most obvious criticism is that any measure of awareness based on subjective confidence alone allows each observer to establish his or her own criteria for awareness (cf. Merikle 1983, 1984). Furthermore, as noted by Eriksen (1960), there can never be any empirical validation of the measure itself, since differences in subjective confidence cannot be distinguished empirically from response bias. Thus, if the awareness threshold is simply equated with the subjective threshold, disagreements concerning perception without awareness will never be resolved because of the impossibility of establishing the validity of the subjective threshold as an adequate measure of awareness.

Given these problems with defining awareness solely in terms of a subjective threshold, at least one additional criterion must be used to distinguish conscious from unconscious processes. Fortunately, the solution to this definitional problem has been expressed several times (Dixon 1971, 1981; Shevrin and Dickman 1980), although the proposed solution has had surprisingly little empirical impact. Simply stated, the additional criterion needed to distinguish conscious and unconscious perceptual processes is a demonstration that a particular independent variable has a qualitatively different effect when information is consciously perceived than when the same information is unconsciously perceived. The demonstration of qualitative differences provides much stronger support for the distinction between conscious and unconscious processes than is provided by an approach based solely on evidence indicating that perceptual information is processed both above and below a particular threshold. In fact, if qualitative differences cannot be established, then it is probably impossible to reach general agreement as to the most appropriate definition of awareness.

A major weakness in the approach exemplified by many of the recent studies presumed to provide evidence for unconscious perceptual processes is that the experimental data have consisted only of demonstrations indicating that priming is produced by stimuli presented above

and below a particular awareness threshold (Balota 1983; Fowler et al. 1981; Marcel 1983a). Thus, the conclusiveness of the reported data depends entirely upon the adequacy with which the awareness thresholds in these studies were defined and measured, and it is the absence of any general consensus concerning the adequacy of the threshold measures used in these studies that has led to the disagreements concerning the importance of the reported findings for the perception-without-awareness hypothesis (Henley 1984; Merikle 1982, 1984; Purcell et al. 1983).

To overcome the problems associated with these recent approaches to the study of unconscious perceptual processes, the approach adopted in the present studies was based on first defining an awareness threshold in terms of an observer's subjective threshold and then attempting to establish that the same perceptual information presented above or below this threshold has qualitatively different behavioural effects. If it can be demonstrated that perceptual information presented below the subjective threshold has a qualitatively different effect than perceptual information presented above the subjective threshold, then strong support would be provided for the claim that the subjective threshold defines the transition between two different perceptual states which may be equated with conscious and unconscious perceptual processing.

The idea that qualitative differences in perceptual processing occur as a function of claimed awareness was tested in the present experiments by using a Stroop colour-word priming task in conjunction with a manipulation that varied the proportion of trials on which the colour-word prime reliably predicted the colour-patch target. In a Stroop task involving the presentation of congruent, control, and incongruent trials, the usual procedure is to administer a block of trials in which each type of trial occurs equally often (i.e., 33.3% of the trials). Under these conditions, both facilitation (control minus congruent trials) and inhibition (incongruent minus control trials) occur. However, it has been demonstrated that both facilitation and inhibition increase when the proportion of congruent trials is increased (Glaser and Glaser 1982, Taylor 1977). Thus, for example, if congruent word-colour combinations occur on 66.7% of the trials and control and incongruent trials each occur on 16.7% of the trials, both facilitation and inhibition are greater than is found when each trial type occurs equally often.

Probability effects, such as the one described above, have been investigated using a variety of tasks, and the results of these studies generally have been interpreted to indicate that observers adopt voluntary processing strategies which utilize the predictive information provided by the primes (Lowe and Mitterer 1982; Neely 1977; Posner and Snyder 1975a,b; Taylor 1977). According to this view, the increased facilitation and inhibition that occurs on a Stroop task when congruent word-colour combinations are presented on a large proportion of the trials is due to the fact that observers become selectively biased towards the most probable response, based on the identity of the prime. This is a reasonable strategy for the task, given that it should facilitate performance on the large proportion of trials involving congruent colour-word combinations, and only disrupt performance on the small number of trials involving incongruent word-colour combinations.

The unique aspect of the present approach is the additional assumption that observers may be able to initiate a predictive strategy only when they are consciously aware of the identity of the primes. This assumption is consistent with views such as those expressed by both Posner and Snyder (1975a,b) and Underwood (1982) who equate the attentional processes underlying strategy effects with consciousness. If this assumption is correct, then a predictive strategy should be adopted in the Stroop priming task only when observers are aware of the words used as primes. On the other hand, when observers claim to have no awareness of the words, then it should be impossible for them to initiate any

strategy to predict a future event such as the presentation of a particular colour patch. A demonstration that predictive strategies are limited to situations in which observers are consciously aware of the primes, as defined by the subjective threshold, would indicate that conscious and unconscious processes are qualitatively different, and it is this type of finding that is needed to support a distinction between conscious and unconscious perceptual processes.

Experiment 1

The purpose of this experiment was to replicate previous findings indicating that changes in the proportion of congruent trials on a Stroop task influence the relative magnitudes of facilitation and inhibition. For this reason, all primes were clearly visible. In addition, there were two probability conditions. In one condition, congruent, control, and incongruent trials were presented equally often, so that the presentation of a colour word could not be used to predict whether the name of the subsequent target would be the same or different. In the other condition, congruent prime-target combinations occurred on 66.7% of the trials, whereas incongruent and control combinations each occurred on 16.7% of the trials. Thus, in this condition, presentation of each colour word predicted the name of the target on four out of every five trials. Based on previous research involving Stroop tasks (Glaser and Glaser 1982, Taylor 1977), the increase in congruent-trial probability from .333 to .667 was expected to decrease congruent-trial naming latency and to increase incongruent-trial naming latency, while leaving control-trial performance relatively unaffected.

Method

Subjects
Twenty volunteers recruited from the University of Waterloo received $5 for participating in a single session. All subjects had normal or

corrected-to-normal visual acuity and claimed to have normal colour vision.

Apparatus and Materials

The stimulus materials were displayed on an Electrohome colour monitor that was interfaced to an Apple II Plus microcomputer via an Electrohome Supercolor board. The monitor was viewed through a hood that physically divided the screen into separate left-eye and right-eye fields; fusion of these fields was aided by viewing the display through a set of rotating prisms. The viewing distance was 65 cm and the luminance of each field measured 32 cd/m^2 when the light beige background colour (colour No. 91) was displayed.

A button box placed in front of the subject was used to initiate display presentations and to record responses on the detection trials. Colour naming latencies were measured by the microcomputer from colour onset to the activation of a voice key. Display timing and millisecond response accuracy were coordinated using a John Bell Engineering 6522-VIA interfaced to the microcomputer (see De Jong 1982; Merikle, Cheesman, and Bray 1982).

Each stimulus display consisted of five separate components: a white fixation rectangle, a colour word (BLUE, GREEN, RED, or YELLOW) or control prime (XXXXX), two pattern masks, and a rectangular colour-patch target (blue, green, red, or yellow). The fixation rectangle was presented centrally and measured 2.2 cm (1.9°)[1] horizontal by 1.1 cm (1.0°) vertical. The primes could appear either above or below the fixation rectangle and were constructed from white uppercase letters using the standard 5 × 7 character font provided by the microcomputer. The dimensions of each letter were approximately 0.4 cm (0.4°) horizontal by 0.6 cm (0.5°) vertical, and the vertical distance from the centre of the fixation rectangle to the centre of the prime was 1.4 cm (1.2°). Each pattern mask was comprised of two rows of 14 white, uppercase letters presented in the same character font as the primes. The 28 characters

were selected randomly with replacement from the following population: A, B, E, G, H, M, N, Q, R, S, and W. The masks formed separate rectangles measuring 6.6 cm (5.8°) horizontal by 1.3 cm (1.1°) vertical, and both masks were displayed on each trial in order to overlap spatially each possible prime location. The colour patches were centred within the fixation rectangle and measured 1.0 cm (0.9°) horizontal by 0.4 cm (0.4°) vertical.

Design

The overall experimental design was a 3 (prime-target relationship) by 2 (congruent-trial probability) within-subjects factorial. The three prime-target relationships were congruent, incongruent, and control. On congruent trials, the prime had the same name as the target, whereas on incongruent trials, the prime and target had different names. The primes on control trials simply consisted of the series of 5 Xs. In one probability condition, congruent, incongruent, and control trials were presented equally often, so that each prime-target relationship occurred on 33.3% of the trials. For the other probability condition, congruent trials were presented on 66.7% of the trials, while incongruent and control trials each occurred on 16.7% of the trials. Colour-naming performance for both probability conditions was evaluated during a single session, and the order in which these conditions were administered was counterbalanced across subjects.

For each probability condition, the stimulus displays were presented in blocks of 48 trials with each of the four targets appearing equally often. Within any trial block, prime-target pairs corresponding to each prime-target relationship were presented in the relative proportions prescribed by the particular probability condition. The congruent trials consisted of the eight unique combinations formed by pairing the four colour patches with the same colour-word prime presented either above or below the fixation rectangle. Similarly, eight different control trial combinations were formed using the control prime. Thus, regardless of the probability condition, complete sets of congruent and control prime-target combinations were administered within every trial block. Since the factorial combination of four targets, three primes, and prime presentation either above or below the fixation rectangle yielded 24 unique incongruent trial combinations, more than one trial block was required to display all the incongruent prime-target combinations. In this case, the incongruent items were sampled exhaustively across trial blocks before any prime-target combination was repeated.

The 48 trials assigned to each trial block were presented randomly with two constraints. First, targets of the same colour were never presented successively. Second, after any particular trial, the number of occurrences of the most frequently presented target never exceeded by more than two the number of occurrences of the least frequently presented target.

In order to ensure that the primes were clearly visible during the experimental trials, a series of detection trials involving lexical decisions was administered prior to the colour-naming trials. The stimuli for these trials consisted of the four primes (BLUE, GREEN, RED, and YELLOW) and four nonword variants of the primes (BUEL, GENER, ERD, and YOLLEW). Each nonword variant was selected to be maximally confusable with its corresponding colour word. The stimuli were presented in blocks of 48 trials consisting of three repetitions of the eight stimuli at the two spatial locations. Within each block, the 48 stimulus displays were presented randomly with the constraint that the same stimulus never appeared three times in succession.

Procedure
Each subject was tested individually during one 90-min. session.

Detection Trials Prior to the colour-naming trials, several blocks of detection trials involving word-nonword decisions were administered.

The subjects were informed that on each trial a colour word or nonword variant would be presented either above or below the fixation rectangle and that they should accurately indicate whether a word or nonword had been presented by pressing the appropriate button. In order to equate the viewing conditions of the detection trials with those of the colour-naming trials, the subjects were also instructed to maintain fixation on the centrally presented rectangle at all times during each trial. In addition, the subjects were asked to provide an estimate of their detection performance after every block of 48 trials. They were told that performance would be 50% correct with complete guessing and that, therefore, their estimates should range between 50% and 100% correct.

At the beginning of each trial, the fixation rectangle was presented to both eyes and remained in view throughout the trial. The subjects fixated the centre of the rectangle and initiated a trial sequence by pressing the start button. After a delay of 250 ms, a colour word or nonword was presented to the left eye for 16.7 ms. Following a constant prime-mask stimulus onset asynchrony (SOA) of 250 ms, the pattern masks were presented to the right eye for 200 ms. After a response button was pressed, the screen went blank for approximately 500 ms before the fixation rectangle for the next trial was presented.

Upon completion of each block of 48 trials, the subjects' performance estimates were recorded, and the pattern masks were changed by selecting a new set of letters. In addition, if subjects indicated that their performance was errorless, they were asked if the stimuli were clearly visible. Additional trial blocks were administered until both the observed and estimated performances were 100% correct, and subjects claimed that all targets were clearly visible.

Colour-Naming Trials The subjects were instructed to fixate the centre of the fixation rectangle continually during each trial and to name, as quickly as possible, the colour patch that appeared within the fixation rectangle. Before each probability condition was administered, the subjects were informed as to the relative proportions of each trial type, but they were cautioned to respond only to the colour patch and to avoid naming the word.

The sequence of events on each trial was similar to the event sequence on the detection trials. The subjects pressed the start button and, following a delay of 250 ms, a colour-word or control prime was presented to the left eye for 16.7 ms. The prime-mask SOA was equal to 250 ms, and both pattern masks were presented to the right eye for 200 ms. Prime presentation was also followed by the presentation of a colour-patch target after a 66.7 ms prime-target SOA. The target remained in view until the subject named the colour, at which point the entire screen went blank. There was a further delay of approximately 500 ms before the fixation rectangle for the next trial appeared.

For each probability condition, four blocks of 48 trials were administered. The first block of trials served as practice, and the remaining three blocks of trials provided the experimental observations. After every block of 48 trials the pattern masks were changed by selecting a new set of letters. Subjects were given a 3-min. rest after each block of trials and approximately 10 min. intervened between the two probability conditions.

Results

Mean naming latencies for correct trials and percentage errors are presented in table 33.1 for each condition. The data in table 33.1 are based on a maximum of 48 observations/subject/condition when congruent trial probability was .33, and maximums of 96, 24, and 24 observations/subject/condition for congruent, incongruent, and control trials, resectively, when congruent trial probability was .66.

Table 33.1

Mean naming latencies and percentage errors in experiment 1

Prime-target relationship	Congruent trial probability			
	.33		.66	
	RT	%E	RT	%E
Congruent	454	0.5	441	0.4
Control	494	2.0	500	2.3
Incongruent	576	13.1	602	19.0

The means in table 33.1 indicate that as congruent trial probability increased from .33 to .66, naming latency for both control and incongruent trials increased while congruent trial naming latency decreased. This pattern of results suggests that the increased probability of congruent trials promoted subjects to utilize the additional predictive information provided by the primes.

The naming latencies were evaluated by a 3 (prime-target relationship) by 2 (congruent-trial probability) analysis of variance. The analysis revealed a significant main effect for prime-target relationship, $F(2, 38) = 74.96$, $p < .001$, and a nonsignificant main effect for congruent trial probability, $F(1, 19) = 0.93$, $p > .20$. Of more importance, though, was the significant interaction between these factors, $F(2, 38) = 11.56$, $p < .001$, indicating that performance for the three prime-target relationships changed differentially as congruent trial probability increased from .33 to .66. Planned comparisons indicated that naming latency increased significantly for incongruent trials, $t(38) = 4.59$, $p < .01$,[2] showed a marginally significant decrease for congruent trials, $t(38) = 2.21$, $p < .10$, and did not change significantly for control trials, $t(38) = 1.07$, $p > .20$. Thus, the naming latency data confirm that an increase in congruent prime probability produces an advantage on congruent trials with a corresponding cost to performance on incongruent trials.

The error data summarized in table 33.1 were also evaluated by a 3×2 analysis of variance. This analysis revealed significant main effects for prime-target relationship, $F(2, 38) = 51.56$, $p < .001$, and congruent trial probability, $F(1, 19) = 6.87$, $p < .025$, as well as a significant interaction between these factors, $F(2, 38) = 6.18$, $p < .01$. Planned comparisons showed a significant increase in errors with increased congruent trial probability for incongruent trials, $t(38) = 4.39$, $p < .01$, but no significant differences for either congruent or control trials, both $ts < 1$. This pattern of results is consistent with the naming latency data in showing that the most robust effect of the probability manipulation involves the incongruent trials. Furthermore, the error data indicate that speedaccuracy trade-offs were not a factor in the experiment, as naming latency and error rates were positively correlated.

Discussion

The results of this experiment indicate that the probability effect reported by other investigators (Glaser and Glaser 1982, Taylor 1977) was successfully replicated. Increased congruent-trial probability produced a marginal decrease in naming latency on congruent trials and a considerable increase in naming latency on incongruent trials. This particular pattern of results indicates that the cost to processing on incongruent trials produced by the increase in congruent-trial probability outweighed the benefit which occurred on congruent trials (cf. Posner and Snyder 1975b). Thus, in general, congruent-trial probability has its most pronounced effect on the naming of targets preceded by incongruent colour words.

The present results are consistent with an interpretation suggesting that the increase in congruent-trial probability led observers to use the identity of the primes to anticipate the presentation of particular targets. Although it is not possible to specify the exact process mediating the strategy induced by the increase in congruent-

trial probability, given that the probability effect was replicated, it is possible to use this variant of a Stroop task to establish if induced strategy changes are limited to conditions in which observers are aware of the primes.

Experiment 2

The question of primary interest in this experiment concerned whether or not the strategy effects observed in experiment 1 would occur when observers claimed to have no awareness of the primes. As discussed previously, it is reasonable to expect that observers can implement a strategy based upon the expectation of a future event only when they are aware of a prime. If this assumption is correct, then no evidence for strategy effects should be found when primes are presented below the awareness threshold. On the other hand, given that awareness was defined in terms of a subjective threshold, an overall Stroop effect should occur even when the primes are presented below this threshold. Thus, when primes are presented below the subjective threshold, priming should occur, but this priming should not vary with changes in the proportion of congruent trials, as occurs when primes are clearly visible.

Two major procedural changes distinguish this experiment from the previous one. First, prior to the priming trials, several blocks of detection trials were administered to establish each observer's subjective threshold. Subjective thresholds were defined in terms of the prime-mask SOA at which an observer consistently claimed to detect the primes at a chance level of accuracy. The second procedural change introduced in the present study was that subjective threshold and suprathreshold conditions were intermixed within each block of priming trials. By randomizing the presentation of the two threshold conditions within each trial block, it was possible to ensure that any observed strategy difference across the two threshold conditions was induced on a trial-by-trial basis and did not result from a general strategy applicable only to a particular threshold condition.

Method

Subjects
Each of 16 volunteers, ranging in age from 19 to 29, received $30 for participating in the study.

Apparatus and Materials
Both the apparatus and stimulus materials were identical to those used in experiment 1.

Design
The overall design was a 3 (prime-target relationship) by 2 (congruent-trial probability) by 2 (threshold condition) factorial. The only change, relative to experiment 1, was that performance was evaluated under two threshold conditions. These threshold conditions were designated as suprathreshold and subjective threshold. Under the suprathreshold condition, a constant prime-mask SOA of 250 ms was used, and this condition served as a replication of experiment 1. Under the subjective threshold condition, the prime-mask SOA was equal to the longest word-mask SOA at which subjects consistently claimed that their word-nonword decision performance approximated a chance level of accuracy.

Colour-naming performance at each level of congruent-trial probability was assessed during a separate session, and the presentation order for these sessions was counterbalanced across subjects. Within each session, colour-naming trials for both threshold conditions were randomly intermixed. Initially, separate blocks of 48 trials were constructed for each threshold condition in exactly the same manner as experiment 1. The trials within these blocks were then intermixed and presented randomly within a single 96-trial block using the same constraints employed in experiment 1.

Procedure
Each subject participated in four 1-hour sessions. During the first two sessions, the word-mask SOAs reflecting subjective threshold were determined. The final two sessions involved the presentation of the colour-naming trials.

Detection Trials The subjects were provided with the same detection trial instructions as in experiment 1. In addition, after each trial block, subjects were also asked to indicate which colour words, if any, they felt were easily detected. This information was used to fine tune the adjustment of the prime-mask SOAs at the subjective threshold.

The sequence and timing of events for each trial was changed only slightly from the detection trials of the previous experiment. The colour word or nonword was presented to the left eye for 16.7 ms, and following the prime-mask SOA the pattern masks were presented to the right eye for 200 ms. In order to equate detection performance across the four primes so as to establish accurately the subjective threshold, the prime-mask SOA was varied independently for each word-nonword pair.

After every block of 48 trials, each pattern mask was changed, and subjects provided both their performance estimates and an indication of the stimuli they saw clearly. Feedback concerning detection performance was not provided.

In the first detection session, subjects were familiarized with the 250-ms suprathreshold prime-mask SOA, and rough estimates of the prime mask SOAs necessary for the subjective threshold condition were established. Once subjects obtained 100% correct detections and indicated that the colour words were clearly visible at the 250-ms SOA, the prime-mask SOAs were reduced by 50 ms per trial block until detection performance fell below 100% correct. Thereafter, the prime-mask SOAs for individual word-nonword pairs were adjusted by either 16.7 or 33.3 ms depending upon the subjects' estimates of their performance and self-reports concerning the visibility of the words. As soon as subjects began to estimate consistently that detection performance was 50% correct, the prime-mask SOAs were noted and the session was terminated.

During the second session, the subjective threshold was carefully calibrated for each word-nonword pair. The prime-mask SOAs were adjusted until the objective detection accuracies for all words were relatively homogeneous (within 15%) and subjects consistently claimed that their performance was less than 55% correct. Individual prime-mask SOAs were adjusted by 16.7 ms after every block of trials until three consecutive blocks of trials requiring no adjustments were completed.

Colour-Naming Trials Subjects were presented with the same instructions and information regarding congruent trial probability as in experiment 1. In addition, subjects were told not to expect to see a prime on every trial.

On each trial, a colour-word or control prime was presented to the left eye for 16.7 ms and then masked via the right eye. The prime-mask SOA was equal to either the appropriate subjective threshold value or 250 ms for the suprathreshold condition. The prime-mask SOA for control trials presented under the subjective threshold condition was equal to an average of the four individual subjective threshold word-mask SOAs. Presentation of the prime was also followed by the presentation of a centrally located target at a prime-target SOA of 66.7 ms. The target remained in view until subjects named its hue.

Each congruent-trial probability condition was tested across 3 blocks of 96 experimental trials. Within each of these trial blocks, the subjective threshold and suprathreshold conditions were tested on an equal number of trials. The experimental trials were preceded by a block of 48 practice trials in which the prime-mask SOA was 250 ms. A 3-min rest was provided after completion of each block of trials.

Results

Detection Trials

For each subject, the percentage correct detection was calculated for each word-nonword pair at the prime-mask SOA established for the subjective threshold. Overall mean detection performance averaged across the four colour words was 64.8% correct ($SD = 5.52$), and the means for individual subjects ranged from 57.0% to 77.5% correct. The mean prime-mask SOA established for the subjective threshold was 34.8 ms, with a range of 16.7–83.3 ms.

Colour-Naming Trials

Table 33.2 presents the mean naming latency and the percentage errors for each condition. The naming latencies for the suprathreshold trials provide a precise replication of experiment 1. As congruent trial probability increased from .33 to .66, naming latency increased substantially for incongruent trials, showed only a small increase for control trials, and decreased for congruent trials. Thus, the strategy effect was evident for the clearly visible primes in this experiment.

In contrast to the results for the suprathreshold condition, the subjective threshold data provide a rather different pattern of results. Although primes in the subjective threshold condition were clearly being perceived, as indicated by the substantial overall difference between incongruent and congruent trials, it appears that congruent-trial probability had virtually no influence on colour-naming performance. As indicated in table 33.2, response latencies on incongruent, congruent, and control trials are very similar at both levels of congruent-trial probability. Thus, the variation in congruent trial probability appears to have no effect when observers claim no awareness for the primes.

The different patterns of results observed in each threshold condition were confirmed by an overall analysis of variance which revealed a three-way interaction involving prime-target

Table 33.2
Mean naming latencies and percentage errors in experiment 2

Prime detectability	Prime-target relationship	Congruent trial probability			
		.33		.66	
		RT	%E	RT	%E
Subjective threshold	Congruent	446	2.1	439	1.7
	Control	464	2.1	470	3.4
	Incongruent	488	3.8	487	4.2
Suprathreshold	Congruent	424	0.8	412	0.4
	Control	465	1.1	469	2.1
	Incongruent	550	9.5	584	13.8

relationship, congruent-trial probability, and threshold condition, $F(2, 30) = 8.01$, $p < .005$. In order to clarify this interaction, the data from each threshold condition were analyzed separately after the control trials had been excluded. This approach was adopted for three reasons. First, since the critical comparison for demonstrating an effect of congruent-trial probability involves only congruent and incongruent trials, the most sensitive analysis requires exclusion of the control trials. Second, separate analyses for each threshold condition were warranted since the variability in the data under the suprathreshold condition was considerably greater than under the subjective threshold condition. Finally, in the subjective threshold condition, the control trials may not have been completely comparable to the other two types of trials. Although separate prime-mask SOAs were determined for each word used on the congruent and incongruent trials, each observer's prime-mask SOA for the control stimulus was based on the average prime-mask SOA for the colour words. Thus, the neutral stimulus may have been more discriminable than the colour words.

The mean congruent and incongruent trial naming latencies for each threshold condition are presented in figure 33.1. As found in experiment 1, the analysis of variance on the data for

the suprathreshold condition revealed a significant main effect for prime-target relationship, $F(1, 15) = 165.73$, $p < .001$, a nonsignificant main effect of congruent-trial probability, $F(1, 15) = 3.14$, $p < .10$, and a significant interaction between these variables, $F(1, 15) = 16.61$, $p < .001$. The interaction indicates that the difference between congruent and incongruent trials increased as congruent-trial probability increased from .33 to .66. In contrast to the results found for the suprathreshold condition, the analysis of the data for the subjective threshold condition revealed a significant main effect only for prime-target relationship, $F(1, 15) = 95.65$, $p < .001$, and neither the main effect for congruent trial probability, $F(1, 15) < 1$, nor the interaction between these variables, $F(1, 15) = 1.32$, were significant sources of variance. Thus, although Stroop priming occurred under both threshold conditions, the increase in congruent-trial probability influenced performance only when the primes were clearly visible in the suprathreshold condition.

A series of planned comparisons evaluating performance on congruent and incongruent trials as a function of congruent trial probability confirmed that different patterns of results occurred under the two threshold conditions. These comparisons indicated that, under the suprathreshold

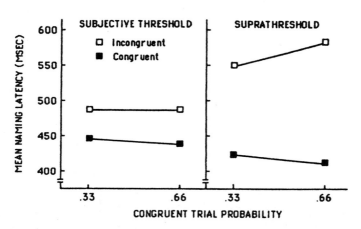

Figure 33.1
Mean naming latencies for congruent and incongruent trials as a function of congruent-trial probability under subjective and suprathreshold conditions in experiment 2.

condition, the increase in congruent-trial probability decreased naming latencies on congruent trials, $t(15) = 2.51$, $p < .05$,[3] and increased naming latencies on incongruent trials, $t(15) = 3.08$, $p < .05$. However, under the subjective threshold condition, no change in naming latency occurred on either congruent trials, $t(15) = 1.20$, or incongruent trials, $t(15) < 1$, when congruent-trial probability was increased.

The error data were also analyzed separately for each threshold condition after excluding the control trials. Each analysis revealed a significant main effect for prime-target relationship, both $Fs(1, 15) > 7.83$, $p < .025$, and the main effect for congruent trial probability was significant under the suprathreshold condition, $F(1, 15) = 6.72$, $p < .025$, but nonsignificant under the subjective threshold condition, $F(1, 15) < 1$. In addition, the interaction between prime-target relationship and congruent-trial probability was significant for the suprathreshold condition, $F(1, 15) = 8.37$, $p < .025$, but failed to reach significance for the subjective threshold trials, $F(1, 15) < 1$. Thus, in general, the error data and the naming latency data are completely consistent.

Discussion

The different patterns of results obtained under the subjective threshold and suprathreshold conditions are consistent with the hypothesis that strategy effects occur only when observers are consciously aware of the primes. Despite the fact that the primes were perceived under both threshold conditions, as indicated by the presence of significant priming effects, the probability effect was observed only in the suprathreshold condition. Given that the observers could capitalize on the predictive relationship between primes and targets only when the primes were clearly visible, the data provide strong support for the assumption that the subjective threshold defines the transition between conscious and unconscious perceptual processing.

The qualitatively different effects found under the suprathreshold and subjective threshold conditions indicate that priming effects, per se, are mediated by a different set of perceptual processes than the probability effect induced by variations in congruent-trial probability. The presence of significant priming under both threshold conditions indicates that both conscious and unconscious processes contribute to the overall magnitude of Stroop priming. However, the absence of a probability effect under the subjective condition suggests that voluntary strategies are adopted only as a consequence of conscious perceptual processing. One possible reason for such processing differences has been proposed by Marcel (1983b), who argues that conscious and unconscious processes are based on qualitatively different representational codes. From this view, it follows that conscious processes should provide a unique contribution to the processing of stimuli, which unconscious processes, by themselves, do not provide. The absence of a probability effect when observers were unaware of the primes is totally consistent with this idea.

Experiment 3

The primary purpose of this experiment was to replicate the results obtained in the previous experiment under slightly different experimental conditions. Even though the previous results are entirely consistent with the view that the subjective threshold provides an appropriate definition of the boundary between conscious and unconscious perceptual processes, a replication of the basic findings under somewhat different conditions would provide additional empirical support for the proposed theoretical position.

Relative to experiment 2, two major procedural changes were introduced in the present experiment. First, the detection trials used to establish subjective thresholds were based on a four-alternative, forced-choice recognition task involving the four colour words used in the subsequent priming task. The forced-choice recognition task provided a direct measure of each observer's ability to assign responses to colour words confidently. For this reason, it provided a better measure of each observer's subjective threshold than the lexical-decision task used in experiment 2. The lexical-decision task did not necessarily ensure that the observers could not

confidently discriminate among the four colour words, since it only required observers to discriminate the four colour words from the four colour-word variants.

The second major procedural change involved the introduction of a more extreme variation in congruent-trial probability. This change was implemented by eliminating the control trials and setting the probability of a congruent trial within a session at either .25 or .75. These two modifications ensured that each prime was followed by each target equally often when congruent-trial probability was set at .25. Thus, there was absolutely no predictive relationship between primes and targets in the .25 probability condition in the present experiment. In experiment 2, on the other hand, the lower congruent-probability condition (i.e., .33) actually involved a small predictive relationship between primes and targets, as primes were presented only on two-thirds of the trials, and each prime was followed by a congruent colour target on one-half of these trials. The more extreme variation in congruent-trial probability studied in the present experiment allowed an assessment of the probability effect under conditions in which there was either no predictability or high predictability between primes and targets.

Method

Subjects
Sixteen volunteers, ranging in age from 18 to 31, received $30 for participating in four sessions.

Apparatus and Materials
The apparatus was the same as used in experiments 1 and 2. However, the arrangement of the stimulus materials was changed in order to allow the primes to be presented and masked within the fixation area.

Each stimulus display consisted of five separate components: a white fixation rectangle, a forward pattern mask (QYGRUEWN), a colour-word prime (BLUE, GREEN, RED, or YELLOW), a backward pattern mask (RYBU-

LOG), and a rectangular colour frame (blue, green, red, or yellow). The fixation rectangle measured 4.8 cm (4.2°) horizontal by 2.1 cm (1.9°) vertical, and the colour words were centred within this area. As in the previous experiments, the pattern masks and the primes were presented in white uppercase letters using the standard 5×7 character font provided by the microcomputer. The length of the forward and backward masks measured 3.8 cm (3.4°) and 3.4 cm (3.0°), respectively, and the length of the colour words ranged from 1.5 cm (1.3°) to 3.2 cm (2.8°). The colour frames completely enclosed the fixation rectangle. Each side of a colour frame was 0.3 cm (0.3°) wide, and the outer dimensions of the frames were 6.6 cm (5.8°) horizontal by 3.9 cm (3.4°) vertical.

Design

The experimental design was a 2 (prime-target relationship) by 2 (congruent-trial probability) by 2 (threshold condition) factorial. The two prime-target relationships were congruent and incongruent, the two threshold conditions were suprathreshold and subjective threshold, and the two levels of congruent-trial probability were either .25 or .75. As in the previous experiment, colour-naming performance for each congruent trial probability condition was evaluated over separate sessions and counterbalanced across subjects. Within each session, displays corresponding to each prime-target relationship and threshold condition were randomly intermixed and administered in blocks of 32 trials.

For each trial block, the displays were equally divided between suprathreshold and subjective threshold presentation conditions, and each target appeared equally often within each threshold condition. When congruent-trial probability was .25, each threshold condition contained 4 congruent trials and 12 incongruent trials, so each unique congruent and incongruent prime-target combination was presented once. When congruent trial probability was .75, each threshold condition contained 12 congruent and 4 incongruent

items. In this case, the 4 unique congruent trials were presented three times each, while 4 of the possible 12 unique incongruent prime-target combinations were selected. Thus, three blocks of trials were required before the entire set of incongruent combinations was exhaustively sampled for each threshold condition. Within each trial block, the 32 trials were presented randomly with the same constraints used in experiments 1 and 2.

The stimuli used on the detection trials were the four colour words. They were presented in blocks of 24 trials consisting of six repetitions of each word. The 24 stimulus displays in each block were randomly presented with the constraint that the same word never appeared three times in succession.

Procedure

The subjects were tested individually over four 1-hour sessions. The prime-mask SOAs corresponding to the subjective threshold for each word were established during the first two sessions, and colour naming performance was evaluated across the final two sessions.

Detection Trials The subjects were informed that one of four colour words would be presented within the fixation rectangle and that responses should be indicated by pressing the button corresponding to the colour word. The subjects were also told that each colour word would appear equally often and therefore their guesses should be distributed across the four possible responses. In addition, the subjects were informed that after every block of 24 trials they would be required to indicate the total number of detection responses they were confident were correct. Since subjects could keep a running total of their confident detection decisions in every block, they found this procedure much easier than estimating overall performance, as subjects were required to do in experiment 2. Finally, the subjects were asked to report after every trial block which colour words were clearly visible.

On each trial, the fixation rectangle was presented to both eyes and remained in view throughout the trial. After the start button had been depressed, there was a 250-ms delay before the forward mask was presented to the right eye for 50 ms. Following a delay of 50 ms after the offset of the forward mask, a word was presented to the left eye for 16.7 ms. The backward mask was subsequently presented to the right eye for 50 ms at the predetermined prime-mask SOA. Once a detection response was made, the screen went blank for approximately 500 ms before the fixation rectangles for the next trial reappeared.

Subjective thresholds were established by basically the same procedures followed in experiment 2. During the first session, the prime-mask SOA for each word was systematically decreased until subjects consistently indicated over three consecutive blocks of 24 trials that less than 3 of the 24 detection decisions were made with confidence. During the second session, the objective detection levels for each word were matched as closely as possible by adjusting the prime-mask SOAs until the criterion of five consecutive trial blocks (i.e., 120 trials) requiring no further adjustments was met.

Colour-Naming Trials With the exception that subjects were instructed to name the colour of the frame surrounding the fixation rectangle, the instructions and information given to subjects at the beginning of each colour-naming session were the same as in experiment 2. The sequence of events on each trial was similar to that which occurred on the detection trials, except that following a 100-ms prime-target SOA, a colour frame was presented and remained in view until subjects responded.

Twelve blocks of 32 trials were administered to each subject during each colour-naming session. The first three blocks were treated as practice and the remaining 288 trials provided the experimental observations. During the first two blocks of practice trials, the primes were always masked at the 300-ms suprathreshold SOA. For the third trial block, the suprathreshold and subjective threshold trials were randomly intermixed as they were during the experimental trials. The subjects were given a short rest after every block of trials.

Results

Detection Trials

For each subject, percentage correct detection was calculated for each colour word at the prime-mask SOA established for the subjective threshold. The mean detection performance averaged across the four colour words was 55.3% ($SD = 5.51$), and the means for individual subjects ranged from 46.7% to 63.3%. The mean word-mask SOA used for subjective threshold presentations was 44.8 ms, and individual word-mask SOAs ranged from 16.7 to 66.7 ms. Despite the relatively high level of detection accuracy obtained using these word-mask SOAs, the overall mean performance estimate was only 32.3% ($SD = 3.7$) correct.

Colour-Naming Trials

The mean naming latencies and percentage errors for each condition are presented in table 33.3. When congruent trial probability was .25, each mean was based on a maximum of 36 observations/subject for congruent trials and 108 observations/subject for incongruent trials. Conversely, when congruent trial probability was .75, congruent and incongruent means were based on a maximum of 108 and 36 observations/subject, respectively.

As indicated by figure 33.2, the pattern of results for the suprathreshold condition is consistent with the results obtained in experiments 1 and 2. As congruent trial probability increased from .25 to .75, naming latency for incongruent trials increased (45 ms) while congruent trial naming latency decreased (36 ms). Thus, changes in the predictability of the primes substantially influenced performance for both congruent and incongruent trials.

Table 33.3
Mean naming latencies and percentage errors in experiment 3

		Congruent trial probability			
		.25		.75	
Prime detectability	Prime-target relationship	RT	%E	RT	%E
Subjective threshold	Congruent	473	1.5	454	2.1
	Incongruent	500	2.7	500	4.2
Suprathreshold	Congruent	445	0.2	409	0.6
	Incongruent	540	5.9	586	12.5

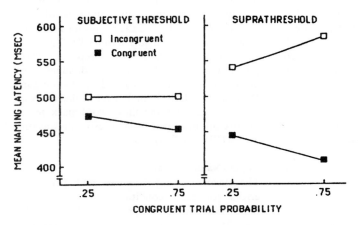

Figure 33.2
Mean naming latencies for congruent and incongruent trials as a function of congruent-trial probability under subjective and suprathreshold conditions in experiment 3.

On the other hand, the data for the subjective threshold condition indicate that the manipulation of congruent-trial probability had considerably different effects on the processing of congruent and incongruent primes. Although the increase in congruent-trial probability produced absolutely no effect on incongruent trial naming latencies, there was a small decrease in congruent trial naming latencies (20 ms) when congruent trial probability increased from .25 to .75. This observation indicates that some component of the processing of congruent primes is influenced

by changes in congruent trial probability despite claimed unawareness.

The data were analyzed using a 2 (prime-target relationship) by 2 (congruent-trial probability) by 2 (threshold condition) analysis of variance. The presence of a significant three-factor interaction, $F(1, 15) = 41.20$, $p < .001$, indicates that a different pattern of results occurred in each threshold condition. For this reason, separate analyses of variance were performed on the data for each threshold condition. Both analyses yielded highly significant main effects for prime-target relationship, both $Fs(1, 15) > 27.08$, $p < .001$, but neither analysis revealed a significant main effect for congruent-trial probability, both $Fs(1, 15) < 2.14$. Furthermore, the interaction between prime-target relationship and congruent-trial probability was a significant source of variance in the data for both the suprathreshold, $F(1, 15) = 19.22$, $p < .001$, and the subjective threshold condition, $F(1, 15) = 14.47$, $p < .005$. Planned comparisons revealed that performance in the suprathreshold condition changed significantly on both congruent, $t(15) = 5.87$, $p < .01$, and incongruent trials, $t(15) = 3.87$, $p < .01$, as congruent-trial probability increased from .25 to .75. In contrast, similar planned comparisons on the data for the subjective threshold condition revealed a significant decrease in performance on the congruent trials, $t(15) = 3.02$, $p < .05$, but no change in performance on the incongruent trials, $t(15) < 1$, as a function of congruent trial probability. Thus, the analyses indicate that the manipulation of congruent-trial probability affected both congruent and incongruent trial performance when the primes were clearly visible, but only performance on congruent trials is affected when the primes were masked so that observers claimed to have no awareness of the stimuli.

The error data were also submitted to a separate 2×2 analysis of variance for each threshold condition. The analysis for the subjective threshold condition revealed no significant differences, all $Fs(1, 15) < 2.90$, $p > .10$. In comparison, the analysis of the errors from the suprathreshold condition revealed significant main effects for prime-target relationship and congruent trial probability, as well as a significant interaction between these factors, all $Fs(1, 15) > 16.99$, $p < .001$. Planned comparisons indicated that the source of the interaction was an increase in incongruent trial error rates as congruent-trial probability increased, $t(15) = 5.08$, $p < .001$, without a corresponding increase in congruent trial error rates, $t(15) = 2.20$, $p > .05$.

Discussion

In general, the results of this experiment replicate, under somewhat different experimental conditions, the findings observed in experiment 2. In both experiments, the increase in congruent-trial probability under the suprathreshold condition produced a large increase in naming latency on the incongruent trials and a relatively smaller decrease in naming latency on the congruent trials. More importantly, under the subjective threshold condition in both experiments, the increase in congruent-trial probability had absolutely no effect on naming latency on the incongruent trials, even though the presence of significant priming effects indicates that the colour words were perceived. These different effects of congruent-trial probability on incongruent trials under the subjective threshold and suprathreshold conditions indicate that the primes were processed in a considerably different manner, depending on whether or not they were presented under conditions leading to claimed awareness. Thus, the results of both experiments provide strong support for the view that the subjective threshold defines the transition between conscious and unconscious perceptual processes.

The one finding in the present experiment that differs from the results of experiment 2 concerns the effect of congruent-trial probability on congruent trials under the subjective threshold condition. In both experiments, the increase in congruent-trial probability produced a small decrease in naming latency under the subjective threshold condition. However, in the present experiment, this small decrease, which was approximately one-half the decrease observed in the suprathreshold condition, was significant, whereas in experiment 2, the comparable decrease was statistically nonsignificant. The slightly larger effect observed in the present experiment is probably due to the more extreme variation in congruent-trial probability. This finding suggests that some component of perceptual processing on congruent trials is selectively influenced by variations in congruent-trial probability even when observers claim not to be aware of the primes.

The present results are entirely consistent with the hypothesis that observers can initiate a strategy based on the predictive relationship between primes and targets only when they are consciously aware of the primes. As indicated by the results obtained in the suprathreshold condition, adoption of this strategy has both costs and benefits. Although the strategy leads to improved performance on congruent trials, it also leads to a considerable decrement in performance on incongruent trials. The results obtained in the subjective threshold condition, on the other hand, indicate that a predictive strategy was not adopted in this condition, as the probability manipulation had absolutely no effect on performance on the incongruent trials. Rather, the results for the subjective threshold condition indicate than an increase in congruent-trial probability produces a small benefit on congruent trials, without an associated cost on incongruent trials when observers are not consciously aware of the primes. This benefit without cost in the subjective threshold condition indicates that there are several components to the effect of the probability manipulation, as has been suggested by other investigators (Glaser and Glaser 1982, Taylor 1977).

Taken together, the results of both this experiment and experiment 2 support the view that the subjective threshold defines the boundary between conscious and unconscious perceptual processes. The different effects of congruent-trial probability observed in the suprathreshold and subjective threshold conditions indicate that the primes were processed in a qualitatively different manner in each condition. Given these differential effects of congruent-trial probability in the two threshold conditions, the present results establish the validity of the subjective threshold as a measure of the boundary between conscious and unconscious processes.

General Discussion

The present studies provide strong support for using the subjective threshold, or the threshold of claimed awareness, to define the boundary between conscious and unconscious perceptual processes. The subjective threshold is an appealing measure of awareness as, intuitively, it seems to capture the phenomenological distinction between conscious and unconscious perceptual experiences. However, by itself, the subjective threshold is a useless measure of awareness. As noted previously (Merikle 1983, 1984), when awareness is defined simply in terms of subjective confidence, it is equivalent to asking observers whether or not they are conscious of a stimulus. Thus, in effect, each observer is asked to provide his or her own definition of awareness. For this reason, before the subjective threshold can be used effectively to define awareness, at least one additional criterion or converging operation is required. In the present studies, this additional criterion was satisfied by the demonstration that variations in congruent-trial probability differentially affected performance under the suprathreshold and subjective threshold conditions. This demonstration of qualitative differences in perceptual processing as a function of claimed awareness supports the conclusion that the subjective threshold defines the transition between conscious and unconscious perceptual processes.

Adoption of this proposed twofold approach based on subjective thresholds and subsequent demonstrations of qualitative differences in perceptual processing has two major advantages. First, demonstrations of qualitative differences in perceptual processing as a function of claimed awareness indicate how conscious and unconscious processes differ, and it is only by establishing qualitative differences that it will ever be possible to specify the critical differences that distinguish conscious from unconscious perceptual processes. In fact, if qualitative differences in perceptual processing cannot be demonstrated, even the need for a distinction between conscious and unconscious perceptual processes becomes questionable. A second advantage of the proposed approach is that it provides a basis for resolving the controversies surrounding recent studies presumed to demonstrate perception without awareness (Balota 1983, Fowler et al. 1981, Marcel 1983a, McCauley et al. 1980). If it is assumed that subjective rather than objective thresholds were inadvertently established in these studies, then the results of these studies are entirely consistent with the present approach. Of course, as previously mentioned, these studies have a major shortcoming in that the data, at best, can only suggest that perceptual information is processed without awareness, since no attempt was made to demonstrate qualitatively different effects for consciously and unconsciously perceived information.

If many of the previous studies which appear to provide evidence for unconscious perceptual processing did involve an evaluation of performance at the subjective threshold, then the results from some of these studies can be interpreted as providing support for unconscious perceptual processing, since the reported data suggest that consciously and unconsciously perceived stimuli are processed in qualitatively different ways. In one important study, Marcel (1980) observed that the interpretation of polysemous or ambiguous words is biased by prior context when the words are clearly visible, but remains relatively unaffected by prior context when the words are masked so that observers claim not to be aware of their presence. Marcel's experiment involved lexical decisions to clearly visible target stimuli that were presented immediately following the presentation of either masked or unmasked polysemous words used as primes. Furthermore, a clearly visible context word which was either neutral with respect to all possible meanings of the polysemous word or closely related to one meaning of the polysemous word was presented prior to the presentation of each prime. The interesting result found in

this study was that lexical decisions to words semantically-related to the biased meaning of a prime were facilitated and lexical decisions to words unrelated to the biased meaning were inhibited when the primes were clearly visible. However, when the primes were masked so that they were presented below the awareness threshold, the prior context had no selective effect, as lexical decisions to words related to either meaning of a polysemous word were facilitated. Thus, Marcel's experiment demonstrates that the same priming stimulus can produce either inhibition or facilitation depending on whether or not it is consciously or unconsciously perceived.

Another important study suggesting that consciously and unconsciously perceived words lead to qualitatively different effects has recently been reported by Forster and Davis (1984). Using a lexical-decision task in conjunction with repetition priming, Forster and Davis found that high and low frequency primes which were unavailable for conscious report produced equivalent priming effects. This finding contrasts with the results observed when the primes were clearly visible since, in this situation, there was a more pronounced repetition priming effect for low frequency than high frequency words. On the basis of these results, Forster and Davis argued that lexical access, per se, occurs unconsciously but that conscious perceptual processing is necessary before the differential effects of word frequency become evident.

Finally, Groeger (1984), using a somewhat different approach, has shown that conscious and unconscious perceptual processes lead to qualitatively different error patterns when observers make subsequent forced-choice decisions. In his study, a word was briefly presented, and observers were then required to select a response from a subsequently-presented matrix of words. These matrices never contained the actual word that had been presented, and they consisted solely of words either semantically or structurally related to a previously-presented target word. When the target words were presented so that the observers claimed not to have seen a stimulus, the words selected from the matrices were semantically related to the target words. However, when the target words were presented at longer exposure durations, the subsequently selected words were visually similar to the target words. Thus, it appears that decisions concerning target words are primarily influenced by meaning when the words are unconsciously perceived and guided by structural characteristics when the words are consciously perceived.

Taken together, the results of these studies are consistent with the proposed approach, as long as it is assumed that unconscious perceptual processing in these studies was evaluated at a level of discriminative responding more similar to a subjective than an objective threshold. In fact, Marcel (personal communication, October 29, 1984) has indicated that the awareness threshold established in his study for each observer probably did reflect a subjective rather than an objective threshold. Likewise, the pilot data presented by Forster and Davis (1984) indicate that their subjects were probably able to respond discriminatively to the primes at a somewhat better than chance level of accuracy. Given that subjective thresholds were probably established in these studies, then the reported results indicating qualitatively different effects for consciously and unconsciously perceived stimuli are entirely consistent with the proposed approach. Furthermore, the nature of these differences provides an indication of how conscious and unconscious perceptual processes may differ.

The present emphasis on the need to establish qualitative differences between conscious and unconscious processes is consistent with Marcel's (1983b) theoretical discussions of the role of conscious experience in perceptual processing. Marcel states that the single most important distinction between conscious and unconscious processes is that they reflect qualitatively different representational codes. According to Marcel, conscious perceptual processing is not merely

a stronger version of unconscious processing. Rather, conscious perceptual processing allows structures and interpretations to be imposed on perceptual information which are unavailable when information is processed unconsciously. Although Marcel, in his model, equated conscious perceptual processing or phenomenological experience with the presence of any form of discriminative responding, it is possible, with relatively minor changes, to revise his model so that conscious perceptual processing is aligned with the subjective threshold rather than an objective threshold (cf. Cheesman and Merikle 1985). With these revisions, Marcel's model becomes consistent with both the recent evidence indicating that discriminative responding provides a completely adequate measure of all perceptual processing (Cheesman and Merikle 1984, Nolan and Caramazza 1982) and the present proposal that the transition from unconscious to conscious perceptual processing is reflected by the subjective threshold, or in other words, the threshold for claimed awareness.

Clearly, the final success of the subjective threshold or other possible related measures of awareness depends upon the success of future research in elucidating additional differences that distinguish conscious from unconscious perceptual processes. The real advantage of the present approach over other approaches that have been used to study unconscious processes is that the subjective threshold emphasizes the importance of distinguishing perceptual processes on the basis of correlated phenomenological experiences, as opposed to distinguishing perceptual processes simply on the basis of discriminative responding. Thus, the present approach provides a basis of resolving the controversies surrounding the use of discriminative responding as an index of awareness (e.g., Merikle 1982). Furthermore, even though the proposed approach implies that discriminative responding, per se, does not provide an adequate measure of awareness, it is entirely consistent with the view that discriminative responding does provide a completely accurate indicator of perceptual processing (e.g., Eriksen 1960). Finally, adoption of the present approach, with its emphasis on establishing qualitative differences between conscious and unconscious processes, changes the important research questions from those that ask whether unconscious perceptual processing occurs to those that ask how conscious and unconscious perceptual processes may differ.

Acknowledgment

This research was supported by a Natural Sciences and Engineering Research Council of Canada Postgraduate Scholarship to the first author and by Grant APA-231 from the Natural Sciences and Engineering Research Council of Canada to the second author.

Notes

1. The visual angle subtended by each stimulus dimension is provided within parentheses following each linear measurement.

2. Each comparison was based upon the pooled error interaction term, and Type I error rates were corrected using the Bonferroni t procedure.

3. Individual error terms were calculated for each comparison and Type I error rates were corrected using the Bonferroni t procedure.

References

Allport, D. A. (1977). On knowing the meaning of words we are unable to report: The effects of visual masking. In S. Dornic (Ed.), *Attention and performance VI* (pp. 505–533). Hillsdale, NJ: Erlbaum.

Balota, D. A. (1983). Automatic semantic activation and episodic memory encoding. *Journal of Verbal Learning & Verbal Behavior*, 22, 88–104.

Cheesman, J., and Merikle, P. M. (1984). Priming with and without awareness. *Perception & Psychophysics*, 36, 387–395.

Cheesman, J., and Merikle, P. M. (1985). Word recognition and consciousness. In D. Besner, T. G. Waller, and G. E. MacKinnon (Eds.), *Reading research: Advances in theory and practice: Vol. 5* (pp. 311–352). New York: Academic Press.

De Jong, M. L. (1982). *Apple II assembly language*. Indianapolis: Howard Sams.

Dixon, N. E. (1971). *Subliminal perception: The nature of a controversy*. London: McGraw-Hill.

Dixon, N. E. (1981). *Preconscious processing*. Chichester: Wiley.

Eriksen, C. W. (1960). Discrimination and learning without awareness: A methodological survey and evaluation. *Psychological Review*, 67, 279–300.

Forster, K. I., and Davis, C. (1984). Repetition priming and frequency attenuation in lexical access. *Journal of Experimental Psychology: Learning, Memory, & Cognition*, 10, 680–698.

Fowler, C. A., Wolford, G., Slade, R., and Tassinary, L. (1981). Lexical access with and without awareness. *Journal of Experimental Psychology: General*, 110, 341–362.

Glaser, M. O., and Glaser, W. R. (1982). Time course analysis of the Stroop phenomenon. *Journal of Experimental Psychology: Human Perception & Performance*, 8, 875–894.

Groeger, J. A. (1984). Evidence for unconscious sematic processing from a forced error situation. *British Journal of Psychology*, 75, 305–314.

Henley, S. H. A. (1984). Unconscious perception re-revisited: A comment on Merikle's (1982) paper. *Bulletin of the Psychonomic Society*, 22, 121–124.

Holender, D. (1986). Semantic activation without conscious identification in dichotic listening, parafoveal vision, and visual masking: A survey and appraisal. *Behavioral and Brain Sciences* 9, 1–66.

Lowe, D. G., and Mitterer, J. O. (1982). Selective and divided attention in a Stroop task. *Canadian Journal of Psychology*, 36, 684–700.

Marcel, A. J. (1974, July). *Perception with and without awareness*. Paper presented at the meeting of the Experimental Psychology Society, Stirling, Scotland.

Marcel, A. J. (1980). Conscious and preconscious recognition of polysemous words: Locating the selective effects of prior verbal context. In R. S. Nickerson (Ed.), *Attention and performance VIII* (pp. 435–457). Hillsdale, NJ: Erlbaum.

Marcel, A. J. (1983a). Conscious and unconscious perception: Experiments on visual masking and word recognition. *Cognitive Psychology*, 15, 197–237.

Marcel, A. J. (1983b). Conscious and unconscious perception: An approach to the relations between phenomenal experience and perceptual processes. *Cognitive Psychology*, 15, 238–300.

McCauley, C., Parmelee, C. M., Sperber, C. D., and Carr, T. H. (1980). Early extraction of meaning from pictures and its relation to conscious identification. *Journal of Experimental Psychology: Human Perception & Performance*, 6, 265–276.

Merikle, P. M. (1982). Unconscious perception revisited. *Perception & Psychophysics*, 31, 298–301.

Merikle, P. M. (1983). Subliminal perception reaffirmed [Review of *Preconscious Processing*]. *Canadian Journal of Psychology*, 37, 324–326.

Merikle, P. M. (1984). Toward a definition of awareness. *Bulletin of the Psychonomic Society*, 22, 449–450.

Merikle, P. M., and Cheesman, J. (1986). Consciousness is a subjective state. *Behavioral and Brain Sciences* 9, 42.

Merikle, P. M., Cheesman, J., and Bray, J. (1982). PET Flasher: A machine-language subroutine for timing visual displays and response latencies. *Behavior Research Methods & Instrumentation*, 14, 26–28.

Neely, J. H. (1977). Semantic priming and retrieval from lexical memory: Roles of inhibitionless spreading activation and limited-capacity attention. *Journal of Experimental Psychology: General*, 106, 226–254.

Nolan, K. A., and Caramazza, A. (1982). Unconscious perception of meaning: A failure to replicate. *Bulletin of the Psychonomic Society*, 20, 23–26.

Posner, M. I., and Snyder, C. R. R. (1975a). Attention and cognitive control. In R. L. Solso (Ed.), *Information processing and cognition: The Loyola symposium* (pp. 55–85). Hillsdale, NJ: Erlbaum.

Posner, M. I., and Snyder, C. R. R. (1975b). Facilitation and inhibition in the processing of signals. In P. M. A. Rabbitt and S. Dornic (Eds.), *Attention and performance V* (pp. 669–682). New York: Academic Press.

Purcell, D. G., Stewart, A. L., and Stanovich, K. E. (1983). Another look at semantic priming without awareness. *Perception & Psychophysics*, 34, 65–71.

Shevrin, H., and Dickman, S. (1980). The psychological unconscious: A necessary assumption for all psychological theory? *American Psychologist*, 35, 421–434.

Taylor, D. A. (1977). Time course of context effects. *Journal of Experimental Psychology: General*, 106, 404–426.

Underwood, G. (1982). Attention and awareness in cognitive and motor skills. In G. Underwood (Ed.), *Aspects of consciousness: Vol. 3. Awareness and self-awareness* (pp. 111–145). London: Academic Press.

34 The Psychological Unconscious: A Necessary Assumption for All Psychological Theory?

Howard Shevrin and Scott Dickman

In a section entitled "Can states of mind be unconscious?" William James (1890), in his classic *Principles of psychology*, presented 10 arguments in favor of unconscious processes and 10 refutations of these arguments. The arguments in favor of unconscious states of mind ranged from unconscious inference, as in perceptual constancy, to unconscious motivation, which has since become so closely identified with psychoanalysis and Freud. To most of the arguments in favor of unconscious processes, James replied that a more parsimonious approach could be based on the assumption of neurophysiological processes unassociated with any psychological counterparts (e.g., "activated brain-tracts") or on the assumption that a psychological state could be briefly conscious and quickly forgotten, a fate suffered by many dreams. He also advanced the argument of a "split-off" cortical consciousness, as in multiple personalities, which sounds very much like a position recently taken by Hilgard (1977). James (1890) warned that "the unconscious is the sovereign means for believing whatever one likes in psychology and of turning what might become a science into a tumbling ground for whimsies" (p. 163).

Historically, American psychology since James has taken extreme positions on the issue of unconscious mental processes. Behaviorism, reacting against the methodological deficiencies of introspection, not only rejected the unconscious but also rid itself of consciousness, a direction hardly agreeable to James, for whom consciousness was the very subject matter of psychology. Psychoanalysis, as reflected in much clinical practice, has continued to base itself on unconscious mental processes, no matter what its particular school—classical Freudian, neo-Freudian, Jungian, Sullivanian, and so forth. Recent popular variants, such as transactional analysis, primal-scream therapy, and gestalt therapy, also share the assumption of unconscious mental processes. In more recent years,

the "black box," into which no Skinnerian would peer, has tempted the voyeuristic impulses of not a few behaviorists. A growing number of behaviorists have begun thinking about thinking, finding it necessary to hypothesize about cognitive factors mediating between stimulus and response. Shallice (1972) has argued against the behaviorists' rejection of consciousness as a pseudoconcept, contending that "concepts such as strategy and rehearsal are ... used as explanatory concepts. Such concepts depend on the theorist reflecting on conscious experience" (p. 383). Others, such as London (1972), Bandura (1974), and Lazarus (1977), have described their own evolution from radical behaviorism, in which cognitive mediating factors play no role, to a view of psychology in which subjective and conscious events are important. As cognition and consciousness have returned to psychology, the concept of unconscious mental processes has received increasing attention (Erdelyi 1974, Neisser 1976, Nisbett and Wilson 1977, Posner 1973).

It is the purpose of this article to show that in a number of different research areas, investigators have developed explanations that incorporate concepts akin to psychological unconscious processes. In fact, the variety and extent of such explanations, touching on several significant areas of investigation, suggest strongly to us the likelihood that no psychological theory can do without the assumption of a psychological unconscious.

Before presenting the models referred to, it will be necessary to offer a definition of unconscious psychological processes.

The Psychological Unconscious: Description and Definition

The clinical phenomena that led to the assumption of unconscious processes often take the form of a patient describing a bothersome condition that the patient can neither account for nor control (e.g., a phobia, a self-destructive pattern of behavior, a depressive mood) (Rapaport 1944/1967, Sherwood 1969). The patient's report in effect conveys a discontinuity in his or her ability to make sense out of some important aspect of experience.[1] Thus, a discontinuity is inferred when the apparent (i.e., consciously accessible) causal factors for a particular thought, feeling, or act are not, in and of themselves, sufficient to explain its occurrence. The psychodynamically oriented clinician then assumes that the disturbance can be accounted for by the existence of certain psychological processes unknown and unavailable to the patient. Underlying the concept of a psychological unconscious is the axiomatic belief that psychological factors are not epiphenomenal but can be causative agents. The psychological unconscious is simply that class of psychological events that are at the time unknown to the patient but that actively affect the patient's behavior. Furthermore, this impact on behavior reveals itself as a discontinuity, in which illogical or irrational relationships are often involved. Thus, the psychodynamic concept of the unconscious can be defined in terms of three characteristics: It is *psychological*, it is *active*, and it can be *different* in character from conscious psychological processes.

By *psychological* we mean simply that all categories of descriptive terminology applicable to conscious experience can also be applied to unconscious processes: perception, judgment, thought, affect, motivation, and so forth.[2] Thus, personally significant, cognitively abstract, and highly idiosyncratic experiences can be unconscious. Moreover, inasmuch as conscious processes are correlated with brain events, the same may be assumed for unconscious processes.

By *active* we mean that unconscious processes affect ongoing behavior and experience, even though the experiencer may be unaware of this influence. From this point of view, a memory trace, indicating some structural modification of the nervous system, would not be considered to belong to the psychological unconscious until such time as it actively influenced psychological events.

By *different* we mean that unconscious processes may follow different principles of organization than those that characterize psychological processes occurring during the normal, waking state of consciousness.

On the basis of this definition, we arrive at two postulates—a weak form and a strong form—for which we shall venture to adduce a range of relevant theory in psychology at large. In the *weak* form of this postulate, we shall assume that psychological unconscious processes exist and actively affect conscious psychological processes. In the *strong* form of the postulate, we shall add only that these psychological unconscious processes follow different laws of organization. It is worth noting that the view of unconscious processes held by psychodynamically oriented clinicians includes an important feature that we have not incorporated into either of the above postulates: We make no reference at this point to the special role of motivational factors (e.g., drives, impulses), which are so important to the psychodynamically oriented clinician. However, in the course of our discussion, we shall attempt to point out the ways in which motivational factors fit within our conceptual framework.

Evidence and Theory in Support of the Psychological Unconscious

We shall now consider a number of different sources of evidence and a variety of theories, all of which appear to involve an implicit assumption of psychological unconscious processes. These areas of research and theory are (a) selective attention, (b) subliminal perception, and (c) certain visual phenomena involving perceptual processing, namely, retinal image stabilization, binocular rivalry, and backward masking. We do not consider these areas to be exhaustive of the areas in psychology that would provide support for our thesis; rather, we consider these particular areas to be of special importance because of the diversity of the methods on which they are based and because of their theoretical significance.

Selective Attention

An individual, at any given time, is confronted with more stimulation from within and from without than can be managed adaptively. Some degree and kind of selection must occur. What is the nature of this selection process? In recent years some interesting answers have emerged, based on a body of highly ingenious experimentation. We shall focus on the general theories that have been advanced to account for the findings emerging from this area of research, rather than reviewing the specific studies themselves. For detailed reviews of selective-attention research, see Moray (1969) and Kahneman (1973).

Inherent in all the major models of attention is the assumption that at least part of the cognition related to attention takes place outside of awareness. Six such models will be described briefly. These models are based on extensive experimental research that has given rise to a literature marked by sharp controversy. For our purposes, however, we need rely only on the noncontroversial and broadly accepted findings, while identifying the controversial issues wherever they are relevant.

The earliest of these models was proposed by Broadbent (1958). In Broadbent's original "filter theory" of attention, signals enter the perceptual system through a number of parallel sensory channels. These parallel sensory inputs feed into a memory store, where they are retained for a few seconds. Beyond this memory store is a single channel that has a much smaller capacity than the combined capacity of all the input channels. A filter, lying between the memory store and the limited-capacity channel, selects one of the input lines and allows the signals that enter through it to gain access to the limited-capacity channel. Signals feeding in from the other channels are held briefly in memory and then lost. Thus, an initial sensory analysis of the stimulus input does occur prior to awareness of the nature of that input. Broadbent indicates that the determination of which signals are allowed access to the limited-capacity channel is based not only on the properties of the stimuli but also on the state of the organism (e.g., its drive state).

While a filtering mechanism of the sort described does involve perceptual processing outside of awareness, it should be noted that the analysis that occurs prior to awareness is a very rudimentary one inasmuch as only sensory information is involved—*meaning* is not a factor. Moreover, there is no provision for those stimuli that do not achieve awareness to be stored in any form. However, because Broadbent uses terms like *memory* to describe processes occurring prior to awareness, it appears that he considers them to be psychological; because they precede awareness, they are unconscious; lastly, because the filtering that occurs outside of awareness affects what will become conscious and because it interacts with the state of the organism at the time, these unconscious psychological processes are not simply latent but are active in our sense. There is also a hint that these unconscious processes work on a different principle from that of conscious processes—input is organized along multiple channels, as contrasted with the single channel for conscious processes. On the whole, however, Broadbent's (1958) model is more consistent with the weak postulate for unconscious processes than with the strong postulate.

Treisman's (1964) theory of perception is similar to Broadbent's in that information enters the system through multiple parallel channels. Treisman's model incorporates two stages of perceptual processing. The initial filter analyzes the incoming signals only on the basis of simple physical properties, such as intensity or frequency. All signals pass through this filter and are processed further; however, this first filter attenuates the signal strength of the nonattended channels to a level below that of the attended channel. The signals then proceed through a second screening process based on more complex characteristics. In this higher order screening process, thresholds differ for different types of signals, so that even though a signal may have been attenuated by the earlier filter, it can still pass through this later screening process if it is of a type for which the threshold is low. In this second-level screening, the mechanisms that respond to biologically (or emotionally) important signals have permanently lowered thresholds; the thresholds for other types of signals may vary, depending on circumstances. In this model, the full import of a signal reaches awareness only after it has passed through the higher order second-stage screening process.

For Treisman, the processing that occurs prior to awareness involves far more complex attributes of the stimulus than is the case in Broadbent's (1958) model. Furthermore, these complex unconscious processes are concurrent (going on in parallel channels), whereas conscious processes are serial (single-channel in nature). Thus, Treisman's (1964) model is strongly consistent with the weak postulate and moderately consistent with the strong postulate.

Deutsch and Deutsch (1963) have propounded a theory of attention similar to Treisman's except that it does not posit an initial analysis on the basis of simple physical characteristics. Instead, all signals reach the higher order analyzers and then undergo complex perceptual analysis. Each signal increases the output of some mechanism for perceptual discrimination to a certain level; only the highest level output enters awareness. Conscious perception, in this scheme, is a response to the output of the higher order analyzing mechanisms; thus complex processing must occur outside of awareness. This model is, for our purposes, essentially similar to the Treisman (1964) model, and the same considerations apply to it as to the latter model.

The fourth model of attention to be discussed is that of Neisser (1967). Neisser's model is similar to the others described in that it posits parallel input processes that feed into a single mechanism of awareness. Neisser differs from the other theorists, however, in his conception of the nature of the processing that occurs without awareness and also in the degree to which he concerns himself with the explication of these perceptual processes in cognitive terms.

According to Neisser (1967), attentive mechanisms come into play only after preliminary processes have already ordered the stimulus field into coherent figural units, because these attentive mechanisms cannot operate on the whole field simultaneously. The preliminary, or preattentive, processes must of necessity be global and holistic in nature, since their function is to separate each figure or object as a whole from the rest of the stimulus field. Attentive processes, in contrast to the preattentive ones just described, are sequential, proceeding in a logical fashion on the basis of what is appropriate in terms of past experience.

Neisser's model allows for the possibility that a crude percept resulting from the preattentive processing may receive no further elaboration within consciousness. He raises the possibility that such elaboration may be deliberately avoided in certain areas and suggests a similarity between this notion and the clinician's concept of repression.

Neisser's (1967) model is clearly consistent with the weak postulate of a psychological unconscious. Complex psychological processes are carried on unconsciously, and there is an active commerce between these unconscious processes and conscious ones. But unconscious psychological processes are also qualitatively different from conscious ones in this scheme. Neisser's model is thus consistent with the strong postulate for unconscious processes as well.

In the fifth model to be described, offered by Posner (1973), a single-channel central-processing capacity is the aspect of attention most closely associated with consciousness.

Consciousness, in this view, involves such mental operations as rehearsal and choosing a response. At least two stages of perceptual processing, encoding and comparison with long-term memory, occur outside of consciousness; that is, they occur before the subject becomes aware of the stimulus.

It would appear that the first stage of processing in Posner's scheme consists in the encoding of the stimulus. There is, in Posner's (1973) view, "simultaneous registration and retention of multiple codes of the same event" (p. 41). The different ways in which a given stimulus can be encoded (e.g., visually, symbolically) represent "isolable subsystems," which develop independently of each other. The later, rehearsal phase (associated with consciousness) is code specific and tends to select one of the codes for dominance. However, even when attention is directed (because of the nature of the task) to only one of the ways in which a stimulus can be coded, the stimulus may nonetheless be coded other ways as well. Posner (1973) gives an example of this phenomenon, drawn from the visual-search literature:

When the subject is presented visually with a list of letters, the names are also activated although they may not be conscious. Similarly, when the subject hears a list of letter names, the visual code is increased in availability. (p. 59)

The next stage of analysis after encoding involves comparison of the stimulus with the contents of long-term memory. According to Posner, the processes involved here also take place outside of awareness. In the studies Posner draws on most, the subject is first presented with a "target" stimulus (e.g., a digit) and is then told to search through a stimulus array to locate that particular stimulus. This stage of processing, in Posner's view, involves a comparison of each stimulus in the array through which the subject is searching with the previously presented stimulus (now stored in long-term memory). This comparison takes place outside of awareness. Posner

(1973), reviewing research bearing on this point, concludes,

The data suggest that both the target and non-target items are subject to a memory search process but only the target item gives rise to the phenomenological experience of jumping out at the subject. Thus, the phenomenal experience occurs rather late in the sequence of processing. (p. 41)

Posner believes that in the course of perceptual processing the stimulus makes contact with long-term memory prior to the point at which awareness occurs. He also argues that the fact that a limited-capacity channel exists in the sequence of perceptual processing does not restrict the range of associations that can be activated by a given stimulus outside of awareness. "Indeed," suggests Posner (1973), "it might require more effort to inhibit such associations than to produce them" (p. 41). This notion fits in well with the strong postulate because it suggests that processing outside of awareness is qualitatively different from processing within awareness.

For Posner and his colleagues, then, consciousness is bound up with those processes that involve the limited-capacity system. "This mechanism," they state, "serves to impose a serial order upon what are essentially widespread parallel processes initiated by a stimulus" (Posner, Klein, Summers, and Buggie 1973, p. 11). They even go so far as to suggest a physiological correlate (an event-related brain potential) for this central processing mechanism: "The mechanism whose activity we have been detecting by interference [i.e., the mechanism of consciousness] is also the one which releases the late positive wave (P_{300})" (Posner et al. 1973, p. 11). Posner's model is consistent with the strong postulate for unconscious psychological processes.

Although not primarily dealing with attention, Sternberg's (1975) research on memory in visual processing is of some relevance. The basic paradigm in Sternberg's studies involves two steps. First, the subject commits to memory a set of stimuli (e.g., letters, digits, figures), which are called the *positive set*. He is then presented with a single test stimulus and must indicate by pressing one of two switches whether or not the test stimulus is a member of the positive set.

The results of Sternberg's reaction-time studies led him to hypothesize that the subject goes through the positive set, comparing each member with the test stimulus, at a rate of about 30 comparisons per second. Sternberg (1975) states specifically that "judging from what subjects report, the search is not accessible to introspection" (p. 5). Furthermore, Sternberg cites evidence that this rate is substantially faster than the rate of covert speech (which might be taken as one index of the rate of conscious processing). And he also states that "even when introspections include a search, it is reported to be slow and self-terminating" (p. 10), by which Sternberg means that the subject stops the search as soon as he or she finds the counterpart of the test stimulus among the comparison stimuli. In other words, there is a qualitative difference between conscious and unconscious processing. Sternberg's model is consistent with the assumption that unconscious psychological processes exist and do, in fact, obey different laws from those governing conscious processes, and thus his model is consistent with the strong postulate.

Summary

All six theorists assume that an initial phase of cognitive activity occurs outside of awareness, and each uses psychological terms to describe the processes involved. Second, these processes outside of awareness interact with and influence ongoing and subsequent conscious psychological processes, at the very least insofar as they determine what enters consciousness. For these reasons, these models are consistent with the weak postulate for unconscious psychological processes. But there is more. All six models posit that cognitive processes outside of awareness are based on a different mode of cognition from that of conscious processes. For five of these models, unconscious processes are multichan-

neled, whereas conscious processes are single channeled. In the sixth model (Sternberg 1975), at least one kind of unconscious process is considered to be exhaustive in nature and much more rapid in execution, as compared with conscious processes. For some theoreticians there are even greater differences. For Neisser (1967), preattentive cognition is global and gestalt in character, though lacking in symbolic significance; for Posner (1973; Posner et al. 1973), multiple codes can be activated outside of awareness even though only a single code may enter consciousness. Posner raises the possibility of the inhibition of associations existing prior to consciousness as well as of a physiological index for consciousness itself. All of these models are based, not on clinical data, but largely on experimental investigations. There is still a considerable gap between the conception of unconscious psychological processes offered by these theorists and the view of the same processes held by psychodynamically oriented clinicians. For instance, none of these theoreticians discusses the possibility that percepts can be stored in long-term memory and can exert an active influence on simultaneous conscious processes, even though they may never enter into awareness or may not do so until long after they were originally perceived. The conception of unconscious motivation and memory held by most psychodynamic theorists, however, does in fact encompass such a possibility.

We shall now turn our attention to the literature on subliminal perception, in which some of these possibilities are considered.

Subliminal Perception

In selective-attention research, the stimuli are either fully conscious or can become conscious once attention is directed to them. In dichotic-listening experiments, for example, on which a considerable amount of attention research is based, stimuli are usually presented separately to each ear. Subjects are instructed to attend to the stimuli in one ear and to repeat them out loud to insure continued attention. Of interest is the finding that, generally, subjects are unaware of the stimuli in the unattended ear, although these stimuli exercise an influence on various response parameters of the attended stimuli. The unattended stimuli remain outside awareness only as long as a subject is attending to the other ear.

There is also an extensive literature on the investigation of stimuli that cannot be consciously perceived, even when attention is directed to them. These are stimuli that are presented so quickly that no matter how alert and focused a subject's attention, the stimuli remain unreportable. Nevertheless, effects of the subliminal stimuli are detectable. Dixon (1971), who has written an extensive evaluation of the subliminal-perception literature and has offered an interesting neurophysiological model, has suggested that selective attention and subliminal perception represent "end points on a single continuum of information processing" (p. 306). At any given time, an individual is presented with a broad array of stimuli of varying intensities and of varying relevance to adaptive tasks. Selection on some basis must occur. Subliminal stimuli are those stimuli that do not become conscious simply because they are too weak in intensity, even though they may be highly relevant.

Subliminal-perception research is relevant to our thesis because this research suggests that complex effects of stimuli that do not enter awareness can persist well beyond a few seconds or minutes, which is the span that the effects of stimuli in selective-attention experiments have thus far been determined to persist. At the same time, subliminal-perception research has been a source of controversy in psychology. In fact, Dixon's (1971) book is subtitled *The nature of a controversy*. The same book presents a strong case in favor of subliminal perception as a valid phenomenon, based on converging evidence from eight bodies of supporting research. More recently, Nisbett and Wilson (1977) have argued,

The basic question of whether people can respond to a stimulus in the absence of the ability to report verbally on its existence would today be answered in the affirmative by many more investigators than would have been the case a decade ago ... largely because of better experimental methods and the convincing theoretical argument that subliminal perception phenomena can be derived ... from the notion of selective attention and filtering. (p. 239)

These comments are of special relevance because much of the controversy has centered on methodological difficulties.[3] Our emphasis in this article, however, is not primarily on the actual research investigations but on the explanations developed to account for a variety of findings. As with the selective-attention literature, controversies within the field may challenge one or another experimental hypothesis, but it can be shown that there is an underlying commonality in the explanations offered that does not depend on any one particular finding. Unlike selective-attention researchers, who did not set out to study unconscious psychological processes but were increasingly compelled to take such processes into account, researchers in the area of subliminal perception have often been interested in such processes from the start and have purposefully studied them experimentally.

Before briefly describing a number of models for explaining subliminal-perception findings, some of which parallel the models just presented for selective attention, we think it may be helpful to formulate what we consider to be the key issues bearing on our thesis for which subliminal-perception studies provide support:

1. Subliminal-perception research is concerned with stimuli too weak to become conscious immediately, no matter how much attention is directed to the stimulus field. No amount of shifting attention, as in dichotic-listening experiments, can bring the stimulus into consciousness.

2. Nevertheless, these stimuli have detectable effects on conscious processes, both immediately and, in some cases, after an interval of time.

3. These effects emerge in changed states of consciousness, as in dreams. By contrast, selective-attention research thus far has been concerned exclusively with one state of consciousness: the usual waking, alert state that most psychological subjects are paid to maintain.

4. Subliminal stimuli can be used to explore differences between unconscious and conscious processes.

The subliminal-perception literature provides an additional line of converging evidence for the necessity of assuming the existence of unconscious psychological processes.

We shall now describe five models developed to explain the various findings in the subliminal-perception literature.

Klein and Holt (1960) postulated that the effects of subliminal stimuli persist only briefly and have to be incorporated quickly into some ongoing cognitive activity or else they will disappear and leave no trace of their presence. They argued that inasmuch as the subliminal stimulus is never cognized as such but is only detected by its indirect effects on conscious processes, it will remain ineffective unless it can be assimilated into some ongoing cognitive activity. This model was based largely on an experimental paradigm in which subliminal stimuli were interspersed among conscious stimuli. The subliminal stimulus was either the word *angry* or the word *happy*, while the conscious stimulus was an ambiguous face that could be judged either way. The investigators determined that the face was seen as happy or angry depending on the particular subliminal word presented (Bach and Klein 1957; Sackeim, Packer, and Gur 1977; Smith, Spence, and Klein 1959). Klein and Holt's model follows closely the findings derived from their particular method. Interestingly, this model is comparable to Broadbent's (1958) view: Stimuli enter a short-term memory system, and unless they become conscious immediately, they have no further effect. The main difference from Broadbent's model is the fact that this inter-

action between short-term memory and attention concerns subliminal stimuli exclusively. Klein and Holt's model is consistent with the weak postulate for unconscious psychological processes.

On the basis of an interesting series of experiments, Spence arrived at a model that is at variance with the model proposed by Klein and Holt: In his research Spence determined that a subliminally presented word can evoke a series of associations based on its meaning (Spence 1961, 1966; Spence and Holland 1962; Spence and Smith 1977). He found that associations could be elicited at some point after the subliminal stimulus had been presented. On the basis of his findings, Spence posited what he called the "restricting effects of awareness." According to Spence, when a stimulus is presented subliminally, as compared to when it is presented supraliminally, a greater variety of associations are elicited. Awareness of the stimulus appears to limit or restrict the range of associations elicited by the stimulus word. This concept appears to be quite similar to the one offered by Posner (1973) when he proposed that stimuli are multicoded (i.e., elicit multiple associations) even though we may be consciously aware of only one of these codes or associations. Again, the significant difference is that Spence is concerned solely with subliminal stimuli, which in themselves never become conscious. Spence's model is consistent with the strong postulate for unconscious psychological processes.

Perhaps the most comprehensive model for subliminal perception has been offered by Fisher (1956). A pioneer in subliminal-perception research, he suggested that it would be useful to assume that all cognitive processes of whatever kind have to start in an unconscious phase; some become conscious almost immediately, while others remain unconscious for longer periods of time and may then appear in various altered states of consciousness such as dreams. Moreover, Fisher interpreted his findings to support the view that unconscious cognition is qualitatively different from conscious cognition. His model is consistent with the strong postulate for unconscious psychological processes.

Dixon (1971) proposed one of the first neurophysiological models attempting to account for subliminal perception. He argued that although certain instances of subliminal perception may involve temporal or spatial summation at the level of peripheral receptor neurons, for complex stimulus arrays the processes involved must lie at higher levels of the nervous system. As evidence for this hypothesis, Dixon cited a study done by Libet, Alberts, Wright, and Feinstein (1967) demonstrating that cortical responses can be evoked by stimuli below the awareness threshold. He also described an experiment by Shevrin and Rennick (1967) which indicated that subliminal stimuli influence both cortical evoked potentials and the subject's free associations. And he discussed a study by Begleiter, Gross, and Kissin (1969) which suggests that it may be the meaning rather than the structure of the subliminal stimulus that determines both the cortical response and subsequent behavior.

Dixon's (1971) proposed physiological model is consistent with these findings and also with results of studies of perceptual defense which suggest that the threshold (in terms of intensity) for emotionally significant stimuli, such as words or pictures, tends to be either higher or lower than the threshold for emotionally neutral stimuli. Dixon argued that the most important mechanism underlying these phenomena probably involves corticofugal influences on the reticular activating system. According to this view, the classical afferent fibers transmit the information that forms the specific content of consciousness, but these fibers do not per se mediate awareness. For awareness to occur, there must be not only sensory input through these afferent fibers but a simultaneous activation of the nonspecific reticular system.

In subliminal perception, then, the intensity of the stimulus is great enough to elicit activity in the sensory fibers but lacks sufficient energy to activate the nonspecific reticular system. Thus information reaches the cortex without awareness of the stimulus itself.

Subliminal perception, according to Dixon, is made possible by the fact that the primary, classical afferent lemniscal system (which conveys sensory information to the cortex) conducts faster than the secondary, nonspecific extralemniscal system (which is involved in reticular activation). As a consequence of this disparity in conduction speeds, it is possible for information to reach the cortex and for the cortex to exert inhibitory control over the reticular system prior to the arrival of the neural impulse that would normally have activated that system and thereby produced awareness of the stimulus.

Inasmuch as this suggests that the underlying neural processes are different for subliminal and supraliminal processes, Dixon's (1971) model is consistent with the strong postulate for unconscious psychological processes. And, whether this particular model is correct or not, the most important contribution Dixon has made with regard to the physiological basis of subliminal perception (as he himself has pointed out) is simply to demonstrate that such a phenomenon is plausible in terms of current neurophysiological knowledge. Such a demonstration, in turn, can serve as a spur to further investigation of the neurophysiological underpinnings of unconscious psychological processes. To the extent that such future research can firmly establish that such neurophysiological measures as cortical evoked potentials index unconscious psychological processes in the same way that evoked potentials have been shown to index conscious perceptual processing, it will provide investigators with an additional tool with which to study these unconscious processes.

On the basis of findings from a series of evoked-potential studies employing a pair of visual stimuli presented sub- and supraliminally, Shevrin (1973) proposed that the evidence strongly suggests that (a) complex unconscious psychological processes have identifiable neurophysiological correlates, (b) these neurophysiological processes are associated with attention to the meaning of the stimulus, (c) different parameters of the evoked potential are associated with different thought processes related to the subliminal stimulus, and (d) subjects characterized as repressive, on the basis of psychological tests, show reduced evoked potentials to the subliminal stimuli but show augmented potentials to the same stimuli when they are supraliminal. Moreover, Shevrin (1978) has suggested that there may, in fact, exist an evoked-potential correlate of consciousness. This correlate may take the form of a critical duration of a late positive evoked-potential component occurring sometime between 150 and 250 ms poststimulus. This model is based in part on Libet's findings demonstrating that a certain critical duration of cortical excitation (0.5 s in actual time) is necessary before consciousness of a stimulus is activated (Libet et al. 1967). Thus, the "weakness" in subliminal stimulation may not be the failure to activate the reticular activating system but may be a failure to activate it for a critical duration. Shevrin's explanation, in particular the point noted in (d) above, is consistent with the strong postulate for unconscious psychological processes.

In partial confirmation of Shevrin's work, Kostandov and Arzumanov (1977) have reported that the average evoked potential associated with emotionally significant verbal stimuli showed systematic changes in latency and amplitude as a function of consciousness.[4] When neutral and emotionally meaningful words were present in consciousness, a positive wave at 300 ms poststimulus (P_{300}) tended to be greater in amplitude for the emotional words at the occipital region and also shorter in latency; no differences were found at the vertex. When neutral and emotionally meaningful words remained unrecognized, latency differences disappeared, but significant amplitude differences were present in favor of the emotional words at both the occipital site and the vertex site for P_{300}. Kos-

tandov and Arzumanov (1977) concluded that "the difference in the amplitude of the evoked potential for neutral and emotional words suggests ... that even if the verbal stimulus is not recognized, the analysis of its semantic content occurs at the cerebral cortex" (p. 321). They have hypothesized that "unspecific impulses" from the limbic system must undergo a different fate depending on whether the emotional stimulus is conscious or not. When it is conscious, the effect of these impulses is restricted to the occipital region; when the stimulus is unconscious, their effect appears to spread to the vertex as well. The possible psychological effects of this spread are not specified, although one can speculate that they may be related to Spence's "restricting effects of awareness" and the "single-channel" conception of consciousness embodied in a number of cognitive models of selective attention. It is also important to note that, as in previous perceptual-defense studies, the recognition threshold for the emotionally meaningful words is higher than the threshold for the neutral words for most subjects but lower for some subjects. Nevertheless, the evoked-potential difference is found regardless of threshold. Thus we can see that there is indeed a prior cognition of semantic properties, as evidenced by the evoked potential, to which the individual responds with either a raising or a lowering of recognition thresholds. The defense or vigilance is subsequent to actual cognition. Insofar as there are differences for unconscious stimuli, we can consider this study to support the strong postulate for unconscious processes. It is also of interest, in view of Posner's (1973) hypothesis concerning the P_{300} amplitude as a possible correlate of consciousness, that the Russian investigators found that the P_{300} amplitude was the critical correlate. For the Russian investigators, however, P_{300} appears to be associated with unconscious processes, whereas Posner has hypothesized that P_{300} might be a correlate of consciousness. Further research will be needed to reconcile this difference.

Summary

In general, the findings and models emerging from subliminal-perception research converge strikingly on the same conclusion that the findings and models emerging from attention research have reached: A great deal of complex cognitive activity can go on without benefit of consciousness. Moreover, this complex activity is characterized by different properties from those present in conscious cognitive activity. Thus, subliminal research supports both the weak and the strong postulates for unconscious psychological processes.

Visual Phenomena Involving Perceptual Processing

Subliminal-perception research generally deals with complex stimuli whose effects are studied over relatively long periods of time. We have cited experiments that show how cortical evoked potentials accompany subliminal cognition. In addition to these experiments, there is a growing body of research which has found that cortical evoked potentials are present when a stabilized retinal image disappears from consciousness, when an image is suppressed in one eye through binocular rivalry with the other, and when a stimulus is masked by a second, succeeding stimulus. For more extensive reviews of the research pertaining to the central mediations of these phenomena, see Turvey (1973), Coren and Porac (1974), and Walker (1978).

For our purposes, a major limitation of these studies lies in the fact that they make no attempt to document any contemporaneous effects on conscious cognition, leaving unanswered the question of whether the psychological processes indexed here can be said to be active (in the sense used in our definition of the weak postulate). Hence, these studies can only be considered to lend indirect support to the weak postulate; they are noted here largely because they represent, potentially at least, a converging line of evidence based on quite different methods from those described heretofore.

Retinal Image Stabilization

When an image is stabilized on the retina in such a way that as the eye moves, the stimulus continues to act on precisely the same area of the retina, the image disappears (although part or all of it may briefly reappear from time to time). Riggs and Whittle (1967) and Lehman, Beeler, and Fender (1967) have reported that there were no changes in the cortical evoked potential when their subjects stated that the image had faded from consciousness. At the same time, the retinal evoked potential indicated that retinal cells were firing, and so the visual stimulus was being propagated along the optic nerve. Riggs and Whittle used an occipital electrode, and Lehman et al. used an occipital-parietal display. In the latter study, the investigators also found that bursts of EEG alpha appeared to precede the reported fading of the image, strongly suggesting that a central "turn-off" of consciousness was at work. The authors of these two studies concluded that the loss of awareness was a cortical and not a peripheral phenomenon. Studies that have used other approaches than examination of cortical evoked potentials to investigate the effect of stabilization of the retinal image have also offered evidence that this phenomenon is central rather than peripheral in origin (e.g., Bennett-Clark and Evans 1963; Blakemore, Muncey, and Ridley 1971). In the one study with less striking results (Keesey 1969), it was still found that an evoked potential was present for the faded image, but it was smaller in size than when associated with a conscious stimulus. Thus, retinal image stabilization seems to represent another experimental paradigm in which the evoked potential serves to index the existence of perceptual processing at a cortical level in the absence of subjective awareness of the stimulus.

Binocular Rivalry

Binocular-rivalry studies offer still another experimental paradigm in which the presence of cortical evoked potentials may be detected in the absence of subjective perception of the eliciting stimulus. The general procedure in these studies is to present different images simultaneously to the two eyes, making certain that the visual fields of the eyes do not overlap. In such a situation, at different times one or the other eye will be dominant; that is, the subject will be aware of the image presented to the visual field of that eye while being unaware of the image presented to the visual field of the other (suppressed) eye. A visual evoked response (VER) will be found for the suppressed image even though this VER may be smaller than the VER associated with the image for the dominant eye (Cobb, Morton, and Ettlinger 1967; Harter, Seiple, and Musso 1974; Harter, Towle, and Musso 1976; Lehman et al. 1967; Lehman and Fender 1968; Riggs and Whittle 1967; Spekreijse, Van Der Tweel, and Regan 1972).

It might also be noted that a number of studies of binocular rivalry using other approaches than evoked-potential recording have also found evidence to suggest that binocular suppression occurs at a central (i.e., cortical) rather than at a peripheral level (Walker 1978). In one particularly interesting study, for instance, Walker (1975) found that a moving visual stimulus that was presented at a subliminal intensity to the suppressed eye (the subject reported no awareness of it whatsoever) reduced the proportion of time the other eye maintained its dominance. In his discussion of his results, Walker argued that this phenomenon can be accounted for only by assuming that information about the moving stimulus reaches the cortex even though it never enters awareness. It would appear, then, that binocular rivalry represents another condition under which perceptual information is processed at a cortical level despite the fact that it is not subjectively perceived.

Backward Masking

Two basic types of backward masking have been demonstrated. In one type, a stimulus is presented, followed by a second stimulus of greater intensity. When the inter-stimulus interval is around 25 ms and the second stimulus is more intense than the first, the subject will perceive only the second stimulus. This phenomenon is sometimes called the *Crawford effect*. The other type of backward masking is termed *metacontrast*. Here, the stimuli used are generally shapes or patterns. They are presented one after the other at equal light intensities. The location of the two stimuli in the subject's visual field is such that if the two stimuli were presented simultaneously, their contours would be adjacent. In this situation, the presentation of the second stimulus "masks" the subject's perception of the first, so that he or she is not aware of it. The Crawford effect appears to be mediated peripherally and will not be pursued further (see Donchin and Lindsley 1965; Donchin, Wicker, and Lindsley 1963; Fehmi, Adkins, and Lindsley 1969). However, there is reason to believe that in metacontrast the masked stimulus—although the subject is not aware of it—elicits a cortical evoked potential.

Andreassi and his coworkers have investigated this metacontrast phenomenon (Andreassi, DeSimone, and Mellers 1976; Andreassi, Mayzner, Beyda, and Davidovics 1971; Andreassi, Stern, and Okamura 1974). The general procedure was to present five X's (or patterns) in a horizontal spatial array: XXXXX. The second and fourth figures were presented simultaneously, followed after a brief interval by the first, third, and fifth figures (presented at the same time). In this way, the first two figures presented were surrounded on either side by the second set of three figures, providing the basis for the metacontrast effect to occur. When the stimulus sets were presented with an interstimulus interval of 40 ms, the subjects perceived the second set of stimuli but not the first. When masking was thus obtained, the amplitude of the visual evoked potential to the first, or masked, stimulus decreased as the disparity in intensity between the two stimuli was increased; however, the evoked potential never entirely disappeared, even in the conditions in which stimulus intensities were most discrepant.

The presence of an evoked potential in the absence of any awareness of the masked stimulus provides another example of perceptual processing outside of awareness.

Discussion and Conclusions

The different avenues of research and theorizing reviewed in this article converge on three fundamental propositions, which can be stated as follows:

1. The initial cognitive stage for all stimuli occurs outside of consciousness.

2. This initial cognitive stage outside of consciousness is psychological in nature, is active in its effect on consciousness, and can be different from conscious cognition in its principles of operation.

3. Consciousness of a stimulus is a later and optional stage in cognition.

These three propositions bring us to an interesting further question: If the initial stage of cognition is unconscious, what factors determine the emergence into consciousness of a particular stimulus? We should like to suggest that there are at least three groups of factors that, working singly or together, determine this final step in cognition:

1. Stimulus factors (e.g., loudness, brightness, figural coherence);

2. State factors (e.g., level of arousal, sleep stage, fatigue, distractibility);

3. Motivational factors (e.g., avoidance of anxiety, guilt, conflict).

Some cognitive theorists, such as Neisser (1967, 1976), have made reference to all three factors. Broadbent's (1958) model allowed for the state of the organism to affect the selection of stimuli that become conscious. Treisman (1964) posited built-in low thresholds for biologically and emotionally important stimuli, which would permit these stimuli to pass through higher filter systems into consciousness. Of special interest to the clinician is the last group of factors, consisting of motivational factors. Several experiments we have cited (Kostandov and Arzumanov 1977, Shevrin 1973) suggest that the specific emotional content of a stimulus may raise the threshold for the perception of that stimulus, with the clear implication that the stimulus is analyzed prior to the individual's awareness of it. As Posner (1973) noted in regard to his research on attentional processes, although an individual may be aware of the fact that a particular stimulus has "popped" into awareness, he may be quite unaware of the preceding complex selection process. Evidence of this kind provides the bridge to the psychoanalytic concept of repression. Repression may be conceptualized as a motivated inhibition of awareness of a particular stimulus. This motivated inhibition may work independently of stimulus strength and state of arousal. It is conceivable that at least some of the forces affecting the preattentive processes are motivational in nature.

In most cognitive research, and, in particular, in research on selective attention, generally only one state of consciousness is considered—the normal waking state. In fact, in many of these studies, consciousness is often tacitly equated with this particular state of normal waking consciousness. The single-channel cognition model of consciousness may be a special case limited to waking consciousness. Dream consciousness, states of intoxication, and psychotic states may not share this single-channel characteristic. These other states of consciousness remain an important area for experimental investigation because they might provide an additional bridge between laboratory research on cognitive processes and the consulting room.

Another important qualification to be borne in mind is that all the research cited in the present article is based on external stimuli. Much clinical thinking, on the other hand, is based on the fate of internal stimuli—for example, wishes and needs. While the evidence presented here does not demonstrate that the processing of internal stimuli is identical to the processing of external stimuli, it does suggest that these two processes are not necessarily dissimilar. Although Freud (1915/1958a) argued, and many clinicians have assumed, that the mechanisms used by the individual to fend off external stimuli differ from those used for internal stimuli (e.g., motor acts for external stimuli vs. repression for internal stimuli), the evidence presented in this article suggests that a much greater similarity exists between the two modes of processing than Freud supposed. In fact, elsewhere in his writings Freud described how attentional processes are involved in symptom formation (Breuer and Freud 1893–95/1958) and in repression itself (Freud 1915/1958b), thus providing a bridge, through the concept of attention, to the models proposed by attention theorists that we have described in this article.

If the thesis we have elaborated here is correct, then James (1890) was mistaken in his rejection of unconscious psychological processes. Rather than being the "sovereign means for believing what one likes in psychology," the assumption of unconscious psychological processes appears to be a conceptual necessity in a variety of models dealing with selective attention, subliminal perception, retinal image stabilization, binocular rivalry, and metacontrast. Ironically, these areas of investigation are entirely experimental, not clinical, in nature and are thus not as likely to be subject to James's concern that the notion of unconscious psychological processes would turn "what might become a science into a tumbling ground for whimsies." Behaviorism, for its part, must accommodate itself to accepting the importance of what goes on inside the "black box," especially since we now have methods for investigating its contents. The clear message from much recent thinking in psychology appears to be that behavior cannot be understood without taking conscious experience into account and that conscious experience cannot be fully under-

stood without taking unconscious psychological processes into account. The laboratory and the consulting room do seem to be sharing at least a common wall, which may in fact turn out to have a door in it.

Finally, if the thesis elaborated in this article is correct, then no psychological model that seeks to explain how human beings know, learn, or behave can ignore the concept of unconscious psychological processes. Moreover, we dare to hope that the present article may provide a basis for a shared task and useful communication between clinician and experimenter.

Notes

1. The reader is referred to Rapaport (1944/1967) for an extended discussion of the concept of discontinuity and its relationship to psychodynamic concepts.

2. We are defining the term *psychological* on the basis of an ostensive definition, comparable to defining the color red by pointing to a series of red objects. In this way we are essentially using a common sense approach, drawing on readily available experience shared by most people. We chose this type of definition rather than an analytic type (e.g., red is defined as that color experience associated with a physical stimulus having the property of so many angstrom units) to avoid getting into a "mind–body" quagmire. For our present purposes we propose to leave open the question whether by such terms as judgment, thought, affect, and the like we are talking about "mind" or "body." We are simply talking about identifiable and reportable phenomena.

3. One important controversial issue has centered around the use of threshold measures in subliminal research, which, according to signal-detection theorists, confounds sensory sensitivity with response parameters. Dixon (1971) has taken up this issue, discussing the theoretical implications as well as citing subliminal-perception research based on signal-detection techniques that have yielded positive results. Nisbett and Wilson (1977) also discuss signal-detection theory and subliminal perception.

4. It is of considerable interest that a growing number of Russian investigators have been conducting inves-

tigations on subliminal and other unconscious processes. The Russians have sponsored an international conference on unconscious processes; three volumes of the proceedings of this conference have been published, containing articles by Russian, American, French, German, and other investigators (Prangishvili, Sherozia, and Bassin 1978).

References

Andreassi, J., DeSimone, J., and Mellers, B. Amplitude changes in the visual evoked cortical potential with backward masking. *Electroencephalography and Clinical Neurophysiology*, 1976, *41*, 387–398.

Andreassi, J., Mayzner, M., Beyda, D., and Davidovics, S. Visual cortical potentials under conditions of sequential blanking. *Perception & Psychophysics*, 1971, *10*, 164–168.

Andreassi, J., Stern, M., and Okamura, H. Visual cortical evoked potentials as a function of intensity variations in sequential blanking. *Psychophysiology*, 1974, *11*, 336–345.

Bach, S., and Klein, G. S. The effects of prolonged subliminal exposure of words. *American Psychologist*, 1957, *12*, 397–398.

Bandura, A. Behavior theory and the models of man. *American Psychologist*, 1974, *29*, 859–869.

Begleiter, H., Gross, M., and Kissin, B. Evoked cortical responses to affective visceral stimuli. *Psychophysiology*, 1969, *5*, 517–529.

Bennett-Clark, H., and Evans, C. Fragmentation of patterned targets when viewed as prolonged afterimages. *Nature*, 1963, *199*, 1215–1216.

Blakemore, C., Muncey, J., and Ridley, R. Perceptual fading of a stabilized retinal image. *Nature*, 1971, *233*, 204–205.

Breuer, J., and Freud, S. Studies on hysteria. *Standard Edition* (Vol. 2) (J. Strachey and A. Strachey, Trans.). London: Hogarth Press, 1958. (Originally published 1893–1895.)

Broadbent, D. *Perception and communication*. Oxford: Pergamon Press, 1958.

Cobb, W., Morton, H., and Ettlinger, G. Cerebral potentials evoked by pattern reversal and their suppression in visual rivalry. *Nature*, 1967, *216*, 1123–1125.

Coren, S., and Porac, C. The fading of stabilized images: Eye movements and information processing. *Perception & Psychophysics*, 1974, *16*, 529–534.

Deutsch, J., and Deutsch, D. Attention: Some theoretical considerations. *Psychological Review*, 1963, *70*, 80–90.

Dixon, F. *Subliminal perception: The nature of a controversy*. London: McGraw-Hill, 1971.

Donchin, E., and Lindsley, D. Visually evoked response correlates of perceptual masking and enhancement. *Electroencephalography and Clinical Neurophysiology*, 1965, *19*, 325–335.

Donchin, E., Wicker, J., and Lindsley, D. Cortical evoked potentials and perception of paired flashes. *Science*, 1963, *141*, 1285–1286.

Erdelyi, M. A new look at the new look: Perceptual defense and vigilance. *Psychological Review*, 1974, *81*, 1–25.

Fehmi, L., Adkins, J., and Lindsley, D. Electrophysiological correlates of visual perceptual masking in monkeys. *Experimental Brain Research*, 1969, *7*, 299–316.

Fisher, C. Dreams, images, and perception: A study of unconscious-preconscious relationships. *Journal of the American Psychoanalytic Association*, 1956, *4*, 5–48.

Freud, S. Instincts and their vicissitudes. *Standard Edition* (Vol. 14) (C. M. Baines, Trans.). London: Hogarth Press, 1958. (Originally published 1915.) (a)

Freud, S. Repression. *Standard Edition* (Vol. 14) (C. M. Baines, Trans.). London: Hogarth Press, 1958. (Originally published 1915.) (b)

Harter, M., Seiple, W., and Musso, M. Binocular summation and suppression: Visually evoked cortical responses to dichoptically presented patterns of different spatial frequencies. *Vision Research*, 1974, *14*, 1169–1180.

Harter, M., Towle, V., and Musso, M. Size specificity and interocular suppression: Monocular evoked potentials and reaction times. *Vision Research*, 1976, *16*, 1111–1117.

Hilgard, E. *Divided consciousness: Multiple controls in human thought and action*. New York: Wiley, 1977.

James, W. *The principles of psychology* (Vol. 1). New York: Holt, 1890.

Kahneman, D. *Attention and effort*. Englewood Cliffs, N.J.: Prentice-Hall, 1973.

Keesey, V. Comparison of human visual cortical potentials evoked by stabilized and unstabilized targets. *Vision Research*, 1969, *11*, 657–670.

Klein, G. A., and Holt, R. R. Problems and issues in current studies of subliminal activation. In J. G. Peatman and E. L. Hartley (Eds.), *Festschrift for Gardner Murphy*. New York: Harper & Row, 1960.

Kostandov, E., and Arzumanov, Y. Averaged cortical evoked potentials to recognized and non-recognized verbal stimuli. *Acta Neurobiologiae Experimentalis*, 1977, *37*, 311–324.

Lazarus, A. Has behavior therapy outlived its usefulness? *American Psychologist*, 1977, *32*, 550–554.

Lehman, D., Beeler, G., and Fender, D. EEG responses to light flashes during the observation of stabilized and normal retinal images. *Electroencephalography and Clinical Neurophysiology*, 1967, *22*, 136–142.

Lehman, D., and Fender, D. Component analyses of human averaged evoked potentials: Dichoptic stimuli using different target structures. *Electroencephalography and Clinical Neurophysiology*, 1968, *24*, 542–553.

Libet, B., Alberts, W. W., Wright, E. W., and Feinstein, B. Responses of human somato-sensory cortex to stimuli below threshold for conscious sensation. *Science*, 1967, *158*, 1597–1600.

London, P. The end of ideology in behavior modification. *American Psychologist*, 1972, *27*, 913–920.

Moray, N. *Attention: Selective processes in vision and hearing*. London: Hutchinson Educational, 1969.

Neisser, U. *Cognitive psychology*. New York: Appleton-Century-Crofts, 1967.

Neisser, U. *Cognition and reality*. San Francisco: Freeman, 1976.

Nisbett, R., and Wilson, T. Telling more than we can know: Verbal reports on mental processes. *Psychological Review*, 1977, *84*, 231–259.

Posner, M. Coordination of internal codes. In W. Chase (Ed.), *Visual information processing*. New York: Academic Press, 1973.

Posner, M., Klein, R., Summers, J., and Buggie, S. On the selection of signals. *Memory & Cognition*, 1973, *1*, 2–12.

Prangishvili, A. S., Sherozia, A. E., and Bassin, F. V. (Eds.), *The unconscious: Nature, functions, methods of study*. Tbilisi, U.S.S.R.: Metsniereba, 1978.

Rapaport, D. The scientific methodology of psychoanalysis. In M. M. Gill (Ed.), *The collected papers of David Rapaport*. New York: Basic Books, 1967. (Originally published 1944.)

Riggs, L., and Whittle, P. Human occipital and retinal potentials evoked by subjectively faded visual stimuli. *Vision Research*, 1967, *7*, 444–451.

Sackeim, H. A., Packer, I. K., and Gur, R. C. Hemisphericity, cognitive set, and susceptibility to subliminal perception. *Journal of Abnormal Psychology*, 1977, *86*, 624–630.

Shallice, T. Dual functions of consciousness. *Psychological Review*, 1972, *79*, 383–393.

Sherwood, M. *The logic of explanation in psychoanalysis*. New York: Academic Press, 1969.

Shevrin, H. Brain wave correlates of subliminal stimulation, unconscious attention, primary- and secondary-process thinking, and repressiveness. *Psychological Issues*, 1973, *8*(2), 56–87. (Monograph 30)

Shevrin, H. Evoked potential evidence for unconscious mental processes: A review of the literature. In A. S. Prangishvili, A. E. Sherozia, and F. V. Bassin (Eds.), *The unconscious: Nature, functions, methods of study*. Tbilisi, U.S.S.R.: Metsniereba, 1978.

Shevrin, H., and Rennick, P. Cortical response to a tactile stimulus during attention, mental arithmetic and free associations. *Psychophysiology*, 1967, *3*, 381–388.

Smith, G. J. W., Spence, D. P., and Klein, G. S. Subliminal effects of verbal stimuli. *Journal of Abnormal Social Psychology*, 1959, *59*, 167–176.

Spekreijse, H., Van Der Tweel, L., and Regan, D. Interocular sustained suppression: Correlations with evoked potential amplitude and distribution. *Vision Research*, 1972, *12*, 521–526.

Spence, D. P. The multiple effects of subliminal stimuli. *Journal of Personality*, 1961, *29*, 40–53.

Spence, D. P. How restricted are the restricting effects?: A reply. *Journal of Personality and Social Psychology*, 1966, *3*, 131–132.

Spence, D. P., and Holland, B. The restricting effects of awareness: A paradox and an explanation. *Journal of Abnormal Social Psychology*, 1962, *64*, 163–174.

Spence, D. P., and Smith, G. W. Experimenter bias against subliminal perception? Comments on a replication. *British Journal of Psychology*, 1977, *68*, 279–280.

Sternberg, S. Memory scanning: New findings and current controversies. *Quarterly Journal of Experimental Psychology*, 1975, *27*, 1–32.

Treisman, A. Selective attention in man. *British Medical Bulletin*, 1964, *20*, 12–16.

Turvey, M. On peripheral and central processes in vision: Inferences from an information-processing analysis of masking with patterned stimuli. *Psychological Review*, 1973, *80*, 1–52.

Walker, P. The subliminal perception of movement and the 'suppression' in binocular rivalry. *British Journal of Psychology*, 1975, *66*, 347–356.

Walker, P. Binocular rivalry: Central or peripheral selective processes? *Psychological Bulletin*, 1978, *85*, 376–389.

35 Brain Stimulation in the Study of Neuronal Functions for Conscious Sensory Experiences

B. Libet

Introduction

Much of the waking brain's activities and responses can proceed at unconscious levels, without subjective experiences directly associated with them (e.g., Libet 1965, 1973, 1981a; Shevrin and Dickmann 1980). This suggests that specifically unique neural actions are required, within the context of the normally functioning brain, to elicit conscious sensory experiences and presumably subjective experiences generally (Libet 1965). To study the causal relationship between specific neural actions and subjective experience requires an ability to manipulate neural function in a controlled manner; direct intracranial electrical stimulation in the conscious human subject is one of the very few approaches available for such purposes. The utilization of intracranial stimulation is of course limited to opportunities presented by invasive neurosurgical procedures for therapeutic purposes and by the risk factors it may introduce; and, in any case, it should only be employed with the properly informed consent and cooperation of the subject. These factors, and the inherent modes by which electrical stimuli can elicit or control neural actions, impose severe limits on the possible scope of meaningful experiments. The acceptably brief electrical pulses presumably excite some axonal elements almost exclusively; the functional effectiveness of the stimulus is then clearly dependent on whether axonal impulses initiated by the stimuli can effectively activate or lead to the activation of an appropriately large and organized spatio-temporal configuration of neural elements needed for eliciting an experience (see Libet 1973 and below).

How Do Electrical Stimuli Initiate or Alter Cortical Cerebral Functions?

In general, electrical stimuli have been found (1) to elicit some organized overt functional response and (2) to interfere with and/or (3) to modulate an ongoing functional activity.

The first type of action defines the "excitable" cortex, most of the cortex being "silent" in this regard (e.g., Penfield 1958). Functional motor and sensory responses are most easily elicitable at the primary motor and sensory areas, respectively; the former is located in precentral gyrus ("area 4") and the latter, in the case of somatic sensibilities, in postcentral gyrus ("areas 3–1–2", also termed SI). These areas are connected to subcortical lower motoneurone (motor) or primary sensory neurones (sensory) by the most direct and fastest "specific" pathways, which also maintain a high degree of topographical, spatial segregation relative to the peripheral effector (muscle) and sensory structures. After the sensory stimulus, the earliest neural messages reach the appropriate primary sensory cortex first, within 10–25 ms; they initiate a characteristic response confined to primary cortex, recordable electrically as the "primary evoked potential"; this is followed by slower event-related potentials exhibiting wider cortical distributions and more related to cognitive aspects of the sensory response. The so-called association cortex, surrounding primary areas and occupying the vast intervening areas, is functionally involved with the more complex aspects of motor and sensory integrations and of higher functions generally. These areas are generally "silent" in response to electrical stimuli, particularly in nonepileptic patients (Libet 1973); some of the important exceptions to this are the ability of stimuli to elicit generalized bodily movements at supplementary motor cortex (located on mesial surface, inside the midline of the brain) and hallucinatory psychic responses termed "experiential" by Penfield (1959) at temporal lobe cortex. However, silent cortex can respond to electrical stimuli with observable responses other than direct motor acts or reports of subjective experiences. These responses include electrophysiological ones, the so called direct cortical responses (DCR); the establishment of conditioned behavioral responses to stimuli applied to virtually any cortical area in cats and monkeys (e.g., Doty 1969); and interference with or modulation of various ongoing functions (see below). It is perhaps more appropriate to view the absence of overt functional responses to stimulation of silent cortex as a reflection of (a) inadequacy of stimuli employed and/or (b) inadequacy of the observations employed to detect changes in behavioral or unconscious psychical processes (Libet 1973).

The second or "interference" effect of electrical stimuli can appear when stimulating excitable cortex, for example by producing an anesthesia for or masking of normal peripheral sensory inputs when applied to primary sensory cortex (see Penfield 1968, Libet 1973). These interference actions appear to require stronger electrical stimuli than those needed for eliciting a near threshold sensory experience (e.g., Libet 1973, Libet et al. 1975; see further below). Stimuli can also interfere with or disrupt normal functional responses even when applied to "silent" cortex; this provides a potentially powerful tool for studying all cortical areas (e.g., Penfield 1959, and more recently Ojemann 1982). The third or modulatory action is represented by some simpler examples, for example, stimulation in the vicinity of postcentral gyrus producing enhancement of a somatic sensation (Libet 1978; see further below); and by more complex psychical changes, for example, illusionary changes in present or ongoing experience induced by temporal lobe stimulations (termed "interpretive" responses by Penfield 1959).

Even with these limited potentialities of brain stimuli, it has been possible to pry out some of the significant parameters of neuronal action involved in eliciting a conscious sensory experience (see Libet 1973), and to obtain evidence for the existence of two remarkable temporal factors governing the relation of neural activity to subjective perception of a sensory stimulus (see Libet 1978, 1981b; Libet et al. 1979). The vari-

ous electrical parameters (e.g., intensity, polarity, electrode size, pulse duration, pulse frequency, train duration), that help determine the effectiveness of a stimulus for this purpose (see Libet 1973, Libet et al. 1964), will not be reviewed in detail here, except for the specific relationship between intensity (peak current) and train duration of a stimulus consisting of repetitive pulses, each of brief duration (0.5 ms or less). This relationship has turned out to be the most interesting and productive one among the significant stimulus parameters.

The Intensity (I)-Train Duration (TD) Relationship

When the intensity (I) of stimulus pulses is adjusted for each train duration (TD), so that the same, just barely threshold, conscious sensory experience is produced by each I-TD combination (figure 35.1), one finds there is a minimum (liminal) intensity below which no sensation can be elicited no matter how long the TD. Conversely, the liminal intensity stimulus elicits no reportable sensory experience at all unless its repetitive pulses are continued for at least an average of 0.5 s (Libet 1966, 1973; Libet et al. 1964). This remarkably long minimum stimulus train duration required at liminal I, termed the *utilization TD*, was relatively independent of changes in pulse frequency or in other stimulus variables. With TD's shorter than the utilization TD, the required I begins to rise steeply (see figure 35.1). The resulting I-TD curve and the approximately 0.5-s value for utilization TD appeared to be a property of the cerebral sensory system generally, and not simply a function of stimulating at the pial surface of cortex. Similar I-TD curves were found with stimuli in the subcortical pathways rostral to the medullary nuclei, for example, in ventroposterolateral nucleus (n.VPL) of thalamus and in medial lemniscus (LM); they were not found at peripheral nerve or skin (Libet 1973; Libet et al. 1964, 1967, 1972), or in the dorsal columns of

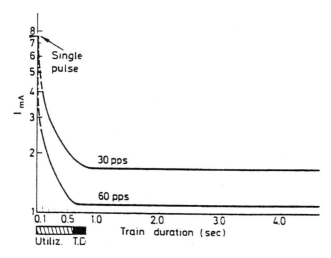

Figure 35.1
Intensity/train duration combinations for stimuli just adequate to elicit a threshold conscious experience of somatic sensation, when applied to primary somatosensory cortex SI (postcentral gyrus). Curves are presented for two different pulse repetition frequencies, employing rectangular pulses of 0.5-ms duration. Bar for "utilization TD" indicates the minimum train duration required (or "utilized") in order to elicit any conscious sensation when intensity is at the minimum effective level ("liminal I"). Note that liminal I remains constant even if TD is increased above the utilization TD. (From Libet 1966.)

spinal cord (Nashold et al. 1972) which of course contain ascending collateral axons of primary afferent fibers.

Qualities of Somatic Sensations Elicited by Cortical Stimuli

When stimulus values are kept to liminal levels, virtually all kinds of the naturally experienced somatosensory qualities, except for pain, can be elicited by stimulating postcentral gyrus (Libet 1973; Libet et al. 1975); see table 35.1. However, when intensity of a given liminal stimulus was raised by 50–100% or more, a naturallike quality of the liminal response could regularly be changed to a paresthesia (tingling, electric shock, pins and needles, numbness, etc.); this could help to explain the preponderance of paresthesia-like sensations generally elicited by others

when stimulating postcentral gyrus (e.g., Penfield 1958). Such findings suggest that not merely spatial localizability but also specific qualities are individually represented in somatosensory cortex, presumably in the form of columnar modules (Mountcastle 1967). The production of the rather nonspecific paresthesialike qualities by supraliminal stimuli could be due to activation of mixed types of columns, as in the case of supraliminal stimulation of a peripheral nerve containing a mixture of sensory fibers (see figure 35.2) (e.g., Libet 1973, Libet et al. 1975).

Neural Responses That Do Not Lead to Sensory Experience

With a surface electrode on primary somatosensory (SI) cortex (postcentral gyrus) stimulus pulses at even below liminal I elicit substantial

Table 35.1

Somatosensory qualities of sensations elicited by stimulation of postcentral gyrus

A) *Incidence of qualities, among 124 non-epileptic subjects*[a]

I. "*Paresthesia-like*" (total)	88
II. "*Natural-like*" (total)	115
a) something "moving inside"	32
b) feeling of movement of part	32
c) deep pressures	20
d) surface mechano-type	12
e) vibration	6
f) warmth	11
g) coldness	2

B) *Subject's descriptions*, within each category of qualities listed in (A).

I. *Paresthesia-like* sensory responses: tingling; electric shocks; pins and needles; prickling; numbness.

II. "*Natural-like*" sensory responses:

a) something "moving inside": wave moving along inside through the affected part; or wavy-like feeling inside; or wavy "like a snake back's" motion; rolling or flowing motion inside; moving back and forth inside; circular motion inside; crawling under the skin, or more deeply.

b) feeling of movement of the part (but with no actual motion observable to outside): quiver; trembling; shaking; flutter; twitching; jumping; rotating; jerking; pushing; pulling; straightening; floating; or sensation of hand raising up, or lifting.

c) deep pressures: throbbing; pulsing; swelling; squeezing; tightening.

d) surface mechano-type: touch; tapping; hairs moving; rolling (a ball, etc.) over surface; water running over surface; talcum powder sprinkling on; light brushing of skin; holding a ball of cotton; rubbing something between thumb and index finger.

e) vibration: vibration, buzzing (distinct from tingling, etc.).

f) warmth, or warming.

g) coldness.

[a] Each type of quality is counted only once for a given subject, even if it was elicited repeatedly by multiple tests in that subject. However, if a given subject experienced more than one type of quality, he was listed in each appropriate category. Referral sites for almost all responses were in the upper extremity, mostly in the regions of the hand and fingers. Stimuli were at liminal I in 60 subjects, and at or somewhat > liminal I in 64 subjects. Stimulus pulse frequencies were between 15 and 120 pps, train durations > 0.5 sec.
Modified from Libet et al. (1975) In: Kornhuber HH (ed) The somatosensory system. Thieme, Stuttgart, pp 291–308

"direct cortical responses" (DCR), recordable at within a few mm of adjacent cortex. At liminal I or above, each pulse may elicit even larger DCR's and other electrophysiological responses, but no conscious sensory experience at all unless TDs are sufficiently long (figure 35.3). Similar DCRs can be elicited at "silent cortex," with no reportable experiences. Initial negative components of DCR's could even be abolished at SI cortex, by surface application of GABA (gamma amino butyric acid), with no effects on the subjective sensory experiences elicited either by direct stimulation of postcentral gyrus or by natural peripheral sensory input (Libet 1973).

Cortical neuronal activities represented by the primary evoked response, to afferent input via the specific projection pathway, also appear *not* to be sufficient for sensory experience. A single pulse stimulus in n.VPL of thalamus or in LM (medial lemniscus) can elicit at SI cortex a large primary evoked potential, apparently identical in its form and neuronal basis with the primary evoked potential elicited by a peripheral stimulus (figure 35.3). But this single pulse in LM is completely ineffective for eliciting conscious sensation, regardless of how high the peak current (I) is raised and of how large the evoked potential elicited by it (Libet et al. 1967). (A sufficiently

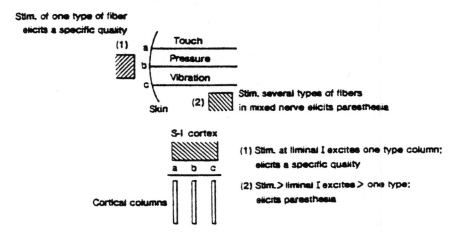

Figure 35.2
Schema of hypothesis to explain conversion of specific quality of sensation to paresthesia, when strength of stimulus to SI cortex is raised above liminal intensity (see table 35.1 and text). The hypothesis states that excitation of one type of sensory unit, whether in periphery or primary SI cortex, elicits a specific "natural" quality; whereas excitation of a mixture of types (not simply numbers) of units elicits a paresthesia. The upper schema shows the similar explanation for the known difference between threshold stimuli at skin (1) versus surface stimulation of the peripheral mixed nerve (2).

strong single pulse at SI cortex can elicit a muscular twitch response, and this may then indirectly generate a sensation by exciting sensory structures.) Even a skin stimulus below threshold level for any conscious sensation can still elicit a small primary evoked potential but no later components (Libet et al. 1967). The association of sensory experience with appearance of later components of evoked potential and the wider cortical distribution of the latter, suggest that the regions as well as the kinds of neuronal activities required to elicit sensation are much broader than those available in primary sensory cortex alone (e.g., Libet et al. 1975).

Clearly, there can be substantial neuronal responses to stimuli in the sensory pathways that are not sufficient, and at least in some cases also not necessary, for eliciting conscious sensory experience. On the other hand, it seems probable that some such responses could be involved in behavioral and psychological detection at unconscious levels (e.g., Libet 1965; Libet et al.

1967, 1972; Shevrin et al. 1971). In this connection, it is essential that behavioral detection not be confused with subjective experience of a stimulus; the former may be manifested with or without the latter (see Libet 1973, 1981a). Indeed, the present evidence (see further below) supports our contention that to elicit subjective experience requires specific and unique kinds and durations of neural activities not essential to "unconscious" forms of detection.

Cerebral Delay in "Neuronal Adequacy" for a Sensory Experience

As indicated above, stimuli at any of the cerebral levels in the somatosensory specific projection system require substantial train durations, varying with intensity, in order to become effective. For example, a subject who requires the usual utilization-TD of about 500 ms at liminal I reports that he feels absolutely nothing with the

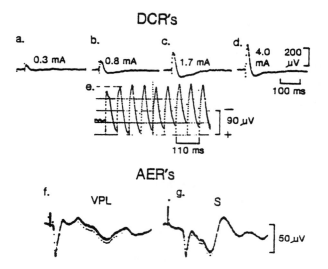

Figure 35.3
Direct cortical responses (DCRs) of human SI cortex of awake and conscious Parkinson patient, evoked by stimulation (with 0.3-ms pulses) of an adjacent site a few millimeters away. Each tracing in (a)–(d) is average of 18 responses; stimulus pulses, 1 per 2 s, peak currents as indicated. Subject reported he did not feel any of these "single pulse" (actually low frequency) stimuli. In (e), the liminal I pulse at 0.8 mA (see (b)) were delivered at 20/s for 0.5 s; each of the 10 separate trains averaged for (e) elicited a conscious sensory response, with utilization TD = 0.5 s. Recordings were made with d.c. amplifier system, positive downwards. Calibrations in (e) differ from those for (a)–(d). *Average evoked responses* (AERs) recorded on SI cortex in response either to ipsilateral thalamic (VPL) or contralateral skin (S) stimuli, in an awake and conscious patient with heredofamilial tremor. Each tracing is average of 250 responses at 1.8 per s; total length of trace is 125 ms. In (f), stimuli applied in VPL (ventro-postero-lateral nucleus); subject reported not feeling any of these stimuli, even though peak currents were 6 times the liminal I that was adequate for sensory experience when a train of 60/s and TD > 0.5 s was applied. In (g), stimuli S (skin of back of hand); peak currents were at 2 times threshold for subjectively feeling a single pulse, and all stimuli were felt. (a)–(d) and (f)–(g) from Libet et al. 1967, reprinted by courtesy of *Science*; (e) from Libet et al. 1972, with permission of *Excerpta Medica*.)

same stimulus train shortened to 400 ms. Since there is no reportable experience after the stimulus unless stimulus TD is raised to 500 ms, in this example, it seems clear that the state of "neuronal adequacy" for eliciting the conscious experience is not achieved until at least the end of the required TD of stimulus pulses. ("Neuronal adequacy" is used in the broad sense of integrated patterns of neural activity needed to mediate the function in question, rather than of stimple uncomplicated excitation—following the example of Jasper 1963.) The possibility that such neuronal adequacy is delayed even beyond the minimum stimulus TD appears to be an unlikely one, in view of further evidence (see below). The question of what is neuronally unique about the activity elicited by the minimum stimulus train remains an open one. One viable hypothesis suggests that it is sufficient duration per se, of appropriate neuronal activities, that gives rise to the emergent phenomenon of subjective experience (Libet 1965, Libet et al. 1972).

For peripheral sensory fibers (in skin, nerve, or ascending collaterals in dorsal columns) a single threshold stimulus pulse is sufficient to elicit a sensory experience. It might, therefore, be argued that the long TDs required of cerebral stimuli may be due to an abnormal processing of such inputs, for example because they may induce cortical inhibitory patterns. (Actually, it would seem very improbable that the very different kinds and patterns of inhibitory and excitatory responses elicited by a surface cortical as opposed to a medial lemniscal, LM, stimulus train would result in the same utilization-TDs, about 500 ms, needed by either one to achieve neuronal adequacy; see Libet 1973). Although more indirect, the evidence obtainable for the case of a peripheral stimulus also indicates that similarly long delays are required to achieve cerebral neuronal adequacy. This evidence has been discussed elsewhere (Libet 1973, 1978, 1981b, Libet et al. 1972, 1979). Only the portion involving retroactive effects of a cortical stimulus on a peripherally-induced sensation will be briefly summarized in the following.

Retroactive Modulatory Effects of a Cortical Stimulus

It had already been shown that a sufficiently strong stimulus to primary sensory cortex could interfere with sensations induced by simultaneous peripheral stimuli (e.g., Penfield 1958, 1959). The hypothesis that suitable cortical activities must persist for up to about 500 ms following a threshold skin pulse, before becoming adequate for conscious sensation, would predict that even when a sufficient cortical stimulus (C) *follows* a skin pulse (S) by some hundreds of milliseconds, C should still be able to interfere with or otherwise modify the peripherally-induced sensation. This was indeed found to be the case (Libet 1978, Libet et al. 1972). Retroactive effects were produced by a delayed "conditioning" C stimulus (applied to postcentral gyrus) even when C did not begin until 200–500 ms after an S pulse.

The effect was one of retroactive masking or inhibition in some subjects, or of retroactive enhancement of the S-induced sensation in others. (Whether one obtained masking or enhancement was thought to be a function of a difference in location of the C stimulus with respect to the most "excitable" sites for a C-induced sensation.) The delayed conditioning "C" stimulus was applied to a relatively large area of postcentral gyrus, via a 10-mm disc electrode. In order to exert retroactive effects, the C stimulus train required a supraliminal intensity (I), at least 1.2–2 times the liminal I needed for C itself to elicit a sensation; this brings the C stimulus into a range that can interfere with responses to peripheral inputs. The C stimulus also required a minimum TD of at least 100 ms for this purpose; this would raise the effective conditioning interval, by which C can follow S, to at least 300–600 ms. The fact that neural inputs (from C) can either interfere with or modulate the S-induced sensory experience, even when delayed by 300–600 ms after an S stimulus, indicates that the S-induced experience is not finally developed neuronally until after such delays.

Subjective Timing versus Time for Neuronal Adequacy

If a brief peripheral sensory stimulus leads to a state of cerebral neuronal adequacy for a sensory experience only after substantial delays of up to about 500 ms, as postulated on the evidence, then one may ask whether the *subjective timing* of the experience is similarly delayed. In a direct test of this question, the subject was asked to report the subjective timing order of skin (S)- and cortically (C)-induced sensations, when an S pulse and a C stimulus were coupled with different time intervals (Libet et al. 1979). It was found that S was experienced before C even when the S pulse was delivered well after the onset of the C stimulus, in fact at any time before the end of the C train of pulses that was required

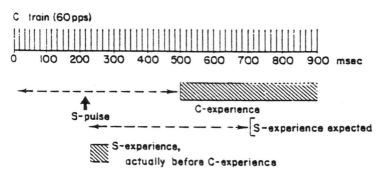

C train (60 pps)

0   100 200 300 400 500 600 700 800 900 msec

S-pulse

C-experience

S-experience expected

S-experience,
actually before C-experience

Figure 35.4
Diagram of experiment on subjective time order of two sensory experiences, one elicited by a stimulus train to SI cortex (C) and one by a threshold pulse to skin (S). C consisted of repetitive pulses (at 60/s) applied to postcentral gyrus, at the lowest (liminal) peak current sufficient to elicit any reportable conscious sensory experience. The sensory experience for C ("C-experience") would not be initiated before the end of the utilization-train duration (average about 500 ms), but then proceeds without change in its weak *subjective* intensity for the remainder of the applied liminal C train (see Libet et al. 1964; Libet 1966, 1973). The S-pulse, at just above threshold strength for eliciting conscious sensory experience, is here shown delivered when the initial 200 ms of the C train have elapsed. (In other experiments, it was applied at other relative times, earlier and later.) If S were followed by a roughly similar delay of 500 ms of cortical activity before "neuronal adequacy" is achieved, initiation of S-experience might have also been expected to be delayed until 700 ms of C had elapsed. In fact, S-experience was reported to appear subjectively before C-experience (see text). (From Libet et al. 1979, by permission of *Brain*.)

at sensory cortex (see schema in figure 35.4). This was true whether S and C stimuli were both at the liminal threshold strengths (when minimum duration of C would be about 500 ms), or S and C were both set for a somewhat greater (matched) intensity at which minimum duration of C was 200 ms. These results indicated (a) that there is essentially no delay in the subjective timing of an S-induced experience (unless one wishes to add the unnecessary assumption that both S- and C-experiences are "postponed" by some similar time that is additional to the train-duration requirement in the case of C); and (b) that neuronal adequacy for the C-experience is achieved at or near the end of the required stimulus TD, whether this be 500 or 200 ms or other tested values.

The foregoing results on subjective timing order for S and C stimuli appeared to be in conflict with the other evidence that strongly supports the proposal for long cortical delays even

after a skin pulse (see above). In view of this, as well as of our reluctance to assign fundamentally different cerebral processes to producing similar sensory experiences induced by different stimuli, we generated a second alternative hypothesis to account for the paradoxical difference between delayed neuronal adequacy and nondelayed subjective timing for the experience (Libet et al. 1979), as is described subsequently.

Subjective Referral of Sensory Experience Backwards in Time

There were two components in the revised hypothesis:

1. After the delayed achievement of neuronal adequacy, there occurs an *automatic referral of the experience backwards in time*, to a time that approximates that for delivery of the stimulus.

2. The initial cortical response to the fast specific (lemniscal) projection message generated by the sensory input, as represented by the *primary evoked potential* at SI cortex, *serves as timing signal* for this backward referral (see figure 35.5).

Latencies for the primary evoked potential are brief enough, 10–20 ms, so that differences among these latent periods cannot be differentiated subjectively (see Libet et al. 1979). The experience would thus be "antedated," and its timing would appear to the subject to occur without the actual substantial delay required for achieving the neuronal adequacy for the experience.

A crucial experimental test of this hypothesis was made possible by the special features of the responses to stimulation of medial lemniscus (LM). Each pulse of the LM stimulus, including the very first one, should and does elicit the same primary evoked potential that the skin pulse elicits; thus the LM stimulus should resemble the skin stimulus in providing the putative timing signal (for referral) at the very start of a train of pulses. On the other hand, the LM stimulus resembles the cortical stimulus in requiring similarly long durations of up to about 500 ms; unlike the skin stimulus, a single LM pulse is completely ineffective in producing a conscious sensory experience (Libet et al. 1967, 1972). The hypothesis for subjective referral thus makes a startling experimental prediction: If a skin pulse (S) is delivered so as to be synchronous with the *beginning* of a stimulus train in medial lemniscus (LM, in brain stem), the subject should report that both of the resulting sensory experiences began at the same time; the subjective timings should be the same in spite of the empirically established fact that the LM stimulus train of pulses, like the cortical stimulus, could not become adequate for eliciting any sensory experience unless allowed to continue for up to about 500 ms (see figure 35.6). (For technical reasons, intensities were set in these experiments so that an absolute minimum of 200 ms or more was required by the LM stimuli.) Related predictions

were made for different S-LM coupling intervals. The experimental results of such tests, even when subjected to a rigorous statistical analysis, clearly confirmed these predictions (Libet et al. 1979). Furthermore, additional independent lines of evidence in support of the hypothesis are already in evidence (Libet et al. 1979).

Some Further Implications in Relating Mind and Brain

The presently generated concept of subjective referral-in-time is analogous to the long recognized subjective referral-in-space. The spatial form of a subjective sensory experience is known to be markedly different from the spatial configuration of the activated cortical neuronal system that gives rise to the experience. A simple direct demonstration of this is routinely obtainable upon stimulating primary sensory cortex, for example, S-I (postcentral) cortex. Stimulation there gives rise to conscious sensations experienced in the contralateral body part, with an inverted vertical orientation and with proportions of the sensory field grossly distorted from the neural representation (homunculus) at the cortex (e.g., Penfield 1958); there is of course no experience located subjectively in the head, where the neural activation is actually occurring. The role of the specific projection system, in providing signals that discriminate functions in the spatial referral process, is now expanded to one that functions also in temporal referral. Both spatial and temporal referrals actually help to "correct," at the subjective level, the distortion that is inherent in the way in which activities of cerebral neurons represent the real spatial and temporal sensory configurations impinging at the peripheral levels (see Libet 1981b). The "corrections" also extend to the experience of subjective synchrony for a number of sensory stimuli, differing in intensity and even modality, when these are delivered synchronously at different bodily sites. The subjective synchrony, or absence of "subjective jitter," is experienced in spite of the

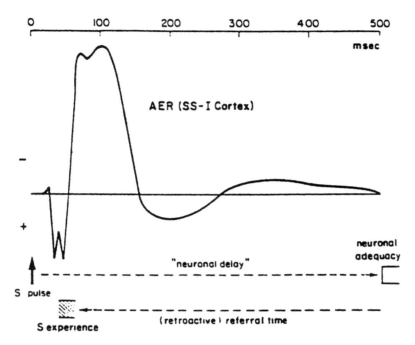

Retroactive referral (antedating) of subjective sensory experience

Figure 35.5
Diagram of hypothesis for subjective referral of a sensory experience backwards in time. The average evoked response (AER) recorded at SI cortex was evoked by pulses just suprathreshold for sensation (at about 1 per s, 256 averaged responses) delivered to skin of contralateral hand. Below the AER, the first line shows the approximate delay in achieving the state of "neuronal adequacy" that appears (on the basis of other evidence) to be necessary for eliciting the sensory experience. The second line shows the postulated retroactive referral of the subjective timing of the experience, from the time of "neuronal adequacy" backwards to some time associated with the primary surface-positive component of the evoked potential. The primary surface-positive component of the evoked potential. The primary component of AER is relatively highly localized to an area on the contralateral postcentral gyrus in these awake human subjects. The secondary or later components, especially those following the surface negative component after the initial 100–150 ms of the AER, are wider in distribution over the cortex and more variable in form even when recorded subdurally (see, e.g., Libet et al. 1975). It should be clear, therefore, that the present diagram is not meant to indicate that the state of "neuronal adequacy" for eliciting conscious sensation is restricted to neurons in primary SI cortex of postcentral gyrus; on the other hand, the primary component or "timing signal" for retroactive referral of the sensory experience would be a function more strictly of this SI cortical area. (The later components of the AER shown here are small compared to what could be obtained if the stimulus repetition rate were lower than 1/s and if the subjects had been asked to perform some discriminatory task related to the stimuli, as seen, for example, in Desmedt and Robertson 1977.) (From Libet et al. 1979, by permission of *Brain*.)

I. P-Cerebral: stim. interval = 0 msec

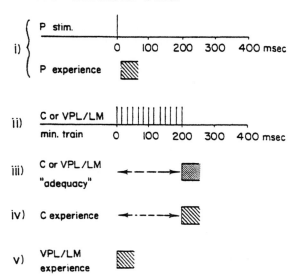

Figure 35.6
Diagram of timing relationships for the two subjective experiences when a peripheral stimulus (P) is temporally coupled with a cerebral stimulus, as predicted by the modified hypothesis. The cerebral stimulus train is applied either to SI cortex (C) or to n.VPL of thalamus (or to medial lemniscus, LM). Therefore, timing relationships may be compared for two types of coupled pairs: (*a*) P paired with SI; and (P) paired with n.VPL/LM. In the set shown here, the train of stimulus pulses at C, or in VPL/LM, *began* at the same time as the P stimulus pulse was delivered; that is, the P-cerebral interval was 0. P usually consisted of a single pulse applied to skin of the hand on the side of body opposite to that in which a referred sensation was elicited by the cerebral stimulus. The P-experience (see line [i]) is timed subjectively to appear within 10–20 ms after the P stimulus (see also figure 35.4). Each cerebral stimulus (in line [ii]) is a train of pulses, usually 60/s, with peak current adjusted so that a minimum train duration of about 200 ms is required in order to produce any conscious sensory experience; this means that the state of "neuronal adequacy" (see line [iii]) with either C or VPL/LM stimuli could not be achieved before 200 ms of stimulus train duration had elapsed. The subjective timing of the beginning of a sensory experience elicited by the C stimulus (line iv) is delayed until the end of the minimum TD (200 ms) of this stimulus. But the experience of VPL/LM (line iv) is timed earlier; that is, the sensation elicited here is subjectively referred, retroactively, to a time associated with the primary evoked cortical response. The latter is elicited even by the first stimulus pulse in VPL/LM and resembles the primary evoked response to a peripheral stimulus (see figure 35.3f–g), but it is not elicited by stimuli to SI cortex (see figure 35.3a–e). (From Libet et al. 1979, by permission of *Brain*.)

probability that, for the different stimuli, the individual delays for neuronal adequacy may differ by hundreds of milliseconds (Libet 1981b, Libet et al. 1979). If sensory experiences are each referred backwards to the time of the early primary evoked potentials elicited by each sensory input, any differences among the times to achieve neuronal adequacy become subjectively irrelevant. It is also noteworthy that subjective referral in time would not have been discovered without the experimental opportunity to directly manipulate neural actions by means of intracranial stimulations.

It is important to realize that these subjective referrals and corrections are apparently taking place at the level of the *mental* "sphere"; they are not apparent, as such, in the activities at neural levels (Libet 1981b, Libet et al. 1979, Sherrington 1951, Eccles 1980). The distinction is based on the observed phenomena; its validity is therefore independent of the theory one may adopt for the mind-brain relationship, whether this be monist-emergent (e.g., Sperry 1980) or dualist (e.g., Popper and Eccles 1977, Eccles 1980). The distinction does not deny that there are orderly relationships between the two spheres, that is, between the inner subjective experience (the "mental") and the externally observable (the "physical") side; but it does imply that a complete knowledge of the "physical" (neural events) could not, in itself, have described or predicted the "mental" (subjective experiences) (Libet 1981b).

The postulated requirement for substantial delays, in achieving cerebral neuronal adequacy for sensory experiences, raises additional potential functional inferences that are separate from the issue of referral in time. These psychologically interesting inferences have been discussed elsewhere (Libet 1965, 1966, 1978, 1981b; Libet et al. 1972). They include the following:

1. Quick responses to a stimulus, as in a reaction time test, are performed initially unconsciously, with the conscious awareness of the stimulus, of its significance and of the response appearing after the cognitive and behavioral motor events.

2. Signal detection may occur without awareness. This is already implicit in item #1, and experimental evidence for it has appeared (e.g., Fehrer and Raab 1962, Shevrin et al. 1971).

3. The provision of substantial time, between the stimulus and the eventual cerebral adequacy for awareness, provides an opportunity for alterations in the eventual nature or appearance of the conscious experience; modulating processes could be exogenous (as in the experiment of retroactive effects of a C stimulus), or endogenous (based upon previous experiences, personality bias, repressive factors, etc.)

4. Finally, a possible neural basis to account for the distinction between conscious experience and unconscious mental operations may be postulated, in terms of durations of neuronal activities (Libet 1965, Libet et al. 1972); in this, the suitable neural activities, wherever they may be occurring in the brain, would have to endure for or appear at sufficiently delayed times, in order to achieve the transition from an unconscious mental operation to a conscious experience.

References

Desmedt JE, Robertson D (1977) Differential enhancement of early and late components of the cerebral somatosensory evoked potentials during forced-paced cognitive tasks in man. J Physiol (Lond) 271:761–782

Doty RW (1969) Electrical stimulation of the brain in behavioral cortex. Ann Rev Physiol 20:289–320

Eccles JC (1980) The Human Psyche. Springer, Berlin Heidelberg New York, 279 pages

Fehrer E, Raab O (1962) A comparison of reaction time and verbal report in the detection of masked stimuli. J Exp Psychol 64:126–130

Jasper HH (1963) Studies of non-specific effects upon electrical responses in sensory system. In: Moruzzi G, Albe-Fessard D, Jasper HH (eds) Progress in brain research, Vol. I Elsevier, Amsterdam, pp 272–293

Libet B (1965) Cortical activation in conscious and unconscious experience. Perspect Biol Med 9:77–86

Libet B (1966) Brain stimulation and the threshold of conscious experience. In: Eccles JC (ed) Brain and conscious experience. Springer-Verlag, Berlin Heidelberg New York, pp 165–181

Libet B (1973) Electrical stimulation of cortex in human subjects and conscious sensory aspects. In: Iggo A (ed) Somatosensory System. Springer, Berlin Heidelberg New York (Handbook of sensory physiology, vol. II, pp 743–790)

Libet B (1978) Neuronal vs. subjective timing, for a conscious sensory experience. In: Buser PA, Rougeul-Buser A (eds) Cerebral Correlates of Conscious Experience. Elsevier/North Holland Biomedial Press, Amsterdam, pp 69–82

Libet B (1981a) ERPs and conscious awareness. In: Galambos R, Hillyard SA (eds) Electrophysiological Approaches to Human Cognitive Processing. (Neurosci Res Program Bull 20:171–175). The MIT Press Journals, Cambridge

Libet B (1981b) The experimental evidence for subjective referral of sensory experience backwards in time. Philos of Sci 48:182–197

Libet B, Alberts WW, Wright EW, Delattre LD, Levin G, Feinstein B (1964) Production of threshold levels of conscious sensation by electrical stimulation of human somatosensory cortex. J Neurophysiol 27:546–578

Libet B, Alberts WW, Wright EW, Feinstein B (1967) Responses of human somatosensory cortex to stimuli below threshold for conscious sensation. Science 158:1597–1600

Libet B, Alberts WW, Wright EW, Feinstein B (1972) Cortical and thalamic activation in conscious sensory experience. In: Somjen GG (ed) Neurophysiology studied in man. Excerpta Medica, Amsterdam, pp 157–168

Libet B, Alberts WW, Wright EW, Lewis M, Feinstein B (1975) Cortical representation of evoked potentials relative to conscious sensory responses and of somatosensory qualities in man. In: Kornhuber HH (ed) The somatosensory system. Thieme, Stuttgart, pp 291–308

Libet B, Wright EW Jr, Feinstein B, Pearl DK (1979) Subjective referral of the timing for a conscious sensory experience: a functional role for the somatosensory specific projection system in man. Brain 102:191–222

Mountcastle VB (1967) The problem of sensing and the neural coding of sensory events. In: Quarton GC, Melnechuk T, Schmitt FO (eds) The neurosciences. Rockefeller University Press, New York, pp 393–408

Nashold B, Somjen G, Friedman H (1972) Paresthesias and EEG potentials evoked by stimulation of the dorsal funiculi in man. Exp Neurol 36:273–287

Penfield W (1958) The Excitable Cortex in Conscious Man. Liverpool University Press, Liverpool, 42 pp

Penfield W (1959) The interpretive cortex. Science 129:1719–1725

Popper KR, Eccles JC (1977) The self and its brain. Springer, Berlin Heidelberg New York, 597 pp

Sherrington CS (1951) Man on his Nature. Cambridge University Press, London, 300 pages (2nd edition)

Shevrin H, Dickman S (1980) The psychological unconscious: a necessary assumption for all psychological theory? Am Psychol 35:421–434

Shevrin H, Smith WH, Fritzler D (1971) Average evoked responses and verbal correlates of unconscious mental processes. Psychophysiology 8:149–162

Sperry RW (1980) Mind-brain interaction: mentalism, yes; dualism, no. Neuroscience 5:195–206

VII CONSCIOUSNESS AND MEMORY

If the senses are naturally intertwined with consciousness, memory is surely the paradigm of unconscious contents, stored over years yet still retrievable. Consciousness interacts with memory especially in the processes of learning and retrieval, that is, with the input and output functions of memory. It also seems likely that when memories are reworked, as in problem solving, creative thinking, and reconstructing the past, consciousness is once again involved.

Long-term memory (LTM) is the store of permanent memories, now believed to include several types, including episodic memory, an autobiographical record of conscious experience, semantic memory, a store of abstract knowledge, and procedural or skill memory. Additionally, long-term memory plausibly includes the lexicon of natural language, enduring perceptual and motor set, and even long-lasting attitudes and personality features.

Explicit and Implicit Memory

Endel Tulving has been one of the consistent advocates for a more open-minded approach to consciousness in cognitive psychology. As he writes, "After its banishment as an epiphenomenon by behaviouristic psychology, consciousness has recently again been declared to be the central problem of psychology.... A few psychologists have taken up the challenge posed by the many problems of consciousness, but contemporary psychology at large has continued to overlook this uniquely human property of the human mind" (Tulving 1985, p. 1; chap. 36, this volume). That neglect is now rapidly fading.

Tulving's advocacy has paid off in terms of scientific findings. In his classic 1985 article (chap. 36, this volume) Tulving outlined several distinct types of memory that are now widely accepted, and which have been found to have distinctive brain correlates. Episodic memory stores memory of lived conscious episodes;

by comparison, procedural (skill) and semantic (abstract meaning) memory is unconscious.

The paper by Schacter et al. (1996; chap. 37, this volume) presents a set of PET scan findings about the hippocampus in the conscious recollection of studied words, in contrast to implicitly retrieved word in response to three-letter cues. Current theory suggests that the hippocampus may not be the locus of episodic memory, but that it is clearly involved in conscious storage and retrieval operations.

Much learning occurs by paying attention to something without being conscious of the details of what is learned (Reber 1989; chap. 38, this volume). Grammar learning is a particularly good example, because children typically do not acquire language by means of explicit rules the way we might learn the rules of algebra or a foreign language. There certainly are rules that appear to operate, but they are not conscious or articulatable explicitly. The existence of such rules is shown by such well-established phenomena as overgeneralization in early childhood of regular past-tense forms, resulting in errors like "see-seed" and "hear-heared." Such overgeneralizations are typical in children of three or four, but they soon disappear. They are evidence for rule learning, but the rules are not explicit.

Instead, there is a sizable body of findings that suggest that linguistic rule learning is often implicit and inarticulate. We hear a series of words, and unconsciously we infer and remember the regularities implicit in them. That does not mean, however, that consciousness plays no role in implicit learning: After all, children do pay attention to the words of their language as well as their ordering, and "paying attention" means to allow oneself to become conscious of something. Likewise, subjects in implicit learning experiments are always asked to pay attention to some set of items. It appears that consciousness is a necessary condition for acquisition of implicit material, but that the details of what is to be learned need not be conscious. Reber (1989;

chap. 38, this volume) presents a classic set of studies of this phenomenon.

One possibility is that consciousness, though limited in capacity at any one moment, nevertheless offers a gateway to much more extensive unconscious knowledge sources in memory. The recognition vocabulary of educated English speakers contains about 100,000 words. Although we do not use all of those words in everyday speech, we can understand each one as soon as it is presented in a sentence that makes sense. Each individual word is already quite complex. The *Oxford English Dictionary* devotes 75,000 words to the many different meanings of the word "set." Yet all we do as humans to access these complex unconscious bodies of knowledge is to become conscious of a target word. It seems that understanding language demands the gateway of consciousness. This is another case of the general principle that consciousness creates widespread access to unconscious sources of knowledge, such as the mental lexicon, meaning, and grammar.

Similarly, the size of long-term episodic memory is unknown, but we do know that simply by paying attention to as many as 10,000 distinct pictures over several days without attempting to memorize them, we can spontaneously recognize more than 90% a week later (Standing 1973). Remarkable results like this are common when we use recognition probes, merely asking people to choose between known and new pictures. Recognition probes apparently work so well because they re-present the original conscious experience of each picture in its entirety. Here the brain does a marvelous job of memory search, with little effort. It seems that humans create memories of the stream of input merely by paying attention; but because we are always paying attention to *something*, in every waking moment, this suggests that autobiographical memory may be very large indeed. Once again we have a vast unconscious domain, and we gain access to it using consciousness. Mere consciousness of some event helps to store a recognizable memory of it, and when we reexperience it, we can distinguish it accurately from millions of other experiences.

Skill and Automaticity

Repeated events typically fade from consciousness. That is true for repetitive stimuli that become habituated, as well as predictable actions, which tend become automatic quite rapidly. There seems to be a close connection between redundancy and loss of conscious access. A stimulus that is significant, such as a memory of a traumatic emotional event, can be repeated with little loss of conscious access. But when the memory becomes truly redundant and empty of useful information, it will tend to fade rapidly. There seems to be a close connection between novelty/informativeness and consciousness (Baars 1988).

Automaticity is characterized by a loss of awareness as well as by "unitization," the tendency to act as a single entity, as in the act of jumping on a bicycle. Learning to ride a bicycle involves learning to balance, move the pedals, and steer, but when the whole sequence become automatic, riding the bicycle seems to become much more like a unitized action—a single chunk of activity.

Richard Shiffrin has made many contributions to the study of automatic functioning, mostly within a framework that made it difficult to deal with consciousness. Thus loss of conscious access seemed to be just one of many features of automaticity, perhaps a side issue, and certainly one that was difficult to deal with. An alternative view might be that loss of conscious access is the core fact about automaticity, and that other aspects (unitization, low capacity use, lack of modifiability, etc.) are consequences of the loss of conscious access (Baars 1988). In this section Shiffrin (1997; chap. 39, this volume) presents a careful review of the evidence regarding these questions.

Along with loss of conscious access, automaticity also involves a loss of control and access to errors. Langer and Imber (1979; chap. 40, this volume) have shown that error detection becomes quite poor when a skill becomes automatic: the less conscious it is, the more difficult it is to monitor. These investigators were pursuing the hypothesis that perceived competence affects performance: the more skilled we think we are, the better we perform. One way in which we lose touch with our own competence is by automatization; when we become skilled readers, musicians, or truck drivers, we lose conscious access to many details of our own actions, and hence we may become more vulnerable to false negative attributions about our own performance. This line of reasoning led Langer and Imber to devise a simple coding task that people could learn to the point of automaticity in a matter of minutes. They found that misleading negative self-labels affected highly practiced subjects (who were automatic in the task) but not the more conscious subjects. If we have no conscious access to our own performance, and if some credible source of information seems to indicate that we are doing badly, we tend to accept misleading feedback because we cannot check reality. With direct conscious access to our own performance we are much less influenced by misleading labels. These results suggest that three things go together: losing voluntary control over action details, losing consciousness of them, and losing the ability to monitor and edit the details. Indeed, the ability to monitor and edit a planned act may be the essence of voluntary control (Baars 1988, 1992).

In another remarkable sign of progress in understanding brain function, Raichle (1998; chap. 41, this volume) describes a series of brain-imaging studies on automatism. It is possible that these studies single out effortful versus automatic activities rather than conscious versus unconscious ones. The kind of consciousness in studied these experiments may not be the same as consciousness in visual cortex (see section 2).

Thus the emphasis in this work is on frontal functions, rather than the posterior cortex that is most directly involved in sensory consciousness. Nevertheless, automaticity does seem to be associated with lack of reportable conscious access to skilled tasks. As Raichle writes, "... it seems possible to make a distinction between brain systems supporting conscious, reflective performance and brain systems supporting the non-conscious, reflexive performance of the same task."

Retrieval, Recall, and Recognition

Memory retrieval is most often spontaneous, though we typically study deliberate recall. Jerome Singer's work (chap. 31, this volume) shows how much spontaneous mentation goes on during our waking hours. Tversky and Kahneman (1973; chap. 42, this volume) have shown that the ease of retrieval to consciousness, called availability, has great influence on our capacity for judgment. Gardiner et al. (1998; chap. 43, this volume) have explored a number of empirical differences between conscious and nonconscious memory retrieval. In general, it seems that deliberate recall of episodic memory is quite different from spontaneous recognition of a familiar face, for example. Indeed, recognition probes of memory rely on familiarity judgments ("Yes, it looks familiar," vs. "No, it doesn't look familiar"). These are often thought of as fringe conscious experiences (see Mangan, chap. 45, this volume).

Jacoby (1991; 1994; chap. 44, this volume) and his coworkers have argued that conscious and unconscious influences in retrieval can be distinguished by way of a "process dissociation" task. Subjects are typically given one list of words to memorize and are then asked to do a process dissociation task, in which they are asked *not* to say out loud words that are presented but which they already know from the previous list. The argument is that if they can successfully avoid saying the previously learned words, they must be remembering that those words were indeed studied before. But if they cannot avoid intrusions from the previous list, that must reflect unconscious influences on the task of retrieval. Process dissociation is still a hotly debated topic, but it is one of the few efforts that seems to promise a distinct improvement in our operational definition of conscious and unconscious processes (see Introduction).

References

Baars, B. J. (1988) *A cognitive theory of consciousness.* New York: Cambridge University Press.

Baars, B. J. (1992) *Experimental slips and human error: Exploring the architecture of volition.* NY: Plenum Press.

Bowers, K., Regehr, G., Balthazard, C., and Parker, K. (1990) Intuition in the context of discovery. *Cognitive Psychology*, 22 (1), 72–110.

Gardiner, J. M., Ramponi, C., Richardson-Klavehn, A. (1998) Experiences of remembering, knowing, and guessing. *Consciousness & Cognition, 7*, 1–26.

Jacoby, L. L. (1991) A process dissociation framework: Separating automatic from intentional uses of memory. *Journal of Memory & Language, 30*, 513–541.

Jacoby, L. L. (1994) Measuring recollection: Strategic versus automatic influences on associative context. In C. Umilta and M. Moscovitch (Eds.) *Attention and Performance XV.* Cambridge, MA: MIT Press. Pp. 661–680.

Langer, E. J., and Imber, L. G. (1979) When practice makes imperfect: debilitating effects of overlearning. *Journal of Personality and Social Psychology, 37* (11), 2014–2024.

Mangan, B. (1993) Taking phenomenology seriously: The "fringe" and its implications for cognitive research. *Consciousness & Cognition, 2* (2), 89–108.

Raichle, M. E. (1998) The neural correlates of consciousness: An analysis of cognitive skill learning. *Phil. Trans. R. Soc. Lond. B*, 353, 1–14.

Reber, A. S. (1993) *Implicit learning and tacit knowledge: An essay on the cognitive unconscious.* NY: Oxford University Press.

Schachter, D. L., Alpert, N. M., Savage, C. R., Rauch, S. L., and Albert, M. S. (1996) Conscious recollection and the human hippocampal formation: Evidence from positron emission tomography. *Proc. Natl. Acad. Sci. USA, 93*, 321–325.

Shiffrin, R. M. (1994) Attention, automatism, and consciousness. In J. D. Cohen and J. W. Schooler (Eds.) *Scientific approaches to consciousness.* Pp. 49–64. Mahwah, N. J.: L. Erlbaum Assoc.

Standing, L. (1973) Learning 10,000 pictures. *Q. J. Exp Psychol., 25*, 207–222.

Tulving, E. Memory and consciousness. *Journal of Canadian Psychology*, 1985, 26:1, 1–12.

Tversky, A., and Kahneman, A. (1973) Availability: A heuristic for judging frequency and probability. *Cognitive Psychology, 2*, 207–232.

36 Memory and Consciousness

Endel Tulving

Of all the mysteries of nature, none is greater than that of human consciousness. Intimately familiar to all of us, our capacity to contemplate the universe and to apprehend the infinity of space and time, and our knowledge that we can do so, have continued to resist analysis and elude understanding.

After its banishment as an epiphenomenon by behaviouristic psychology, consciousness has recently again been declared to be the central problem of psychology (Hilgard 1980, Miller 1980, Neisser 1979). A few psychologists have taken up the challenge posed by the many problems of consciousness, but contemporary psychology at large has continued to overlook this uniquely human property of the human mind.

Nowhere is the benign neglect of consciousness more conspicuous than in the study of human memory. One can read article after article on memory, or consult book after book, without encountering the term "consciousness." Such a state of affairs must be regarded as rather curious. One might think that memory should have something to do with remembering, and remembering *is* a conscious experience. To remember an event means to be consciously aware now of something that happened on an earlier occasion. Nevertheless, through most of its history, including the current heyday of cognitive psychology, the psychological study of memory has largely proceeded without reference to the existence of conscious awareness in remembering.

The literature on consciousness is rich, with many contributions by philosophers (e.g., Dennett 1969), psychologists (e.g., Gray 1971; Mandler 1975; Natsoulas 1978, 1981; Posner and Klein 1973; Shallice 1972; Underwood 1982; Underwood and Stevens 1979, 1981), neuroscientists (e.g., Eccles 1977, Sperry 1969), and others (e.g., Globus, Maxwell, and Savodnik 1976; Griffin 1976, 1984; Josephson and Ram-achandran 1980). But much of it consists of "epistemological, metaphysical, and existential" theorizing—to borrow the apt phrase from Peter Dodwell (1975)—without corresponding empirical facts. Even when attempts are made to relate consciousness to the activity of the brain, the situation is not much better, as observed by Gazzaniga and LeDoux:

> When the inevitable topic of consciousness is approached in the light of modern brain research, the experienced student has come to brace himself for the mellifluous intonations of someone's personal experience and ideas on the matter, as opposed to data. (1978, p. 141)

The psychological literature relevant to the problem of the relation between memory and consciousness differs from the larger literature on consciousness by the dearth of both ideas and facts. There has been little apart from the idea that primary memory can be identified with consciousness (e.g., Craik and Jacoby 1975, James 1890), the idea that rehearsal of information in primary memory is a conscious process (e.g., Atkinson and Shiffrin 1971, Wickelgren 1977), and the idea that latent memory traces are unconscious, whereas activated ones are conscious (e.g., Underwood 1979). And just about the only facts concerning memory and consciousness come from shadowing experiments in which the level of conscious awareness of to-be-tested materials has been manipulated (e.g., Eich 1984, Moray 1959, Norman 1969).

The present paper describes an attempt to relate memory to consciousness in terms of data obtained through clinical observation and laboratory experiment. Its basic pretheoretical assumption is that progress in the scientific understanding of consciousness—as against its epistemological, metaphysical, or experiential understanding—requires not only the postulation and identification of different *kinds* of consciousness but also their *measurement* as an aspect of experience, or as a dependent variable.

The paper consists of six parts. First, a hypothetical scheme is described in which different varieties of memory are related to different varieties of consciousness. Second, clinical observations from a case study, together with relevant evidence and ideas from other sources, are used to describe and characterize a particular kind of consciousness and conscious awareness, referred to as autonoetic (self-knowing) consciousness. Third, the concept of autonoetic conscious awareness is further elaborated. In the fourth part, autonoetic consciousness is related to the synergistic ecphory model of recall and recognition (Tulving 1982, 1983). In the fifth part, two demonstration experiments are described in which autonoetic awareness was measured and shown to vary systematically with conditions under which recall and recognition were observed. Finally, the question of the biological utility of episodic memory and autonoetic consciousness is briefly discussed.[1]

Varieties of Memory and Consciousness

Let us assume that there are three different kinds of memory, or three memory systems: procedural, semantic, and episodic (Tulving 1983). They are alike in that they all make possible the utilization of acquired and retained knowledge. But they differ in the kind of knowledge that they handle, and in the ways in which different kinds of knowledge are acquired or used.

Procedural memory (Anderson 1976, Tulving 1983, Winograd 1975) is concerned with how things are done—with the acquisition, retention, and utilization of perceptual, cognitive, and motor skills. Semantic memory—also called generic (Hintzman 1978) or categorical memory (Estes 1976)—has to do with the symbolically representable knowledge that organisms possess about the world. Episodic memory mediates the *remembering* of personally experienced events (Tulving 1972, 1983).

Ideas about the relations between the three systems have varied. Not too long ago (Tulving 1983), I thought of the three systems as representing two different levels in a hierarchy: memory as a whole subdivided into two general types, procedural and propositional, with episodic and semantic constituting two *parallel*, albeit interacting and overlapping, subsystems of propositional memory. Recently, however, I was led by a number of critics to the view that a more reasonable assumption concerning the relation between the episodic and semantic system is one according to which episodic memory constitutes a single distinct subsystem of semantic memory (Tulving 1984).

It seems reasonable to extend this idea to cover all three systems and to assume that they constitute a class-inclusion hierarchy in which procedural memory entails semantic memory as a *specialized* subcategory, and in which semantic memory, in turn, entails episodic memory as a specialized subcategory. According to this scheme, it is impossible for an organism to possess episodic memory without the corresponding semantic memory, and impossible for it to possess semantic memory without the corresponding procedural memory, although semantic memory systems can exist independently of episodic systems, and procedural systems independently of semantic systems.

Each of the three memory systems, in addition to other ways in which it differs from others, is characterized by a different kind of consciousness. I will refer to the three kinds of consciousness as anoetic (non-knowing), noetic (knowing), and autonoetic (self-knowing). Their relation to each other and to the three memory systems is schematically depicted in table 36.1.[2]

The procedural memory system is characterized by anoetic consciousness. Anoetic consciousness is temporally and spatially bound to the current situation. Organisms possessing only anoetic consciousness are conscious in the sense that they are capable of perceptually registering, internally representing, and behaviourally

Table 36.1
A schematic diagram of the relations between memory systems and varieties of consciousness

Memory system		Consciousness
Episodic	$\longleftrightarrow$	Autonoetic
$\downarrow$		$\downarrow$
Semantic	$\longleftrightarrow$	Noetic
$\downarrow$		$\downarrow$
Procedural	$\longleftrightarrow$	Anoetic

responding to aspects of the present environment, both external and internal. Anoetic consciousness does not include any reference to nonpresent extraorganismic stimuli and states of the world.

Semantic memory is characterized by noetic consciousness. Noetic consciousness allows an organism to be aware of, and to cognitively operate on, objects and events, and relations among objects and events, in the absence of these objects and events. The organism can flexibly act upon such symbolic knowledge of the world. Entering information into, and retrieval of information from, semantic memory is accompanied by noetic consciousness.

Of special interest in the present paper is autonoetic consciousness, correlated with episodic memory. It is necessary for the remembering of personally experienced events. When a person remembers such an event, he is aware of the event as a veridical part of his own past existence. It is autonoetic consciousness that confers the special phenomenal flavour to the remembering of past events, the flavour that distinguishes remembering from other kinds of awareness, such as those characterizing perceiving, thinking, imagining, or dreaming.

Evidence for autonoetic consciousness will be drawn from clinical observations of an amnesic patient, to be described presently. The distinction between the other two kinds of consciousness is based on conjecture. But it is not without precedent. Consider, for instance, a classification of different kinds of memory proposed by Hermann Ebbinghaus, who is usually thought of as the inventor of the nonsense syllable and as responsible for psychology's long preoccupation with rote learning. Ebbinghaus distinguished between three kinds of effects of "mental states which were at one time present in consciousness and then have disappeared from it" (1885, p. 1). In the first place, he suggested, we call back into consciousness a seemingly lost state that is then "immediately recognised as something formerly experienced" (1885, p. 1): that is, we *remember*. In the second case—Ebbinghaus said it occurs when we reproduce a mental state "involuntarily"—this accompanying consciousness may be lacking and "we know only indirectly that the 'now' is identical with the 'then'" (1885, p. 2). In the third case, earlier processes leave consequences or effects that facilitate "the occurrence and progress of similar processes," although these effects "remain concealed from consciousness" (1885, p. 2). Ebbinghaus's first case can be thought to correspond to autonoetic, the second to noetic, and the third to anoetic consciousness.

A Man without Autonoetic Consciousness: A Case Study

Evidence pertinent to autonoetic consciousness comes from a case study of an amnesic patient whom I and my colleague, Daniel Schacter, have been observing at our Unit for Memory Disorders in Toronto. This young man, here referred to as N. N., suffered a closed head injury a few years ago as a result of a traffic accident.

N. N.'s amnesia for personal events is profound. It covers the time both before and after his accident. When he is distracted, he forgets something said to him almost immediately. Although his immediate memory span is eight digits, on a picture-memory recognition test on which normal subjects score 60–70% correct, his score is zero. On a cued-recall test of categorized words, he does not distinguish between correct responses and category intrusions. Although he knows a few things about his past—for instance, what year the family moved into the house where they live now, the names of the schools he went to, or where he spent his summers in his teens—he cannot recall a single event or incident from the past. Like the patient S. S. described by Cermak and O'Connor (1983), N. N.'s knowledge of his own past seems to have the same impersonal experiential quality as his knowledge of the rest of the world.

His language skills and general knowledge are relatively intact. He can define words such as "evasive," "perimeter," and "tangible"; he can provide a reasonably good verbal description of the "script" of going to a restaurant or making a long-distance telephone call; he can describe the typical daily activities of a university student; he knows what the North American continent and the Statue of Liberty look like, and can draw their outlines. He also knows the meaning of the term "consciousness." When asked what consciousness is, he says, "It's being aware of who we are and what we are, and where we are."

N. N. has no difficulty with the concept of chronological time. He knows the units of time and their relations perfectly well, and he can accurately represent chronological time graphically. But in stark contrast to his abstract knowledge of time, his awareness of subjective time seems to be severely impaired. When asked what he did before coming to where he is now, or what he did the day before, he says that he does not know. When asked what he will be doing when he leaves "here," or what he will be doing "tomorrow," he says he does not know.

Here is part of the transcript of an interview, with me as the interviewer:

E. T.: "Let's try the question again about the future. What will you be doing tomorrow?"

(There is a 15-second pause.)

N. N.: smiles faintly, then says, "I don't know."

E. T.: "Do you remember the question?"

N. N.: "About what I'll be doing tomorrow?"

E. T.: "Yes. How would you describe your state of mind when you try to think about it?"

(A 5-second pause.)

N. N.: "Blank, I guess."

When asked, on different occasions, to describe the "blankness" that characterizes his state of mind when he tries to think about "tomorrow," he says that it is "like being asleep" or that "it's a big blankness sort of thing." When asked to give an analogy, to describe what it is like, he says, "It's like being in a room with nothing there and having a guy tell you to go find a chair, and there's nothing there." On another occasion he says, "It's like swimming in the middle of a lake. There's nothing there to hold you up or do anything with." When asked to compare his state of mind when he is trying to think about what he will be doing tomorrow with his state of mind when he thinks about what he did yesterday, he says it is the "*same kind of blankness.*" N. N. makes all these observations calmly and serenely, without showing any emotion. Only when he is asked whether he is not surprised that there is "nothing there" when he tries to think about yesterday or tomorrow, does he display slight agitation for a moment and utter a soft exclamation of "Wow!"

N. N. clearly is conscious and he clearly has a good deal of preserved memory capability. At the same time his consciousness and memory are severely impaired, and impaired highly selectively. He knows many things about the world, he is aware of this knowledge, and he can express it relatively flexibly. In this sense he is not greatly different from a normal adult. But he seems to have no capability of experiencing extended subjective time, or chronognosia (Bouman and Grunbaum 1929): even if he feels that he has a personal identity, it does not include the past or the future; he cannot remember any particular episodes from his life, nor can he imagine anything that he is likely to do on a subsequent occasion. He seems to be living in a "permanent present." In terms of the threefold classification of consciousness proposed here, we could say that N. N. possesses both anoetic and noetic consciousness but not autonoetic consciousness, and that his procedural and semantic memory systems are relatively unimpaired whereas his episodic memory is severely damaged.

We must obviously be very cautious when we generalize from observations of individual cases, particularly since no two amnesic patients are ever exactly alike. Nevertheless, it is reasonable to believe that N. N. does not represent an isolated occurrence of a severe impairment in the ability to apprehend and contemplate extended subjective time. His case tells us that amnesia can be characterized as a derangement of consciousness and not just a derangement of memory for past events.

Autonoetic Consciousness, Subjective Time, and Episodic Memory

Students of amnesia have noted before that some amnesic patients live in a "permanent present" (e.g., Barbizet 1970, p. 33). The context of the discussion of relevant cases usually implies that such patients are unaware of their *past*. But writers on amnesia have sometimes pointed out that because the patients cannot utilize the past, their future too must remain hazy, vague, and confused, leaving them "marooned in the moment" (e.g., Lidz 1942, p. 596). Our observations of N. N. corroborate the idea that the lack of conscious awareness of personal time encompasses both the past and the future. A normal healthy person who possesses autonoetic consciousness is capable of becoming aware of her own past as well as her own future; she is capable of mental time travel, roaming at will over what has happened as readily as over what might happen, independently of physical laws that govern the universe. N. N. seems to be completely incapable of doing so. It is this fact that provides the basis for the conclusion that he is severely or completely lacking in autonoetic consciousness.

David Ingvar has measured regional cerebral blood flow in normal people in a resting state, and has observed a "hyperfrontal" pattern of cortical activation (Ingvar 1979). He has interpreted such hyperfrontality as reflecting properties of a consciousness that embraces the past, the present, and the future:

On the basis of previous experiences, represented in memories, the brain—one's mind—is automatically busy with extrapolation of future events and, as it appears, constructing alternative hypothetical behaviour patterns in order to be ready for what may happen. (Ingvar 1979, p, 21)

Ingvar has also suggested that the frontal lobes constitute the anatomical basis for people's "memory for the future" (Ingvar, personal communication; see also Ingvar 1983). It seems reasonable to assume, however, that the kind of consciousness that Ingvar is concerned with is more like autonoetic consciousness than consciousness at large.

The lessons learned from N. N. and the ideas suggested by Ingvar make it possible to speculate about the general nature of autonoetic consciousness and to make up a tentative list of its properties. A summary of these properties is as follows:

1. Encompasses personal time: past and future

2. Necessary component of remembering of events

3. Appears late in development

4. Selectively impaired or lost in brain damage

5. Varies across individuals and situations

6. Can be measured

We have already discussed the first idea: autonoetic consciousness encompasses extended subjective time, an individual's ability to apprehend her personal past and future. Although

N. N. is conscious in many ways, he does not perceive the present moment as a continuation of his own past and as a prelude to his future. N. N. is like one of Jaynes's bicameral men, who did not have feelings of personal identity in our sense and "who could not reminisce because they were not fully conscious" (Jaynes 1976, p. 371).

The second suggestion is that autonoetic consciousness is a *necessary correlate* of episodic memory. According to the scheme I am describing, there is no such thing as "remembering without awareness" (cf. Eich 1984, Jacoby and Witherspoon 1982, Masson 1984). Organisms can behave and learn without (autonoetic) awareness, but they cannot *remember* without awareness. Nor can nonliving matter remember anything, even if it can act upon previously stored information (e.g., Robinson 1976). Like many other amnesic patients described in the literature who can acquire a variety of new skills (Moscovitch 1982, Cohen and Squire 1980, Parkin 1982), N. N. shows normal learning of the kind referred to as priming effects in word-fragment completion (Schacter 1984; Tulving, Schacter, and Stark 1982). He can also learn new words, and new meanings of old words, although at a rather slow rate, as shown in ongoing research conducted by Elizabeth Glisky at the Unit for Memory Disorders. But he does not seem to be able to remember anything.

Third, autonoetic consciousness appears later in an individual's development than do other forms of consciousness (e.g., Knapp 1976). Many writers have suggested that very young children have neither episodic memory nor (autonoetic) consciousness (e.g., MacCurdy 1928, Neisser 1978, Nelson and Gruendel 1981). Nelson and Gruendel's observations are representative:

There is no evidence that the young child who remembers an episode remembers it as having taken place at a particular time in a particular temporal context—that is, that it constitutes an autobiographical memory of the type that older children and adults can draw on. (1981, p. 149)

And Neisser has suggested that a young child may be conscious of an object when he perceives it, but "he is not aware that he, a person with a particular history and character and probable future," is seeing the object (1978, p. 172). Every young child is an extremely capable learner: her behaviour and experiences can have readily identifiable consequences for her future behaviour and experiences. Yet she need not have any (autonoetic) conscious awareness as to the origin of these consequences: there need be no remembering (Lockhart 1984, Schacter and Moscovitch 1984). As episodic memory follows semantic memory in normal development (Kinsbourne and Wood 1975), so autonoetic consciousness emerges from noetic consciousness.

The fourth property of autonoetic consciousness is its selective dependence on particular brain processes: the case of N. N. shows that certain kinds of brain damage may result in its impairment, or loss, without comparable impairment in other forms of consciousness. Correlation with brain mechanisms must be regarded as one of the more important criteria for distinguishing between different kinds of consciousness. If such correlations did not exist, and if differential impairment of different kinds of consciousness had never been observed, classification of consciousness into distinct varieties would remain yet another metaphysical exercise.

The fifth property of autonoetic consciousness concerns its variability among individuals and its variable occurrence in different situations (e.g., Roth 1980). Individuals presumably vary in the extent to which they "possess" and benefit from autonoetic consciousness in their daily activities, as they vary with respect to other mental characteristics. Similarly, autonoetic consciousness can be expected to vary systematically with the conditions under which it is observed.

Finally, autonoetic consciousness is measurable. Although perhaps a trite point in some ways, it is worth making because of the current state of research on consciousness. If it were not possible to make quantitative statements about autonoetic consciousness, its usefulness as a scientific concept would be greatly diminished.

Recovery of Knowledge about Past Events

I have argued that N. N. possesses neither episodic memory nor autonoetic consciousness. Yet it is a fact that he can make veridical statements about his past. The resolution of this apparent contradiction between the argument and the fact lies in the assumption that people can have and can express knowledge about things that have happened to them even if they can rely only on their semantic memory (Schacter and Tulving 1982; Schacter, Harbluk, and McLachlan 1984). That is, even when a person does not *remember* an event, she may *know* something about it. Such knowledge is created in the same way, and it is of the same quality, as the knowledge about the temporally and spatially extended world and its abstract features existing independently of the person.

If it is possible to recover knowledge about past events from either the episodic system or the semantic system, then the phenomenal experience that accompanies the recovery of such information may be one of remembering (autonoetic awareness) or knowing (noetic awareness), or a mixture of the two. It follows, then, that one way of measuring autonoetic awareness could take the form of asking people, when they recall or recognize a previously encountered item, whether they *remember* the event or whether they *know* in some other way that it occurred. The probability of the "remember" judgement can serve as an index of the extent to which autonoetic consciousness is involved in recovery of knowledge about past events in a particular situation.

Different situations in which autonoetic consciousness can be expected to vary and where its measurement may be informative can be specified in terms of the synergistic ecphory model of recall and recognition (Tulving 1982, 1983). The central assumption of the model is that both the

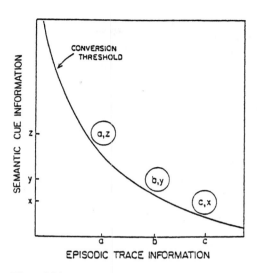

Figure 36.1
Schematic diagram of the synergistic ecphory model of retrieval.

general nature and specific characteristics of recollective experience (the phenomenal experience of remembering a past event) are determined jointly by episodic and semantic information. A schematic representation of the model is shown in figure 36.1. The horizontal axis of the coordinate system represents episodic trace information, the vertical axis represents semantic retrieval information, and the two-dimensional space defined by the two axes represents so-called ecphoric information. It is this ecphoric information, an amalgam of episodic and semantic information, that determines the general nature as well as specific content of recollective experience.

The curved line in the diagram represents the *conversion threshold* for a particular level of overt behaviour that serves as an indicant of the rememberer's mental state. This overt behaviour, or memory *performance*, can take different forms. One such form, for instance, is recall of the name of a previously observed event. Another one is recognition, such as identification of a test item as "old." Each type of performance has its own conversion threshold, although only one is shown in figure 36.1. The conversion threshold divides the space of ecphoric information into two regions. Ecphoric information above the threshold is sufficient for the required performance, whereas that below the threshold is not.

The model shows how overt memory performance can be supported by different combinations of episodic trace information and semantic retrieval information. A trade-off relation exists between these two kinds of information such that impoverished episodic traces can be compensated for by richer retrieval cues, and vice versa. From the hypothesized correlation between episodic memory and autonoetic consciousness it follows that the kind of conscious awareness that characterizes an act of recollection varies with the nature of the "mix" of trace and cue information—that is, with the location of the bundle of ecphoric information in the sketch in figure 36.1.

That the three bundles of ecphoric information designated as a, z, b, y, and c, x, representing combinations of corresponding bundles of trace information (A, B, C) and retrieval information (X, Y, Z), are all above the conversion threshold indicates that the behavioural response (e.g., correct recall) would be equally possible in all three cases. Yet, according to the logic outlined here, the recollective experience underlying or accompanying memory performance corresponding to ecphoric information c, x would be expected to be characterized by a greater degree of autonoetic consciousness than b, y, which in turn would be expected to represent a greater degree of autonoetic consciousness than a, z.

Measurement of Autonoetic Consciousness

We will next discuss two experiments in which (a) situations were created corresponding to different points above the conversion threshold in the ecphoric space of figure 36.1, and (b) auton-

oetic conscious awareness accompanying retrieval in these different situations was assessed.

In the first experiment, 79 university students heard, on a single presentation trial, a list of 27 category names and single category instances (e.g., *musical instrument*—VIOLA; *a fruit*—PEAR). The students' memory performance was subsequently tested in three successive tests that yielded *three sets* of recalled items. The first test was a free-recall test: subjects were asked to recall as many instances as they could, in any order. The second was a cued-recall test: names of categories to which the studied instances belonged were given as specific retrieval cues. The third was a cued-recall test: the initial letter of each category instance was given as a cue in addition to the name of the category to which the word belonged.

The logic here is as follows: The ecphoric information (mixture of trace and cue information) of the first set of items, those recalled in *free* recall, corresponds to the ecphoric bundle c, x in figure 36.1: relatively rich episodic trace information combined with relatively impoverished retrieval information. The ecphoric information of the second set of items, those recalled in the category-cued recall *but not recalled in free recall*, corresponds to the ecphoric bundle b, y in figure 36.1: richer retrieval information combined with poorer trace information. The trace information of the second set of items can be assumed to be of lower quality than that of the first set because otherwise these items too would have been accessible for retrieval in free recall. Extending the same logic to the third set of items, those recalled to category names and initial letters, *but not recalled in the other two tests*, we can think of ecphoric information of these items as represented by the bundle a, z in figure 36.1: rather plentiful retrieval information combined with relatively impoverished trace information.

The extent to which subjects' recollective experience was characterized by autonoetic awareness for the three sets of items was assessed by asking subjects, in each of the three tests, to in-

Table 36.2
Recall and "remember" judgements in Experiment 1

	Free recall	Category recall	Letter recall
Probability of recall	.51	.35	.10
Probability of recall conditionalized on remaining items	(.51)	.54	.74
Probability of "remember" judgement	.88	.75	.48

Table 36.3
Recognition data and "remember" judgements in Experiment 2

Test items	Measure	Test	
		Day 1	Day 8
Old	Hit rate	.86	.62
	p("remembered")	.83	.55
New	FA rate	.17	.27
	p("remembered")	.45	.40

dicate, for each item they recalled, whether they actually "remembered" its occurrence in the list or whether they simply "knew" on some other basis that the item was a member of the study list. The proportion of recalled items for which subjects made "remember" judgements was calculated separately for the three sets of recalled items, and taken as an estimate of the presence of autonoetic awareness in recollection. The expectation was that the proportion of "remember" judgements would be greatest for free-recall items, next highest for items recalled in response to category names but not previously recalled in free recall, and lowest for items recalled only in response to both category names and initial-letter cues.

The results of the first experiment are summarized in table 36.2. The three sets of recalled items—those given in free recall, those given in category-cued recall but not in free recall, and those given in the category- and initial-letter-cued condition but not in the other two conditions—are designated as free-recall items, category-recall items, and letter-recall items in table 36.2.

Three descriptive statistics were calculated for each of the three sets of recalled items: (a) proportion of items in the set, (b) this proportion expressed with respect to the items *remaining* to be recalled after the first, or the second, test, and (c) the mean proportion of the items in the set that were judged as having been "remembered" by the subjects. The important

data for our present purposes are given by the latter measures.

As table 36.2 shows, the proportion of "remembered" items was highest for free-recall, next highest for category-recall, and lowest for letter-recall items. These data suggest that the involvement of autonoetic consciousness in recall of past events varies directly with the contribution of the episodic (trace) information to ecphoric information on which recall is based.

The second experiment can be summarized briefly, since its logic was very much the same as that used in the first experiment. "Remember" and "know" judgements were collected from a small group of 10 subjects in two recognition tests, one (for half the items) given in the same experimental session in which 36 to-be-remembered words were presented for study, the other (for the other half) given seven days later. The logic here is based on the assumption that the episodic trace information would be reduced in "richness" over the seven-day retention interval, with corresponding decreases in autonoetic awareness, and that, therefore, bundles of ecphoric information underlying recognized items would be more heavily weighted with semantic retrieval information after the longer than after the shorter retention interval. Thus, the expectation was that the proportion of "remember" judgements would decline with the retention interval.

As the data summarized in table 36.3 show, these expectations were borne out: With the

Table 36.4

Distributions of confidence judgements for items judged "remembered" and items judged "known" in Experiment 2

Recognized items	Confidence judgements			
	1	2	3	Mean
"Remembered"	9	40	143	2.74
"Known"	25	63	35	2.08

hit rates decreased and the false-alarm rate increased over the seven-day retention interval, the proportion of "remember" judgements for correctly recognized words was lower on Day 8 than on Day 1. We conclude that autonoetic conscious awareness is more clearly present in the recollection of recently encountered events than in that of events encountered a longer time ago.

In the second experiment we also collected conventional confidence judgements from the subjects. As shown in table 36.4, in which the data for "old" test items are pooled over both short and long retention intervals, there was a tendency for subjects to be more confident about their recognition of those items that they classified as "remembered" than those classified as "known": a positive correlation between confidence and "remember" judgements.

Adaptive Value of Autonoetic Consciousness

The results of the two experiments have shown that the distinction between "knowing" and "remembering" previous occurrences of particular events is meaningful to people, that people can make corresponding judgements about their memory performance, and that these judgements vary systematically with conditions under which retrieval of information takes place. The success of the experiments in conforming to the expectations derived from the hypothesized correlation between episodic memory and autonoetic consciousness, and from the synergistic ecphory

model, provides support for the assumption that people can retrieve information about personally experienced events without autonoetic "remembering" of the event, simply on the basis of their noetic "knowledge" that the event happened. A new problem arises, however. If recovery of information about past events can occur independently of episodic memory and autonoetic consciousness, why should the episodic system and autonoetic consciousness have emerged at all in the course of evolution? Wherein lies their adaptive advantage?

One possible answer to this question, supported by the data showing positive correlation between confidence ratings and "remember" judgements in our second experiment, is that the adaptive value of episodic memory and autonoetic consciousness lies in the heightened subjective certainty with which organisms endowed with such memory and consciousness believe, and are willing to act upon, information retrieved from memory. Knowledge about environmental regularities certainly has adaptive value. By enhancing the perceived orderliness of an organism's universe, episodic memory and autonoetic consciousness lead to more decisive action in the present and more effective planning for the future (cf. Griffin 1976, Lachman and Naus 1984). In this connection, it is worth noting that amnesia has been frequently characterized by the patients' lack of subjective certainty about the mnemonic knowledge that they do in fact possess (e.g., Lidz 1942, Talland 1965, Weiskrantz 1978).

We have often been told that the human brain is the most complicated piece of matter in the universe. We could also say that human consciousness is the most enigmatic manifestation of this piece of matter. Understanding consciousness, its emergence from the brain and its role in human intelligence and in human affairs, can only come, if it ever does come, at the end of a very long scientific journey. What I have tried to do in this paper is to discuss some of the steps with which the journey might begin.

Acknowledgments

This article is a somewhat modified version of an invited paper presented at the meeting of the Canadian Psychological Association, Ottawa, June 1984, in connection with the 1983 CPA Award for Distinguished Contributions to Canadian Psychology as a Science.

Research reported in the article has been supported by the Natural Sciences and Engineering Research Council, Grant No. A8632, and by a Special Research Program Grant from the Connaught Fund, University of Toronto.

The author is grateful for collaboration to Janine Law and Daniel Schacter.

Notes

1. Although the terms "consciousness" and "conscious awareness" (or simply "awareness") are closely related, and sometimes used interchangeably, in the present discussion they are used in different senses. "Consciousness" refers to a particular capability of living systems, whereas "awareness" refers to the internally experienced outcome of exercising this ability in a particular situation. (Another closely related term, "attention," even though not used in this paper, would refer to the control that the organism, or environmental events, can exert over the direction of consciousness in the selection of "contents" of awareness.)

2. The terms "anoetic consciousness" (Vol. 1, p. 50) and "noetic consciousness" (Vol. 2, p. 11) have been used by Stout (1896) in somewhat different, but related, senses from those used here.

References

Anderson, J. R. (1976). *Language, memory, and thought*. Hillsdale, N.J.: Erlbaum.

Atkinson, R. C., and Shiffrin, R. M. (1971). The control of short-term memory. *Scientific American, 225*(2), 82–90.

Barbizet, J. (1970). *Human memory and its pathology*. San Francisco: Freeman.

Bouman, L., and Grünbaum, A. A. (1929). Eine Störung der Chronognosie und ihre Bedeutung in dem betreffenden Symptomenbild [A disturbance of chronognosia and its meaning in the corresponding syndrome]. *Monatsschrift für Psychiatrie und Neurologie, 73*, 1–40.

Cermak, L. S., and O'Connor, M. (1983). The anterograde and retrograde retrieval ability of a patient with amnesia due to encephalitis. *Neuropsychologia, 21*, 213–234.

Cohen, N. J., and Squire, L. R. (1980). Preserved learning and retention of pattern analyzing skill in amnesia: Dissociation of knowing how and knowing that. *Science, 210*, 207–209.

Craik, F. I. M., and Jacoby, L. L. (1975). A process view of short-term retention. In F. Restle (Ed.), *Cognitive theory* (Vol. 1). Potomac, Md.: Erlbaum.

Dennett, D. C. (1969). *Content and consciousness*. New York: Humanities Press.

Dodwell, P. C. (1975). Contemporary theoretical problems in seeing. In E. C. Carterette and M. P. Friedman (Eds.), *Handbook of perception* (Vol. 5). New York: Academic Press.

Ebbinghaus, H. (1885). *Über das Gedächtnis* [On memory]. Leipzig: Duncker und Humblot. (English translation. New York: Dover Press).

Eccles, J. C. (1977). *The understanding of the brain* (2nd ed.). New York: McGraw Hill.

Eccles, J. C. (1980). *The human psyche*. Berlin: Springer Verlag.

Eich, E. (1984). Memory for unattended events. Remembering with and without awareness. *Memory and Cognition, 12*, 105–111.

Estes, W. K. (1976). The cognitive side of probability learning. *Psychological Review, 83*, 37–64.

Gazzaniga, M. S., and LeDoux, J. E. (1978). *The integrated mind*. New York: Plenum.

Globus, G. G., Maxwell, G., and Savodnik, I. (Eds.). (1976). *Consciousness and the brain*. New York: Plenum.

Gray, J. A. (1971). The mind-brain identity theory as a scientific hypothesis. *Philosophical Quarterly, 21*, 247–252.

Griffin, D. (1976). *The question of animal awareness*. New York: Rockefeller University Press.

Griffin, D. (1984). *Animal thinking*. Cambridge, Mass.: Harvard University Press.

Hilgard, E. R. (1977). *Divided consciousness: Multiple controls in human thought*. New York: Wiley.

Hilgard, E. R. (1980). Consciousness in contemporary psychology. *Annual Review of Psychology, 31*, 1–26.

Hintzman, D. L. (1978). *The psychology of learning and memory*. San Francisco: Freeman.

Ingvar, D. (1979). "Hyperfrontal" distribution of the general grey matter flow in resting wakefulness: on the functional anatomy of the conscious state. *Acta Neurologica Scandinavica, 60*, 12–25.

Ingvar, D. (1983). Hjärnan, tiden och metvetandet [Brain, time and consciousness]. *Forskning och Framsteg, 39–45*.

Jacoby, L. L., and Witherspoon, D. (1982). Remembering without awareness. *Canadian Journal of Psychology, 36*, 300–324.

James, W. (1890). *Principles of psychology*. New York: Holt.

Jaynes, J. (1976). *The origin of consciousness in the breakdown of the bicameral mind*. Boston: Houghton Mifflin.

Josephson, B. D., and Ramachandran, V. S. (Eds.). (1980). *Consciousness and the physical world*. Oxford: Pergamon.

Kinsbourne, M., and Wood, F. (1975). Short-term memory processes and the amnesic syndrome. In D. Deutsch and J. A. Deutsch (Eds.), *Short-term memory*. New York: Academic Press.

Knapp, P. H. (1976). The mysterious "split": A clinical enquiry into problems of consciousness and brain. In G. G. Globus, G. Maxwell, and I. Savodnik (Eds.), *Consciousness and the brain*. New York: Plenum.

Kuhlenbeck, H. (1965). The concept of consciousness in neurological epistemology. In J. R. Smythies (Ed.), *Brain and mind*. London: Routledge & Kegan Paul.

Lachman, R., and Naus, M. (1984). The episodic/semantic continuum in an evolved machine. *Behavioral and Brain Sciences, 7*, 244–246.

Lidz, T. (1942). The amnestic syndrome. *Archives of Neurology and Psychiatry, 47*, 588–605.

Lockhart, R. S. (1984). What do infants remember? In M. Moscovitch (Ed.), *Infant memory*. New York: Plenum.

MacCurdy, J. T. (1928). *Common principles in psychology and physiology*. London: Cambridge University Press.

Mandler, G. (1975). Consciousness: Respectable, useful, and necessary. In R. L. Solso (Ed.), *Information processing and cognition*. Hillsdale, N.J.: Erlbaum.

Masson, M. E. J. (1984). Memory for the surface structure of sentences: Remembering with and without awareness. *Journal of Verbal Learning and Verbal Behavior, 23*.

Miller, G. A. (1980). Computation, consciousness, and cognition. *Behavioral and Brain Sciences, 3*, 146.

Moray, N. (1959). Attention in dichotic listening: Affective cues and the influence of instructions. *Quarterly Journal of Experimental Psychology, 11*, 56–60.

Moscovitch, M. (1982). Multiple dissociations of function in amnesia. In L. S. Cermak (Ed.), *Human memory and amnesia*. Hillsdale, N.J.: Erlbaum.

Natsoulas, T. (1978). Consciousness. *American Psychologist, 33*, 906–914.

Natsoulas, T. (1981). Basic problems of consciousness. *Journal of Personality and Social Psychology, 41*, 132–178.

Neisser, U. (1978). Anticipations, images, and introspection. *Cognition, 6*, 169–174.

Neisser, U. (1979). Review of *Divided Consciousness* by E. R. Hilgard. *Contemporary Psychology, 24*, 99–100.

Nelson, K., and Gruendel, J. (1981). Generalized event representations: Basic building blocks of cognitive development. In M. E. Lamb and A. L. Brown (Eds.), *Advances in developmental psychology*. Hillsdale, N.J.: Erlbaum.

Norman, D. A. (1969). Memory while shadowing. *Quarterly Journal of Experimental Psychology, 21*, 85–93.

Parkin, A. (1982). Residual learning capability in organic amnesia. *Cortex, 18*, 417–440.

Posner, M. I., and Klein, R. M. (1973). On the functions of consciousness. In S. Kornblum (Ed.), *Attention and performance IV*. New York: Academic Press.

Robinson, A. L. (1976). Metallurgy: Extraordinary alloys that remember their past. *Science, 191*, 934–936.

Roth, M. (1980). Consciousness and psychopathology. In B. D. Josephson and V. S. Ramachandran (Eds.), *Consciousness and the physical world*. Oxford: Pergamon.

Schacter, D. L. (1984). Priming of old and new knowledge in amnesic patients and normal subjects. *Annals of N. Y. Academy of Sciences.*

Schacter, D. L., Harbluk, J. L., and McLachlan, D. R. (1984). Retrieval without recollection: An experimental analysis of source amnesia. *Journal of Verbal Learning and Verbal Behavior, 23.*

Schacter, D. L., and Moscovitch, M. (1984). Infants, amnesics, and dissociable memory systems. In M. Moscovitch (Ed.), *Infant memory.* New York: Plenum Press.

Schacter, D. L., and Tulving, E. (1982). Memory, amnesia, and the episodic/semantic distinction. In R. L. Isaacson and N. E. Spear (Eds.), *Expression of knowledge.* New York: Plenum.

Shallice, T. (1972). Dual functions of consciousness. *Psychological Review, 79*, 383–393.

Shallice, T. (1978). The dominant action system: An information-processing approach to consciousness. In K. S. Pope and J. L. Singer (Eds.), *The stream of consciousness.* New York: Plenum.

Sperry, R. W. (1969). A modified concept of consciousness. *Psychological Review, 76*, 532–536.

Stout, G. F. (1896). *Analytic psychology* (Vols. 1 and 2). London: Swan Sonnenschein.

Talland, G. A. (1965). *Deranged memory.* New York: Academic Press.

Tulving, E. (1972). Episodic and semantic memory. In E. Tulving and W. Donaldson (Eds.), *Organization of memory.* New York: Academic Press.

Tulving, E. (1982). Synergistic ecphory in recall and recognition. *Canadian Journal of Psychology, 36*, 130–147.

Tulving, E. (1983). *Elements of episodic memory.* Oxford: Clarendon Press.

Tulving, E. (1984). Relations among components and processes of memory. *Behavioral and Brain Sciences, 7*, 257–268.

Tulving, E., Schacter, D. L., and Stark, H. A. (1982). Priming effects in word-fragment completion are independent of recognition memory. *Journal of Experimental Psychology: Learning, Memory and Cognition, 8*, 336–342.

Underwood, G. (1979). Memory systems and conscious processes. In G. Underwood and R. Stevens (Eds.), *Aspects of consciousness: Vol. 1. Psychological issues.* London: Academic Press.

Underwood, G. (Ed.). (1982). *Aspects of consciousness: Vol. 3. Awareness and self-awareness.* London: Academic Press.

Underwood, G., and Stevens, R. (Eds.). (1979). *Aspects of consciousness: Vol. 1. Psychological issues.* London: Academic Press.

Underwood, G., and Stevens, R. (Eds.). (1981). *Aspects of consciousness: Vol. 2. Structural issues.* London: Academic Press.

Weiskrantz, L. (1978). A comparison of hippocampal pathology in man and other animals. In *Functions of the septohippocampal system. CIBA Foundation Symposium.* Oxford: Elsevier.

Wickelgren, W. A. (1977). *Learning and memory.* Englewood Cliffs, N.J.: Prentice-Hall.

Winograd, T. (1975). Understanding natural language. In D. Bobrow and A. Collins (Eds.), *Representation and understanding.* New York: Academic Press.

37 Conscious Recollection and the Human Hippocampal Formation: Evidence from Positron Emission Tomography

Daniel L. Schacter, Nathaniel M. Alpert, Cary R. Savage, Scott L. Rauch, and Marilyn S. Albert

Understanding the role of the hippocampal formation in learning and memory constitutes an enduring problem in cognitive neuroscience. Studies of brain-damaged amnesic patients implicate the hippocampal formation in explicit or conscious memory for past events. By contrast, the hippocampal formation is thought to be uninvolved in a nonconscious or implicit form of memory known as priming (1–4). Yet previous attempts to test these ideas directly by studying the normal human brain with positron emission tomography (PET) have yielded inconclusive results.

In an early PET study by Squire et al. (5), subjects studied a list of familiar words (e.g., GARNISH) and were then tested with three-letter word stems (e.g., GAR__). When subjects were instructed to provide a word from the study list on a cued recall test (explicit memory), there were significant blood flow increases in the vicinity of the right hippocampal formation compared with a baseline condition in which subjects responded to stems of nonstudied words. In a separate scan conducted in the same experimental session, subjects were instructed to complete stems of previously studied words with the first word that comes to mind (implicit memory), and a priming effect was observed: subjects preferentially completed the stems with words from the study list. Compared with the baseline condition, priming was associated with decreased blood flow in extrastriate occipital cortex and increased blood flow in the right hippocampus/parahippocampal gyrus. Because amnesic patients with hippocampal damage show intact priming effects (6–8), the former finding is consistent with the idea that such effects are mediated by brain systems outside the hippocampal formation. But the latter finding is inconsistent with this idea.

However, performance in the priming condition may have been "contaminated" by some form of explicit memory (9): subjects may have intentionally or unintentionally remembered the primed words (5). If such contamination accounts for hippocampal activation in the priming condition, then it should be possible to abolish hippocampal activation by eliminating explicit retrieval. Yet several PET experiments have failed to find hippocampal activation even in association with explicit retrieval (10–13). Most critically, Buckner et al. (14) reported a follow-up of the Squire et al. experiment in which subjects were given three-letter word beginnings and attempted to remember words that had been studied previously either in the auditory modality or in a different typographic case. Buckner et al. observed no evidence of hippocampal activations in either condition (14). Because subjects were attempting to remember target items in both the different-modality and different-case conditions, the absence of blood flow changes in the hippocampal formation suggests that trying to retrieve a past event is not sufficient to activate the hippocampus. Hippocampal activation may be more closely related to some aspect of the actual recollection of an event. By contrast, Buckner et al. (14) found that areas in prefrontal cortex showed blood flow increases in both the different-case and different-modality conditions, thus raising the possibility that frontal activations, which have been observed frequently in PET studies of explicit retrieval (5, 10, 12–16), are related to the effort involved in trying to remember recently studied items (11).

To test these hypotheses, we performed a priming experiment in which we attempted to eliminate conscious recollection and an explicit memory experiment in which we attempted to separate out the effort to recall an event from the actual recollection of it.

Methods

Experimental Procedure

In the priming experiment, subjects studied target words in a way that ensured that they would later have poor explicit memory for them (6). Specifically, subjects performed a shallow, nonsemantic study task that requires them to indicate the number of T-junctions in a word. After the subjects had studied 24 familiar words (20 target plus 4 nontested buffers), PET scans were carried out while subjects responded to three-letter word stems, with separate blocks of stems for studied words (priming) and nonstudied words (baseline). During each 1-min. scan, subjects were instructed to respond with the first word that came to mind and to do their best to complete each stem. We refer to the nonscanned study task, the scanned priming condition, and the scanned baseline condition as a "study-test unit." The volunteers were then given two additional study-test units, thus yielding a total of three scans for primed words and three scans for baseline words. Order of conditions and items assigned to conditions was counterbalanced across subjects.

For the explicit memory experiment, one condition was designed to yield high levels of explicit recall and the other was designed to yield low levels of explicit recall. We accomplished this by manipulating how subjects studied a series of target words. Forty-eight different words (40 targets plus 8 buffers) were shown for 5 s each; no scanning was performed during this study phase. The High Recall condition consisted of 20 target words that were presented four times each, with presentations distributed randomly throughout the list; each time one of these words appeared, subjects made a semantic judgment (they counted the number of meanings associated with each word). We reasoned that on a later memory test, subjects would easily recollect many of these words. The Low Recall con-

dition consisted of 20 words that were presented only once; subjects made a nonsemantic judgment about each word (the T-junction counting task used in our first experiment). We reasoned that on a later test, subjects would recall few of these words despite trying hard to do so.

Two separate 90-s blocks of three-letter stems, separated by a 10-min. rest or study period, were presented on a computer monitor. One block contained stems that could be completed with the High Recall words and the other contained stems that could be completed with the Low Recall words; subjects were instructed to try to remember a study-list word that fit each stem. If they could not recall a study-list target, they were told to guess. Subjects were allowed up to 5 s to respond to each stem. Immediately after their response, the next stem appeared. After subjects completed the two test scans, two further study-test units were administered. Prior to the first study-test unit and after the third, subjects performed the baseline task used in the previous experiment, in which they completed stems of nonstudied words with the first word that came to mind. Order of conditions and items assigned to conditions was completely counterbalanced across subjects.

Subjects

Six healthy male and two healthy female volunteers (mean age = 19.6 yr) participated in the priming experiment; five healthy male and three healthy female volunteers (mean age = 20.5 yr) participated in the explicit memory experiment. All subjects were screened to rule out the presence of medical, psychiatric, or neurological disorders.

PET Scanning

A gantry held the computer monitor, tilted so that the screen was readily visible from within the PET camera. PET data were acquired while subjects inhaled oxygen-15-labeled carbon dioxide ($[^{15}O]CO_2$) for 1 min. Each scan proceeded as follows:

1. Subjects were reminded of the instructions to lie still, breathe normally, and to perform either the stem completion or cued recall task

2. The PET camera was started at time zero, and continued acquiring data for 90 s

3. The stem completion (or cued recall) task started at time zero, preceded by four buffer items, and continued until completion of the block of 24 trials (all subjects required >90 s to finish the stem completion or cued recall tasks)

4. The final 60 s of PET camera data acquisition (i.e., time 30–90 s) coincided with the 60-s period of active tracer inhalation

5. At the end of this period, PET data acquisition and radiolabeled gas flow were terminated

6. Following a 10-min. tracer-washout period, the next scan was performed, until the series of eight scans was completed.

The PET facilities and procedures were very similar to those previously described (e.g., refs. 17 and 18). A General Electric–Scanditronix (Uppsala) model PC4096 15-slice whole-body tomograph was used (19). An individually molded thermoplastic face mask (True Scan, Annapolis, MD) was used to minimize head motion. Transmission measurements were made by using an orbiting pin source.

All brain images were corrected for interscan movement, by realignment with respect to the first scan, prior to further image processing. An automated motion-correction algorithm was employed (after ref. 20). Motion-corrected PET brain images were then transformed to the standard Talairach coordinate system (21) as previously described (e.g., refs. 17 and 22). Blood flow images were normalized to 50 ml/min. per 100 g and were rescaled and smoothed with a 20-mm Gaussian filter.

Once the transformations of the PET data were performed and the data were expressed in stereotaxic space, statistical parametric maps (SPMs) were created. Each SPM was inspected for regions of activation with Z scores ≥ 3.00 for unplanned comparisons ($P < 0.001$, uncorrected for multiple comparisons), and >2.58 ($P < 0.005$) for planned comparisons involving hippocampal formation, prefrontal cortex, and extrastriate occipital cortex.

Results

Analysis of behavioral data from the priming experiment revealed that a significantly larger percentage of stems was completed with study-list words in the priming condition than in the baseline condition (30% vs. 17%; $F(1, 7) = 41.81$, $P < 0.0001$). The magnitude of priming is comparable to similar effects obtained in conditions where explicit memory has been effectively eliminated (23, 24), but it is much smaller than the priming effect reported in the PET study of Squire et al. (5), reflecting the explicit contamination that likely occurred in that experiment. Analysis of priming effects separately for each study-test unit revealed nearly identical levels of priming in the first, second, and third test blocks ($F < 1$), providing additional evidence that subjects did not engage in intentional retrieval strategies, which would have inflated priming in later test blocks.

To examine relevant changes in regional cerebral blood flow, data from the three study-test units were combined to yield a single baseline condition and a single priming condition. When we compared these two conditions, we found that priming was associated with significant blood flow decreases in bilateral extrastriate occipital cortex (Brodmann area 19; table 37.1/figure 37.1). The decrease on the right was in approximately the same location as in the previous study, whereas the decrease on the left had a more superior focus. By contrast, there were no significant blood flow changes in the vicinity of the hippocampal formation (maximum Z

Table 37.1

Primary regions of interest exhibiting significant change in blood flow associated with the priming and explicit memory conditions [all additional findings ($Z \geq 3.00$) listed in text]

Contrast	Region	Z score (max pixel value)*	Max pixel coordinates[†]
Priming contrasts			
Priming minus Baseline	Right area 19	−3.10	33, −74, 0
	Left area 19	−3.23	−33, −79, 24
Explicit memory contrasts			
Low Recall minus High Recall	Left prefrontal (area 10/46)	3.81	−31, 43, 8
	Left anterior cingulate	3.25	−7, 15, 32
	Right precuneus (area 19)	3.70	5, −72, 32
High Recall minus Low Recall	Right hippocampal	2.82	25, −34, 0
High Recall minus Baseline	Left hippocampal	3.38	−19, −39, −4
	Right hippocampal	3.96	15, −37, 0
Low Recall minus Baseline	Right orbitofrontal (area 11)	3.25	5, 35, −12
	Right anterior cingulate	3.77	7, 34, 0
	Left prefrontal (area 10)	3.47	−35, 54, 8
	Right prefrontal (area 10)	3.12	30, 46, 8
	Right prefrontal (area 9)	4.04	12, 47, 28

*Values represent the maximum pixel value (Z score units) within the region of interest from the statistical parametric map.

[†] Coordinates in Talairach space (21), expressed as x, y, z; $x > 0$ is right of the midsagittal plane, $y > 0$ is anterior to the anterior commissure, and $z > 0$ is superior to the anterior commissure–posterior commissure plane.

score $= 0.33$ for available points z axis $= -12$ to $+4$). In addition to the predicted blood flow changes in the extrastriate regions, we also observed other significant ($Z > 3.0$) decreases and increases in association with priming that will be discussed in a separate report. Baseline minus priming [decreases]: right insular cortex (39, −26, 0), right thalamus (7, −30, 4), right putamen (16, 2, 8), right motor/premotor cortex (61, −8, 28), and right parietal cortex (area 7; 30, −55, 52). Priming minus baseline [increases]: left prefrontal cortex (area 47; −39, 30, −8), left precuneus (area 7; −13, −51, 56). All findings are expressed in Talairach coordinates as x, y, z.

In the explicit memory experiment, behavioral data confirmed that subjects remembered many more words in the High Recall condition (79%)

than in the Low Recall condition (35%; $F(1, 7) = 205.74$, $P < 0.0001$). However, the percentage of words recalled did not differ significantly across the three test blocks ($F < 1$). To examine associated blood flow changes, we compared the High and Low Recall conditions directly to one another, collapsing across the three test blocks. The logic of the comparison holds that brain regions that are specifically associated with the conscious recollection of a word should show significant blood flow increases in the High Recall minus Low Recall comparison, whereas regions that are specifically associated with the effort involved in trying to retrieve a recently studied word should show significant blood flow increases in the Low Recall minus High Recall comparison. Consistent with our hypothesis that

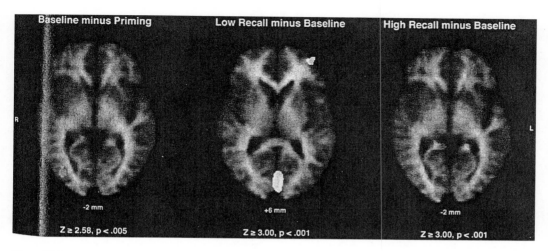

Figure 37.1
PET statistical maps show territories of activation superimposed over averaged magnetic resonance images, transformed to Talairach space. Activations are thresholded to a Z score ≥ 2.58 for the Baseline minus Priming image and 3.00 for the Low Recall minus Baseline and High Recall minus Baseline images. Images are transverse sections, with z coordinates reflecting distance in millimeters from the anterior commissure–posterior commissure plane. The Baseline minus Priming image shows a region of significantly decreased blood flow (green) associated with priming in right visual association cortex (area 19). The Low Recall minus Baseline image shows regions of significantly increased blood flow (yellow) associated with high effort and low explicit recall (35% accuracy) in the left prefrontal cortex (area 10) and secondary visual cortex (area 18). The High Recall minus Baseline image shows regions of significantly increased blood flow (red) associated with high levels of explicit recall (79% accuracy) in bilateral hippocampal regions.

prefrontal regions are related to retrieval effort, the Low Recall minus High Recall comparison revealed a significant blood flow increase in the left dorsolateral prefrontal cortex (Brodmann areas 10 and 46; table 37.1). Previous studies have implicated this region in generating words and semantic associations (25–28). It is likely that attempts to generate candidate word responses occurred more frequently in the Low Recall condition than in the High Recall condition. This comparison also revealed significant increases in the left anterior cingulate and the right precuneus, which have been implicated previously in attentional processes, such as target selection (29, 30), that should have been more relevant to the Low Recall than the High Recall condition.

Consistent with our hypothesis that the hippocampus is involved in some aspect of conscious recollection, the High Recall minus Low Recall comparison yielded only a single significant increase, in the right hippocampal formation (table 37.1). The locus of this activation is nearly identical to the locus of the activation reported in the same-case condition of the earlier stem-cued recall study (5, 14).

To examine further the consistency of our results, we compared the High Recall and Low Recall conditions, with the Baseline condition in which subjects completed stems of nonstudied words with the first word that came to mind (table 37.1/figure 37.1). The logic was similar to our reasoning in the previous comparisons: brain regions associated with conscious recollection should show significant blood increases in the High Recall minus Baseline comparison, whereas regions associated with retrieval effort should show increases in the Low Recall minus Baseline comparison. In the High Recall minus Baseline comparison, there were extensive bilateral blood flow increases in the hippocampal formation, but no significant activations in the vicinity of the frontal lobes. The Low Recall minus Baseline comparison yielded extensive bilateral blood flow increases in the prefrontal cortex, especially in Brodmann area 10, but none in the vicinity of the hippocampal formation. Prefrontal cortex, particularly on the right side, has been activated in numerous previous PET studies of explicit retrieval (5, 10–14, 16), and the increases that we observed are close to previously reported ones. These results, together with the finding of significant left frontal activation in the Low Recall minus High Recall comparison, imply that the pervasive activation of frontal regions in previous memory studies reflects the effort involved in attempting to retrieve a past event. Both the High Recall and Low Recall minus Baseline comparisons yielded a number of other significant ($Z > 3.0$) blood flow increases that will be discussed in a separate report. High Recall minus Baseline: left cerebellum (-26, -68, -12), right cuneus (area 17; 3, -71, 8), bilateral supramarginal gyrus (area 40; -47, -28, 20; 47, -22, 20), and right visual association cortex (area 19; 26, -82, 24). Low Recall minus Baseline: left brain stem (-10, -13, -12), left cerebellum (-24, -50, -12), left secondary visual cortex (area 18, -3, -76, 4), right supramarginal gyrus (area 40; 41, -3, 16), left insular cortex (-34, -16, 16), and right cuneus (area 18; 7, -82, 24). All findings are expressed in Talairach coordinates as x, y, z.

Discussion

Our major findings—that the hippocampal formation showed significant blood flow increases in the High Recall condition compared with the Low Recall and Baseline conditions, but no such increases during priming—provide new information about the role of the hippocampal formation in implicit and explicit memory. We first consider several puzzles that are clarified by our findings, and then we consider issues that remain to be clarified.

In view of our results, it now seems likely that previous findings of hippocampal activation during priming on the stem completion test were due to the influence of conscious recollection (5). Because frontal regions were not active during priming in the experiment of Squire et al., this "contamination" from explicit memory probably reflects incidental or unintentional conscious recollection of words studied twice, under semantic encoding conditions, several minutes prior to the priming task. Our data support the idea that priming occurs independently of the hippocampal formation and depends instead on brain systems involved with the perceptual representation of words and objects (1–4).

Our data also help to clarify why the previous experiment by Buckner et al. (14) using the stem-cued recall test failed to detect significant blood flow increases in the vicinity of the hippocampus during explicit retrieval in both a different-case condition and a different modality condition. Our results suggest that hippocampal activation is more closely associated with the actual recollection of a past event than with the effort involved in attempting to remember the event. Simply instructing subjects to try to remember an event is probably not sufficient to produce significant blood flow increases in the hippocampal formation. These observations suggest that in the different-case and different-modality conditions of the experiments of Buckner et al., the way in which subjects recollected studied items differed from the manner in which they recollected them in the same-case condition. Note that the absolute levels of recall in the different-case condition (73%) and different-modality condition (62%) of Buckner et al.

are closer to the levels of performance in our High Recall condition (79%) than in our Low Recall condition (35%). Although we must be cautious about between-experiment comparisons, these results suggest that the absolute level of recall may be less important in determining whether hippocampal activation is observed than the qualitative manner in which target events are remembered. Further research will be needed to specify exactly which features of recollection are most relevant to hippocampal activation.

This account is also consistent with the results of a study in which subjects studied and later tried to recognize structurally possible and structurally impossible novel visual objects (15). Right hippocampal activation was observed in association with explicit recognition of possible objects, but there was no corresponding activation in association with recognition of impossible objects. The possible objects were remembered more accurately than were the impossible objects. Our results thus suggest that differences in either the level or type of recollection associated with possible and impossible objects, respectively, account for the differential activation of the right hippocampal region during explicit recognition of the two types of objects.

Our hypotheses regarding conscious recollection and the hippocampus do not explain all relevant findings, however. We note first that factors other than conscious recollection, such as the novelty of a stimulus, can produce hippocampal activation (15, 31). The response of the hippocampal formation to a novel stimulus may be associated with its role in encoding and consolidation of new memories, whereas activations related to conscious recollection indicate a role for the hippocampus in memory retrieval.

However, in several studies that are quite similar to ours, where subjects presumably consciously recollected recently studied verbal materials, no hippocampal activations were observed (10–13). We make several observations. First, our study-test unit design used three separate replications for each subject of all critical comparisons to maximize power to detect hippocampal and other activations. Several of the experiments that failed to detect any evidence of hippocampal activation used only a single replication of critical comparisons (10–12), perhaps resulting in insufficient power to detect blood flow increases associated with hippocampal activity. Second, because the exact features of conscious recollection that are most relevant to hippocampal activation remain to be determined, it is possible that aspects of recollection that are most relevant to hippocampal activation played a more prominent role in our paradigm than in others. For instance, in one experiment that failed to observe hippocampal activation, some nonstudied items were presented with studied items during a single scan, possibly diluting the overall level of recollection (10). Other experiments used auditory presentation and test (12, 13, 16). Given the previously observed absence of hippocampal activation when modality and typographic case of stimuli differed at study and test (14), it is possible that reinstating visual information about a studied item, plus a high level of remembering, both contribute to blood flow increases in the hippocampal formation during explicit retrieval (see refs. 32 and 33 for data concerning visual information and recollective experience). Also, several experiments that failed to detect hippocampal activation used recognition tests (10, 11, 13, 16), whereas we used recall. Although the hippocampus was activated during recognition of novel visual objects in a study noted earlier (15), conscious recollection during recall and recognition may differ, such that it is more difficult to detect hippocampal blood flow increases in association with recognition than with recall. Additional studies will be needed to determine which of these factors, if any, are relevant to hippocampal activations in PET studies.

In contrast to inconsistent activation of the hippocampal formation in PET experiments, lesion studies with experimental animals and studies of human amnesic patients with hippocampal damage indicate a broader role for the hippocampus in explicit memory (for reviews, see refs. 3 and 34), which may reflect in part the hippocampal contribution to encoding and consolidation of memories alluded to earlier. By contrast, our results and the other PET evidence described in the preceding paragraph all bear on the role of the hippocampus in memory retrieval. The hippocampal formation may play a more limited role in retrieval than it does in encoding and consolidation. Alternatively, limitations on PET measurement techniques may account for some previous failures to detect hippocampal activity. While the exact role of the hippocampal formation in human memory retrieval remains to be specified, our study indicates that further exploration of specific aspects of conscious recollection is likely to be revealing.

Finally, our results also bear on the role of prefrontal cortex in explicit retrieval. Consistent with other recent PET data, they suggest that frontal regions play an important role in the retrieval effort associated with attempts to recall past events (11). The right anterior prefrontal cortex (area 10) in particular has been especially active during explicit retrieval (16). We observed activation of this area in the Low Recall minus Baseline comparison, but not in the Low Recall minus High Recall comparison, whereas left prefrontal cortex was active in both comparisons. One interpretation of this pattern is that right area 10 is especially relevant to shifting from semantic or lexical retrieval, which was required when subjects completed stems with the first word that came to mind in the baseline condition, to explicit or episodic retrieval, which was required when subjects tried to recall study list words. If so, it is curious that we did not see right frontal activity in the High Recall minus Baseline comparison, since the former involves episodic retrieval and the latter does not. This may be because words that have been studied four times in a semantic encoding condition, as in our High Recall condition, came to mind with little retrieval effort during the cued-recall test.

An important problem for future research is to specify the conditions under which both right and left prefrontal regions play a greater or lesser role in efforts to retrieve recently experienced episodes.

Acknowledgments

We thank Kimberly Nelson for help with preparation of the manuscript and Brian Rafferty for experimental assistance. This research was supported by grants from the Charles A. Dana Foundation, Grant RO1 AG08441-06 from the National Institute on Aging, Grant T32 CA09362 from the National Cancer Institute, and Grants MH01215 and MH01230 from the National Institute of Mental Health.

References

1. Moscovitch, M. (1994) in *Memory Systems 1994*, eds. Schacter, D. L. and Tulving, E. (MIT Press, Cambridge, MA), pp. 269–310.

2. Schacter, D. L. (1994) in *Memory Systems 1994*, eds. Schacter, D. L. and Tulving, E. (MIT Press, Cambridge, MA), pp. 233–268.

3. Squire, L. R. (1992) *Psychol. Rev.* 99, 195–231.

4. Tulving, E. and Schacter, D. L. (1990) *Science* 247, 301–306.

5. Squire, L. R., Ojemann, J. G., Miezin, F. M., Petersen, S. E., Videen, T. O. and Raichle, M. E. (1992) *Proc. Natl. Acad. Sci. USA* 89, 1837–1841.

6. Graf, P., Squire, L. R. and Mandler, G. (1984) *J. Exp. Psychol. Learn. Mem. Cognit.* 10, 164–178.

7. Schacter, D. L. (1987) *J. Exp. Psychol. Learn. Mem. Cognit.* 13, 501–518.

8. Shimamura, A. P. (1986) *Q. J. Exp. Psychol.* 38A, 619–644.

9. Schacter, D. L., Bowers, J. and Booker, J. (1989) in *Implicit Memory: Theoretical Issues*, eds. Lewandowsky, S., Dunn, J. C. and Kirsner, K. (Erlbaum, Hillsdale, NJ), pp. 47–69.

10. Andreasen, N. C., O'Leary, D. S., Arndt, S., Cizadio, T., Hurtig, R., Rezai, K., Watkins, G. L.,

Boles, Ponto, L. L. and Hichwa, R. D. (1995) *Proc. Natl. Acad. Sci. USA* 92, 5111–5115.

11. Kapur, S., Craik, F. I. M., Jones, C., Brown, G. M., Houle, S. and Tulving, E. (1995) *NeuroReport* 6, 1880–1884.

12. Shallice, T., Fletcher, P., Frith, C. D., Grasby, P., Frackowiak, R. S. J. and Dolan, R. J. (1994) *Nature (London)* 368, 633–635.

13. Tulving, E., Kapur, S., Markowitsch, H. J., Craik, F. I. M., Habib, R. and Houle, S. (1994) *Proc. Natl. Acad. Sci. USA* 91, 2012–2015.

14. Buckner, R. L., Petersen, S. E., Ojemann, J. G., Miezin, F. M., Squire, L. R. and Raichle, M. E. (1995) *J. Neurosci.* 15, 12–29.

15. Schacter, D. L., Reiman, E., Uecker, A., Polster, M. R., Yun, L. S. and Cooper, L. A. (1995) *Nature (London)* 29, 587–590.

16. Tulving, E., Kapur, S., Craik, F. I. M., Moscovitch, M. and Houle, S. (1994) *Proc. Natl. Acad. Sci. USA* 91, 2016–2020.

17. Rauch, S. L., Savage, C. R., Alpert, N. M., Miguel, E. C., Baer, L., Breiter, H. C., Fischman, A. J., Manzo, P. A., Moretti, C. and Jenike, M. A. (1995) *Arch. Gen. Psychiatry* 52, 20–28.

18. Kosslyn, S. M., Alpert, N. M., Thompson, W. L., Chabris, C. F., Rauch, S. L. and Anderson, A. K. (1994) *J. Cognit. Neurosci.* 5, 263–287.

19. Kops, E. R., Herzog, H., Schmid, A., Holte, S. and Feinendegen, L. E. (1990) *J. Comput. Assist. Tomogr.* 14, 437–445.

20. Woods, R. P., Cherry, S. and Mazziotta, J. (1992) *J. Comput. Assist. Tomogr.* 16, 620–633.

21. Talairach, J. and Tournoux, P. (1988) *Co-Planar Stereotaxis Atlas of the Human Brain* (Thieme, New York).

22. Alpert, N. M., Belrdichevsky, D., Weise, S., Tang, J. and Rauch, S. L. (1993) *Quantification of Brain Function: Tracer Kinetics and Image Analysis in Brain PET* (Elsevier, Amsterdam), pp. 459–463.

23. Graf, P., Mandler, G. and Haden, P. (1982) *Science* 218, 1243–1244.

24. Bowers, J. S. and Schacter, D. L. (1990) *J. Exp. Psychol. Learn. Mem. Cognit.* 16, 404–416.

25. Petersen, S. E., Fox, P. T., Posner, M. I., Mintum, M. and Raichle, M. E. (1988) *Nature (London)* 331, 585–589.

26. Frith, C. D., Friston, K., Liddle, P. F. and Frackowiack, R. S. J. (1991) *Neuropsychologia* 29, 1137–1148.

27. Kapur, S., Craik, F. I. M., Tulving, E., Wilson, A. A., Houle, S. and Brown, G. M. (1994) *Proc. Natl. Acad. Sci. USA* 91, 2008–2011.

28. Raichle, M. E., Fiez, J. A., Videen, T. O., MacLeod, A. M., Pardo, J. V., Fox, P. T. and Petersen, S. E. (1994) *Cereb. Cortex* 4, 8–26.

29. Frith, C. D., Friston, K., Liddle, P. F. and Frackowiak, R. S. J. (1991) *Proc. R. Soc. London B* 244, 241–246.

30. Posner, M. I. and Dehaene, S. (1994) *Trends Neurosci.* 17, 75–79.

31. Tulving, E., Markowitsch, H. J., Kapur, S., Habib, R. and Houle, S. (1994) *NeuroReport* 5, 2525–2528.

32. Brewer, W. F. (1988) in *Remembering Reconsidered: Ecoloical and Traditional Approaches to the Study of Memory*, eds. Neisser, U. and Winograd, E. (Cambridge Univ. Press, New York), pp. 21–90.

33. Dewhurst, S. A. and Conway, M. A. (1994) *J. Exp. Psychol. Learn. Mem. Cognit.* 20, 1088–1098.

34. Milner, B. (1972) *Clin. Neurosurg.* 19, 421–466.

38 Implicit Learning and Tacit Knowledge

Arthur S. Reber

Some two decades ago the term *implicit learning* was first used to characterize how one develops intuitive knowledge about the underlying structure of a complex stimulus environment (Reber 1965, 1967). In those early writings, I argued that implicit learning is characterized by two critical features: (a) it is an unconscious process, and (b) it yields abstract knowledge. Implicit knowledge results from the induction of an abstract representation of the structure that the stimulus environment displays, and this knowledge is acquired in the absence of conscious, reflective strategies to learn. Since then, the evidence in support of this theory has been abundant, and many of the details of the process have been sharpened. This article is an overview of this evidence and an attempt to extend the general concepts to provide some insight into a variety of related processes such as arriving at intuitive judgments, complex decision making, and, in a broad sense, learning about the complex covariations among events that characterize the environment.

Put simply, this is an article about learning. It seems curious, given the pattern of psychological investigation of the middle decades of this century, that the topic of learning should be so poorly represented in the contemporary literature in cognitive psychology. The energies of cognitive scientists have been invested largely in the analysis and modeling of existing knowledge rather than in investigations of how it was acquired. For example, in an important recent article on the general topic of unconscious memorial systems, Schacter (1987) never came to grips with the distinction between implicit learning and implicit memory. The latter, the focus of his review, was dealt with historically, characterized, outlined, and analyzed, but virtually no attention was paid to the processes by which these implicit memories "got there." This general lack of attention to the acquisition problem may

be one of the reasons why much recent theorizing has been oriented toward a nativist position (e.g., Chomsky 1980; Fodor 1975, 1983; Gleitman and Wanner 1982). Failure to explicate how complex knowledge is acquired invites the supposition that "it was there all the time."

What follows is an exploration of implicit learning from the point of view that the processes discussed are general and universal. Implicit acquisition of complex knowledge is taken as a foundation process for the development of abstract, tacit knowledge of all kinds. The stepping-off place is the presumption that there is, at this juncture, no reason to place any priority on particular biological determinants of a specific kind. All forms of implicit knowledge are taken as essentially similar at their deepest levels. This position needs to be pushed as far as it can go; it has considerably more explanatory power than has been generally recognized.

Experimental Procedures

Research on implicit learning is properly carried out with arbitrary stimulus domains with complex, idiosyncratic structures. In order to obtain insight into a process such as implicit learning, it is essential to work with novel, synthetic systems and to focus on the capacity of one's subjects to induce knowledge of a deep sort from such stimulus fields. Over the years, a number of different techniques have been used. My colleagues and I have chosen, in our laboratory, to work with two procedures that we have found to be extremely useful: artificial grammar learning and probability learning. The former is well known in the literature and has been used by many; the latter is somewhat obscure but, as will become clear, is an extremely sensitive technique that has provided some intriguing data. It is useful to provide a short overview of each here and to outline the general procedures for its use. Various other techniques that have found their way into the laboratory, such as the various procedures developed by such workers as Lewicki (see 1986a) and Broadbent (see Broadbent, Fitz-Gerald, and Broadbent 1986), are introduced later.

Grammar Learning

Figure 38.1 shows one of the first synthetic grammars used along with the basic types of "sentences" that it can generate. This grammar was first used by Reber (1965, 1967). It is a Markovian system derived from a simpler system that formed the basis of George Miller's *Project Grammarama* (see Miller 1967) and has subsequently been used to generate the stimuli for a number of other studies (Howard and Ballas 1980, Millward 1981, Reber and Lewis 1977, Roter 1985). It can be taken as representative of the grammars used in a variety of other experiments.

Although there have been many variations on a theme here, the basic procedure used in

these grammar learning studies is to have an acquisition phase, during which subjects acquire knowledge of the rules of the grammar, and a testing phase, during which some assessment is made of what they have learned. Additional details are supplied as follows when needed.

Several points, however, need to be kept clear about these synthetic languages and how they have been used to examine implicit, unconscious cognitive processes. First, they are complex systems, too complex to be learned in an afternoon in the laboratory, as Miller (1967) noted. Miller saw this as a liability, which it is if one wishes to examine explicit concept learning. This complexity, however, should be regarded as a virtue in the current context, for a rich and complex stimulus domain is a prerequisite for the occurrence of implicit learning. If the system in use is too simple, or if the code can be broken by conscious effort, then one will not see implicit processes. Second, the grammars given here are finite-state systems that generate strings of symbols in a left-to-right, nonhierarchical fashion. This fact should not be taken as reflecting any prejudices about the structural underpinnings of natural languages or their acquisition. We elected to use finite-state grammars for several reasons independent of theoretical issues in linguistics or natural language learning: They are mathematically tractable; they have an intrinsic probabilistic structure that is well known; they can generate a relatively large number of strings to use as stimuli; and, as mentioned, they are sufficiently complex so that the underlying formal structure is not within the conscious memorial domain of the typical subject upon the subject's entering the laboratory. Finally, as will become clear, there is nothing special about these stimulus generators in any interesting psychological sense. The basic components of implicit learning emerge in a wide variety of different empirical settings with a range of different stimulus environments.

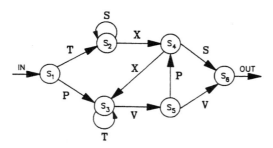

Figure 38.1
Schematic diagram of a finite-state grammar. (Stimuli are generated by following any path of arrows leading from the initial State 1 to the terminal State 6. The following are the five basic strings of the grammar with the loops or recursions in brackets: 1. T[S]XS; 2. T[S]XX[[T]VPX]VV; 3. T[S]XX[[T]VPX]VPS; 4. P[[T]VPX]VV; 5. P[[T]VPX]VPS.)

Probability Learning (PL)

The format that we adopted departs noticeably from the traditional two-choice procedure in which each trial consists of a "ready" signal, a prediction response, and an outcome event. The procedure used to explore implicit processes derives from the proposition that the essential nature of a PL experiment has little to do with the explicit learning of probabilities of events. Rather, what passes in the literature for probability learning is actually a much more subtle process in which subjects learn implicitly about the stochastic structure of an event sequence to which they have been exposed. In the course of making predictions, they mimic its structure and thereby generate a sequence of responses, one by-product of which is an approximate matching of the probabilities of the events—that is, *probability learning*.

Accordingly, the PL procedure was modified as follows (Reber 1966, Reber and Millward 1968). The subject begins an experimental session simply by observing the occurrence of a sequence of rapidly presented events. There is no ready signal, and the subject makes no prediction responses. In this situation, a passively observed event is functionally equivalent to a traditional trial, and a learning session consisting of 2 or 3 min. of observing events at a rate of two per second is sufficient to put a subject at an asymptotic rate of responding; that is, subsequent prediction responses made by subjects who have had this learning experience show all of the characteristics of ordinary subjects who have had an equivalent number of traditional trials. We dubbed this procedure the *instant asymptote* technique.

The typical experiment with this modified PL procedure consists of an acquisition phase, during which subjects observe event sequences that may have any of a variety of stochastic structures, and a testing phase, during which subjects make prediction responses. As with the grammar learning studies, there are many variations on this basic theme; they are introduced later as needed.

Despite the many superficial differences between the probability learning paradigm and the grammar learning experiment, there are two essential commonalities. First, in both cases the subject is confronted with a stimulus environment about which knowledge must be acquired in order to respond effectively during the testing session. Second, neither of the structural systems being used is part of or even remotely similar to the epistemic contents of the typical subject's long-term memory. These points are fundamental; the whole purpose of examining implicit learning in the laboratory is to develop understanding of how rich and complex knowledge is initially obtained independently of overt, conscious strategies for its acquisition. This process is ubiquitous in human experience and yet, as a focus of psychological inquiry, it is largely ignored.

What follows is a brief review of our work with these two procedures presented in the form of basic issues that the literature addresses. These issues are integrated with the growing body of literature on unconscious, nonreflective, implicit processes and, finally, summed up in a systematic attempt to see how such cognitive systems could evolve and how they fit into contemporary struggles with a number of classic problems in pure and applied psychology.

The work in our laboratory that is the focus of this overview (beginning with the very first studies by Reber 1965, 1966) was carried out with a particular research strategy: to use a limited number of techniques to examine a wide variety of effects. The virtue of this approach is that by developing a few techniques and building a robust data base, one can explore a large number of issues and not be terribly concerned about the vagaries that get introduced with alternative procedures. Given that the problems of implicit learning and tacit knowledge can be explored through these two procedures, this heuristic says that they should be used in as many circumstances as makes scientific sense. Biological fans of *E. coli* will recognize this strategy.

There is, of course, an alternative strategy: to examine these nonconscious cognitive and perceptual processes in as wide a variety of experimental environments as possible. The virtue of this strategy is that one is not likely to be seduced by idiosyncratic properties of particular procedures; generalizations come easier. If implicit learning is real, it should emerge in contexts conceptually remote from synthetic grammars and structured event sequences. Ideally, both strategies should be carried out. As will become clear, those whose research programs have taken the latter tack, such as Lewicki (1985, 1986a,b; Lewicki, Czyzewska, and Hoffman 1987), have typically produced data that are congruent and complementary.

Empirical Studies of Implicit Learning

On the Exploitation of Structure

When a stimulus environment is structured, people learn to exploit that structure in the sense that they come to use it in order to behave in a relevant fashion in its presence. This proposition seems noncontroversial as a generalization about human cognition; in fact it lies at the core of several approaches to perception (Gibson 1966, 1979; Mace 1974), decision making, and information processing (Garner 1974, Hasher and Zacks 1984) and can be seen as underlying, in a broad sense, any of a number of general theoretical analyses such as Anderson's (1983) production systems, Nelson's (1986) and Schlesinger's (1982) models of natural language acquisition, Fried and Holyoak's (1984) model of category induction, Lewicki's (1986a) analysis of socialization, and, interestingly, Holland, Holyoak, Nisbett, and Thagard's (1986) model of induction and Rumelhart and McClelland's (1986) connectionist systems. The latter two are of spe-

cial importance because each can be seen as advances in the cognitive sciences' hopefully awakened interest in knowledge acquisition.

In an early study on this general problem (Reber 1967), subjects were shown to become interestingly sensitive to the constraints of a synthetic grammar simply from exposure to exemplary strings. In that experiment, subjects were not informed that they were working with rule-governed stimuli. They were merely requested to memorize strings of letters in what was touted as a rote memory experiment. With practice they became increasingly adept at processing and memorizing strings, whereas a control group working with nonordered letter strings showed no such improvement. Furthermore, after this neutral learning task, subjects were able to use what they had apprehended of the rules of the grammar to discriminate between new letter strings that conformed to the grammatical constraints and letter strings that violated one or more of the rules of the grammar. In simplest terms, these subjects can be said to have been exploiting the structure inherent in the stimulus display. This basic finding is a robust one and has been reported by numerous authors (e.g., Brooks 1978; Dulany, Carlson, and Dewey 1984; Howard and Ballas 1980; Mathews et al. 1989; Millward 1981; Morgan and Newport 1981).

Similar observations concerning the exploitation of structure have been made in somewhat different contexts by other researchers. Broadbent and his coworkers showed that knowledge of complex rule systems governing simulated economic/production systems is also acquired and used in an implicit fashion (Berry and Broadbent 1984, Broadbent and Aston 1978, Broadbent et al. 1986). In those studies, subjects were presented with an imaginary manufacturing situation such as a sugar production plant and instructed simply to maneuver variables such as wages, labor peace, worker output, and the like to yield a particular overall production standard. The systems, in fact, operate according to sophisticated, complex rule systems that relate these factors to each other. Achieving the required production standards requires that the rules be "known," in some sense of that word. Broadbent and his colleagues consistently reported that subjects induced the rule systems implicitly and made appropriate adjustments in the relevant variables and did so in the absence of conscious knowledge of the rules themselves. The pattern of these findings strongly parallels those in the synthetic grammar learning studies.

Several of the PL studies have also yielded analogues of this process. Reber and Millward (1971) found evidence that subjects can accurately anticipate the changing probabilities of events even when the anticipatory response requires an integration of information across 50 preceding events. In this particular case, the probability of each individual event on any trial n was systematically increased and decreased as n moved through a period of 50 trials. Subjects were first given 1,000 instant asymptote trials with this sawtooth event sequence and then requested to predict successive events. Under these conditions, rather than shadowing the changing event probabilities, subjects ultimately learned to anticipate the shifts in the likelihood of events so that their predictions of events rose and fell coincidentally with the actual event sequences. They had learned the underlying structure of the stimulus environment and were capable of exploiting it to direct their choices.

Millward and Reber (1972), using event sequences with short- and long-range contingencies between events, reported an even more impressive ability of subjects to exploit stochastic structures. Subjects were exposed to sequences that contained event-to-event dependencies such that the actual event that appeared on any trial n was stochastically dependent on the event that had occurred on some previous trial $n - j$, where $j = 1, 3, 5,$ or 7. Training consisted of several hundred trials of the instant asymptote procedure with the particular stochastic dependency for that session. During the first session, $j = 1$; during the second, $j = 3$; and so forth.

During testing, subjects displayed a clear sensitivity to these dependencies, a sensitivity that reflected an ability to exploit structure that required knowledge of event dependencies as remote as seven trials. What makes this finding interesting is that this capacity appears to be beyond what were found in earlier work (Millward and Reber 1968, Reber and Millward 1965) to be limits on explicit recall. In those experiments, subjects were asked to recall which event had occurred on a specified previous trial. Beyond five trials, they were virtually reduced to guessing.

Parallel findings were recently reported by Lewicki and his coworkers (Lewicki et al. 1987; Lewicki, Hill, and Bizot 1988), who, using reaction time measures, showed that subjects implicitly knew the future location of a stimulus event even though, when they were asked to report explicitly where the event would occur, their performances were no better than chance. Lewicki and his colleagues used a complex rule that specified which of four quadrants of a field would contain a target number. The actual location was based on the pattern of quadrants in which the number had appeared on particular earlier trials. The situation, like the PL studies, was based on an arbitrary relationship between events. With extended practice, subjects showed dramatic decreases in reaction time to respond to the location of the target number. The improvement was clearly due to tacit knowledge of the stochastic relationship and not simply to increased facility with the task. Changing the rules produced an abrupt increase in reaction time, but when, in a postexperimental debriefing session, subjects were given an opportunity to consciously predict the critical quadrants, their performances were no better than chance. An intriguing element in these studies was that all of Lewicki et al.'s (1988) subjects were faculty members in a department of psychology, and all knew that the research they were involved in was oriented toward the study of nonconscious cognitive processes.

Clearly, subjects learn to use the structural relationships inherent in these various complex stimulus domains. No real surprises here. In many ways these various studies function basically as complicated existence demonstrations; they show that it is possible to obtain this kind of unconscious, nonreflective, implicit learning in a controlled laboratory setting, that it can occur in a relatively short time span, and that it can be seen to emerge when the stimulus is a structured domain whose content is arbitrary and distinctly remote from typical day-to-day experiences with the real world.

On Implicit Versus Explicit Processes

The experiments reviewed were all run under instructional sets in which subjects were unaware that the stimuli were structured or rule defined. In these cases, the point was to maximize the emergence of implicit learning.

It is important to be clear about this issue and the kinds of manipulations that have been used. It is universally accepted that the college undergraduate whose cognitive processes form (for better or worse) the foundations of our science is an active and consciously probing organism, especially in regard to things with structure and patterns. The aforementioned researchers carried out their experiments by carefully circumventing this pattern-searching tendency. In Reber and Millward's PL studies and in Lewicki's target location experiments, they accomplished this by "blitzing" the subjects with information at rates beyond those at which conscious codebreaking strategies could operate. The grammar learning studies and Broadbent's production system experiments were successful because the structure of the stimuli was highly complex and the instructions to the subjects were calculated to be vague. An obvious question is, What effect would explicit instructions have? What happens when subjects are informed, at the outset, that the materials that they will be working with reflect regularities and patterns?

The first manipulation of the factor of explicitness used the PL technique (Reber 1966, Reber and Millward 1968). The procedure consisted simply of telling some of the subjects exactly what was going on in the experiment. Specifically, by informing one group of subjects of the relative probabilities of the two events, the researchers gave them concrete instructions about the frequency characteristics of the event sequence that they would be asked to predict. These subjects were then run in a standard PL procedure and compared with a control group run with the same event sequences but without the explicit information.

The information about the event frequencies had virtually no effect on behavior. The two groups were statistically indistinguishable from each other, even on the first block of 25 prediction trials in which the impact of the instructions would have been most likely to be felt. Clearly, probability learning is more than the learning of probabilities. Rather, what really goes on is the apprehension of deep information about the structure of the sequence of events.

Postexperimental debriefings were revealing. Subjects were quite clear about knowing which light would be the dominant one, and all said that they believed the instructions. But, in virtually every case, they claimed that somehow the specific information lacked meaning that they felt they could use. It took real experience with the event sequence to acquire a knowledge base that was usable for directing choices on individual trials. This experiment used Bernoulli sequences; there was no "structure" in the usual sense of the word. Nevertheless, subjects reported achieving a sense of the nature of the event sequence from experience with events that they did not derive from the explicit instructions. Of importance is that this occurred despite the fact that, in principle, there is nothing to be extracted from the event sequence other than the relative frequencies of the two events.

Several studies using the grammar learning procedure have also explored the boundary between implicit and explicit knowledge. In the first experiment, Reber (1976) used the simple device of encouraging one group of subjects to search for the structure in the stimuli while a comparable group was run under a neutral instructional set. Both groups were given the same learning phase, during which they had to memorize exemplars from a synthetic grammar, and an identical testing phase, during which they were asked to assess the well-formedness of novel letter strings. *Well-formedness* is defined by whether the grammar could generate the string. Informed subjects were told only about the existence of structure; nothing was said about the nature of that structure.

The explicitly instructed subjects in this study performed more poorly in all aspects of the experiment than did those given the neutral instructions. They took longer to memorize the exemplars, they were poorer at determining well-formedness of test strings, and they showed evidence of having induced rules that were not representative of the grammar in use. The suggestion is that at least under these circumstances, implicit processing of complex materials has an advantage over explicit processing.

However, as gradually became clear, what this study actually showed is that explicit processing of complex materials has a decided disadvantage in relation to implicit processing. This is no mere play on words. The implicit/explicit distinction is rather more complex than it first appeared. Analysis of the fine grain of the data from Reber's (1976) article revealed that the explicit instructions seemed to be having a particular kind of interference effect. Specifically, subjects were being encouraged to search for rules that, given the nature of finite-state grammars with their path-independent, Markovian properties and given the kinds of attack strategies that the typical undergraduate possesses, they were not likely to find. Moreover, they tended to make improper inductions that led them to hold rules about the stimuli that were, in fact, wrong. The simplest conclusion seems to be

the right one: Looking for rules will not work if you cannot find them.

In a number of other studies, instructions of various kinds have been shown to have any of a number of effects. Brooks (1978) used finite-state grammars similar to the one used by Reber (1976) and a paired-associates learning procedure in which strings of letters from grammars were paired with responses of particular kinds (e.g., animal names, cities). He found that informing subjects about the existence of regularities in the letter strings lowered overall performance. Reber, Kassin, Lewis, and Cantor (1980) found poorer performance with explicit instructions when the stimuli were presented in a large, simultaneous array in which letter strings were posted on a board in haphazard fashion. Howard and Ballas (1980) reported detrimental effects of explicit instructions with structured sequences of auditory stimuli when there was no systematically interpretable pattern expressed by the stimulus sequences. In all these cases, the original finding was basically replicated.

However, Millward (1981) found no difference between explicitly and implicitly instructed subjects in an experiment that, in principle, looked like a replication of Reber's (1976) with the seemingly modest variation that the strings used during learning were up to 11 letters long, whereas in Reber's study stimuli were no longer than 8 letters. Abrams (1987), using a strict replication of Reber's procedure with the exception that the study was run on a computer, failed to find the instructional effect. Dulany et al. (1984) reported no significant differences between the two instructional sets, although in this case a rather different testing procedure may have masked differences. Mathews et al. (1989) found a complex pattern of differences between instructional groups, depending on whether the letter set used to instantiate the grammar was modified over the several days of the experiment. They also used a grammar somewhat more complex than is typical. Danks and Gans (1975) reported no differences when they used a synthetic system that was considerably simpler than the Markovian systems used by others.

Last, several studies showed an advantage for the explicitly instructed subjects. Howard and Ballas (1980) reported that the explicit instructions that debilitated performance when introduced under conditions of semantic uninterpretability could also function to facilitate performance when the stimuli expressed semantically interpretable patterns. Reber et al. (1980) showed that it was possible to shift performance about rather dramatically by intermixing instructional set with the manner of presentation of the stimulus materials and with the time during learning when the explicit instructions were introduced.

There are two factors here that help make these data somewhat less haphazard than they appear to be. The first is psychological salience; the second is the circumstances under which the instructions are given to the subjects. The first of these is the more interesting and the one from which insight into process can be gained.

In two of the instances in which explicit instructions facilitated performance, the manner of presentation of the stimuli was such that the underlying factors that represent the grammar were rendered salient. In Howard and Ballas's (1980) study, the semantic component focused the subjects on the relevant aspects of the patterned stimuli. The effectiveness of such a semantic component has often been noted in artificial grammar learning studies (Moeser and Bregman 1972, Morgan and Newport 1981). In Reber et al.'s (1980) study, the simple expedient of arranging the exemplars of the grammar according to their underlying form produced the instructional facilitation. Moreover, several other researchers apparently arranged matters, inadvertently, so that structural properties became more salient. In Millward's (1981) study, for example, the use of longer strings provided many opportunities for subjects to be exposed to the loops or recursions in the grammar (see fig-

ure 38.1) and thereby increased the psychological salience of the underlying structure. In Danks and Gans's (1975) study, the relatively simple nature of the stimuli likely acted to equate the mode of processing of the stimuli in both groups; that is, both groups were likely using a reasonably explicit mode independently of the instructions. Hence the converse of the earlier conclusion: Looking for rules will work if you can find them.

Some cases appear to be genuine failures to replicate the original finding: specifically, those of Dulany et al. (1984) and Abrams (1987). In Dulany et al.'s study, the procedure used during learning should, in principle, have yielded a difference during testing. These are some interesting aspects of this experiment, but there are no obvious reasons why the effect failed to emerge. On the surface, Abrams's study, which was carried out in our laboratory, should also have produced an instructional effect. In that study, however, there were reasons for suspecting the computer used to run the study as the culprit. This remains to be explored, but simply presenting the explicit instructions on the computer screen may not have the compelling quality that a "real" experimenter reading them has. As other work suggests (Reber and Allen 1978), implicit learning is the default mode; therefore, if the subjects do not understand or do not believe the instructions, then no differences would be expected. This suggests a possible important methodological factor that has gone largely unnoticed: the sophisticated equipment that we use commonly in our laboratories may be having untoward effects on our studies.

In any event, the literature on the implicit/ explicit problem is clearly complex, and it takes but a moment's reflection to appreciate the fact that there are still other important issues lurking behind these findings. First, it seems clear that any number of confounding factors may influence, either positively or negatively, the impact of explicit instructions (cf. Lewicki 1986a). Such instructions may introduce an element of stress or anxiety, may evoke a sense of motivation, may encourage one or another conscious strategy, and the like. To date, few of the researchers mentioned have taken such factors into account, and not much is known about how conscious, explicit processing systems interact with the implicit and unconscious. For example, a recent study suggests that using instructions that engage the explicit system may also elicit anxiety and that anxiety may be related to poor performance on a standard grammar learning task (Rathus, Reber, and Kushner 1988).

Second, it seems clear that we are still dealing with a rather limited kind of analysis of complex learning, particularly if one wishes to view this research in its constrained laboratory setting as representing a general metaphor for real-world acquisition processes. In the real world nearly all complex skills are acquired with a blend of the explicit and the implicit, a balance between the conscious/overt and the unconscious/covert. There is surely a difference between simply informing a learner that the stimulus materials have structure, as researchers in the aforementioned experiments did, and telling the learner something definitive about that structure. The next section deals with this issue.

Effects of Providing Specific Information

This issue concerns the impact of giving subjects precise information about the nature of the stimulus display that they will be exposed to. This is an important question for a number of reasons. For one, this issue broaches on some of the classic questions in pedagogic theory about how best to convey highly complex and richly structured information to students. It also emerges in various studies on the acquisition of expertise in such areas as medical diagnosis, in which the relationship between specific knowledge presented to medical students and their emergent tacit knowledge base is turning out to be most complex (see, e.g., Carmody, Kundel, and Toto 1984).

Reber et al. (1980) attempted to address this issue by using the standard grammar learning procedure. In that study, subjects were presented with the actual schematic structure of the grammar; that is, they were presented with figure 38.1. Each subject was handed the diagram and given a 7-min. "course" in how such a structure can be used to generate strings of symbols. This procedure was supported by an observation period during which a set of exemplars was shown to the subjects. In this training format a maximally explicit learning procedure was thus mixed with a maximally implicit one.

Reber et al. (1980) explored the manner of interaction between these two modes of apprehension by introducing the explicit training at different points in the observation period. One group of subjects received the explicit instruction at the outset before any exemplars were seen; one group received it part way through the observation period; and for a third group, the explication of structure was delayed until after they observed the full set of exemplars. As in the typical grammar learning study, knowledge acquired during learning was assessed by means of a well-formedness task.

The key finding was that the earlier during the observation training the explicit instructions were given, the more effective they were. From the previous discussions it is clear that increasing the salience of the relationships between symbols increases the effectiveness of subjects' attentional focus. It is also clear that instructions that encourage the subject to deal with the stimuli in ways that are discoordinate with underlying structure have detrimental effects on acquisition. Thus the explication of the precise nature of the structure underlying the stimuli must have differential impact on learning, depending on which of these two processes is encouraged.

The most plausible interpretation, and the one that has interesting implications for theories of instruction, is that the function of providing explicit instructions at the outset is to direct and focus the subjects' attention. It alerts them to the kinds of structural relations that characterize the stimuli that follow and permits appropriate coding schemes to be implemented. These instructions did not teach the grammar in any full or explicit fashion; rather, they oriented the subjects toward the relevant invariances in the display that followed so that the subjects, in effect, taught themselves.

Accordingly, when such explicit instruction is introduced later in the observation period, its effects are different because two sources of difficulty are introduced. First, it imposes a formalization of structure that is, in all likelihood, discoordinate with the tacit system that was in the process of being induced. Second, it reduces the number of exemplars that can be used as a base for extracting invariance patterns. In the extreme case in which the instructions were delayed until the completion of the observation period, this informational base is virtually eliminated.

These points can use some further exploration. There is every reason to suspect that subjects' tacit representation of rules is idiosyncratic in various characteristics. The induction routines hypothesized by Holland et al. (1986) predict this personalized aspect at the outset. From earlier work, it is clear that subjects are known to use a wide variety of coding schemes in focusing their attention on the stimuli (see Allen and Reber 1980, Reber and Allen 1978, and Reber and Lewis 1977, for details). So long as these schemes do not entail inappropriate rule formation, their impact is superficial. Independently of individualistic mnemonics, attentional focusing priorities, or preferred rehearsal strategies, the implicit learner will emerge from the training session with a tacit, valid knowledge base coordinate with the structure of the stimulus environment.

The degree to which the explicit instructions introduce difficulties will thus be dependent on the extent to which the subject's tacit representation of structure matches the formalization provided by the schematic of the grammar and the accompanying characterization of its generational properties. In Dulany et al.'s (1984) terms, subjects are learning "correlated grammars" whose properties are, in all likelihood, not commensurate in any simple way with the Markovian system in use. Recent results from Mathews et al. (1989) strongly corroborate this interpretation.

The deep difficulty here is that there is a potentially infinite number of formalizations that could account for the structure displayed in any given subset of strings from one of these grammars; present the "wrong" one to a subject, and the instructions will not have a salutary effect. The problem is apparent: How much can we expect a subject to benefit from the specific information that the set of exemplars just observed and tacitly coded as, say, bigram covariation patterns is "in reality" to be formalized as a Markovian process? To take an obvious analogy, most of us with our extensive observation and generation of utterances in English have failed to derive any facilitative effect of explicit instruction with transformational grammar that, at least in principle, can be posed as a legitimate formalization of our tacit knowledge. Moreover, such explicit awareness of structure can actually be a nuisance when one tries to fulfill the kinds of demands placed on subjects in these experiments, as in the discrimination of well-formed, novel instances from instances that contain some violation of the formal system.

In a study that addressed this point directly, Bialystok (1981) found that subjects learning French as a second language could rapidly and accurately detect ungrammatical sentences and could do so largely independently of the complexity of the grammatical rules violated. However, when asked to characterize the nature of the violated rules, the complexity factor played a significant role. Complexity, of course, is defined in such cases by the kinds of grammars that are taught in "French as a second language" courses.

In summary, although there are not a lot of hard empirical data here, those that are available point toward an interesting conclusion. Specific instruction concerning the materials to be learned in complex situations will be maximally beneficial when it is representationally coordinate with the tacit knowledge derived from experience. Because this issue is ultimately critical for theories of instruction, it is one much in need of close examination.

On Deep and Surface Structure

The issue here is the degree to which implicit learning can be seen as acquisition of knowledge that is based on the superficial physical form of the stimuli or as knowledge of the deeper, more abstract relations that can, in principle, be said to underlie them.

In an early article, Reber (1969), reported evidence for the proposition that implicit knowledge is abstract and not dependent in any important way on the particular physical manifestations of the stimuli. This study consisted of two sessions during which subjects memorized letter strings from a grammar. When the second session began, the stimulus materials were, without warning, modified. For some subjects the same letters continued to be used, but the rules for letter order were now those of a different grammar (the "syntax" was altered). For other subjects the underlying structure was not tampered with, but the letters used to represent the grammar were replaced with a new set (the "vocabulary" was changed). The two obvious control groups, one for which both aspects were altered and one for which neither was changed, were also run. The various manipulations had systematic effects on subjects' ability to memorize stimuli in the second session. Modification of the rules for letter order produced decrements

in performance; modifications of the physical form had virtually no adverse effects. So long as the deep rules that characterized the stimuli were left intact, their instantiations in the form of one or another set of letters was a factor of relatively little importance.

The recent study by Mathews et al. (1989) supported this general finding. Their experiment was run over a 4-week period. Subjects who received a new letter set each week (which was based on the same underlying syntax) performed as well as subjects who worked with the same letter set throughout the course of the experiment. The effect was quite striking; the transfer from letter set to letter set occurred smoothly and apparently without the need for any conscious translation.

Reber and Lewis (1977) reported an equally striking example of the abstract nature of tacit knowledge. They assessed knowledge of the grammar by having subjects solve anagram problems. After a standard training session during which subjects memorized exemplars from the language, they solved anagrams from the synthetic language over a 4-day period. For reasons to be discussed, it is convenient to code letter strings in the form of bigrams and to note the rank order of frequency of occurrence of each possible bigram. For example, the string PTTTVV contains bigrams PT, TV, and VV once each and TT twice. Given how this experiment was run, three rank orders of frequency of occurrence of bigrams exist: (a) one based on the actual solutions offered by the subjects (corrected, of course, for guessing), (b) one based on the frequency of occurrence of each acceptable bigram within the artificial language itself (within the string lengths used), and (c) one based on the actual bigrams that appeared in the learning stimuli.

Rank-order correlations among these three were revealing. The correlation between (a) and (b) was .72, whereas that between (a) and (c) was only .04. The interesting point about these results is that the comparison between (a) and (b) is a comparison between subjects' usable knowledge and a deep representation of the frequency patterns of the grammar. Rank-order (b) was formed on the basis of the full set of acceptable strings that the grammar could, in principle, generate within the specific string lengths. Subjects, however, never saw this full set of strings; they were exposed only to the exemplars chosen for the training sessions. These particular strings were selected to ensure that each subject saw at least one string of each possible length and, for each length when it was possible, at least one example of each of the grammar's three loops. This procedure yielded a set of strings that displayed all of the deep structural characteristics of the finite-state language but, in terms of specific frequency of bigrams, was distinctly idiosyncratic.

The comparison between (a) and (c) is a reflection of the degree to which subjects are simply keying on the raw frequency data as displayed in the exemplars. The failure for this correlation to be different from zero suggests that subjects were not solving the anagrams on the basis of superficial knowledge of frequency of bigrams or on the basis of a fixed set of memorized instances. They clearly acquired knowledge that can be characterized as deep, abstract, and representative of the structure inherent in the underlying invariance patterns of the stimulus environment.

This finding is analogous to Posner and Keele's (1968, 1970) oft-cited abstraction of prototype effect. The underlying prototypes that their subjects extracted from the exemplary dot patterns are specifiable only in terms of an averaging of the spatial relations among the various components of the patterns. But, psychologically, such an averaging is not just a simple piling up of the features of the exemplars. If memory behaved like that, the resulting representation would be, not distinct prototypes that Posner and Keele found, but a blob.

The induction routine that appears to be operating in situations such as these is necessarily one that results in an abstract representation. Moreover, it is one that is applicable to the classification of novel instances and not specifically characterizable by a raw compilation of experienced instances.

This issue is one of considerable complexity. The point of the preceding argument is not that all memorial systems must be viewed as founded on induced abstractions. The evidence of Brooks (1978) and others (cf. Smith and Medin 1981) shows that memories are frequently based on instantiations, fairly uninterpreted representations of the stimulus inputs. The point is that when implicit acquisition processes are operating the resulting memorial system is abstract. As was shown elsewhere (Allen and Reber 1980, Reber and Allen 1978), the same subjects working with the same grammars can emerge from a learning session with either an instantiated memory system or an abstract one, depending on the learning procedures used. In those articles, that old war horse *functionalism* was shown to provide the best characterization of this issue; that is, the specific functions that need to be carried out invite the learner to assume a cognitive stance that is functional, that will accomplish the task at hand. Under some circumstances (such as the paired-associates learning procedure used by Brooks 1978 and by Reber and Allen 1978), a rather concrete, instantiated memorial system will be established; under others (the instant asymptote technique in the PL studies by Reber and Millward 1968 and the observation procedure in Reber and Allen's 1978 study), a distinctly abstract representation will emerge. In the pure implicit, unconscious acquisition mode, the default position is abstraction.

On Mental Representation

As Rosch and Lloyd (1978) pointed out, sooner or later every discourse on mental process and structure must come to grips with the problem of the form of the representation of knowledge held. Such discussions must begin with some presumptions. The ones introduced here are, of course, open to emendation as understanding processes. They are taken as the starting point simply because they have considerable explanatory power, more than most contemporary cognitivists have granted.

First, the general argument put forward by such diverse theorists as Gibson (1966, 1979), Garner (1974, 1978), and Neisser (1976), that the stimulus is more than the physical setting for the occurrence of a response, is taken as a given. This point is more than a simplistic swipe at behaviorism; it is an argument that stresses that the stimulus domain within which we function is extraordinarily rich and complex and, in all likelihood, much more so than most cognitivists have been willing to recognize. The underlying causative nature of the stimulus environment is rarely explored; most theorists are satisfied with characterizations that are theory driven.

Second, there is general agreement with the arguments put forward (in rather different forms, to be sure) by Palmer (1978) and Anderson (1978, 1979, 1983) to the effect that most theoretical attempts to deal with the representation issue are misguided. Palmer maintained that the confusion derives from a failure to deal directly with metatheoretical factors concerning existing models. Anderson argued that in principle, there are no ways in which behavioral data can be used to identify uniquely any one particular mental representation. There are some reasons for perhaps disputing these claims (see, e.g., Hayes-Roth 1979; Pylyshyn 1979, 1980), but they are not a concern here.

From the point of view that I take as presumptive here, it matters not at all whether the following interpretations of mental representation are supported by a well-structured consideration of metarepresentational factors or whether they can be shown to be uniquely speci-

fiable. The point of view that I take reflects that of classical functionalism as introduced in the preceding section. Functional theories are typically regarded these days as formulations (abstract, to be sure) of what is possible for a person to process and why. This seems right, and as has been argued elsewhere (Allen and Reber 1980, Reber and Allen 1978), the main consideration should be with characterizing representations, in terms of how the individual can be seen as behaving in an adaptive fashion, rather than in terms of pure representational theory. For example, as discussed earlier, there are good empirical reasons for regarding the functional representation of the mental content of a finite-state grammar as an ordered set of bigrams (and trigrams; see Mathews et al. 1989) and not as a formal Markovian system.

Third, the oft-dismissed position of representational realism is accepted as a first approximation. What is in the stimulus world is what ends up in the mind of the perceiver/cognizer. The point is that a good way to start dealing with the representation problem is with the physical stimulus itself. Under various constraints of processing and various task demands, enrichment and/or elaborative operations are certainly used, and the resulting coded representation may very well not be isomorphic with the stimulus field. Nevertheless, as Mace (1974) put it, a good initial strategy is to "ask not what's inside your head, ask what your head's inside of."

Several findings from studies with artificial grammars are relevant to the issue of representation. Table 38.1 gives the summary data from 14 separate experiments that reveal some interesting patterns. Some details on procedure are needed: In all of these studies, knowledge acquired during learning was assessed through the well-formedness task in which subjects are presented with a number of test strings (typically 100) that must be classified as either grammatical or nongrammatical. In the typical experiment, the 100 trials consist of 50 unique items, each of

Table 38.1
Correct (C) and Error (E) response patterns to individual items during well-formedness tasks

Condition/training procedure	Pattern				Consistency
	CC	CE	EC	EE	
Reber (1967)					
1. Simple memorization	.69	.07	.12	.12	.81
Reber (1976)					
2. Simple memorization	.66	.10	.11	.13	.79
3. Memorization/rule search	.53	.12	.12	.23[a]	.76
Reber and Allen (1978)					
4. Simple observation	.73	.08	.09	.11	.84
5. Paired associates	.65	.12	.07	.16[a]	.81
Reber, Kassin, Lewis, and Cantor (1980, Experiment 1)					
6. Random display/implicit instructions	.51	.16	.14	.19	.70
7. Random display/explicit instructions	.48	.12	.14	.25[a]	.73
8. Structured display/implicit instructions	.52	.16	.16	.16	.68
9. Structured display/explicit instructions	.68	.10	.10	.11	.79
Reber, Kassin, Lewis, and Cantor (1980, Experiment 2)					
10. Rules at beginning of observation	.67	.11	.12	.11	.78
11. Rules in middle of observation	.58	.12	.14	.16	.74
12. Rules at end of observation	.57	.13	.15	.16	.73
13. Rules only	.54	.11	.16	.18[a]	.72
14. Observation only	.48	.15	.13	.24[a]	.72

[a] EE value significantly higher than the mean of the CE and EC values.

which is presented twice without feedback about the correctness of the response.

This procedure yields data that directly address the representational issue. The logic of the analysis is simple. There are four possible outcomes for each individual item for each subject: The subject may classify it correctly on both presentations (CC), classify it correctly on only one of the two (CE or EC), or misclassify it on both presentations (EE). Assume that the subject operates by using a simple decision-making strategy: When the status of the item is known, it is always classified correctly; when it is not known, a guess is made. This simple model is quite powerful and allows for a surprisingly deep analysis of the representation problem.

Specifically, under this model, (a) the values of CE, EC, and EE should be statistically indistinguishable from each other, and all should be significantly lower than the value of CC. This pattern is expected on the grounds that the items that contribute to CE, EC, and EE are those about which the subject's knowledge base is not relevant. (b) A value of EE significantly greater than the values of EC and CE is prima facie evidence for the elaboration of nonrepresentative rules on the part of subjects. Thus if subjects emerge from the learning phase with rules (either explicit or implicit) that are not accurate reflections of the grammar, this knowledge base will consistently lead them to misclassify particular items. (c) The robustness of representative knowledge can be assessed from the relationship between the values of EC and CE. If the value of CE is detectably larger than EC, we can reasonably suspect that forgetting was occurring during testing; correspondingly, if EC is larger than CE, we can infer that learning was occurring during testing. (d) One can estimate knowledge of the grammar by looking at the value of CC, which contains only those items whose status was known by the subjects plus those guessed correctly on both presentations. Last, (e) one can derive an overall measure of consistency of responding by taking the sum of CC and EE.

Of the values from 14 experimental conditions (see table 38.1), the uninteresting ones can be dispensed with first. There are no cases in which the values of CE and EC are significantly different from each other. Thus there is no evidence of loss of knowledge during the well-formedness task and no evidence that any additional learning was taking place.

The interesting results are those concerning comparisons between the values of EE and those of EC and CE. When no difference is found between EE and the mean of CE and EC, it is reasonable to conclude that there was no evidence of nonrepresentative rules in use. Values of EE that are large in relation to those of EC and CE indicate that subjects were using rules that are not representative of the grammar. The footnoted values in table 38.1 are the five conditions that yielded evidence that subjects emerged from the learning phase with notions about structure that were not commensurate with the stimulus display.

It is instructive to look closely at these five cases. In condition 13, the subjects were given only the schematic diagram of the grammar but no opportunity to observe exemplars. It appears that, not surprisingly, such a procedure encourages subjects to invent specific rules for letter order and, in the absence of complete learning, to elaborate rules about permissible letter sequences that are not reflective of the grammar.

Conditions 3 and 7 illustrate what happens when subjects are under an instructional set that encourages the use of rule search strategies but in which the letter strings are given to them in a haphazard order. Such a set of demand characteristics encourages subjects to invent a sufficient number of inappropriate rules to inflate the EE values.

In condition 5 a paired-associate task was used to impart knowledge. As is discussed elsewhere (Allen and Reber 1980, Reber and Allen 1978), the very nature of such a task leads subjects to set up an instantiated memorial system composed of parts of items and some whole items along with their associated responses. Hence the inflated EE value is not due to the application of inappropriate rules; rather, it is due to subjects' tendency to misclassify test strings because inappropriate analogies exist in instantiated memory. The fifth condition with an inordinately high EE value was 14. There is no obvious explanation for this outcome. This datum is an anomaly; 1 such outcome out of 14, however, is not bad at all.

The remaining nine conditions all yielded response patterns that fit with the proposition that whatever subjects are acquiring from the training sessions can be viewed as basically representative of the underlying structure of the stimulus domains. These consist of "neutral set" conditions, in which the subjects are led to approach the learning task as an experiment in memory or perception and no mention is made of the rule-governed nature of the stimuli (conditions 1, 2, 4, 6, and 8), and "structured set" conditions, in which subjects are provided with information concerning rules for letter order but in a manner than ensures that conscious rule searching will be coordinate with the kinds of rules in use (conditions 9, 10, 11, and 12).

Taken together, these experiments lend general support to the proposition that implicit learning functions by the induction of an underlying representation that mirrors the structure intrinsic to the environment. Such an induction

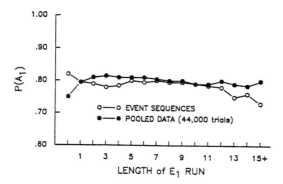

Figure 38.2
Pooled recency data from five separate probability learning experiments. (The open circles give the average probability that the more frequent event will occur over all event sequences used; filled circles give the average probability that the subjects will make the more frequent response, adjusted for overshooting. The data are based on 44,000 trials from 88 asymptotic subjects tested with the probability of the more frequent event set at .80.)

process takes place naturally when one is simply attending in an unbiased manner to the patterns of variation in the environment or when one is provided with an orientation that is coordinate with these variations.

This characterization of the appropriateness of mental representation entails nothing about the sheer amount of knowledge that one takes out of a learning session. In fact, it is relatively easy to show that there is little to enable one to distinguish explicit from implicit processes here. The consistency values in table 38.1 reveal surprisingly little variation from condition to condition, particularly when compared with the range of CC and EE values. These consistency values can be seen as a raw estimate of the total number of rules that subjects can be said to be using during decision making, for they are simply the sums of the CC and EE values. Taking a simple (and only quasi-legitimate) average across conditions reveals that the overall mean consistency values for the footnoted conditions and the nonfootnoted ones are .75 and .76, respectively. Thus there is no evidence that either set of conditions produces more rule learning; the difference is that explicit learning results in the emergence of

a number of inappropriate rules, whereas implicit learning tends to yield representative, veridical rules.

This same model of representation is supported by data from other tasks. In Reber and Lewis's (1977) anagram solution task, subjects worked with the same problem sets over 4 days. In that study there was improvement over time, so a stochastic model was fit to the data and used to predict the pattern of error and correct responses to individual test items that would be expected under the assumption that subjects were not using inappropriate rules. (For details on the model, see the original article.) The results were in keeping with the general theme here. The EEEE value (the proportion of items solved incorrectly on all 4 days of the study) was no higher than would be expected under the assumption that subjects either knew the solution to a particular anagram or made nonsystematic guesses for problems not within the domain of their knowledge base.

Several experiments in which the PL procedure was used are also of interest. The relevant data are the recency curves. In the standard analysis of a PL experiment, a recency curve represents the probability of a given response plotted against the length of the immediately preceding run of that event. Recency curves may take on any of a number of shapes, depending on the conditions of the experiment. Negative recency is most common, particularly early in an experiment. Under various circumstances, however, even positive recency may be observed (see Friedman et al. 1964 for details). The concern here is with the recency curves from experiments with 500 or more trials with a Bernoulli event sequence with probability of the more likely event set at .80.

Figure 38.2 presents the pooled recency data from five such experiments (see Reber 1967, Reber and Millward 1968). All subjects were run though a learning period with either the traditional PL or the instant asymptote technique. The subject-generated curve has been adjusted downward by exactly .04 at all points to correct for a ubiquitous overshooting effect that is observed in all of these many-trial experiments (see Rebel and Millward 1968 for a discussion of this issue). This adjustment in no way modifies the startling aspect of these two curves.

With few exceptions, the curves sit on top of each other. There is no evidence whatsoever for either the positive recency predicted by the early conditioning models or the negative recency reported by many. There is, however, overwhelming evidence for a mental representation that reflects the structure of the stimulus environment. The simplest characterization of this curve, which is based on a total of 44,000 responses, is that it reveals that subjects mimic the structure of the event sequence. Subjects' prediction responses show flat recency curves because the event sequences themselves display flat recency curves—as they must, being Bernoulli in nature.

This is not a new point; it was made earlier by Derks (1963) and by Jones and Meyers (1966), who showed that experiments can encourage either positive or negative recency by presenting event sequences with either many long or many short runs of events. But the precision with which subjects' response patterns can reflect the event patterns has never really been appreciated. To take this point to a further extreme, data like those in figure 38.2 are so robust that they can actually be used as a check on one's experimental procedure. In one PL study (Millward and Reber 1972), the subjects' overall response proportions were .523 and .476 for the two events, a result that was perplexing because each event had been programmed to occur in exactly half of the trials. The anomaly turned out to be in the computer program used to generate the sequences. A check revealed that the two events had actually been presented to subjects with proportions of .520 and .480!

Although the preceding analyses seem to provide support for the representational realist position, it is still unclear just how far one can legitimately push such a proposition. In many of the experiments reported here and in other related areas of study (see Schacter 1987), subjects respond in ways that indicate that their mental content may not be quite so neatly isomorphic with that of the stimulus field. However, it also seems reasonably clear that when such transforms or constructions of representations are observed, "secondary" processes are responsible; that is, the "primary" process of veridical representation of environmental structure becomes colored either by elaborative operations, as in experiments in which instructional sets encouraged invention of inappropriate rules (Howard and Ballas 1980, Reber 1976), or by restrictive operations, as in studies in which task demands led to the narrowing of attentional focus (Brooks 1978, Cantor 1980, Reber et al. 1980). Also, careful scrutiny of the EE values in table 38.1 reveals that even in the nonfootnoted conditions there was a tendency for some nonrepresentational elaboration to take place. In all nine of these cases, the EE value is equal to or higher than the EC or CE values ($p < .05$ by a sign test).

The problem of mental representation is clearly no easy nut to crack. The position taken here seems to be a reasonable one, although it will probably be shown to be wrong in the final analysis. Tacit knowledge is a reasonably veridical, partial isomorphism of the structural patterns of relational invariances that the environment displays. It is reasonably veridical in that it reflects, with considerable accuracy, the stimulus invariances displayed in the environment. It is partial in that not all patterns become part of tacit knowledge. It is structural in that the patterns are manifestations of abstract generative rules for symbol ordering.

On the Availability of Tacit Knowledge

The conclusion reached in the first studies on implicit learning (Reber 1965) was that the knowledge acquired was completely unavailable to consciousness. The many experiments carried out since have shown that position to have been an oversimplification. The picture that is emerging, though perhaps somewhat less striking, is certainly more interesting. Specifically, knowledge acquired from implicit learning procedures is knowledge that, in some raw fashion, is always ahead of the capability of its possessor to explicate it. Hence although it is misleading to argue that implicitly acquired knowledge is completely unconscious, it is not misleading to argue that the implicitly acquired epistemic contents of mind are always richer and more sophisticated than what can be explicated.

In Reber and Lewis's (1977) study, data were first presented to support this position. Over the 4 days of that study, during which subjects solved anagram puzzles on the basis of the syntax of an artificial grammar, there was a general increase in the ability of subjects to communicate their knowledge of the rule system in use. There was also an increase in the ability to solve the anagrams, but the former never caught up with the latter, that is, as subjects improved in their ability to verbalize the rules that they were using, they also developed richer and more complex rules. Implicit knowledge remained ahead of explicit knowledge.

In a recent study, Mathews et al. (1989) used a novel yoked-control technique to explore this issue. Subjects were interrupted at intervals during a well-formedness judgment task and asked to explicate the rules that they were using. The information was then given to yoked-control subjects, who were then tested in the same well-formedness task. So equipped, these control subjects managed to perform at roughly half the level of accuracy of the experimental subjects. Moreover, as the experiment progressed and each experimental subject improved, so did each yoked control, but the controls never caught up with the experimental subjects.

The most direct attempt to deal with the issue of the degree to which implicitly acquired knowledge is available to consciousness was carried out by Dulany et al. (1984). After a standard learning procedure, subjects were asked to mark each well-formedness test item as acceptable or not and to specify what features of that item led them to classify it as they did. Dulany et al. argued that the features so marked accounted for the full set of decisions that each subject made, a result that, if correct, supports the notion that used knowledge of the grammar was held consciously. Reber, Allen, and Regan (1985), however, argued that the nature of the task that Dulany et al. used carried its own guarantee of success; that is, the task forced the data to appear as though they carried the implication of consciousness, whereas actually the subjects were reporting only vague guesses about the appropriateness or inappropriateness of letter groups. The issue continues to be disputed. Dulany, Carlson, and Dewey (1985) presented reasons for doubting Reber et al.'s analysis, whereas Hayes (unpublished) recently produced evidence in support of the interpretation of Reber and his coworkers.

One of the problems with this line of research is that it fails to distinguish between knowledge that is available to consciousness after attempts at retrieval and knowledge that is present in consciousness at the time that the decisions themselves are being made. Carmody et al. (1984) noted this problem in assessing the knowledge base that physicians are taught to use versus what they actually use in diagnosis, and Schacter (1987) argued that conclusions reached about the availability of implicit information must take account of a variety of task constraints that have their own impacts. Nevertheless, if it is not yet clear, the discussions that follow will emphasize even further the central thesis of this line of research. To wit: A considerable portion of memorial content is unconscious, and, even more important, a goodly amount of knowledge acquisition takes place in the absence of intent to learn.

Entailments and Implications

The preceding discussion is a reasonably thorough review of the current state of affairs as regards the general issues of the acquisition, usage, representation, and availability of tacit knowledge. As Schacter (1987) pointed out recently, one of the intriguing aspects of the history of work on this issue is that there is such an amazing variety of implicit processes that have been observed and yet there is nothing approaching a satisfactory theoretical account of them. What follows may or may not improve on this state of affairs. The following is a small flurry of speculation concerning the possible entailments and implications of the research. Each of the topics is touched upon only briefly; the point here is to provoke new avenues of study, not to draw any hard conclusions.

On the Origins of Unconscious Cognition

Usually the header here is the "Origins of *Conscious* Cognition," not "*Unconscious*." Tradi-

tionally, the focus has been on consciousness with the implication that defining and characterizing consciousness will solve the problem; unconscious processes will be handled by the invoking of exclusionary clauses. The history of the variety of ways in which the unconscious has been represented (Ellenberger 1970) shows this clearly. Consciousness assumes epistemic priority because it is so introspectively obvious, whereas the unconscious must be struggled with in derivative fashion.

The point to be defended here is that this ordering of priorities has been an error. The theoretically important exercise should be on the origins of unconscious cognitive processes. Consciousness, evolutionarily speaking, is a late arrival on the mental scene. Perhaps it is not of such recent origin as some have argued (Jaynes 1976), but surely it postdates a number of fairly rich and elaborative cognitive processes that functioned and still function in our phylogenetic predecessors (Griffin 1981, 1984). There is, moreover, absolutely no reason to suppose that these presumably adaptive mental capacities ought to have been lost. In fact, there are a number of reasons for supposing that they continue to flourish interpenetrated by an emerging executive system, conscious mentation.

Taking such a perspective gives unconscious cognition the empirical and theoretical priority that it deserves but has not enjoyed since the era of the philosophical emergentists. Unconscious cognitive functions should not have to be defended against arguments that deny their role in action (see the debate between Dulany et al. 1984, 1985, and Reber et al. 1985). The proper stance is to assume that unconscious mental processes are the foundations upon which emerging conscious operations are laid. The really difficult problem, then, is to discern how these components of mind interact.

This perspective has some interesting entailments. One is that it suggests a novel way to see how the work on implicit learning fits in with a good deal of other research on the cognitive unconscious. Another is that it allows for a new framework for:

Parsing the Cognitive Unconscious

A conspicuously large number of processes and functions have been assigned to the unconscious over the past century or so. They have come in a variety of forms, some concerned with perceptual processes, some with dynamic, some with motivational and emotional, and some with cognitive. A number of schemata have also been proposed for defining and classifying the subcategories of unconscious functions and operations (see Ellenberger 1970, Erdelyi 1985). Herein is one more.

As a first approximation, assume a relatively high-level parse that separates unconscious mentation into two classes, one that most aptly can be called the *primitive* and one that, for reasons to be spelled out, can be thought of as the *sophisticated*. The primitive unconscious encompasses a variety of basic functions, all of which are carried out more or less automatically and are more or less devoid of meaning, affect, or interpretation. Included here is a range of processes such Gibson's (1979) direct pickup of information in perception, Hasher and Zacks's (1984) automatic encoding of information about the frequency of events as they occur, Lewicki's (1985, 1986a,b) studies showing unconscious apprehension of feature covariation, Broadbent and his coworkers' (Berry and Broadbent 1984, Broadbent and Aston 1978, Broadbent et al. 1986) studies on simulated economic and manufacturing systems, and, of course, the studies reviewed on implicit learning of complex covariations displayed by synthetic grammars and structured event sequences.

The operations of this primitive unconscious seem to be about as fundamental for a species' survival as any nonvegetative function could be. Virtually every organism must be able to perform a basic Hasher and Zacks's (1984) type

of counting of the occurrences of ecologically important events. Ground squirrels presumably count small holes and keep a kind of log of their locations, and lions count gnus and their various properties. Rats, pigeons, dogs, and other laboratory subjects count covariations between events even in the most basic circumstances. The essence of Pavlovian conditioning is the apprehension of a genuine covariation between the conditioned stimulus and the unconditioned stimulus (Rescorla 1967, 1988). The reason that the work of such researchers as Hasher and Zacks, Lewicki, and others is typically regarded as cognitive in nature and somehow different from Rescorla's is that it is typically carried out with mature adult subjects and with materials that have a rich cognitive underpinning, such as words, sentences, and pictures. Yet, there is no a priori reason to regard these high-level cognitive "counts" as different in any fundamental way from the very simple countings of Rescorla's subjects. What is different is the process by which each organism comes to categorize the items whose frequency and covariation patterns are being logged, not the mechanism for representing the raw data.

From this perspective, the grammar learning experiments, the PL studies, and the rest of the literature on implicit learning can be viewed as epistemic kin of the most basic of the primitive unconscious functions. For example, Lewicki (1985) showed that in the limiting case, only one exposure to a target person with a salient personality characteristic (e.g., kindness, capability) and particular physical characteristic (e.g., long or short hair) is sufficient to set up a tacit knowledge base that reflects these covariations and affects decisions made about novel people. In cases with a richer data base, such as the structured event sequences of the synthetic languages and the probability learning experiments, the kinds of structural covariations that are apprehended are deeper and more abstract. Yet, they can be viewed as categorical extensions in that the basic process is, in principle, still one of counting, only what is being counted are complex interdependent covariations among events—or, as they are commonly known in the literature, *rules*.

These various manifestations of the functions of the primitive unconscious have a number of additional factors in common. First, and most basic, the pickup of information takes place independently of consciousness or awareness of what is picked up. Put another way, adding the factor of consciousness changes the very nature of the process (Reber 1976, Reber and Allen 1978, Reber et al. 1980). As stated at the outset, this may be taken as the defining feature of implicit learning.

Second, although much of what is acquired may eventually be made available to conscious expression, what is held or stored exceeds what can be expressed. This is displayed in one of two fashions: Either predictions of performance made on the basis of available knowledge fall short of actual performance (Mathews et al. 1989, Nisbett and Wilson 1977; Reber and Lewis 1977) or differential effects of variables are seen when the implicit–explicit instructional set is varied (Graf and Mandler 1984, Reber 1976, Reber et al. 1980, Schacter and Graf 1986). Schacter (1987) noted that this inequality between implicit knowledge that is inaccessible and implicit knowledge that can be articulated explicitly may have to do with the degree of elaborative encoding that is allowed. Indeed, most of the studies in which a substantial proportion of once-tacit knowledge is made available to consciousness are those in which considerable overt encoding is carried out (e.g., Dulany et al. 1984).

Third, the memorial content of the primitive unconscious has a causal role to play in behavior. This proposition goes almost without saying, given the preceding discussion, but it needs to be specified; if there were no causal component to unconscious cognition, we might as well simply return to a radical behaviorism. Put simply, the primitive unconscious processes are for learning

about the world in very basic ways. They are automatic and ineluctable; they function to pick up critical knowledge about categories and about covariations of aspects of categories. They do not, however, have any functions that involve meaning or affect; these are the province of the *sophisticated* unconscious.

In this latter class are included such phenomena as unconscious perception of graphic and semantic information (Marcel 1983), perceptual vigilance and perceptual defense (Erdelyi 1974), the implicit pickup of affective information that is based on phonological factors (Corteen and Wood 1972) or geometric features (Kunst-Wilson and Zajonc 1980; Seamon, Brody, and Kauff 1983; Seamon, Marsh, and Brody 1984), and repetition priming effects with various linguistic and nonlinguistic materials (Jacoby and Dallas 1981; Scarborough, Cortese, and Scarborough 1977; Scarborough, Gerard, and Cortese 1979, among many others). In some ways the evidence for the unconscious element is stronger here than it is with the primitive unconscious. The use of forced-choice recognition tests as a measure of sensitivity in the work of Marcel (1983), Kunst-Wilson and Zajonc (1980), Seamon et al. (1983), and Seamon et al. (1984) supports the strong claim that these processes are occurring virtually independently of awareness. Although there may be some problems with methodology (see Holender 1986), this procedure is, in principle, superior to that used by most researchers, who mainly browbeat their subjects into telling what they know (Allen and Reber 1980, Berry and Broadbent 1984, Brooks 1978, Reber and Allen 1978).

What makes these various processes intriguing and what differentiates these sophisticated processes from the primitive is that all share a basic operating property: They all depend on a rich, abstract knowledge base that asserts itself in a causal manner to control perception, affective choice, and decision making independently of consciousness. This component of the cognitive unconscious depends on previously acquired knowledge, as opposed to the primitive component, which operated to acquire such knowledge. The very epistemic base that makes these sophisticated processes functional can be seen as that derived from the primitive processes.

These sophisticated systems also differ from the primitive in other ways. First, they are components of mind that are generally available to consciousness. In other words, there is awareness of the knowledge base itself; a subject in one of Marcel's (1983) experiments surely knows the target word and, moreover, surely knows that he or she knows it. What is crucial is that this overt knowledge base has a higher threshold for engagement than the covert one does. Second, they are based on knowledge systems that have become highly automatized. They share this automatic quality with the primitive functions in the limit, but there are good reasons for thinking that much of this interpretive and semantic knowledge derived from explicit processes that became automatic only after pained, conscious action. Interestingly, this line of argument parallels that taken by Dulany et al. (1984, 1985) in their criticism of the synthetic grammar learning studies; however, Dulany et al. targeted the wrong level for invoking it. Last, these systems all function on a symbolic level. All of the critical components of the sophisticated unconscious involve semantic and affective properties of stimuli. This aspect seems to be largely missing in the primitive domain. It seems that these sophisticated processes are more uniquely the stuff of humanity than are the primitive processes, which are operating systems that we share with virtually all corticated species and are found rather far down the phylogenetic scale.

The Robustness of Implicit Processes

There has been a good deal of work to suggest that implicit systems are robust in the face of disorders that are known to produce serious deficits in conscious, overt processes. Support for this functional separation of conscious and un- conscious cognitive processing has come from the study of various patient populations. Classic cases are amnesia (see Milner, Corkin, and Teuber 1968 for the early work and Schacter 1987 for a recent overview), blindsight (Weiskrantz 1986), prosopagnosia (Bauer 1984), and alexia (Shallice and Saffran 1986). In all these cases there is compelling evidence of effective performance in the absence of awareness.

The model of mental parsing suggested earlier provides a novel interpretation of this work. There is a standard heuristic in evolutionary biology that older primitive systems are more robust and resistant to insult than are newer, more complex systems. The hypothesis that the implicit cognitive processes are the functional components of the evolutionarily older, primitive system predicts that they should show greater resistance than should explicit processes. By extension, all of the various phenomena that have been cited as manifestations of primitive unconscious processes would be expected to display similar robustness under conditions in which parallel explicit processes have been diminished or even lost entirely.

The strongest evidence in support of such an interpretation comes from cases in which direct comparison between implicit and explicit processes has been made in clinical settings. In an extended series of studies, Warrington and Weiskraniz (see 1982 for an overview) found no deficits in amnesics when the task involved memory for words based on word-stem and word-fragment cues, but performance was seriously impaired when overt word recognition and recall procedures were used. A similar pattern emerged with Hasher and Zacks's frequency encoding task, in which performance was found to be robust in the face of clinical depression (Hasher and Zacks 1979, Roy 1982) and even Korsakoff's syndrome (Strauss, Weingartner, and Thompson 1985). Last, a recent study of Abrams and Reber (1989) suggested that even the acquisition of knowledge is undiminished so long as the task is a nonreflective, unconscious one. They used an implicit grammar learning task and an explicit short-term memory task with a mixed population of institutionalized depressives, schizophrenics, and alcoholics with organic brain damage. The patients performed more poorly than a normal control group on the memory task, but the performances of the two groups were statistically indistinguishable on the implicit learning task. This last study is particularly important, for it is one of the few that shows that implicit *learning* is robust in the face of serious psychological and/or neurological disorders (see Graf and Schacter 1985 for another example involving a word-completion task).

On Intuition

One of the gains of this line of research on implicit processes is that it provides the opportunity to reclaim intuition for cognitive psychology. There is probably no cognitive process that suffers from such a gap between phenomenological reality and scientific understanding. Introspectively, intuition is one of the most compelling and obvious cognitive processes; empirically and theoretically, it is one of the processes least understood by contemporary cognitive scientists.

The basic argument is simple: The kinds of operations identified under the rubric of implicit learning represent the epistemic core of intuition; that is, the introspective qualities that most people—from Bergson (1913) and Croce (1922) to Jung (1926), Polanyi (1958), and Westcott (1968)—identify when discussing intuition are those processes that have emerged in the studies of implicit acquisition of complex knowledge. Perhaps the most compelling aspect of intuition, and the one most often cited in the various definitions that have been given (see Westcott 1968), is that the individual has a sense of what is right or wrong, a sense of what is the appropriate or inappropriate response to make in a given set of circumstances, but is largely ignorant of the reasons for that mental state. This, of course, is how the typical subject has been

characterized after a standard acquisition session in an implicit learning experiment.

The point is that intuition is a perfectly normal and common mental state/process that is the end product of an implicit learning experience. In other words, intuition ought not to be embedded in personality theory as it was with Jung (1926), and although it is a topic of some philosophical interest, it is probably best not dealt with as an a priori topic as it was by Croce (1922). It is a cognitive state that emerges under specifiable conditions, and it operates to assist an individual to make choices and to engage in particular classes of action. To have an intuitive sense of what is right and proper, to have a vague feeling of the goal of an extended process of thought, to "get the point" without really being able to verbalize what it is that one has gotten, is to have gone through an implicit learning experience and have built up the requisite representative knowledge base to allow for such judgment.

Summary

This article is an attempt to come to grips with an essential, although oft-ignored, problem in contemporary cognitive psychology: the acquisition of complex knowledge. At the heart of the presented thesis is the concept of implicit learning wherein abstract, representative knowledge of the stimulus environment is acquired, held, and used to control behavior. The operations of implicit learning are shown to take place independently of consciousness; their mental products have been demonstrated to be held tacitly; their functional controlling properties have been shown to operate largely outside of awareness. The strong argument is that implicit learning represents a general, modality-free Ur-process, a fundamental operation whereby critical covariations in the stimulus environment are picked up.

The key problem in all of this is to specify, as clearly as possible, the boundary conditions on the process of implicit learning—that is, to outline the circumstances under which it emerges and those under which it is suppressed or overwhelmed. A substantial part of the empirical work reviewed here should be seen in that light. Last, there has been an attempt to show how such a process can be seen as functioning in the context of other, complex cognitive operations and to speculate on how it might be viewed in a variety of other frameworks, from that of evolutionary theory to those of various clinical syndromes affecting cognitive function to those of some novel considerations of intuition.

Acknowledgments

Preparation of this article was supported in part by a grant from the City University of New York PSC-CUNY Research Awart Program.

Special thanks go to Rhianon Allen, Ruth Hernstadt, Paul Lewicki, and Robert McCauley for suggestions, insights, and gentle criticisms (which I probably should have paid more attention to).

References

Abrams, M. (1987). *Implicit learning in the psychiatrically impaired.* Unpublished doctoral dissertation, City University of New York.

Abrams, M., and Reber, A. S. (1989). Implicit learning in special populations. *Journal of Psycholinguistic Research, 17*, 425–439.

Allen, R., and Reber, A. S. (1980). Very long term memory for tacit knowledge. *Cognition, 8*, 175–185.

Anderson, J. R. (1978). Arguments concerning representations for mental imagery. *Psychological Review, 85*, 249–277.

Anderson, J. R. (1979). Further arguments concerning representations for mental imagery. *Psychology Review, 86*, 395–406.

Anderson, J. R. (1983). *The architecture of cognition.* Cambridge, MA: Harvard University Press.

Bauer, R. M. (1984). Autonomic recognition of names and faces in prosopagnosia: A neuropsychological application of the guilty knowledge test. *Neuropsychologia, 22*, 457–469.

Bergson, H. (1913). *Introduction to metaphysics.* New York: Liberal Arts Press.

Berry, D. C., and Broadbent, D. E. (1984). On the relationship between task performance and associated verbalizable knowledge. *Quarterly Journal of Experimental Psychology, 36*, 209–231.

Bialystok, E. (1981). Some evidence for the integrity and interaction of two knowledge sources. In R. Anderson (Ed.), *New directions in research on the acquisition and use of a second language.* Rowley, MA: Newbury.

Broadbent, D. E., and Aston, B. (1978). Human control of a simulated economic system. *Ergonomics, 21*, 1035–1043.

Broadbent, D. E., FitzGerald, P., and Broadbent, M. H. P. (1986). Implicit and explicit knowledge in the control of complex systems. *British Journal of Psychology, 77*, 33–50.

Brooks, L. R. (1978). Nonanalytic concept formation and memory for instances. In E. Rosch and B. B. Lloyd (Eds.), *Cognition and categorization* (pp. 169–211). New York: Wiley.

Cantor, G. W. (1980, April). *On symbol string-type and the generalization of the implicit learning paradigm.* Paper presented at the annual meeting of the Eastern Psychological Association, New York.

Carmody, D. P., Kundel, H. L., and Toto, L. C. (1984). Comparison scans while reading chest images: Taught, but not practiced. *Investigative Radiology, 19*, 462–466.

Chomsky, N. (1980). *Rules and representations.* New York: Columbia University Press.

Corteen, R. S., and Wood, B. (1972). Autonomic responses to shock-associated words in an unattended channel. *Journal of Experimental Psychology, 94*, 308–313.

Croce, B. (1922). *Aesthetic* (2nd ed.). New York: Norwood.

Danks, J. H., and Gans, D. L. (1975). Acquisition and utilization of a rule structure. *Journal of Experimental Psychology: Human Learning and Memory, 1*, 201–208.

Derks, P. L. (1963). Effect of run length in the gambler's fallacy. *Journal of Experimental Psychology, 65,* 213–214.

Dulany, D. E., Carlson, R. A., and Dewey, G. I. (1984). A case of syntactical learning and judgment: How conscious and how abstract? *Journal of Experimental Psychology: General, 113,* 541–555.

Dulany, D. E., Carlson, R. A., and Dewey, G. I. (1985). On consciousness in syntactical learning and judgment: A reply to Reber, Allen, and Regan. *Journal of Experimental Psychology: General, 114,* 25–32.

Ellenberger, H. F. (1970). *The discovery of the unconscious.* New York: Basic Books.

Erdelyi, M. H. (1974). A new look at the New Look: Perceptual defense and vigilance. *Psychological Review, 81,* 1–25.

Erdelyi, M. H. (1985). *Psychoanalysis: Freud's cognitive psychology.* New York: Freeman.

Fodor, J. A. (1975). *The language of thought.* Cambridge, MA: Harvard University Press.

Fodor, J. A. (1983). *Modularity of mind: An essay on faculty psychology.* Cambridge, MA: MIT Press.

Fried, L. S., and Holyoak, K. J. (1984). Induction of category distributions: A framework for classification learning. *Journal of Experimental Psychology: Learning, Memory, and Cognition, 10,* 234–257.

Friedman, M. P., Burke, C. J., Cole, M., Keller, L., Millward, R. B., and Estes, W. K. (1964). Two-choice behavior under extended training with shifting probabilities of reinforcement. In R. C. Atkinson (Ed.), *Studies in mathematical psychology* (pp. 250–291). Stanford, CA: Stanford University Press.

Garner, W. R. (1974). *The processing of information and structure.* Hillsdale, NJ: Erlbaum.

Garner, W. R. (1978). Aspects of a stimulus: Features, dimensions, and configurations. In E. Rosch and B. B. Lloyd (Eds.), *Cognition and categorization* (pp. 99–133). Hillsdale, NJ: Erlbaum.

Gibson, J. J. (1966). *The senses considered as perceptual systems.* Boston: Houghton Mifflin.

Gibson, J. J. (1979). *The ecological approach to visual perception.* Boston: Houghton Mifflin.

Gleitman, L. R., and Wanner, E. (1982). Language acquisition: The state of the art. In E. Wanner and L. R. Gleitman (Eds.), *Language acquisition: The state of the art* (pp. 3–48). New York: Cambridge University Press.

Graf, P., and Mandler, G. (1984). Activation makes words more accessible but not necessarily more retrievable. *Journal of Verbal Learning and Verbal Behavior, 23,* 553–568.

Graf, P., and Schacter, D. L. (1985). Implicit and explicit memory for new associations in normal and amnesic subjects. *Journal of Experimental Psychology: Learning, Memory, and Cognition, 11,* 501–518.

Griffin, D. R. (1981). *The question of animal awareness: Evolutionary continuity of mental experience.* New York: Rockefeller University Press.

Griffin, D. R. (1984). *Animal thinking.* Cambridge, MA: Harvard University Press.

Hasher, L., and Zacks, R. T. (1979). Automatic and effortful processes in memory. *Journal of Experimental Psychology: General, 108,* 356–388.

Hasher, L., and Zacks, R. T. (1984). Automatic processing of fundamental information. *American Psychologist, 39,* 1372–1388.

Hayes, N. A. Consciousness cannot explain syntactical judgment: A rebuttal of Dulany, Carlson, and Dewey. Unpublished ms.

Hayes-Roth, F. (1979). Distinguishing theories of representation: A critique of Anderson's "Arguments Concerning Mental Imagery." *Psychological Review, 86,* 376–392.

Holender, D. (1986). Semantic activation without conscious identification in dichotic listening, parafoveal vision, and visual masking: A survey and appraisal. *The Behavioral and Brain Sciences, 9,* 1–66.

Holland, J. H., Holyoak, K. J., Nisbett, R. E., and Thagard, P. R. (1986). *Induction: Processes of inference, learning and discovery.* Cambridge, MA: MIT Press.

Howard, J. H., and Ballas, J. A. (1980). Syntactic and semantic factors in the classification of nonspeech transient patterns. *Perception and Psychophysics, 28,* 431–439.

Jacoby, L. L., and Dallas, M. (1981). On the relationship between autobiographical memory and perceptual learning. *Journal of Experimental Psychology: General, 110,* 306–340.

Jaynes, J. (1976). *The origins of consciousness in the breakdown of the bicameral mind.* Boston: Houghton Mifflin.

Jones, M. R., and Myers, J. L. (1966). A comparison of two methods of event randomization in probability learning. *Journal of Experimental Psychology*, 72, 909–911.

Jung, C. (1926). *Psychological types* (H. G. Baynes, Trans.). London: Routledge & Kegan Paul.

Kunst-Wilson, W. R., and Zajonc, R. B. (1980). Affective discrimination of stimuli that cannot be recognized. *Science*, 207, 557–558.

Lewicki, P. (1985). Nonconscious biasing effects of single instances on subsequent judgments. *Journal of Personality and Social Psychology*, 48, 563–574.

Lewicki, P. (1986a). *Nonconscious social information processing*. New York: Academic Press.

Lewicki, P. (1986b). Processing information about covariations that cannot be articulated. *Journal of Experimental Psychology: Learning, Memory, and Cognition*, 12, 135–146.

Lewicki, P., Czyzewska, M., and Hoffman, H. (1987). Unconscious acquisition of complex procedural knowledge. *Journal of Experimental Psychology: Learning, Memory, and Cognition*, 13, 523–530.

Lewicki, P., Hill, T., and Bizot, E. (1988). Acquisition of procedural knowledge about a pattern of stimuli that cannot be articulated. *Cognitive Psychology*, 20, 24–37.

Mace, W. M. (1974). Ecologically stimulating cognitive psychology: Gibsonian perspectives. In W. Weimer and D. Palermo (Eds.), *Cognition and the symbolic processes*. Hillsdale, NJ: Erlbaum.

Marcel, A. J. (1983). Conscious and unconscious perception: Experiments on visual masking and word recognition. *Cognitive Psychology*, 15, 197–237.

Mathews, R. C., Buss, R. R., Stanley, W. B., Blanchard-Fields, F., Cho, J.-R., and Druhan, B. (1989). The role of implicit and explicit processes in learning from examples: A synergistic effect. *Journal of Experimental Psychology: Learning, Memory, and Cognition*, 15, 1083–1100.

Miller, G. A. (1967). *The psychology of communication*. New York: Basic Books.

Millward, R. B. (1981). Models of concept formation. In R. E. Snow, P. A. Frederico, and W. E. Montague (Eds.), *Aptitude, learning, and instruction: Cognitive process analysis*. Hillsdale, NJ: Erlbaum.

Millward, R. B., and Reber, A. S. (1968). Event-recall in probability learning. *Journal of Verbal Learning and Verbal Behavior*, 7, 980–989.

Millward, R. B., and Reber, A. S. (1972). Probability learning: Contingent-event sequences with lags. *American Journal of Psychology*, 85, 81–98.

Milner, B., Corkin, S., and Teuber, H. L. (1968). Further analysis of the hippocampal amnesic syndrome: 14-year follow-up study of H.M. *Neuropsychologia*, 6, 215–234.

Moeser, S. D., and Bregman, A. S. (1972). The role of reference in the acquisition of a miniature artificial language. *Journal of Verbal Learning and Verbal Behavior*, 11, 759–769.

Morgan, J. L., and Newport, E. L. (1981). The role of constituent structure in the induction of an artificial language. *Journal of Verbal Learning and Verbal Behavior*, 20, 67–85.

Neisser, U. (1976). *Cognition and reality*. San Francisco: Freeman.

Nelson, K. (1986). *Making sense: The acquisition of shared meaning*. New York: Academic Press.

Nisbett, R. E., and Wilson, T. D. (1977). Telling more than we know: Verbal reports on mental processes. *Psychological Review*, 84, 231–259.

Palmer, S. E. (1978). Fundamental aspects of cognitive representation. In E. Rosch and B. B. Lloyd (Eds.), *Cognition and categorization* (pp. 259–303). Hillsdale, NJ: Erlbaum.

Polanyi, M. (1958). *Personal knowledge: Toward a post-critical philosophy*. Chicago: University of Chicago Press.

Posner, M. I., and Keele, S. W. (1968). On the genesis of abstract ideas. *Journal of Experimental Psychology*, 77, 353–363.

Posner, M. I., and Keele, S. W. (1970). Retention of abstract ideas. *Journal of Experimental Psychology*, 83, 304–308.

Pylyshyn, Z. (1979). Validating computational models: A critique of Anderson's indeterminacy of representation claim. *Psychological Review*, 86, 383–394.

Pylyshyn, Z. (1980). Computation and cognition: Issues in the foundation of cognitive science. *The Behavioral and Brain Sciences*, 3, 111–169.

Rathus, J., Reber, A. S., and Kushner, M. (1988). *Implicit learning and anxiety levels*. Unpublished ms.

Reber, A. S. (1965). *Implicit learning of artificial grammars*. Unpublished master's thesis, Brown University.

Reber, A. S. (1966). *A perceptual learning analysis of probability learning.* Unpublished doctoral dissertation, Brown University.

Reber, A. S. (1967). Implicit learning of artificial grammars. *Journal of Verbal Learning and Verbal Behavior, 77,* 317–327.

Reber, A. S. (1969). Transfer of syntactic structure in synthetic languages. *Journal of Experimental Psychology, 81,* 115–119.

Reber, A. S. (1976). Implicit learning of synthetic languages: The role of instructional set. *Journal of Experimental Psychology: Human Learning and Memory, 2,* 88–94.

Reber, A. S., and Allen, R. (1978). Analogy and abstraction strategies in synthetic grammar learning: A functionalist interpretation. *Cognition, 6,* 189–221.

Reber, A. S., Allen, R., and Regan, S. (1985). Syntactical learning and judgment, still unconscious and still abstract: Comment on Dulany, Carlson, and Dewey. *Journal of Experimental Psychology: General, 114,* 17–24.

Reber, A. S., Kassin, S. M., Lewis, S., and Cantor, G. W. (1980). On the relationship between implicit and explicit modes in the learning of a complex rule structure. *Journal of Experimental Psychology: Human Learning and Memory, 6,* 492–502.

Reber, A. S., and Lewis, S. (1977). Toward a theory of implicit learning: The analysis of the form and structure of a body of tacit knowledge. *Cognition, 5,* 333–361.

Reber, A. S., and Millward, R. B. (1965). Probability learning and memory for event sequences. *Psychonomic Science, 3,* 431–432.

Reber, A. S., and Millward, R. B. (1968). Event observation in probability leaning. *Journal of Experimental Psychology, 77,* 317–327.

Reber, A. S., and Millward, R. B. (1971). Event tracking in probability learning. *American Journal of Psychology, 84,* 85–99.

Rescorla, R. A. (1967). Pavlovian conditioning and its proper control procedures. *Psychological Review, 74,* 71–80.

Rescorla, R. A. (1988). Pavlovian conditioning: It's not what you think it is. *American Psychologist, 43,* 151–160.

Rosch, E., and Lloyd, B. B. (1978). Representations. In E. Rosch and B. B. Lloyd (Eds.), *Cognition and categorization* (pp. 213–215). Hillsdale, NJ: Erlbaum.

Roter, A. (1985). *Implicit processing: A developmental study.* Unpublished doctoral dissertation, City University of New York.

Roy, F. A. (1982). Action and performance. In A. W. Ellis (Ed.), *Normality and pathology in cognitive functions.* New York: Academic Press.

Rumelhart, D. E., and McClelland, J. L. (Eds.) (1986). *Parallel distributed processing.* Cambridge, MA: MIT Press.

Scarborough, D. L., Cortese, C., and Scarborough, H. S. (1977). Frequency and repetition effects in lexical memory. *Journal of Experimental Psychology: Human Perception and Performance, 3,* 1–17.

Scarborough, D. L., Gerard, L., and Cortese, C. (1979). Accessing lexical memory: The transfer of word repetition effects across task and modality. *Memory & Cognition, 7,* 3–12.

Schacter, D. L. (1987). Implicit memory: History and current status. *Journal of Experimental Psychology: Learning, Memory, and Cognition, 13,* 501–518.

Schacter, D. L., and Graf, P. (1986). Effects of elaborative processing on implicit and explicit memory for new associations. *Journal of Experimental Psychology: Learning, Memory, and Cognition, 12,* 432–444.

Schlesinger, I. M. (1982). *Steps to language: Toward a theory of native language acquisition.* Hillsdale, NJ: Erlbaum.

Seamon, J. G., Brody, N., and Kauff, D. M. (1983). Affective discrimination of stimuli that are not recognized: Effects of shadowing, masking, and cerebral laterality. *Journal of Experimental Psychology: Learning, Memory, and Cognition, 9,* 544–555.

Seamon, J. G., Marsh, R. L., and Brody, N. (1984). Critical importance of exposure duration for affective discrimination of stimuli that are not recognized. *Journal of Experimental Psychology: Learning, Memory, and Cognition, 10,* 465–469.

Shallice, T., and Saffran, E. (1986). Lexical processing in the absence of explicit word identification: Evidence from a letter-by-letter reader. *Cognitive Neuropsychology, 3,* 429–458.

Smith, E. E., and Medin, D. L. (1981). *Categories and concepts.* Cambridge, MA: Harvard University Press.

Strauss, M. E., Weingartner, H., and Thompson, K. (1985). Remembering words and how often they occurred in memory-impaired patients. *Memory & Cognition, 13,* 1507–1510.

Warrington, E. K., and Weiskrantz, L. (1982). Amnesia: A disconnection syndrome? *Neuropsychologia, 20,* 233–248.

Weiskrantz, L. (1986). *Blindsight.* New York: Oxford University Press.

Westcott, M. R. (1968). *Toward a contemporary psychology of intuition.* New York: Holt, Rinehart & Winston.

39 Attention, Automatism, and Consciousness

Richard M. Shiffrin

A good part of my professional life has been spent exploring data and theory bearing on two related dichotomies: short-term memory/long-term memory, and attention/automatism. These dichotomies provide the most obvious choices for the mapping of consciousness to concepts in cognition. But, up to now, I have largely refrained from discussing these possibilities. This chapter focuses on the possible relation between attention and consciousness.

The relations between attention, automatism, and consciousness were a fundamental concern of the field of philosophy/psychology around the turn of the century (e.g., James 1890, 1904; Pillsbury 1908), and have remained an abiding topic of interest in these fields to the present day, probably because attention heightens consciousness of events and thoughts. Indeed, there is little question that when a high level of attention is directed at some event, the event will be high in consciousness, and when something is at a high level of consciousness, it will tend to hold attention. Numerous books and articles on this theme appear on a regular basis (not always expressing novel views). However, the test of the relation lies not in the cases that are clear and uncontroversial, but in the possibility that it will clarify the ambiguous cases that abound in our cognitive systems.

This chapter is concerned with the degree to which we can implicate attentive processing in consciousness, and conversely, identify automatic processing with the failure to reach consciousness. One of the difficulties of drawing such analogies lies in the fact that both conceptual frameworks are imprecisely defined, though for somewhat different reasons. In the case of consciousness, we have a large collection of subjectively defined experiences and perceptions constituting a rather fuzzy, and not necessarily internally consistent, representation. In the case of attention, we have an enormous empirical and theoretical literature, but no one theory comes very close to encompassing the range of findings, and there is no accepted method for distinguishing attentive and automatic processing.

To elaborate on this last point, there is no simple and generally agreed on set of necessary or sufficient conditions, and no generally accepted empirical test for distinguishing attentive and automatic processes. Such criteria are sometimes available in certain restricted paradigms, like search tasks. The difficulty of generating universally applicable criteria may well be rooted in the fact that the concepts of attention and automatism are omnipresent in cognition, producing an enormous range of domains of applicability. Nonetheless, in order to make headway, a collection of empirical and theoretical criteria for distinguishing attentive and automatic processing are outlined. These criteria were presented in Shiffrin (1988; see also Shiffrin and Schneider 1977). The criteria are rooted in a theory distinguishing the two forms of processing. Though controversial in a number of features, this conceptual framework is shared in large part by researchers going back to the 1800s, and accepted (with some caveats concerning details) by a majority of present theorists. With these criteria as a reference point, this chapter discusses relations with the more subjectively defined concept of consciousness. Keep in mind that consciousness is often viewed through the window of attention. Something unconscious before attentional focus may become conscious during or after. This fact is in good part responsible both for the appeal of the attention/consciousness mapping, as well as for the conceptual fuzziness of the consciousness construct.

A framework for human information processing in terms of automatic and attentive components is described elsewhere (Shiffrin 1988), and thus it is not repeated here. The crucial point is

Table 39.1
Criteria for distinguishing attentive and automatic processing

Capacity and resource use
Preparation
Rate of learning and unlearning
Depth of processing
Modifiability
Effort
Precedence and speed
Awareness and consciousness
Control and intentionality
Level of performance and parallel processing
Memory effects

that tasks are never wholly automatic or attentive, and are always accomplished by mixtures of automatic and attentive processes. With this in mind, consider the following criteria for distinguishing attentive from automatic processing, and the relation of each to consciousness. The criteria are listed in table 39.1.

Capacity and Resource Use

It is generally agreed that attentive processing requires a share of limited processing resources, and a process that does not require resources is automatic.

In practice, resource demands are often measured by interference tasks, because two attentive processes must interfere with each other in any situation where system capacity is stressed and the subject tries to employ both. In addition, the subject can eliminate the interference at will, by choosing to stop one or the other process. On the other hand, a process is surely automatic if interference is produced despite attempts to drop or ignore the process.

It is not clear how this distinction bears on consciousness. Consciousness is surely limited in content and extent, but the boundaries are not

clearly obtainable. Nonetheless, we might ask whether stimuli that produce interference can be defined as conscious, and stimuli that do not as unconscious.

As discussed elsewhere (e.g., Klinger and Greenwald 1995; Merikle, Joordens, and Stolz 1995), there are numerous demonstrations that stimuli failing to reach awareness, in the sense that they cannot be identified and perhaps cannot even be reported to have been present, nevertheless produce quite measurable effects on performance, both positive and negative. In visual studies, such stimuli are typically produced by using a brief presentation followed by a mask. In such cases, the apparently below-threshold stimulus can produce priming effects on the response to an immediately following stimulus, both positive and negative, depending on the relation between the prime and target. We would not want to define such primes as conscious.

There is another sense in which this correspondence may fail: Stimuli at an unattended location (or on an unattended perceptual dimension) can call attention automatically and indirectly produce interference as a result (e.g., a sudden loud noise). Such calls for attention can be trained, as shown by Shiffrin and Schneider (1977) and MacCleod and Dunbar (1988), and are often found in vision when one part of a display is quite perceptually different from all the other parts of the display, as summarized by Yantis (1993).

Certainly, automatic processes that call attention produce effects on consciousness. For example, in the study reported by Shiffrin and Schneider (1977), subjects were instructed to attend to two characters along a specified diagonal of a four-character display, ignoring the irrelevant diagonal. When characters previously trained to attract attention appeared on the ignored diagonal, subjects had an increased tendency to miss targets on the relevant diagonal. This performance criterion suggests subjects were unaware of the missed targets. However, the implications for consciousness are not this clear: It is possible that subjects would claim they were continuously conscious of the stream of characters on the relevant diagonal, but simply had too little time to carry out the decision operations necessary to produce a correct response. Although we did not systematically ask subjects for verbal reports, such reasoning is bolstered by the fact that in some of our studies using successively presented displays of four characters, many targets were missed at speeds of 800 ms per display, which is sufficient time to read aloud the four characters in each display. This occurred in conditions where the subject had to search each display for multiple targets. Most people would be reluctant to claim lack of conscious perception of the displayed characters in such a situation. This example also illustrates the oft-made point that consciousness of one quality of a stimulus (in this example, the name of a character) may take place when consciousness of other qualities does not occur (in this example, the classification of the character as a target).

Conversely, one can ask whether some process not requiring capacity (measured by a lack of interference) is necessarily unconscious. Here the answer is surely no. For example, Schneider and Fisk (1982) showed that the requirement to detect a well-trained target on one diagonal of a four-character display did not interfere with an attention-demanding simultaneous task: detection of not-so-well-trained targets on the other diagonal of the display. This situation differs from the previous one because this result occurred at times when the well-trained target did not actually appear. The subjects were conscious of the characters on the automatic diagonal at some level, and were effectively classifying them as nontargets, so the lack of interference seems a poor or arguable criterion for consciousness. More generally, and loosely, would anyone want to claim lack of consciousness of the ordinary evident contents of our sensory environment (say

the visual field) because some task was not hindered (e.g., if we perform an auditory task as well with eyes open as closed)?

To look at this another way, it is clear that many stimuli of which we are aware do not produce interference in a given task setting (e.g., the shape of the CRT screen used to display the materials for an experiment). Thus, the claim would have to be that in order to be classified as conscious, such stimuli would have to be able to produce interference in some as-yet-unknown task to be discovered later. Aside from the issue of appropriate experimental controls and interpretation if interference in a task variation were to be found, it is obvious that such a criterion for consciousness could never be of any practical help, because one could never be sure that the set of possible task variations with which to demonstrate interference had been exhausted. Thus, any very tight link between an interference criterion and the presence or absence of consciousness would not seem possible.

Nonetheless, there are incontrovertible links between attention and consciousness: Not only do both exhibit capacity limitations, but these limitations are positively correlated. If nothing else, the positive correlations are produced by the fact that attention can be used to move information into and out of the forefront of consciousness. So we may be unaware of a minor leg pain, or our breathing, when attending to an interesting article (perhaps not this one), become quite aware of these when asked to attend to them, and become unaware again when our attention returns to another domain. We can probably not say much more than this: Despite a great deal of research, the measurement of attentional capacity is still in its infancy, and questions concerning as whether there are one or several capacity limits are still being investigated. To draw precise comparisons between attentional capacity and the even more imprecise notion of limited consciousness is not presently possible.

Preparation

Suppose a process is triggered by some stimulus event. If the presence of that event triggers the process, but no attentive process or preparation is required to do so, the process might be considered automatic (e.g., a reaction to a sudden noise). However, such a process or its immediate consequences might well be entered into consciousness, so a process judged to be automatic by this criterion could not be classified unconscious, at least without splitting millisecond-length hairs.

Rate of Learning and Unlearning

Automatic processes are generally learned gradually, or, if already learned (or innate) are difficult (or impossible) to unlearn or modify. Attentive processes can be turned on or off at the whim of the subject. Although cases exist where learning of an automatic process can occur very quickly (e.g., a learned aversion to a smell/taste that produces an immediate and strong, noxious, systemic reaction), subsequent unlearning will generally be slow. Earlier (Shiffrin 1988) I considered the rate of learning criterion without giving sufficient consideration to rate of unlearning. At the present time, the slow rate of unlearning provides the single best criterion for an automatic process.

There are certainly interesting relations between rate of learning and consciousness. It seems that extensive consistent practice often produces two correlated effects: a learning of an automatic behavior, and a tendency for the behavior to drop out of consciousness. For example, when learning to drive, pressing the accelerator may require attention and consciousness, but after learning this activity takes place automatically and unconsciously. The relation between attention and consciousness early in learning is at least partly due to the fact that

high degrees of attention do tend to produce consciousness (as described earlier). Training sometimes produces an automatic call for attention, and an associated conscious perception, but sometimes does not produce an automatic call for attention. In this latter case, there does seem to be a tendency for the trained stimuli to return to the state of consciousness that held prior to training. This state will be less conscious than that during early stages of training, and will sometimes be unconscious.

Nonetheless, rates of learning and unlearning are almost useless as a basis for defining conscious activity. First, as a practical concern, such a criteria defines the status of a process in terms of its past history of training, or the possible future course of training, rather than its present behavior. It would be difficult, to say the least, to define something as unconscious because its use in some task is unlearned slowly. More important, such criterion cannot be applied universally: Some automatic processes are learned quickly (e.g., the taste aversion reaction used in the previous example), and may or may not be conscious. Even slowly learned automatic processes sometimes involve calls to attention and hence may produce consciousness. Conversely, slow unlearning is not helpful, because the process unlearned slowly may or may not have been conscious (in part depending on whether a call to attention had been involved).

Depth of Processing

One view of processing of sensory inputs limits automatic processing to informationally and temporally early stages of processing. Such automatic processing is sometimes termed *pre-attentive* because it is followed by attentive selection. Often the automatic processing in such theories is limited to primitive and simple sensory features. This is not the prevailing view; the evidence points to automatic and attentive processing coexisting in parallel, with sometimes deep processing of information without attention. Nonetheless, does either view provide a useful approach to the problems of consciousness?

The pre-attentive approach would presumably lead one to ascribe unconsciousness to early stages of sensory processing, and consciousness to late stages of processing. However, a great deal of research has shown that a stimulus can be presented, processed to late or deep stages, and yet be out of the subject's awareness. A typical study involves the presentation of a word masked so quickly that subjects are near chance reporting whether anything had been presented, and hence is not in consciousness. Yet the meaning of the masked word can affect responding to a related word that is subsequently presented, showing that the word had been processed to a deep level (as in the work by Marcel 1983a,b; Fowler, Wolford, Slade, and Tassinary 1981; see also Merikle 1992). In other cases, the processing can be shown to be deep because abstracted qualities of a stimulus are involved, as when reports of "liking" a presented stimulus are modified by the masked stimulus (e.g., Niedenthal 1990).

Such findings show that deep processing does not always produce conscious awareness. Can it be argued that shallow enough processing never leads to awareness? This question is either unanswerable, or the answer is clearly no. We are often conscious of very early stages of stimulus processing, such as color or shape, even if the awareness itself arises at subsequent levels of processing. We also know that very primitive sorts of processing can attract attention (see Yantis 1993 for one summary). Making this whole issue even more difficult to assess is the role played by attention in studies of subliminal perception: Although studies show that stimuli can affect subsequent behavior even when their existence is not reported, in most studies the subject is trying to attend to the region in sensory space containing the subliminal stimulus. It would be useful to have well-controlled studies examining the subliminal effects of stimuli appearing in sensory regions that are not attended.

A correlated question concerns stimuli that do appear to enter consciousness: At what level are they conscious? An extreme example is, say, a fragmented picture of a Dalmatian: Before the "dog" appears to perception, one is conscious of patches of black on a white background; afterward, one has a fairly clear visual percept of a particular dog, as well as the awareness of the lower level patches. (This could be viewed as another case of the early/late dichotomy, the "dog" entering consciousness late, whether due to automatic processing, attentive processing, or both.) Thus, the depth or level of processing does not provide a good basis for predicting what is and is not conscious.

The distinction between consciousness and automaticity, and how these vary with depth of processing, is perhaps best brought out by research carried out to study perceptual unitization (Lightfoot and Shiffrin 1992). This study trained initially novel characters, characters whose encoding required attention, to the point where they were encoded automatically as single, integral, units. But, how do these training changes affect conscious perception? To make the point clearly, the tasks and results are described in some detail.

Examples of the stimuli are shown in figure 39.1. Subjects were trained to search for such stimuli in a visual field of many similar stimuli. We arranged matters so a conjunction of at least two features was required to carry out each comparison (each pair of stimuli shared exactly one feature). The rate of search is initially slow, as shown in figure 39.2.

Each character comparison takes about 250 ms, as if three separate comparisons (one for each feature) were occurring at rates of about 80 ms per feature. Over 35 sessions of training (800 trials per session), search rates dropped to 60–70 ms per comparison, as if a single com-

Set 1a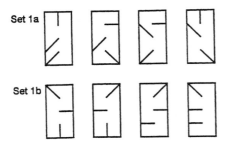

Set 1b

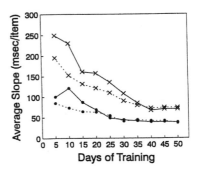

Figure 39.1
Examples of novel stimuli used in the search task of Lightfoot and Shiffrin 1992. One row of stimuli was used in blocks of trials under varied mapping training: One stimulus was chosen at random in each trial to be the target, and the others were distractors. The other row was used in blocks of trials with consistent mapping training: One stimulus was always the target, and the others always distractors.

Figure 39.2
Slopes (given as ms/display item) of the function relating search time to display size for the stimuli and conditions illustrated in figure 39.1, as a function of days of training.

parison per character was taking place. After training, response time showed the typical linear functions with 2:1 slope ratios (and consistent and varied training made no difference). Thus, at asymptote, the usual limited-capacity, terminating, attentive, search was being utilized. The improvement shown in figure 39.2 was not just due to generalized practice. When *S*s were switched after training to a new set of conjunction stimuli, sharing no features with the first set, their performance reverted back to that seen at the outset of training. What had been learned was specific to these stimuli.

We carried out a number of investigations to establish that the operative features for these stimuli, before training, were the three internal line segments. For example, we transferred to stimuli that did or did not contain the external frames, and were able to show that conjunctions of the frames and the internal segments were not being used. Quite a number of transfer tasks were then carried out to demonstrate that after training a comparison involved a single holistic step. For example, the task was switched to one

still using trained stimuli, but with the target sharing no feature with any distractor. For three sessions or so, performance did not change at all, as if single holistic comparisons were being used, suggesting the training was not specific to particular pairings, and that performance depended only on the use of integral units as stimuli. The fact that performance did not improve suggests that single feature search, which produces better performance in this situation, is not being utilized at the outset of the transfer trials. If subjects had been using feature comparisons prior to transfer, rather than holistic unit comparisons, then there should have been an immediate improvement. The idea, then, is that training produced automatic classification of such stimuli as particular known units.

Suppose we now ask, what is in consciousness when a display of known or unknown characters is presented to the visual field? If trained characters are presented, then the coded, unitary, representations are likely in consciousness, starting from a point relatively early in processing, even when attention is not aimed at a particular stimulus, analogous to what we imagine to be the case when alphabetic characters are presented. If untrained characters are presented, as is the case early in training, then the case may be more ambiguous. Consider first the encoding given to the target presented prior to the trial; it has not yet been trained and thus is almost certainly encoded (slowly) with attentional processing. It seems likely that such attentional processing produces a perception of the target as a unit. This view is suggested by the work, say, of Ankrum and Palmer (1991), who showed that unknown figures acted as unitary objects in short-term memory for the purpose of part–whole matching.

Consider next the encoding of the (untrained) display characters early in training. They appear to the subject's consciousness to be unitary characters, or wholes. However, the evidence collected suggests they are compared feature by feature—that what is conscious are separate features placed together in a particular configuration rather than a single unit. This distinction is not obvious to the subject, and only shows up in the observed behavior. In one sense this does no more than provide another demonstration of the failure of the attentive–automatic distinction to map onto the concept of consciousness. Looked at another way, however, the result suggests that researchers in consciousness must carefully specify the "level of awareness" of the stimuli that appear to be conscious.

In summary, depth of processing does not provide a promising vehicle for distinguishing consciousness from unconsciousness (just as depth of processing should not be used as a criterial attribute for distinguishing automatic and attentive processes; e.g., Shiffrin 1988). Because unaware stimuli can produce fairly deep processing as measured by subsequent responses to other stimuli, deep processing can be unconscious. Conversely, shallow processing can at least sometimes be conscious, although it is generally not possible to be sure whether one is aware of the processing itself, or of the attention to the results of the processing.

Modifiability of Automatic Processing

As discussed earlier, automatic processes are either difficult to learn, or to unlearn, or both. Perhaps all automatic processes can only be unlearned quite slowly. However, the degree of response that is engendered in such cases, at a given level of learning, is often modifiable through the application of attention. Interpretation of such findings is made difficult because we generally do not know what subprocesses are being affected by attention. Thus, modifiability of processing is not of much use in distinguishing automatic from attentive processing. For similar reasons, this criterion could not be of help if applied to the question of consciousness.

As a theoretical point, however, one might ask: What would be the relation of modifiability of component processes to consciousness, assuming that techniques were available to assess at a fine enough grain of analysis the automaticity of component processes? Presumably, we would learn that automatic component processes were sometimes slow to develop and always difficult or slow to modify. Would those processes be unconscious and, conversely, the remaining components conscious? I rather doubt this would be a useful view because consciousness is likely a quality characteristic of macroevents rather than microprocesses. A good example is found in memory search (e.g., Sternberg 1966), one of the tasks for which information about the status of component processes is available. There is good reason to believe that in memory search tasks where targets and distractors exchange roles from trial to trial, the comparison stage is an attention-demanding process (e.g., Schneider and Shiffrin 1977). This conclusion is based on the high slopes of the search function. In fact, the inconsistent mapping prevents automatization of this stage, judging from the fact that the slopes do not decrease with practice. However, other components of the task (perhaps such as the

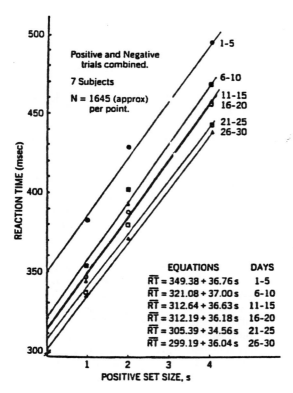

Figure 39.3
Mean response time as a function of positive set size, as a function of days of training, using varied mapping memory search. From Kristofferson 1972. © 1972 by Canadian Psychological Association. Reprinted with permission.

manual response) do improve with practice, because the intercept of the search function drops. These components are undoubtedly becoming increasingly automatic. These slope and intercept results are nicely illustrated by Kristofferson (1972), as indicated in figure 39.3. On the other hand, consistent mapping leads to a lowering of slopes, probably due to what Schneider and Shiffrin (1977) called the development of automatic categorization. Although the automatization of memory search is certainly accompanied by a considerable reduction in perceived effort

and task difficulty, it does not seem that the task itself is any less conscious to the subject. The general problem is that these changes and lack of changes in automaticity of the component processes are not reflected in changes in task consciousness. Memory search happens quite rapidly and consciousness of the component processes does not seem to be available to the subject.

Of course, the import of these results goes beyond the specific issue of modifiability. The fact that components of a task can vary in degree of automaticity without affecting consciousness provides a compelling reason to doubt the analogy between attention/automatism and conscious/unconscious.

Effort

Attentive processing is sometimes said to be *effortful*, a concept relating in part to the notions of capacity limitations (see Kahneman 1973). In the attempts to use this concept as a criterial measure for distinguishing automatic and attentive processing, one runs into some major problems: first, the issue of finding an appropriate method to measure effort. One approach is to define effort by subjective report. This approach does not map onto the consciousness dimension particularly well, as illustrated by the memory search findings discussed in the previous section. More simply, we often seem aware of things that do not require effort, such as the contents of the visual or auditory environment. Another approach defines effort in terms of capacity utilization: Effortful activity should reduce capacity to carry out simultaneous tasks. In other words, effort is defined functionally through observations of interference. A major problem with this approach has been discussed earlier: Automatic processes can call attention, thereby producing interference, and producing what may seem to be effortful results.

Additional problems arise when trying to use effort to classify states of consciousness. Is effort required to produce consciousness? I suspect almost everyone would answer no, in part because of a belief that automatic processing can be used to enter information into consciousness. Other questions relating to this issue could be raised (e.g., Does maintaining information in consciousness require effort?). It is doubtful that the edges and measures of consciousness are clearly enough defined to answer such questions.

Precedence and Speed

More often than I would like to admit, researchers have proposed or assumed implicitly that automatic processes are faster that attentive processes, and precede attentive processes in time and processing order. This is a misconception caused largely by the fact that attentive processes tend to be spread out in time (due to limited capacity), so an automatic process operating in parallel has a speed advantage. However, for any given automatic process operating in a task in which the processing load is low, attentive processing can operate as efficiently, or more efficiently. Schneider and Shiffrin (1977) gave many demonstrations of this point in the context of visual and memory search tasks. For example, with a load of one item, attentive search (produced by varied mapping) results in performance measured in response time and accuracy as good as, or better than, the performance seen in automatic search (produced by consistent mapping). One would expect such demonstrations to be even more evident in cases where the automatic process is not so well learned, but the subject induced to utilize it anyway, perhaps by the presence of a dual task (e.g., see the early stages of training in the study of Schneider and Fisk 1982).

Regardless of the value of the processing speed criterion for distinguishing automatic from attentive processing, one can ask whether processing speed is related to consciousness (e.g., Are fast thoughts unconscious, and slow ones conscious?). If it becomes possible to define these terms well enough to permit investigation, then this will prove to be a question worth pondering.

Awareness and Consciousness

We need not dwell on this criterion because it is the subject of this chapter. Shiffrin (1988) did not try to distinguish these terms when considering possible criteria for distinguishing automatic from attentive processing. Although other authors (e.g., Dulany 1997; Johnson and Reeder 1997) discuss the difference between awareness and consciousness, I have not found such a distinction helps to establish an analogy between attention/automatism and either awareness/unawareness or conscious/unconscious.

Control and Intentionality

When a process operates on the basis of preset parameter values and/or parameter values set by the environmental input, it may be characterized as automatic; if the parameter values are set by choice of the subject, then the process may be characterized as attentive. This has not proved a useful criterion in practice, partly because the environmental stimuli generally include the results of prior attentive processes, partly because automatic processes can call attention, and partly because some attentive processes operate so quickly that moment-to-moment control is unlikely.

The relation to consciousness is even less clear. Control of behavior is sometimes conscious and sometimes unconscious (e.g., walking vs. mountain climbing). Also, the process of controlling behavior, and controlling attention, is sometimes conscious and sometimes not (e.g., moving visual attention systematically across a field in a visual search vs. attention moving to a location containing a sudden evident movement).

Level of Performance and Parallel Processing

Level of performance was discussed earlier (in the section "Precedence and Speed") and therefore it need not be repeated here. This section points out that consideration of parallel versus serial processing does not help us make an appropriate distinction in either the attentive or consciousness domain.

There can be no doubt that much automatic processing is limited, even if parallel in character: To take an obvious example, two different stimuli may each be trained to call for attention automatically, but a limitation will appear if both stimuli appear simultaneously, one to the right and one to the left of fixation. Sometimes parallel processing produces an advantage for automatic processing, but not always (as discussed in an earlier section). Attentive processing is limited in capacity, but not necessarily serial in character. Thus the distinction between parallel and serial processing does not map well onto the distinction between automatic and attentive processing.

It is not evident how one asks whether consciousness is serial or parallel in character. Thoughts high in consciousness often seem serial, probably because they are associated with language, but at other times consciousness seems parallel, as when we attend to the visual scene before us. So the distinction between parallel and serial processing does not seem to map well onto the distinction between the conscious and unconscious.

Memory Effects

One can discourse at length on possible links between consciousness and memory, on the identification of short-term memory with conscious thought, on the possible consciousness of information in very short-term sensory memories, on whether one should assess the presence of memories using implicit or explicit tests, and on ways to distinguish memory from conscious perception. Such questions would be the subject of some other work (e.g., see Jacoby, Yonelinas, and Jennings 1997). For the moment, consider only the possibility that attentive processes can be identified because they invariably leave a residue that can be found in explicit, episodic, memory tests, whereas automatic processes may not necessarily leave a memory trace that can be found in explicit memory tests, and/or may always leave a trace that can be found in implicit memory tests.

One key question, then, is whether or not one can be certain that attentive processes leave explicit memory traces, in at least some sort of memory (we know that retrieval failure, amnesias, and forgetting can occur, so that a memory at one point in time may be missing at another). This is not easy to answer, especially for stimuli near or below threshold, or stimuli embedded in massive amounts of other information. So this criterion is not used in practice to distinguish automatic from attentive processes.

The relation to consciousness is not very straightforward. The subliminal perception literature is concerned with demonstrations that unaware stimuli affect memory only on implicit tests. We might therefore ask: Is attention necessary to produce explicit memory? This is not established, because attention is typically given in at least small amounts to all stimuli in the perceptual surround; thus, we really know little about the memorial fate of unattended stimuli, whether tested implicitly or explicitly.

A second key question is whether or not implicit memories can occur without attention, and if so, do they always do so? The subliminal attention literature does not tell us, because the subject is trying to attend to the sensory region containing the subliminal stimulus. A rather different approach is found in the process-dissociation technique of Jacoby and his colleagues (e.g., Jacoby et al. 1997). Although impressive indirect evidence has been collected in many studies that one component of storage is automatic and perhaps unconscious, and results in information storage accessible through implicit tests, all the studies occur in situations where attention is certainly being given at study to the stimuli in question. The same point makes it difficult to say much about consciousness and unconsciousness: At the time of storage, the stimuli are certainly given conscious processing. At the time of implicit test, the subject is some-

times clearly unaware that the test stimulus had been studied, but it is not clear whether this is always the case. It is also clear that one could not use a positive indication of memory using an implicit test to infer whether original storage had been carried out using attention.

In summary, there is no good case for relating the distinction between attentive and automatic processing to that between the conscious and unconscious. Despite the positive correlation between attention and consciousness, the mapping between the two conceptual frameworks is quite poor. This conclusion in no way detracts from the strong positive correlation between these frameworks, and it would be interesting in some other setting to explore or model the nature of the connection. Steps in this direction can be seen, for example, in the work by Jacoby et al. (1997).

References

Ankrum, C., and Palmer, J. (1991). Memory for objects and parts. *Perception and Psychophysics, 50*(2), 141–156.

Dulaney, D. E. (1997). Consciousness in the explicit (deliberative) and implicit (evocative). In *Scientific approaches to consciousness: The XXVth Carnegie Symposium on Cognition* (pp. 179–212). Mahwah, NJ: Lawrence Erlbaum Associates.

Fowler, C. A., Wolford, G., Slade, R., and Tassinary, L. (1981). Lexical access with and without awareness. *Journal of Experimental Psychology: General, 110,* 341–362.

James, W. (1890). *The principles of psychology.* New York: Holt.

James, W. (1904). Does "consciousness" exist? *Journal of Philosophy, Psychology and Scientific Methods, 1*(18), 477–491.

Johnson, M. K., and Reeder, J. A. (1997). Consciousness as meta-processing. In *Scientific approaches to consciousness: The XXVth Carnegie Symposium on Cognition.* Mahwah, NJ: Lawrence Erlbaum Associates.

Kahneman, D. (1973). *Attention and effort.* Englewood Cliffs, NJ: Prentice-Hall.

Klinger, M. R., and Greenwald, A. G. (1995). Unconscious priming of association judgments. *Journal of Experimental Psychology: Learning, Memory, and Cognition, 21,* 569–581.

Kristofferson, M. W. (1972). Effects of practice on character classification performance. *Canadian Journal of Psychology, 26,* 54–60.

Lightfoot, N., and Shiffrin, R. M. (1992). On the unitization of novel, complex visual stimuli. In *Proceedings of the 14th Annual Conference of the Cognitive Science Society* (pp. 277–282). Hillsdale, NJ: Lawrence Erlbaum Associates.

MacLeod, C. M., and Dunbar, K. (1988). Training and Stroop-like interference: Evidence for a continuum of automaticity. *Journal of Experimental Psychology: Learning, Memory, and Cognition, 14,* 126–135.

Marcel, A. (1983a). Conscious and unconscious perception: An approach to the relations between phenomenal experience and perceptual processes. *Cognitive Psychology, 15,* 238–300.

Marcel, A. (1983b). Conscious and unconscious perception: Experiments on visual masking and word recognition. *Cognitive Psychology, 15,* 197–237.

Merikle, P. M. (1992). Perception without awareness: Critical issues. *American Psychologist, 47,* 792–795.

Merikle, P. M., and Joordens, S. (1997). Measuring unconscious influences. In *Scientific approaches to consciousness: The XXVth Carnegie Symposium on Cognition.* Mahwah, NJ: Lawrence Erlbaum Associates.

Merikle, P. M., Joordens, S., and Stolz, J. A. (1995). Measuring the relative magnitude of unconscious influences. *Consciousness and Cognition: An International Journal, 4,* 422–439.

Niedenthal, P. M. (1990). Implicit perception of affective information. *Journal of Experimental Social Psychology, 26,* 505–527.

Pillsbury, W. B. (1908). *Attention.* New York: Macmillan.

Schneider, W., and Fisk, A. D. (1982). Concurrent automatic and controlled visual search: Can processing occur without resource cost? *Journal of Experimental Psychology: Learning, Memory, and Cognition, 8,* 261–278.

Schneider, W., and Shiffrin, R. M. (1977). Controlled and automatic human information processing: I. Detection, search, and attention. *Psychological Review, 84,* 1–66.

Shiffrin, R. M. (1988). Attention. In R. A. Atkinson, R. J. Herrnstein, G. Lindzey, and R. D. Luce (Eds.), *Stevens' handbook of experimental psychology: Vol. 2. Learning and cognition* (pp. 739–811). New York: Wiley.

Shiffrin, R. M., and Schneider, W. (1977). Controlled and automatic human information processing: II. Perceptual learning, automatic attending, and a general theory. *Psychological Review, 84,* 1127–1190.

Sternberg, S. (1966). High-speed scanning in human memory. *Science, 153,* 652–654.

Yantis, S. (1993). Stimulus-driven attentional capture. *Current Directions in Psychological Science, 2*(5), 156–161.

Ellen J. Langer and Lois G. Imber

In a recent article (Langer and Benevento 1978) it was argued that decrements in performance may result from negative interpersonal contextual factors, like labels that connote inferiority relative to another person (e.g., assistant vs. boss), regardless of the outcome one experiences. It was suggested that, if salient, the inferior label may lead the individual to an erroneous inference of incompetence, resulting in performance decrements.[1] This effect was termed self-induced dependence. It is self-induced in that individuals who are given low status labels relative to other people, for example, may draw unnecessary inferences from those labels that they then generalize to new situations without any external inducement to do so. Self-induced dependence was originally proposed in contrast to learned helplessness (see Seligman 1975) where a perception of incompetence is clearly externally induced through prior exposure to uncontrollable aversive outcomes.

If people become dependent on labels when performing tasks with which they have had a good deal of prior experience, as was the case in the Langer and Benevento studies, one might assume that they would be even more vulnerable with respect to tasks with which they have had little practice. However, recent research on the "mindlessness of ostensibly thoughtful action" (Langer 1978, 1979; Langer, Blank, and Chanowitz 1978; Langer and Newman 1979) suggests that the reverse may occur. That is, repeated experience with a task actually may *increase* an individual's vulnerability to an experience such as being provided with a label that connotes inferiority.

When an individual first approaches a task she/he is necessarily attentive to the particulars of the task. With each repetition of the task, less and less attention to those particulars is required for successful completion of that task. As "mindlessness" is achieved, the components of the task may drop out or coalesce to form a whole. Learning, then, in a sense is learning what elements of the task may be ignored (see Langer 1978). Repeated practice with the task as a whole rather than with the individual parts may lead to a strange turn of events. The person who has overlearned the task, the expert, may be in a position of knowing that he/she can perform the task, without any longer knowing *how* he or she performs it, that is, without knowing the steps or components that make up the performance. If external factors like labels then led the individual to question his or her competence on these overlearned tasks, the individual would have difficulty supplying information about the solution process as evidence of competence and could erroneously infer incompetence.

The present research was designed to assess this relationship between amount of task experience and vulnerability to an inferior label.

In Phase 1 of the paradigm used, baseline measures are taken as pairs of subjects individually perform a task successfully. In Phase 2 subjects perform a different task together, with one in the role of a "worker" and the other as the "boss." In Phase 3, subjects return to the original task. To test the relationship between vulnerability to external factors like labels and amount of task experience, task experience was also varied in the present investigation. In Phase 1 subjects either were given an opportunity to overlearn a novel task or were given only a moderate amount of practice with that task. In Phase 2, a no practice group was introduced, and all subjects performed a second task under one of three labeling conditions (assistant, boss, no label). In Phase 3 all subjects returned to the original task. A curvilinear relationship between the amount of practice and susceptibility to labels connoting relative inferiority was predicted. Since the vulnerability is presumed to be a function of people losing sight of the intervening steps of the task, it was expected that individuals who had no prior task experience and those for whom the task had become overlearned would show the performance decrement in the inferior label conditions. However, it was predicted that since moderate practice groups would be necessarily attentive to the components of the target task, they would not show the decrement.

Experiment 1

The first study employed a 3×3 design where the variables of interest were label (no label, assistant, boss) and amount of practice (no practice, moderate practice, overpractice).

Method

Subjects

One hundred twenty-six adults were recruited from Boston and New York airport lounges to participate in a study concerned with developing methods to improve task performance. Since there were far more women at the airports than men, either waiting for their own planes or for the departures or arrivals of friends and relatives, we recruited only females.[2] They were informed that for our research we needed people to perform different tasks for us, individually and in pairs. Once one subject agreed to participate in the study, a second subject, a stranger to the first, was recruited to be her partner. Thus all subjects were run in pairs, and there were 14 subjects per cell. The experiment was conducted by one female and five male experimenters. Experimenters who administered the tasks were blind to the label assignment.

Task

A novel task was employed so that both extremes of task experience, no practice and overpractice, could be compared. It was also necessary for the task to have several parts so that it could be determined whether, as predicted, overpractice results in obfuscation of the task components. To this end a coding task was devised that involves translating English sentences into a different language where every letter is represented by a corresponding symbol and number. Letters were alphabetically arranged in groups (two groups of nine and one of eight letters); each group had a different symbol (a triangle, circle, or square), and each letter in each group had a number from one to nine (eight). (Punctuation marks had only symbols, rather than symbols and numbers). For example, the letter A had as the corresponding symbol a triangle and the number 1, and the letter J had as the symbol a circle and the number 1. Subjects were given computer cards on which sentences had been typed, and they were required to transcribe these sentences into the new language. They were to write the symbol below each letter and circle the corresponding number in the column for each letter of the sentence. This task permits subjects to chunk the various elements into fewer and fewer units, thereby facilitating overlearning with repeated practice.

For practical purposes it was important to determine a criterion for overpractice in advance. To that end, the task was pretested on 18 adult female subjects. Subjects were instructed to inform us when they felt as though they could perform the task automatically. After coding two sentences, none of the subjects had overlearned the task. After coding six sentences all subjects were performing the task at least 50% more quickly and more accurately than they had done originally: they no longer referred to the coding reference sheet, their performance reached an asymptote, and by this time they had all reported that the task had become automatic. Therefore, the overpracticed group in the present experiment was given six practice sentences, whereas the moderate practice group was given only two.

Procedure

In Phase 1 of the study subject pairs were randomly divided into three groups: no practice, moderate practice, and overpractice on the coding task. After the task was explained and demonstrated, the overpracticed group was instructed to code six sentences, the moderate practice group was instructed to code two sentences, and the no practice group did no coding. This group went immediately to Phase 2 of the study. Each sentence appeared on a separate computer card. While one experimenter administered this task, a second experimenter, who was hidden from view, recorded the amount of time it took subjects to complete the first sentence. The amount of time it took to complete this sentence and the number of errors made were used as baseline measures for the moderate and overpractice groups.

All subjects now participated in Phase 2 of the research. They were each told that the task they would be asked to perform next required a joint effort: One of them would be the assistant and one the boss (one-third of the pairs performed this task without labels indicating relative status). Subjects were asked to examine a picture and find objects that were hidden in it. One person was to find the objects, and the other was to record the objects found. To control for task effects, for half of the pairs the boss did the searching and the assistant the recording, whereas for the remaining half the tasks were reversed. The experimenter handed subjects the envelope with instructions to place the task materials back in the envelope when they had finished. At that time she/he would return to give them further instructions. In the meantime she/he was purportedly going to recruit two more subjects. Subjects chose a slip of paper from the envelope that indicated both whether they would be in the boss, assistant, or no label condition and what their task would be. When the second experimenter, whose presence was unknown to the subject, observed that the task had been completed she/he signaled the first experimenter, who then returned to complete the final phase of the experiment and thus was blind to the labeling condition.

In the last phase of the study, subjects were told that an individual effort rather than a joint effort again was required. All subjects then were asked to code another sentence. (This, of course, was the first sentence for the no practice group.) Once again the second experimenter timed their performance. Both speed and accuracy served as dependent measures.

At the end of the task, all subjects were asked to complete a brief questionnaire. They were asked to make a list of the components of the task. Specifically, subjects were told, "To do the coding task, certain steps were involved. For instance, you had to look at the letter to be coded. Please list as many steps as you can think of which you used to perform the coding task." When subjects completed this questionnaire, they were completely debriefed.

Results and Discussion

Before examining the effects of the label, it is important to verify group comparability at the start of the experiment. Therefore scores for all of the groups that performed the prelabel task were compared. As expected, the analysis of variance of prelabel scores (the amount of time it took subjects to code the first sentence and the number of errors they made) showed no differences among the six groups for which this measure was relevant: the no label, assistant, and boss, moderate practice and overpracticed groups. Speed scores ranged from 5.56 to 5.89, and accuracy scores ranged from 2.36 to 3.07.

It was expected, however, that differences would emerge on postlabel measures. A 3 (No Label, Assistant, Boss) × 3 (No Practice, Moderate Practice, Overpractice) analysis of variance was performed on both the speed and accuracy of the postlabel coding task. The analysis performed on speed scores yielded highly significant main effects for practice, $F(2, 117) = 133.82$, $p < .001$, and label, $F(2, 117) = 25.05$, $p < .001$, as well as a highly significant interaction, $F(4, 117) = 8.96$, $p < .001$.[3] Table 40.1 presents

Table 40.1

Mean number of minutes to complete the postlabel coding task

Condition	Label		
	Assistant	No label	Boss
No practice	7.10$_a$	5.50$_b$	5.40$_b$
Moderate practice	4.50$_b$	4.54$_b$	4.72$_b$
Overpractice	4.40$_b$	3.28$_c$	3.10$_c$

Note: All cell $ns = 14$. Cells bearing different subscripts are significantly different from each other: subscript a differs from all other cells at $p < .001$, and subscript c differs from b cells at $p < .05$.

Table 40.2

Mean number of errors made in postlabel coding task

Condition	Label		
	Assistant	No label	Boss
No practice	5.35$_a$	2.36$_c$	2.00$_c$
Moderate practice	1.64$_c$	1.93$_c$	1.50$_c$
Overpractice	4.93$_b$	1.07$_c$	1.14$_c$

Note: The cell bearing subscript a differs from those bearing subscript c at $p < .001$. Cell b differs from cells c at $p < .01$. Cells a and b do not differ from each other.

the mean number of minutes it took to complete the postlabel coding task for each group. A Newman–Keuls test was performed to understand better the relationships among these means and thus the nature of these significant effects. Cells bearing different subscripts in the table are significantly different from each other by this test. As may be gleaned from the table, subjects in the no practice/assistant condition took longer to complete the postlabeling task than did subjects in all other conditions ($p < .001$), whereas subjects in the no label/overpracticed and boss/overpracticed group performed most quickly ($p < .05$). It is, of course, not surprising that subjects who have had enough practice to overlearn a task perform that task faster than subjects do who have had very little practice. What is interesting is the comparison of the assistant and the no label groups within each practice condition. As predicted, the label *assistant* had a detrimental effect for both the no practice and the overpracticed groups but had no effect on the moderate practice condition.

The analysis performed on the number of errors made by subjects on this task yielded very similar results. The analysis yielded highly significant main effects for practice, $F(2, 117) = 12.02$, $p < .001$, and for label, $F(2, 117) = 35.85$, $p < .001$, and a highly significant interaction, $F(4, 117) = 9.80$, $p < .001$. The mean number

of errors made by each group is shown in table 40.2. A Newman–Keuls test revealed that the means that bear different subscripts in the table are significantly different from each other. Once again, in contrast to the moderate practice group, the label assistant seems to have had a detrimental effect for both the no practice and overpracticed groups. Subjects in both of these groups made at least twice as many errors as subjects in the other conditions did. Although 86% of the overpracticed/assistant group showed a decrement in performance from Phase 1 to Phase 3, only from 7% to 14% of the remaining relevant groups performed more poorly, $\chi^2(2) = 6.08$, $p < .05$.

Although decrements were expected on the target task, subjects in the assistant groups should not show a decrement in performance on the intervening hidden objects task because this task has been defined as one that is consistent with their label, that is, it is an "assistant" task. The analysis of these scores in fact revealed no group differences. This further suggests that the assistant subjects took the task as seriously as the other groups of subjects did (see Langer and Benevento 1978).

Although subjects in all assistant groups apparently took the label seriously, only those who had no prior experience with the target task and those who were overpracticed on it were debilitated by the inferior status label. It was hypothesized and indeed found that this label would not adversely affect subjects in the moderate practice group. This group was expected to be protected from the potentially debilitating effects of the label because their experience with the task, in contrast to that of the no practice group, has taught them the components of the task, but not so much as to obscure them, in contrast to the overpracticed group. After performing the last task, subjects in each group were asked to list all the components or steps they could think of that were involved in performing the coding task. The mean number of steps listed for the no practice and overpracticed groups ranged from 3.07 to 4.43, whereas the means for the moderate practice groups ranged from 6.07 to 6.21. The analysis of variance revealed a significant main effect for the amount of practice, $F(2, 117) = 30.95$, $p < .001$. A Newman–Keuls test confirmed the prediction: The moderate practice groups listed significantly more steps than either the no practice or overpractice groups, which were not different from each other.

If the components of a task do indeed become obscured with practice, this should be revealed not only in the number of steps listed but also in their degree of specificity. To assess this, each subject's list was rated by two blind raters ($r = .92$) on a 10-point scale that ranged from very specific to very global. The analysis revealed a significant group difference, $F(2, 123) = 31.38$; $p < .001$. A Newman–Keuls test showed that the responses of the no practice group ($M = 7.5$) were equivalent in specificity to the overpracticed group ($M = 6.57$) and that both were far more global than the moderate practice group ($M = 3.6$). Typical steps listed by the no practice and overpracticed groups were "Look at the letter and write in the code." In contrast, typical steps listed by the moderate practice group included such things as "Fill in the circle if it is a capital and check for punctuation." Of course, the more specific one is, the more steps

are available to be listed. Therefore, although both measures are interesting, they should not be viewed as independent of one another.

The performance decrements found in this study occur for tasks for which the components are not salient (a novel task and an overlearned task), after the individual had experience in an inferior status position. Therefore one may ask whether these decrements can be prevented by making components of the task salient. The next study was undertaken with this in mind.

Experiment 2

This experiment used basically the same paradigm as that described in experiment 1. Subjects in Phase 1 performed a task successfully, in Phase 2 they performed a different task in one of three label conditions (assistant, no label, boss), and in Phase 3 they returned to the original task. In this experiment, however, only one level of practice was used. A task was selected that subjects, in all likelihood, already performed automatically. To see whether the debilitation could be prevented by making components of the task salient, task components were listed for half of the subjects before they began Phase 1 of the experiment. Thus the study utilized a 2 (Components Salient/Nonsalient) × 3 (Assistant, No Label, Boss) design. It was predicted that relative to the no label condition, the assistant condition would show a decrement in performance, and the boss condition would either show an increment in performance (as in the Langer and Benevento 1978 study) or would be equivalent to the no label group (as in experiment 1 reported in this paper). It was predicted, however, that the performance decrement would occur only in the components-nonsalient condition. That is, it was expected that the salience manipulation would prevent the debilitation, since these subjects now would have a set of task components recently used and verified to supply as evidence if they questioned their ability.

Method

Subjects

Seventy-two adult females were recruited to serve as subjects from the lounges of Logan Airport in Boston. They were asked to participate in a study on developing educational methods where subjects would be asked to perform different tasks either individually or with another person. Once one subject agreed to participate, a second person, who was a stranger to her, was recruited to be her partner. Thus, as in experiment 1, subjects were run in pairs.

Task

The target task was a proofreading task. This was selected because it is a task that almost all literate people have performed—for example, when reading one's term paper for school, in reading over a letter before sending it, and so forth—and because it is a task where many rules may be employed without the individual's necessarily knowing what they are. That is, the individual can locate errors without being able to articulate why the error is an error. Two articles were chosen from popular women's magazines for this task. Their titles accurately reflect their content: One was entitled "Is your doctor overcharging you?" and the other was "Energy savers' guide." The articles were edited so that each contained 40 errors distributed evenly throughout each article. There were 13 spelling errors, 9 errors of capitalization, 12 punctuation errors, and 6 grammatical errors in each article.

Procedure

All subjects were initially told that one task found helpful for developing educational methods is proofreading.

Virtually everyone has done this task although they do not necessarily call it proofreading. For example, if you ever read over a paper for school before handing it in, you were proofreading. Or if you ever read over a letter you wrote before sending it to see if it said what you intended it to say, you were proofreading. Therefore we would like you to proofread a story for us.

Components-Salient Condition   For this condition the experimenter went on to say,

Most people can do this task even though they are not aware of just how they do it. That is, they are not always aware of the rules they are using. For instance, if you knew the word "susan" should be typed "Susan," you would be using the rule that the first letter of proper nouns is always capitalized. We would like you to make a list of *at least* three things which you would need to know in order to correct a story for errors.

After subjects completed their lists, they were told that we would like them to remember these rules when they read the story we were about to give them to proofread.

When you find an error, try to recall the rule you used, and then circle the error. You are only given 3 minutes to read the story, so do not expect to finish it. Most people who do this task can find six errors in 3 minutes. If you are able to do this, you should consider yourself successful at this task.

The time allotted for this task was intentionally brief in order to prevent overlearning of the components.

Components-Nonsalient Condition   Subjects in this condition were also told that proofreading is a task that most people can do. In addition, they were told,

In order to proofread a story for errors, you should at least glance at each word in the story to see if it is correctly written. For instance, if the word "susan" appeared, you would know it is an error because the word should read "Susan." First, we would like you to make a list of at least three ways in which proofreading is used. We would like you to read this story and circle any errors that you find. You are only given 3 minutes to read the story, so do not expect to finish it. Most people who do this task can find six errors in 3 minutes. If you are able to do this, you should consider yourself successful at this task.

Thus both groups were led to expect success on the task. Instructions encouraged both to pay attention to the story, both were given an example of an error, and both were asked to make task-relevant lists. The difference was that rules for determining errors were generated only by the components-salient group. The task was pretested on a similar group of subjects to ensure that all experimental subjects would be successful at the task, that is, that each subject would find at least six of the errors.

After subjects successfully completed this task, they were told that the second task required a joint effort. One person was to solve a cryptogram task while the other person used the stopwatch provided to keep track of the solution times. The cryptogram task consisted of four lists of five words each that were written in number form. Each number had a corresponding letter ($A = 1$, $B = 2$, and so on). The subjects' task was to transcribe the numbers into their alphabet equivalents with the use of a code. Two-thirds of the subject pairs from each of the two conditions described above were told that the task thus "required" someone to be the boss and someone to be the assistant. One-third of the subject pairs performed this task without reference to relative status (no label condition). Task effects were controlled for by varying the label assigned to the particular task (timing vs. solving). That is, for example, for half of the bosses the task was solving and for half the task was timing. After one subject in each pair had been asked to indicate the task she wanted to perform, the pair was informed which task was the boss task and which was the assistant task. Subjects worked together on the cryptogram task for approximately 5 min. and then were informed that their joint participation was concluded. All subjects then were asked to proofread another story. As in Phase 1 of the study, they were given 3 min. to locate as many errors in the story as they could. These scores, in comparison with the prelabel proofreading scores, comprised the primary dependent measure.

At the end of the proofreading task, subjects were asked to complete a brief questionnaire. They were asked to make a list of the components of the proofreading task. Specifically, subjects were asked to "make a list of rules that you know about writing which helped you to identify errors in the stories." The time it took each subject to make the list was recorded. When subjects had completed the questionnaire, they were completely debriefed.

Results

An analysis of the prelabel scores revealed no difference among the groups. Thus there was group comparability at the start of the experiment. Although the prelabel scores were equivalent across the groups (ranging from 13.33 errors found to 14.67), a very different picture emerges when one examines the postlabel scores. Table 40.3 shows the mean number of proofreading errors located by each of the six experimental groups. The analysis of these scores yielded a highly significant main effect for label, $F(2, 66) = 8.09$, $p < .001$, and a highly significant interaction, $F(2, 66) = 7.74$, $p < .001$.[4] A Duncan test was computed to reveal the nature of this interaction. As may be ascertained from the subscripts in the table, the major hypothesis of the study was supported. The components-

Table 40.3

Mean number of postlabel proofreading errors correctly located

| Condition | Label | | |
	Assistant	No label	Boss
Components salient	14.33_a	13.99_a	14.41_a
Components nonsalient	8.92_b	13.00_a	17.42_c

Note: All cell ns = 12. Cells bearing different subscripts are significantly different from each other: subscript b differs from all other cells at $p < .005$, and subscript c differs from all a cells at $p < .05$.

nonsalient group replicated the Langer and Benevento (1978) finding such that, relative to the no label condition, the assistant group showed a severe decrement in performance, whereas the boss group showed a facilitation effect. However, the salience manipulation was successful in wiping out the differences among the groups. The scores for the components-salient condition are virtually identical to the prelabel scores. The correlation for the components-salient groups between their performance on the prelabel and postlabel stories was .83. Similarly, the correlation between prelabel and postlabel stories for the nonlabeled subjects in the components-nonsalient group was .95. Although these groups found as many errors in the second story as in the first, the assistants in the components-nonsalient group found on the average 5.75 *fewer* errors in the second story. The bosses in this group found 2.67 *more* errors on the average than they had in the prelabel story.

Of those subjects in the components-nonsalient/assistant group, 92% showed a decrement from Phase 1 to Phase 3. In contrast to this only 25–33% of the remaining groups showed a decrement in performance. Both 2×2 comparisons are significant [salient/nonsalient by assistant/boss: $\chi^2(1) = 4.48$, $p < .05$; salient/nonsalient by assistant/no label: $\chi^2(1) = 3.89$, $p < .05$].

To test again that subjects who were labeled *assistant* took the task in Phase 2 seriously, scores for the intervening cryptogram task were compared. As predicted, there were no differences among the groups. Assistants solved the puzzles as quickly as the remaining groups. (Solution times ranged from 43.18 to 47.37 s).

Further evidence that the salience manipulation was responsible for restoring subjects to their prelabel performance comes from the number of rules subjects reported using in the proofreading task and the time it took them to compose this list. Subjects in the salience condition, if they were keeping the rules in mind while performing the task as instructed, should have

been able to list more rules more quickly than the components-nonsalient group could. The analysis of the number of components listed (salient $M = 3.56$ vs. nonsalient $M = 2.78$, $t = 2.98$, $p < .005$) and the analysis of time to compose these lists (salient $M = 44.56$ vs. nonsalient $M = 73.81$, $t = 6.39$, $p < .001$) suggest that this was the case.

One might argue that subjects' ability to generate components of the activity both before and after the task suggests that counter to the position presented here, the components are not inaccessible. However, although subjects in the components-nonsalient condition listed rules after the task, that does not mean that they used those rules (i.e., identified errors as a function of realizing why they were errors) while performing the proofreading task (see Dweck and Gilliard 1975). In fact, it is important to demonstrate that they did *not* use the rules, whereas the components-salient group *did*. To do this, the next analysis was conducted to see the relationship between the ability to list certain rules and the actual use of those rules. Since all subjects made a list at the end of the last proofreading task, this list was used for the first comparison. Table 40.4 shows the correlation coefficients for the type of rule listed by the proportion of errors found for each type of error. Correlation coefficients bearing asterisks are significant at $p < .001$. As may be seen in the table by looking at the diagonals, the relationship between listing and finding particular errors was significant for the components-salient group, but there was no such relationship for the components-nonsalient group. That is, for example, subjects who listed spelling found more spelling errors than subjects who did not list spelling in the components-salient condition, and this was not the case for the components-nonsalient group.

As may be seen in the top portion of Table 40.4, the correlations between rules listed at the beginning of the experiment and the proportion of errors found (these correlations are reported in parentheses in the table) are also significant

Table 40.4

Between-subjects correlation coefficients for rules listed at end of experiment (yes/no) by proportion of errors found

Type of rule	Errors found/total errors			
	1	2	3	4
Components-salient condition				
1. Spelling	.69* (.72)	−.40 (.08)	−.20 (−.08)	.22 (.15)
2. Capitalization	−.30 (.01)	.68* (.60)	−.01 (.15)	−.40 (−.32)
3. Punctuation	.00 (.14)	−.01 (−.10)	.67* (.70)	−.46 (−.49)
4. Grammar	.37 (.34)	−.05 (−.18)	−.34 (−.26)	.82* (.63)
Components-nonsalient condition				
1. Spelling	−.35	.07	−.13	.01
2. Capitalization	.09	−.13	.04	.14
3. Punctuation	−.05	.10	−.16	−.14
4. Grammar	.34	.13	.21	−.25

Note: All cell $ns = 36$. Numbers in parentheses represent correlations between rules listed at the start of the experiment by proportion of errors found.
*$p < .001$.

at $p < .001$. This strongly suggests that the salience manipulation was effective in providing subjects with rules to use while they performed the proofreading task.

To explore further the relationship between rules listed and errors found, a second correlational analysis was performed on *within*-subjects scores. This analysis yielded a coefficient that represented, for every subject, the relationship between rules listed and the proportion of errors of each type that were found. These correlation coefficients were then transformed into Z scores, and the resulting analysis yielded a significant effect for salience, $F(1, 66) = 71.12$, $p < .001$. The mean correlations between the types of rules listed and the types of errors found ranged from −.29 to −.01 for the components-nonsalient conditions and from .77 to .86 for the components-salient groups. Clearly there was a strong relationship between rules listed and the rules used for the components-salient group that was absent for the components-nonsalient group.

Discussion

Both experiments provide strong support for the assumption that overlearning may lead to increased vulnerability to labels that connote relative inferiority. In the paradigm used, the effect of the label reveals itself in the final phase of the experiments. Subjects in the second phase of both studies are performing what is deemed by the label *assistant* to be a low status task. There is no reason, therefore, for them to question their ability to perform it. However, the original and final tasks are not assistant tasks. To the extent that subjects accept the validity of the label, they may question their competence with regard to tasks that may now be perceived as psychologically inconsistent with that label. Such questioning will not necessarily have negative consequences, if the individual can convince himself or herself that he or she in fact can perform the task. This evidence must be lacking with respect to a novel or unfamiliar task. If, as the present studies suggest, overlearning results in the obfuscation of the individual components of the task, evidence also will be lacking in this case. Therefore only groups with moderate experience should be able to proceed with the task unhampered by the label. Experiment 1 showed this to be true. Performance decrements resulted after the label assignment for the no practice and the overpracticed groups but not for the moderate practice groups.

Since the overpracticed group was able to generate task components when asked to do so, it is important to consider why this information did not protect them from the label's influence. The present research suggests two reasons for this. First, the overpracticed subjects did not list very specific task components. One might reasonably assume that global knowledge of what a task consists of should not be very confidence inducing. If one wanted to teach the task to someone else, for example, these global components alone would be inadequate. Second, the untreated overpracticed group in experiment 2 showed no relationship between the steps generated and the steps they actually used in performing the task. Being able to list components that *could* possibly be used to complete a task should not be as confidence inducing as knowing steps that *were* experienced successfully.

The second experiment provides evidence that the decrement in performance that may occur on overlearned tasks may be prevented. It will be recalled that this experiment compared two overpracticed groups: a group that, except for the tasks used, basically was treated just as the overpracticed group in the first experiment had been and a second group for whom the components of the task were made salient. The performance decrement occurred again for subjects bearing the inferior label in the untreated group. Making the components of the task salient, however, apparently inoculated the comparison group of subjects against the potential effects of the label.

One may question how the salience manipulation in experiment 2 could have been effective in

light of the assumption, for which all of us can summon anecdotal support, that renewed attention to that which is overlearned is disruptive (cf. Kimble and Perlmutter 1970, Langer 1978). The salience manipulation made subjects attend to an overlearned task, yet their performance was not hampered. The reason for this is likely to lie in the fact that subjects were asked to generate steps necessary to perform the task *before* performing it. Subjects in the components-salient group showed a strong relationship between the components they generated initially and the components they attended to while performing the task, whereas subjects in the group left to their own devices (the components-nonsalient group) showed no relationship between the components they generated afterward and the components they attended to while performing the task. This suggests that the salience manipulation led subjects in some sense to follow a new set of rules for themselves. Therefore if they were approaching the task with a new set of rules (thereby changing the task to a nonoverlearned task), attention to those rules (which was revealed in the high correlation between the rules cited and the ones actually used) should not be disruptive. And of course performance on an overlearned task also would not be disrupted if it simply were performed automatically without bringing competence into question. The proficiency manifested by subjects in the overpracticed/no label and boss groups in experiment 1 bears this out. Thus although negative external factors like pejorative labels may be quite debilitating, they, of course, are not necessarily so. What about positive external factors? The data from the present studies do not permit any clear conclusions with respect to the label "boss." More research on situational and individual difference variables is necessary before any conclusions about positive labels can be drawn.[5]

In addition to exploring the potentially facilitating effects of positive external influences like labels, additional research is also required to understand more fully the relationship between particular task characteristics and performance debilitation of this sort. The present analysis would suggest that tasks that have only one step, tasks whose performance requires the articulation of steps (e.g., learning the alphabet), or tasks that are so complex as to preclude complete mastery would not render the individual vulnerable to external influences. Vulnerability may be evident for many, if not most, other tasks, however.

It is clear that overlearning is adaptive, since it frees limited attention to be paid elsewhere. It would seem from their daily interactions that most people in the world are aware that overlearning serves this function, since they appear to be constantly adding familiarity, predictability, and structure to their lives, which facilitate overlearning. While acknowledging the adaptive function mindlessness or overlearning may serve in freeing limited capacity, the present article supports previous work (Langer 1978, 1979; Longer, Blank, and Chanowitz 1978; Langer and Newman 1979; Langer 1981; Langer and Weinman 1979) in demonstrating the ways in which mindlessness may also be maladaptive.

Although the detrimental effects of overlearning may be pervasive, it is also likely that some subject populations are more susceptible to these effects than others are. For example, the elderly are a group who for many reasons (see Langer 1978, 1979, Note 1) probably have more experience with overlearned tasks than the nonelderly do. Children probably have more experience with no practice tasks relative to nonchildren. Thus these two groups should be most susceptible to external factors, such as pejorative labels, that may lead one to question one's competence. Although the groups may look similar, they are of course quite different in that the elderly can in fact do the tasks in question. Similarly, people who chronically occupy low status jobs are likely to be particularly susceptible. However, most interesting, perhaps, would be the inclusion of experts on this list.

Although one probably does not want to discourage overlearning or the attainment of mindlessness because of its general advantage in fast and efficient performance, educating people as to the potential side effects would seem fruitful. However, the present research suggests another, more direct way in which potential performance decrements may be prevented. Stated generally, focusing on process rather than on outcome may reduce vulnerability to debilitation of this kind.

Acknowledgments

This research was supported by a grant from the William F. Milton Fund of Harvard University and by Grant MH32946-01 from the National Institute of Mental Health to the first author.

The authors are grateful to Herb Kelman and Ross Rizley for their helpful comments and to Rob Rubin, Marty Richardson, Howard Botwinick, and Paul Levitt for their help in conducting the studies.

Notes

1. Other interpersonal factors that are hypothesized to result in unnecessary performance decrements include no longer performing tasks that others continue to perform, engaging in a demeaning task, or simply allowing someone else to help you.

2. Although the subjects in these studies were all females, there is no reason to assume that the results would not generalize to males. Further investigation is required before this can be determined conclusively, however.

3. Because subjects were run in pairs, there may be a loss of degrees of freedom. A more conservative test that uses the degrees of freedom based on the number of pairs within groups shows that each of the Fs in this study are still significant at the $p < .001$ level.

4. An analysis using the degrees of freedom based on the number of pairs within groups shows that this more conservative test lowers the p value for these measures to .01.

5. In the original Langer and Benevento studies, the label "boss" had a facilitating effect such that relative to the no label conditions, these groups performed significantly better. Although this was also true for experiment 2 in the present investigation, it was not true for the first experiment. Here subjects labeled *boss* within each level of practice were equivalent to the no label groups. The fact that the "boss" group across all four studies did not show a decrement in performance suggests that the majority of subjects in this condition are not questioning their ability to perform the task, for such questioning for the overlearned and no practice groups would reveal to them an inability to find evidence to support the label. If one goes back to the original studies (Langer and Benevento 1978), one finds that whereas the boss groups on the average performed better than the no label groups, the proportion of subjects who performed this way is the same for both groups. Although most subjects are unquestioningly accepting the label and trying to live up to it, it would appear that a few are not so accepting. The relative proportions from experiment to experiment of this latter minority group would determine whether the aggregate measures reveal equivalence, facilitation, or perhaps even debilitation.

References

Dweck, C. S., and Gilliard, D. Expectancy statements as determinants of reactions to failure: Sex differences in persistence and expectancy change. *Journal of Personality and Social Psychology*, 1975, *32*, 1077–1084.

Kimble, G., and Perlmutter, L. The problem of volition. *Psychological Review*, 1970, *77*, 361–384.

Langer, E. J. Rethinking the role of thought in social interaction. In J. Harvey, W. Ickes, and R. Kidd (Eds.), *New directions in attribution research.* Hillsdale, N.J.: Erlbaum, 1978.

Langer, E. J. The illusion of incompetence. In L. Perlmutter and R. Monty (Eds.), *Choice and perceived control.* Hillsdale, N.J.: Erlbaum, 1979.

Langer, E. J. *Old age: An artifact?* Washington, D.C.: National Research Council, 1981.

Langer, E. J., and Benevento, A. Self-induced dependence. *Journal of Personality and Social Psychology*, 1978, *36*, 886–893.

Langer, E. J., Blank, A., and Chanowitz, B. The mindlessness of ostensibly thoughtful action: The role of "placebic" information in interpersonal interaction. *Journal of Personality and Social Psychology*, 1978, *36*, 635–642.

Langer, E. J., and Newman, H. M. The role of mindlessness in a typical social psychological experiment. *Personality and Social Psychology Bulletin*, 1979, *5*, 295–298.

Langer, E. J., and Weinman, C. *Mindlessness, confidence, and accuracy.* Unpublished manuscript, Harvard University, 1979.

Seligman, M. E. P. *Helplessness.* San Francisco: Freeman, 1975.

41 The Neural Correlates of Consciousness: An Analysis of Cognitive Skill Learning

Marcus E. Raichle

Introduction

Two components of human conscious behaviour are *content* and *arousal* (Plum and Posner 1980). One of the great challenges of modern neurobiology is to identify the brain systems responsible for these components. As Damasio (1995) has recently stated "... knowing how [the brain engenders consciousness], to a considerable extent, requires that we first know where."

Much work points to systems ascending from the reticular core of the brainstem via the thalamus to the cortex as responsible for arousal or alert wakefulness (Steriade 1996a,b). We are much less certain, once alert wakefulness has been achieved, which cortical systems are responsible for the content of our consciousness. One of the difficulties in identifying these cortical systems is distinguishing them from those concerned with the many non-conscious cognitive, attentional and emotional processes that occur in support of our conscious experiences. Several approaches have been used.

One approach is to examine patients with lesions that deprive them of some aspect of their normal conscious experience. Typical of such an approach is the study of patients with blindsight (Weiskrantz 1986, 1997). Such patients, fully awake and otherwise alert, have lost the conscious perception of visual information presented to their blind hemifield. However, information entering the blind hemifield still influences behaviour. The inference to be drawn is that the area of the brain damaged by the lesion contributes to the content of conscious experience.

A second approach is to examine normal activities in which consciousness is transiently suspended. Francis Crick and Christof Koch have provided a recent review of this approach (Crick and Koch 1998). A typical experiment might involve an analysis of the suppression of conscious visual experience during eye movements or so-called saccadic suppression (Bridgeman et al. 1994). During saccadic suppression, visual perception is suspended yet information presented during this period of time influences behaviour. By identifying changes in the neural circuitry that occur when a conscious visual perception is momentarily suspended, one would hope to identify regions that contribute to conscious experience. Functional brain imaging with positron emission tomography (PET) has recently been used to identify changes during saccadic suppression in humans (Paus et al. 1995).

William James once aptly said, "habit diminishes the conscious attention with which our acts are performed" (James 1890). This comment captures the essence of a third approach. In some ways analogous to the second, this approach would be to identify the brain systems supporting a task when it is novel and effortful and compare these systems with those engaged when the task is routine and reflexive. The performance demands of such a task must necessarily be sufficient to require conscious attention (or "willed action"; Frith et al. 1991) for its initial performance. The brain systems unique to the novel state, if identified by comparison with the practised state, then become candidate systems necessary for conscious experience.

Because tasks involving motor as well as cognitive skills can be transformed from reflective, effortful tasks to reflexive, seemingly effortless tasks within a short period of time (Petersen et al. 1998) it is feasible to employ this third approach together with modern functional imaging techniques. We already know from such functional imaging studies in normal humans that this transformation is accompanied by dramatic changes in the underlying brain circuitry concerned with the task (Raichle et al. 1994). These transformations provide important insights into those brain systems concerned with conscious elements of naive task performance.

It is the purpose of this paper to explore the use of this approach in the context of a simple word-reading paradigm involving cognitive skill learning in normal human subjects. As will become apparent, the results present a complex picture of widely distributed change (both increases and decreases) in the activity of brain systems uniquely associated with naive task performance. The richness of the information provided should stimulate, as well as constrain, theories about brain systems serving consciousness.

The Paradigm

Studies of word reading have played a central role in functional brain-imaging studies of language over the past decade (for recent reviews, see Fiez and Petersen 1998, Posner and Pavese 1998). This work has benefited from the large amount of information already known about this skill (for review, see Rayner and Pollatsek 1989). These extant behavioural data on word reading have provided the basis for the design of many imaging experiments with both positron emission tomography (PET) and functional magnetic resonance imaging (fMRI).

Beginning in the 1980s, the author and his colleagues Steven E. Petersen, Michael I. Posner, Peter T. Fox, Julie Fiez, and Mark Mintun began their own imaging and behavioural experiments of word reading (Petersen et al. 1988, 1989, 1990; Raichle et al. 1994; Shulman et al. 1997b). It is from these published experiments that the data to be presented in this paper have in part been culled.

A key feature of the experiments to be discussed in this paper is their hierarchical design. In concert with most other functional imaging studies, the strategy here compares images of blood flow obtained with PET in a control state with those obtained when the brain is engaged in a task of interest (for a more detailed review of the strategy and its physiological basis see Raichle 1998) The five behavioural states include:

1. awake, alert with eyes closed performing no task

2. maintaining visual fixation on a television monitor containing only a fixation point

3. maintaining visual fixation on a television monitor while common English nouns are presented just below the point of fixation

4. reading aloud the nouns as they are presented

5. speaking aloud an appropriate use or verb for each noun as it is presented.

In the initial experiments (Petersen et al. 1988, 1989) the words were presented 60 times per minute and were on the monitor for 500 ms. In the later experiments (Raichle et al. 1994) the words were presented 40 times per minute, again for 500 ms each. English was the native language of the subjects and they were all skilled readers. The behavioural-state subtractions to be discussed in this paper include 2–1, 3–2, 4–3, 5–4 and $5_{\text{practised}} - 5_{\text{naive}}$.

Observations

Figure 41.1 illustrates, in horizontal sections, the areas of the brain that *increase* their activity (i.e., blood flow) in association with incremental increases in the complexity of a simple word-reading task. Figure 41.2 is a sagittal representation of the information in figure 41.1 and more clearly depicts the changes occurring along the midline in parietal and frontal cortices.

As shown in the first row of figure 41.1, opening the eyes and maintaining fixation on a small crosshair on an otherwise blank television monitor results in activation of the visual cortex compared with resting quietly with eyes closed. The images in the second row of figures 41.1 and 41.2 represent those additional areas of the brain that become active when common English nouns appear on the screen. The subjects' instructions

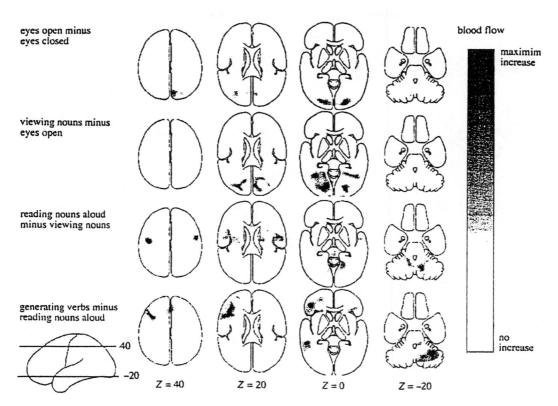

Figure 41.1
Four different hierarchically organized conditions are represented in these mean blood flow difference images obtained with PET. All of the changes shown in these images represent increases over the control state for each task. A group of normal subjects performed these tasks involving common English nouns (Petersen et al. 1988, 1989; Raichle et al. 1994). These horizontal images are oriented with the front of the brain on top and the left side to the reader's left. $Z = 40$ indicates millimetres above and below a horizontal plane through the brain marked $Z = 0$ (Fox et al. 1985).

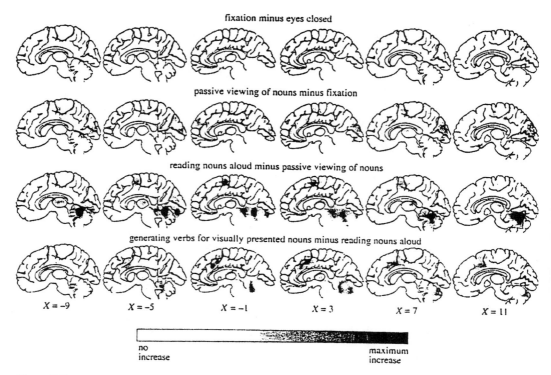

fixation minus eyes closed

passive viewing of nouns minus fixation

reading nouns aloud minus passive viewing of nouns

generating verbs for visually presented nouns minus reading nouns aloud

$X = -9$ $X = -5$ $X = -1$ $X = 3$ $X = 7$ $X = 11$

no increase   maximum increase

Figure 41.2
Data identical to those shown in figure 41.1 except that they are presented in the sagittal plane. These images begin 9 mm to the left of the midline ($X = -9$) and end 11 mm to the right of the midline ($X = 11$).

were simply to maintain fixation. Multiple areas within visual cortices become active when words are presented even though no specific processing of these words has been requested. Much effort has been devoted to an analysis of changes such as these (Fiez and Petersen 1998; Howard et al. 1992; Petersen et al. 1990; Price et al. 1994, 1996) but the results have so far been inconclusive.

The images in the third row of figures 41.1 and 41.2 reflect those areas of the brain associated with the motor aspects of reading words aloud. Not surprisingly, these include the primary motor cortices bilaterally, the supplementary motor cortex (best seen along the anterior midline in

figure 41.2) and the paramedian cerebellum. There was also prominent activity over Sylvian-insular cortices bilaterally (figure 41.1, row 3, $Z = 20$).

Finally, the images in the fourth row of figures 41.1 and 41.2 reflect those additional areas of the brain active during verb generation. These include the anterior cingulate cortex (best seen in figure 41.2), the left prefrontal cortex, the left temporal cortex and the right hemisphere of the cerebellum. The latter finding was a particular surprise because the subtraction producing this image had eliminated all of the motor aspects of speech production.

Reviewing all of the changes in figures 41.1 and 41.2 it is possible to appreciate those associated with the perfected skill of word reading (i.e., the first three rows) and those changes associated with the much more difficult and novel task of verb generation. It should be noted that all subjects performing verb generation initially found it difficult. This was reflected in a much slower voice onset latency and a failure to supply a verb for all nouns in order to keep pace with the task (Raichle et al. 1994).

The data presented in figures 41.1 and 41.2 illustrate nicely a hierarchical dissection of word reading in terms of regions of the brain increasing their activity in support of the component processes involved. In keeping with the thesis of this paper it would be attractive to assume that areas of the brain added in support of the verb-generation task (i.e., fourth row, figures 41.1 and 41.2) become candidates for those concerned with task-associated consciousness. However, before making such an assumption it is important to appreciate, rather more fully, additional changes taking place in brain organization not revealed in these two figures. To set the stage for a presentation of these changes, we should first examine one of the major criticisms of the subtractive logic leading to the images in figures 41.1 and 41.2.

The strategy employed in the experiments depicted in figures 41.1 and 41.2 was first introduced by the Dutch physiologist Franciscus C. Donders in 1868 (reprinted in Donders 1969). Donders proposed a general method to measure thought processes based on a simple logic. He subtracted the time needed to respond to a light (say, by pressing a key) from the time needed to respond to a particular colour of light. He found that identifying the colour of trun the light required about 50 ms. In this way, Donders isolated and measured a mental process for the first time by subtracting a control state (i.e., responding to a light regardless of its colour) from a task state (i.e., discriminating the colour of the light). It is this logic that is now applied in the experiments presented in figures 41.1 and 41.2.

One criticism of this approach has been that the time necessary to press a key after a decision to do so has been made is affected by the nature of the decision process itself. By implication, the nature of the processes underlying key pressing, in this example, may have been altered. Although this issue (known in cognitive science jargon as the assumption of pure insertion) has been the subject of continuing discussion in cognitive science, it finds a resolution in functional brain imaging, where changes in any process are directly signalled by changes in observable brain states.

Careful analysis of the changes in the functional images reveals whether processes (e.g., specific cognitive operations) can be added or removed without affecting ongoing processes (e.g., motor processes). This is accomplished by examining the data not only for areas activated during the course of a particular cognitive paradigm but also for those that become deactivated. An analysis of regional deactivations is presented in figures 41.3 and 41.4. Figure 41.4 is a sagittal representation of the information in figure 41.3 and more clearly presents changes occurring along the midline of the brain in the parietal and orbital frontal cortices. By examining the images in figures 41.1–41.4, together, a much more complete picture emerges of the dramatic changes taking place in the word-reading paradigm under analysis here.

Finally, to exploit fully the paradigm depicted in figures 41.1–41.4 for the purpose of identifying candidate regions of the brain concerned with task-related consciousness, it is important to assess the effect of practice on the regions uniquely recruited in the verb-generation task (row 4, figure 41.1). As we have previously demonstrated (Raichle et al. 1994) a brief period of practice on the verb-generation task results in a significant reduction in voice onset latency (i.e., subjects are able to respond more quickly when

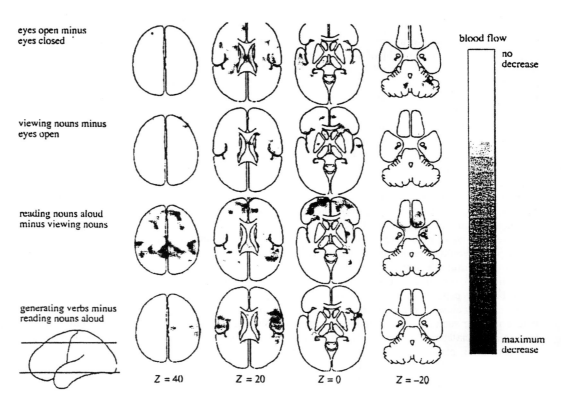

eyes open minus
eyes closed

viewing nouns minus
eyes open

reading nouns aloud
minus viewing nouns

generating verbs minus
reading nouns aloud

Z = 40   Z = 20   Z = 0   Z = -20

blood flow

no
decrease

maximum
decrease

Figure 41.3
Hierarchically organized subtractions involving the same task conditions as shown in figure 41.1, the difference being that these images represent areas of decreased activity in the task condition compared with the control condition.

they see the same noun on multiple occasions). In addition, responses become stereotyped, with the same verb being chosen each time a particular noun is presented. These changes in performance are associated with dramatic changes in the brain regions supporting task performance. The brain changes associated with practice are illustrated in figures 41.5 and 41.6. In these two figures it can be seen that the anterior cingulate cortex (and associated medial frontal cortices), the left prefrontal cortex (including the left as well as the right frontal operculum), the

left temporal cortex and the right cerebellum (not as well shown; see Raichle et al. 1994 for more details), which are all active during naive verb generation, return to their baseline level of activity.

Activity in the ventral medial frontal cortex, reduced in the naive condition (see figure 41.3, rows 3 and 4) is reduced even further after practice. Regional activity within Sylvian-insular cortices, active during word reading (figure 41.1, row 3, $Z = 20$) yet inactivated during naive verb generation (figure 41.3, row 4, $Z = 20$), are now

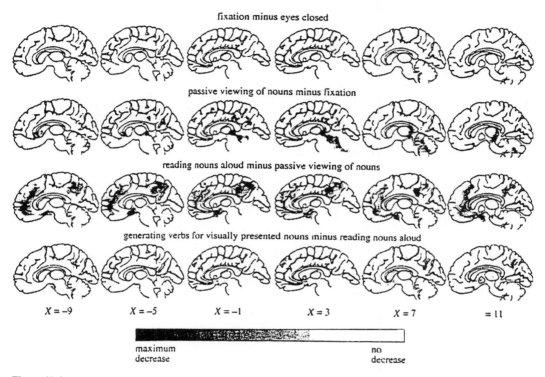

Figure 41.4
Data identical to those shown in figure 41.3 except that they are presented in the sagittal plane. The slices are positioned as noted in figure 41.2.

reactivated, especially on the right side. Finally, midline activity within the region of the precuneus and posterior cingulate cortex, reduced from baseline during naive word reading and verb generation (figure 41.4), increases in association with increased activity in visual cortices as the result of practice on the verb generation task (figure 41.6, row 2).

Discussion

The purpose of this exercise was to identify brain activity changes associated with task-related conscious behaviour. The strategy involved comparing PET images of blood flow change obtained in a novel reading task (verb generation) with those obtained during a well-practised task with identical perceptual and motor requirements (word reading). Additionally, comparisons were made between the naive and practised performance of the verb-generation task itself. On these comparisons, it was hypothesized that regions of the brain concerned with conscious task performance could be isolated and identified. Consistent with this hypothesis, regional changes in brain activity associated with conscious, effortful performance

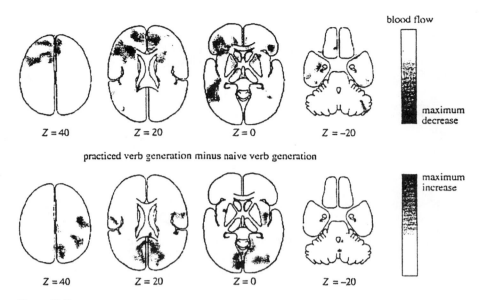

Figure 41.5
Changes in activity resulting from practice on the verb-generation task include decreases (top row) and increases (bottom row) in brain activity.

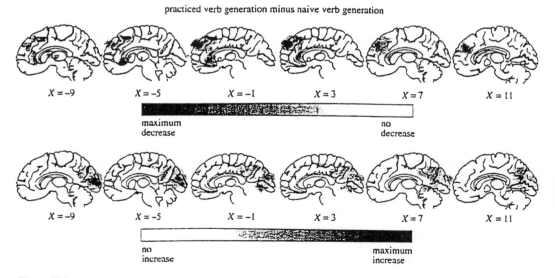

Figure 41.6
Data identical to those shown in figure 41.5 except that they are presented in the sagittal plane. The slices are positioned as noted in figure 41.2.

of the verb-generation task were identified. These included widely distributed regions of both increases and decreases in brain activity.

Regions of Increased Activity

When naive performance of the verb-generation task was compared with word reading, regions in the anterior cingulate cortex, left prefrontal cortex, left temporal cortex, and right cerebellar hemisphere were found to exhibit increased activity. Consistent with our hypothesis that these regions were uniquely associated with the conscious performance of this task, their activity ceased with practice that both produced significant improvement in performance and elicited stereotyped responses (Raichle et al. 1994). Further support for the unique role of these regions in conscious task performance was given by changes in the opposite direction in Sylvian-insular cortices bilaterally (Raichle et al. 1994). Thus, regions active during naive task performance disappeared with practice whereas regions within Sylvian-insular cortices bilaterally, inactive during naive task performance, become active with practice. The reciprocal nature of these changes make it unlikely that practice simply results in a more efficient use of regions always devoted to task performance.

Thus, reading aloud familiar words uses a pathway from word-perception regions to speech-production regions via regions in Sylvian-insular cortices bilaterally. Before practice, a completely different pathway connects word-perception regions to speech-production regions. How are we to think about these two pathways and the circumstances under which they are used? What is their relationship, if any, to the several instances of dual route ideas in speech production? What, if anything, does this have to say about conscious versus non-conscious behaviours?

To begin, the two routes revealed by our studies of the verb-generation task (Petersen et al. 1988, 1989; Raichle et al. 1994) would qualify for the two routes envisioned in Lichtheim's original theoretical formulation (Lichtheim 1885; McCarthy and Warrington 1984). Although probably first suggested by John Hughlings Jackson (Jackson 1874), the idea of two pathways was first advanced most clearly by Lichtheim, a Swiss neurologist. In an attempt to provide a conceptual framework for the various forms of aphasia reported by Broca, Wernicke, and others, he devised a scheme centred around three brain systems: an auditory word-form area concerned with the perceptual aspects of language; a centre for the motor representations of words, or a motor centre of speech; and a very distributed system "for the elaboration of concepts." As he envisioned it, information coming from the auditory word-form system could advance to the motor centre for speech either directly, or via the concept system. The latter route via the concept system he characterized as more 'conscious' and less fluent than the former (see Lichtheim 1885, p. 474). One pathway used a direct route from perception to production whereas the other used a more indirect route involving a distributed system of widely separated areas of the cerebral cortex.

In a very telling discussion Lichtheim (1885, p. 474) said:

[I]t would appear as if, in naming objects, the auditory representations once found had to react in consciousness. This variety of language is a much more "conscious" one than fluent speaking, in which *we are aware of the sense of what we are saying, rather than of every word we say* [italics added]. Under certain circumstances conversational language is carried on in a similar way to naming, as, for instance, when we use an idiom not quite familiar to us. Here we must seek the words by the complicated process just mentioned; the direct communication between concept and motor center without cooperation of sound-representation does not exist; the subconscious act of speaking is not yet possible. A greater psychical exertion is obviously required, and consequently more fatigue is entailed.

Lichtheim also envisioned, presciently, that acquisition of language occurred by imitation, "as observed in the child, and upon the reflex arc which this process presupposes." He went on to say "when intelligence of the imitated sounds is superimposed, a connection is established between the auditory center (for word-representations) and the part (of the brain) where concepts are elaborated."

Shallice and Norman (see Shallice 1988) formulate such issues more generally in terms of what they call contention scheduling and a supervisory attention system. Contention scheduling is the process by which selection is made of routine actions or thought processes. It is considered to be a decentralized process involving a very large but finite set of discrete programmes, hierarchically organized. Routine activities of our daily lives, such as driving a car back and forth to work, are managed in a non-conscious manner through contention scheduling (Lichtheim, I am sure, would have used spontaneous speech as an example). A particular set of programmes or schema has a level of activation dependent upon the triggering inputs it receives. Summarized nicely in the model of Norman and Shallice (Shallice 1988), this general idea has much support in the psychological literature (see summary discussion in Shallice 1988, p. 333). We would suggest that, in the verb-generation paradigm (Raichle et al. 1994), regions within Sylvian-insular cortices represent some of the regions involved in the process of contention scheduling as formulated by Norman and Shallice (Shallice 1988).

The above formulation of the functional organization of our mental lives is obviously incomplete. A moment's reflection suggests that, useful as they may be under a majority of circumstances, routine actions and thought processes are sometimes inappropriate, occasionally embarrassing and, even, potentially dangerous (Reason and Mycielska 1982). Therefore, there has to exist a means by which routine, reflexive behaviours and thoughts can be inhibited and replaced, either transiently or permanently, by more appropriate behaviours and thoughts

(Reason and Mycielska 1982). Norman and Shallice (Shallice 1988) postulate the existence of a second system to accomplish this, which they call the supervisory attention system.

The supervisory attention system of Norman and Shallice (Shallice 1988) provides a mechanism whereby elements or schemas within the lower-level contention-scheduling system for routine, reflexive behaviours and thoughts can be temporarily modified by activating or inhibiting particular elements within it. This facilitates coping with novel situations in which the routine selections are unsatisfactory. As Shallice (1988, p. 345) states, "the primary function of the Supervisory System is that of producing a response to novelty that is planned rather than one that is routine or impulsive." In a general sense this fits nicely with Lichtheim's concept of a centre for the elaboration of concepts.

Whereas Lichtheim (1885) and Norman and Shallice (1985) envisioned a superimposition of higher centres for the conscious guidance of behaviour over more routine, reflexive responses, our data would suggest a substitution of regions. In our example, regions guiding non-automatic or conscious speech acts are preferentially selected, by a process yet to be defined, over those areas concerned with automatic or non-conscious speech acts when a well-learned, reflexive response such as word reading is not appropriate. As a corollary, one must also envision circumstances in which the reverse is true: automatic responses are preferred and, hence, selected. As Sutherland (1996) has pointed out, "[w]hen confronted by a predator, it is surely better to climb a non-optimal tree than to be eaten while weighing the respective merits of different trees." The manner in which the brain is biased either way (i.e., towards or away from automatic behaviours) remains a most important and challenging question.

Lichtheim (1885) did not specify the neural correlates of his higher centres but he was quite clear that he did not believe them to be housed in a single area.

Though in the diagram point B [see Lichtheim (1885), diagram 1, p. 436] is represented as a sort of center for the elaboration of concepts, this has been done for simplicities sake; with most writers, I do not consider the function to be localized in one spot of the brain, but rather to result from the combined action of the whole sensorial sphere. Hence, the point B should be distributed over many spots. (Lichtheim 1885, p. 477)

Shallice and Norman (Shallice 1988) were much more specific in drawing attention to the role of the frontal lobe in their supervisory attention system. They reviewed extensive evidence, primarily from neuropsychology, showing that patients with frontal-lobe injury often act in an impulsive and reflexive manner as if they lacked a supervisory attention system.

Reviewing the evidence that has now been gained from functional imaging studies in normal subjects, one would have to conclude that both Lichtheim and Norman and Shallice were correct in anticipating brain regions uniquely involved in conscious, reflective behaviour as distinct from regions concerned with reflexive, habitual performance. It is clear from the data presented in this paper that multiple, widely distributed areas of the normal human brain, including the cerebellum, are involved in the performance of a novel speech-production act, as Lichtheim (1885) would have predicted. Likewise, it is also clear that the frontal lobe plays a role, although not an exclusive one, as Norman and Shallice (Shallice 1988) implied.

The experiments used for illustrative purposes in this paper and the work of Lichtheim (1885) focus specifically on language. The work of Norman and Shallice (Shallice 1988) as well as others (see, for example, Passingham 1993, Shiffrin and Schneider 1977) suggest that the issues involved transcend any single domain of human performance. What other evidence do we have? Are the general principles of neural organization emerging from imaging studies of language in normal subjects applicable to other domains of human performance, as others would suggest? Several examples are illustrative.

The data most directly comparable to the data reviewed in this paper are those from a PET functional imaging study of maze learning in strongly right-handed subjects by van Mier and colleagues (for a recent summary, see Petersen et al. 1998). In the maze-learning study, subjects, with their eyes closed, used a stylus to trace a complex maze etched on the surface of a bit pad. Two groups of subjects were studied: those who used their right hand and those who used their left hand to perform the maze task. Performance was recorded in the naive state, after a period of practice and then with a novel maze. The tasks were designed to parallel directly the design of the word-reading and verb-generation studies reviewed in this paper (Raichle et al. 1994). The objective of the maze-tracing study was to determine whether the differences in brain organization distinguishing naive and practised verb generation applied also to naive and practised maze tracing.

The results of the maze-tracing study clearly support the hypothesis that naive and practised performance of a task are distinguished by qualitative differences in brain organization. Independent of the hand used, some brain regions (right premotor cortex, right parietal cortex, and left cerebellum) were only active during a novel maze-tracing task. Other brain regions, in particular the supplementary motor cortex, were only active after practice. These are not the same areas that alternate activity when one compares naive and practised verb generation as illustrated in figures 41.5 and 41.6. Thus, when one thinks of a supervisory attention system (Shallice 1988) it must be envisioned as many regions (i.e., a distributed system) that are, importantly, task-specific.

Do we have other instances of this type of neural organization that distinguishes naive from practised performance? Two illustrative examples come to mind: acquisition of conditional motor associations in the monkey (Chen and Wise 1995a,b; Mitz et al. 1991) and song learning in birds (for review see Nottebohm 1991).

In a series of innovative experiments Wise and his colleagues (Chen and Wise 1995a,b; Mitz et al. 1991) studied conditional motor responses in the monkey, correlating unit activity in the cerebral cortex with performance. In these studies monkeys learned to saccade to specific targets in their visual field based on an association between the appearance of a visual cue and a particular target location. In the naive state the monkeys had to guess which locus in their visual field was indicated by a particular stimulus. Correct guesses were rewarded with juice. Performance was measured as the number of correct responses. As expected, performance improved with practice as the monkeys learned the correct association between target location and a particular stimulus. Unit recording of neuronal activity was performed in two cortical locations, the supplementary eye field (SEF) and the frontal eye field (FEF).

The results of these studies in monkeys show a remarkable parallel to the studies of word reading reviewed in this paper (Petersen et al. 1988, 1989; Raichle et al. 1994) and the maze-learning experiments discussed above (Petersen et al. 1998). In the SEF of the monkey, Chen and Wise (1995a) identified two populations of neurons that they termed, respectively, learning-selective and learning-dependent. The learning-selective neurons were only active in the presence of a novel cue. As the monkey learned the relationship between novel cue and its associated saccade location, activity in the learning-selective neurons ceased. The converse was true for the learning-dependent cells, which only became active as the monkey learned the correct association between target and cue. Similar classes of neurons were also found in the FEF but their proportions were much less (Chen and Wise 1995b). This difference suggested that the roles of the SEF and the FEF in conditional motor responses differed significantly.

Another illustrative example of alternative neural organizations underlying the performance of the same task is singing in birds such as canaries and zebra finches. Work by a variety of groups (Nottebohm 1991) has provided a detailed description of the areas within the songbird brain responsible for the acquisition and production of song. Central to this organization is an area known as the higher vocal centre or HVC. This area plays an important role in the acquisition and production of song. Two pathways emerge from the HVC. One pathway projects directly from the HVC to the robust nucleus of the archistriatum or RA. It is known as the "direct pathway." From the RA, fibres pass through a series of areas and lead to brainstem nuclei that control the vocal apparatus responsible for the actual production of song. The second pathway also leaves the HVC on its way to the RA but only arrives at the latter location after passing through a number of intermediate areas in the songbird brain. This is known as the "recursive loop." Thus, there are two pathways from the HVC to the RA: a short, direct one and the long, recursive one. The recursive loop is of particular interest because it is critical for song learning but not for the production of learned song. Alternatively, the direct loop is quite capable of supporting a song after the skill has been mastered but is not capable of supporting the learning process.

The similarities in neural organization supporting these very different tasks (verb generation and maze tracing in humans, conditional oculomotor responses in monkeys, and singing in birds) are striking. Brain regions as well as local populations of neurons active in naive task performance, especially where it competes with a more reflexive or habitual response to the same stimulus or instruction, are replaced by other brain regions and populations of neurons in the practised (i.e., routine, habitual, or reflexive) performance of the same task. From these data it seems possible to make a distinction between brain systems supporting conscious, reflective performance and brain systems supporting the non-conscious, reflexive performance of the same task. The general organizational principles underlying such a distinction appear to transcend species, levels of organization (general systems as well as local neuronal networks seem similarly organized) and tasks. The detailed organization surrounding individual tasks, however, appears to be unique to each task.

Many analyses might conclude at this point with comments about the potential role of brain regions that increase their activity during reflective or novel task performance. However, the data presented in this paper suggest that there is more to the story. While some regions of the brain increase their activity during novel task performance, others, just as dramatically, decrease their activity.

Regions of Decreased Activity

When subjects become actively involved in word reading, both reading aloud and verb generation, multiple regions across both cerebral hemispheres show a significant decrease in activity (figures 41.3–41.6). These include regions along the midline in the orbitofrontal cortex, posterior cingulate cortex and precuneus that have been noted to decrease in a wide variety of tasks (for details of a large meta-analysis of such changes see Shulman et al. 1997b). Characteristic of the experiments in which these particular decreases are regularly seen are ones in which subjects must actively process a visual stimulus. The control state is one in which the same stimulus is passively viewed. Additionally, decreases should also be noted in Sylvian-insular cortices bilaterally. These appear only in naive verb generation and not in word reading, where increases are observed (figure 41.1, row 3, $Z = 20$).

What are we to make of these reductions? Physiologists have long recognized that individual neurons in the cerebral cortex can both increase or decrease their activities from a resting, baseline firing pattern depending on task conditions. Decreases, however, seem to have received somewhat less attention. Nevertheless, examples of decreases abound in the neuro-physiological literature (see, for example, Georgopoulos et al. 1982). A parsimonious view of these decreases in neuronal activity is that they reflect the activity of inhibitory interneurons acting within local neuronal circuits of the cerebral cortex. Because inhibition is energy-requiring (Ackerman et al. 1984, Batini et al. 1984, Biral et al. 1984), it should be impossible to distinguish inhibitory from excitatory cellular activity on the basis of changes in either blood flow or metabolism. Thus, on this view, a local increase in inhibitory activity is just as likely to increase blood flow and the fMRI BOLD signal (see below) as a local increase in excitatory activity. How, then, might decreases in blood flow as seen with PET (figures 41.3–41.6) or the fMRI BOLD signal arise?

To understand the significance of the decreases in blood flow in a functional imaging experiment it is important to distinguish two separate conditions in which they might arise. The usual circumstance accounting for reductions in activity arises when two images are compared, one containing a regional increase in blood flow caused by some type of task-induced activity and the other not.

Let us consider, for example, the increase in activity over the Sylvian-insular cortices that occur when individuals read aloud a word compared with viewing the same word passively. This is seen bilaterally in figure 41.1, row 3 at $Z = 20$. Turning to figure 41.2, row 4, note that we now observe a reduction in activity in almost the same region as subjects perform, naively, verb generation compared with reading aloud. What has occurred is that images in which the region is activated (i.e., word reading) are subtracted from images in which the region is not activated (i.e., verb generation). These results suggest that this region is used in automatic speech production such as word reading, not for a novel reading task such as verb generation. However, as verb generation becomes more automatic this region is reactivated (figure 41.4, row 2, $Z = 20$ and $Z = 0$).

The second circumstance in which decreases in blood flow and the fMRI BOLD signal are observed are not due to data manipulations of the type just described. Rather, blood flow and the fMRI BOLD signal decrease regionally from a baseline state for that region. The immediate question that arises in the mind of most is how such a baseline state is defined. How, for instance, is it to be distinguished from just another activation state? The definition arises from a consideration of the metabolic and circulatory events surrounding the activation of a typical cortical region (for a recent review, see Raichle 1998) and how these differ from the metabolism and circulation of the baseline state of the awake human brain.

Measurements in the normal, adult, awake human reveal a brain that consumes approximately 0.27 μm of glucose and 1.54 μm of oxygen per gram of tissue per minute (Siesjo 1978). This is supplied by a blood flow of approximately 0.55 ml of blood per gram of tissue per minute (Siesjo 1978). Although these values vary from one region of the brain to another (for example, the average value in white matter is typically one one-quarter that of grey matter) the relation among them remains remarkably constant. As a consequence, the fraction of available oxygen removed by the cerebral cortex of the resting brain from circulating blood (i.e, the so-called oxygen extraction fraction or OEF) is quite uniform.

What is so distinctive about areas of increased activity are the deviations from these baseline relations. One might have assumed that when there is an increase in local cellular activity in the cerebral cortex it would be accompanied by a proportionate increase in blood flow and oxygen consumption. This would be reflected in an unchanged OEF. However, this is not observed (Fox and Raichle 1986, Fox et al. 1988). Blood flow actually increases substantially in excess of any increase in oxygen consumption, leading to a significant decrease in the OEF. The

direct correlate of this is a local increase in the ratio of oxyhaemoglobin to deoxyhaemoglobin as oxygen supply exceeds demand. It is the local increase in the oxyhaemoglobin: deoxy-haemoglobin ratio that forms the basis for the fMRI signal. This fMRI signal usually is referred to as the BOLD or blood oxygen level-dependent contrast (Kwong et al. 1992; Ogawa et al. 1990, 1992).

Positive BOLD contrast is now routinely seen by investigators worldwide doing functional brain imaging studies with fMRI. There is a remarkable correspondence between the location of BOLD contrast and changes in blood flow measured with PET when the same tasks are studied (for recent review, see Raichle 1998). This correspondence has become routine confirmation of the fact that blood flow changes in excess of any change in oxygen consumption during changes in the functional activity of the cerebral cortex.

Given the above information, we are now in a position to ask a rather obvious question. What is the baseline-state metabolic and circulatory status of brain regions that exhibit a reduction in blood flow and a negative BOLD contrast when subjects actively engage in task performance? The regions of particular interest are those seen along the midline in figures 41.3–41.6 and previously noted to behave similarly across a wide variety of visual attention tasks (Shulman et al. 1997b). For these medial regions of orbital–frontal and posterior cingulate or parietal cortex, the OEF does not differ significantly from the overall brain average in the baseline state (data from 20 normal adult controls; M. E. Raichle, A.-M. MacLeod, W. Drevets, and W. J. Powers, unpublished observations) whereas the blood flow, oxygen consumption and glucose utilization significantly exceed the brain average. Remarkably, the region of the posterior cingulate cortex and adjacent precuneus is actually the metabolically most active region of the cerebral cortex in the resting brain (data from 20 normal adult controls; M. E. Raichle, A.-M. MacLeod, W. Drevets, and W. J. Powers, unpublished observations).

The above analysis leads to the inescapable conclusion that anterior as well as posterior regions of the cerebral hemispheres, particularly prominent but not exclusively along the midline, are intensely active during the baseline state of the awake brain (such as when the eyes are closed or during passive viewing of a television monitor and its contents). With focused attention on a variety of tasks (see, for example, Shulman et al. 1997b), as well as figures 41.3–41.6 these regions exhibit a conspicuous reduction in activity. What makes the active state of these regions so distinctive is that it is characterized by metabolic and circulatory relationships that typify baseline, not functionally activated, cerebral cortex. It is as though these areas of the brain are uniquely active as a default baseline state of the conscious resting brain.

Several additional general comments about these decreases from a baseline state should be made. First, they are not, as some have informally suggested, merely the haemodynamic consequence of increases elsewhere (i.e., an intracerebral steal phenomenon). Such a hypothesis is very unlikely to be correct because of the tremendous haemodynamic reserve of the brain (Heistad and Kontos 1983) and also because there is no one-to-one spatial or temporal correlation between increases and decreases (figures 41.1–41.6).

Second, these decreases are not confined to regions of the brain whose baseline activity significantly exceeds that of the overall brain average. For example, it has been shown that, in anticipation of stimulation, areas of somatosensory cortex outside the representation of the skin area that is the target of the expected stimulation exhibit marked reductions in activity as measured with PET (Drevets et al. 1995). These observations are thought to reflect a model of spatial attention in which potential signal enhancement relies on a generalized suppression or filtering of background activity (Whang et al. 1991).

Third, the relatively large spatial extent of these regional decreases suggests the inactivation of specific systems within the cerebral cortex. The mechanism(s) by which this is achieved remain(s) to be determined. What is most important for our present purpose is identifying the functions with which these regions are associated. Whatever the functions, it seems reasonable to suggest that they must be suspended for proper task execution.

With regard to the posterior cingulate cortex and adjacent precuneus, animal studies suggest that it is involved in orientation within and interpretation of the environment (for a recent review, see Vogt et al. 1992). The response of posterior cingulate neurons to visual stimuli, for example, is crucially dependent upon the physical characteristics of the stimulus. Small spots of light to which a monkey may be attending and responding do not elicit neuronal responses in this area. In contrast, large, brightly textured stimuli elicit responses even if they are totally irrelevant to tasks the animal is performing. Lesions of the posterior cingulate cortex also disrupt spatial working memory. From the studies reviewed by Vogt and his colleagues (Vogt et al. 1992), it is not possible to separate, cleanly, spatial working memory functions from functions concerned with evaluation and interpretation of the environment.

Additional light is shed on the function of the posterior cingulate cortex and adjacent precuneus by the work of Carol Colby (Colby et al. 1988), John Allman (Baker et al. 1981) and their colleagues. Both of these studies call attention to the fact that elements of the dorsal stream of extrastriate visual cortex (area M in the owl monkey and area PO in the macaque) are part of a network of areas concerned with the representation of the visual periphery. These areas are primarily located along the dorsal midline and can be distinguished experimentally in various ways from those areas of the visual system of the monkey that represent the fovea (i.e., the central ten degrees of the visual field). From these data and those reviewed by Vogt et al. (1992) emerges a specific hypothesis. Activity within the posterior cingulate cortex and adjacent precuneus in the baseline state in humans is associated with the representation (monitoring) of the world around us (i.e., our environment or our visual periphery). The hypothesis further predicts that efficient processing of items in the centre of our visual field requires generalized suppression or filtering of this background activity (Whang et al. 1991). This is operationally achieved by reducing activity of the posterior cingulate cortex and precuneus. As has been shown by Shulman et al. (1997a), attention to centrally presented stimuli is accompanied by enhanced responses in areas of the visual system concerned with their processing at the same time that posterior cingulate and precuneus are shut down (Shulman et al. 1997b).

Behavioural evidence in humans provides additional support for the above hypothesis. Mackworth (1965) has shown that increased foveal load leads to decreased extrafoveal information acquisition. He termed this phenomenon "tunnel vision." This work has been confirmed and extended by a number of workers (see, for example, Henderson and Ferreira 1990). Older adults are more affected by foveal load than younger adults (Owsley et al. 1995). Although no studies have been done to relate this decrement in performance with normal aging to reductions in the activity of the posterior cingulate and adjacent precuneus, recent studies in patients with Alzheimer's disease provide in intriguing perspective.

As reported recently by Kuhl and associates (Minoshima et al. 1994, 1997), reduction in the activity of the posterior cingulate gyrus is the earliest metabolic abnormality detected in patients with Alzheimer's disease with PET. Abnormalities in the processing of extrafoveal information have been noted in patients with dementia of the Alzheimer's type (Benson et al. 1988) but no systematic study has been performed on this group of patients in the light of the recent findings of Kuhl and associates (Minoshima et al. 1994, 1997).

Finally, severe damage to the parietal cortex, when it extends medially to include the precuneus and the posterior cingulate region, produces a condition known as Balint's syndrome (Hecaen and Ajuriaguerra 1954) whose cardinal feature is the inability to perceive the visual field as a whole (i.e., severe tunnel vision). This is known as simultanagnosia (Rizzo and Robin 1990). It is of interest that simultanagnosia has been reported in patients with dementia of the Alzheimer's type (Benson et al. 1988). Of interest would be a study of the relationship between decrements in baseline metabolic activity in this region in patients with Alzheimer's disease and the development of simultanagnosia.

Thus, the posterior cingulate cortex and adjacent precuneus can be hypothesized as a region of the brain associated with the continuous gathering of information about the world around us. It would appear to be a default condition of the brain with rather obvious evolutionary significance. Successful performance on tasks requiring focused attention demand that such broad information-gathering is curtailed. We see this reflected in marked decreases in this region during focused attention. As a task becomes easier and requires less focused attention, activity in this area predictably resumes (figure 41.6, row 1).

The other midline region of the cortex exhibiting prominent decreases in activity during focused attention is the orbitofrontal cortex. As with the posterior cingulate and adjacent precuneus, these changes have not only been observed in the tasks discussed in this paper but also in a wide variety of other tasks requiring focused attention (Shulman et al. 1997b). In contrast to the behaviour of the posterior cingulate and adjacent precuneus, the decreases we observe in the orbitofrontal cortex not only decrease initially when reading tasks are novel and require focused attention, but actually decrease even further with practice (figure 41.6, row 2). Further analysis of these changes (Simpson et al. 1997) reveals a number of important features. First, the reductions observed in this region, as they increase with practice, are significantly correlated with improved performance as measured by improved reaction times on the verb-generation task. Secondly, these changes represent correlated responses within a group of areas in the orbital and medial inferior prefrontal cortex and the hypothalamus. This is consistent with the connectional anatomy of this region known from non-human primates (Carmichael and Price 1994, 1995, 1996). Third, the likelihood that these changes are related to the emotional aspects of novel task performance is supported by a parallel study of anticipatory anxiety in normal subjects (Simpson et al. 1997). Reductions similar to those seen in the verb-generation task were correlated with the degree of anxiety reported by the subjects. Less anxious subjects showed greater reductions in activity.

These observations occur against a background of considerable clinical and experimental data suggesting that the orbital and medial prefrontal cortex play an important role in emotional behaviour (Drevets et al. 1997), especially fear (for review, see LeDoux 1996) and decision-making (Bechara et al. 1997, Damasio et al. 1994). These activities are based on converging information from multiple sensory modalities (Rolls and Baylis 1994) and connections to the amygdala, hypothalamus, brain-stem, and basal ganglia (Carmichael and Price 1996). Puzzling, of course, is the fact that the changes we observe are seen as reductions and, as discussed in detail earlier, they begin from a baseline level of activity that is significantly above the brain mean.

A broad view of the function of the prefrontal cortex suggests that it is active when new rules need to be learned and older ones rejected (Dias et al. 1997; Wise et al. 1996). The activation of

regions within the prefrontal cortex during the naive performance of the verb-generation task (figure 41.1, row 4) would certainly be consistent with that view. When this same reasoning is applied to the orbital and medial prefrontal cortex one must confront the fact that activity in this region may be greatest in the baseline state. Thus, as we come to associate general monitoring of incoming sensory information with the posterior cingulate cortex and adjacent precuneus, we may also come to associate an evaluation of this information with the medial and orbital frontal cortices.

Conclusions

The main purpose of this paper was to present a functional brain-imaging strategy that isolates neural correlates of consciousness in humans. This strategy is based on skill learning. In the example presented (rapidly generating verbs for visually presented nouns) a cognitive skill is examined before and after practice. As shown, there are marked qualitative differences in the neural circuitry supporting performance of this task in the naive and practised state. William James succinctly captures the interpretation we wish to place on this transformation in performance and neural circuitry: "habit diminishes the conscious attention with which our acts are performed" (James 1890). Areas active during naive performance become candidate neural correlates of consciousness.

The neural correlates of consciousness for one task may not correspond, region for region, to those for another task. This is most directly demonstrated in our own data when comparisons are made between verb generation and maze tracing (Petersen et al. 1998). Thus, although a common theme emerges from the work reviewed here in terms of principles governing the neural instantiation of conscious and non-conscious behaviour of the same task, differences do exist among tasks in terms of the specific brain regions involved. Put another way, no single, unique architecture emerges as a unifying feature of conscious, reflective performance (see also Shulman et al. 1997b). The cerebral cortex appears like the sections of a symphony orchestra. No one section or individual is at all times necessary for the production of the music. Likewise, in the brain, no one region (system) is necessary for consciousness under all circumstances. Rather, it is a distributed process with changing participants, some of which are identified through the strategy described. Relationships determine performance and performance can be infinitely variable.

The continuity of consciousness must also be kept in mind in pursuing the type of analysis presented in this paper. Consciousness does not cease when task performance changes from a naive, effortful, attention-focusing experience to a practised, effortless one requiring little attention. It is in this regard that it is important to consider the role of those regions of the brain whose activity ceases during naive task performance only to resume under baseline conditions. These task-induced deactivations from a baseline state provide important clues concerning neural correlates of consciousness in the baseline state. The recognition of these decreases probably represents a unique contribution of functional brain imaging to our understanding of human cortical physiology and should stimulate increased interest in the manner in which brain resources are allocated on a large systems level.

Acknowledgments

The material in this paper was presented, in part, as the 1997 Thomas William Salmon Lecture of the New York Academy of Medicine. I thank my many colleagues whose published data I have reviewed in this paper and, for generous support over many years, the National Institutes of Health of the USA, The McDonnell Center for Studies of Higher Brain Function of Washington University School of Medicine, The John T. and Katherine T. MacArthur Foundation, and the Charles A. Dana Foundation.

References

Ackerman, R. F., Finch, D. M., Babb, T. L. and Engel, J. Jr 1984 Increased glucose metabolism during long-duration recurrent inhibition of hippocampal cells. *J. Neurosci.* 4, 251–264.

Baker, J. F., Petersen, S. E., Newsome, W. T. and Allman, J. M. 1981 Visual response properties of neurons in four extrastriate visual areas of the owl monkey (*Aotus trivirgatus*): a quantitative comparison of medial, dorsomedial, dorsolateral, and middle temporal areas. *J. Neurophysiol.* 45, 397–416.

Batini, C., Benedetti, F., Buisseret-Delmas, C., Montarolo, P. G. and Strata, P. 1984 Metabolic activity of intracerebellar nuclei in the rat: effects of inferior olive inactivation. *Expl Brain Res.* 54, 259–265.

Bechara, A., Damasio, H., Tranel, D. and Damasio, A. R. 1997 Deciding advantageously before knowing the advantageous strategy. *Science* 275, 1293–1295.

Benson, D. F., Davis, J. and Snyder, B. D. 1988 Posterior cortical atrophy. *Archs Neurol.* 45, 789–793.

Biral, G., Cavazzuti, M., Porro, C., Ferrari, R. and Corazza, R. 1984 [^{14}C]Deoxyglucose uptake of the rat visual centres under monocular optokinetic stimulation. *Behav. Brain Res.* 11, 271–275.

Bridgeman, B., Hijiden, A. H. C. V. d. and Velichovsky, B. M. 1994 A theory of visual stability across saccadic eye movements. *Behav. Brain Sci.* 17, 247–292.

Carmichael, S. T. and Price, J. L. 1994 Architectonic subdivision of the orbital and medial prefrontal cortex in the macaque monkey. *J. Comp. Neurol.* 346, 366–402.

Carmichael, S. T. and Price, J. L. 1995 Limbic connections of the orbital and medial prefrontal cortex of macaque monkeys. *J. Comp. Neurol.* 368, 615–641.

Carmichael, S. T. and Price, J. L. 1996 Connectional networks within the orbital and medial prefrontal cortex of macaque monkeys. *J. Comp. Neurol.* 371, 179–207.

Chen, L. L. and Wise, S. E. 1995a Neuronal activity in the supplementary eye field during acquisition of conditional oculomotor associations. *J. Neurophysiol.* 73, 1101–1121.

Chen, L. L. and Wise, S. E. 1995b Supplemetary eye field contrasted with frontal eye field during acquisition of conditional oculomotor associations. *J. Neurophysiol.* 73, 1121–1134.

Colby, C. L., Gattass, R., Olson, C. R. and Gross, C. G. 1988 Topographic organization of cortical afferents to extrastriate visual area PO in the macaque: a dual tracer study. *J. Comp. Neurol.* 238, 1257–1299.

Crick, F. and Koch, C. 1998 Consciousness and neuroscience. *Cerebr. Cortex* 8, 97–107.

Damasio, A. R. 1995 Knowing how, knowing where. *Nature* 375, 106–107.

Damasio, H., Grabowski, T., Frank, R., Galaburda, A. M. and Damasio, A. R. 1994 The return of Phineas Gage: clues about the brain from the skull of a famous patient. *Science* 264, 1102–1105.

Dias, R., Robbins, T. W. and Roberts, A. C. 1997 Dissociable forms of inhibitory control within prefrontal cortex with an analog of the Wisconsin Card Sort Test: restriction to novel situations and independence from "on-line" processing. *J. Neurosci.* 17, 9285–9297.

Donders, F. C. 1969 On the speed of mental processes. *Acta Psychol.* 30, 412–431.

Drevets, W. C., Burton, H., Videen, T. O., Snyder, A. Z., Simpson, J. R., Jr and Raichle, M. E. 1995 Blood flow changes in human somatosensory cortex during anticipated stimulation. *Nature* 373, 249–252.

Drevets, W. C., Price, J. L., Simpson, J. R. Jr, Todd, R. D., Reich, T., Vannier, M. and Raichle, M. E. 1997 Subgenual prefrontal cortex abnormalities in mood disorders. *Nature* 386, 824–827.

Fiez, J. A. and Petersen, S. E. 1998 Neuroimaging studies of word reading. *Proc. Natn. Acad. Sci. USA* 95, 914–921.

Fox, P. T. and Raichle, M. E. 1986 Focal physiological uncoupling of cerebral blood flow and oxidative metabolism during somatosensory stimulation in human subjects. *Proc. Natn. Acad. Sci. USA* 83, 1140–1144.

Fox, P. T., Perlmutter, J. S. and Raichle, M. E. 1985 A stereotactic method of anatomical localization for positron emission tomography. *J. Comput. Assist. Tomogr.* 9, 141–153.

Fox, P. T., Raichle, M. E., Mintun, M. A. and Dence, C. 1988 Nonoxidative glucose consumption during focal physiologic neural activity. *Science* 241, 462–464.

Frith, C. D., Friston, K., Liddle, P. F. and Frackowiak, R. S. J. 1991 Willed action and the prefrontal cortex in man: a study with PET. *Proc. R. Soc. Lond.* B 244, 241–246.

Georgopoulos, A. P., Kalaska, J. F., Caminiti, R. and Massey, J. T. 1982 On the relations between the direction of two-dimensional arm movements and cell discharge in primate motor cortex. *J. Neurosci.* 2, 1527–1537.

Hecaen, H. and Ajuriaguerra, J. 1954 Balint's syndrome (psychic paralysis of gaze) and its minor forms. *Brain* 77, 373–400.

Heistad, D. D. and Kontos, H. A. 1983 Cerebral circulation. In *Handbook of physiology. The cardiovascular system*, vol. 3 (ed. J. T. Sheppard and F. M. Abboud), pp. 137–182. Bethesda, MD: American Physiological Society.

Henderson, J. M. and Ferreira, F. 1990 Effects of foveal processing difficulty on the perceptual span in reading: implications for attention and eye movement control. *J. Exp. Psychol.: Learn. Mem. Cogn.* 16, 417–429.

Howard, D., Patterson, K., Wise, R., Brown, D., Friston, K., Weiller, C. and Frackowiak, R. 1992 The cortical localizations of the lexicons: positron emission tomography evidence. *Brain* 115, 1769–1782.

Jackson, J. H. 1874 On the nature of the duality of the brain. *Med. Press Circ.* 1, 19, 41, 63.

James, W. 1890 *Principles of psychology*. New York: Henry Holt & Company.

Kwong, K. (and 12 others) 1992 Dynamic magnetic resonance imaging of human brain activity during primary sensory stimulation. *Proc. Natn. Acad. Sci. USA* 89, 5675–5679.

LeDoux, J. 1996 *The emotional brain*. New York: Simon & Schuster.

Lichtheim, L. 1885 On aphasia. *Brain* 7, 433–484.

McCarthy, R. and Warrington, E. K. 1984 A two-route model of speech production: evidence from aphasia. *Brain* 107, 463–485.

Mackworth, N. H. 1965 Visual noise causes tunnel vision. *Psychonom. Sci.* 3, 67–70.

McCarthy, R. and Warrington, E. K. 1984 A two-route model of speech production: Evidence from aphasia. *Brain* 107, 463–485.

Minoshima, S., Foster, N. L. and Kuhl, D. E. 1994 Posterior cingulate cortex in Alzheimer's disease. *Lancet* 344, 895.

Minoshima, S., Giordani, B., Berent, S., Frey, K. A., Foster, N. L. and Kuhl, D. E. 1997 Metabolic reduction in the posterior cingulate cortex in very early Alzheimer's disease. *Ann. Neurol.* 42, 85–94.

Mitz, A. R., Godschalk, M. and Wise, S. P. 1991 Learning-dependent neuronal activity in the premotor cortex: activity during the acquisition of conditional motor associations. *J. Neurosci.* 11, 1855–1872.

Norman, D. A. and Shallice, T. 1986 Attention to action: willed and automatic control of behavior. In *Consciousness and self-regulation*, pp. 1–18. New York: Plenum Press.

Nottebohm, F. 1991 Reassessing the mechanisms and origins of vocal learning in birds. *Trends Neurosci.* 14, 206–211.

Ogawa, S., Lee, T. M., Kay, A. R. and Tank, D. W. 1990 Brain magnetic resonance imaging with contrast depedent on blood oxygenation. *Proc. Natn. Acad. Sci. USA* 87, 9868–9872.

Ogawa, S., Tank, D. W., Menon, R., Ellermann, J. M., Kim, S.-G., Merkle, H. and Ugurbil, K. 1992 Intrinsic signal changes accompanying sensory stimulation: functional brain mapping with magnetic resonance imaging. *Proc. Natn. Acad. Sci. USA* 89, 5951–5955.

Owsley, C., Ball, K. and Keeton, D. M. 1995 Relationship between visual sensitivity and target localization in older adults. *Vision Res.* 35, 579–587.

Passingham, R. E. 1993 *The frontal lobes and voluntary action.* (Oxford Psychology Series.) Oxford University Press.

Paus, T., Marrett, S., Worsley, K. J. and Evans, A. C. 1995 Extraretinal modulation of cerebral blood flow in the human visual cortex: implications for saccadic suppression. *J. Neurophysiol.* 74, 2179–2183.

Petersen, S. E., Fox, P. T., Posner, M. I., Mintum, M. and Raichle, M. E. 1988 Positron emission tomographic studies of the cortical anatomy of single-word processing. *Nature* 331, 585–589.

Petersen, S. E., Fox, P. T., Posner, M. I., Mintun, M. A. and Raichle, M. E. 1989 Positron emission tomo-

graphic studies of the processing of single words. *J. Cogn. Neurosci.* 1, 153–170.

Petersen, S. E., Fox, P. T., Snyder, A. Z. and Raichle, M. E. 1990 Activation of extrastriate and frontal cortical areas by visual words and word-like stimuli. *Science* 249, 1041–1044.

Petersen, S. E., Mier, H. v., Fiez, J. A. and Raichle, M. E. 1998 The effects of practice on the functional anatomy of task performance. *Proc. Natn. Acad. Sci. USA* 95, 853–860.

Plum, F. and Posner, J. B. 1980 *The diagnosis of stupor and coma.* (Contemporary Neurology Series.) Philadelphia, PA: F. A. Davis Company.

Posner, M. I. and Pavese, A. 1998 Anatomy of word and sentence meaning. *Proc. Natn. Acad. Sci. USA* 95, 899–905.

Price, C. J., Wise, R. J. S., Watson, J. D. G., Petterson, K., Howard, D. and Frackowiak, R. S. J. 1994 Brain activity during reading: the effects of exposure duration and task. *Brain* 117, 1255–1269.

Price, C. J., Wise, R. J. S. and Frackowiak, R. S. J. 1996 Demonstrating the implicit processing of visually presented words and pseudowords. *Cerebr. Cortex* 6, 62–70.

Price, C. J., Wise, R. J. S., Watson, J. D. G., Petterson, K., Howard, D. and Frackowiak, R. S. J. 1994 Brain activity during reading: the effects of exposure duration and task. *Brain* 117, 1255–1269.

Raichle, M. E. 1998 Behind the scenes of function brain imaging: a historical and physiological perspective. *Proc. Natn. Acad. Sci. USA* 95, 765–772.

Raichle, M. E., Fiez, J. A., Videen, T. O., MacLeod, A. M., Pardo, J. V., Fox, P. T. and Petersen, S. E. 1994 Practice-related changes in human brain functional anatomy during nonmotor learning. *Cerebr. Cortex* 4, 8–26.

Rayner, K. and Pollatsek, A. 1989 *The psychology of reading.* Englewood Cliffs, NJ: Prentice-Hall.

Reason, J. and Mycielska, K. 1982 *Absent-minded? The psychology of mental lapses and everyday errors.* Englewood Cliffs, NJ: Prentice-Hall.

Rizzo, M. and Robin, D. A. 1990 Simultanagnosia: a defect of sustained attention yields insights on visual information processing. *Neurology* 40, 447–455.

Rolls, E. T. and Baylis, L. L. 1994 Gustatory, olfactory, and visual convergence within the primate orbitofrontal cortex. *J. Neurosci.* 14, 5437–5452.

Shallice, T. 1988 *From neuropsychology to mental structure.* Cambridge University Press.

Shiffrin, R. and Schneider, W. 1977 Controlled and automatic human information processing. II. Perceptual learning, automatic attending and a general theory. *Psychol. Rev.* 84, 127–190.

Shulman, G. L., Corbetta, M., Buckner, R. L., Raichle, M. E., Fiez, J. A., Miezin, F. M. and Petersen, S. E. 1997a Top-down modulation of early sensory cortex. *Cerebr. Cortex* 7, 193–206.

Shulman, G. L., Fiez, J. A., Corbetta, M., Buckner, R. L., Miezin, F. M., Raichle, M. E. and Petersen, S. E. 1997b Common blood flow changes across visual tasks. II. Decreases in cerebral cortex. *J. Cogn. Neurosci.* 9, 648–663.

Siesjo, B. K. 1978 *Brain energy metabolism.* New York: Wiley.

Simpson, J. R. J., MacLeod, A. K., Fiez, J. A., Drevets, W. C. and Raichle, M. E. 1997 Blood flow decreases in human medial inferior prefrontal cortex and hypothalamus correlate with anxiety self-rating and with practice-related changes on a cognitive task. *Soc. Neurosci. Abstr.* 23, 1317.

Steriade, M. 1996a Arousal: revisiting the reticular activating system. *Science* 272, 225–226.

Steriade, M. 1996b Awakening the brain. *Nature* 383, 24–25.

Sutherland, N. S. 1996 The biological causes of irrationality. In *Research and perspectives in neursciences* (ed. Y. Christen), pp. 145–156. Berlin: Springer.

Vogt, B. A., Finch, D. M. and Olson, C. R. 1992 Functional heterogeneity in cingulate cortex: the anterior executive and posterior evaluative regions. *Cerebr. Cortex* 2, 435–443.

Weiskrantz, L. 1986 *Blindsight. A case study and implications.* (Oxford Psychology Series No. 12.) Oxford University Press.

Weiskrantz, L. 1997 *Consciousness lost and found. A neuropsychological exploration.* Oxford University Press.

Whang, K. C., Burton, H. and Shulman, G. L. 1991 Selective attention in vibrotactile tasks: detecting the presence and absence of amplitude change. *Percept. Psychophys.* 50, 157–165.

Wise, S. P., Murray, E. A. and Gerfen, C. R. 1996 The frontal cortex–basal ganglia system in primates. *Crit. Rev. Neurobiol.* 10, 317–356.

42

Availability: A Heuristic for Judging Frequency and Probability

Amos Tversky and Daniel Kahneman

Introduction

Much recent research has been concerned with the validity and consistency of frequency and probability judgments. Little is known, however, about the psychological mechanisms by which people evaluate the frequency of classes or the likelihood of events.

We propose that when faced with the difficult task of judging probability or frequency, people employ a limited number of heuristics which reduce these judgments to simpler ones. Elsewhere we have analyzed in detail one such heuristic—representativeness. By this heuristic, an event is judged probable to the extent that it represents the essential features of its parent population or generating process. Evidence for representativeness was obtained in several studies. For example, a large majority of naive respondents believe that the sequence of coin tosses HTTHTH is more probable than either HHHHTH or HHHTTT, although all three sequences, of course, are equally likely. The sequence which is judged most probable best represents both the population proportion (1/2) and the randomness of the process (Kahneman and Tversky 1972). Similarly, both naive and sophisticated subjects evaluate the likelihood that an individual will engage in an occupation by the degree to which he appears representative of the stereotype of that occupation (Kahneman and Tversky 1973). Major biases of representativeness have also been found in the judgments of experienced psychologists concerning the statistics of research (Tversky and Kahneman 1971).

When judging the probability of an event by representativeness, one compares the essential features of the event to those of the structure from which it originates. In this manner, one estimates probability by assessing similarity or connotative distance. Alternatively, one may estimate probability by assessing availability, or associative distance. Life-long experience has taught us that instances of large classes are recalled better and faster than instances of less frequent classes, that likely occurrences are easier to imagine than unlikely ones, and that associative connections are strengthened when two events frequently co-occur. Thus, a person could estimate the numerosity of a class, the likelihood of an event, or the frequency of co-occurrences by assessing the ease with which the relevant mental operation of retrieval, construction, or association can be carried out.

For example, one may assess the divorce rate in a given community by recalling divorces among one's acquaintances; one may evaluate the probability that a politician will lose an election by considering various ways in which he may lose support; and one may estimate the probability that a violent person will "see" beasts of prey in a Rorschach card by assessing the strength of association between violence and beasts of prey. In all these cases, the estimation of the frequency of a class or the probability of an event is mediated by an assessment of availability.[1] A person is said to employ the availability heuristic whenever he estimates frequency or probability by the ease with which instances or associations could be brought to mind. To assess availability it is not necessary to perform the actual operations of retrieval or construction. It suffices to assess the ease with which these operations could be performed, much as the difficulty of a puzzle or mathematical problem can be assessed without considering specific solutions.

That associative bonds are strengthened by repetition is perhaps the oldest law of memory known to man. The availability heuristic exploits the inverse form of this law, that is, it uses strength of association as a basis for the judgment of frequency. In this theory, availability is a mediating variable, rather than a dependent variable as is typically the case in the study of memory. Availability is an ecologically valid clue for the judgment of frequency because, in general, frequent events are easier to recall or imagine than infrequent ones. However, availability is also affected by various factors which are unrelated to actual frequency. If the availability heuristic is applied, then such factors will affect the perceived frequency of classes and the subjective probability of events. Consequently, the use of the availability heuristic leads to systematic biases.

This paper explores the availability heuristic in a series of ten studies.[2] We first demonstrate that people can assess availability with reasonable speed and accuracy (section 2). Next, we show that the judged frequency of classes is biased by the availability of their instances for construction (section 3), and retrieval (section 4). The experimental studies of this paper are concerned with judgments of frequencies, or of probabilities that can be readily reduced to relative frequencies. The effects of availability on the judged probabilities of essentially unique events (which cannot be reduced to relative frequencies) are discussed in the fifth and final section.

Assessments of Availability

Study 1: Construction

The subjects ($N = 42$) were presented with a series of word-construction problems. Each problem consisted of a 3×3 matrix containing nine letters from which words of three letters or more were to be constructed. In the training phase of the study, six problems were presented to all subjects. For each problem, they were given 7 s to estimate the number of words which they believed they could produce in 2 min. Following

each estimate, they were given two minutes to write down (on numbered lines) as many words as they could construct from the letters in the matrix. Data from the training phase were discarded. In the test phase, the construction and estimation tasks were separated. Each subject estimated for eight problems the number of words which he believed he could produce in 2 min. For eight other problems, he constructed words without prior estimation. Estimation and construction problems were alternated. Two parallel booklets were used, so that for each problem half the subjects estimated and half the subjects constructed words.

Results

The mean number of words produced varied from 1.3 (for XUZONLCJM) to 22.4 (for TAPCERHOB), with a grand mean of 11.9. The mean number estimated varied from 4.9 to 16.0 (for the same two problems), with a grand mean of 10.3. The product-moment correlation between estimation and production, over the sixteen problems, was 0.96.

Study 2: Retrieval

The design and procedure were identical to study 1, except for the nature of the task. Here, each problem consisted of a category, for example, *flowers* or *Russian novelists*, whose instances were to be recalled. The subjects ($N = 28$) were given 7 s to estimate the number of instances they could retrieve in 2 min., or 2 min. to actually retrieve the instances. As in study 1, the production and estimation tasks were combined in the training phase and alternated in the test phase.

Results

The mean number of instances produced varied from 4.1 (city names beginning with F) to 23.7 (four-legged animals), with a grand mean of 11.7. The mean number estimated varied from

6.7 to 18.7 (for the same two categories), with a grand mean of 10.8. The product–moment correlation between production and estimation over the 16 categories was 0.93.

Discussion

In the above studies, the availability of instances could be measured by the total number of instances retrieved or constructed in any given problem.[3] The studies show that people can assess availability quickly and accurately. How are such assessments carried out? One plausible mechanism is suggested by the work of Bousfield and Sedgewick (1944), who showed that cumulative retrieval of instances is a negatively accelerated exponential function of time. The subject could, therefore, use the number of instances retrieved in a short period to estimate the number of instances that could be retrieved in a much longer period of time. Alternatively, the subject may assess availability without explicitly retrieving or constructing any instances at all. Hart (1967), for example, has shown that people can accurately assess their ability to recognize items that they cannot recall in a test of paired-associate memory.

Availability for Construction

We turn now to a series of problems in which the subject is given a rule for the construction of instances and is asked to estimate their total (or relative) frequency. In these problems—as in most estimation problems—the subject cannot construct and enumerate all instances. Instead, we propose, he attempts to construct some instances and judges overall frequency by availability, that is, by an assessment of the ease with which instances could be brought to mind. As a consequence, classes whose instances are easy to construct or imagine will be perceived as more frequent than classes of the same size whose instances are less available. This prediction is tested in the judgment of word frequency, and in the estimation of several combinatorial expressions.

Study 3: Judgment of Word Frequency

Suppose you sample a word at random from an English text. Is it more likely that the word starts with a *K*, or that *K* is its third letter? According to our thesis, people answer such a question by comparing the availability of the two categories, that is, by assessing the ease with which instances of the two categories come to mind. It is certainly easier to think of words that start with a *K* than of words where *K* is in the third position. If the judgment of frequency is mediated by assessed availability, then words that start with *K* should be judged more frequent. In fact, a typical text contains twice as many words in which *K* is in the third position than words that start with *K*.

According to the extensive word-count of Mayzner and Tresselt (1965), there are altogether eight consonants that appear more frequently in the third than in the first position. Of these, two consonants (*X* and *Z*) are relatively rare, and another (*D*) is more frequent in the third position only in three-letter words. The remaining five consonants (*K, L, N, R, V*) were selected for investigation.

The subjects were given the following instructions:

The frequency of appearance of letters in the English language was studied. A typical text was selected, and the relative frequency with which various letters of the alphabet appeared in the first and third positions in words was recorded. Words of less than three letters were excluded from the count.

Yor will be given several letters of the alphabet, and you will be asked to judge whether these letters appear more often in the first or in the third position, and to estimate the ratio of the frequency with which they appear in these positions.

A typical problem read as follows:

Consider the letter *R*.
Is R more likely to
appear in   ____ the first position?
                             ____ the third position?
                             (check one)
My estimate for the ratio of these two values
is _____ : 1.

Subjects were instructed to estimate the ratio of the larger to the smaller class. For half the subjects, the ordering of the two positions in the question was reversed. In addition, three different orderings of the five letters were employed.

Results

Among the 152 subjects, 105 judged the first position to be more likely for a majority of the letters, and 47 judged the third position to be more likely for a majority of the letters. The bias favoring the first position is highly significant ($p < .001$, by sign test). Moreover, each of the five letters was judged by a majority of subjects to be more frequent in the first than in the third position. The median estimated ratio was 2:1 for each of the five letters. These results were obtained despite the fact that all letters were more frequent in the third position.

In other studies we found the same bias favoring the first position in a within-subject design where each subject judged a single letter, and in a between-subjects design, where the frequencies of letters in the first and in the third positions were evaluated by different subjects. We also observed that the introduction of payoffs for accuracy in the within-subject design had no effect whatsoever. Since the same general pattern of results was obtained in all these methods, only the findings obtained by the simplest procedure are reported here.

A similar result was reported by Phillips (1966) in a study of Bayesian inference. Six editors of a student publication estimated the probabilities that various bigrams, sampled from

their own writings, were drawn from the beginning or from the end of words. An incidental effect observed in that study was that all the editors shared a common bias to favor the hypothesis that the bigrams had been drawn from the beginning of words. For example, the editors erroneously judged words beginning with *re* to be more frequent than words ending with *re*. The former, of course, are more available than the latter.

Study 4: Permutations

Consider the two structures, A and B, which are displayed below.

(A)									(B)	
x	x	x	x	x	x	x	x		x	x
x	x	x	x	x	x	x	x		x	x
x	x	x	x	x	x	x	x		x	x
									x	x
									x	x
									x	x
									x	x
									x	x
									x	x

A path in a structure is a line that connects an element in the top row to an element in the bottom row, and passes through one and only one element in each row.

In which of the two structures are there more paths?
How many paths do you think there are in each structure?

Most readers will probably share with us the immediate impression that there are more paths in A than in B. Our subjects agreed: 46 of 54 respondents saw more paths in A than in B ($p < .001$, by sign test). The median estimates were 40 paths in A and 18 in B. In fact, the number of paths is the same in both structures, for $8^3 = 2^9 = 512$.

Why do people see more paths in A than in B? We suggest that this result reflects the differential availability of paths in the two structures. There are several factors that make the paths in A more available than those in B. First, the most immediately available paths are the columns of the structures. There are eight columns in A and only two in B. Second, among the paths that cross columns, those of A are generally more distinctive and less confusable than those in B. Two paths in A share, on the average, about one-eighth of their elements, whereas two paths in B share, on the average, half of their elements. Finally, the paths in A are shorter and hence easier to visualize than those in B.

Study 5: Combinations

Consider a group of ten people who have to form committees of r members, where r is some number between 2 and 8. How many different committees of r members can they form? The correct answer to this problem is given by the binomial coefficient $\binom{10}{r}$ which reaches a maximum of 252 for $r = 5$. Clearly, the number of committees of r members equals the number of committees of $10 - r$ members because any elected group of, say, two members defines a unique nonelected group of eight members.

According to our analysis of intuitive estimation, however, committees of two members are more available than committees of eight. First, the simplest scheme for constructing committees is a partition of the group into disjoint subsets. Thus, one readily sees that there are as many as five disjoint committees of two members, but not even two disjoint committees of eight. Second, committees of eight members are much less distinct, because of their overlapping membership; any two committees of eight share at least six members. This analysis suggests that small committees are more available than large committees. By the availability hypothesis, therefore, the small committees should appear more numerous.

Four groups of subjects (total $N = 118$) estimated the number of possible committees of r members that can be formed from a set of ten people. The different groups, respectively, evaluated the following values of r: 2 and 6; 3 and 8; 4 and 7; 5.

Median estimates of the number of committees are shown in figure 42.1, with the correct values. As predicted, the judged numerosity of committees decreases with their size.

The following alternative formulation of the same problem was devised in order to test the generality of the findings:

In the drawing below, there are ten stations along a route between Start and Finish. Consider a bus that travels, stopping at exactly r stations along this route.

START [ ] [ ] [ ] [ ] [ ] [ ] [ ] [ ] FINISH

What is the number of different patterns of r stops that the bus can make?

The number of different patterns of r stops is again given by $\binom{10}{r}$.

Here too, of course, the number of patterns of two stops is the same as the number of patterns of eight stops, because for any pattern of stops there is a unique complementary pattern of non-stops. Yet, it appears as though one has more degrees of freedom in constructing patterns of two stops where "one has many stations to choose from" than in constructing patterns of eight stops where "one must stop at almost every station." Our previous analysis suggests that the former patterns are more available: more such patterns are seen at first glance, they are more distinctive, and they are easier to visualize.

Four new groups of subjects (total $N = 178$) answered this question, for $r = 2, \ldots, 8$, following the same design as above. Median estimates of the number of stops are shown in figure 42.1. As in the committee problem, the appar-

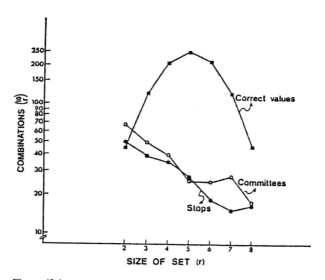

Figure 42.1
Correct values and median judgements (on a logarithmic scale) for the Committees problem and for the Stops problem.

ent number of combinations generally decreases with *r*, in accordance with the prediction from the availability hypothesis, and in marked contrast to the correct values. Further, the estimates of the number of combinations are very similar in the two problems. As in other combinatorial problems, there is marked underestimation of all correct values, with a single exception in the most available case, where *r* = 2.

The underestimation observed in experiments 4 and 5 occurs, we suggest, because people estimate combinatorial values by extrapolating from an initial impression. What a person sees at a glance or in a few steps of computation gives him an inadequate idea of the explosive rate of growth of many combinatorial expressions. In such situations, extrapolating from an initial impression leads to pronounced underestimation. This is the case whether the basis for extrapolation is the initial availability of instances, as in the preceding two studies, or the output of an initial computation, as in the following study.

Study 6: Extrapolation

We asked subjects to estimate, within 5 s, a numerical expression that was written on the blackboard. One group of subjects (*N* = 87) estimated the product $8 \times 7 \times 6 \times 5 \times 4 \times 3 \times 2 \times 1$, while another group (*N* = 114) estimated the product $1 \times 2 \times 3 \times 4 \times 5 \times 6 \times 7 \times 8$. The median estimate for the descending sequence was 2,250. The median estimate for the ascending sequence was 512. The difference between the estimates is highly significant ($p < .001$, by median test). Both estimates fall very short of the correct answer, which is 40,320.

Both the underestimation of the correct value and the difference between the two estimates support the hypothesis that people estimate 8! by extrapolating from a partial computation. The factorial, like other combinatorial expressions, is characterized by an ever-increasing rate of growth. Consequently, a person who extrapolates from a partial computation will grossly underestimate factorials. Because the results of the first few steps of multiplication (performed from left to right) are larger in the descending sequence than in the ascending sequence, the former expression is judged larger than the latter. The evaluation of the descending sequence may proceed as follows: "8 times 7 is 56 times 5 is already above 300, so we are dealing with a reasonably large number." In evaluating the ascending sequence, on the other hand, one may reason: "1 times 2 is 2 times 3 is 6 times 4 is 24, and this expression is clearly not going very far...."

Study 7: Binomial—Availability versus Representativeness

The final study of this section explores the role of availability in the evaluation of binomial distributions and illustrates how the formulation of a problem controls the choice of the heuristic that people adopt in intuitive estimation.

The subjects ($N = 73$) were presented with these instructions:

Consider the following diagram:

```
X  X  0  X  X  X
X  X  X  X  0  X
X  0  X  X  X  X
X  X  X  0  X  X
X  X  X  X  X  0
0  X  X  X  X  X
```

A path in this diagram is any descending line which starts at the top row, ends at the bottom row, and passes through exactly one symbol (X or 0) in each row.

What do you think is the percentage of paths which contain

6 X's and no 0 _____%
5 X's and 1 0 _____%
⋮
No X and 6 0's _____%

Note that these include all possible path-types and hence your estimates should add to 100%.

The actual distribution of path-type is binomial with $p = 5/6$ and $n = 6$. People, of course, can neither intuit the correct answers nor enumerate all relevant instances. Instead, we propose, they glance at the diagram and estimate the relative frequency of each path-type by the ease with which individual paths of this type could be constructed. Since, at every stage in the construction of a path (i.e., in each row of the diagram) there are many more X's than 0's, it is easier to construct paths consisting of six X's than paths consisting of, say, five X's and one 0, although the latter are, in fact, more numerous. Accordingly, we predicted that subjects would erroneously judge paths of 6 X's and no 0 to be the most numerous.

Median estimates of the relative frequency of all path-types are presented in figure 42.2, along with the correct binomial values. The results confirm the hypothesis. Of the 73 subjects, 54 erroneously judged that there are more paths consisting of six X's and no 0 than paths consisting of five X's and one 0, and only 13 regarded the latter as more numerous than the former ($p < .001$, by sign test). The monotonicity of the subjective distribution of path-types is apparently a general phenomenon. We have obtained the same result with different values of p (4/5 and 5/6) and n (5, 6 and 10), and different representations of the population proportions (e.g., four X's and one 0 or eight X's and two 0's in each row of the path diagram).

To investigate further the robustness of this effect, the following additional test was conducted. Fifty combinatorially naive undergraduates from Stanford University were presented with the path problem. Here, the subjects were not asked to estimate relative frequency but merely to judge "whether there are more paths containing six X's and no 0, or more paths containing five X's and one 0." The subjects were run individually, and they were promised a $1 bonus for a correct judgment. The significant majority of subjects (38 of 50, $p < .001$, by sign test) again selected the former outcome as more

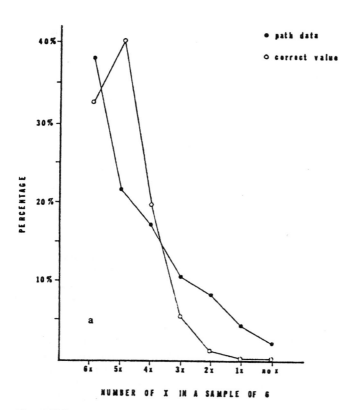

Figure 42.2
Correct values and median judgments: Path problem.

frequent. Erroneous intuitions, apparently, are not easily rectified by the introduction of monetary payoffs.

We have proposed that when the binomial distribution is represented as a path diagram, .people judge the relative frequency of the various outcomes by assessing the availability of individual paths of each type. This mode of evaluation is suggested by the sequential character of the definition of a path and by the pictorial representation of the problem. Consider next an alternative formulation of the same problem.

Six players participate in a card game. On each round of the game, each player receives a single card drawn blindly from a well-shuffled deck. In the deck, 5/6 of the cards are marked X and the remaining 1/6 are marked 0. In many rounds of the game, what is the percentage of rounds in which

6 players receive X and no player receives
0 _____%
5 players receive X and 1 player receives
0 _____%
                              ⋮
No player receives X and 6 players receive
0 _____%

Note that these include all the possible outcomes and hence your estimates should add to 100%.

This card problem is formally identical to the path problem, but it is intended to elicit a different mode of evaluation. In the path problem, individual instances were emphasized by the display, and the population proportion (i.e., the proportion of X's in each row) was not made explicit. In the card problem, on the other hand, the population proportion is explicitly stated and no mention is made of individual instances. Consequently, we hypothesize that the outcomes in the card problem will be evaluated by the degree to which they are representative of the composition of the deck rather than by the availability of individual instances. In the card problem, the outcome "five X's and one 0" is the most representative, because it matches the population proportion (see Kahneman and Tversky 1972). Hence, by the representativeness heuristic, this outcome should be judged more frequent than the outcome "six X's and no 0," contrary to the observed pattern of judgments in the path problem. The judgments of 71 of 82 subjects who answered the card problem conformed to this prediction. In the path problem, only 13 of 73 subjects had judged these outcomes in the same way; the difference between the two versions is highly significant ($p < .001$, by a χ^2 test).

Median estimates for the card problem are presented in figure 42.3. The contrast between figures 42.2 and 42.3 supports the hypothesis that different representations of the same problem elicit different heuristics. Specifically, the frequency of a class is likely to be judged by availability if the individual instances are emphasized and by representativeness if generic features are made salient.

Availability for Retrieval

In this section we discuss several studies in which the subject is first exposed to a message (e.g., a list of names) and is later asked to judge the frequency of items of a given type that were included in the message. As in the problems studied in the previous section, the subject can-

not recall and count all instances. Instead, we propose, he attempts to recall some instances and judges overall frequency by availability, that is, by the ease with which instances come to mind. As a consequence, classes whose instances are readily recalled will be judged more numerous than classes of the same size whose instances are less available. This prediction is first tested in a study of the judged frequency of categories. Next, we review previous evidence of availability effects on the judged frequency of repetitions. Finally, the role of the availability heuristic in judgments of the frequency of co-occurrences is discussed.

Study 8: Fame, Frequency, and Recall

The subjects were presented with a recorded list consisting of names of known personalities of both sexes. After listening to the list, some subjects judged whether it contained more names of men or of women, others attempted to recall the names in the list. Some of the names in the list were very famous (e.g., Richard Nixon, Elizabeth Taylor), others were less famous (e.g., William Fulbright, Lana Turner). Famous names are generally easier to recall. Hence, if frequency judgments are mediated by assessed availability, then a class consisting of famous names should be judged more numerous than a comparable class consisting of less famous names.

Four lists of names were prepared, two lists of entertainers and two lists of other public figures. Each list included 39 names recorded at a rate of one name every 2 s. Two of the lists (one of public figures and one of entertainers) included 19 names of famous women and 20 names of less famous men. The two other lists consisted of 19 names of famous men and 20 names of less famous women. Hence, fame and frequency were inversely related in all lists. The first names of all personalities always permitted an unambiguous identification of sex.

The subjects were instructed to listen attentively to a recorded message. Each of the four lists was presented to two groups. After listening

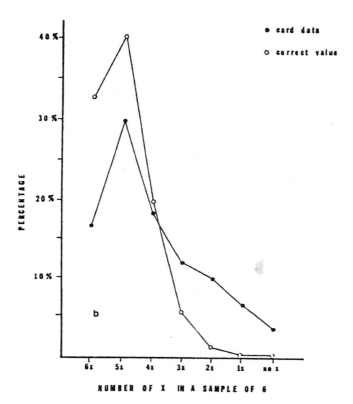

Figure 42.3
Correct values and median judgments: Card problem.

to the recording, subjects in one group were asked to write down as many names as they could recall from the list. The subjects in the other group were asked to judge whether the list contained more names of men or of women.

Results

Recall On the average, subjects recalled 12.3 of the 19 famous names and 8.4 of the 20 less famous names. Of the 86 subjects in the four recall groups, 57 recalled more famous than nonfamous names, and only 13 recalled fewer famous than less famous names ($p < .001$, by sign test).

Frequency Among the 99 subjects who compared the frequency of men and women in the lists, 80 erroneously judged the class consisting of the more famous names to be more frequent ($p < .001$, by sign test).

Frequency of Repetitions

The preceding study supported the notion that people judge the frequency of a class by assessed availability, that is, by the ease with which the relevant instances come to mind. In that study, subjects judged the frequency of classes which consisted of distinct instances, for example, female entertainers or male politicians. Most research on judged frequency, in contrast, has been concerned with the frequency of repetitions, for example, the number of times that a particular word was repeated in a list.

When the number of repetitions is relatively small, people may attempt to estimate the frequency of repetitions by recalling specific occurrences. There is evidence (see, e.g., Hintzman and Block 1971) that subjects retain some information about the specific occurrences of repeated items. There are situations, however, in which occurrences cannot be retrieved, e.g., when the total number of items is large, when their distinctiveness is low, or when the retention interval is long. In these situations, subjects may resort to a different method for judging frequency.

When an item is repeated several times in a list, the association between the item and the list is strengthened. Thus, a subject could use the strength of this association as a clue to the frequency of the item. Hence, one could judge the frequency of repetitions either by assessing the availability of specific occurrences or by a more global assessment of the strength of the item-list association. As a consequence, factors which either enhance the recallability of specific occurrences or strengthen the association between item and list should increase the apparent frequency of the item. This analysis of frequency judgments is closely related to the theoretical treatments proposed by Hintzman and Block (1971) and by Anderson and Bower (1972). A somewhat different analysis has been offered by Underwood (1969a).

The general notion that factors which affect availability have a corresponding effect on the apparent frequency of repetitions has been supported in several studies. For example, the occurrences of an item are more likely to be stored and recalled as distinct units when they are widely spaced. Indeed, Underwood (1969b) showed that items are judged more frequent under conditions of distributed rather than massed practice, and Hintzman (1969) showed that the apparent frequency of an item increases with the spacing between its repetitions in the list. An-

other factor which enhances the memorability of repetitions is vocal rehearsal. Correspondingly, Hopkins, Boylan, and Lincoln (1972) showed that items that were pronounced were perceived as more frequent than items that were read silently.

According to the present analysis, the judgment of frequency is often mediated by an assessment of item-list associations. In many situations, however, the items to which the list is most strongly associated are also the items that are most likely to be retrieved when the subject attempts to recall the list. Hence, the recallability of items from a list provides an indirect measure of the strength of the association from these items to the list. As a consequence, there should be a positive correlation between the recallability of items and their apparent frequency. Indeed, the studies of Leicht (1968) and Underwood, Zimmerman, and Freund (1971) showed that, at any level of actual frequency, items that were better recalled were judged more frequent.

In concluding the discussion of the apparent frequency of repetition, it is important to emphasize that the availability heuristic is not the only method by which frequency of repetition can be estimated. In some contexts, people may have access to a "frequency counter" (see Underwood 1969a). In other contexts, when the number of repetitions is large (see, e.g., Howell 1970), frequency judgments may be mediated by an assessment of rate of occurrence, or inferred from a schema of the relevant structure. For example, in estimating the number of trials in which the red light came on rather than the blue or the green, in a 1000-trial probability-learning experiment, the subject probably infers the estimate from his schema of the statistical structure of the sequence. Frequency estimates obtained from studies of binary and multiple probability learning show that, in general, people are quite accurate in judging relative frequencies of events (see Vlek 1970 for a review). To the extent that availability plays a role in these judgments, it is probably by affecting the schema to which the subject refers in estimating frequency.

Frequency of Co-occurrence

Some recent research has been concerned with judgment of the frequency with which pairs of items have occurred together. The strategies employed to estimate the frequency of a single item can also be employed to estimate the frequency of an item-pair. In addition, the repetition of a pair strengthens the association between its members. The subject may, therefore, use the strength of the association between the members of a pair as a clue to its frequency.

An interesting bias in the judgment of the frequency of co-occurrence has been reported by Chapman (1967) and Chapman and Chapman (1967, 1969). In the initial study, Chapman used two sets of words, and constructed a list in which each word in the first set was paired with each word in the second set. All pairs were visually presented an equal number of times. The subjects were told in advance that they would be required to report how often each word was paired with each other word. In spite of this warning, they made consistent errors in their subsequent judgments of frequency. The frequency of the co-occurrence of related words was overestimated, creating an *illusory correlation* between such words. For example, *lion–tiger* was incorrectly judged to have been shown more often than *lion–eggs*, and *bacon–eggs* was judged more frequent than *bacon–tiger*. A similar illusory correlation was found between unusually long words. For example, *blossoms–notebook* was erroneously judged to have been shown more often than *boat–notebook*. Chapman attributed this result to the distinctiveness of the long words.

In subsequent studies, Chapman and Chapman (1967, 1969) investigated the significant implications of the phenomenon of illusory correlation to impression formation and clinical judgment. They presented naive judges with clinical test material and with clinical diagnoses for several hypothetical patients. Later, the judges evaluated the frequency of co-occurrence of various symptoms and diagnoses in the data to which they had been exposed. Illusory correlation was again observed. The judges markedly overestimated the co-occurrence of pairs that were judged to be natural associates by an independent group of subjects. For example, "suspiciousness" had been rated as calling to mind "eyes" more than any other part of the body. Correspondingly, the judges greatly overestimated the frequency of the co-occurrence of suspiciousness with peculiar drawing of the eyes in the Draw-a-Person test. An ominous finding in the Chapmans' study was that naive judges erroneously "discovered" much of the common but unvalidated clinical lore concerning the interpretation of the Draw-a-Person and the Rorschach tests. Furthermore, the illusory correlation effect was extremely resistant to contradictory data. It persisted even when the actual correlation between the associates was negative. Finally, the illusory correlation effect prevented the judges from detecting correlations that were in fact present in the test material (see also Golding and Rorer 1972).

Availability provides a natural explanation for illusory correlation. We propose that an assessment of the associative bond between two items is one of the processes that mediate the judged frequency of their co-occurrence. The association between two items is strengthened whenever they co-occur. Thus, when a person finds that the association between items is strong, he is likely to conclude that they have been frequently paired in his recent experience. However, repetition is not the only factor that affects associative strength. Factors other than repetition which strengthen the association between the members of a pair will, therefore, increase the apparent frequency of that pair. According to this account, illusory correlation is due to the differential strength of associative bonds. The strength of these bonds may reflect prior association between the items or other factors, such as pair-distinctiveness, which facilitate the formation of an association during learning. Thus, the various sources of illusory correlation can all be explained by the operation of a single mechanism—the assessment of availability or associative strength. The proposed account of the judgment of the frequency of co-occurrences is tested in the last two studies.

Study 9: Illusory Correlation in Word Pairs

This study essentially replicates Chapman's (1967) original result and establishes the relation between judgments of the frequency of pairs and cued recall, i.e., the recall of the second word of the pair, called response, given the first, called stimulus.

A set of twenty pairs of words was constructed. Ten of the pairs consisted of highly related (HR) words, the other ten consisted of unrelated (UR) words. In five of the HR pairs, stimulus and response were natural associates: *knife–fork, hand–foot, lion–tiger, table–chair, winter–summer.* (The first three pairs were taken from Chapman's list.) In five other pairs, stimulus and response were phonetically similar: *gown–clown, cake–fake, blade–blame, flight–fleet, spoon–spanner.* The ten UR pairs were obtained by replacing the stimulus word in each of the above ten pairs, respectively, by the words: *head, lamp, house, paper, dish, bread, box, pencil, book, phone.* Thus, the entire set of pairs was constructed so that each response word appeared with two stimulus words, one which was highly related to it and one which was not. A message

which included these word-pairs was recorded on tape at a rate of one pair every 5 s. Ten of the twenty pairs were repeated three times in the message and the other ten pairs were repeated twice. Pairs that shared the same response word (e.g., *knife–fork, head–fork*) were repeated the same number of times. The order of the pairs was randomized. To minimize the effects of primacy and recency, the same two filler pairs were recorded both at the beginning and at the end of the message.

All subjects ($N = 98$) were instructed to listen attentively to the message. Following the recording, one group of 30 subjects was asked for cued recall: each subject was given a list of all twenty stimulus words (in one of four random orders) and was asked to write the corresponding response words. A second group of 68 subjects was asked for frequency judgments: each subject was given a list of all twenty pairs (again, in one of four random orders) and was asked to judge whether each of the pairs had appeared twice or three times in the message.

Results

Cued Recall For each subject, the number of response words correctly recalled was counted, separately for the HR and the UR pairs under each of the two repetition levels (i.e., 2 and 3). Table 42.1a presents the mean probability of recall for each of the four conditions. A 2×2 analysis of variance showed that subjects recalled

Table 42.1
Mean probability of recall and mean judged frequency

(a) Cued recall				(b) Judged frequency				
		Relatedness					Relatedness	
		Low	High				Low	High
Actual frequency	3	.41	.85		Actual frequency	3	2.45	2.63
	2	.31	.77			2	2.26	2.42

significantly more words from the HR pairs than from the UR pairs ($t = 9.4$, 29 df, $p < .001$), and that they recalled significantly more words from the pairs that had been repeated more often ($t = 2.44$, 29 df, $p < .05$). The interaction between the two factors was not significant.

Judged Frequency Table 42.1b presents the mean judged frequency of the HR and the UR pairs for the two levels of actual frequency. A 2×2 analysis of variance showed that the HR pairs were judged more frequent than the UR pairs ($t = 4.62$, 67 df, $p < .001$), although they were, in fact, equally frequent. The effect of actual frequency was also significant ($t = 7.71$, 67 df, $p < .001$). The interaction between the two factors was not.

Further analyses showed that the differences between HR and UR pairs, in both cued recall and judged frequency, were significant separately for the natural associates and for the phonetically similar pairs.

Study 10: Illusory Correlation in Personality Traits

Chapman's original study, as well as study 9, employed a correlational design where each response was paired with more than one stimulus. According to the present analysis, however, the illusory correlation effect is due to differences among item pairs in the strength of the associative bond between their members. Consequently, the same effect should also occur in a noncorrelational design, where each response is paired with a single stimulus, and vice versa. The present study tests this prediction. In addition, it shows that people can assess the availability of associates, that is, the degree to which the response word is made available by the stimulus word.

A set of sixteen pairs of personality traits was constructed. Eight of the pairs—the highly related pairs—consisted of traits which tend to be associated with each other. The other eight pairs—the unrelated pairs—consisted of traits which are not generally associated with each other. The highly related (HR) pairs were: *kind–honest, poised–relaxed, passive–withdrawn, alert–witty, selfish–greedy, meek–silent, brutal–nasty, healthy–active.* The unrelated (UR) pairs were: *nervous–gentle, lucky–discreet, eager–careful, clever–prudent, humble–messy, nice–anxious, casual–thrifty, clumsy–mature.* In a pilot study designed to validate the classification of the pairs, 36 subjects assessed, for each pair, the probability that a person who has the first trait of that pair also has the second (e.g., the probability that an alert person is witty). The average estimated probabilities for each of the HR pairs exceeded the average estimates for all the UR pairs.

A message which included all pairs was recorded on tape at a rate of one pair every 5 s. Two HR and two UR pairs appeared in the list at each of four levels of frequency, from a single occurrence to four occurrences. The order of the pairs in the message was randomized and five filler pairs were recorded at the beginning and the end of the message.

All subjects were told to listen attentively to a recorded message. Following the recording, subjects were assigned one of three different tasks. The subjects in the *recall* group ($N = 62$) were given a list consisting of all 16 stimulus-traits and were asked to recall the response member of each pair. The subjects in the *assessed-recall* group ($N = 68$) were presented with the 16 trait-pairs and were asked to indicate, on a seven-point scale, the likelihood that they would have been able to recall each response-trait if they had been given the stimulus-trait, immediately after hearing the list. The subjects in the *judged-frequency* group ($N = 73$) were given a list of all the 16 trait-pairs and were asked to judge how often each pair appeared in the message. Four lists with different orders were employed for each of the three tasks.

Results

Recall The number of items that were correctly recalled by each subject was recorded separately for the HR and the UR pairs. On the average, subjects correctly completed 41% of the HR pairs, and only 19% of the UR pairs. The difference is highly significant ($t = 9.27$, 61 *df*, $p < .001$).

Assessed Recall The mean rating of assessed recall was computed for each of the trait-pairs. The product–moment correlation, over the 16 pairs, between mean assessed recall and the proportion of correct responses in the recall group was 0.84. Apparently, people can assess the recallability of associates with reasonable accuracy.

Judged Frequency Figure 42.4 shows mean judged frequency as a function of actual frequency, separately for the HR and the UR pairs. The difference between the two curves is highly significant ($t = 3.85$, 72 *df*, $p < .001$).

Although judgments of frequency were generally accurate, a slight but highly systematic bias favoring related pairs was present. The results support the proposed account of judgment of frequency in terms of the availability of associations, and demonstrate the presence of "illusory correlation" in a non-correlational design.

Retrieval of Occurrences and Construction of Scenarios

In all the empirical studies that were discussed in this paper, there existed an objective procedure

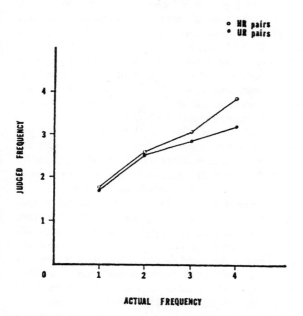

Figure 42.4
Average judged frequency as a function of actual frequency for highly related (HR) and unrelated (UR) trait-pairs.

for enumerating instances (e.g., words that begin with K or paths in a diagram), and hence each of the problems had an objectively correct answer. This is not the case in many real-life situations where probabilities are judged. Each occurrence of an economic recession, a successful medical operation, or a divorce, is essentially unique, and its probability cannot be evaluated by a simple tally of instances. Nevertheless, the availability heuristic may be applied to evaluate the likelihood of such events.

In judging the likelihood that a particular couple will be divorced, for example, one may scan one's memory for similar couples which this question brings to mind. Divorce will appear probable if divorces are prevalent among the instances that are retrieved in this manner. Alternatively, one may evaluate likelihood by attempting to construct stories, or scenarios, that lead to a divorce. The plausibility of such scenarios, or the ease with which they come to mind, can provide a basis for the judgment of likelihood. In the present section, we discuss the role of availability in such judgments, speculate about expected sources of bias, and sketch some directions that further inquiry might follow.

We illustrate availability biases by considering an imaginary clinical situation.[4] A clinician who has heard a patient complain that he is tired of life, and wonders whether that patient is likely to commit suicide may well recall similar patients he has known. Sometimes only one relevant instance comes to mind, perhaps because it is most memorable. Here, subjective probability may depend primarily on the similarity between that instance and the case under consideration. If the two are very similar, then one expects that what has happened in the past will recur. When several instances come to mind, they are probably weighted by the degree to which they are similar, in essential features, to the problem at hand.

How are relevant instances selected? In scanning his past experience does the clinician recall patients who resemble the present case, patients who attempted suicide, or patients who resemble the present case *and* attempted suicide? From an actuarial point of view, of course, the relevant class is that of patients who are similar, in some respects, to the present case, and the relevant statistic is the frequency of attempted suicide in this class.

Memory search may follow other rules. Since attempted suicide is a dramatic and salient event, suicidal patients are likely to be more memorable and easier to recall than depressive patients who did not attempt suicide. As a consequence, the clinician may recall suicidal patients he has encountered and judge the likelihood of an attempted suicide by the degree of resemblance between these cases and the present patient. This approach leads to serious biases. The clinician who notes that nearly all suicidal patients he can think of were severely depressed may conclude that a patient is likely to commit suicide if he shows signs of severe depression. Alternatively, the clinician may conclude that suicide is unlikely if "this patient does not look like any suicide case I have met." Such reasoning ignores the fact that only a minority of depressed patients attempt suicide and the possibility that the present patient may be quite unlike any that the therapist has ever encountered.

Finally, a clinician might think only of patients who were both depressed and suicidal. He would then evaluate the likelihood of suicide by the ease with which such cases come to mind or by the degree to which the present patient is representative of this class. This reasoning, too, is subject to a serious flaw. The fact that there are many depressed patients who attempted suicide does not say much about the probability that a depressed patient will attempt suicide, yet this mode of evaluation is not uncommon. Several studies (Jenkins and Ward 1963, Smedslund 1963, Ward and Jenkins 1965) showed that contingency between two binary variables such as a symptom and a disease is judged by the frequency with which they co-occur, with little or no regard for cases where either the symptom or the disease was not present.

Some events are perceived as so unique that past history does not seem relevant to the evaluation of their likelihood. In thinking of such events we often construct *scenarios*, that is, stories that lead from the present situation to the target event. The plausibility of the scenarios that come to mind, or the difficulty of producing them, then serve as a clue to the likelihood of the event. If no reasonable scenario comes to mind, the event is deemed impossible or highly unlikely. If many scenarios come to mind, or if the one scenario that is constructed is particularly compelling, the event in question appears probable.

Many of the events whose likelihood people wish to evaluate depend on several interrelated factors. Yet it is exceedingly difficult for the human mind to apprehend sequences of variations of several interacting factors. We suggest that in evaluating the probability of complex events only the simplest and most available scenarios are likely to be considered. In particular, people will tend to produce scenarios in which many factors do not vary at all, only the most obvious variations take place, and interacting changes are rare. Because of the simplified nature of imagined scenarios, the outcomes of computer simulations of interacting processes are often counter-intuitive (Forrester 1971). The tendency to consider only relatively simple scenarios may have particularly salient effects in situations of conflict. There, one's own moods and plans are more available to one than those of the opponent. It is not easy to adopt the opponent's view of the chessboard or of the battlefield, which may be why the mediocre player discovers so many new possibilities when he switches sides in a game. Consequently, the player may tend to regard his opponent's strategy as relatively constant and independent of his own moves. These considerations suggest that a player is susceptible to the *fallacy of initiative*—a tendency to attri-

bute less initiative and less imagination to the opponent than to himself. This hypothesis is consistent with a finding of attribution-research (Jones and Nisbett 1971) that people tend to view their own behavior as reflecting the changing demands of their environment and others' behavior as trait-dominated.

The production of a compelling scenario is likely to constrain future thinking. There is much evidence showing that, once an uncertain situation has been perceived or interpreted in a particular fashion, it is quite difficult to view it in any other way (see, e.g., Bruner and Potter 1964). Thus, the generation of a specific scenario may inhibit the emergence of other scenarios, particularly those that lead to different outcomes.

Images of the future are shaped by the experience of the past. In his monograph *Hazard and choice perception in flood plain management*, Kates (1962) writes:

A major limitation to human ability to use improved flood hazard information is a basic reliance on experience. Men on flood plains appear to be very much prisoners of their experience.... Recently experienced floods appear to set an upper bound to the size of loss with which managers believe they ought to be concerned. (p. 140)

Kates attributes much of the difficulty in achieving more efficient flood control to the inability of individuals to imagine floods unlike any that have occurred.

Perhaps the most obvious demonstration of availability in real life is the impact of the fortuitous availability of incidents or scenarios. Many readers must have experienced the temporary rise in the subjective probability of an accident after seeing a car overturned by the side of the road. Similarly, many must have noticed an increase in the subjective probability that an accident or malfunction will start a thermonuclear war after seeing a movie in which such an occurrence was vividly portrayed. Continued preoccupation with an outcome may increase its availability, and hence its perceived likelihood. People are preoccupied with highly desirable outcomes, such as winning the sweepstakes, or with highly undesirable outcomes, such as an airplane crash. Consequently, availability provides a mechanism by which occurrences of extreme utility (or disutility) may appear more likely than they actually are.

A Final Remark

Most important decisions men make are governed by beliefs concerning the likelihood of unique events. The "true" probabilities of such events are elusive, since they cannot be assessed objectively. The subjective probabilities that are assigned to unique events by knowledgeable and consistent people have been accepted as all that can be said about the likelihood of such events.

Although the "true" probability of a unique event is unknowable, the reliance on heuristics such as availability or representativeness, biases subjective probabilities in knowable ways. A psychological analysis of the heuristics that a person uses in judging the probability of an event may tell us whether his judgment is likely to be too high or too low. We believe that such analyses could be used to reduce the prevalence of errors in human judgment under uncertainty.

Acknowledgments

This work was supported by NSF grant GB-6782, by a grant from the Central Research Fund of the Hebrew University, by grant MH 12972 from the National Institute of Mental Health and Grants 5 S01 RR 05612-03 and RR 05612-04 from the National Institute of Health to the Oregon Research Institute.

We thank Maya Bar-Hillel, Ruth Beyth, Sundra Gregory, and Richard Kleinknecht for their help in the collection of the data, and Douglas Hintzman and Paul Slovic for their helpful comments on an earlier draft.

Notes

1. The present use of the term "availability" does not coincide with some usages of this term in the verbal learning literature (see, e.g., Horowitz, Norman, and Day 1966, Tulving and Pearlstone 1966).

2. Approximately 1500 subjects participated in these studies. Unless otherwise specified, the studies were conducted in groups of 20–40 subjects. Subjects in studies 1, 2, 3, 9, and 10 were recruited by advertisements in the student newspaper at the University of Oregon. Subjects in study 8 were similarly recruited at Stanford University. Subjects in studies 5, 6, and 7 were students in the tenth and eleventh grades of several college-preparatory high schools in Israel.

3. Word-construction problems can also be viewed as retrieval problems because the response-words are stored in memory. In the present paper we speak of retrieval when the subject recalls instances from a natural category, as in studies 2 and 8. We speak of construction when the subject generates exemplars according to a specified rule, as in studies 1 and 4.

4. This example was chosen because of its availability. We know of no reason to believe that intuitive predictions of stockbrokers, sportscasters, political analysts, or research psychologists are less susceptible to biases.

References

Anderson, J. R., and Bower, G. H. Recognition and retrieval processes in free recall. *Psychological Review*, 1972, 79, 97–132.

Bousfield, W. A., and Sedgewick, C. H. An analysis of sequences of restricted associative responses. *Journal of General Psychology*, 1944, 30, 149–165.

Bruner, J. S., and Potter, M. C. Interference in visual recognition. *Science*, 1969, 144, 424–425.

Chapman, L. J. Illusory correlation in observational report. *Journal of Verbal Learning and Verbal Behavior*, 1967, 6, 151–155.

Chapman, L. J., and Chapman, J. P. Genesis of popular but erroneous psychodiagnostic observations. *Journal of Abnormal Psychology*, 1967, 73, 193–204.

Chapman, L. J., and Chapman, J. P. Illusory correlation as an obstacle to the use of valid psychodiagnostic signs. *Journal of Abnormal Psychology*, 1969, 74, 271–280.

Forrester, J. W. *World dynamics.* Cambridge, Mass.: Wright-Allen, 1971.

Golding, S. L., and Rorer, L. G. "Illusory correlation and the learning of clinical judgment." *Journal of Abnormal Psychology*, 1972, 80, 249–260.

Hart, J. T. Memory and the memory-monitoring process. *Journal of Verbal Learning and Verbal Behavior*, 1967, 6, 689–691.

Hintzman, D. L. Apparent frequency as a function of frequency and the spacing of repetitions. *Journal of Experimental Psychology*, 1969, 80, 139–145.

Hintzman, D. L., and Block, R. A. Repetition and memory: Evidence for a multiple-trace hypothesis. *Journal of Experimental Psychology*, 1971, 88, 297–306.

Hopkins, R. H., Boylan, R. J., and Lincoln, G. L. Pronunciation and apparent frequency. *Journal of Verbal Learning and Verbal Behavior*, 1972, 11, 105–113.

Horowitz, L. M., Norman, S. A., and Day, R. S. Availability and associative symmetry. *Psychological Review*, 1966, 73, 1–15.

Howell, W. C. Intuitive "counting" and "tagging" in memory. *Journal of Experimental Psychology*, 1970, 85, 210–215.

Jenkins, H. M., and Ward, W. C. Judgment of contingency between responses and outcomes. *Psychological Monographs*, 1965, 79, (1, Whole No. 594).

Jones, E. E., and Nisbett, R. E. The actor and the observer: Divergent perceptions of the causes of behavior. In E. E. Jones, D. Kanouse, H. H. Kelley, R. E. Nisbett, S. Valins, and B. Weiner. *Attribution: Perceiving the causes of behavior.* General Learning Press, 1971.

Kahneman, D., and Tversky, A. Subjective probability: A judgment of representativeness. *Cognitive Psychology*, 1972, 3, 430–454.

Kahneman, D., and Tversky, A. On the psychology of prediction. *Psychological Review*, 1973, in press.

Kates, R. W. Hazard and choice perception in flood plain management. Department of Geography Research Paper No. 78, University of Chicago, 1962.

Leicht, K. L. Recall and judged frequency of implicitly occurring words. *Journal of Verbal Learning and Verbal Behavior*, 1968, 7, 918–923.

Mayzner, M. S., and Tresselt, M. E. Tables of single-letter and bigram frequency counts for various word-length and letter-position combinations. *Psychonomic Monograph Supplements*, 1965, 1(2), 13–32.

Phillips, L. D. Some components of probabilistic inference. Technical Report No. 1, Human Performance Center, University of Michigan, 1966.

Smedslund, J. Note on learning, contingency, and clinical experience. *Scandinavian Journal of Psychology*, 1966, 7, 265–266.

Tulving, E., and Pearlstone, Z. Availability versus accessibility of information in memory for words. *Journal of Verbal Learning and Verbal Behavior*, 1966, 5, 381–391.

Tversky, A., and Kahneman, D. Belief in the law of small numbers. *Psychological Bulletin*, 1971, 76, 105–110.

Underwood, B. J. Attributes of memory. *Psychological Review*, 1969, 76, 559–573. (a)

Underwood, B. J. Some correlates of item repetition in free-recall learning. *Journal of Verbal Learning and Verbal Behavior*, 1969, 8, 83–94. (b)

Underwood, B. J., Zimmerman, J., and Freund, J. S. Retention of frequency information with observations on recognition and recall. *Journal of Experimental Psychology*, 1971, 87, 149–162.

Vlek, C. A. J. Multiple probability learning: Associating events with their probabilities of occurrence. *Acta Psychologica*, 1970, 33, 207–232.

Ward, W. C., and Jenkins, H. M. The display of information and the judgment of contingency. *Canadian Journal of Psychology*, 1965, 19, 231–241.

43

John M. Gardiner, Cristina Ramponi, and Alan Richardson-Klavehn

In recent years there has been a revival of interest in experiential, or phenomenal, aspects of memory (e.g., Brewer 1992, 1996; Conway, Collins, Gathercole, and Anderson 1996; Gardiner 1988; Jacoby 1988, 1991; Johnson 1988; Johnson, Foley, Suengas, and Raye 1988; Larsen 1998; Tulving 1983, 1985). One experiential approach, introduced by Tulving (1985), requires subjects when retrieving an item to make "remember" responses if they are able to bring back to mind some recollection of what occurred at the time the item was encoded, and to make "know" responses if they are aware only of the item's prior occurrence. In Tulving's theory (for recent reviews, see also Nyberg and Tulving 1996; Wheeler, Stuss, and Tulving 1997), remember and know responses measure autonoetic and noetic consciousness, which respectively characterize retrieval from episodic and semantic memory systems.

These responses have been interpreted by other dual-component theories, including one that relates them to recollection and familiarity, conceived as two independent processes (e.g., Jacoby 1991), and another in which remember responses reflect distinctiveness of processing and know responses reflect processing fluency (Rajaram 1996). And, in contrast with these dual-component views, remembering and knowing have also been interpreted by a unitary signal detection model that maps the two responses onto a continuum of trace strength with two different response criteria (e.g., Donaldson 1996).

Since the publication of Tulving's (1985) article, it has been discovered that remember and know responses are dissociable in quite predictable and systematic ways. Indeed, it has been shown that remembering and knowing are functionally independent, in that all possible relations between these two states of awareness have been observed (see Gardiner, Kaminska, Dixon, and Java 1996). There are variables that influ-

ence only remember responses and variables that influence only know responses. There are variables that have opposite effects on remember and know responses. And there are variables that have similar effects on remember and know responses. (For reviews, see Gardiner and Java 1993; Rajaram and Roediger 1997; Richardson-Klavehn, Gardiner, and Java 1996.)

Other recent studies, in which subjects are in addition instructed to report guesses, have found that when subjects report guesses, their responses reveal no memory for studied items —unlike either know or remember responses— even in two-alternative forced-choice tests (Gardiner et al. 1996; Gardiner, Java, and Richardson-Klavehn 1996; Gardiner, Richardson-Klavehn, and Ramponi 1997). These findings not only show that guess responses to studied words generally do not exceed guess responses to unstudied words, but that sometimes subjects make significantly more guesses to unstudied words than studied ones. Apparently, this latter finding in part merely reflects greater response opportunity for unstudied than for studied items, when guessing, and it is most likely to occur when subjects guess very freely.

In the present article we present and describe a database of transcripts of subjects' reported experiences of remembering, knowing, and guessing, following a yes/no recognition test. The transcripts were collected in an experiment by Gardiner et al. (1997), but they were not reported along with that experiment because they were not strictly relevant to the theoretical issues with which that experiment was concerned nor had we at that time envisaged reporting them.

In the article by Gardiner et al. (1997), 48 subjects studied a mixed list of 24 low- and 24 high-frequency words. The recognition test, which took place on the following day, consisted of the studied words together with another unstudied set of 24 low- and 24 high-frequency words. In a replication of Strack and Forster's (1995) experiment 1, response bias was also manipulated. Half the subjects were told (correctly) that 50% of the test words were studied, and half the subjects were told that only 30% of the test words were studied. Low-frequency words were more likely to be recognized than high-frequency words and the word frequency effect occurred in remembering, not in knowing, as has been consistently found before (Gardiner and Java 1990; Huron et al. 1995; Kinoshita 1995; Strack and Forster 1995). The manipulation of response bias had no effects on either measures of discriminability or on measures of criterion in either remember or know responses. This manipulation affected only guess responses, which were significantly greater in the 50% response bias condition, but only for unstudied words. Strack and Forster (1995) had found response bias affected know responses, but their subjects had not been instructed to report guesses. The implication is that their subjects included in their know responses responses that otherwise would have been reported as guesses, had the subjects been allowed that option, and that is why they showed effects of response bias in know responses, whereas our subjects did not.

After each subject in the Gardiner et al. (1997) experiment had finished the recognition test, the experimenter chose at random two responses of each kind and asked subjects to explain them. Although this was done only to confirm that subjects were obeying instructions, and has frequently been done in previous studies, this time the experimenter recorded detailed transcripts of the explanations that subjects provided. Transcripts were not recorded for the first three subjects tested. There were therefore up to 90 transcripts for each of the three kinds of response (not every subject made two responses of each kind). These transcripts are appended in a database (Appendix 1) that other researchers may find interesting and useful. Before describing these transcripts, we provide fuller details of the methodology used in obtaining them.

Methodology

During the yes/no recognition test, subjects first reported whether they recognized each test word, which was presented individually on the screen of a Macintosh Powerbook, as one of the words presented in the study phase. They did this by pressing either a button labeled "YES" if they recognized the word or a button labeled "NO" if they did not recognize it. If they pressed the button labeled "YES," three additional buttons appeared on the screen. These three buttons were labeled "Remember," "Know," and "Guess." Subjects made remember, know, or guess responses by pressing the corresponding button. The instructions for these responses were similar to those used in previous studies and are provided in Appendix 2. The responses were recorded by the computer.

At the end of the recognition test, the word "END" was displayed on the screen for 3 s. After the 3 s had elapsed, the computer displayed a window containing a subset of words from the recognition test, in the order in which they had tested. Test words that had elicited a positive response were followed by the word "remember," "know," or "guess," depending on the button the subject had pressed after the initial response.

Because of the limited size of the window displayed by the computer, it was programmed to randomly select for display about a quarter of the test words, in a "scrolling field." The particular position of the selected subset within the whole test list varied from subject to subject. The rest of the list could be viewed by scrolling through the field; the scrolling was under the experimenter's control.

At this stage subjects were informed that what they could see on the screen were their recognition responses. The experimenter then arbitrarily chose two words for which the subject had reported remember responses, two words for which the subject had reported know responses, and two words for which the subject had reported guess responses. For each arbitrarily selected word, subjects were asked what it was that led them to recognize the word as one they had studied. The emphasis was on what led to the recognition decision. Subjects were not asked to justify their remember, know, or guess responses as such, nor were they informed that the appropriateness of their responses was being evaluated. When discussing their recognition responses with the experimenter, the subjects were more interested in saying why they recognized the word than in justifying the state of awareness they reported.

Sometimes the window displayed did not include the required number of responses of each kind, and when that happened the experimenter scrolled up or down the screen to bring another part of the test list into view. In a few cases, particularly from the earlier part of the test list, subjects did not recall recognizing the word (presumably because of the longer retention interval). If this happened, another word was arbitrarily chosen. It should also be noted that the chosen words were selected arbitrarily with respect to word frequency, and blindly with respect to whether they were studied or unstudied, since their old/new status was not displayed. Also, transcripts from two subjects who were replaced for not obeying the instructions are not included.

The random determination of the parts of the test list displayed, and the arbitrary selection of the chosen words, had the advantage of minimizing any experimenter bias, but also inevitably resulted in an uneven sampling of the actual words and of the extent to which these words elicited each kind of response from different subjects. More systematic sampling might have been attempted but it would have proved difficult, given the lack of experimenter control over subjects' responses; and it could have involved other biases, so that more random sampling

seemed preferable. We doubt that the general characteristics of the recorded transcripts reflect any particular selection biases.

Another potential methodological problem is that of confabulation. There are several reasons, however, for thinking that confabulation is unlikely to have occurred to any appreciable extent. Subjects were under no pressure to justify their reported states of awareness, only their recognition decision, and subjects did occasionally report that they did not recall making the recognition decision. Moreover, there was little evidence of confabulation in a related study by Java, Gregg, and Gardiner (1997) in which some similar explanations of remember and know responses were recorded by subjects at the time they made the recognition decisions. In Java et al.'s second experiment, the validity of these responses was confirmed directly by showing that, following a level of processing manipulation at study, only remember responses reflected level of processing, and they did so accurately. Finally, the possibility of confabulation is rendered less likely by the systematic relations these responses showed with respect to word frequency effects in recognition performance (Gardiner et al. 1997), relations that have been consistently replicated in other studies (e.g., Gardiner and Java 1990, Huron et al. 1995, Kinoshita 1995).

The Transcripts

We next discuss the transcripts for recognition decisions associated with remember, know, and guess responses. Following that, we provide a brief historical and theoretical overview of some interpretations of the states of awareness measured by these responses.

Remembering: Recollections of Recent Encounters

For the most part, subjects had very little difficulty in recalling the reasons for making recog-

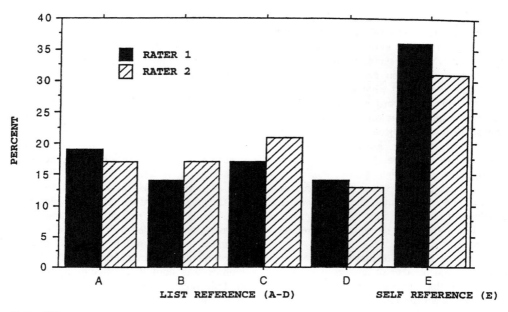

Figure 43.1
Mean percentage of remember responses classified as (*a*) intra-list associations, (*b*) extra-list associations, (*c*) item-specific images, (*d*) item's physical features, and (*e*) self-related.

nition decisions that were followed by remember responses. It is possible to classify these data according to what seem to be the most salient characteristics of the responses (see also Huron et al. 1995; Java et al. 1997; Curran, Schacter, Norman, and Galluccio 1997; Strong 1913). Two broad kinds of response are readily apparent. One is generally to do with subjects' attempts to memorize the study list. These responses typically involve intra-list and extra-list associations, imagery, and occasionally something about the more superficial features of a word, such as its spelling, or its position in the list. For the most part, these responses seem to reflect the use of effortful strategies, associations, and imagery, as mnemonic aids during the study phase.

The second broad kind of response appears to reflect occasions when the presentation of the word in the study list automatically triggered

awareness of some personal memory from everyday life. These experiences apparently came to mind without any there having been any intention of bringing them to mind. This involuntary reminding seems to be the equivalent, at study, of what has been called *involuntary conscious memory* at test (see Richardson-Klavehn et al. 1996).

It is possible to classify remember responses in a more detailed way, and our classification is summarized in figure 43.1. Each of two raters studied the transcripts and independently assigned the 90 responses available into the following categories: (a) intra-list association, (b) extra-list association, (c) item-specific image, (d) item's physical features, and (e) self-reference. Both raters excluded 4 responses on the grounds that they did not seem to fit this classification. Of the remaining 86 responses, one rater judged 5 to be split across two classes, and the other rater judged 14 to be split across two classes. These responses were rated 0.5% for each class, so that the percentage scores in figure 43.1 sum to 100%. The two raters agreed on the classification of 81% of all 90 responses, a reasonably good degree of concordance.

Examples of the responses for each category are as follows:

- Subject 19 *President.* Yesterday I associated this word with the word "minister." Today I automatically remembered about that association. (Intra-list association)
- Subject 43 *Kilt.* I remembered that I thought of a Scottish man. (Extra-list association)
- Subject 6 *Gun.* When I saw it yesterday I had an image of a gun and I thought it was a strange word to put in. (Item-specific image)
- Subject 18 *Sauerkraut.* I remembered it because I could not pronounce it yesterday! (Item's physical features)
- Subject 29 *Harp.* On Friday I was in a restaurant with a harpist. I remember thinking of that yesterday. (Self-reference)

These categories accord well with Huron et al.'s (1995) findings. They classified by far the majority of remember responses as either elaborative inter-item associations or as "personal." Interestingly, they found that schizophrenic patients, for whom remember responses, but not know responses, were impaired in recognition memory, reported very few elaborative inter-item associations. In contrast, these patients reported a similar number of personal associations to normal subjects.

These categories also correspond with those adopted by Curran et al. (1997), who similarly distinguished responses involving "autobiographical reference" from others involving "reference to the study phase" and to associations. In a further parallel, they found that, compared with control subjects, a patient with a right frontal lobe infarction reported very few references to the study phase, but a similar or greater number of autobiographical references.

In sum, a distinction between remembering at test that results from the voluntary use of particular strategies at study, and remembering at test that results from involuntary reminding about oneself at study (cf. Conway and Dewhurst 1995) seems important because of the evidence that certain kinds of patients with memory disorders are impaired with respect to the former, but not with respect to the latter (Curran et al. 1997, Huron et al. 1995).

In a recently completed experiment (Gardiner and Moran 1997), we have found that normal elderly adults showed a similar pattern of results, compared with younger adults. That is, older and younger adults showed at test similar amounts of remembering that appeared to reflect involuntary reminding at study, but older adults showed much less remembering that appeared to reflect the voluntary use of particular encoding strategies.

These findings support a distinction between voluntary and involuntary conscious memory at study, as well as at test (Richardson-Klavehn et al. 1996), and they indicate that involuntary conscious memory may be relatively unimpaired in various groups of individuals who show overall memory impairments. Regardless of this distinction, however, what seems critical for the experience of remembering in the test is that the occurrence of the word in the study list engaged consciousness in a very specific way, one that led to more than simply being aware only of the presence of the word.

Finally, we note that although remember responses to unstudied words are usually quite rare, they do occur. Averaged across all conditions of this experiment, the remember false alarm rate was .02; the corresponding proportion of hits was .33. We interpret these false alarms to mean that occasionally subjects either recollect details of other recent encounters and mistakenly attribute them to the study context, or they recollect details from the study context but incorrectly associate them with that particular item.

Knowing: Attributions of Recent Unremembered Encounters

Eliciting the reasons for recognition decisions followed by know (and guess) responses sometimes required a little more encouragement by the experimenter, because at times subjects found it more difficult to express these reasons. This is reflected by the rather limited vocabulary in these transcripts. The fact that subjects found it harder to articulate the reasons for these recognition decisions is itself significant, and contrasts markedly with the ease with which subjects explained recognition decisions followed by remember responses.

Conspicuously absent from these transcripts of know responses is any indication that they involved recollection of any specific contextual details. Also conspicuously absent from these transcripts of know responses is any indication that they were based on perceptual experiences (cf. Jacoby and Dallas 1981). These responses included quite a few claims of "just knowing," of having feelings of familiarity, or of thinking the word occurred. Some of them are also characterized by the reported absence of the kinds of information present in transcripts of remember responses. Examples are as follows:

- Subject 37 *Gun.* I just knew that I knew it.
- Subject 29 *Kilt.* It seemed familiar but I wondered.
- Subject 3 *Butterfly.* It was one of those words that rang a bell.
- Subject 25 *Gun.* There was no association, I just had a feeling that I saw it, I was sure.
- Subject 8 *Professor.* It was not in any of the little stories I made up to remember the words, but I had a strong feeling of familiarity.
- Subject 34 *Squirrel.* I remembered something about squirrels, but I cannot remember what.

In making know responses subjects are aware of a recent encounter that they cannot remember. Because words are encountered frequently, in many different contexts, attributions to the study context may typically be more difficult in the absence of remembering. This may be why know false-alarm rates generally tend to be higher than remember false-alarm rates, as they were in this experiment. But know responses still revealed an ability to select more studied than unstudied words. Averaged over all conditions of the experiment, the proportion of know responses to studied words was .22, and to unstudied words it was .10. These false alarms, like remember false alarms, may either reflect awareness of other recent encounters that are misattributed to the study context, or of encounters that are correctly attributed to the study context but mistakenly associated with the particular item.

It is also important to note that there is evidence (which we discuss again later) that in certain circumstances recognition performance may be associated largely with knowing, and with little or no remembering (Gardiner and Gregg 1997; see also Conway et al. 1997; Gregg and Gardiner 1994). For example, in the Gardiner and Gregg (1997) study, a very rapid perceptual and incidental orienting task was used at study largely to prevent any elaborative or distinctive processing of the studied words. In the subsequent recognition tests, there were very few remember responses, and many more know responses, compared with those obtained under more usual experimental conditions.

Guessing: Speculations about Recent Encounters Neither Remembered nor Known

By contrast, guess responses in this experiment did not reveal any ability to distinguish between studied and unstudied words (Gardiner et al. 1997; see also Gardiner et al. 1996; Gardiner, Java, and Richardson-Klavehn 1996). Averaged over all conditions of the experiment, the proportion of guess responses to studied words was

.11, and the proportion of guess responses to unstudied words was .13.

The most striking characteristic of the transcripts of the reasons for recognition decisions followed by guess responses is that, unlike the other transcripts, they clearly show various inferences and other judgmental strategies that have nothing directly to do with memory for a studied word (cf. Strack and Forster 1995). The inferences include some to do with memory for the types of words that occurred in the study list. There were two or three clear examples where the reports are based on previous response rates and on what subjects had been told about the appropriate response rate. There were also cases where subjects reported difficulties in distinguishing things that were "on their mind" from what actually occurred (cf. Johnson et al. 1988).

Examples of these transcripts are as follows:

- Subject 33 *Officer*. It was just a guess.

- Subject 1 *Slipper*. I saw this word somewhere recently at some point, but I am not sure whether it was there yesterday.

- Subject 11 *Father*. I kept saying "no" so I just guessed it was there because you said that 50% of the words were there.

- Subject 5 *Harp*. It seemed that there were quite a few musical instruments, so I took a guess that it came up.

- Subject 36 *Holiday*. I am eager to go on holiday so I am not sure whether I saw it here or whether I was thinking about it.

Another striking feature about the transcripts of the know and guess responses concerns the degree of confidence expressed. Table 43.1 shows the results of two raters independently assessing the number of know and guess responses that indicated uncertainty about the accuracy of the response, using lenient criteria based on the presence of phrases such as "not sure," "not confident," or "I think." Percentage scores here are based on the number of available responses,

Table 43.1

Mean percentage of know responses and guess responses classified as indicating uncertainty

Response	Rater 1	Rater 2
Know	11	20
Guess	72	77

since there were a few cases where subjects reported only one response or none. Both raters agreed that very few know responses indicated uncertainty, whereas by far the majority of guess responses did. Their overall agreement rate, for all the responses, was 83%. Both raters also counted the frequency with which know responses indicated that subjects felt sure the words had occurred in the study list, and concurred completely in finding 25% of these responses (the same responses for each rater) could be so classified. As one would expect, there were no such responses among the guesses.

There is also evidence of similar phrases in the transcripts for know responses and guess responses, such as "I had a feeling it was there," "it seemed likely it could have been there," and "it was familiar." This continuity at the experiential level contrasts with the difference between the accuracy of know and guess responses, and it suggests that though subjects rightly felt less confident about their guess responses than about their know responses, they were probably not aware that when they reported guessing they were actually unable to discriminate between studied and unstudied words.

In more naturalistic situations, however, there is evidence that subjects sometimes report guesses that do reveal some accuracy. For example, with forced-choice tests in a long-term diary study of memory for real and imagined events, Conway et al. (1996) found that guess responses were sometimes accurate. Successful guessing in memory for real events presumably reflects some awareness of the relative likelihood of alternative events, which can then be used to exclude events that are less likely. And in a study by Conway et al. (1997) of the acquisition of knowledge by psychology undergraduate students, which also had forced-choice tests, it was found that students who scored relatively high marks in examinations sometimes reported guessing the correct answers, though students who scored relatively low marks did not do this. Presumably, the more knowledgeable students were more aware of other conceptual knowledge relating to the incorrect alternatives, and could sometimes use this knowledge to exclude them. In conventional laboratory studies, the experimental design precludes this kind of strategy because the targets and lures are usually counterbalanced and, a priori, equally likely.

Historical and Theoretical Overview

Remember and know responses measure subjective reports of autonoetic and noetic consciousness. They therefore represent an experiential (or first-person rather than third-person) approach, and are best conceived as one source of evidence about subjective states of awareness, one that can be used in conjunction with other kinds of converging evidence (see, e.g., Nyberg and Tulving 1996, Wheeler et al. 1997). Given the evidence that remembering and knowing can be systematically manipulated, it is also important to discover how, and why, variables have different effects on them, because people base their actions and decisions upon their experiences and their experiences cannot be reliably inferred from conventional, third-person measures of performance (Tulving 1989). However, though the present experiential approach relies on subjective report, it should not be confused with classical introspection, as exemplified in a rather similar article to the present one by Strong (1913).

Strong (1913; see also Strong and Strong 1916) did not of course measure remember, know, and guess responses, let alone attempt to manipulate them. But he did ask subjects to report their experiences in a recognition test. And there are some interesting parallels between his evidence and our evidence (see also Java et al. 1997). Among his examples were:

- *Pressure.* Associated it with tank. Did it now and then remembered doing it before.

- *Period.* Knew it was in list.

- *Marvel.* Have thought of marvel recently, can't think of any possible connection except the list.

- *Divorce.* Mere guess.

Strong (1913) classified responses in terms of their associations. He also distinguished responses based on some specific association coming into consciousness from those made without any association coming into consciousness. He remarked on other recognition responses based on feelings of familiarity without any apparent cause. Indeed, Strong and Strong (1916, p. 341) cited Lehmann (1889) for pointing out "that recognition has two meanings in daily life: (1) to recognize, knowing you have seen previously, but not knowing where; and (2) to recognize, knowing you have seen previously and knowing where, when, etc."

There are at least two fundamental differences between recent experiments in which remember and know responses have been measured, and classical introspection as exemplified in Strong's (1913) article. The first is that remember and know responses measure *states* of awareness, not the "contents" of any particular mental experience. The transcripts presented and discussed in this article are examples of the contents of particular mental experiences, as are the responses in Strong's (1913) article, but the measures apply at the level of qualitatively distinct kinds of experience, as defined by the distinction between autonoetic, noetic, and anoetic consciousness. The contents of any particular mental experience are idiosyncratic. But the states of awareness are lawful.

The second fundamental difference is that remember and know responses are not used as the sole means for making claims about hypothetical information processing constructs. The distinction between episodic and semantic memory systems, for example, is based on many different kinds of evidence, not just on subjective reports (see, e.g., Nyberg and Tulving 1996, Wheeler et al. 1997). The logic in the chain of argument is (a) there are reasons to suppose that there are separate episodic and semantic memory systems in the brain; (b) these systems appear to be associated with two different kinds of consciousness; (c) awareness reflecting these two different kinds of consciousness can be measured by remember and know responses; and (d) it is therefore possible to check, using these measures, whether remembering and knowing behave in the kind of way we would expect, on the basis of all the other evidence.

The logic of this kind of argument is very far removed from simply accepting these responses at face value without any corroborative or converging evidence, or from believing that subjects can actually introspect about the systems (or processes) that give rise to their mental experiences (see Gardiner et al. 1997; Strack and Forster 1995). This logic may not always have been transparent when interpretations of remembering and knowing have been discussed, but it is important not to lose sight of this crucial difference between the present approach and classical introspection.

Remembering and knowing have been linked to other dual-component theories. For example, they have been linked to the constructs of recollection and familiarity in the application of Jacoby's (1991) process dissociation procedure to recognition memory (see, e.g., Jacoby, Yonelinas, and Jennings 1997; see also Mandler 1980). But remembering and knowing do not correspond with recollection and familiarity in the process dissociation procedure, because recollection and familiarity are conceived as independent processes, not as states of awareness. The two procedures differ even in their definitions of consciousness. Recollection in the process dissociation procedure is defined in terms of the ability to bring to mind critical "diagnostic" attributes that allow one set of studied items to be discriminated from another. It is also equated with conscious control. Remembering is defined more broadly, in terms of any recollective experiences associated with studied items, not just those experiences that permit one set of studied items to be discriminated from another. Nor is remembering identified with conscious control, since remembering can occur involuntarily, as well as voluntarily (Richardson-Klavehn et al. 1996). Hence nondiagnostic or "noncriterial" recollection, which in the remember/know procedure should be captured in remember responses, contributes to estimates of the familiarity process in the process dissociation procedure. This familiarity process includes "irrelevant" recollection (Yonelinas and Jacoby 1996). By the same token, this familiarity process does not correspond with knowing in the remember/know procedure because knowing is defined to exclude any recollective experiences.

Nonetheless, there may sometimes be interesting parallels between the remember/know and process dissociation procedures, as well as differences, particularly when remembering is identified with the recollection process, knowing is assumed to reflect the independent familiarity process, and know responses are accordingly adjusted for the amount of remembering to give an estimate of this process (for more discussion, see Jacoby et al. 1997; Richardson-Klavehn et al. 1996; Yonelinas et al. 1996). Presumably, converging conclusions are most likely when remember responses generally include awareness of those attributes that are necessary, in the process dissociation procedure, for successful discrimination between the two sets of items.

Remember and know responses have also been related to the transfer appropriate processing approach, which distinguishes between conceptual and perceptual processes (e.g., Rajaram

1993; see also Gardiner 1988). The initial suggestion was that remembering is largely driven by conceptual processing and that knowing is largely driven by perceptual processing. More recently, Rajaram (1996, 1998) has proposed a distinctiveness/fluency framework, on the basis of evidence that remembering is sometimes influenced by perceptual, as well as by conceptual factors, and that what seems critical in each case is the distinctiveness of the encoding. There is also evidence that knowing is influenced by conceptual as well as by perceptual factors (see Conway et al. 1997; Mantyla 1997), so that the situation now appears to be that there is an orthogonal relation between conceptual and perceptual processing and the states of awareness. This relation can be accommodated by a distinctiveness/fluency framework, if it is granted that fluency may occur conceptually, as well as perceptually (see also Jacoby 1991).

Note that here too the distinction between conceptual and perceptual processing, like the distinction between episodic and semantic memory, is based on much other evidence that is quite independent of the distinction between remembering and knowing. Remembering and knowing are not simply used introspectively to infer the kind of processing. The theoretical arguments here are about how, and why, the different kinds of processing influence the states of awareness (see Rajaram 1996, 1998; Rajaram and Roediger 1997).

Another theoretical model has recently been provided by extensions of signal detection theory (Donaldson 1996; Hirshman and Master 1997; Inoue and Bellezza 1998). This model assumes that mnemonic information differs only along a continuum of familiarity or "trace strength." Remembering and knowing reflect two criteria, a more conservative one for remember responses and a more lenient one for overall recognition, which includes know responses. (Presumably a third, even more lenient criterion could be added to include guess responses.)

Such criteria differences clearly exist, as do differences in the degree of confidence associated with the different responses, though remember and know responses are not equivalent to judgments of high and low confidence (Gardiner and Java 1990). So the critical question is whether know responses merely reflect a more lenient criterion, or whether they also reflect an additional source of memory. The most important prediction of the detection model is that bias-free estimates of discriminability should be equivalent whether derived from overall recognition hit and false-alarm rates or from remember hit and false-alarm rates.

Gardiner and Gregg (1997) argue that this prediction lacks convincing support. One problem is that in meta-analyses of many different experimental conditions, Donaldson (1996) has found that, although the effect size is small, A' estimates of discriminability are consistently greater for overall recognition than for remembering. The use of A' rather than d' estimates is predicated on the assumption that though both estimates are theoretically bias-free, in practice A' estimates are less vulnerable to differences in response criteria than d' estimates, and are therefore more appropriate for a model in which such differences are essential.

A second problem is that Gardiner and Gregg (1997) also consistently found similar, and much larger, differences between A' estimates for overall recognition and for remembering in individual subject data, under the experimental conditions we described earlier, which led to little or no remembering. In fact, from a total of 52 individual subjects, in 47 out of 51 cases in which the two A' estimates differed, A' was greater when derived from overall recognition than when derived from remember responses (Gardiner and Gregg, 1997). Thus there is evidence counter to the model's most important prediction both at the level of meta-analyses of experimental conditions and at the level of individual subject data.

Other findings that present difficulties for a unitary trace strength model discussed by Gardiner and Gregg (1997) include some particularly compelling physiological evidence for the two states of awareness. Düzel et al. (1997) measured event-related potentials (ERPs) associated with remember and know responses in an extended version of the false-recognition paradigm introduced by Deese (1959) and revived by Roediger and McDermott (1995). Remember and know responses gave rise to distinct ERPs, and these ERP patterns of activity were quite similar both for the studied target words and for the nonstudied target words of which they are associates and which led to the false-recognition effect. That these physiological measures of brain activity do not reveal any differences between studied and nonstudied target words suggests that the old/new status of the words is irrelevant to the states of awareness that subjects experience. This outcome supports the interpretations of remember and know false alarms that we suggested earlier.

Of course, it is conceivable that vastly more complex mind-brain systems could be collapsed onto a continuum of trace strength, and that such a continuum could in turn give rise to discrete states of awareness. But, at least as presently formulated, the detection model gives little indication as to how both these translations might be accomplished. And the limitations of the detection model have to be taken in conjunction with behavioral, experiential, and physiological sources of evidence, all of which converge on a dual-component view.

Summing up, in this article we have presented and described a database of transcripts of what subjects said when they were questioned about recognition decisions associated with remember, know, and guess responses. These transcripts confirm the different states of awareness that subjects experience and report, and they are of additional theoretical interest. Of the current interpretations of remembering and knowing that we discuss, the distinction between episodic and semantic systems and the distinctiveness/fluency framework provide the most direct accounts. They also have the advantage that the evidence for the theoretical constructs they employ is relatively independent of evidence from the reported states of awareness but relies on other sources of evidence. The process dissociation procedure is less concerned with the states of awareness as such than with recollection and familiarity, conceived very differently from remembering and knowing, as controlled and automatic processes. A unitary trace strength model seems less viable than any of these alternatives, though it has certainly been of some heuristic value and it has drawn attention to some previously neglected aspects of the decisions that subjects must make when reporting their states of awareness.

Appendix 1: Transcripts of Subjects' Responses

Ss	Remember	Know	Guess
1	*Green.* I felt that when I saw it yesterday, I remembered that it was my favourite colour.	*Road.* I felt I saw this word but could not find the exact feelings of when I saw the word, but I am sure I saw the word, I could though not find the background.	*Slipper.* I saw this word somewhere recently at some point, but I am not sure whether it was there yesterday.
	Policeman. I remembered that it closely followed the word "gun," one came after the other.	*Boy.* I reckon I saw it yesterday, I felt that I saw it yesterday, but I am not *extremely* sure.	*Blossom.* I felt the same as for "slipper," I saw this word recently.
2	*Cider.* I associated it with "outsider" when I saw it yesterday, today I remembered the association.	*Paper.* It was as if I had seen it, I am sure it was there yesterday, but I cannot remember seeing it.	*Party.* I think it was familiar but I was not sure.
	Hotel. My stepfather owns a hotel, yesterday I have tried to associate the words with people I knew and that is what came to my mind today.	*Pickle.* Same as paper, I do not remember seeing it, but I remember it was there.	*Apricot.* Again it looked kind of familiar.
3	*Pickle.* I was thinking of cheese and pickle sandwiches when it came up yesterday.	*Hotel.* It is one of the words I thought it was there yesterday, but there was no particular reason ...	*Telephone.* I was less sure that telephone was there than I was of butterfly for example.
	Puppy. Because I am from Belgium, we call my father Puppy (nickname) so I could not forget that word.	*Butterfly.* It was one of those words that rang a bell.	*Raspberry.* I was not sure whether it was me going to pick raspberries, or whether the word was there yesterday.
4	*Furniture.* I think that when I was trying to remember the words, it was one of the first words that came up.	*Emerald.* It looked familiar I remember maybe repeating it when I was memorising it, but I was not 100% sure.	*Ring.* I thought I recognised it but I was not sure. Because "ring" is familiar but I was not sure whether it was for that or whether I actually saw it.
	Piano. When I saw it yesterday I remember saying. "Oh I can remember that because I can see myself playing the piano."	*Father.* I thought I saw the word father with another word, but I was not sure.	*Zipper.* It was just a guess. I guessed when I recognised things but I was not sure that they were in the list, with "know" I was sure it was there ...
5	*Sofa.* A girl I know is called Sofia. When I saw the word yesterday it made me think of her.	*Zipper.* I just remember it coming up, it was an unusual word, it seemed it came up before, but I did not recall anything about it, no thought was associated with it.	*Furniture.* It seemed familiar, but it was just me thinking of furniture in the room, or was it there? Also up to the point when "furniture" came up, I said I remembered all of them, so I thought they cannot all be right.

Appendix 1
(continued)

Ss	Remember	Know	Guess
	Surf. It was one of the first words that came up, so I was trying to memorise all the first words, so I remember that one.	*Piano.* I am sure that it came up, but I do not remember anything in particular about it.	*Harp.* It seemed that there were quite a few musical instruments, so I took a guess that it came up.
6	*Athlete.* I had an outline of a cartoon image of an athlete when I saw it yesterday, and it all popped back into my mind when I saw it today.	*Grasshopper.* I did not have any images, it did not come up with any images, I remember it just being there.	*Furniture.* It could have been one of the words, but I am not sure, so a guess seemed an appropriate response.
	Gun. When I saw it yesterday I had an image of a gun and I thought it was a strange word to put in.	*Magazine.* One of a few words that I knew I had seen it before and it was familiar.	*Road.* Same as above, it was possible that I have seen it before.
7	*Surf.* I answered "Remember" because it reminded me of living in Plymouth when I saw the word yesterday, so I remembered it this morning.	*Tangerine.* I literally had a feeling that it was there yesterday but I could not remember anything else.	*Limousine.* It seemed likely it could have been there, I could not remember it being there but I had a feeling that it might have been.
	Cranberry. Yesterday I was trying to use strategies to remember things. So I associated it with Delia Smith's book, which has recipes full of cranberries.	*Gondola.* I just thought it was there.	*Cider.* Again, likely to have been there.
8	*Leopard.* Yesterday I was making associations when I saw the words, and I remembered those.	*Professor.* It was not in any of the little stories I made up to remember the words, but I had a strong feeling of familiarity.	*Thorn.* It was not definitely in my head that it was there, but it seemed vaguely familiar.
	Rainbow. Same reason, I remembered a multicoloured telephone box outside the hospital.	*Crucifix.* I was not 100% sure of a connection, but I was pretty sure it was there. It was definitely in my head.	*Holiday.* I guessed that it was there as I made some connections with summer which I knew it was there, but no memories about it.
9	*Tangerine.* I thought of food when I saw it and today that came back to me.	*Cigarette.* Pretty sure it was there, but I cannot go back to an image or anything that happened yesterday.	NO GUESSES.
	Tornado. I thought of an actual "tornado" when I saw it yesterday, so I remembered it today.	*Grasshopper.* Like "cigarette," no association only a feeling of familiarity.	

Appendix 1
(continued)

Ss	Remember	Know	Guess
10	*Mother.* It was near the beginning; it was the second word.	*Record.* I do think it had familiarity, I did not know whether it was because I had seen it before.	*Library.* I thought that was one of the words but I was not sure at all.
	Road. I have tried to relate the words to summer, I know I saw it because of the way I remember it, running down the road in the summer.	*Magazine.* I am sure it was there but I could not place it.	
11	*Piano.* I used to play the piano, so yesterday I thought of that, when I saw the word today I just remembered it from yesterday.	*Athlete.* I am sure I saw it, but I can't remember why I think I saw it.	*Father.* I kept saying "no" so I just guessed it was there because you said that 50% of the words were there.
	Magazine. My friends laugh at me because I buy 5 magazines each week! This is the thought I had when I first saw the word.	*Gun.* I remember it was there, I was sure it was there, it was familiar.	*Church.* Same reason.
12	*Tangerine.* I remembered it. It was the second one up yesterday.	*Grasshopper.* I just thought that when I saw it I recognised it and I thought it was there, but it triggered nothing.	*Claw.* I thought that was there but I was not sure.
	Eye. It was one of the first ones yesterday.	*Squirrel.* I thought it was there, but no thoughts associated. Either that or we were talking about "squirrels" yesterday.	*Horse.* I was not certain but I thought I recognised it.
13	*Hospital.* I remembered it because of my father's condition; he is in a hospital. Seeing the word reminded me that I thought of that, it triggered a connection of thoughts.	*Boy.* It is familiar because it is connected to my children. But I could not find any feelings or thought that I had yesterday that were associated with it.	*Letter.* I was not sure whether it was there or not.
	Mother. I remember that word strongly, the word is still in my memory in the way I saw it yesterday.	*Leopard.* I do not remember seeing words of animals, but the word is familiar, I cannot place it exactly, I knew I read it but I could not relate it to anything.	*Road.* I was not sure, but I thought it was in one of my connections.
14	*Sofa.* I had an image of people sitting on it. I remembered it because I remember thinking about that image.	*Island.* It seemed familiar, I was not aware of other things.	*Gondola.* It seemed that I could recall an image of Venice, but I was not sure whether I was imagining it or whether the word was there.
	Piano. I used to play the piano. I thought of that when I saw the word yesterday.	*Whale.* I did not form any associations, it just seemed familiar.	*Library.* The word was familiar to me but the familiarity was not very strong.

Appendix 1
(continued)

Ss	Remember	Know	Guess
15	*Sauerkraut.* It was probably the way it was spelled, I remember looking at it yesterday and saying; "What does that say!?"	*River.* I answered "Know" because I was pretty sure it was there yesterday, but I couldn't remember, I could not specifically remember seeing it.	*Limousine.* It could have been there, I was not certain whether it was or not.
	Gondola. Because I remember relating it to skiing, that thought came back to me as I saw it today.	*Road.* In a similar way as for "river," I was pretty certain, but I cannot fix in my mind when I saw the word.	*Puppy.* It was more the situation that I have heard that word pretty recently, but I was not sure whether it was here or not.
16	*Kite.* When I read it yesterday I thought of another word, so that is what I remembered today.	*Church.* I felt as if I saw it yesterday.	*Squirrel.* It just seemed as if it was one of the words that would have been there, I have quite a recent image of the word but I was not sure whether it was there yesterday.
	Orchid. It was close to the word "cider," so I made a connection between the two words.	*Cigarette.* I felt as if I have seen that word, I was sure that the word was there yesterday.	*Sky.* It was a short word, so I believed that it was there as there were a number of short words.
17	*Ape.* I remembered that word with another word. I formed a picture of it. I knew as soon as I saw it because I remember thinking of the picture of monkeys at the time.	*River.* I felt I knew it was there as soon as I saw it.	*Hospital.* I thought it might have been there but I was not sure.
	Butterfly. I remember seeing it. Making an image and a picture of it.	*Sauerkraut.* I remembered it because it was an unusual word. I knew it was there.	*Camera.* I thought it might have been there.
18	*Bluebell.* Yesterday it came up close to the word ring. I remembered that.	*Plum.* I think I remembered it, but I was not sure as nothing came back to me about seeing it, but I knew it was there, it was sort of familiar.	*Harp.* I remember that yesterday I was thinking about "music," so I took a guess that the word was there.
	Sauerkraut. I remembered it because I could not pronounce it yesterday!	*Sea.* I remember something about "sea" but I was not sure whether it was related to "surf" or "sea." I was not sure, but I remember thinking about sea, but did not know whether it was because of seeing the word sea or not.	*Log.* I was not sure, there was nothing associated.

Appendix 1
(continued)

Ss	Remember	Know	Guess
19	*President.* Yesterday I associated this word with the word "minister." Today I automatically remembered about that association.	*Grasshopper.* I just knew it was there, there were no thoughts associated.	*Athlete.* I was not sure, I kind of recognised it but I was not sure.
	Tornado. Yesterday I studied something about "hazards" so I associated the word with that.	*Sofa.* I was just sure of seeing the word here and I knew I had seen it.	*Gondola.* I kind of remember it, but I did not know whether it was here that I saw it or elsewhere.
20	*Gondola.* I remember saying to myself. "What on earth is that?!" when I saw it yesterday.	*Harbour.* It was familiar, but I was confused. I knew it was there but could not be sure.	*Flea.* I am almost certain that it was there. But not entirely.
	Policeman. My brother is a policeman. I thought of that.	—	—
21	*Tornado.* I remember watching a program on television about it. I thought of that yesterday, and today the word reminded me of the program.	*Harp.* I just felt that I saw the word yesterday. There was something about musical instruments.	*Rainbow.* I think I saw some word similar to "rainbow" yesterday.
	Piano. The word "house" came before it, so I had an image of a house with a piano inside.	*Car.* I just knew it was there, nothing came back to my mind.	*Sea.* I thought I saw it but I was not sure.
22	*Furniture.* When I first saw it I thought about "chairs" and "tables". That was brought back when I saw the word today.	*Surf.* I had a feeling that I had seen that word, I kind of remember the word: when it came up just before it reminded me that I had seen it somewhere.	*Broom.* I felt I had seen it, but I was not sure, I thought guessing was the appropriate answer.
	Horse. I had an image of an horse.	*Hospital.* I have also been to a hospital recently so that could be why the word is so familiar to me, but I believed it was there.	*Gondola.* It was the sound of the word that had some familiarity.
23	*Cigarette.* Because I smoke. I remember seeing it yesterday because of the image that it conjured. The same thoughts came back to me yesterday.	*Tangerine.* I recognised it as a word from yesterday, but I cannot really remember what I thought, I could not remember seeing it on the screen but I was sure it was there yesterday.	*Bluebell.* It was a pure guess. I had a very slight feeling that it was there. I am not sure whether I saw it yesterday or before.
	Rectangle. Yesterday as it came on the screen I imagined a rectangle against an orange background and that image came back to me.	*River.* I could imagined it written across the screen, I thought I might have seen it yesterday. I felt it was there, but I do not know why.	*Clown.* I remembered an image but it could have been my imagination, I do not know whether it was there, so I just guessed.

Appendix 1
(continued)

Ss	Remember	Know	Guess
24	*Kilt.* It reminded me of going to Scotland when I saw it yesterday.	*Car.* I just knew I had seen it yesterday, there was no story connected to it, it was just very familiar.	*Weed.* I was not sure at all!
	Ape. When it came up I remember thinking that there were lots of words with three letters.	*Summer.* I knew I had seen it, I had thought about summer but I could not remember what my thoughts were, it was just a feeling of seeing the word.	*Uniform.* It was sort of familiar but I was not sure, maybe I had seen it somewhere else.
25	*Harp.* I remembered when I saw the word I quickly saw a harp in a church. The same picture came back.	*Sea.* When I saw the word it was familiar, I just thought it was there but there was nothing else.	*Uniform.* When I saw the word I thought I recognised it, I had a feeling it might have been there.
	Kilt. I had a picture of someone standing on a hill in a kilt. That picture came back today.	*Gun.* There was no association, I just had a feeling that I saw it, I was sure.	*Water.* I had a feeling that it was there but I was not sure.
26	*Surf.* At the time I was counting the number of "S" words and I remembered that "surf" was one of them and it was short.	*Cranberry.* It was an unusual word. I thought I recognised it as soon as I saw it. I could not remember thinking about it, but I thought I had seen it, I could not think where else I would have seen it.	*Ring.* I seemed to keep pressing the "yes" button a lot. So I thought it was better saying that it was a guess, because of the 30%. But it seemed familiar.
	Grasshopper. Because I help this group of children, I thought about that yesterday and that stuck in my mind.	*Furniture.* I just thought I had seen it, I recognised it and I was sure it was there. But also because I saw the word chair I thought maybe I was wrong but it was familiar.	*Harp.* It was a short word and an object, so maybe it could have been one of them.
27	*Grasshopper.* I think the word boulder was there and I imagined a boulder with a grasshopper.	*Rectangle.* It just sounded familiar, I couldn't remember anything about it I just had a vague idea that it was there yesterday.	*Water.* I remember that there were lots of things to do with sea, or words to do with water, so I imagined that it was there.
	Blood. It conjured a strong image, so I remember seeing that word yesterday.	*Cranberry.* It was just familiar.	*Hotel.* Another one like "water."
28	*Athlete.* I remembered having a conversation with a friend of mine.	*Sea.* I thought I remembered it but there were no thoughts regarding the word, perhaps just the feeling of seeing it yesterday.	*City.* I was not sure.
	Harp. I remembered being present at a concert where music was playing.	*Magazine.* I had a feeling of familiarity.	*Car.* I was not sure. I had a very vague feeling that perhaps I saw it.

Appendix 1
(continued)

Ss	Remember	Know	Guess
29	*Athlete.* I had a picture of the Olympics.	*Sea.* I do not remember seeing it but it felt familiar.	*Cranberry.* I thought that there were lots of fruit-words yesterday, so I thought it was one of them.
	Harp. On Friday I was in a restaurant with a harpist. I remember thinking of that yesterday.	*Kilt.* It seemed familiar but I wondered.	*Furniture.* There were a few long words, I thought it could have been one of them.
30	*Sofa.* I remember picturing a sofa yesterday and relating it to furniture.	*Ring.* I think I remember seeing it, but there was no link or image. I can't remember feeling anything.	*Harp.* I was not sure about it, it could have been there just as well as it could have not been there.
	Cranberry. It was the first word on the list.	*Emerald.* I think I remember linking it to something, but I cannot remember what to.	*Church.* I think I tried picturing a church, but also someone was talking to me about churches the other day, so I might have confused the two things.
31	*President.* When I saw it on the screen yesterday I was thinking of presidents' faces.	*Church.* I felt there was a strong familiarity with it, I thought I saw the word but it was not connected to anything.	*Piano.* I felt a that there wasn't such strong familiarity. Maybe I saw it, but there were no strong feelings.
	Tornado. When I saw it yesterday it reminded me of the "Rover" advert.	*Rectangle.* I think I saw this word (but maybe it was triangle!), I do not remember visualising a rectangle but I saw it.	*Father.* I think I saw it but I was not sure.
32	*Kilt.* I saw it yesterday for definite, I remember seeing the word on the screen.	*Magazine.* I was pretty sure it came out, but I could not identify the word.	*Puppy.* I was not sure that the word was there.
	Sauerkraut. I remember I had to look at it closely yesterday.	*Bluebell.* I am sure about that one, there were a couple of words which were similar and where part of the category flower.	*Leopard.* Not sure.
33	*Furniture.* I thought of a chair when I saw it.	*Library.* I think it came back to me but I cannot pinpoint actually seeing it.	*Rainbow.* I really do not know, it was a guess.
	Cider. I saw a program on under-age drinking recently; so I thought of that when I saw the word.	*Party.* I think it came up but it triggered nothing.	*Officer.* It was just a guess.

Appendix 1
(continued)

Ss	Remember	Know	Guess
34	*Blood.* That word came almost directly after I created an image of the "musician" playing the "piano."	*Squirrel.* I remembered something about squirrels, but I cannot remember what.	*Eye.* There were basically 3 groups of association, and this may not have been the key word, but maybe it was part of the association.
	Nun. I made a connection in my head: it came just after kids and the kids were on the sofa. Nun came after that.	*Kite.* Because it was something to do with the sky. I was fairly confident it was there but there was no direct connection.	*President.* There was no real association, but I remember something about seeing the word "president" recently!
35	*Piano.* I remembered it because "musician" came up first and also I have a friend who plays the piano so I linked the two together.	*Nun.* I could not remember the situation but I knew I saw the word somewhere.	NO GUESSES.
	Grasshopper. Where I work the boss has a tarantula and locusts were fed to them, so I made that connection with grasshoppers.	*Tablespoon.* It was a familiar word to me.	
36	*Butterfly.* I thought of a Greek song about butterflies when I saw the word.	*Magazine.* I think I remember seeing it, but it was not associated with anything, actually I was not sure whether it was "magazine" or "newspaper."	*Telephone.* I was not sure whether I saw the word yesterday or I was thinking that I had to call someone.
	Ring. I was playing with my rings when I saw it yesterday.	*Body.* A lot of words flashed very quickly yesterday and I was not always concentrating, so I thought I saw that one.	*Holiday.* I am eager to go on holiday so I am not sure whether I saw it here or whether I was thinking about it.
37	*Car.* I created all this story surrounding the word "policeman" and the car was part of it, I remembered the story.	*Summer.* Nothing connected to it, it was just part of the whole thing yesterday.	*Clarinet.* It seemed the sort of word you would remember, so I just had a feeling it was one of those words.
	Magazine. This was also part of the story, I remembered an image of a magazine.	*Gun.* I just knew that I knew it.	*Shrimp.* It was a total guess.
38	*Broom.* When this word appeared I remember saying to myself that I had to try and remember that word.	*Furniture.* I just felt sure that it was there but I could not remember seeing it at the time.	*Surf.* I was not sure, I thought it was there.
	Log. I was thinking of "logging" in to the computer.	*Cigarette.* It was the same as for furniture.	*Piano.* It could have been there.

Appendix 1
(continued)

Ss	Remember	Know	Guess
39	*Emerald.* I used a story: grasshopper was before it and I connected it with a green emerald.	*Log.* I just thought I recognised it, I felt that it was there, but there was no story connected to it.	*Tornado.* I thought I recognised it, but I was not sure. I recognised it in the way that I thought it was more there than not. For example, with gun I knew that it was definitely not there.
	Furniture. My friend was moving, I remember thinking of that.	*Cigarette.* I just thought it was there, but again no story, but I knew it was there.	
40	*Green.* I remember thinking of nature straightaway yesterday.	*Car.* I had a feeling that it was there; I think car was there.	*Body.* I remember there was something to do with clothing, so I had a vague thought that it was there.
	Raspberry. I remember associating it with "apricot" and "plum."	*Shrimp.* I knew it was there, I do not remember seeing it but it was familiar.	*Blood.* I think it was there but I was not sure.
41	*Sauerkraut.* It reminded me of my German lessons. It looked odd as one of the words in the list.	*Sea.* It looked sort of as if I saw it, but there was nothing associated to it.	*Gun.* It could have been there but I was not sure.
	Boy. I remember it appearing on the screen.	*Emerald.* I remembered that there was a jewel, but I cannot remember when I saw the word.	*Island.* I was not sure if I saw it.
42	*Surf.* It came up at the beginning and I associated it with "island."	*Cider.* I was sure I had seen it, but I could not remember seeing it.	*Nun.* I was not sure whether I had seen it or not, but I thought I did.
	Horse. I remember thinking about my horse.	*Rectangle.* I am sure it was there but I do not remember thinking about it.	*Paper.* I thought that I might have seen it.
43	*Kilt.* I remembered that I thought of a Scottish man.	*Bluebell.* I could remember that there was a flower, but I could not remember the specific flower.	*River.* I could remember thinking of the word, it seemed as if I recollected it, but it was to vague to say I was sure.
	Body. I could remember thinking that it was an easy word to remember.	*Summer.* I could not remember it, but it sounded familiar, I think I did see it yesterday.	*Record.* It could have possibly been there yesterday.
44	*Emerald.* I recently bought a ring. I had this thought yesterday and it came back to me when I saw the word again.	*Father.* There was something about father, mother and child that seemed familiar.	*Island.* I come from an island, so it could have been that I saw the word on the list or that the word was familiar because I come from an island.

Appendix 1
(continued)

Ss	Remember	Know	Guess
	Piano. I remembered that there were a few musical instruments that came up and "piano" was one of those.	*Church.* I just thought it came up yesterday.	*Log.* I was really guessing with that word.
45	*Piano.* When that word came up I thought of me playing the piano.	*Keg.* It was a feeling that it was there. I was not sure whether it was at work or here that I came across that word.	*Harbour.* I lived by the sea all my life, so I was not sure whether I have encountered that word here or whether it is to do with home.
	Cranberry. I remembered it because when it came up it reminded me that we need more cranberry juice in the union bar where I work.	*Orchid.* I really just recognised without remembering it appearing yesterday.	*Car.* I was not sure.

Appendix 2: Instructions

Written Test Instructions

In this test you will see a series of words, one word at a time. Some of the words are those that you saw yesterday. Others are not. For each word, click the YES button if you recognize the word as one you saw yesterday and click the NO button if you do not think the word was one you saw yesterday.

Recognition memory is associated with two different kinds of awareness. Quite often recognition brings back to mind something you recollect about what it is that you recognise, as when, for example, you recognize someone's face, and perhaps *remember* talking to this person at a party the previous night. At other times recognition brings nothing back to mind about what it is you recognise, as when, for example, you are confident that you recognise someone, and you *know* you recognise them, because of strong feelings of familiarity, but you have no recollection of seeing this person before. You do not remember anything about them.

The same kinds of awareness are associated with recognising the words you saw yesterday. Sometimes when you recognize a word as one you saw yesterday, recognition will bring back to mind something you remember thinking about when the word appeared then. You recollect something you consciously experienced at that time. But sometimes recognizing a word as one you saw yesterday will not bring back to mind anything you remember about seeing it then. Instead, the word will seem familiar, so that you feel confident it was one you saw yesterday, even though you don't recollect anything you experienced when you saw it then.

For each word that you recognize, after you have clicked the YES button, please then click the REMEMBER button, if recognition is accompanied by some recollective experience, or the KNOW button, if recognition is accompanied by strong feelings of familiarity in the absence of any recollective experience.

There will also be times when you do not remember the word, nor does it seem familiar, but you might want to guess that it was one of the words you saw yesterday. Feel free to do this, but if your YES response is really just a guess, please then click the GUESS button.

Lastly, when you are doing this test you may find it helpful to bear in mind that 30%–50% of the words are actually words that you saw yesterday.

Supplementary Oral Instructions

As usual in experiments of this kind, the written test instructions are followed by an oral briefing, in which the differences between the responses are explained again and then explanations and examples of them are elicited from the subjects, to check their understanding of them. The extent of this oral briefing is quite variable, depending on the particular individual. The following paragraphs exemplify what subjects were told at this time:

When you see these words today, if a word triggers something that you experienced when you saw it previously, like, for example, something about its appearance on the screen or the way it was spelled, or the order in which the word came in, I would like you to indicate this kind of recognition, by clicking the REMEMBER button. In other instances the word may remind you of something you thought about when you saw it previously, like an association that you made to the word, or an image that you formed when you saw the word, or something of personal significance that you associated with the word; again if you can recollect any of these aspects of when the word was first presented I would like you to click the REMEMBER button.

Instead, at other times you will see a word and you will recognize it as one you saw yesterday, but the word will not bring back to mind anything you remember about seeing it then, the word will just seem extremely familiar. When you feel confident that you saw the word yesterday, even though you do not recollect anything you experienced when you saw it, I would like

you to indicate this kind of recognition, by clicking the KNOW button.

With know responses you are sure about seeing the word yesterday but cannot remember the circumstances in which the word was presented, or the thoughts elicited when the word was presented. With a guess response, you think it possible that the word was presented but you are not sure that it was. For some reason, you think there was a chance that the word was presented. Some people say "it looks like one of those words that could have possibly have been there." When you think your response was really just a guess, I would like you to click the GUESS button.

Acknowledgments

This research was supported by Grant R000-23-6225 from the Economic and Social Research Council (ESRC) of Great Britain and we are grateful to them for their support. We also thank Martin Conway, Vernon Gregg, and Rosalind Java for comments on an earlier version of the manuscript.

References

Brewer, W. F. (1992). Phenomenal experience in laboratory and autobiographical memory. In M. A. Conway, D. C. Rubin, H. Spinnler, and W. A. Wagenaar (Eds.), *Theoretical perspectives on autobiographical memory* (pp. 31–51). Dordecht, NL: Kluwer.

Brewer, W. F. (1996). What is recollective memory? In D. C. Rubin (Ed.), *Remembering our past: Studies in autobiographical memory* (pp. 19–66). Cambridge: Cambridge University Press.

Conway, M. A., and Dewhurst, S. A. (1995). The self and recollective experience. *Applied Cognitive Psychology*, 9, 1–19.

Conway, M. A., Collins, A. F., Gathercole, S. E., and Anderson, S. J. (1996). Recollections of true and false autobiographical memories. *Journal of Experimental Psychology: General*, 125, 69–95.

Conway, M. A., Gardiner, J. M., Perfect, T. J., Anderson, S. J., and Cohen, G. (1997). Changes in memory awareness during learning: The acquisition of knowledge by psychology undergraduates. *Journal of Experimental Psychology: General*, 126, 393–413.

Curran, T., Schacter, D. L., Norman, K. A., and Galluccio, L. (1997). False recognition after a right frontal lobe infarction: Memory for general and specific information. *Neuropsychologia*, 35, 1035–1049.

Deese, J. (1959). On the prediction of occurrence of particular intrusions in immediate recall. *Journal of Experimental Psychology*, 58, 17–22.

Düzel, E., Yonelinas, A. P., Mangun, G. R., Heinze, H.-J., and Tulving, E. (1997). Event-related brain potential correlates of two states of conscious awareness in memory. *Proceedings of the National Academy of Science*, 94, 5973–5978.

Donaldson, W. (1996). The role of decision processes in remembering and knowing. *Memory & Cognition*, 24, 523–533.

Gardiner, J. M. (1988). Functional aspects of recollective experience. *Memory & Cognition*, 16, 309–313.

Gardiner, J. M., and Gregg, V. H. (1997). Recognition memory with little or no remembering: Implications for a detection model. *Psychonomic Bulletin & Review*, 4, 474–479.

Gardiner, J. M., and Java, R. I. (1990). Recollective experience in word and nonword recognition. *Memory & Cognition*, 18, 23–30.

Gardiner, J. M., and Java, R. I. (1993). Recognising and remembering. In A. Collins, S. Gathercole, M. Conway, and P. Morris (Eds.), *Theories of memory* (pp. 163–188). Hillsdale, NJ: Erlbaum.

Gardiner, J. M., and Moran, H. M. (1997). Unpublished experiment.

Gardiner, J. M., Java, R. I., and Richardson-Klavehn, A. (1996). How level of processing really influences awareness in recognition memory. *Canadian Journal of Experimental Psychology*, 50, 114–122.

Gardiner, J. M., Kaminska, Z., Dixon, M., and Java, R. I. (1996). Repetition of previously novel melodies sometimes increases both remember and know responses in recognition memory. *Psychonomic Bulletin & Review*, 3, 366–371.

Gardiner, J. M., Richardson-Klavehn, A., and Ramponi, C. (1997). On reporting recollective experiences

and "direct access to memory systems". *Psychological Science*, 8, 391–394.

Gregg, V. H., and Gardiner, J. M. (1994). Recognition memory and awareness: A large effect of study-test modalities on "know" responses following a highly perceptual orienting task. *European Journal of Cognitive Psychology*, 6, 137–147.

Hirshman, E., and Master, S. (1997). Modeling the conscious correlates of recognition memory: Reflections on the remember-know paradigm. *Memory & Cognition*, 25, 345–351.

Huron, C., Danion, J.-M., Giacomoni, F., Grange, D., Robert, P., and Rizzo, L. (1995). Impairment of recognition memory with, but not without, conscious recollection in schizophrenia. *American Journal of Psychiatry*, 152, 1737–1742.

Inoue, C., and Bellezza, F. S. (1998). The detection model of recognition using know and remember judgements. *Memory & Cognition*, 26, 299–308.

Jacoby, L. L. (1988). Memory observed and memory unobserved. In U. Neisser and E. Winograd (Eds.), *Remembering reconsidered: Ecological and traditional approaches to the study of memory* (pp. 145–177). Cambridge, UK: Cambridge University Press.

Jacoby, L. L. (1991). A process-dissociation framework: Separating automatic from intentional uses of memory. *Journal of Memory and Language*, 30, 513–541.

Jacoby, L. L., and Dallas, M. (1981). On the relationship between autobiographical memory and perceptual learning. *Journal of Experimental Psychology: General*, 110, 306–340.

Jacoby, L. L., Yonelinas, A. P., and Jennings, J. M. (1997). The relation between conscious and unconscious (automatic) influences: A declaration of independence. In J. D. Cohen and J. W. Schooler (Eds.), *Scientific approaches to the question of consciousness* (pp. 13–47). Hillsdale, NJ: Erlbaum.

Java, R. I., Gregg, V. H., and Gardiner, J. M. (1997). What do people actually remember and know in "remember/know" experiments? *European Journal of Cognitive Psychology*, 9, 187–197.

Johnson, M. K. (1988). Reality monitoring: An experimental phenomenological approach. *Journal of Experimental Psychology: General*, 117, 390–394.

Johnson, M. K., Foley, M. A., Suengas, A. G., and Raye, C. L. (1988). Phenomenal characteristics of memories for perceived and imagined autobiographical events. *Journal of Experimental Psychology: General*, 117, 371–376.

Kinoshita, S. (1995). The word frequency effect in recognition memory versus repetition priming. *Memory & Cognition*, 23, 569–580.

Larsen, S. F. (1998). What is it like to remember? On phenomenal qualities of memory. In C. P. Thompson, J. D. Read, D. Bruce, D. G. Payne, and M. P. Toglia, (Eds.), *Autobiographical and eyewitness memory: Theoretical and applied perspectives*, (pp. 163–190). New York: Erlbaum.

Lehmann, A. (1889): Ueber Wiedererkennen. *Philos. Studien*, V, 95–156.

Mandler, G. (1980). Recognizing: The judgment of previous occurrence. *Psychological Review*, 87, 252–271.

Mantyla, T. (1997). Recollections of faces: Remembering differences and knowing similarities. *Journal of Experimental Psychology: Learning, Memory, and Cognition*, 23, 1203–1216.

Nyberg, L., and Tulving, E. (1996). Classifying human long-term memory: Evidence from converging dissociations. *European Journal of Cognitive Psychology*, 8, 163–183.

Rajaram, S. (1993). Remembering and knowing: Two means of access to the personal past. *Memory & Cognition*, 21, 89–102.

Rajaram, S. (1996). Perceptual effects on remembering: Recollective processes in picture recognition memory. *Journal of Experimental Psychology: Learning, Memory, and Cognition*, 22, 365–377.

Rajaram, S. (1998). The effects of conceptual salience and perceptual distinctiveness on conscious recollection. *Psychonomic Bulletin & Review*, 5, 71–78.

Rajaram, S., and Roediger, H. L., III (1997). Remembering and knowing as states of consciousness during recollection. In J. D. Cohen and J. W. Schooler (Eds.), *Scientific approaches to the question of consciousness* (pp. 213–240). Hillsdale, NJ: Erlbaum.

Richardson-Klavehn, A., Gardiner, J. M., and Java, R. I. (1996). Memory: Task dissociations, process dissociations, and dissociations of consciousness. In G. Underwood (Ed.), *Implicit cognition* (pp. 85–158). Oxford: Oxford Univ. Press.

Roediger, H. L., and McDermott, K. B. (1995). Creating false memories: Remembering words not pre-

sented in lists. *Journal of Experimental Psychology: Learning, Memory, and Cognition*, 21, 803–814.

Strack, F., and Forster, J. (1995). Reporting recollective experiences: Direct access to memory systems? *Psychological Science*, 6, 352–358.

Strong, E. K. J. (1913). The effect of time interval on recognition memory. *Psychological Review*, 20, 339–372.

Strong, M. H., and Strong, E. K. J. (1916). The nature of recognition memory and of the localization of recognitions. *American Journal of Psychology*, 27, 341–362.

Tulving, E. (1983). *Elements of episodic memory*. Oxford: Oxford University Press.

Tulving, E. (1985). Memory and consciousness. *Canadian Psychologist*, 26, 1–12.

Tulving, E. (1989). Memory: Performance, knowledge, and experience. *European Journal of Experimental Psychology*, 1, 3–26.

Wheeler, M. A., Stuss, D. T., and Tulving, E. (1997). Towards a theory of episodic memory: The frontal lobes and autonoetic consciousness. *Psychological Bulletin*.

Yonelinas, A. P., and Jacoby, L. L. (1996). Noncriterial recollection: Familiarity as automatic, irrelevant recollection. *Consciousness and Cognition*, 5, 131–141.

Yonelinas, A. P., Dobbins, I., Szymanski, M. D., Dhaliwal, H. S., and King, L. (1996). Signal detection, threshold, and dual process models of recognition memory: ROCs and conscious recollection. *Consciousness and Cognition*, 5, 418–441.

44 Measuring Recollection: Strategic versus Automatic Influences of Associative Context

Larry L. Jacoby

Introduction

How should one measure an amnesiac's ability to recollect memory for a prior event? An obvious means of measuring recollection would be to question the person directly about memory for the event; for example, a test of cued recall might be used. However, there are problems for measuring recollection in that way. To illustrate, consider difficulties for interpreting an amnesiac's performance on a test of recall cued by presentation of word stems. Suppose that amnesiacs were presented with a long list of words that they were told to remember, and then memory was tested by providing word stems that were to be used as cues for recall of the words presented earlier (e.g., mot_____ as a cue for recall of *motel*). To measure memory, the probability of completing stems with old words is compared with the base rate probability of completing those stems. A measure of base rate is gained by presenting stems that can be completed only with words not presented earlier.

Experiments using these sorts of procedures have shown that amnesiacs' recall performance is sometimes nearly as good as that of subjects with normal functioning memory (Graf, Squire, and Mandler 1984; Warrington and Weiskrantz 1974). Consequently, it might be concluded that given word stems as cues, amnesiacs preserve an almost normal ability to recollect memory for a prior experience (Warrington and Weiskrantz 1974). However, amnesiacs might achieve their high level of cued recall performance by a means other than recollection. They may complete word stems with the first word that comes to mind without being aware that their completions are the words that they were instructed to recall. Indeed, amnesiacs' cued recall performance sometimes does not differ greatly from what would be observed if they were given an indirect test of memory.

For an indirect test, people are not asked to report on memory for an event as they would be for a direct test, such as a test of recognition memory or recall. Rather, they engage in some task that can indirectly reflect memory for the occurrence of that event. Word stem and fragment completion tasks are among the most popular indirect tests of memory (Warrington and Weiskrantz 1974; Tulving, Schacter, and Stark 1982; Graf and Mandler 1984). Dissociations between performance on direct and indirect tests supply examples of effects of the past in the absence of remembering (Richardson-Klavehn and Bjork 1988, Hintzman 1990). Some of the most striking examples of dissociations come from the performance of patients suffering a neurological deficit. Korsakoff amnesiacs, for example, show near-normal effects of memory in their performance of a stem completion task, although their performance on direct tests of memory is severely impaired (for reviews, see Ostergaard and Jernigan 1993; Shimamura 1986).

The problem for gaining an accurate measure of recollection (a strategic, consciously controlled use of memory) is that performance of a direct test may be contaminated by automatic influences of the sort reflected by performance on indirect tests of memory. Automatic influences of memory increase the probability of correct guessing. This informed guessing inflates estimates of recollection and may be largely responsible for accurate memory reports produced by amnesiacs (Gabrieli et al. 1990). Guessing could be discouraged by instructions, but it is unlikely that it could be fully eliminated. Rather than attempting to eliminate guessing, it would be better to measure its effects.

How should one correct for informed guessing on a direct test so as to gain an accurate measure of recollection? One answer to that question is to measure recollection as the difference between performance on a direct test and that on an indirect test of memory. For example, stem-completion performance might be subtracted from recall cued with word stems to gain a measure of recollection. However, that solution is unlikely to be satisfactory. Performance on indirect tests is sometimes contaminated by strategic uses of memory and so cannot be treated as a pure measure of automatic influences of memory (Richardson-Klavehn and Bjork 1988). Another problem for measuring recollection and automatic influences with different tasks is that processes may be qualitatively different across tasks. The issue here is something like the commonplace belief that people express what they "truly believe" when drunk. It is possible that what people believe when drunk is qualitatively different from what they believe when sober. Similarly, the automatic influences revealed by an indirect test may be different from those that are in play on a direct test of memory.

Rather than identify processes with tasks, as is done by use of the contrast between indirect and direct tests, I have used a "process-dissociation procedure" to separate the within-task contributions of consciously controlled and automatic uses of memory (Jacoby 1991). Elsewhere we (e.g., Jacoby and Kelley 1991, Jacoby et al. 1992) have written much about the advantages of the process-dissociation procedure over indirect tests as a means of investigating automatic influences of memory. Here, I change focus by describing the advantages of the process-dissociation procedure over the use of direct tests as a means of measuring recollection.

Reliance on direct tests of memory to measure recollection fails to separate strategic and automatic influences of memory and, consequently, can lead to erroneous conclusions. Failure to distinguish between automatic and strategic influences might account for the disarray in the literature concerning the effects of some variables on performance of direct tests. I present evidence to illustrate problems for interpreting performance on direct tests of memory. After describing advantages of the process-dissociation procedure, I propose a distinction between strategic and automatic influences of associative context and report new experiments to show the utility of that distinction.

Measuring Recollection

The problem of correcting measures of recollection for guessing is as important for measuring normal memory as for measuring the memory performance of amnesiacs. It is classic test theory that motivates the common practice of correcting for guessing by subtracting the probability of false recall from the probability of correct recall or, for measuring recognition memory performance, subtracting false alarms from hits (see Kintsch 1970 for a discussion of high-threshold models). Similar to classic test theory, we assume that guessing is independent of true remembering (recollection). Unlike classic test theory, we assume that memory influences guessing. That is, guessing is informed by automatic influences of memory.

When Recollection Is Zero

The first case that I consider is one in which the process-dissociation procedure shows recollection to be zero, and the absence of recollection could not be detected by use of either classic test theory or signal detection theory. After describing an example to show the use of those standard means of correcting for guessing, I describe the process-dissociation procedure.

In an experiment done by Jacoby, Toth, and Yonelinas (experiment 1b, 1993), people studied a set of words under conditions of full or divided attention and were later given the first three letters of the words as cues for recall. Subjects in a full-attention condition were told to read the words aloud and remember them for a later test of memory. Subjects in a divided-attention condition read aloud the same list of words while simultaneously engaging in a listening task. For the listening task, a long series of numbers was presented, and subjects were to indicate when they heard a sequence of three odd numbers in a row (e.g., 3 9 7). Subjects were told that the task of reading words aloud was designed to interfere with performance on the listening task; no mention was made of the fact that subjects' memory for the read words would later be tested. By confounding attention condition with the deletion of instructions to remember, we hoped to eliminate the possibility of later recollection in the divided-attention condition so as to mimic results one would expect to be produced by amnesia (Craik 1982).

For an inclusion test (later contrasted with an exclusion test), a list of word stems was presented, and subjects were instructed to use each stem as a cue for recall of an earlier-presented word that could be used to complete the stem. If their attempt at recall was unsuccessful, they were to complete the stem with the first word that came to mind. That inclusion test is the same as a standard test of cued recall with instructions to guess when recollection fails. Within the test list were some stems that could be completed only with a new word. Completion of those stems served as a measure of base rate or "false recall." A standard means of correcting cued recall performance for guessing is to subtract the probability of false recall from that of correct recall (Weldon, Roediger, and Challis 1989).

Results showed that cued recall performance in the divided-attention condition was poorer than that in the full-attention condition (.62 versus .46). However, in the divided-attention condition, the probability of completing a stem with an old word was well above base rate (.46 versus .35). Should it be concluded that dividing attention did not fully eliminate the possibility of later recollection, or does the above-base-rate level of performance in the divided-attention condition only reflect guessing informed by automatic influences of memory? Neither classic test theory nor signal detection theory (Swets, Tanner, and Birdsall 1961) helps to answer that question because neither distinguishes between recollection and automatic influences of memory.

The process-dissociation procedure can be used to show that dividing attention during study reduced later recollection to zero and left only automatic influences of memory. An important difference between recollection and automatic influences of memory is that recollection affords a level of strategic, conscious control over responding that is not afforded by automatic influences. Suppose that for an exclusion test, subjects were instructed to complete stems with words that were not presented earlier. For that test, recollection would serve to exclude earlier-presented words as completions for word stems, an effect opposite to that for the inclusion test. To the extent that subjects recollected earlier-presented words, they should be more likely to complete stems with those old words when trying to (inclusion test) than when trying not to (exclusion test) respond with old words. That is, recollection can be measured as the difference between performance in the inclusion and exclusion test conditions, a measure of control. In contrast to recollection, automatic influences of memory are assumed not to support such selective responding. Automatic influences of memory act to increase the probability of completing stems with old words regardless of whether an exclusion or an inclusion test is given.

Subjects in the experiment described were given an exclusion test as well as an inclusion test. For the exclusion test, they were instructed to use the stems as cues for recall of words presented earlier but not to give a recalled word as a completion for a stem. That is, for the exclusion test, subjects were told to complete stems with words that were not presented earlier. Results from the inclusion and exclusion test conditions are shown in the left half of table 44.1. Looking at results for the exclusion test, subjects in the divided-attention condition were less able to use recollection to exclude old words than were subjects in the full-attention condition. Indeed, after

Table 44.1
Probabilities of responding with an old word and estimates of recollection (R) and automatic influences (A)

Attention	Probabilities test		Estimates	
	Inclusion	Exclusion	R	A
Full	.61	.36	.25	.47
Divided	.46	.46	0	.46

Note: Base rate = .35.

divided attention, the probability of completing a stem with an old word for the exclusion test was identical to that for the inclusion test. That identity in performance provides evidence that dividing attention during the study presentation of words reduced later recollection to zero. It can be concluded that responding with an old word did not result from a strategic, consciously controlled use of memory, because such responding was as likely when subjects were trying not to as when they were trying to respond with an old word. After divided attention to study, all that remained were automatic influences of memory.

Performance in the divided-attention condition provides clear evidence of automatic influences. Although the probability of responding with an old word was equal for the inclusion and exclusion tests, that probability was above the base rate gained from stems that could only be completed with new words (.46 versus .35). When recollection can be shown to be zero, subtracting base rate or false recall from correct recall gives a measure of automatic influences.

How can automatic influences be measured when recollection is greater than zero, as in the full-attention condition? Translating the above arguments into a set of simple equations that describe performance in the inclusion and exclusion test conditions provides a means of estimating the separate contributions of automatic and strategic processes. Stated formally, the probability of responding with a studied word in the inclusion test condition is the probability

of recollection (R) plus the probability of the word's automatically coming to mind when there is a failure of recollection, $A(1 - R)$:

$$\text{Inclusion} = R + A(1 - R). \qquad (1)$$

For the exclusion test, a studied word will be produced only when a word automatically comes to mind and there is a failure to recollect that it was on the list, or more formally:

$$\text{Exclusion} = A(1 - R). \qquad (2)$$

In the inclusion test, automatic and intentional influences act in concert. Performance in that condition clearly overestimates recollection and does not provide unambiguous evidence even for its existence. The exclusion test places recollection and automatic influences in opposition. If the probability of completing stems with studied words in that condition is higher than base rate, then one can be sure that automatic influences exist. However, if the probability of recollection is above zero, performance in the exclusion condition underestimates the magnitude of automatic influences.

The probability of recollection (R) can be estimated as the probability of responding with a studied word in the inclusion condition minus the probability of responding with a studied word in the exclusion condition:

$$R = \text{Inclusion} - \text{exclusion}. \qquad (3)$$

Once an estimate of conscious recollection has been obtained, unconscious or automatic influences can be estimated by simple algebra:

$$A = \text{Exclusion}/(1 - R). \qquad (4)$$

We call this the process-dissociation procedure because what we are looking for are factors that produce dissociations in their effects on the estimates of the different types of processes. Equations 1–4 can be applied to the data in table 44.1 to separate recollection and automatic influences. Doing so (right half of table 44.1) shows that dividing attention produced a process dissociation. Although dividing attention reduced the probability of recollection to zero, the estimated contribution of automatic influences was near identical for the full- and divided-attention conditions.

It is important to be able to find such process dissociations. One of the strongest assumptions underlying the procedure is that automatic and strategic uses of memory are independent. If this assumption is valid, we should be able to identify factors that have large influences on one process but leave the other process unchanged. The strategy is analogous to that used by proponents of signal detection theory to justify the assumed independence of discriminability and bias. For signal detection theory, if discriminability and bias are independent, it should be possible to vary bias and leave d' (the estimate of discriminability) unchanged (Snodgrass and Corwin 1988) or vice versa. For our approach, the process dissociation produced by dividing attention during study provides support for the assumption of independence of recollection and automatic influences. Jacoby, Toth, and Yonelinas (1993) further describe the assumptions underlying the process-dissociation procedure and review data that provide support for those assumptions. Process dissociations such as those produced by dividing attention during study have been found in several other experiments.

Even when giving a correct memory response, amnesiacs often deny having the subjective experience of remembering and claim to be only guessing (Moscovitch, Winocur, and McLachlan 1986). For amnesiacs, the probability of recollection is likely very low and, so the probability of completing a stem with an old word should be nearly the same in inclusion and exclusion test conditions. Results consistent with that prediction have been obtained recently (Cermak et al. 1992). The process-dissociation procedure holds an important advantage over other means of measuring memory in that it allows one to separate recollection, an ability that is largely lost by amnesiacs, and, when attention is divided, from automatic or unconscious influences, a use of memory that is preserved by amnesiacs and when attention is divided.

Offsetting Effects of Recollection and Automatic Influences

The above example shows that reliance on standard means of correcting for guessing can overestimate recollection. The next case I consider shows an even more serious error in conclusions that can result from reliance on such standard procedures. A manipulation can have effects on strategic uses of memory that are fully offset by its opposite effects on automatic uses of memory. Given such offsetting effects, reliance on standard procedures for measuring memory leads to the mistaken conclusion that the manipulation had no effect.

Among the effects most intensely investigated using direct tests of memory is the finding that words generated in response to a question are later better remembered than are words that were simply read (Slamecka and Graf 1978; Jacoby 1978; for a review, see Hintzman 1990). Jacoby, Toth, and Yonelinas (experiment 3, 1993) examined this generation effect in recall cued with word stems. In their experiment, words were presented as anagrams to be solved or in their normal form to be read, and then word stems were presented as cues for recall. The test of cued recall took the same form as the inclusion test described in the preceding section. A generation effect would be shown by recall of words presented as anagrams being superior to that of words that were read. The results failed to show an effect of that sort. Instead, the probability of correctly recalling words that had been presented as anagrams was identical to that of recalling words that had been read.

If we had relied on cued recall performance, we would have concluded that the read/generate manipulation had no effect. However, by use of the process-dissociation procedure, we were able

Table 44.2
Probabilities of responding with an old word and estimates of recollection (R) and automatic influences (A)

Study	Probabilities test		Estimates	
	Inclusion	Exclusion	R	A
Read	.82	.49	.33	.73
Anagram	.82	.25	.57	.59

Note: Base rate = .56.

to show that the manipulation produced opposite and perfectly offsetting effects on recollection and automatic influences of memory. The experiment made use of both an exclusion and an inclusion test condition, just as did the experiment described in the preceding section. Although the read/generate manipulation had no effect on performance when an inclusion test was given, there was a large effect on performance when an exclusion test was given (left half of table 44.2). For the exclusion test, subjects were much more successful at avoiding responding with an old word when the word had earlier been produced as a solution for an anagram rather than simply read.

Equations 1–4 can be used to separate the contributions of recollection and automatic influences. Doing so allows one to see the differential effects of the read/anagram manipulation (right half of table 44.2). By use of the process-dissociation procedure, one sees that generating a word as a solution for an anagram produced an advantage in recollection that was perfectly offset by a disadvantage in automatic influences of memory.

The pattern of results found using the process-dissociation procedure parallels dissociations found between performance on indirect and on direct tests of memory. For example, Jacoby (1983) showed that words generated as an antonym of a presented word were later better recognized as old but were less likely to be perceptually identified as compared to words that were read earlier. Jacoby interpreted those results as showing that perceptual identification primarily relies on prior data-driven processing, whereas recognition memory primarily relies on prior conceptually driven processing. Roediger (1990) has extended that argument to account for a variety of dissociations between performance on indirect and direct tests.

Results of the above experiment show that a dissociation of the form found between tasks can also be found between processes within a task. The read/generate effect found for automatic influences in stem-completion performance is the same as found using indirect tests and the effect in recollection is the same as found using direct tests. Consequently, one might conclude that automaticity reflects data- or stimulus-driven processing (Posner and Snyder 1975) and that only recollection is enhanced by prior conceptually driven processing of the sort required to solve anagrams. However, it is important to note that for automatic processes in recognition memory, the read/generate effect is the opposite of that found for automatic processes in stem completion (Jacoby 1991). Because of differences in cues provided for retrieval and differences in task demands, automatic influences on stem-completion performance are more reliant on perceptual characteristics than are automatic influences on recognition-memory performance. I have used differences of that sort to argue for the task dependency of automaticity. Jacoby, Ste-Marie, and Toth (1993) provide a discussion of the relativity of automaticity that draws on theorizing done by Neumann (1984).

Some might object that our inclusion test condition is not a standard test of cued recall but, rather, a mix of a direct and an indirect test because we encouraged guessing. Further, it might be argued that had we instructed subjects to report only words that they were certain were old, we would have found an advantage in cued recall of anagram over read words in the experiment just described and, perhaps, found that cued recall performance was near zero in the divided-attention condition in the experiment described earlier. However, instructing subjects not to guess does not reliably eliminate guessing. So long as guessing is not fully eliminated, automatic influences of memory on guessing do contaminate standard measures of recollection. By encouraging guessing and using the process-dissociation procedure, we gain a measure of automatic influences of memory on guessing and, so, also better measure recollection.

Comparison of Assumptions Underlying Different Measures of Recollection

The standard practice of subtracting false recall from correct recall so as to remove the effects of guessing (Weldon, Roediger, and Challis 1989) derives from classic test theory and is based on assumptions that are likely seldom examined. The assumptions underlying that procedure are that guessing is uncorrelated with true recollection and that memory influences only recollection. The assumed independence of recollection and of guessing is used to separate their effects.

It is assumed that correct recall can be accomplished either by recollecting an old item (R_o) or by producing the old item as a guess (G) when recollection fails ($1 - R_o$):

$$\text{Correct recall} = R_o + G(1 - R_o). \tag{5}$$

In contrast, false recall of the same item, if it were not presented, would require that the item be given as a guess (G) and not be recollected as being new ($1 - R_n$):

$$\text{False recall} = G(1 - R_n). \tag{6}$$

Subtracting false recalls (equation 6) from correct recalls (equation 5) to measure recollection, as is standard, rests on the assumption that R_o equals R_n. That is, it is assumed that the probability of recollecting that an item was presented (R_o) is the same as the probability of recollecting that an item was not presented (R_n). That assumption is probably seldom valid and is

particularly problematic when assessing the effects of study manipulations. For example, consider the use of that assumption in the context of examining the effects of the read/generate manipulation.

An advantage of generated words in correct recall would be described as reflecting a higher probability of recollecting that an item was old (R_o) for generated as compared to read words. The problem comes when one corrects for guessing by subtracting false recalls (base rate) from correct recalls. Reliance on stems that can be completed only with new words to measure false recall forces one to use the same base rate to "correct" recall of read words and recall of anagrams. Doing so requires the contradictory assumptions that R_n for new words is equal to R_o for anagrams and R_o for read words but that R_o is different for the two classes of words. What is needed is separate measures of false recall for read and anagram words.

The exclusion condition used in the process-dissociation procedure provides separate measures of false recall for different classes of studied words. The equations for the process-dissociation procedure (equations 1 and 2) are identical to equations 5 and 6, except for the change from two parameters (R_o and R_n) to one parameter (R) to represent recollection. For the process-dissociation procedure, we assume that the recollection used for inclusion is the same as that used for exclusion. Although the validity of that assumption might sometimes be arguable, it is much more tenable than the standard assumption that R_o equals R_n. Our use of the exclusion test condition allowed us to see that recollection was different for anagram and read words. That difference would not have been revealed had we relied on a test of cued recall (the inclusion test condition) and corrected for guessing by subtracting base rate from correct recall of anagram and read words.

Another difference between the process-dissociation approach and classic test theory is that unlike classic test theory, we assume that memory influences guessing. Without separating the different influences of memory, the memory preserved by amnesiacs and after divided attention might be mistaken for recollection rather than correctly being seen as an automatic influence of memory. Also, a failure to distinguish between different influences of memory can lead to the false conclusion that a factor had no effect when, in actuality, there were two offsetting effects.

Strategic and Automatic Influences of Associative Context

The effectiveness of a recall cue depends on the relation between the cue and the study encoding of the item that is to be recalled. For example, presentation of an associate of a studied word as a cue for its recall is much more effective if the associate and the to-be-remembered word were studied together (Tulving and Thomson 1973). Such "encoding-specificity effects" might be interpreted as showing the importance for recollection of the compatibility of the retrieval cue and the study encoding of the target word. However, encoding-specificity effects might also originate from automatic influences of memory. In line with that possibility, Shimamura and Squire (1984) found that amnesiacs show "associative priming" effects. They presented word pairs, such as *table-chair*, to amnesiacs and control subjects. After presentation, subjects were shown the first word of each pair and were asked to say the first word that came to mind. The likelihood of subjects' responding with the second member of the pair was found to be almost three times above baseline level for amnesiacs as well as for control subjects (For a review of similar results from other experiments, see Moscovitch 1994, Shimamura 1986.)

How should recall cued with associates be corrected for guessing? The problem is the same as described for recall cued with word stems. The standard procedure of subtracting a baseline

level obtained using new items from correct recall does not take automatic influences into account and, consequently, can overestimate the probability of recollection. Further, manipulations of the compatibility of retrieval cues and study encoding likely affect both recollection and automatic influences of memory. To measure effects on recollection accurately, one needs to separate effects on recollection from those on automatic influences.

Experiment 1: Placing Strategic and Automatic Influences in Opposition

A first experiment was done to demonstrate that associative context affects both recollection and automatic influences of memory. In phase 1 of that experiment, associatively related words were presented in pairs (e.g., *talk-chat, eat-drink*) or were repaired and presented as pairs of unrelated words (e.g., *turtle-cider, apple-shell*). Subjects judged whether words in each pair were related or unrelated. Subjects in one condition devoted full attention to making those judgments, whereas subjects in a second condition engaged in a listening task while simultaneously judging whether words were related. For an exclusion test, the first member of each studied pair was presented as a cue along with the initial letter of the associatively related target word (e.g., *eat-d*). Subjects were instructed to produce a word that was associatively related to the cue and began with the presented letter but had not been presented earlier (acceptable responses would be *dine* or *devour*, for example).

Recollection that a word was presented earlier allowed subjects to avoid giving that word as a response. Automatic influences, in contrast, would have the opposite effect by acting to increase the probability of responding with an old word. Only when words were presented in related pairs did the cues provided at test reinstate the associative context of studied words. Consequently, words presented in related pairs were expected to produce both better recollection and larger automatic influences of memory as compared to words presented in unrelated pairs. Based on results of the sort described earlier, dividing attention during the study presentation of pairs was expected to reduce later recollection but leave automatic influences of memory unchanged. Because of the effect on recollection, the probability of mistakenly responding with an old word was expected to be higher in the divided- than in the full-attention condition. The obtained pattern of results was such as to allow one to be certain that associative context affected both automatic and strategic influences of memory.

Subjects

Subjects were volunteers from a first-year introductory psychology course at McMaster University who participated in the experiment for course credit. Eighteen subjects were randomly assigned to each of two experimental conditions created by a manipulation of full versus divided attention at study.

Materials and Design

A pool of 220 related word pairs was selected from *The Connecticut Free Associational Norms* (Bousfield et al. 1961), *The University of South Florida Associative Meaning Norms* (McEvoy et al., n.d.), and the *Norms of Word Association* (Postman and Keppel 1970). The associated words were chosen from a range of association frequencies, with the majority being from the medium range. The highest-frequency associates were not selected, and an additional criterion was that there must be at least one other associate beginning with the same letter as the selected associate (e.g., *burial—coffin, casket, ceremony, crypt*). From the selected pairs, three sets of forty pairs each were formed, and those sets were used to represent the three presentation conditions: presented in related pair, presented in unrelated pair, and new at test. Unrelated pairs were formed by repairing words in related pairs. Each set was balanced with regard to the probability

of the selected associates being given as a response when new. Across formats, the sets were rotated through experimental conditions. Remaining pairs were used as fillers for the study list or for the test list.

The study list contained 120 pairs, with the first 20 pairs and the last 20 pairs in the list serving as fillers. Of those fillers, half were related and the other half were unrelated pairs. The order of items in the study list was random, with the restriction that not more than 3 pairs of the same condition could appear in a row. The test list contained 200 pairs, 80 of them fillers. The first 40 pairs in the test list were fillers (20 pairs of which had been presented during study). The fillers at the beginning of the list were used to allow subjects to become acquainted with the task before data were collected. The remaining 40 fillers were words from new pairs and were spread through the list so as to make the number of cues that would only allow responding with a new word equal to the number of cues that would allow responding with an old word.

Procedure

In the study phase, the word pairs were presented on a monitor for 2 s each with a 0.5-s delay, during which the screen was blank, between the presentation of pairs. For each pair, subjects pressed one key to indicate that the pair of words was related or another key to indicate that they were unrelated. Subjects in the divided-attention condition engaged in a listening task while simultaneously judging whether words were related. The listening task was one previously used by Craik (1982). Subjects monitored a tape-recorded list of digits to detect target sequences of three odd numbers in a row (e.g., 9 3 7). Digits were recorded at a 1.5-s rate. Subjects signaled their detection of a target sequence by saying "now."

For the test, the first word from each pair was presented followed by two spaces and then the first letter of its selected associate. The cue remained on the screen until the subject gave a response or until 15 s elapsed; then the next test item was presented. Subjects were told that they were to produce a word that was associatively related to the cue and began with the provided first letter but had not been presented earlier. They were told that if they were able to recall a previously presented, related word, even if the word had not been paired with the cue word, they were not to use that old word as a response.

The significance level for all tests was set at $p < .05$.

Results

The probability of mistakenly responding with an old word is shown in table 44.3 for words presented in related and unrelated pairs along with the baseline probability of responding with those words when they were new. Analysis of those probabilities revealed a significant interaction between prior presentation and full versus divided attention ($F(2, 68) = 11.62$, $MS_e = .005$).

Results from the full-attention condition provide evidence that reinstating associative context improved recollection. After full attention to judging pairs, words presented in related pairs were given as a response less frequently than were new words and were also less likely to be mistakenly given as a response than were words presented in unrelated pairs. That pattern of results shows that recollection of words presented in related pairs was often sufficiently good to allow subjects to exclude those words as per-

Table 44.3
Probabilities of responding with an "old" word on an exclusion test

Attention	Pair type		
	Related	Unrelated	New
Full	.21	.30	.29
Divided	.36	.33	.27

Note: New pairs provide a measure of base rate.

missible responses. In contrast, results from the divided-attention condition provide evidence of automatic influences of memory. After divided attention, old words from related pairs were more likely to be given as a response than were new words. This increased probability must have resulted from an automatic influence of memory, because an intentional use of memory (recollection) would have produced an opposite effect. Weak evidence of an effect of associative context on automatic influences is provided by the finding that after divided attention, words from related pairs were slightly more likely to be mistakenly given as a response than were words from unrelated pairs.

Experiment 2: Separating Strategic and Automatic Influences

The results of experiment 1 provide evidence that reinstating associative context affects both recollection and automatic influences of memory. However, the design of that experiment was not sufficient to allow one to separate effects of associative context fully on the two types of processes. To accomplish that goal, experiment 2 made use of the process-dissociation procedure.

Materials and Procedure

The materials and procedure for experiment 2 were the same as those for experiment 1, except an inclusion test condition was added. Inclusion and exclusion test items were randomly intermixed, with the color of test items (green or red) signaling their type. For green test items, subjects were instructed to use the presented cue word and first letter to recall an earlier-presented word that was associatively related to the cue word and began with the provided first letter. If subjects were unable to recall a suitable old word, they were told to respond with the first word that came to mind that fit the restrictions. For red stems, in contrast, subjects were instructed not to respond with old words. The instructions for that exclusion test were the same as for experiment 1.

The procedure of randomly intermixing inclusion and exclusion test items was used to equate the interval between prior presentation of an item and type of test. The addition of the inclusion test condition reduced by half the number of words representing each combination of experimental conditions as compared to experiment 1. The only other difference between the two experiments is that pairs were presented for 1.5 s in phase 1 for subjects to judge whether words were related in experiment 2 but for 2 s in experiment 1.

Results

The baseline probability of producing the selected associates when new did not differ significantly across type of test (inclusion versus exclusion) or attention condition (full versus divided attention), and averaged .29. For words presented in related or unrelated pairs, an analysis of the probability of responding with an old word revealed a significant interaction among type of pair (related versus unrelated), type of test, and attention condition ($F(1, 34) = 16.57$, $MS_e = .008$). The results in the left half of table 44.4 show that effects for the exclusion test were similar to those of experiment 1 in that dividing

Table 44.4
Probabilities of responding with an old word and estimates of recollection (R) and automatic influences (A)

Pair type	Probabilities test		Estimates	
Attention	Inclusion	Exclusion	R	A
Related				
Full	.60	.24	.36	.37
Divided	.48	.36	.12	.40
Unrelated				
Full	.37	.30	.07	.32
Divided	.37	.29	.08	.31

Note: Base rate = .29.

attention increased the probability of subjects' mistakenly responding with words from related pairs. For the inclusion test condition, in contrast, dividing attention decreased the probability of subjects' correctly responding with words from related pairs. That pattern of results is what would be expected if dividing attention reduced the probability of recollection.

So as to better examine differential effects of dividing attention and associative context, the equations presented earlier were used to estimate the separate contributions of automatic and strategic uses of memory (right half of table 44.4). The estimates of recollection reveal that words from related pairs were more likely to be recollected than were words from unrelated pairs. Dividing attention reduced recollection of words from related pairs but did not affect recollection of words from unrelated pairs, perhaps because recollection of words from unrelated pairs was near zero even in the full-attention condition. Thus, the results provided strong evidence that dividing attention reduced recollection, whereas reinstating associative context improved recollection.

An analysis of the estimated automatic influences showed that dividing attention did not produce a significant main effect or a significant interaction with type of pair. This result agrees with those from earlier experiments in showing that although dividing attention radically reduces later recollection, automatic influences of memory are left unchanged. More interesting, reinstating associative context increased automatic influences of memory. Estimated automatic influences for words presented in related pairs were larger than for words presented in unrelated pairs ($F(1, 34) = 10.99$, $MS_e = .008$). The estimated automatic influence for words presented in unrelated pairs was not significantly larger than baseline. That is, the results provided no evidence that presenting words in unrelated pairs had the automatic influence of increasing the likelihood of those words being given as a response. Data-driven processing required to read the words earlier was not enough to produce such automatic influences of memory. Rather, to produce automatic influences, it was necessary that words be presented in related pairs so that the associative relation dealt with during study was the same as that used at test.

Effects of Providing Environmental Support

The estimates of recollection gained by use of the process-dissociation procedure differ from estimates that would result if false recall (baseline) was subtracted from correct recall, as is standard. For the full-attention condition, the standard measure of recollection underestimates recollection of words from related pairs ($.60 - .29 = .31$ versus $.36$), whereas for the divided-attention condition, the standard measure overestimates recollection ($.48 - .29 = .19$ versus $.12$). In part, this difference results because the standard measure rests on the contradictory assumptions that the probability of recollecting that an item was not earlier presented (R_n) is the same for the full- and divided-attention conditions and equal to the probability of recollecting that an item is old (R_o), which is assumed to differ for the two attention conditions. In contrast, the process-dissociation procedure provides different baselines (measures of exclusion) for the full- and divided-attention conditions and takes effects of automatic influences of memory on guessing into account.

The results of the experiments provide clear evidence for the utility of a distinction between strategic and automatic influences of associative context. Reinstating associative context has the separate effects of improving recollection and increasing the probability that an old item will be given as a guess. The two effects work in concert to improve performance on direct tests of memory such as a test of cued recall. Because they work in concert for those tests, it is impossible to separate the two effects of associative context or even to see that there are separate

effects. Much of the disarray in results from experiments using direct tests might be produced by the two effects of associative context being mistakenly treated as if they originate from a single source. The contradictory results from experiments examining the memory effects of providing environmental support serve as an example.

Craik (1983, 1986) proposed an environmental support hypothesis to account for variation across situations in the severity of the memory deficit suffered by the elderly. The primary assumptions of that hypothesis are that age-related deficits are at least partially due to deficiencies in self-initiated processing and information present in the environment (environmental support) can have effects that compensate for deficient self-initiated processing. A prediction of the environmental support hypothesis is that age differences in performance on direct tests of memory should decrease as environmental support is increased. Craik and Jennings (1992) reviewed the relevant literature and concluded that the results of some experiments agree with the environmental support hypothesis, whereas results of other studies conflict with that hypothesis by showing that age differences are constant across different levels of environmental support or even larger when greater environmental support is provided. That is, all possible patterns of results have been obtained.

Such mixed results are easily explained if providing environmental support has separate effects on recollection and automatic influences of memory. The aged may suffer a deficit in self-initiated processing and, consequently, show smaller effects of enviromental support (e.g., associative context) on recollection. Indeed, reinstating associative context may affect only automatic uses of memory for the aged but both automatic and strategic uses of memory for younger subjects. The overall effect of providing environmental support would then depend on whether automatic or strategic uses of memory were given the heavier weight by the particular test situation. To examine this possibility, effects on strategic and automatic uses of memory must be separated, as is done by the process-dissociation procedure.

Conclusions

Findings of dissociations between performance on direct and indirect tests of memory have been cause for a great deal of excitement and have resulted in renewed interest in automatic or unconscious influences of memory. A widely recognized problem for interpreting performance on indirect tests comes from the possibility that performance on indirect tests is contaminated by intentional uses of memory. Much less attention has been given to the possibility that performance on direct tests of memory is contaminated by automatic influences of memory.

Rather than identify processes with tasks, I have used the process-dissociation procedure to separate the contributions of strategic and automatic influences within a task. The results reported here weigh on theorizing about automatic influences of memory. For example, the experiments examining the effects of associative context on automatic influences could have been described as showing the advantage of the process-dissociation procedure over the use of indirect tests as a means of measuring effects of conceptually driven processing. Elsewhere (Jacoby et al. 1992; Toth, Reingold, and Jacoby 1994) we provide discussions of that sort and argue that the process-dissociation procedure holds important advantages over indirect tests as a means of investigating automatic influences of memory. Jacoby, Toth, and Yonelinas (1993) discuss the relation between the "direct retrieval" assumptions that underlie the equations presented here and the "generate/recognize" assumptions (Jacoby and Hollingshead 1990) that are often used to describe cued recall performance. They argue that the invariance in automatic influences across

manipulations of attention cannot be predicted by a generate/recognize model of cued recall performance.

The process-dissociation procedure can be applied in a wide range of situations. Debner and Jacoby (1994) have extended the procedure to separate conscious and unconscious effects of perception. The arguments for "seeing" are the same as for recollection in the case of separating conscious and unconscious influences of memory. Supposed demonstrations of unconscious perception that have relied on indirect tests have been dismissed by critics (Holender 1986) on the grounds that performance on the indirect test may have been contaminated by the effects of conscious perception. Here, too, we turn the tables by showing that performance on direct tests, which is usually taken at face value as measuring conscious perception, is sometimes badly contaminated by the effects of unconscious perception.

The implications of the distinction between strategic and automatic uses of memory are, in some ways, even more important for direct than for indirect tests of memory. It is performance on direct tests of memory such as tests of cued recall that has been the traditional focus of investigations of memory. The measures of memory gained using those standard, direct tests do not distinguish between recollection and automatic influences of memory. The results described here show that by failing to distinguish between those two effects of memory, one risks serious errors in conclusions that are drawn.

References

Bousfield, W. A., Cohen, B. H., Whitmarsh, G. A., and Kincaid, W. D. (1961). *The Connecticut Free Associational Norms*. Technical Report 35. Storrs, CT: University of Connecticut. November.

Cermak, L. S., Verfaellie, M., Sweeney, M., and Jacoby, L. L. (1992). Fluency versus conscious recollection in the word completion performance of amnesic patients. *Brain and Cognition, 20*, 367–377.

Craik, F. I. M. (1982). Selective changes in encoding as a function of reduced processing capacity. In F. Klix, J. Hoffman, and E. van der Meer (Eds.), *Cognitive research in psychology*, 152–161. Berlin: Deutscher Verlag der Wissenschaffen.

Craik, F. I. M. (1983). On the transfer of information from temporary to permanent memory. *Philosophical Transactions of the Royal Society, B302*, 341–359.

Craik, F. I. M. (1986). A functional account of age differences in memory. In F. Klix and H. Hapendorf (Eds.), *Human memory and cognitive capabilities, mechanisms and performances*, 409–422. Amsterdam: North-Holland.

Craik, F. I. M., and Jennings, J. M. (1992). Human memory. In F. I. M. Craik and T. A. Salthouse (Eds.), *The handbook of aging and cognition* 51–110. Hillsdale, NJ: Erlbaum.

Debner, J., and Jacoby, L. L. (1994). Unconscious perception: Attention, awareness, and control. *Journal of Experimental Psychology: Learning, Memory, and Cognition, 20*, 304–317.

Gabrieli, J. D. E., Milberg, W., Keane, M. W., and Corkin, S. (1990). Intact priming of patterns despite impaired memory. *Neuropsychologia, 28*, 417–428.

Graf, P., and Mandler, G. (1984). Activation makes words more accessible, but not necessarily more retrievable. *Journal of Verbal Learning and Verbal Behavior, 23*, 553–568.

Graf, P., Squire, L. R., and Mandler, G. (1984). The information that amnesic patients do not forget. *Journal of Experimental Psychology: Learning, Memory, and Cognition, 10*, 164–178.

Hintzman, D. L. (1990). Human learning and memory: Connections and dissociations. *Annual Review of Psychology, 41*, 109–139.

Holender, D. (1986). Semantic activation without conscious identification in dichotic listening, parafoveal vision, and visual masking: A survey and appraisal. *Behavioral and Brain Sciences, 9*, 1–23.

Jacoby, L. L. (1978). On interpreting the effects of repetition: Solving a problem versus remembering a solution. *Journal of Verbal Learning and Verbal Behavior, 17*, 649–667.

Jacoby, L. L. (1983). Remembering the data: Analyzing interactive processes in reading. *Journal of Verbal Learning and Verbal Behavior, 22*, 485–508.

Jacoby, L. L. (1991). A process dissociation framework: Separating automatic from intentional uses of memory. *Journal of Memory and Language, 30*, 513–541.

Jacoby, L. L., and Hollingshead, A. (1990). Toward a generate/recognize model of performance on direct and indirect tests of memory. *Journal of Memory and Language, 29*, 433–454.

Jacoby, L. L., and Kelley, C. M. (1991). Unconscious influences of memory: Dissociations and automaticity. In D. Milner and M. Rugg (Eds.), *The neuropsychology of consciousness*, 201–233. London: Academic Press.

Jacoby, L. L., Ste-Marie, D., and Toth, J. P. (1993). Redefining automaticity: Unconscious influences, awareness and control. In A. D. Baddeley and L. Weiskrantz (Eds.), *Attention, selection, awareness and control: A tribute to Donald Broadbent*, 261–282. London: Oxford University Press.

Jacoby, L. L., Toth, J. P., Lindsay, D. S., and Debner, J. A. (1992). Lectures for a layperson: Methods for revealing unconscious processes. In R. Bornstein and T. Pittman (Eds.), *Perception without awareness*, 81–120. NY: Guilford Press.

Jacoby, L. L., Toth, J. P., and Yonelinas, A. P. (1993). Separating conscious and unconscious influences of memory: Measuring recollection. *Journal of Experimental Psychology: General, 122*, 139–154.

Kintsch, W. (1970). *Learning, memory, and conceptual processes*. New York: Wiley.

McEvoy, C. M., Oth, J. E., Walling, J. R., Wheeler, J. W., and Nelson, D. (n.d.). The University of South Florida Associative Meaning Norms. Tampa, FL: University of South Florida. Unpublished.

Moscovitch, M., Winocur, G., and McLachlan, D. (1986). Memory as assessed by recognition and reading time in normal and memory-impaired people with Alzheimer's disease and other neurological disorders. *Journal of Experimental Psychology: General, 115*, 331–347.

Neumann, O. (1984). Automatic processing: A review of recent findings and a plea for an old theory. In W. Prinz and A. F. Sanders (Eds.), *Cognition and motor processes*, 255–293. Berlin: Springer-Verlag.

Ostergaard, A. L., and Jernigan, T. L. (1993). Are word priming and explicit memory mediated by different brain structures? In P. Graf and M. Masson (Eds.),

Implicit memory: New directions in cognition, development and neuropsychology, 327–349. Hillsdale, NJ: Erlbaum.

Posner, M. I., and Snyder, C. R. R. (1975). Attention and cognitive control. In R. L. Solso (Ed.), *Information processing in cognition: The Loyola Symposium*, 55–85. Hillsdale, NJ: Erlbaum.

Postman, L. J., and Keppel, G. (1970). *Norms of word association*. New York: Academic Press.

Richardson-Klavehn, A., and Bjork, R. A. (1988). Measures of memory. *Annual Review of Psychology*, *39*, 475–543.

Roediger, H. L. (1990). Implicit memory: Retention without remembering. *American Psychologist*, *45*, 1043–1056.

Shimamura, A. P. (1986). Priming effects in amnesia: Evidence for a dissociable memory function. *Quarterly Journal of Experimental Psychology*, *38A*, 619–644.

Shimamura, A. P., and Squire, L. R. (1984). Paired-associate learning and priming effects in amnesia: A neuropsychological study. *Journal of Experimental Psychology: General*, *113*, 556–570.

Slamecka, N. J., and Graf, P. (1978). The generation effect: Delineation of a phenomenon. *Journal of Experimental Psychology: Human Learning and Memory*, *4*, 592–604.

Snodgrass, J. G., and Corwin, J. (1988). Pragmatics of measuring recognition memory: Applications to dementia and amnesia. *Journal of Experimental Psychology: General*, *117*, 34–50.

Swets, J. A., Tanner, W. P., and Birdsall, T. G. (1961). Decision processes in perception. *Psychological Review*, *68*, 301–340.

Toth, J. P., Reingold, E. M., and Jacoby, L. L. (1994). Towards a redefinition of implicit memory: Process dissociations following elaborative processing and self-generation. *Journal of Experimental Psychology: Learning, Memory, and Cognition*, *20*, 290–303.

Tulving, E., Schacter, D. L., and Stark, H. A. (1982). Priming effects in word-fragment completion are independent of recognition memory. *Journal of Experimental Psychology: Learning, Memory, and Cognition*, *8*, 336–342.

Tulving, E., and Thomson, D. M. (1973). Encoding specificity and retrieval processes in episodic memory. *Psychological Review*, *80*, 352–373.

Warrington, E. K., and Weiskrantz, L. (1974). The effect of prior learning on subsequent retention in amnesic patients. *Neuropsychologia*, *12*, 419–428.

Weldon, M. S., Roediger, H. L., and Challis, B. H. (1989). The properties of retrieval cues constrain the picture superiority effect. *Memory and Cognition*, *1*, 95–105.

VIII UNCONSCIOUS AND "FRINGE" PROCESSES

Continuous Interplay between Degrees of Consciousness

Conscious and unconscious events are in constant interaction with each other, and with "fringe states," which are somewhere in between strictly conscious and entirely unconscious states. William James thought that perhaps one-third of our conscious lives may be spent in conscious but vague states of mind, which he called "the fringe." (1890/1983) Mangan's chapter (1999; chap. 45, this volume) supports the case that we would miss something important if we only dealt with focal consciousness, just as we would miss something vital in human vision if we studied only foveal information, at the very center of the retina. These phenomena are often not describable in detail, like foveal objects in vision, but they are frequently verifiable and receive high confidence ratings. There are many quasi-conscious states that allow for verification, such as feelings of rightness, recognition, coherence, mismatch, wrongness, familiarity, attraction/repulsion, and the like. There is a growing experimental literature on these phenomena, under such headings as intuition, feelings of familiarity and knowing, and the tip-of-the-tongue state. In one of the most interesting studies, Bowers, Rehger, Balthazard, and Parker (1990) examined subjects during a gestalt closure task and two word-search tasks. They demonstrated that subjects could respond discriminatively to coherence that they could not identify, and that this tacit perception of coherence guided subjects gradually to an explicit representation of it in the form of a hunch or hypothesis. (p. 72).

Conscious experiences are continually shaped by unconscious sources of information. One of the most common finding in experimental psychology is that unconscious factors that were presumed to be irrelevant to the question being tested turn out to shape the subjects' experiences and responses in unanticipated ways. Although the evidence for unconscious shaping of consciousness is pervasive, it is rarely discussed as a topic, and there is no generally used terminology for it. Baars (1988; chap. 46, this volume) suggested using the term "context" to refer to those unconscious elements that shape conscious experience. Contextual effects extend from sensory perception to memory, judgment, problem solving, beliefs, emotion, motivation, and action control. This selection from Baars (1988; chap. 46, this volume) gives an overview. It seems that all human experience and action is "contextualized," in the sense defined here.

Dissociations from Consciousness

Kihlstrom (1987; chap. 47, this volume) provides an unusually broad introduction to the "cognitive unconscious," including subliminal perception, automatic processing, implicit memory, and hypnotic alterations in consciousness. Hypnosis has been studied since about 1800 (see James 1890/1983), and since the 1950s a great deal of modern research has been performed on hypnotic analgesia and amnesia.

Hilgard, Morgan, and MacDonald (1975; chap. 48, this volume) performed a classic study of hypnotic analgesia, a well-established phenomenon in which normally painful stimuli seem to be experienced as quite acceptable. For a small percentage of highly hypnotizable subjects, however, they showed that the perceived pain of the cold pressor task "leaked out" through a different response modality. When selected subjects were asked not to say, but rather to press a key to indicate whether the cold actually hurt, the keypress response expressed more intense pain. The idea of a hypnotized person disavowing pain by speech while complaining about it by pressing a key seems utterly out of the ordinary.

It is comparable to split-brain dissociations (Sperry 1968; chap. 11, this volume; and Galin 1974; chap. 50, this volume). But findings like that are fairly common among the most hypnotizable few percent of the population. Since these are apparently normal and well-functioning individuals, Hilgard has suggested that multiple dissociative controls may indeed be part of the normal structure of mental life (see James 1890/1983).

Another kind of dissociation is explored by Ramachandran (1995; chap. 49, this volume), in a study of right parietal neglect patients. Neglect typically involves a visual loss of the left half of objects and scenes, often along with anosognosia—lack of conscious knowledge of the deficit—and alien limb syndrome—a denial of ownership of left limbs that are usually paralyzed by the right parietal damage. Initially Ramachandran asked whether the lost part of visual consciousness was still represented in the brain. He devised three different tests, all indicating that unconscious visual information still reaches the brain. The third test is perhaps the most interesting. Neurologists have known that irrigating the left ear with cold water in neglect patients will often lift the left visual loss temporarily. Would it also remove their anosognosia, their denial of knowledge about the disorder? In one patient Ramachandran reported that irrigation, surprisingly, made available her "repressed" knowledge that she was paralyzed, and she then affirmed that she had been paralyzed for several days. Ramachandran attributed the repression to an arsenal of grossly exaggerated Freudian defense mechanisms these patients use to account for their paralysis. Many of these defense mechanisms can be viewed as creative rationalizations, explanations that defy ordinary common sense but which seem plausible to neglect patients, even when their general intelligence and knowledge of the world is not otherwise impaired.

Freudian defense mechanisms like denial, rationalization, and displacement have an everyday plausibility, especially in medical emergencies where most victims may deny the reality of a major disorder for a time, or explain it away, or blame others for their troubles. In the scientific world at large, such defense mechanisms have a controversial reputation at best (see Shevrin and Dickman 1980, chap. 34, this volume; and Baars 1988, chap. 46, this volume). Ramachandran's discovery suggests that some types of brain damage (e.g., parietal neglect) may provide an important scientific paradigm for studying such adaptive cognitive mechanisms.

A similar set of questions is suggested in a classic paper by Galin (1974; chap. 50, this volume) in connection with split-brain syndrome. Patients with severe and uncontrollable epilepsy can sometimes only function after a partial or complete cutting of the corpus callosum, a bridge of neuronal fibers that connects the two hemispheres. Under these circumstances the left hemisphere (in most patients) retains the capacity to control speaking, and both hemispheres have some speech perception. The right hemisphere may be dominant in terms of certain emotional functions, like understandings jokes and irony, whereas the left retains literal meaning. Galin suggests that even in people with intact brains, this division of labor between the two hemispheres may go on, continuing a "life of their own," and, further, that some neurophysiological mechanism is responsible for at least some instances of repression to support this division of labor.

References

Bowers, Kenneth S.; Regehr, Glenn; Balthazard, Claude; and Parker, Kevin. (1990) Intuition in the context of discovery. *Cognitive Psychology*, 22, 72–110.

Bruce Mangan

To get a sense of fringe experience, we only need to repeat an experiment most of us carried out when we were seven or eight years old: saying the same word over and over again rapidly. After 10 or 20 repetitions, *something* in the experience of the word definitely begins to change. What were unobtrusive overtones of felt meaning begin to disappear, becoming evident in their absence. In these cases we typically say that the repeated word has become a "mere sound" and has "lost its meaning."[1] Even at the level of folk psychology we naturally distinguish a sensor and nonsensory component in experience.

The fringe includes virtually every feeling in consciousness that is not a sensory experience in the narrowest sense. Familiarity is a feeling in the fringe. All expressive feelings that can envelop or fuse with conscious sensations—the sorrowfulness of the willow, the joyfulness of sunshine in spring, the friendliness of a smile—are fringe feelings. Free-floating anxiety, the feeling of causal connection, the sense of "mineness" underlying our concept of self—these, too, are fringe feelings—as are intuitions and hunches. The "Aha!" experience of finding the right solution to a problem is a fringe experience (I will call it "rightness"), as is the opposite feeling that something is wrong, out of place, problematic ("wrongness").

Today when people consider the subjective character of consciousness, they often talk about "qualia." The term "qualia" has come to refer to protypically clear and vivid experiences, experiences that are easily inspected in the focus of attention, and that belong to a specific sensory modality—for example, the experience of a sharp pain or the color red. Unlike qualia in this sense, fringe experiences have no vivid sensory content.[2] Fringe experiences are indistinct, hazy, diaphanous; they are like pervading field states in consciousness rather than a specific localized point. Unlike qualia, fringe experiences cannot be grasped and brought into the focus of attention.

William James is now coming back into style. But most of his work on the fringe is still ignored—even though James himself took the fringe to be fundamental for understanding cognition in consciousness. Probably the chief reason that people continue to overlook the fringe is because of its peculiar phenomenology. Any yet there is reason to believe that the investigation of fringe phenomenology will tell us as much about the cognitive operation of consciousness as qualia, perhaps more.

This paper has three related but distinct aims. The first is simply to help bring the topic of the fringe back into cognitive research. The one feature of the fringe that *is* often discussed today is the continuity of consciousness. And yet for James the feeling of continuity plays a subsidiary role in cognition. Continuity is in large part a *consequence* of other and more fundamental aspects of the fringe, as we will see.

The second aim of this paper is to extend James's analysis of the fringe in new ways. To a degree, James goes beyond a simple description of the fringe and begins to analyze it in functional terms, specifying the cognitive role individual fringe experiences play within consciousness and linking fringe phenomenology in general with the structure of neural activity (see Mangan 1991). I have tried to move a step or two further along this path, offering a functional analysis of the fringe that treats it as one part in a much more inclusive cognitive system. Among other things, this means considering the relation of the fringe to nonconscious processing—a line of investigation that James actively resisted.[3]

The fringe itself is completely conscious. But in some respects the fringe functions as if it were a sort of semipermeable membrane, separating conscious and nonconscious processes and selectively mediating the flow of information between them. In general, the function of the fringe is to represent huge amounts of nonconscious context information in consciousness in *radically summarized or condensed* form. This is the basis of the relatively specific fringe functions we will examine of metacognitive monitoring and voluntary retrieval.

The fringe is an overlay of many analytically distinct experiences. From a cognitive standpoint, probably the most important single feeling in the fringe is the experience I call rightness. Rightness and its polar opposite, wrongness, appear to be the evaluative foundation of virtually all complex cognitive activity in consciousness— for these experiences represent the most crucial of all cognitive conclusions: Yes/Accept or No/Reject. By linking this analysis to a slight extension of connectionist theory, we open up the possibility of finding specific neural mechanisms in the brain that determine when rightness is to be experienced in consciousness as well as its intensity level. This may have implications far beyond the study of consciousness, because these neural networks, if they do exist, probably also determine global accept/reject evaluations for the (many more) cognitive processes that do *not* feed into consciousness.[4]

We will also go beyond James by trying to explain *why* consciousness has a fringe/focus structure. The vague, diaphanous, indistinct character of fringe experience appears to be the result of a biological adaptation—a trade-off strategy that is all but mandated by the remarkably limited capacity of consciousness to articulate experience. The fringe is apparently a device to radically *condense* context information in consciousness and in a sense *finesse* the limited capacity of consciousness. The fringe makes minimal demands on the overall articulation resources of consciousness, freeing most of these resources for the representation of detailed focal experience. This analysis lets us explain the overall fringe/focus structure of our phenomenology, and it follows the same general lines biol-

ogists use to explain many other aspects of organic structure.

The third aim of this paper is to link up the fringe and experimental research. It is remarkable that some of the most significant lines of evidence for the fringe already emerged during the early years of the cognitive revolution. Ulric Neisser's groundbreaking *Cognitive psychology* (1967) probably contained more findings related to the fringe than any other single work before Mangan 1991. There is also a direct (if forgotten) line of decent from James's analysis of the fringe to the current study of metacognition. The first prominent work on feeling-of-knowing and metacognition is Hart's (1965). His experiments not only produced early evidence for the operation of rightness, but they were based explicitly on James's discussion of the tip-of-the-tongue phenomenon (TOT). For James, a TOT was a prime example of the fringe in operation. The experimental literature on TOT also derives from Hart via Brown and McNeil (1966). Beyond this, more recent literature on various aspects of tacit or implicit cognition (e.g., Marcel 1983; Lewicki 1988; Janowsky, Shimamura, and Squire 1989; Bowers et al. 1990; Weiskrantz 1992) contains much evidence for the fringe, as will be shown.

With a few hints, one could almost deduce the existence of the fringe from these findings. In any case, the notion of the fringe offers a wide-ranging theoretical unification—one that is able to tie together objective empirical findings from many lines of cognitive research and, at the same time, address some of the most intimate and subjective aspects of our conscious life.

James's Phenomenology of the Fringe

Terms and Methodology

Normally, fringe experiences surround and interpenetrate what James calls the "definite sensorial images" in the focus of attention—that is, qualia in its current sense. For better or worse, James was never one to stick to a single term when ten evocative synonyms were available. He used many other at least roughly equivalent names and phrases for the fringe such as "the free water of consciousness," "feelings of relation and tendency," the "penumbra or halo" of consciousness, "transitive experience," and "vague experience." James's basic contrasting term for fringe experience is clear experience, but he gives clear experience, too, many synonyms such as "substantive experience," "definite sensorial images," and the "nucleus" of consciousness.

James used many different techniques for distinguishing fringe experiences from the sensory contents in the focus of attention. Probably the most recurrent was to look at cases in which the sensory component or nucleus remained the same over time but the overall quality of the experience changed. That which changed was the nonsensory or fringe aspect of the full experience in question. We come to recognize the character of fringe feelings after the fact via a contrast carried out in memory, and so introspection in these cases is indirect. This is how we recognize the fringe sense of meaningfulness that normally envelops the sound of a word by recognizing its absence when we repeat the same word rapidly.

The fringe experience of familiarity also becomes evident by way contrast. As James says:

What is the strange difference between an experience tasted for the first time and the same experience recognized as familiar, as having been enjoyed before, though we cannot name it or say where or when? (p. 252)[5]

Familiarity is certainly a feeling in consciousness, but it has a vary different character from a focal sensory content. The experience of familiarity is diffuse, enveloping; it eludes our introspective grasp. The experience of familiarity can deliver the same message ("encountered before") about an indefinite number of different sensory contents; this is what allows us to distinguish the feeling of familiarity from the various contents it can envelop over time. But familiarity is only one of the virtually infinite number of possible fringe experiences.

The Stream Metaphor

Few today remember the core point James himself wanted to make with the stream of consciousness metaphor: that consciousness is saturated with fringe experiences.

The Crucial Insight: Feelings of Imminence or Potential Accessibility

"What a thought is, and what it may be developed into, or explained to stand for, and be equivalent to, are two things, not one" (p. 279). This is the axis on which James's phenomenology of the fringe turns. Miss it, and most of what James has to say will be lost. Fringe experiences are *not* simply blurred or unfocused versions of more detailed experiences that have just occurred or are just about to occur. A vague experience is simply itself, just as it happens, just as it seems. We will see that *both phenomenologically and functionally, the fringe is a completely distinct domain of consciousness with a completely distinct cognitive role.* Furthermore, many fringe experiences (e.g., familiarity, rightness) do not even feel as if they have a clear sensory aspect that can be elaborated brought in the focus of attention.

The fringe uses just a few gossamer wisps of experience to create the sense of imminence. At any given moment, far more detailed information is potentially accessible *to* consciousness than, in fact, is actually *in* consciousness. This is the trick that lets consciousness finesse its otherwise severely limited capacity to represent information.

Transitive/Substantive Cycling

The relative proportion of vague to clear experience in consciousness is not constant; it varies over time, going through a kind of cycle, with the fringe sense of imminence more pronounced in the transition between one clear content and the next.

When discussing fringe experience in its dynamic role, James often employs yet another set of synonyms: "substantive experience" refers to the clear sensory core or nucleus, whereas "transitive experience" refers to the fringe aspects of consciousness which strengthen when they are between one clear experience and the next.

If we take a general view of the wonderful stream of our consciousness, what strikes us first is the different pace of its parts. Like a bird's life, it seems to be made of an alternation of flights and perching. The rhythm of language expresses this, where every thought is expressed in a sentence and every sentence closed by a period. The resting places are usually occupied by sensorial imaginations of some sort whose peculiarity is that they can be held by the mind for an indefinite time, and contemplated without changing; the places of flight are filled with thoughts of relation, the matters contemplated in the periods of relative rest. Let us call the resting places the "substantive parts" and the places of flight the "transitive parts" of the stream of thought. (p. 243)

During the transition from one substantive content to the next, fringe experiences occupy, briefly, a larger portion of consciousness: the clear content that had occupied the focus of attention begins to become a fringe representation, and the clear content that is about to occupy the focus of attention is represented by fringe experience as imminent. Again, it is a fundamental mistake to conflate fringe representations that something was, or is about to be, a clear and delineated content in consciousness, with that clear content.

The Elusive Fringe

In addition to its vague or unarticulated character, fringe experiences are also elusive. By this I mean that even if we do recognize their presence in consciousness and actively try to "grasp"

them (i.e., bring them into the focus of attention), they instantly transform into something else. What had been a vaguely felt presence becomes something entirely different—a clear experience.

It is very difficult, introspectively, to see the transitive parts for what they really are. . . . Let anyone try to cut a thought across in the middle and get a look at its section, he will see how difficult the introspection of the transitive tract is. The rush of thought is so headlong that it almost always brings us up to the conclusion before we can arrest it. Or if our purpose is nimble enough and we do arrest it, it ceases forthwith to be itself. As a snowflake crystal caught in the warm hand is no longer a crystal but a drop, so, instead of catching the feeling of relation moving to its term, we find we have caught some substantive thing, usually the last word we are pronouncing, statically taken, and with its function, tendency and particular meaning quite evaporated. The attempt at introspective analysis in these cases is in fact like seizing a spinning top to catch its motion, or trying to turn up the gas quickly enough to see how the darkness looks. (pp. 243–244)

The *attempt* to grasp a fringe experience gives us instead "some substantive thing." James does not, so far as I know, consider the much broader implications of this for understanding mechanisms of voluntary conscious retrieval. James's point here is to use various examples to show that fringe experiences do exist in their own right, and at the same time explain why standard introspective approaches had ignored them. James could hardly claim to have found a vast realm of experience overlooked by traditional introspective psychology if he did not also explain how the oversight occurred.

Rightness and Wrongness

James offers only a few remarks, made in passing, about feelings of evaluation in the fringe. But what he does say is pregnant and will help us go beyond James to see how the different elements of the fringe work together as a larger cognitive system. James mentions feelings of evaluation as he points out how we often experience the nonsensory germ of an intention before its sensory content arrives:

How much of [an intention] consists of definite sensorial images, either of words or of things? Hardly anything! Linger, and the words and the things come into the mind; the anticipatory intention, the deviation is no more. But as the words that replace it arrive, it welcomes them successively *and calls them right if they agree with it, and calls them wrong if they do not.* (p. 253, my emphasis)

The most basic and pervasive feelings of relation in consciousness are the signals "right" and "wrong."[6] In the above passage, as elsewhere, James considers the evaluative relation that obtains between and among different aspects of *experience*, often the overall fit between the totality of a given fringe state and substantive content or nucleus it surrounds. For a fringe may or may not harmonize with its nucleus. In effect, James makes the same point while discussing TOT:

Suppose we try to recall a forgotten name. The state of our consciousness is peculiar. There is a gap therein; but no mere gap. It is a gap that is intensely active. A sort of a wraith of a name is in it, beckoning us in a given direction, making us at moments tingle with the sense of closeness, and then letting us sink back without the longed for term.... If wrong names are proposed to us, this singularly gap acts immediately to negate them. (p. 251)

In a TOT, consciousness seems to attempt to pull in a specific substantive element that, for some reason, does not materialize. The fringe aspects of consciousness stands out more strongly without the normally overpowering substantive content. This "gap" that we feel in consciousness is pure nonsensory experience, pure fringe experience—a kind of structured vacancy that certainly is not void and that certainly seems to be doing cognitive work.

On James's account the fringe delivers very general evaluative signals—feelings that tell us to accept or reject this or that specific sensorial content as it materializes. Certainly we can all attest that although these yes/no, right/wrong feelings in the fringe have no sensory content, they can be a strongly felt, in their way as strongly felt as the sensory pain of stubbing a toe.

It is odd that James says so little about evaluative signals in consciousness, given that at one point he tells us they are the most important components in the fringe: "T*he most important feeling in these fringes* ... is the mere feeling of harmony or discord, of a right or a wrong direction in the thought" (p. 261; my emphasis).

Relation, then, to our topic or interest is constantly felt in the fringe, and particularly the relation of harmony and discord, of furtherance or hindrance of the topic. When the sense of furtherance is there, we are "all right"; with the sense of hindrance we are dissatisfied and perplexed, and cast about us for other thoughts. Now *any* thought the quality of whose fringe lets us feel ourselves "all right" is an acceptable member of our thinking, whatever kind of thought it may otherwise be. (p. 259; James's emphasis)

For James, then, the feelings of rightness and wrongness are among the most pervasive feelings in consciousness, able to indicate the success or failure of innumerably different kinds of ongoing cognitive activity. Again, James uses a variety of evocative terms for the same basic facts of experience, and this gives us some idea of the many cognitive domains they invest. He also calls the sense of "right direction" the "feeling of rational sequence" and "dynamic meaning." And dynamic meaning "is usually reduced to the bare fringe we have described of felt stability or unfitness to the context and conclusion" (p. 265).

Here is a final example, one that shows both how strong the experience of rightness or wrongness can be and how completely distinct these experiences are from the sensory content with which they merge. Read the entire paragraph through at normal speed:

A newspaper is better than a magazine. A seashore is a better place than the street. At first it is better to run than to walk. You may have to try several times. It takes some skill but it is easy to learn. Even young children can enjoy it. Once successful, complications are minimal. Birds seldom get too close. Rain, however, soaks in very fast. Too many people doing the same thing can also cause problems. One needs lots of room. If there are no complications it can be very peaceful. A rock will serve as an anchor. If things break loose from it, however, you will not get a second chance. (Klein 1981)

When most people read this for the first time, it makes no sense. No thread of meaning connects one sentence with the next. The objective fact that our organism doesn't understand this paragraph is represented in consciousness by a certain kind of subjective fringe feeling—a jagged, disjoint sense of "wrong" movement from sentence to sentence. And even when the fringe feeling of wrongness is intense, it is still diffuse as it seethes around and through the purely sensory aspect of the experience—the look of the words or the sound they make. Note that although fringe experiences in the average are probably less intense than focal experiences, this is by no means always the case. A vague experience can be extremely intense. Vagueness and intensity fall on different phenomenological dimensions. Fringe and focal experience can both vary over the full range of the intensity continuum.

Now the reader should look again at the seemingly disjoint paragraph above. But first let me remind him or her of the word "kite." Now the clouds will lift, instantly. *Before* rereading the paragraph, the reader will experience a strong, diffuse sense of rightness flooding consciousness. Here rightness functions as a feeling of imminence: we feel with certainty that *when* we reread the paragraph, it will make perfect sense, that each sentence will fit together into a larger, integrated, meaningful whole. And during the actual rereading this does turn out to be the case; as we move from sentence to sentence, the fringe feeling is of integration, coherence, right fit among all the individual parts. Here rightness

constitutes what James calls our sense of "rational sequence" or "dynamic meaning."

Explaining the Fringe and Its Functions

It should now be evident that fringe feelings exist, that they are distinct from sensory contents, and that they play a role in conscious cognition. On this basis, we can now move the analysis of the fringe further into new ground, and to a degree explain *why* our phenomenology has the character that it does. This will apply basic principles of biological explanation to consciousness. My most inclusive point is this: the phenomenology of the fringe is an adaptive response to the limited capacity of consciousness to articulate experience.

To avoid confusion, the reader should always keep one point in mind: Fringe and focal experiences differ even more radically in their respective cognitive *functions* than they do in their *phenomenology*. As we have seen, fringe and focal experiences normally merge seamlessly in the flow of consciousness and often can only be distinguished indirectly. Experiences in the fringe or the focus of consciousness differ only by degree along a single phenomenological dimension that I will call the high articulation/low articulation continuum. (This gives us a more precise way to characterize the difference between clear and vague experience as James uses these terms.) Functionally, however, fringe and focus differ in many ways, and they differ hugely.

Context Representation, Monitoring, and Voluntary Retrieval

Overall, the fringe functions to represent context information in consciousness, to monitor the flow of information as it moves through consciousness, and to mediate the willful retrieval of nonconscious information into consciousness. These functions are closely related and they can all be found, if we look carefully, in James's analysis of the fringe. But James himself does not isolate them, and in the case of voluntary retrieval, he apparently misses a crucial implication of his own findings.

James seems to recognize that feelings of relation and tendency, of meaning, of temporal connection with the past and the expected future all involve context information. We saw James say above that fringe experiences contain feelings of "stability or unfitness to the context and conclusion."[7] To understand the nature of context information is arguably the main challenge for cognitive research today. The standard assumption is that contextual processes operate exclusively at the nonconscious level. Yet if James is right, *the fringe represents some context information directly* in *consciousness*, albeit in an extremely condensed form.

The fringe experiences of rightness and wrongness are the most inclusive of all evaluative signals in consciousness. In functional terms, they signal the degree to which the other contents of consciousness (in both the fringe and focus) are or are not compatible with a vast amount of relevant nonconscious context information.

Rightness and wrongness operate in virtually all cognitive domains. In monitoring, when the overall flow of contents (what I will call at times the "trajectory" of consciousness) is going well, we feel rightness; when the flow or trajectory is going ill, we feel wrongness. These feelings vary in intensity and thereby signal innumerable degrees of cognitive success or failure in consciousness. These fringe feelings are able to represent as imminent the future success or failure of a trajectory. In trying to solve, say, a demanding math problem, rightness/wrongness gives us the sense of more or less promising directions long before we have the actual solution in hand.

Rightness considered in its monitoring function (i.e., as representing the positive evaluation of the overall direction or trajectory of experience occurring over at least a few substantive/transitive cycles) envelops the string of individual

nuclei as they move through consciousness with the feeling of smooth, integrated flow. This functions as our basal "all is well" signal, indicating that our potential capacity to handle the material in question is strong. Wrongness, of course, represents the opposite message in consciousness, that potential cognitive capacity is weak.

When we read the kite-flying paragraph for the first time, the feeling of wrongness indicated that if we were called on to handle this material (say, answer questions about the subject of the paragraph), we would have serious cognitive problems. On the other hand, the sense of smooth, coherent movement from sentence to sentence signals consciousness that we do have the capacity to deal with the paragraph. The entire genre of nonsense literature (e.g., Lewis Carroll's "Jabberwocky") rests on the fact that our general signal of cognitive coherence, the feeling of rightness in its monitoring function, can be tricked in various ways to envelop verbal material that, when analyzed substantively, makes no literal sense.

Rightness/wrongness monitoring is ubiquitous, providing a generalized and subtly shifting evaluative ground over which virtually all specific cognitive activity in consciousness plays—in guiding the trajectory of complex problem solving, for example, or giving us a sense of how well a conversation is conforming to, or violating, its many tacit constraints (social, grammatical, syntactical, etc.). In general, this means that much of what people call the continuity of consciousness—the sense of smooth transition from content to content—derives from rightness in its monitoring function. In aesthetic experience, maximizing the feeling of rightness is an end in itself.[8]

In cases ranging from aesthetic "ineffability" to feeling-of-knowing experiments and in some instances of blindsight, people are often unable to identify the precise phenomenological basis for their judgments, even though they can make these judgments with consistency and, often, with conviction. To explain this capacity, people talk about "gut feelings," "just knowing," hunches, and intuitions. By identifying the fringe and its component experience of rightness, we may be able to demystify the notion of intuition. From the standpoint of consciousness, *intuition is simply a conspicuous, if heretofore puzzling, example of fringe feelings doing cognitive work in the absence of a sensory content.* We can link intuition to an inclusive cognitive system, one that operates in virtually all cases of complex conscious cognition. As discussed in the section "Contemporary Research and the Fringe," isolating the experience of rightness may open up a new window on neural processing, a window that may, among other things, let us see how our organism can determine the likely direction in which a solution lies *before* the solution is found.

In general, if we consider the operation of consciousness over time, rightness works as a feedback device, guiding the local and specific activity of focal attention toward increasing conformity with antecedent and unconsciously encoded context demands. This process leads to a reciprocal interaction between conscious and unconscious processing: the process of detailed conscious analysis will usually change the context, and this in turn will change the evaluative signal that rightness manifests, and so on.

In addition to context representation and monitoring, the fringe is also part of the mechanism that apparently allows consciousness to actively retrieve nonconscious information into focal attention. Again the tip-of-the-tongue example is a useful case. When we expect the right word to come into consciousness and it doesn't, we experience a kind of tantalizing vacancy. We grasp at this vacancy almost as if we were trying to squeeze a specific content out of it. When the right word doesn't manifest, we feel what James calls the "wraith" of the word: the sense of the word is as a *potential* sensory content but without the actual sensory content. Our frustration in such cases *presupposes* that normally mental grasping of this sort *will* yield the right word quickly and effortlessly.

Cognitive processes are not designed to be evident but to be useful. Normally, fringe retrieval is so fast and error free that we overlook it. Only when the system malfunctions, and the ghost of the word does not incarnate, do we begin to see that the act of *attempting* to focus on an aspect of the fringe is a voluntary "call" command that initiates the conversion of information implied by the fringe into detailed experience in the nucleus.

Explaining Fringe Phenomenology

Before taking up the general question of why consciousness has a fringe/focus structure. Let me first try to explain two relatively specific features of fringe phenomenology that James simply described—substantive/transitive cycling and the elusive or ungraspable quality of fringe experiences.

So far as I know, James did not extrapolate from the atypical case of a tip-of-the-tongue experience to typical cases of voluntary retrieval into consciousness. But as we saw above, James's account certainly implies that a TOT is just an instance of normal retrieval that has become stuck in midcycle, and that the fringe is an important link in the process that normally "calls" new information into consciousness. The command that actually triggers this call being the *attempt* to focus attention on the fringe or, more precisely, to focus on that aspect of the fringe that implies the detailed information to be retrieved. The vague fringe feeling that something is imminent or *potentially* accessible for focal inspection is a very different experience from the subsequent representation of that something in the focus of attention.

If so, we can explain the elusive, ungraspable character of fringe experience as *a consequence of its call function.* This is the "design" reason fringe experiences thwart attempts at direct (i.e., focal) introspection. The cognitive purpose of focusing on a vague experience in the fringe is not to make *that* experience a stable entity in attention, but to bring a far more articulated (informative) experience into focal inspection. If the attempt to attend to fringe experiences *themselves* simply brought them unchanged into the focus of attention, the ability of the fringe to execute its retrieval function would be severely undercut. We will return to this point with the "menu bar" analogy for the fringe below.

It is primarily the call function of the fringe that creates the impression that fringe experiences are "nothing but" fleeting, preliminary forms of clear experiences. In the section "Contemporary Research and the Fringe," I show that this is probably the chief reason that researchers today recognize many aspects of fringe phenomenology but still miss the overall cognitive role fringe experiences play in conscious cognition.

We can explain transitive/substantive cycling between vague and clear experience as the macro consequence of a series of individual acts of retrieval. In each case of voluntary retrieval, the attempt to focus attention on the fringe produces a brief pulse of transitive "flight" before the retrieved articulated content constitutes a point of "rest" in attention. In other words, transitive states are (in part) the result of a series of acts of retrieval, substantive states are the relatively stable experiences that result from this retrieval.

To turn now to perhaps the most inclusive question: Why should consciousness have a fringe/focus structure in the first place? Can we generate a scientifically plausible hypothesis able to account for the overall phenomenological character of the fringe/focus structure of consciousness beyond its elusive quality? In other words, can we go beyond a *description* of fringe phenomenology as vague, ill defined, and diaphanous to an *explanation* of this phenomenology?

First a conceptual point. In order to explain why a biological entity (say, our heart) is the way it is, we identify the various factors that have shaped it. These factors fall into at least two categories: (1) the function or functions that the entity in question executes and (2) the par-

ticular systemic factors that have *constrained* or otherwise *limited* the entity's ability to execute these functions. In general, it is only after we have been able to identify both general functions *and* the particular systemic constraints on a biological system or subsystem that we are able to move toward a full explanation of its *particular* character—that is, as the joint outcome of particular constraints and functional demands.

For example, to explain why our heart has the particular character it has, we need to know that it functions as a pump. But in itself this abstract functional information is hardly enough to enable us to explain why the human heart is constituted as it is. We also need to understand the various specific constraints to which the heart had adapted in its coevolution with our overall physiological system: for example, constraints on its design imposed by the nature of muscle contraction, the need to maintain blood pressure within certain limits, the particular viscosity of the blood and the need to pump blood without damaging it, and so on.

We can apply the same general method of biological explanation to the fringe. We have already reviewed some of the fringe's cognitive functions—context representation, monitoring, voluntary retrieval. Let us now consider one of the apparent constraints on consciousness that, co-evolving with its functions, may have produced the fringe/focus structure in our phenomenology.

At any given moment, consciousness is extremely limited or "narrow." This has been a recurring theme since the dawn of the cognitive revolution. Standard examples include our inability to attend to more than a single source of novel input such as a conversation at any given moment, and our inability to apprehend more than a few perceptual objects simultaneously. This limit on consciousness can be expressed in various ways, and some of this research will be reviewed in the next section.

Here I will consider how we can capture this limitation in subjective, phenomenological terms. I propose that the most inclusive way to describe the subjective limitation on consciousness is as a limit on its *articulation or resolution* capacity. In other words, consciousness is only able to resolve itself to a certain level of detail at any given moment.

This is nothing more than a slight generalization from George Miller's (1956) classic observation that the capacity of consciousness is limited to about seven distinct "chunks" of experience. One virtue of Miller's formulation is that the concept of a chunk applies naturally to both our subjective phenomenology and to objective empirical findings about the limitations on conscious processing. But in experience a single chunk itself as some residual articulation, notably texture. And the blurred quality of peripheral experience, as well as the nonsensory aspects of the fringe are also part of our experience but are not handled by the notion of a delineated chunk in the focus of attention.

The notion of articulation, then, is able to include that of chunking, but it goes beyond chunking by capturing the more general character phenomenological detail that we find in the experience of texture and the blurred quality of peripheral experience. The general notion of articulation capacity subsumes experience in or out of focal attention, chunked or not chunked.

We can then formalize the subjective *limitation* under which consciousness labors as a limitation of its articulation capacity. Put in these terms, it is evident that the fringe uses only a small amount the total articulation resources of consciousness. Most of consciousness's limited resources are devoted to articulating detailed entities in focal attention. The vague, amorphous, and diaphanous character of fringe experience places the fringe very much on the low end of the articulation continuum.

Intersecting this way to formalize our phenomenology with the functions the fringe executes, we get the following picture: The fringe works, in effect, to radically *condense* information in consciousness. By representing infor-

mation indistinctly, the fringe frees up more of consciousness's resources to articulate the contents in the focus of attention. It is inefficient to burden consciousness with detailed information if simply informing it of a summary conclusion will do.

The fringe/focus structure of consciousness therefore appears to be the result of a trade-off strategy between the need to articulate information in detail, and the need to represent the larger context in which that information is embedded. To maximize the efficiency of conscious cognition, a fringe experience need only be distinct enough to deliver its message, and thereby minimally impinge on consciousness's articulation capacity. The current equilibrium between the allocation of limited articulation capacity to focus and fringe is presumably the result of a long biocognitive evolution.

The fringe, then, responds to a fundamental cognitive paradox: On one hand, consciousness is extremely limited in its representational capacity, however conceived. On the other hand, consciousness interfaces with extremely complex bodies of nonconscious information that transcend consciousness's capacity for direct representation by many orders of magnitude. Consciousness cannot possibly represent in detail anything distantly approaching the totality of information that bears on its cognitive activity. The fringe is able to finesse the limited capacity of consciousness by using just a few wisps of vague experience to represent summary facts about states of nonconscious information that are otherwise far too complex for direct conscious representation.

The Fringe as Menu Bar

There is a useful analogy (if not pressed too far) between the fringe and the user interface devices of menu and status bars found on many computer screens. The analogy applies to passive display of information as well as to its active retrieval. Both consciousness and a CRT labor under a basic articulation limitation, and both employ similar trade-off strategies to circumvent this limitation.

Over time, a virtual infinity of different images can occupy a computer screen, as they can occupy consciousness. But at any given moment, there is only so much resolution or articulation capacity available for representation in either medium.[9] The minimum grain size is fixed. In the case of a computer screen, resolution is limited by the size and number of pixels built into the screen. The menu bar works to finesse the pixel limitation, because it indicates the existence of massive amounts of information not actually displayed on the screen but represented as *potentially* available if needed.

Menu bars (and status bars) come at a cost. The pixels devoted to the display of peripheral information cannot at the same time articulate the immediate task at hand that occupies most of the screen. But while peripheral displays reduce the maximum resolution capacity available for the main display, they allow, in compensation, for the representation of relevant "context" information, albeit in radically summarized form. For a standard word-processing program, these include simple formatting information, the document page number, the "help," and "view" boxes, and so on.

The second point of analogy between a computer screen and the structure of consciousness should help us see why fringe experience is so elusive—why, when we attempt to focus on fringe experience, a very different experience actually manifests in the focus of attention.

What is the standard command we use to call detailed information to the screen, information that is otherwise only represented implicitly by a menu bar? We simply move the cursor to the relevant box and click the mouse. This move-and-click procedure is a crucial link in the process that converts potential off-screen information into an actual on-screen representation. The direct analogy to consciousness is, of course, that when we attempt to attend to a vague experience in the fringe, the normal outcome is the presence of articulated information in the focus of attention. Why does the fringe refuse to itself come into the focus? For the same reason, by analogy, that menu bars don't themselves occupy the center of the screen when we click them. The retrieval function of the icon would thereby cease.

One point in which this analogy breaks down is that each pixel on a CRT screen is the same size, and though small, icons are still displayed with some clarity on the screen. The vague, diaphanous character of the fringe is, as it were, created by "fat" pixels (Mangan 1993c). In this regard, consciousness has something like the structure of the receptive fields in the eye; the "pixels" of consciousness become larger and larger the further they are from the focus of attention.

Contemporary Research and the Fringe

The notion of the fringe can be used to link up many findings in the current cognitive literature; this linkage gives empirical support to the phenomenological and theoretical analysis proposed so far. At the same time, this linkage bring out an underlying connection among a number of findings in metacognition, the limitations of conscious processing, and the phenomenology present or absent in various dissociations, among other areas.

Aspects of fringe phenomenology have already been detected in current cognitive research. But these feelings have been interpreted as simply a fuzzy or preliminary form of clear experiences, thus missing much of the fringe's unique functional role in conscious cognition. The chief mistake is what I will call the "fleetingness fallacy"—that fringe experiences do not differ from sensory experience in the focus of attention, except that fringe experiences come and go quickly and occur in the periphery.

General Anticipations of the Fringe

The extreme "narrowness" or the limited capacity of consciousness is of course one of the earliest findings of the cognitive revolution. It remains a fundamental orchestrating fact for the empirical study of consciousness, as Baars (1988) has shown in some detail. The cognitive revolution virtually began with the dichotic listening experiments of Cherry (1953) and Broadbent (1954), who showed that consciousness can usually handle only one complex stream of novel information at a time—the so-called cocktail party effect. And within a single stream, consciousness labors under the further restriction of its chunking limits, first set out in the contemporary literature in Miller's (1956) now classic paper, "The magical number seven, plus or minus two" (chap. 23, this volume).

To handle these findings, researchers also appeal to the explanatory principle used in the previous section—the efficient allocation of a scarce cognitive resource. Broadbent (1958) argued that the single source limitation could be explained as an efficient way to husband limited processing capacity. Miller (1956, 1962) explained the operations of packing and unpacking as a cognitive strategy that worked, over time, to circumvent the chunking limit. Early in his career, Neisser (1967) held that the distinction between preattentive processes and focal attention was the result of a trade-off of limited cognitive resources, with the narrowness and selectivity of focal attention "simply an allotment of analyzing mechanisms to a limited region of the field" (p. 89).

Neisser's early work on preattentive processes probably came the closest to rediscovering the fringe experimentally. According to Neisser (who tried to avoid the term "consciousness"; see Mandler this volume) the preattentive realm contains "shadowy and impalpable experiences" (p. 303) that represent "crude and global properties" (p. 301) of the articulated contents in the focus of attention. To a degree, preattentive processes work as a context in which attentive acts take place: "Attentive acts are carried out in the context of the more global properties already carried out at the preattentive level" (p. 90).

But there are significant differences between the fringe and Neisser's notion of preattention. He uses "preattention" to refer to both conscious and unconscious elements. The term refers indiscriminately to vague, inarticulate, and peripheral experiences on the one hand, and to completely unconscious, extremely complex, and parallel processes on the other. And his main interest in preattention is on preliminary figural segmentation, not on the representation of context information in consciousness; nor does he consider the role of "preattentive" experience in voluntary acts of retrieval. Nor does Neisser take the elusive aspect of preattentive experience to be a positive structural characteristic in its own right but rather explains it as the result of its supposedly fleeting and preliminary character.

Another experimental approach to the fringe (if taken as James's sense of directly felt significance or meaning) is to recognize it by contrast when it is relatively absent. After "semantic satiation" a rapidly repeated word will lose its cognitive savor; we naturally say a word in this case has "lost its meaning." The effect is familiar to most children. It is quite amenable to experiment, and it has been called since Severance and Washburn (1907) a "lapse of meaning." This sort of meaning lapse is a completely introspective phenomenon, but its experimental manipulation yields consistent results. So, for example, Wertheimer (1958) reported that image related words retain their feeling of meaning longer than abstract words.

Crick and Koch (1990), coming from a very different theoretical direction, develop a notion of "working awareness," which they feel corresponds roughly to a "spotlight of attention" model. But they suspect that, by itself, a clearly defined content may not be sufficient to capture the reality of conscious experience:

Can a spotlight of attention, moving over the visual field from one "salient" location to the next, explain the perceptual richness of our [conscious] environment? Would such a mechanism not lead to a sort of tunnel vision?... We suggest very tentatively that this richness may be mediated by another form of awareness that is very transient.... (p. 272)

Again we find research groping toward fringe phenomena but restricted by the presumption that the phenomenological character of these experiences is simply a consequence of the rapidity of its occurrence.

The connectionists have also tried to explain vague experiences. For Rumelhart et al. (1986), a stable content in consciousness as a fully settled or "relaxed" parallel network. However, if "the relaxation process is especially slow, consciousness will be the time average over a dynamically changing set of patterns and thus would be expected to lead to 'fuzzy' or unclear impressions" (p. 39). Here again vague experiences are presumed to have no cognitive function. They are explained as artifacts produced by many overlapping patterns, each one of which could also occupy consciousness in clear form.

A far more sophisticated account of (in effect) fringe mechanisms is offered by Rock and Gutman (1981). They give us what I believe is the single best experimentally based account that, in effect, distinguishes the fringe's ability to (1) signal the *availability* of detailed conscious information and (2) mediate the retrieval of that information into consciousness. These are two related but very different cognitive functions, availability being signaled far more often than the occurrence of actual retrieval. Rock and Gutman point out that what they call "inattentive" experience (this term, by the way, avoids the conscious/nonconscious confound in "preattentive") provides functional information in consciousness that is not a specific, identifiable form or object. The experimental situation is arranged so that subjects viewing stimuli of two superimposed figures (say, a tree and a house) will only attend to one of them. Nevertheless,

subjects are still able to report some general information about the nonattended figure, for instance, that it was red and had curvy lines.

From findings of this sort, Rock and Gutman derive a fundamental conclusion

In daily life ... [when] we are not attending to a pattern at which we are looking, there is the distinct impression nevertheless that something is there and has certain phenomenal characteristics.... By virtue of the iconic representation, we as observers recognize that the *potential* to transmute this impression is there. (their emphasis)

Information experienced "inattentively" is still conscious, although it lacks the overall specifiable organization we find in an object in the focus of attention. Inattentive experience serves two crucial functions—it implies that detailed information is available *if* attention were to be directed toward it, and provides a target toward which attention can be focused in order to actually bring the detailed information into consciousness.

Rightness

Under various guises, some recognition of the feeling of rightness can also be found in the cognitive literature. But for the most part, these remain veiled. Perhaps because Neisser (1967) did recognize a kind of proto-fringe, he was also able to move closer than most to recognizing monitoring and control experiences. Neisser thought he had isolated a preattentive feeling of "familiarity," and for the moment we will use this term to explain his findings as he did. But we will see that in fact Neisser found experimental evidence of rightness and not familiarity.

Familiarity is treated as a preattentive experience (p. 97), and Neisser asserts that the feeling of familiarity *by itself* can be a datum in target search experiments. No experience of a specific content is necessary. Neisser reports that, on occasion, subjects will be able to recognize that one of a possible set of prespecified targets is present in an array of other letters (e.g., either the letter "D" or "W") without being able to say *which* target was present (p. 99). This finding can be interpreted as a sort of dissociation of the feeling of "familiarity" from a specific content. The feeling is taken to be a sufficient datum for subjects to perform the target search task, even when the specific "familiar" content is not experienced. If we look closely at Neisser's experiment, it seems that it was rightness, and not familiarity, that allowed subjects to know that a target letter was present without knowing what specific target it was. For Neisser's target search experiments did not manipulate familiarity levels. Subjects were to respond as quickly as possible when the designated target was present (i.e., to the "right" target).

Rightness and familiarity are at least as functionally distinct as they are phenomenologically distinct. This point is crucial, but rarely made. One of the few to note the difference between the two is Walter Kintch (1970): "Obviously, 'appropriateness within a given context' as well as 'perceived oldness' may serve as the basic datum for a subject's decision" in some recognition tasks (p. 276). We can feel strongly that something is right, even if it is unfamiliar—for example, when we recognize the solution to a math problem for the first time. Or when Archimedes discovered the principle of specific gravity, his "Eureka" hailed the recognition of the *right*, but absolutely *unfamiliar*, solution. And who knows how many far more familiar facts Archimedes considered and judged to be wrong before he hit on his discovery.

In the study of cognition, rightness is far more important than familiarity, even though rightness receives far less consideration. Survival depends on finding the right response, which may or may not be the familiar response. Especially for the study of consciousness, rightness and not familiarity is the crucial datum. Consciousness generally deals with novel information, familiar information tending to leave consciousness via habituation (Baars 1988).

To feel we have the right solution is to feel that we know the solution. There is now a growing literature on the feeling of knowing, but apparently lingering behaviorist prejudices are still at work. For even when the phenomenon is given the name "feeling of knowing" (FOK), virtually no attempt is made to work out the precise phenomenological character of the feeling. This is especially ironic, given that FOK research grows directly from the experimental investigation of TOT; the original paper by Hart (1965) makes explicit reference to James's discussion of TOT. And as we saw, the heart of a TOT for James is the sense that the *right* answer is imminent. The phenomenological datum in a FOK is, I would maintain, rightness.

Typically, a feeling of knowing experiment elicits TOTs by asking questions like "What is the capital of Vermont?" or "Name the Union general who was in command at the battle of Gettysburg." When a TOT occurs, subjects estimate the likelihood that they know the right answer, which produces a FOK measure. Typically, subjects respond well above chance, and among the most interesting TOT/FOK findings is that the strength of the feeling of knowing judgment is positively correlated with the amount of time a subject spends searching for an inaccessible memory (Nelson, Gerler, and Narens 1984). The finding that the FOK influences search time is of some importance, because it is evidence that the design and operation of consciousness itself presupposes its functional efficacy, as does the fringe structure generally. Nelson, Gerler, and Narens further note that for Korsakoff's syndrome amnesiacs, search times are very short, which implies that the disruption in the FOK system may also contribute to retrieval failure in this type of amnesia. Janowsky, Shimamura, and Squire (1989) also found low feeling of knowing for Korsakoff's amnesiacs, but not for non-Korsakoff amnesiacs, which suggests that the FOK deficit is associated with pathology of the frontal lobe.

To the degree that the FOK and TOT literature is concerned with the *feeling* of knowing, we again encounter another version of the fleetingness hypothesis. In this case, the presumption that the specific word is somehow coming into and then out of consciousness too quickly to be recognized directly. The possibility of a generalized control experience of rightness—a signal of (potential or actual) context-fit—in other words, a recurring experiential component in common to TOT and FOK—is overlooked. So Brown and McNeill (1966), in one of the classic studies of TOT, offer this interpretation:

We know from the Sperling phenomenon . . . that people can have fleeting access to many details in visual memory that they cannot retrieve a fraction of a second later. . . . There are other sources of support for the idea of fleeting conscious events. In the tip-of-the-tongue phenomenon people often report a fleeting conscious image of the missing word "going by too quickly to grasp." Often we are sure that the momentary image *was* the missing word, and indeed if people in such a state are presented with the correct word, *they can recognize it very quickly and distinguish it from incorrect words*, suggesting that the fleeting conscious "flash" was indeed accurate. (my emphasis)

There are many difficulties with this analysis, and Brown and McNeill indirectly note the chief one themselves but without seeing its import: the crucial datum is the evaluative recognition that the *right* configuration is potentially available, or now manifest, in focal attention. Certainly the general evaluation of right-fit must be made at some cognitive level, and this evaluation is something over and above the specific word taken by itself, be it represented inside or outside consciousness. The heart of a TOT is the *recognition of rightness*, and that recognition is antecedently specified by the particular context, which is of course largely unconscious at any given moment. We all know that occasionally a TOT can last for quite a few, sometimes agonized, seconds, plenty of time to introspectively recognize the specific content—if that were really the heart of the process. *All fleeting experiences may be vague, but not all vague experiences are fleeting.* Given that a TOT can be relatively long-lasting, I do not see how we can explain its vague character by an appeal to fleetingness alone.

The subliminal perception literature also yields evidence of rightness, and here the fringe aspect of the experience lets us demystify the notion of intuition, in which we have a hunch. So Marcel (1983) remarks on the phenomenon of "gut feelings." In his unconscious priming experiments, one effect was most significant on so-called passive subjects, who, Marcel reports, were more inclined to select (unconsciously primed) words "which 'felt' right" even though they had no conscious criterion for their judgment and could not explain it (p. 204). But here, as I suspect in so many other cases of tacit or implicit cognition, we would seem to have behavior mediated by fringe experience dissociated from a sensory content that would normally occupy the focus of attention.

There is a lingering puzzle about what it is that can guide subjects to recognize that something is right, when they are unable to identify any specific criterion for their judgment. So Weiskranz (1992) wonders how "one can deal quantitatively with the phenomenon of 'switched' or 'gut' awareness? For example G. Y., a blindsight subject, sometimes says (but this is not true of all blindsight nor G. Y., under all conditions) that he 'knows' that a stimulus has occurred, but insists that he definitely does not 'see'." Here again, simply having right/wrong information in the fringe is by itself quite sufficient for successfully performing blindsight tasks; and subjects do at times report correlative experiences of "just knowing."

Although the situation is complex, and anomalies abound, it is worth noting that an evaluative signaling system in the fringe bears an intriguing relation to an analysis of pathological states of consciousness made by D. L. Schacter (1990). Certain amnesiacs are unaware of information that they nevertheless use implicitly; those afflicted with anosognosia are unaware of a cognitive or physical deficit. Schacter suspects that these two kinds of "unawareness" are quite different and need to be accounted for. The implicit knowledge/anosognosia contrast does seem to reflect a cognitive distinction in consciousness. Some amnesiacs with only implicit knowledge have apparently lost the ability to feel retrieval accessibility over a certain cognitive domain, and in consequence the "target" experience toward which attention would otherwise focus is gone. Similarly, in anosognosia, the pathological inability to feel wrongness in a given domain would interfere with the conscious recognition of deficits and, at the same time, remove the natural target used to call detailed information about a deficit into consciousness.

If fringe experience is distinct from focal attention and the fringe itself is able to manifest distinguishable component experiences like rightness and familiarity, it should be possible to find cases where these cognitive elements do not operate in their normal, integrated fashion, but are disrupted by neurological malfunctions, or can be teased apart experimentally. If the analysis so far is correct, we should expect to find at least some cases where fringe components operate in the absence of focal consciousness and, conversely, where focal consciousness can occur in the absence of the context information normally encoded in the fringe.

Connectionism and Rightness

Let us return to Weiskrantz's question about how to deal quantitatively with gut feelings and the like. Using connectionism, we *can* attempt to quantify conscious intuitions (and the more explicit serial processes which build on them) by modeling, on a computer, versions of the nonconscious/conscious process that produces these feelings. It would seem that the most important of these feelings is rightness, as the most fundamental positive evaluative component of the fringe, and that rightness can be modeled by goodness-of-fit.

Remember the basic structural limitation on consciousness/nonconscious interaction: If consciousness does perform the cognitive functions it appears to, it must somehow take into account vast amounts of unconscious information that it cannot itself contain; the articulation limitations of consciousness make detailed representation of context information impossible. Rightness represents, in consciousness, perhaps the single most important mechanism controlling conscious/nonconscious interaction: rightness would seem to represent the degree to which an explicit content in consciousness is compatible with its vast unconscious context; rightness links these two cognitive subsystems into a constant and reciprocal interaction.

If the last 30 years of cognitive research have taught us anything, it is that the structure of unconscious context information is massively parallel and distributed; far more like a connectionist network than any serial model currently available. Hopfield's (1982) discovery of goodness-of-fit (see Rumelhart et al. 1986 for a technical discussion of goodness-of-fit) shows that in many cases it is possible to condense into a single metric or index the level of global coherence resulting from an immense number of mutually interacting, neuronlike nodes. And if the connectionist model of nonconscious processing is roughly correct, we can simulate it, to a degree, on a computer, using goodness-of-fit as the interacting link between parallel (nonconscious) and serial (focal attentive) aspects.

Rightness, in consciousness, does seem to behave like a goodness-of-fit metric: that is, it does seem to signal the degree to which a given conscious content is compatible with its parallel and distributed nonconscious context. I believe I have shown that many lines of evidence and theory indicate that the feeling of rightness exists, that it is a distinct entity, and that it is not to be confused with any focal content in consciousness. Rightness signals a coherence relation between *whatever* content may occupy consciousness and *whatever* nonconscious con-

text the content is embedded in. Ignoring habituation, as the content in consciousness becomes
more integrated with its (presumably) parallel
and distributed nonconscious context, the rightness "metric" should increase in intensity.

We would expect this process, for example,
to be evident in early stages of problem solving. Equating rightness with a goodness-of-fit
metric, then, gives us a coherent picture of how
"hunches" and "intuitions" work at both the
conscious and nonconscious level. Rightness is
able to guide conscious activity before any clear
content has appeared as an explicit evaluative
criterion. The findings of Bowers et al. (1990)
illustrate just such a process: In the context of
discovery:

tacit perception of coherence guided Ss gradually to an
explicit representation ... in the form of a hunch or
hypotheses. Clues to coherence may automatically
activate the problem solvers relevant mnemonic and
semantic networks, and eventually the level of patterned activation is sufficient to cross a threshold of
consciousness. At this point it represents a hunch or
hypothesis. (p. 72)

See McGovern 1993 for an extended discussion
of this point.

From the standpoint of current connectionist
theory, however, there is a serious problem with
my analysis to this point. In their present form,
networks do not themselves "compute" goodness-of-fit in order to settle into a stable,
maximum goodness interpretation. An actual
goodness-of-fit computation is carried out for
secondary, descriptive purposes, and uses a
standard sequential summation. The computation of the goodness-of-fit of a network is *not*, at
the moment, itself carried out by a network.

But because, as I believe I have shown, there is
strong reason to hold that rightness exists, we
can assume that rightness must be produced
somehow by our cognitive system. The complexity of determining context fit mandates an
unconscious process, and our best current understanding of unconscious processing at the

moment is that it be networklike. Therefore, this
line of thought predicts that some as yet unrecognized "secondary" network architecture must
be able to determine the goodness-of-fit of the
"primary" network, which settles into coherent
state as a direct consequence of the immediate
content of consciousness. Some secondary process must tell us how coherent the primary network configuration is. It has been shown that
FOK may have its locus in the frontal lobes
(Janowsky, Shimamura, and Squire 1989), and
so perhaps the secondary network system is
much more in evidence there.

To search for secondary, goodness-of-fit
determining networks, of course, neuroscience
needs to have some idea what network architectures are able to do the job (a rough and
ready version is good enough for now). So, a
search for secondary networks in the brain
would do well to enlist connectionist computer
scientists to work out some likely versions of
secondary networks. And perhaps neuroscientist
and computer scientist will mutually sharpen
one another's ideas if the investigation proves
justified.

A final implication of the fringe to be dealt
with now touches on the question of the efficacy
of consciousness. If the fringe is indeed like a
menu bar, then the structure of consciousness *itself* implies that consciousness, qua consciousness, is doing cognitive work, just as it already
appears to be. Looking carefully at the function
of the fringe provides a new piece of evidence
against epiphenomenalism. For in addition to
our feelings of undertaking willful action, the
functional analysis of the fringe implies that
consciousness is equipped with a set of controls
that seem to be designed precisely *for* willful
action.

Acknowledgments

This paper reports selected findings from Mangan 1991, some of which were presented with

additional supporting evidence in Mangan 1993b,c.

Notes

1. This effect, sometimes called semantic satiation, has been confirmed objectively by many experimental studies going back to Severance and Washburn (1907). See section "Contemporary Research and the Fringe" for further discussion.

2. Later I will extend the notion of the fringe to include certain cases of peripheral and low articulation *sensory* experiences as treated, for example, by Rock and Gutman (1981). These must not be confused with peripheral and/or low articulation signals that arise from the structure of our perceptual organs (e.g., from the wide receptive fields in the eye). James's discussion of the fringe is limited to nonsensory experience.

3. Theories dealing with an intermediate domain of cognitive processing "below" consciousness and "above" neurons did not appeal to James. For instance, James ridiculed Kant's notion of cognition, calling it (rightly) an "elaborate internal machine shop" (p. 368). Yet of all traditional theories of the mind, Kant's comes closest to the current view of nonconscious processing and its relation to consciousness (see Bechtel 1988 and Flanagan 1991). Mangan (1991) devotes two chapters to Kant's view of cognition, emphasizing Kant's final position on the constitution and operation of cognitive processes as found in the *Critique of judgement.*

4. This follows Ewald Hering's use of phenomenology to develop hypotheses about specific neural structures (see Mangan 1993b).

5. All page references without further specification are to the standard pagination of James's *Principles of psychology*; these follow the 1890 edition.

6. James says feelings of relation are "numberless." They range from fringe feelings corresponding to specific logical relations such as "a feeling of *and*, a feeling of *if*, a feeling of *but*, a feeling of *by* ..." (pp. 245–246) to much more all purpose feelings such as familiarity and rightness. From a cognitive standpoint, the feeling of familiarity is much *less* important than the feelings of rightness and wrongness. See section "Contemporary Research and the Fringe."

7. James's notion of context was relatively narrow. He held what I would call a "horizontal" view of context: The context for a given experience consists of a set of other past or projected *experiences*. Consistent with his rejection of a Kantian approach to nonconscious processing, James did not seem to hold a modern "vertical" sense of context information as including vast amounts of information processing that never enter consciousness.

8. This point may be key to understanding the cognitive basis and phenomenology of aesthetic experience. Mangan (1991) develops this idea in some detail.

9. See Mangan 1993a for a brief analysis of consciousness as an information bearing medium and the problems this raises for functionalism.

References

Baars, B. (1988). *A cognitive theory of consciousness.* New York: Cambridge University Press.

Bechtel, W. (1988). *Philosophy of mind: An overview for cognitive science.* Hillsdale, NJ: Erlbaum.

Bowers, K., Regehr, G., Balthazard, C., and Parker, K. (1990). Intuition in the context of discovery. *Cognitive Psychology*, 22, 72–110.

Broadbent, C. D. (1954). The role of auditory localization in attention and memory span. *Journal of Experimental Psychology*, 47, 191–196.

Broadbent, C. D. (1958). *Perception and communication.* Elmsford, NY: Pergamon Press.

Brown, R., and McNeill, D. (1966). The "tip-of-the-tongue" phenomenon. *The Journal of Verbal Learning and Verbal Behavior*, 5, 325–337.

Crick, F., and Koch C. (1990). Towards a neurobiological theory of consciousness. *Seminars in the Neurosciences*, 2, 263–275.

Flanagan, O. (1991). *The science of the mind.* Cambridge, MA. MIT Press.

Hart, J. T. (1965). Memory and feeling-of-knowing experience. *Journal of Educational Psychology*, 56, 208–216.

Hopfield, J. (1982). Neural networks and physical systems with emergent collective computational abilities. *Proceedings of the National Academy of Sciences, USA*, 79, 2554–2558.

James, W. (1890). *The principles of psychology*. New York: Holt.

Janowsky, J., Shimamura, A., and Squire, L. (1989). Memory and metamemory: Comparisons between patients with frontal lobe lesions and amnesic patients. *Psychobiology*, 17, 2–11.

Klein, M. (1981). In L. T. Benjamin, Jr. and K. D. Lowman (eds.) *Activities handbook for the teaching of psychology*, p. 83. Washington, DC: American Psychological Association.

Kintch, W. (1970). *Learning, memory, and conceptual processes*. New York: Wiley.

Lewicki, P. (1988). *Nonconscious social information processing*. New York: Academic Press.

McGovern, K. (1993). Feelings in the fringe. *Consciousness and Cognition*, 2, 119–125.

Mangan, B. (1991). *Meaning and the structure of consciousness: An essay in psycho-aesthetics*. Doctoral dissertation. University of California, Berkeley.

Mangan, B. (1993a). Dennett, consciousness, and the sorrows of functionalism. *Consciousness and Cognition*, 2, 1–17.

Mangan, B. (1993b). Taking phenomenology seriously: The "fringe" and its implications for cognitive research. *Consciousness and Cognition*, 2, 89–108.

Mangan, B. (1993c). Some philosophical and empirical implications of the fringe. *Consciousness and Cognition*, 2, 142—154.

Mandler, G. (1975). Consciousness: Respectable, useful, and probably necessary. In R. Solso (ed.), *Information processing and cognition: The Loyola Symposium*. Hillsdale, NJ: Erlbaum.

Marcel, A. (1983). Conscious and unconscious perception: An approach to relations between phenomenal experience and perceptual processes. *Cognitive Psychology*, 15, 238–300.

Miller, G. (1956). The magical number seven, plus or minus two. *Psychology Review*, 63, 81–97.

Miller, G. (1962). *Psychology: The science of mental life*. New York: Harper & Row.

Neisser, U. (1967). *Cognitive psychology*. New York: Appleton-Century-Crofts.

Nelson, T., Gerler, D., and Narens, L. (1984). Accuracy of feeling of knowing judgements for predicting perceptual identification and relearning. *Journal of Experimental Psychology*, 133, 286–300.

Rock, I., and Gutman, D. (1981). The effect of inattention on form perception. *Journal of Experimental Psychology: Human Perception and Performance*, 7, 275–285.

Rumelhart, D., Smolensky, P., McClelland, J., and Hinton, G. (1986). Schemata and sequential thought processes in PDP models. In D. Rumelhart and J. McClelland (eds.), *Parallel distributed processing: Explorations in the microstructure of cognition*, Vol. 2. Cambridge, MA: MIT Press.

Schacter, D. (1990). Toward a cognitive neuropsychology of awareness: Implicit knowledge and anosognosia. *Journal of Clinical and Experimental Psychology*, 12, 155–178.

Severance, E., and Washburn, M. (1907). The loss of associative power in words after long fixation. *American Journal of Psychology*, 18, 182–186.

Weiskrantz (1992). Introduction: Dissociated issues. In A. Milner and M. Rugg (eds.) *The neuropsychology of consciousness*. New York: Academic Press.

Wertheimer, M., and Gillis, W. M. (1958). Satiation and the rate of lapse of verbal meaning. *Journal of General Psychology*, 59, 79–85.

46 The Fundamental Role of Context: Unconscious Shaping of Conscious Information

Bernard J. Baars

Introduction

As we walk, run, turn, sit, dance, or climb on dry land, specialized components of the nervous system make running predictions to compensate for our changing relationship to gravity and to the visual surround. The world is experienced as stable only when this remarkable feat of prediction is successful. These orientational predictions are entirely unconscious, but they profoundly influence our conscious experience. As long as they are successful, these *contextual* predictions give no sign of their existence. That may change for a time when we step on a small sailboat, but in a curious way: we still do not experience the change in the framework of our experience; we just notice an instability in the entire perceptual field. Stepping on the sailboat we experience the novel, unpredictable movements of our body as a change in the world, even though we know full well that the world has not changed; only our relationship to it has. The real world does not sway with the motion of the deck. The same thing happens for a moment when we step back on dry land after "gaining our sea legs": unconsciously we now predict a regular yawing and rolling, so that the relationship between reality and expectation has once more gone awry. This experience of an unstable world causes the contextual orientation system to revise its predictions again, and because we are experienced land walkers, we soon regain our feet.

The system that computes our orientation to gravity and the visual world is part of the context of our experience. We continually benefit from a host of such contextual processes, without experiencing them as objects of conscious experience. Their influence can be inferred from many sources of evidence. The example of the sailing trip involves perceptual-motor context, but much the same argument can be made for the contexts of thinking, belief, and communication. A great deal of the research literature in perception and cognition provides evidence for the pervasive influence of unconscious contexts.

"Context" is a key idea, defined as a system that shapes conscious experience without itself being conscious at that time. It is a close modern relative of "set" and "adaptation level" in perception, and of various proposals for knowledge structures and "frames" in cognitive science. Contexts are equivalent to currently unconscious expectations that shape conscious experiences and to currently unconscious intentions that shape voluntary actions. The observations supporting this idea were well known to pre-behavioristic psychologists in Europe and the United States, including Wundt, James, the Würtzburg School, Brentano, and Gestalt psychology. The word "context" is often used in current psychology to mean the physical surround, but in this chapter it only refers to the inner world that shapes our experience. After all, the physical environment affects our experiences and actions only if it is represented in the inner world. Thus the context-in-the-world inevitably shapes our experience by way of the context-in-the-head. Further, the inner context preserves important information from the past, which is not available from our current surroundings at all. It makes more sense, therefore, to locate the psychological context inside the nervous system.

Why add one more term to the current rash of words that mean much the same thing? The reason is simple. For us, the word "context" is not just any mental representation—it is an unconscious representation that acts to influence another, conscious representation. This special meaning is not captured by any of the other terms.

This chapter will look into some of the characteristics of stable contexts. I begin with a survey of the great amount of evidence for contextual knowledge, specify some common properties of contexts, and explore the interaction between conscious contents and unconscious contexts.

Sources of Evidence

Contexts are a bit tricky to think about because by definition we do not experience them directly. For this reason, we begin with four pervasive sources of evidence for unconscious contexts that shape conscious experience.

1. The existence of priming effects, where one conscious experience alters the processing of another, although the first experience is gone by the time the second arrives

2. The universal phenomenon of fixedness, where one cannot escape the influence of unconscious contextual assumptions that stand in the way of solving a problem, or of perceiving an alternative

3. The case of top-down unconscious influences, which change our conscious experience of any event that is ambiguous, unknown, degraded, fragmentary, isolated, unpredictable, or partly forgotten

4. The case of strong violations of contextual expectations, which can cause a part of the unconscious context to become conscious and reportable

Table 46.1 summarizes the contrast between conscious and unconscious phenomena connected with context.

I will give examples of each case.

Priming Effects: Conscious Experiences Generally Improve Receptivity to Related Conscious Experiences

When one experience affects the likelihood of a similar experience, we can say that the first event has "primed" or shaped the context for the second event. This is a phenomenon of extreme

Table 46.1
Contexts of a single conscious event

Conscious cases	Comparable unconscious cases
1. Percepts, images, inner speech, and bodily feelings.	Contextual factors that shape and evoke these conscious events.
Readily accessible concepts.	Conceptual presuppositions.
2. Input that can be interpreted within a currently dominant context.	"Acontextual" input for which the appropriate context is not currently dominant.
3. Previously unattended events interrupting the attended stream (e.g., the subject's name).	Unattended events that affect the interpretation of attended events (e.g., disambiguating words).
4. Strong violations of unconscious contexts. (decontextualization)	Weak violations of unconscious contexts (e.g., proofreader effect).

generality. Blumenthal (1977) quotes Fraisse (1963, p. 88), for example:

When I listen to speech, I perceive the clause being pronounced by the speaker, but I interpret it in accordance with all the sentences which I no longer perceive and of which I have only retained a general idea. When I listen to music, I perceive again and again a short, rhythmic structure, but this is integrated with a melodic whole to which it owes its affective resonance.

Music and speech are indeed very good examples. Psycholinguistic research has now amassed extensive evidence for widespread discourse relations that are necessary to understand even a single word in a conversation, although those relationships are of course not focally conscious. Similarly, in a piece of music the key, the initial statement of the themes, their development and variations, all must shape the way we experience a single phrase in the middle of a symphony. But none of that is conscious when we have that experience.

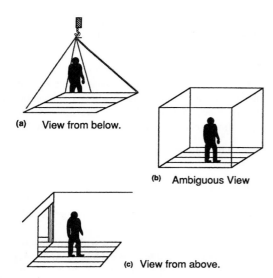

(a)   View from below.

(b)   Ambiguous View

(c)   View from above.

Figure 46.1
Priming effects: Conscious events increase access to similar events. One of the many hundreds of demonstrations of priming effects, the ambiguous Necker cube allows one to interpret the middle figure (b) as seen either from above or below. Which interpretation will be chosen is influenced by previous conscious experiences. The construction worker being lifted on a platform by a crane (a) provides one imaginable framework in which we view from below a person standing on a floor. Viewing (a) for a little while will tend to prime the view from below, whereas contemplating (c) will tend to prime the view from above. Because we more commonly experience the top view (c), there is an overall bias toward it, which may be considered a long-term priming effect.

Figure 46.1 gives an example of a short-term priming effect. The middle figure (46.1b) is an ambiguous Necker cube. By paying attention to figure 46.1a for several seconds and then going back to figure 46.1b, we tend to interpret the ambiguous figure as if we are looking at the bottom of the cube. The experience of figure 46.1a structures the experience of figure 46.1b, even though figure 46.1a is not conscious when it

does so. Now we can pay attention to figure 46.1c for a while; now we are more likely to see the ambiguous cube from the top.

We can easily show linguistic priming. Compare the next two examples, in which the first word primes an interpretation of the second:

(1)   volume: book

(2)   arrest: book

The conscious interpretation of "book" will tend to differ depending on the prime.

In general, a conscious priming event:

• decreases reaction time to similar conscious events

• lowers the threshold for related material that is near the perceptual threshold, or is ambiguous, vague, fleeting, degraded, badly understood, or isolated from its surround. Indeed any task that has an unconscious choice-point in the flow of processing is sensitive to priming for the relevant alternative (Baars 1985).

• a prime increases the likelihood of similar events emerging in memory, through free association, cued recall, and recognition tasks.

• finally, a conscious prime stimulates the probability of actions and speech related to the priming stimulus (Baars 1985).

Priming effects are ubiquitous in sensation, perception, comprehension, and action. In an older psychological vocabulary, priming creates set. Indeed, the Psychophysical Law, the oldest and one of the best-established findings in psychology, states that the experienced intensity of any stimulus depends on the intensity of preceding stimuli. This can be thought of as a temporal priming effect with universal application.

Priming effects are not always momentary; they can last as least as long as a conversation, and there may indeed be conscious formative experiences that shape human lives for years. So we are not talking merely of momentary events. Even a single conscious experience may trigger a short term change in context; in the case of traumatic experiences, the effects can last for years.

The similarity of a prime and a primed event can be either perceptual or conceptual. The similarity between "book" and "volume" in the example above is not perceptual but semantic or conceptual; the similarity between the two views of the Necker cube in figure 46.1 is more perceptual.

The following subsection discusses another extremely general phenomenon in which unconscious knowledge helps to shape conscious events.

Fixedness: Being Blind to "the Obvious"

The four sentences below are normal, coherent English sentences:

(3)   The ship sailed past the harbor sank.

(4)   The building blocks the sun shining on the house faded are red.

(5)   The granite rocks by the seashore with the waves.

(6)   The cotton clothing is made of grows in Alabama. (Milne 1982).

On first reading these sentences, most of us feel "stuck"; they do not cohere, they do not work somehow. We may be driven to try rather farfetched ideas to make sense of them: maybe sentence (3) is really two conjoined clauses, such as "The ship sailed past and the harbor sank"? But harbors do not sink, so that interpretation does not work either. If we truly believe that these are normal English sentences, the experience of trying to understand them can be intensely frustrating and annoying.

What is going on? Consider the following context for sentence (3):

A small part of Napoleon's fleet tried to run the English blockade at the entrance to the harbor. Two ships, a sloop and a frigate, ran straight for the harbor while a third ship tried to sail past the harbor in order to draw enemy fire. The ship sailed past the harbor sank.

If you have just encountered sentence (3) for the first time, this little story should help solve the problem. We could, of course, insert the subordinate clause marker "which" to create:

(3′)   The ship which sailed past the harbor sank.

But this use of "which" is optional in English, though we tend to insert it when needed for clarity. When our contextual knowledge is sufficient, it can be dropped.

The problem we encountered with sentence (3) is one kind of fixedness. We tend to approach sentences in English with the contextual assumption that the first verb will be the main verb, barring contrary semantic or syntactic information (viz., Milne 1982). If "sailed" is assumed to be the main verb, then we do not know what to do with the verb "sank." But "sailed" may also be the verb of a subordinate clause, as in the following examples:

(7)   a.   The ship sailed by the commodore was a beautiful sight.
       b.   The ships sailed at Newport are racing sloops.
       c.   To my surprise, a ship sailed by a good crew sank.

Here the main verbs always come later in the sentence. The trouble with sentence (3) is that we tend to become committed to one syntactic interpretation before all the evidence is in, and we may find it impossible to back away from it. In the most general terms, we are captured by one unconscious interpretation of the beginning of the sentence—we are fixated by the wrong syntactic context.

Fixedness can be found in all kinds of problem solving. It is found in vision, language perception, in solving puzzles, in science, literature, politics, and warfare. American policy during the Vietnam War may have been an example of fixedness, given that it followed certain assumptions about international relations that were widely accepted at that time, across the political spectrum. In retrospect, some of those assumptions are questionable. But that is just the point about fixedness: seen in retrospect or from "the outside," it is hard to believe that the fixated person cannot see the "obvious" solution. But within the fixating context, the solution is not obvious at all: it is literally impossible to perceive.

Yet fixedness is a completely normal part of learning. Whenever we try to learn something before we have the knowledge needed to make sense of the material, we may find ourselves interpreting it in the wrong context. McNeill (1966) cites the example of a mother trying to teach her child something about English negation—a bit prematurely:

Child: Nobody don't like me.

Mother: No, say "Nobody likes me."

Child: Nobody don't like me.

Mother: No, say "Nobody likes me."

(*Eight* repetitions of this dialogue.)

Mother: No, now listen carefully, say, "Nobody likes me."

Child: Oh! Nobody don't likes me.

A year later the same child would laugh at the error, but when the dialogue was recorded he or she was not prepared to perceive the difference. In learning, as in life, readiness is all.

A major point is to realize that our notion of "fixedness" depends critically on having an outside point of view in which the mistake is a mistake. That is to say, as adults we can find the above example comfortably amusing because we know the right answer. But for the child the error is no error at all. The "flawed" sentence is not experienced as erroneous; in terms of the child's internalized rules, it is not an error at all.

Selective Attention as a Contextual Fixedness Effect

One powerful implication is that "fixedness" exists in states of mind that we consider to be perfectly correct. For example, one can plausibly argue that selective attention is a fixed state of mind—after all, in shadowing speech in one ear we are utterly oblivious to the unattended stream of speech, as much as the child in the language example is oblivious to the "correct" sentence. Thus the remarkable ability of one stream of speech to capture our conscious experience to the exclusion of any other looks like a contextual fixedness effect. Notice that structural similarities between the two streams of speech will cause leakage between them; that is, when they share context, the "unconscious" stream tends to affect the conscious stream (e.g., Norman 1976). Normally we can hear the acoustical qualities of the unattended ear, perhaps because these qualities match the acoustical contexts of the attended ear. After all, the attended ear must detect a range of sounds as well. Further, when the semantic context of the attended involves an ambiguous word like "bank," it is open to influences from the unattended ear to the extent those influences are consistent with the semantic ambiguity (MacKay 1973; chap. 16, this volume). In table 46.1 this point is made by listing "acontextual" information on the unconscious side of the contrastive table. When there is potentially conscious input, but the right context is not brought to bear on it, it does not become conscious.

Similarly, in absorbed states of mind—in reading a fine novel or watching an entrancing motion picture—we are deaf and blind to the world. In absent-minded states we are likewise captured by one train of thought to the exclusion of others (Reason 1983). One plausible supposition is that all these states are initiated, shaped, and bounded by powerful context hierarchies that permit no interruption for the time being.

Only a change in the fixating context, or giving up on the task, can release us from fixedness. Above, this change in context is created by the little story about Napoleon's ships running the English blockade. This creates a new context that works, but that no doubt has its own fixating properties. This is the normal case, of course: we may change to more a effective context, but we cannot undo context as such. Inevitably we are condemned to both its advantages and drawbacks.

The existence of fixedness provides extensive evidence for the power of contexts. Next, we consider the case in which context actually enters into conscious experience.

Top-Down Influences and the Pervasiveness of Ambiguity

Many domains of experience are full of local ambiguities. This is obvious in some cases and not so obvious in others. For some obvious examples, there are many times when information about the world is degraded, inadequate, or forgotten. Examples include listening to a conversation in a noisy room, trying to see an oncoming bus at a great distance, or walking through a dark room at night. In all these cases we rely more than usual on the inner context to constrain conscious experience. In the social realm, it is terribly important for us to know other people's minds—their intentions, beliefs, and attitudes toward us. But we cannot read their minds directly. The evidence we have is ambiguous, and hence vulnerable to our own goals and expectations, wishes, and fears. We often make inferences about other people's minds with a degree of confidence that is simply not justified by the evidence (Nisbett and Wilson 1977). In this case, inner context controls our experience far too often. Political convictions show this even more graphically. A glance at the editorial pages of a newspaper shows how people with different convictions use the same events to support opposite beliefs about the world, about

other people, and about morality. Or take the domain of "the future." Human beings are intensely concerned about the future, and we often have strong beliefs about it, even when future events are inherently probabilistic (Tversky and Kahneman 1973). The evidence is inadequate or ambiguous, and hence we rely more and more on internal contextual constraints.

Those examples are fairly obvious, but there are many ambiguous domains in which we experience events with great confidence, though careful experiments show that there is much more local uncertainty than we realize. There is extensive evidence that our own bodily feelings, which we may use to infer our emotions, are often ambiguous (Schachter and Singer 1962, Valins 1967). Further, our own intentions and reasons for making decisions are often inaccessible to introspection, or at least ambiguous (Nisbett and Wilson 1977). Our memory of the past is often as poor as our ability to anticipate the future, and it is prone to be filtered through our present perspective (Bransford 1979, Mandler 1984). Historians must routinely cope with the universal tendency of people to reshape the past in light of the present, and lawyers actively employ techniques designed to make witnesses change their memory of a crime or accident (see Bransford 1979).

Even perceptual domains that seem stable and reliable are actually ambiguous when we isolate small pieces of information. Every corner in a normal rectangular room can be interpreted in two ways, as an outside or an inside corner. To see this, the reader can simply roll a piece of paper into a tube and look through it to any right-angled corner of the room. Every room contains both two- and three-dimensional ambiguities in its corners, much like the Necker cube and bookend illusions (figure 46.1). Similarly, the experienced brightness of surfaces depends upon the brightness of surrounding surfaces (Gelb 1932, Gilchrist 1977). Depth perception is controlled by our contextual assumptions about the direction of the incoming light, about the shape and size of objects, and the like (Rock 1983). These ambiguities emerge when we isolate stimuli—but it is important to note that in normal visual perception, stimulus input is often isolated. In any single eye fixation we only take in a very small, isolated patch of information. Normal detailed (foveal) vision spans only 2 degrees of arc; yet when people are asked about the size of their own detailed visual field, they often believe it must be about 180 degrees. Even the visual world, which seems so stable and reliable, is full of local ambiguities (Marr 1982).

Language provides a great many examples of ambiguity. Indeed, every level of linguistic analysis has its own kind of ambiguity. Thus:

1. Ambiguities of sound. The English /l/ is perceived as either /r/ or /l/ by Japanese speakers, whereas the unaspirated /k/ (as in "cool") is freely exchanged by English speakers with the aspirated /kʰ/ (as in "keel"). In Arabic this difference marks very different words. Most English speakers simply do not hear the tones that are critical in languages like Chinese. Further, there are many identical strings of sounds in every language that are divided up differently, as in "ice cream" and "I scream" in English. We typically become conscious of these ambiguous sound sequences only in learning a new language.

2. Morphemic ambiguity. The final /s/ in English has four different morphemic interpretations. It can be plural ("the books"), third-person singular verb ("he books the tickets"), possessive ("the book's cover"), and plural possessive ("the books' covers").

3. Lexical ambiguity. A glance at the dictionary should convince anyone that each word has more than one meaning. More common words tend to have more meanings.

4. Syntactic ambiguity. There are numerous syntactic ambiguities. The best-known ones are the surface- and deep-structure ambiguities of Chomskyan theory (Chomsky 1957, 1965). Thus, "old men and women" is a surface ambiguity that involves grouping: one can have "old

(men and women)" or "(old men) and women." Sentences like "Flying planes can be dangerous" and "They are eating apples" have ambiguities that cannot be represented in a single tree diagram; they involve ambiguity in underlying subjects and objects.

5. Discourse ambiguity. Consider the following example:

(8) a. The glass fell off the table.
    b. It broke.
    b′. It was always a little unstable.

The referent of "it" changes between (8b) and (8b′). It can only be determined by an appeal to context and to the subject's knowledge about glasses and tables. Such ambiguities are extremely common.

6. Referential ambiguities. This occurs when we refer to "that chair" in an auditorium full of chairs or to "that book" in a library.

7. Semantic ambiguity. All too often, concepts do not relate clearly to other concepts. What really is consciousness? What is an atom, or a physical force, or a biological species? All unresolved scientific questions involve deep semantic ambiguity.

8. Topical uncertainty and ambiguity. Consider the following paragraph (Bransford 1979):

The procedure is actually quite simple. First you arrange items into different groups. Of course one pile may be sufficient depending upon how much there is to do. If you have to go somewhere else due to lack of facilities that is the next step; otherwise, you are pretty well set. It is important not to overdo things. That is, it is better to do too few things at once than too many. In the short run this may not seem important but complications can easily arise. A mistake can be made as well. At first, the whole procedure will seem complicated. Soon, however, it will become just another facet of life. It is difficult to foresee any end to the necessity for this task in the immediate future, but then, one never can tell. After the procedure is completed one arranges the materials into different groups again. Then they can be put into their appropriate places. Eventually they will be used once more and the whole cycle will have to be repeated. However, that is part of life.

Confused? Here is the context: the paragraph is about washing clothes. If you read it again, it will be much more comprehensible, details will clarify in experience, and memory for the material will improve greatly.

What is the point of this litany of ambiguities? It is true that ambiguity is pervasive; but the conscious experience of ambiguity is quite rare. We generally gain information about a world that is locally ambiguous, yet we usually experience a stable, coherent world. This suggests that before input becomes conscious, it interacts with numerous unconscious contextual influences to produce a single, coherent, conscious experience. Consciousness and context are twin issues, inseparable in the nature of things.

Global Workspace architecture was originally developed to deal precisely with the problem of unifying many ambiguous or partial sources of information into a single, unified solution (Baars 1988, 1998).

Another source of evidence on contexts is considered next.

Decontextualization: Strong Violations of Context Can Become Consciously Accessible

Unconscious contextual assumptions can become consciously accessible. Every statement we hear or read has presupposed (contextual) information that must be understood before it can make sense. The "washing machine" paragraph shown earlier is an example. But these contextual presuppositions remain unconscious unless they are violated. If we suddenly speak of putting a five-pound weight into the washing machine, we tend to become conscious of one contextual assumption. We will call this process decontextualization. It is a theoretically central phenomenon. Consider the following little story, which is quite normal, so that presupposed ideas tend to remain unconscious:

(9) It was a hot day. Johnny walked to the store and bought some ice cream to eat.

Then he brought home a snow cone for his mother.

But now consider the following version. (It will help to read slowly):

(10) a. It was a hot day in December.
      b. Johnny walked three hours to the town store.
      c. He was completely broke but not very hungry.
      d. He bought a gallon of ice cream and ate to his heart's content.
      e. He also brought a snow cone home to his mother.

The second story makes implausible a number of conditions in the presupposed context of the event "buying ice cream," so that we find this normally unconscious knowledge becoming conscious. The story in (9) probably left unconscious the fact that "walking to the store to get ice cream" is usually assumed to take a matter of minutes, not three hours; that hot days are likely in summer, not in December; that buying involves money, and thus "being broke" excludes buying anything; that one can eat ice cream even without being very hungry, but that one would certainly not eat a gallon of ice cream if one were not very hungry; and that walking home for three hours on a hot day, carrying a snow cone, would cause it to melt. When these implausible claims are presented, the contradicted context tends to come to mind spontaneously.

We can think of this presupposed context as a set of stable, predictable constraints on normal discourse (see figure 46.2) (Foss 1982). As long as a piece of presupposed knowledge remains predictable, it also tends to remain unconscious. But when it is strongly violated, its consequences tend to become conscious in some way. This is similar to the pattern we find with violated expectations in stimulus habituation, with obstacles created in automatic tasks, and with increases in task difficulty for habituated mental images. In all these cases, novel information is

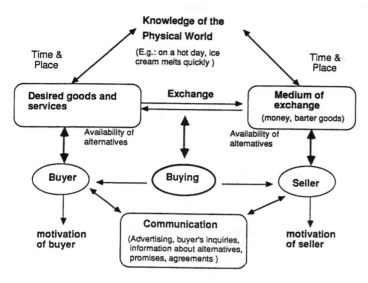

Figure 46.2
Presuppositions of the concept of "buying" that may become conscious upon violation. The knowledge necessary to understand and everyday concept like "buying" shown in the form of a semantic network. "Buying" presupposes other concepts, such as time, space, exchange, movement, transportation, communication, money or another valued medium of exchange, motivation, anticipated gain for both buyer and seller, and so on. It is incomprehensible, or something very different, without these concepts. But these presupposed concepts are not conscious in a routine act of buying. Some of the presupposed concepts may become consciously accessible when they are violated or when there is some uncertainty about them. Thus, the idea of carrying an ice cream cone for an hour on a hot day violates some presuppositions, which may then be broadcast via the global workspace. In Global Workspace theory, the presupposed network of concepts needed to understand a consciously accessed concept is called a conceptual context.

created by the violation of established, predictable properties of the situation. Of course, when we make parts of a conceptual context conscious, this places the newly conscious material in its own unconscious context. Becoming conscious of contextual knowledge while it is acting as context is like chasing one's tail; it is ultimately impossible.

A Summary of the Evidence for Unconscious Contexts

First, conscious experiences change later, related experiences long after the earlier ones have be-

come unconscious. Presumably, the first experience creates a context within which the later one is shaped and defined.

Second, the universal phenomenon of fixedness suggests that all conscious and deliberate processes are bounded by assumptions that are unconscious to the subject, though they may be obvious to outside observers. Selective attention and aborbed states may be variations on this theme of fixedness.

Third, there is extensive evidence for local ambiguity in all areas of life—the past, the future, other people's minds, our own feelings, visual and auditory perception, language understanding, and so on. All these domains are rife with ambiguity. Yet ambiguities are rarely experienced as ambiguities. Normally, many different contexts interact to create a single conscious interpretation of reality.

Fourth, strong violations of our contextual assumptions can become conceptually conscious—that is, we can refer to these surprises as objects of experience, and by becoming conscious, we can sometimes change our previous contextual way of thinking about them.

We can assess contexts in two convenient ways. First, priming tasks can be designed to be sensitive to the information contained in a dominant context. Current cognitive psychology has dozens of examples of the use of such priming techniques (e.g., Swinney 1979, Baars 1985). Second, one can observe the occurrence of surprise to events that violate contextual expectations. Thus changes in heart rate—a measure of surprise—have been used to assess the existence of phoneme boundaries in infants who could not possibly tell us about their experience. Surprise could be used much more often with adults, because there is little reason to think that adult voluntary report of contextual structures is accurate; hence we may miss contextual events in adults rather often because of our reliance on verbal report.

Several Kinds of Contexts

We can talk about several kinds of contexts: first, the context of perception/imagery; next, the context of conceptual thought; third, goal contexts, which evoke and shape actions; and finally, the context of communication that is shared by two people talking with each other, or by ourselves talking to ourselves. Notice that some of these contexts actually shape conscious experience as such, whereas others evoke conscious thoughts and images, or help select conscious percepts. Perceptual/imaginal contexts clearly enter into the conscious qualitative experience. A

goal context may simply serve to recall a word or evoke a mental image. That is, not all contexts necessarily enter into the experience itself. Naturally these different kinds of contexts interact with each other. Perceptual events and images have a lot of influence on conceptual thinking; concepts influence inner speech, images, and the selection of perceptual events; goals influence concepts, and vice versa. Let us now examine the types of context in a little more detail.

The Context of Perception

Imagine sitting in a tiny, well-lit movie theater, looking at a metallic disk instead of a movie screen. The disk appears to be white. But now someone lights a cigarette, and as the smoke curls upward you see it floating through a slender but powerful light beam, coming from the rear of the theater, and aimed precisely at the metal disk. You look back at the disk, and suddenly you notice that it isn't white at all, but black. This is the Gelb Effect (Gelb 1932) and can be summarized by saying that the color of a surface is a function of the perceived incoming light. If we are never conscious of the incoming light, we will attribute the brightness of the disk to its surface color and not to the light. Once having seen the cigarette smoke intersecting the light beam, the disk is seen to be black. Similarly, if we turn a picture of the moon's craters upside down, the experience of depth is reversed, so that craters are seen as hills. This is because scenes are interpreted under the assumption that light comes from above, as indeed it usually does. When the photo of the moon is turned upside down, the light is still assumed to come from the top of the picture, and concavities are turned into convexities (Rock 1983).

Perceptual research since the nineteenth century has uncovered hundreds of such phenomena. All of them can be summarized by saying that complex and subtle unconscious systems, which we call contexts, shape and define conscious perceptual experiences.

The Context of Imagery

Imagery has not been studied as extensively as perception, but over the past decade very interesting findings have emerged, suggesting constraints on visual imagery of which we are generally unconscious. These constraints tell us both about the format and the content of imagery (Kosslyn and Schwartz 1981). The "field" of visual imagery has a close resemblance to vision: it has the same flat elliptical shape as the visual field, it presents us with one perspective on a potentially three-dimensional spatial domain, and the scanning time needed to move from one point to another in the mind's eye is a linear function of the distance between the two points, just as we might expect of the visual field.

Clearly, as we learn more about mental imagery, we will continue to find more of these constraints, which are largely unconscious until they are brought to mind.

The Conceptual Context: Conceptual Presuppositions Are Often Unconscious

Anyone who has tried to think very clearly about some topic must know from experience that our stable presuppositions tend to become unconscious. Whatever we believe with absolute certainty, we tend to take for granted. More accurately perhaps, we lose sight of the fact that alternatives to our stable presuppositions can be entertained. Indeed, scientific paradigm shifts generally take place when one group of scientists begins to challenge a presupposition that is held to be immutable (and hence is largely unconscious) in the thinking of an older scientific establishment. In his autobiography, Albert Einstein described this phenomenon in nineteenth-century physics (1949):

... all physicists of the last century saw in classical mechanics a firm and final foundation for all physics, yes, indeed, for all natural science ... Even Maxwell and H. Hertz, who in retrospect appear as those who demolished the faith in mechanics as the final basis of all physical thinking, in their conscious thinking adhered throughout to mechanics as the secured basis of physics. (p. 21; italics added)

Some pages later he recalls how he gained the insight which led to the Special Theory of Relativity:

... After ten years of reflection such a principle resulted from a paradox upon which I had already hit at the age of sixteen: If I pursue a beam of light with the velocity c (the velocity of light in a vacuum), I should observe such a beam of light as a spatially oscillatory electromagnetic field at rest. However, there seems to be no such thing.... One sees that in this paradox the germ of the special relativity theory is already contained. Today everyone knows, of course, that all attempts to clarify this paradox satisfactorily were condemned to failure as long as the axiom of the absolute character of time, viz., of simultaneity, *unrecognizedly was anchored in the unconscious.* (p. 53; italics added)

Kuhn (1962) quotes Charles Darwin to much the same effect:

Darwin, in a particularly perceptive passage at the end of his Origin of Species, wrote, 'Although I am fully convinced of the truth of the views given in this volume ... I by no means expect to convince experienced naturalists whose minds are stocked with a multitude of facts all viewed, during a long course of years, from a point of view directly opposite to mine.... (B)ut I look with confidence to the future—to young and rising naturalists, who will be able to view both sides of the question with impartiality.' (italics added, p. 125)

Darwin observed that many older naturalists were simply unable to consciously think consistently of the alternatives to their own, stable presuppositions. In psychology this phenomenon is easy to observe today, because the field has recently passed through something much like a paradigm shift (see Baars 1986a). It is still remarkably easy to find psychologists who find it impossible to take the existence of consciousness seriously. For these people, the implications of consciousness as something scientifically real and important remain hidden and unconscious.

It would be interesting to find out why conceptual presuppositions tend to become conscious so readily in a simple story like the one cited above, compared to the case of scientific change, where Darwin, Einstein, and many others have complained so much about the inability of other scientists to entertain alternatives to their own presuppositions. Was it because these scientists were emotionally invested in their customary way of viewing the world? Or do more complex knowledge domains make it more difficult to see contextual alternatives and their consequences? Or both?

Scientific Paradigms as Largely Unconscious Contexts

Communication problems occur when people try to exchange ideas under different contextual assumptions. This is especially clear in the case of paradigmatic differences in a scientific community. One might expect science at least to be free of such communication problems, because scientists deal with a shared, observable empirical domain and because mature sciences make use of explicit formal theories. Not so. Historians have long remarked on the frequency of communication problems in science, but it is only with Thomas Kuhn's seminal monograph *The structure of scientific revolutions* (1962/1970) that these communication problems have come to be widely acknowledged as part of the fundamental nature of science. Kuhn described two kinds of evolution in the history of science: within a certain framework, or "paradigm," development is cumulative, because scientists share common tools, goals, typical problems, and assumptions about reality. Thus physics enjoyed a shared paradigm in the two centuries after Newton's *Principia Mathematica*, until the late nineteenth century, when the paradigm began to develop difficult internal contradictions. Einstein's relativity theory solved some of those problems, giving rise to a new framework within which physicists could again communicate without se-

rious problems for some time; but Einsteinian physicists had great difficulty communicating with those who continued to view the world in Newtonian terms. Kuhn calls this phenomenon "the incommensurability of competing paradigms":

Since new paradigms are born from old ones, they ordinarily incorporate much of the vocabulary and apparatus, both conceptual and manipulative, that the traditional paradigm had previously employed. But they seldom employ these borrowed elements in quite the traditional way. Within the new paradigm, old terms, concepts, and experiments fall into new relationships with the other. The inevitable result is what we must call, though the term is not quite right, a misunderstanding between the two competing schools. The laymen who scoffed at Einstein's general theory of relativity because space could not be "curved"—it was not that sort of thing—were not simply wrong or mistaken. Nor were the mathematicians, physicists, and philosophers who tried to develop a Euclidian version of Einstein's theory. What had previously been meant by space was necessarily flat, homogeneous, isotropic, and unaffected by the presence of matter. If it had not been, Newtonian physics would not have worked. To make the transition to Einstein's universe, the whole conceptual web, whose strands are space, time, matter, force, and so on, had to be shifted and laid down again on nature whole.... Communication across the revolutionary divide is inevitably partial. Consider, for another example, the men who called Copernicus mad because he proclaimed that the earth moved. They were not either just wrong or quite wrong. Part of what they meant by "earth" was fixed position. Their earth, at least, could not be moved. Correspondingly, Copernicus' innovation was not simply to move the earth. Rather, it was a whole new way of regarding the problems of physics and astronomy, one that necessarily changed the meaning of both "earth" and "motion." Without those changes the concept of a moving earth was mad....

These examples point to the ... most fundamental aspect of the incommensurability between competing paradigms. In a sense that I am unable to explicate further, the proponents of competing paradigms practice their trades in different worlds. One contains constrained bodies that fall slowly, the other pendulums that repeat their motions again and again. In one, (chemical) solutions are compounds, in the other mixtures. One is embedded in a flat, the other in a curved, matrix of space. Practicing in different worlds, the two groups of scientists see different things when they look from the same point in the same direction. Again, that is not to say that they can see anything they please. Both are looking at the world, and what they look at has not changed. But in some areas they see different things, and they see them in different relations one to the other. That is why a law that cannot even be demonstrated to one group of scientists may occasionally seem intuitively obvious to another. Equally, it is why, before they can hope to communicate fully, one group or the other must experience the conversion we have been calling a paradigm shift. Just because it is a transition between incommensurables, the transition between competing paradigms cannot be made a step at a time, forced by logic and neutral experience.... (Kuhn 1962/1970, pp. 149–151)

Why is it so difficult for committed scientists to change paradigms? From our model, it would seem that change is hard, at least in part because at any single moment the bulk of a paradigm is unconscious. In our terms, paradigms are conceptual contexts. If one tried to make a paradigm conscious, one could only make one aspect of it conscious at any one time because of the limited capacity of consciousness. But typically paradigm differences between two groups of scientists involves not just one, but many different aspects of the mental framework simultaneously. This may also be why conversion phenomena in science (as elsewhere) tend to be relatively rapid, all-or-none events that seem to have a not-quite-rational component. In fact, Kuhn compares the experience of conversion to a "Gestalt switch" such as we observe with the Necker cube.

Intentions as Goal Contexts

Thus far we have talked about two kinds of context—the qualitative (perceptual-imaginal) context and the conceptual context. Conscious experiences also interact with a third kind of unconscious context, which I will call the goal context. Goal contexts are useful in understanding problem solving, intentions, and voluntary control. It is important at this point to introduce the concept of an ordered goal hierarchy— simply, the idea that goals are ordered in significance at any point in time, and that higher (more significant) goals will tend to predominate over lower ones. This is by no means a new idea; it has been suggested by numerous motivational and cognitive psychologists (e.g., Maslow 1970), and the computational implications of goal hierarchies have been worked out in some detail by artificial intelligence researchers. My emphasis at this point is on the control of conscious events by such contextual goal hierarchies, which are diagrammed in figure 46.3.

Note that goal hierarchies cannot be rigid over time. For instance, the goal of eating must rise higher in the hierarchy after food deprivation. But at any one moment the hierarchy is ordered. That is, at any particular time we will prefer food over sex over watching TV. Some goals are more stable over time: generally, survival has a higher priority than avoiding boredom. I will not develop this notion here; I simply suggest that a set of ordered goals act as context for the flow of conscious experience.

Other Types of Context

Social and cultural contexts usually operate unconsciously. The sociologist Ervin Goffman writes,

When the individual in our Western society recognizes a particular (social) event, he tends ... (to) employ one or more frameworks or schemata of interpretation ... to locate, perceive, identify, and label a seemingly infinite number of concrete occurrences defined in its terms. He is likely to be unaware of such organized features as the framework has and unable to describe the framework with any completeness if asked, yet these handicaps are no bar to his easily and fully applying it. (1974, p. 21)

Anthropologists often encounter their own cultural presuppositions in a dramatic way when

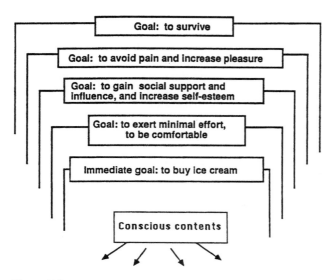

Figure 46.3
A significance hierarchy of goal contexts. A hypothetical set of ordered goal contexts (a goal hierarchy) that together influence conscious contents without themselves being entirely conscious when they do so. Notice that high-level goal contexts are more significant than lower-level ones. No claim is made about the particular goals chosen. Under different conditions the hierarchy might be somewhat different—surely, the goal of eating becomes more significant after a long, involuntary fast. Such goals are largely contextual by definition; they will tend to become conscious when violated in some way, but not in the normal course of events.

they enter a culture that violates those presuppositions; as usual, unconscious presuppositions can become conscious when they are severely violated. A member of another culture may seem to thrust his face toward a Westerner in a conversation at an unacceptable eight inches away. This experience may be shocking or offensive, but it makes conscious what is normally taken for granted: namely the fact that we, too, adopt a typical social distance. Thus unconscious customs and habits come to the foreground. Custom leads to adaptation and loss of consciousness; this is why children, novices, and strangers can guide us to become conscious again of things we have lost touch with in the process of becoming adults, experts, and members of various ingroups. These properties of context have major

implications for sociology and anthropology. For instance, all cultures have periodic ceremonies, festivals, and initiation rites using dramatic or even traumatic symbolism; a major function of these events may be to create and renew memorable conscious experiences that invoke and reinforce the unconscious contextual assumptions of the society.

Conclusion

The notion of unconscious "contextual" shaping of conscious experience is extremely widespread, but it is rarely stated as a general hypothesis. In the study of conscious and unconscious functions, this very general idea is nearly indispensible.

Acknowledgment

With thanks to The Neurosciences Institute and The Neurosciences Research Foundation.

References

Baars, B. J. (1985) Can involuntary slips reveal a state of mind? With an addendum on the conscious control of speech. In M. Toglia and T. M. Shlechter (eds.) *New directions in cognitive science*. Norwood, NJ: Ablex.

Baars, B. J. (1986) *The cognitive revolution in psychology*. New York: Guilford Press.

Baars, B. J. (1993) *A cognitive theory of consciousness*. New York: Cambridge University Press.

Baars, B. J. (1998) Metaphors of consciousness and attention in the brain. *Trends in Neuroscience*, 21, 58–62.

Blumenthal, A. L. (1977) *The process of cognition*. Englewood Cliffs, NJ: Prentice-Hall.

Bransford, J. D. (1979) *Human cognition*. Belmont, California: Wadsworth.

Chomsky, N. (1965) *Aspects of the theory of syntax*. Cambridge, MA: MIT Press.

Chomsky, N. (1957) *Syntactic structures*. The Hague: Mouton.

Einstein, A. (1949) Autobiographical notes. In P. A. Schilpp (ed.), *Albert Einstein—Philosopher-scientist*, Vol. I. New York: Harper & Row.

Foss, D. J. (1982) A discourse on semantic priming. *Cognitive Psychology*, 14, 590–607.

Fraisse, P. (1963) *The psychology of time*. New York: Harper & Row.

Gelb, A. (1932) Die Erscheimungen des simultanen Kontrastes und der Eindruck del Feldbeleuchtung. *Zeitschrift fur Psychologie*, 127, 42–59.

Gilchrist, A. (1977) Perceived lightness depends upon perceived spatial arrangement. *Science*, 195, 185–187.

Goffman, E. (1974) *Frame analysis: An essay on the organization of experience*. New York: Harper & Row.

Kosslyn, S. M. and Schwartz, S. P. (1981) Empirical constraints on theories of visual imagery. In J. Long and D. Baddeley (eds.), *Attention and Performance IX*, pp. 241–260. Hillsdale, NJ: Erlbaum.

Kuhn, T. S. (1962/1970) *The structure of scientific revolutions*. Chicago: University of Chicago Press.

MacKay, D. G. (1973) Aspects of a theory of comprehension, memory, and attention. *Quarterly Journal of Experimental Psychology*, 25, 22–40.

Mandler, G. A. (1984) *Mind and body: Psychology of emotion and stress*. New York: Norton.

Marr, D. (1982) *Vision*. San Francisco: Freeman.

Maslow, A. (1970) *Motivation and personality*. 2nd. ed. New York: Harper & Row.

McNeill, David (1966) Developmental psycholinguistics. In F. Smith and G. A. Miller (eds.), *The Genesis of Language*. Cambridge, MA: MIT Press.

Milne, R. W. (1982) Predicting garden-path sentences. *Cognitive Science*, 6, 349–374.

Nisbett, R. E. and Wilson, T. D. (1977) Telling more than we can know: Verbal reports on mental processes. *Psychological Review*, 84, 231–259.

Norman, D. A. (1976) *Memory and Attention*. New York: Wiley.

Reason, J. (1983) Absent-mindedness and cognitive control. In J. Harris and P. Morris (eds.), *Everyday memory, actions, and absentmindedness*. New York: Academic Press.

Rock, I. (1983) *The logic of perception*. Cambridge, MA: MIT Press.

Schachter, S. and Singer, J. E. (1962) Cognitive, social, and physiological determinants of emotional state. *Psychological Review*, 69, 379–399.

Swinney, D. (1979) Lexical access during sentence comprehension. (Re)consideration of context effects. *Journal of Verbal Learning and Verbal Behavior*, 18, 645–660.

Tversky, A. and Kahneman, A. (1973) Availability: A heuristic for judging frequency and probability. *Cognitive Psychology*, 2, 207–232.

Valins, S. (1967) Cognitive effects of false heart-rate feedback. *Journal of Personality and Social Psychology*, 4, 400–408.

47 The Cognitive Unconscious

John F. Kihlstrom

Scientific psychology began as the study of consciousness. Wundt, Titchener, and others who founded the earliest psychological laboratories generally assumed that the mind was able to observe its own inner workings. For this reason they relied on the method of introspection, by which trained observers attempted to analyze their percepts, memories, and thoughts, and reduce them to elementary sensations, images, and feelings (1). Quite quickly, however, observations in both the laboratory and the clinic suggested that mental life is not limited to conscious experience. For example, Helmholtz concluded that conscious perception was the product of unconscious inferences based on the individual's knowledge of the world and memory of past experiences. Somewhat later, Freud asserted that our conscious mental lives are determined by unconscious ideas, impulses, and emotions, as well as defense mechanisms unconsciously arrayed against them. These nineteenth-century ideas exemplify the notion of the cognitive unconscious—mental structures and processes that, operating outside phenomenal awareness, nevertheless influence conscious experience, thought, and action.

Scientific inquiry on conscious and nonconscious mental life was interrupted by the radical behaviorism of Watson and his followers, who argued that consciousness was nonexistent, epiphenomenal, or irrelevant to behavior. Beginning in the 1950s, however, psychology abandoned a radically behaviorist point of view in what has since come to be known as the "cognitive revolution" (2). Cognitive psychology comes in various forms, but all share an abiding interest in describing the mental structures and processes that link environmental stimuli to organismic responses and underly human experience, thought, and action. In this manner, cognitive theories are distinct from biological theories, whose conceptual vocabulary is limited to the structures and processes of the brain and other portions of the nervous system, and from the approach of radical behaviorism, which thinks of the behaving organism as a "black box" whose internal workings, biological or cognitive, can remain unknown (3, 4). Recently, cognitive psychologists have joined with colleagues from anthropology, neurobiology, computer science, linguistics, philosophy, and other fields to form cognitive science, an interdisciplinary effort to unravel the mysteries of the human mind.

One of the most salutary by-products of the development of cognitive science has been a revival of interest in consciousness (1, 5). Still, many psychologists who are committed to the study of conscious perception, memory, and thought have been reluctant to admit that nonconscious mental structures and processes are psychologically important. This article discusses some strands of theory and research in cognitive psychology that offer new insights into the workings of nonconscious mental structures and processes.

The Information-Processing Perspective

The classic information-processing conception of human cognition, modeled after the modern high-speed computer, includes a set of structures for storing information, as well as a set of processes by which information is transferred from one structure to another (6). In this model, information from the environment, transduced into a pattern of neural impulses by the sensory receptors, is briefly held in the sensory registers, one for each modality. Information in the sensory registers is then analyzed by processes known as feature detection and pattern recognition. By means of attention, information that has been identified as meaningful and relevant to current goals is then transferred to a structure known as primary or short-term memory where it is subject to further analysis. At this stage perceptual information is combined with information retrieved from secondary or long-term memory. Primary memory, which has an extremely limited capacity to process information, is considered the staging area of the cognitive system, where processes such as judgment, inference, and problem-solving take place. Information resides in primary memory only so long as it is rehearsed. On the basis of an analysis of the meaning of the stimulus input, some response is generated; and finally, a trace of the event is permanently encoded in secondary memory.

In such an approach, the term "unconscious" describes those products of the perceptual system that go unattended or unrehearsed, and those memories that are lost from primary memory through decay or displacement before they can be encoded in secondary memory. In a more substantial sense, however, consciousness is identified either with attention and rehearsal, or with the cognitive staging area that holds those percepts, memories, and actions to which attention is being directed. Thus, nonconscious mental life is identified with early preattentive perceptual processes such as feature detection and pattern recognition; or with those latent memory traces that have not been retrieved from secondary storage and transferred to primary memory. The implication of this view is that unattended percepts and unretrieved memories make no contact with higher mental processes, and thus cannot influence conscious experience, thought, and action. Thus, the classic information-processing model, by regarding attention and rehearsal as prerequisites for a full-fledged cognitive analysis of the stimulus, and by implicitly identifying consciousness with higher mental processes, leaves little or no room for the psychological unconscious.

Quite a different perspective on nonconscious mental life is provided by more recent revisions of information processing theory, such as Anderson's ACT* (7). Models such as ACT*

(which stands for Adaptive Control of Thought, the asterisk marking the final version) assume a single, unitary memory store. The contents of memory are then classified into declarative knowledge structures that represent the individual's fund of general and specific factual information, and the procedural knowledge repertoire of skills, rules, and strategies that operate on declarative knowledge in the course of perception, memory, thought, and action. Furthermore, declarative knowledge can be classified as either episodic or semantic in nature. Episodic memory is autobiographical in character, and contains more or less explicit reference to the self as the agent or experiencer of some event, and the unique environmental and organismic context in which that event occurred; semantic memory is the "mental lexicon" of abstract knowledge, stored without reference to the circumstances in which it was acquired.

Whether episodic or semantic in nature, declarative knowledge is represented by a graph structure, with nodes representing concepts and associative links representing the relations between them. Nodes in this network are activated by perceptual processes that encode mental representations of external stimulus events, or by internal thought mechanisms. In either case, activation then spreads from one cognitive unit to another along the associative links, activating still other nodes in the memory network. Similarly, procedural knowledge is represented as a system of productions consisting of nodes representing the person's processing goals and the conditions under which some cognitive or behavioral action will meet them. When declarative memory structures corresponding to relevant goals and conditions are activated, any procedure that includes them will be executed. The product of such a procedure is represented in memory as another activated declarative knowledge structure.

According to models such as ACT*, consciousness is identified with a temporary storage structure known as working memory, which is similar to the primary memory of the classic model but with a much larger capacity. Working memory contains activated representations of the organism in its current environment, currently active processing goals, and preexisting declarative knowledge structures activated by perceptual inputs or by the operations of various procedures. Thus, the revised model holds that people can become aware of declarative knowledge (about themselves, their environments and processing goals, and other relevant information), and that this awareness depends on the amount of activation possessed by the representations in question. However, it also holds that procedural knowledge is not available to introspection under any circumstances. Thus, procedural knowledge appears to be unconscious in the strict sense of the term. We are aware of the goals and conditions of procedures, and the products of their execution, but not of the operations themselves. In this way, ACT* and similar revisionist models afford a much wider scope for the cognitive unconscious than did the classic statements.

Similarly, a major place for nonconscious mental structures and processes has been created by a recent variant on information-processing theory known as connectionism or parallel distributed processing (PDP) (8). In PDP models the conceptual analog for the human information-processing system is provided by the brain itself, and especially the synaptic connections among neurons, rather than the microchips of the high-speed computer. Whereas ACT* and similar models assume the existence of a single central processing unit (such as primary or working memory), PDP models postulate the existence of a large number of processing units, each devoted to a specific but simple task. Each unit, when activated, excites and inhibits others along a rich network of associative links. This pattern of mutual influence continues until the entire system relaxes to a steady state of activation that represents the information being processed.

It is assumed in PDP models that information about an object or event is distributed widely across the processing system, rather than localized in any particular unit. Moreover, the activation of individual processing units can vary continuously as opposed to discretely. For these reasons, it is not necessary for an object to be fully represented in consciousness before information about it can influence experience, thought, and action. In addition, traditional information-processing theories tend to assume that various perceptual-cognitive functions are bound together in a unitary processing system operating under a single set of rules and under the control of a central executive. By contrast, PDP models assume that various systems (such as those supporting perception and language, for example) operate independently and under different rules. Only some modules are assumed to be accessible to awareness and subject to voluntary control. Finally, PDP models abandon the traditional assumption that information is processed in a sequence of stages. Parallel processing permits a large number of activated units to influence each other at any particular moment in time, so that information can be analyzed very rapidly. Both the number of simultaneously active processing units and the speed at which they pass information among themselves may exceed the span of conscious awareness.

In the final analysis, PDP models of information processing assert that consciousness is a matter of time rather than activation. By virtue of massive parallelism, processing systems tend to reach a steady state very rapidly, within about a half second. At this point of relaxation the information represented by the steady state becomes accessible to phenomenal awareness. Information may also reach consciousness if the relaxation process is slowed by virtue of ambiguity in the stimulus pattern; in this case, however, the contents of consciousness will shift back and forth between alternative representations. In either case, the clear implication of the PDP framework is that unconscious processing is fast and parallel, while conscious processing is slow and sequential. Originally formulated to account for certain phenomena in perception, PDP models have also been developed for domains of language, memory, and inference in which models such as ACT* have been so successful. Although the PDP framework is relatively new, these models are important precisely because they provide a unified theoretical account of a number of psychological phenomena that have heretofore been considered to be unrelated. In contrast to multistore information-processing theories that restrict the cognitive unconscious to elementary sensory-perceptual operations, PDP models seem to consider almost all information processing, including the higher mental functions involved in language, memory, and thought, to be unconscious.

It is not possible, on the basis of data available at present, to choose between these two approaches to human information processing. Models like ACT* and PDP may apply at different levels of the cognitive system. In any event, the important point is that both classes of models appear to agree that the cognitive unconscious encompasses a very large portion of mental life. With these theoretical perspectives in mind, we may turn to specific experimental studies that illustrate the cognitive unconscious at work.

Automatic Processes

Certainly a good deal of mental activity is unconscious in the strict sense of being inaccessible to phenomenal awareness under any circumstances (9). In conversational speech, for example, the listener is aware of the meanings of the words uttered by the speaker but not of the phonological and linguistic principles by which the meaning of the speaker's utterance is decoded. Similarly, during perception the viewer may be aware of two objects in the external environment but not of the mental calculations performed to determine that one is closer or larger than the other. Although we have conscious access to the products of these mental processes—in that we are aware of the meaning of the utterance or the size and distance of the objects, and can communicate this knowledge to others—we have no conscious access to their operations.

Unconscious procedural knowledge of this sort appears to be innate. In fact, Fodor has proposed that the mind consists of a number of innate, domain-specific cognitive modules controlling such activities as language and visual perception, hardwired in the nervous system and operating outside of conscious awareness and voluntary control (10). However, other cognitive procedures appear to be acquired through experience. In the case of skill learning, the process is initially accessible to consciousness—as indicated, for example, by the novice sailor's overt or covert rehearsal of the steps involved in tying a knot—and later becomes unconscious by virtue of practice—as indicated by the inability of many musicians, athletes, and typists to describe their skills to others, and by the fact that conscious attention to them actually interferes with their performance. In other words, skills that are not innate may become routinized through practice, and their operations thereby rendered unconscious. Employing a metaphor derived from computer science, this process is described as knowledge compilation, suggesting that the format in which the knowledge is represented has been changed (1, 11). In this way, both innate and acquired cognitive procedures may be unconscious in the strict sense of the term.

Unconscious procedural knowledge has also been described as automatic as opposed to controlled or effortful (12, 13). Automatic processes are so named because they are inevitably engaged by the presentation of specific stimulus inputs, regardless of any intention on the part of the subject. In addition, automatic processes consume little or no attentional resources. It is a fundamental premise of cognitive psychology that the amount of attention that can be allocated to various activities is limited, producing a bottleneck in information processing (14). Thus, our ability to perform two or more tasks simultaneously is limited by the demands they make on available attentional resources. If attentional demands exceed attentional resources, the tasks will interfere with each other. Nevertheless, routinized processes consume little or no attentional capacity (13). For this reason, it is possible for expert typists to carry on a conversation while transcribing even complicated material, or for skilled drivers to negotiate the road while listening to the radio news.

Nevertheless, automatic processing may have some negative consequences as well. The typist may not remember what he has typed, and the driver may not remember landmarks that she has passed along the way. Effective memory depends to a great extent on the amount and type of cognitive activity devoted to the event at the time of perception, and some automatized processes—however well suited they are for other tasks—may not encourage good encodings. For example, Spelke and her colleagues performed an experiment in which subjects were asked to read unfamiliar prose material and take dictation at the same time (15). On initial trials, performance on both tasks was quite poor. After 6 weeks of practice, however, the subjects were able to take accurate dictation and read simultaneously with at least 80 percent comprehension. Nonetheless, later tests showed that the subjects were generally unable to recall the words they had transcribed, and had little or no awareness of how the word lists had been structured. Thus, the dictation task, once automatized, no longer interfered with reading for comprehension; but neither did it yield highly memorable encodings of the dictated material.

The fact that automatized processes consume little or no attentional capacity has important consequences for consciousness. In the first place, of course, automatic processes are themselves unconscious, in that the person has no introspective access to their principles of operation—or even the fact that they are in operation at all. Thus, fluent speakers of English agree that the phrase "the big red barn" is grammatically better than the phrase "the red big barn," even though they are unable to articulate the underlying syntactical rule that guides such decisions. Similarly, in the social domain, speakers may like one face more than another, while being unable to say exactly why they have that preference. A large number of social judgments and inferences, especially those guiding first impressions, appear to be mediated by such unconscious processes (16).

Experiments on automaticity are important because they indicate that a great deal of complex cognitive activity can go on outside of conscious awareness, provided that the skills, rules, and strategies required by the task have been automatized. They expand the scope of unconscious preattentive processes, which were previously limited to elementary perceptual analyses of the physical features of environmental stimuli. Now it is clear that there are circumstances under which the meanings and implications of events can be unconsciously analyzed as well. Thus, people may reach conclusions about events—for example, their emotional valence (17)—and act on these judgments without being able to articulate the reasoning by which they were reached. This does not mean that cognitive activity is not involved in such judgments and inferences; it only means that the cognitive activity, being automatized, is unconscious in the strict sense of that term and thus unavailable to introspective awareness.

Subliminal Perception

Although the procedural knowledge structures guiding thought and action are unconscious, the declarative knowledge structures on which they operate are ordinarily available to consciousness. Thus, it should be possible for people to notice and describe the salient features of an object or event, even if they cannot articulate the way in which those features have been integrated to form certain judgments made about it. However, another implication of automatization is that the processes in question may operate on declarative knowledge structures that are not themselves fully conscious. According to the classic information-processing model, preattentive processes act on stimulus information before it has been encoded in short-term memory—which, according to the model, is the locus of conscious awareness. But, in the classic model, complex analyses of meaning were excluded from this domain. However, it now appears that complex analyses, once routinized, take on many of the properties of preattentive feature detection and pattern recognition. Accordingly, it may be possible to perform meaning analyses on information, which is not itself accessible to conscious awareness, by means of automatized, unconscious procedural knowledge.

This possibility raises the question of subliminal perception. Researchers in classic psychophysics assumed that each modality was associated with an absolute threshold (or limen), represented by the weakest detectable stimulus. By means of the method of limits, in which the intensity of a weak stimulus is increased until it is reliably detectable, and the intensity of a strong stimulus is decreased until it is no longer detectable, the limen is given by the smallest intensity that can be detected 50 percent of the time. However, the probability of detection is directly related to stimulus intensity both above and below the threshold, suggesting that subthreshold stimuli are still processed by the sensory-perceptual system. Subliminal perception refers to the possibility that stimuli too weak to be consciously detected nonetheless have an impact on perceptual and cognitive functioning.

Subliminal perception is often studied by means of a tachistoscope, which can present stimuli for intervals (for example, less than 5 ms) that are too brief to be consciously perceived. A number of investigators have found that such stimuli reappear in the subject's subsequent dreams (the Poetzel phenomenon) and otherwise affect the person's performance on some experimental task. Subliminal perception is also at the root of the so-called New Look in perception, which attempted to integrate the study of perception with that of personality and motivation. For example, Bruner and his colleagues, among others, reported that subjects had different thresholds for identifying "taboo" and neutral words (18). The clear implication of these findings was that stimuli could be analyzed for their emotional significance as well as for certain physical features and patterns before they reached awareness. This aspect of mental life may be called preconscious processing (19). However, it is not the processing itself that is preconscious. Rather, the term preconscious describes the declarative knowledge that is subject to cognitive processing.

For obvious reasons, subliminal perception is of considerable interest to the advertising community; it has also been of considerable interest to psychoanalysts and others who believe that people defend against potentially threatening percepts, memories, ideas, and impulses by excluding them from awareness (20). It has also been very controversial. Almost since the beginning, a variety of methodological critiques have sought to demonstrate that stimuli cannot be processed for meaning unless they have been consciously identified (1, 21). Recently, however, a number of compelling demonstrations of preconscious processing have appeared in the literature. For example, investigators have employed a priming protocol in which a stimulus word (called the prime) is followed by another word (called the target), and the subject has to decide whether the target is a meaningful word. Such judgments are facilitated when the prime is also a word. However, Marcel and others arranged to present the prime followed by a second stimulus (called the mask) consisting of randomly arranged letters, before the target appeared. The timing is such that subjects are unable to reliably detect masked primes. Nevertheless, such preconscious primes facilitate performance on the judgment task (22). Since lexical decisions obviously require some degree of semantic processing, it appears that meaning analyses are performed on stimuli that are themselves outside of conscious awareness.

Studies by Kunst-Wilson and Zajonc, among others, indicate that preconscious processing affects emotional as well as semantic judgments (23, 24). Many of these demonstrations rely on the mere exposure effect, which refers to the fact that repeated presentation of a previously unfamiliar stimulus tends to increase its attractiveness (contrary to folklore, familiarity does not necessarily breed contempt). Although the original effect was obtained with clearly perceptible stimulus materials, the finding holds even though the presentations are so brief (as little as 1 ms) as to render the stimuli undetectable by the subjects. Thus, by virtue of prior preconscious presentation, subjects come to prefer stimuli that they do not recognize as familiar.

It may be that preconscious declarative knowledge can only be subject to processing by unconscious, automatized procedures. After all, it seems contradictory to suggest that people can intentionally and deliberately process information of which they are unaware. Conscious awareness should be a logical prerequisite of conscious control. But it does seem that preconscious declarative knowledge is subject to analysis by unconscious procedural knowledge. Such information-processing activity would be nonconscious in a double sense: neither the stimuli themselves, nor the cognitive processes that operate on them, are accessible to phenomenal awareness. Such doubly nonconscious processes nevertheless exert an important impact on social interaction. Through the operation of routinized procedures for social judgment, for example, we may form impressions of people without any conscious awareness of the perceptual-cognitive basis for them.

Results such as these are important for cognitive theory because they indicate that a great deal of information processing takes place outside of working memory. Apparently, perceptual processing automatically activates preexisting semantic memory structures corresponding to the features of the stimulus event, as well as related nodes by virtue of spreading activation. If some of these nodes correspond to the goals and conditions of various production systems, certain procedures will be executed as well. However, none of this requires the involvement of working memory. Thus, in contrast to the implications of the classic model for human information processing, a great deal of complex cognitive activity can be devoted to stimuli that are themselves outside of phenomenal awareness.

Preconscious processing can influence the ease with which certain ideas are brought to mind, and the manner in which objects and events are perceived and interpreted. For example, priming influences perceptual fluency by facilitating the perception of prime related features in the target stimulus. Thus, when a prime and a target are identical it is easier to identify the target than when they are different; similarly, identification is easier when the prime and the target belong to the same conceptual category or are otherwise semantically related. A similar sort of influence may obtain when other judgments are to be made about the target. Consider, for example, a complex target (say, the name of a familiar person) some of whose features are socially desirable (for example, kind and warm) while others might be considered socially undesirable (for example, dull and unintelligent). Now, assume that presentation of the target has been preceded by a prime carrying wholly negative connotations. Activation from the memory node representing the prime will spread to nodes representing other undesirable attributes. Then, when the target is presented, activation will spread to nodes representing both desirable and undesirable features. However, more activation will accrue to nodes representing socially undesirable features, leading to a more negative impression of the target than would otherwise have occurred. Moreover, if the nodes representing the various features are also conditions of production systems whose goals have been activated in working memory, perceptual fluency may have tangible effects on the perceiver's actions with respect to the target.

Although the recent demonstrations of preconscious processing seem compelling, they do not necessarily constitute an empirical argument in favor of subliminal advertising and other forms of surreptitious social influence. On the affirmative side, it seems that preconscious processing can activate automatized procedural knowledge, and thus affect the way that consumers think about products, or perhaps even their actual buying behavior. The magnitude of these effects even may be increased because preconscious processing obviates the possibility of conscious countercontrol of these effects. Priming occurs automatically regardless of whether the prime is accessible to conscious awareness, but the automatic effects of consciously perceptible stimuli may be obviated by whatever processing strategies are deliberately deployed to analyze and respond to them.

On the negative side, many priming effects are extremely short-lived—activation dissipates as fast as it spreads—so that they may not last long enough for the person who views an advertisement on television, say, to get to the grocery store. Furthermore, the effects of preconscious stimulation may be mitigated to some degree by restrictions on the nature of the cognitive processing that it can instigate. For example, a recent series of experiments by Greenwald and his colleagues required subjects to evaluate the affective connotations of various target words (24). Preconscious presentation of positive and negative words speeded judgments when the prime and target were congruent (that is, both positive or both negative); however, no facilitation was obtained when the prime consisted of a positively toned phrase consisting of two negatively toned words (for example, "enemy fails"). Thus,

preconscious processing may be limited to relatively simple meaning analyses, and may only operate to amplify preexisting tendencies. Finally, in order for preconscious processing to affect action it is necessary that relevant goal structures be activated in procedural memory. Thus, even if subliminal perception were theoretically possible, consumers would not be led to choose a particular brand of soft drink unless they were thirsty and intended to purchase some refreshments.

Implicit Memory

Because preconscious processing appears to be mediated by the activation of relevant mental representations already stored in memory, the question is raised whether analogous effects may be observed in memory itself. That is, just as there are palpable effects on experience, thought, and action of stimuli that cannot be consciously perceived, so there may be similar effects of events that cannot be consciously remembered. One such effect was observed in an experiment by Nelson on savings in relearning (25). The subjects were asked to memorize a list of paired associates consisting of a number and a word arbitrarily linked together. Four weeks later they were given tests of cued recall and recognition for these items. When forgotten pairs were presented along with entirely new pairs on a second set of learning trials, previously seen items that were not consciously recognized nonetheless had an advantage measured in performance on subsequent learning and memory tasks.

Some of the most dramatic instances of nonconscious memory appear in cases of the amnesic syndrome (sometimes called Korsakoff's syndrome), which results from bilateral damage to the medial temporal lobe (including the hippocampus) and diencephalon (including the mammiliary bodies) of the brain. Patients suffering from this disorder (which may reflect a number of different etiologies, including chronic alcoholism) manifest a gross anterograde amnesia, meaning that they cannot remember events that occurred since the onset of the brain damage; other intellectual functions remain relatively intact. Although it was originally thought that amnesic patients were unable to encode traces of new experiences, it now appears that their memory deficit is much more selective. For example, amnesic patients can learn new cognitive and motor skills, as well as new vocabulary items and other factual information; however, they appear unable to remember the episodes in which they acquired this knowledge (26, 27). In other words, the amnesic syndrome appears to impair the encoding of new episodic memories, while sparing procedural knowledge and semantic memory (28).

More recent evidence suggests that some aspects of episodic memory are preserved in these patients (29). Consider a case in which subjects are asked to study a list of familiar words and are asked to recall the words shortly thereafter. Compared to the performance of intact subjects, amnesic patients show gross impairments in memory. Different results are obtained when the subjects are asked to identify briefly presented words or to complete a word stem or other fragment with a meaningful word. Not surprisingly, intact subjects show superior performance on trials where the correct response is a word that had appeared on the previously studied list, compared to trials where the correct response is an entirely new word. This advantage of old over new items reflects a sort of priming effect of the previous learning experience. However, amnesic subjects also show normal levels of priming, despite the fact that they cannot remember the words they studied. In addition, Schacter and his colleagues provided amnesic patients with obscure factual information in a question-and-answer format (for example, "What job did Bob Hope's father have?—Fireman"). On later test trials, the patients were able to correctly answer questions on the material, but could not remember the circumstances under which they had acquired the information—a phenomenon known as cryptomnesia or source amnesia (30).

Priming and source amnesia show that task performance may be affected by residual memories of prior experiences, even though those experiences are not accessible to conscious recall. On the basis of results such as these, Schacter and others have drawn a distinction between explicit and implicit memory (29, 31). Explicit memory requires the conscious recollection of a previous episode, whereas implicit memory is revealed by a change in task performance that is attributable to information acquired during such an episode. An increasingly large literature from both patient and nonpatient populations indicates that people can display implicit memory without having any conscious recollection of the experiential basis of the effect. Implicit memory effects are conceptually similar to subliminal perception effects, in that both reveal the impact on experience, thought, and action of events that are not accessible to conscious awareness. However, the two effects should be distinguished. In contrast to subliminal perception, the events contributing to implicit memory effects were clearly detectable by the subject, attention was devoted to them, and they were represented in phenomenal awareness at the time they occurred. Still, both sets of phenomena illustrate the psychological unconscious, by showing perception and memory outside of phenomenal awareness.

Hypnotic Alterations of Consciousness

Although the domain of the psychological unconscious would seem to be exhausted by automatic processes, subliminal perception, and implicit memory, a somewhat different perspective is offered by the phenomena of hypnosis (32–34). Hypnosis is a social interaction in which one person, the subject, responds to suggestions offered by another person, the hypnotist, for experiences involving alterations in perception, memory, and action. One common aspect of these experiences is an alteration in phenomenal awareness, but the changes in consciousness are not precisely the same as those seen in automaticity, subliminal perception, and implicit memory.

For example, in hypnotic analgesia, hypnotized subjects may fail to experience discomfort from a normally painful stimulus (35). This reduction in pain is not mediated by placebo effects, endogenous opiates, or by the tranquilizing effects of hypnotic relaxation. Given the traditional models of human information processing, hypnotic analgesia might be interpreted as involving a failure to attend to and process normally painful stimuli. However, a number of findings indicate that the pain stimulus has been adequately registered by the sensory-perceptual system. For example, psychophysiological indices such as heart rate respond to painful stimuli, even though the subject reports feeling little or no pain. Similarly, perceptual representations of the pain stimulus may be accessed by the hidden observer technique developed by Hilgard (36). After analgesia has been successfully established, the hypnotist attempts to communicate with a "hidden part" of the person that may have recorded the actual stimulus state of affairs. Under these circumstances, many analgesic subjects give pain reports comparable to those collected under normal conditions. The hidden observer is a metaphor for these nonconscious mental representations of stimulus input, and the means by which they may be accessed. The success of the technique indicates that analgesic subjects may be unaware of stimuli that have been thoroughly processed by the sensory-perceptual system.

Within the domain of memory, similar anomalies of awareness may be noted in posthypnotic amnesia (37). Following appropriate suggestions, subjects may fail to remember the events and experiences that transpired while they were hypnotized. However, the critical memories may be recovered after administration of a prearranged signal to cancel the amnesia suggestion. This property of reversibility clearly shows that posthypnotic amnesia reflects a disruption of memory retrieval, rather than a failure of encoding or loss from storage. However, the retrieval disruption is selective. For example, amnesic subjects may still make use of procedural and semantic knowledge acquired during hypnosis, even though—as in the phenomenon of posthypnotic source amnesia (30)—they do not remember the circumstances under which this knowledge was acquired. Even within the domain of episodic memory the effects of amnesia are selective. For example, subjects who are amnesic for a word list memorized during hypnosis will nonetheless be more likely to produce list items as word associations, category instances, or in word-fragment completion tasks, compared to carefully matched words that had not been memorized (38). Thus, amnesic subjects are affected by memories that have been adequately encoded, but are not accessible to conscious retrieval.

Alterations in subjective awareness occur in other hypnotic phenomena as well. For example, it may be suggested that after hypnosis has been terminated, the subject will engage in a particular action in response to a prearranged cue. Subjects responding to such posthypnotic suggestions often exhibit a dual lack of awareness: they may be unaware of the fact that they are performing the behavior that has been suggested; or, in the event that they do notice the activity, they may be unaware of the origins of their behavior in the hypnotist's prior suggestion (39). Although such behavior often strikes an observer as compulsive and involuntary, it is not automatic in the technical sense used in information-processing theory (40). In a recent experiment, for example, subjects were asked to search for two different digits simultaneously in strings of numbers presented on a computer screen. One search task was given as a posthypnotic suggestion and covered by amnesia, the other as a nonhypnotic instruction without amnesia. Even on trials where the suggestion and instruction were not in conflict, the subjects showed a tradeoff such that each search task interfered with the other. Thus, although the posthypnotic suggestion was executed outside of awareness, it nonetheless consumed attentional capacity.

The interpersonal and motivational context in which hypnotic phenomena arise renders interpretation of them difficult. From the perspective of information-processing approaches to cognitive psychology, they seem to make a prima facie case for a different type of nonconscious mental structures and processes than those indicated by automatic processing, subliminal perception, and implicit memory. For example, posthypnotic suggestion seems superficially similar to unconscious procedural memory, at least insofar as it shares the IF (cue)–THEN (response) structure of other procedural knowledge. However, posthypnotic responses are obviously not innate stimulus-response connections; nor have they had the opportunity to become automatized through routinization and practice; finally, their execution consumes attentional resources. Still, response to posthypnotic suggestions takes place outside of phenomenal awareness. Thus it appears that there are circumstances in which complex, deliberate, attention-consuming processes may operate nonconsciously.

Just as posthypnotic suggestion seems to expand the domain of nonconscious mental processes, hypnotic analgesia and posthypnotic amnesia appear to expand the domain of nonconscious mental structures. Although the registration of the pain stimulus outside phenomenal awareness would seem somewhat analogous to subliminal perception, it is important to note that the stimulus itself is in no sense subliminal. Analgesic subjects fail to feel the pain of stimuli whose intensity and duration are more than sufficient to produce that experience under nonhypnotic conditions. Similarly, the results of experiments on posthypnotic amnesia are reminiscent of the distinction between explicit and implicit memory. Again, however, there is a difference. In the standard demonstrations of implicit memory, the memories involved often are permanently inaccessible to conscious recollection: for example, there are no known circumstances in which patients suffering the amnesic syndrome are able to remember the experiences they have forgotten. In contrast, posthypnotic amnesia is easily reversible, so that the inaccessibility of the critical memories is only temporary.

Unconscious, Preconscious, and Subconscious

The results of these and other experiments, conducted in a wide variety of circumstances and with many different types of subjects, lead to a provisional taxonomy of nonconscious mental structures and processes constituting the domain of the cognitive unconscious (34, 41). One thing is now clear: consciousness is not to be identified with any particular perceptual-cognitive functions such as discriminative response to stimulation, perception, memory, or the higher mental processes involved in judgment or problem-solving. All of these functions can take place outside of phenomenal awareness. Rather, consciousness is an experiential quality that may accompany any of these functions. The fact of conscious awareness may have particular consequences for psychological function—it seems necessary for voluntary control, for example, as well as for communicating one's mental states to others. But it is not necessary for complex psychological functioning.

More specifically, there are, within the domain of procedural knowledge, a number of complex processes that are inaccessible to introspection in principle under any circumstances. By virtue of routinization (or perhaps because they are innate), such procedures operate on declarative knowledge without either conscious intent or conscious awareness, in order to construct the person's ongoing experience, thought, and action. These mental processes, which can be known only indirectly through inference, may be described as unconscious in the strict sense of that term.

In principle, declarative knowledge is available to phenomenal awareness, and can be known directly through introspection. Traditional information-processing analyses seem to imply that conscious access to declarative knowledge is a matter of activation. If a knowledge structure is activated above some threshold, it is conscious; if not, it is not conscious. There is the further implication that declarative knowledge structures activated at subthreshold levels are essentially latent. However, it is now clear that procedural knowledge can interact with, and utilize, declarative knowledge that is not itself accessible to conscious awareness. The phenomena of subliminal perception and implicit memory, then, suggest a category of preconscious declarative knowledge structures. Unlike automatized procedural knowledge, these percepts and memories would be available to awareness under ordinary circumstances. Although activated to some degree by current or prior perceptual inputs, and thus able to influence ongoing experience, thought, and action, they do not cross the threshold required for representation in working memory, and thus for conscious awareness.

In addition to unconscious cognitive rules and skills operating on declarative representations and preconscious declarative representations that serve as sources of spreading activation, the phenomena of hypnosis and related states seem to exemplify a category of subconscious declarative knowledge. These mental representations, fully activated by perceptual inputs or acts of thought, above the threshold ordinarily required for representation in working memory, and available to introspection under some circumstances, seem nevertheless inaccessible to phenomenal awareness. In the nineteenth century, Janet described such structures as dissociated from conscious awareness (32, 34, 42). On the basis of his clinical studies of hysteria and other forms of psychopathology, he developed a theory of psychological automatism that anticipated in many respects current notions of modularity and parallelism. Such dissociative phenomena are of theoretical interest wherever they occur, because they imply that high levels of activation, although presumably necessary for residence in working memory, are not sufficient for conscious awareness.

Writing in the *Principles of psychology* almost a century ago, William James suggested that the key to the consciousness is self-reference: "The universal conscious fact is not 'feelings exist' and 'thoughts exist' but '*I* think' and '*I* feel'" ((43), p. 226, emphasis added). In other words, in order for ongoing experience, thought, and action to become conscious, a link must be made between its mental representation and some mental representation of the self as agent or experiencer—as well, perhaps, as some representation of the environment in which these events take place. These episodic representations of the self and context reside in working memory, but apparently the links in question are neither automatic nor permanent, and must be actively forged. In cases of subliminal perception and the amnesic syndrome they appear not to be encoded in the first place; in cases of implicit memory observed in normal subjects, they appear to have been available at one time, but no longer; in certain phenomena of hypnosis, they appear to be temporarily set aside. Without such linkages certain aspects of mental life are dissociated from awareness, and are not accompanied by the experience of consciousness.

One achievement of contemporary cognitive psychology is a clear theoretical framework for studying the nonconscious mental structures and processes that interested Helmholtz, Freud, James, and Janet. Such theories have led to the development of new experimental paradigms, and the improvement of old ones, that tentatively reveal a tripartite classification of nonconscious mental life that is quite different from the seething unconscious of Freud, and more extensive than the unconscious inference of Helmholtz. Now work must begin to clarify the nature of the processes by which cognitive and motoric procedures are automatized, the scope of preconscious processing of subliminal percepts and implicit memories, the process of self-reference, and the nature of dissociation.

Acknowledgments

This work is based on research supported in part by National Institute of Mental Health grant MH-35856, an H. I. Romnes Faculty Fellowship from the University of Wisconsin, and the Program on Conscious and Unconsious Mental Processes of the John D. and Catherine T. McArthur Foundation. I thank J. C. Chorny, L. A. Cooper, W. Fleeson, K. I. Forster, M. F. Garrett, R. Hastie, E. R. Hilgard, I. P. Hoyt, L. Canter Kihlstrom, S. B. Klein, L. Nadel, R. Nadon, L. A. Otto, P. A. Register, D. L. Schacter, D. Tataryn, B. A. Tobias, and J. Wood for helpful discussions and comments during the preparation of this manuscript.

Notes and References

1. K. A. Ericsson and H. A. Simon, *Protocol Analysis: Verbal Reports as Data* (MIT Press, Cambridge, MA, 1984).

2. H. Gardner, *The Mind's New Science: A History of the Cognitive Revolution* (Basic Books, New York, 1985); M. Hunt, *The Universe Within: A New Science Explores the Human Mind* (Simon and Schuster, New York, 1982).

3. J. R. Anderson, *Cognitive Psychology and Its Implications* (Freeman, San Francisco, 1985); G. H. Bower and E. R. Hilgard, *Theories of Learning* (Prentice-Hall, Englewood Cliffs, NJ, 1981); S. E. Palmer and R. Kimchi, in *Approaches to Cognition: Contrasts and Controversies*, F. J. Knapp and L. C. Robertson, Eds. (Erlbaum, Hillsdale, NJ, 1986), pp. 37–77.

4. R. Hastie, in *Political Cognition*, R. R. Lau and D. O. Sears, Eds. (Erlbaum, Hillsdale, NJ, 1986), pp. 11–40.

5. K. S. Bowers and D. Meichenbaum, Eds., *The Unconscious Reconsidered* (Wiley-Interscience, New York, 1984); E. R. Hilgard, *Annu. Rev. Psychol.* 31, 1 (1980); *American Psychology in Historical Perspective* (Harcourt Brace Jovanovich, San Diego, 1987); R. L. Klatzky, *Memory and Awareness: An Information-Processing Perspective* (Freeman, San Francisco, 1984); G. Mandler, in *Information Processing and Cognition*, R. Solso, Ed. (Erlbaum, Hillsdale, NJ, 1975), pp. 229–254; J. L. Singer and J. Kolligian, *Annu. Rev. Psychol.* 38, 533 (1987); E. Tulving, *Can. Psychol.* 26, 1 (1986).

6. R. C. Atkinson and R. M. Shiffrin, in *The Psychology of Learning and Motivation*, K. S. Spence and J. T. Spence, Eds. (Academic Press, New York, 1968), vol. 2, pp. 89–195; D. E. Broadbent, *Perception and Communication* (Pergamon, London, 1958); A. N. Newell, *Cognit. Sci.* 4, 135 (1980).

7. J. R. Anderson, *Language, Memory, and Thought* (Erlbaum, Hillsdale, NJ, 1976); *The Architecture of Cognition* (Harvard Univ. Press, Cambridge, MA, 1983); see also G. H. Bower, in *Handbook of Learning and Cognitive Processes*, W. K. Estes, Ed. (Erlbaum, Hillsdale, NJ, 1975), vol. 1, pp. 25–80; A. Newell and H. A. Simon, *Human Problem Solving* (Prentice-Hall, Englewood Cliffs, NJ, 1972); E. Tulving, *Elements of Episodic Memory* (Oxford Univ. Press, Oxford, 1984).

8. G. E. Hinton and J. A. Anderson, Eds., *Parallel Models of Associative Memory* (Erlbaum, Hillsdale, NJ, 1981); D. E. Rumelhart, J. L. McClelland, and the PDP Research Group, *Parallel Distributed Processing: Explorations in the Microstructures of Cognition* (MIT Press, Cambridge, MA, 1986), two volumes.

9. N. Chomsky, *Rules and Representations* (Columbia Univ. Press, New York, 1980); J. Hochberg, *Perception* (Prentice-Hall, Englewood Cliffs, NJ, ed. 2, 1978); L. Kaufman, *Sight and Mind: An Introduction to Visual Perception* (Oxford Univ. Press, New York, 1974); I. Rock, *The Logic of Perception* (MIT Press, Cambridge, MA, 1983).

10. J. Fodor, *The Modularity of Mind* (MIT/Bradford, Cambridge, MA, 1983).

11. J. R. Anderson, *Psychol. Rev.* 89, 369 (1982).

12. L. Hasher and R. T. Zacks, *J. Exp. Psychol. Gen.* 108, 365 (1979); D. LaBerge and S. J. Samuels, *Cognit. Psychol.* 6, 293 (1975); G. D. Logan, ibid. 12, 523 (1980); M. I. Posner and C. R. R. Snyder, in *Information Processing and Cognition*, R. Solso, Ed. (Erlbaum, Hillsdale, NJ, 1975).

13. W. Schneider and R. M. Shiffrin, *Psychol. Rev.* 84, 1 (1977); R. M. Shiffrin and W. Schneider, ibid., p. 127; ibid. 91, 269 (1984).

14. H. Egeth, in *The Psychology of Learning and Motivation* (Academic Press, New York, 1977), vol. 11, pp. 277–320; D. Kahneman and A. Triesman, in *Varieties of Attention*, R. Parasuraman and D. R. Davies, Eds. (Academic Press, New York, 1984), pp. 29–61.

15. E. A. Spelke et al., *Cognition* 4, 215 (1976).

16. J. A. Bargh, in *Handbook of Social Cognition*, R. S. Wyer and T. K. Srull, Eds. (Erlbaum, Hillsdale, NJ, 1984), vol. 3, pp. 1–43; R. H. Fazio et al., *J. Pers. Soc. Psychol.* 50, 229 (1986); P. Lewicki, *Nonconscious Social Information Processing* (Academic Press, New York, 1986); R. E. Nisbett and T. D. Wilson, *Psychol. Rev.* 84, 231 (1977); E. R. Smith, ibid. 91, 392 (1984); L. Winter et al., *J. Pers. Soc. Psychol.* 49, 904 (1985).

17. R. B. Zajonc, *Am. Psychol.* 35, 151 (1980); ibid. 117, 39 (1984).

18. J. Bruner and L. Postman, *J. Pers.* 16, 69 (1947).

19. N. F. Dixon, *Subliminal Perception* (McGraw-Hill, New York, 1971); *Preconscious Processing* (Wiley, London, 1981).

20. M. H. Erdelyi, *Psychol. Rev.* 81, 1 (1974); T. Moore, *J. Marketing* 46, 38 (1982); H. Shevrin and S. Dickman, *Am. Psychol.* 35, 421 (1980).

21. C. Eriksen, in *Nebraska Symposium on Motivation*, M. R. Jones, Ed. (Univ. of Nebraska Press, Lincoln, 1958), pp. 169–227; D. Holender, *Behav. Br. Sci.* 9, 1 (1986).

22. D. A. Balota, *J. Verb. Learn. Verb. Behav.* 22, 88 (1983); K. S. Bowers, in *The Unconscious Reconsidered*, K. S. Bowers and D. Meichenbaum, Eds. (Wiley-Interscience, New York, 1984), pp. 227–272; J. Cheesman and P. M. Merikle, *Can. J. Psychol.* 40, 343 (1986); K. I. Forster, *Lang. Cognit. Proc.* 1, 87 (1985); C. A. Fowler et al., *J. Exp. Psychol. Gen.* 110, 341 (1981); A. J. Marcel, *Cognit. Psych.* 15, 197, 238 (1983).

23. W. R. Kunst-Wilson and R. B. Zajonc, *Science* 207, 557; J. G. Seamon et al., *J. Exp. Psych. Learn. Mem. Cognit.* 9, 544 (1983); *Bull. Psychon. Soc.* 21, 187 (1983); *J. Exp. Psych. Learn. Mem. Cognit.* 10, 465 (1984).

24. A. S. Greenwald and T. J. Liu, *Bull. Psychon. Soc.* 23, 292 (1985).

25. T. O. Nelson, *J. Exp. Psychol. Hum. Learn. Cognit.* 4, 453 (1978).

26. D. N. Brooks and A. D. Baddeley, *Neuropsychogia* 14, 111 (1967); N. J. Cohen and L. R. Squire, *Science* 210, 207 (1980); E. L. Glisky et al., *J. Clin. Exp. Neuropsychol.*, 1986; D. L. Schacter et al., *J. Verb. Learn. Verb. Behav.* 23, 593 (1984).

27. P. Graf et al., *J. Exp. Psychol. Learn. Mem. Cognit.* 10, 164 (1984).

28. D. L. Schacter and E. Tulving, in *The Expression of Knowledge*, R. L. Isaacson and N. E. Spear, Eds. (Plenum, New York, 1982), pp. 33–65; L. R. Squire, *Science* 232, 1612 (1986).

29. D. L. Schacter and P. Graf, *J. Exp. Psychol. Learn. Mem. Cognit.* 12, 432 (1986).

30. F. J. Evans and W. A. F. Thorn, *Int. J. Clin. Exp. Hypn.* 14, 162 (1966); F. J. Evans, *J. Abnorm. Psychol.* 88, 556 (1979).

31. D. L. Schacter, *J. Exp. Psychol. Learn. Mem. Cognit.*, 1987; L. L. Jacoby, in *Remembering Reconsidered: Ecological and Traditional Approaches to the Study of Memory*, U. Neisser and E. Winograd, Eds. (Cambridge Univ. Press, Cambridge, in press); E. Eich, *Mem. Cognit.* 12, 105 (1984).

32. E. R. Hilgard, *Divided Consciousness: Multiple Controls in Human Thought and Action* (Wiley-Interscience, New York, rev. ed., 1986).

33. J. F. Kihlstrom, in *Repression, Dissociation, and the Warding-Off of Conflict-Related Cognitions*, J. L. Singer, Ed. (Univ. of Chicago Press, Chicago, 1990). For alternative social-psychological interpretations of hypnotic phenomena, see T. R. Sarbin and W. C. Coe, *Hypnosis: A Social Psychological Analysis of Influence Communication* (Holt, Rinehart, and Winston, New York, 1972); N. P. Spanos, *Behav. Brain Sci.* 9, 449 (1986).

34. J. F. Kihlstrom, in *The Unconscious Reconsidered*, K. S. Bowers and D. Meichenbaum, Eds. (Wiley-Interscience, New York, 1984), pp. 149–211.

35. E. R. Hilgard and J. R. Hilgard, *Hypnosis in the Relief of Pain* (Kaufman, Los Altos, CA, rev. ed. 1983).

36. H. J. Crawford, et al., *Am. J. Psychol.* 92, 193 (1979); E. R. Hilgard, *Psychol. Rev.* 80, 396 (1973); E. R. Hilgard et al., *J. Abnorm. Psychol.* 87, 239 (1978); E. R. Hilgard et al., ibid. 84, 280 (1975); V. J. Knox et al., *Arch. Gen. Psychol.* 30, 840 (1974).

37. J. F. Kihlstrom and F. J. Evans, in *Functional Disorders of Memory*, J. F. Kihlstrom and F. J. Evans, Eds. (Erlbaum, Hillsdale, NJ, 1979), pp. 179–218; J. F. Kihlstrom, in *The Psychology of Learning and Motivation*, G. H. Bower, Ed. (Academic Press, New York, 1985), vol. 19, pp. 131–178.

38. J. F. Kihlstrom, *Cognit. Psychol.* 12, 227 (1980); J. A. Williamsen et al., *J. Abnorm. Psychol.* 70, 123 (1965).

39. P. W. Sheehan and M. T. Orne, *J. Nerv. Ment. Dis.* 146, 209 (1968).

40. K. S. Bowers and H. A. Brenneman, *J. Abnorm. Psychol.* 90, 55 (1981); V. J. Knox et al., *Int. J. Clin. Exp. Hypn.* 23, 305 (1975); J. A. Stevenson, *J. Abnorm. Psychol.* 85, 398 (1976).

41. J. F. Kihlstrom, *Can. Psychol.* 28, 116 (1987).

42. H. F. Ellenberger, *The Discovery of the Unconscious: The History and Evolution of Dynamic Psychiatry* (Basic Books, New York, 1970).

43. W. James, *Principles of Psychology* (Holt, New York, 1890).

48

Pain and Dissociation in the Cold Pressor Test: A Study of Hypnotic Analgesia with "Hidden Reports" Through Automatic Key Pressing and Automatic Talking

Ernest R. Hilgard, Arlene H. Morgan, and Hugh Macdonald

Suggestions of analgesia following hypnotic induction have long been known to be effective in subjects responsive to hypnosis. The question of what happens to the perception of pain in hypnotic analgesia, however, has continued to challenge investigators. The bulk of experimental evidence suggests that whereas hypnotically analgesic subjects report much less pain than in normal waking (and occasionally none at all), the cardiovascular concomitants of the pain response continue as usual (Hilgard et al. 1974).

It appears that some amnesialike process may conceal from the hypnotized person his or her own perception of the pain; the amnesia differs from ordinary posthypnotic amnesia in that the perception of pain is diverted from consciousness before it has ever become conscious. This concealed perception of pain can be brought to light if the amnesia is broken by the familiar technique of automatic writing, or by a related technique known by analogy as automatic talking. Preliminary evidence was presented by Hilgard (1973), and subsequent experimental evidence within ischemic pain by Knox, Morgan, and Hilgard (1974). The metaphor of a "hidden observer" was used to describe the reporting of the pain as concealed under the amnesic barrier, but of course no homunculus is implied. The point is that while the subject is honestly reporting no felt pain, some cognitive system within him is registering and processing the pain in a form that can be revealed by the adopted procedures for breaking the amnesic barrier. The existence of such a hidden report of pain has been known for many years, but systematic studies have been lacking (Estabrooks 1957, James 1889, Kaplan 1960).

The study by Knox et al. (1974) relied on concurrent reports through the ordinary verbal reports of the hypnotically analgesic subject alternating with hidden reports through automatic talking. The automatic talking procedure

temporarily broke the amnesic barrier, but the barrier was quickly restored. Such vacillations within hypnosis can be produced readily, as Blum (1972) has frequently demonstrated. Knox and her colleagues found that during the period of suggested analgesia with eight highly susceptible subjects, there was no felt pain or suffering at all within ischemia, whereas the hidden reports revealed both pain and suffering of approximately the same level as found in normal waking ischemia. This was coherent with the preliminary data reported by Hilgard (1973), except that the expected reduction in suffering was not found. The intermittent reports may have caused a sampling of the pain and suffering, with the suffering following the intermittently sampled sensory pain before it was again concealed by amnesia, but further experimentation is required on the issue of pain versus suffering. Some subsequent pilot subjects in ischemia, in which the pain and suffering reports were obtained retrospectively (i.e., after the amnesia was broken when the painful stress had already been terminated), have reported essentially normal pain with an absence of suffering. The pain–suffering differentiation is therefore somewhat uncertain, and this report adds a few data relative to that distinction.

This study differs from that of Knox et al. (1974) by using the pain of circulating ice water (cold pressor test) as the source of laboratory pain, and by using automatic key pressing (the equivalent of automatic writing) as a means of regularly breaking the amnesia while the subject is also giving a verbal report, followed by retrospective reports when the amnesic barrier has been broken by automatic talking.

The total investigation involved other features, such as the suggestion of analgesia with and without a prior induction of hypnosis and two methods of suggesting analgesia, which will be made the basis of a separate report. We are here concerned primarily with the differences between the usual report and the hidden report within hypnotic analgesia, based on data from subjects larger in number and not quite as highly selected as those in the previous experiment. The selection criteria were relaxed slightly to determine, if possible, some of the limiting conditions bearing on the feasibility of the hidden report methods.

Method

Subjects

Subjects were 20 university students, half male and half female, who had been tested on hypnotic susceptibility scales and had scored at least 9 on a 10-point modification of the Harvard Group Scale of Hypnotic Susceptibility (HGSHS) (Shor and Orne 1962) and a 10-point individual modified form of the Stanford Scale of Hypnotic Susceptibility, Form C (SHSS-C) (Weitzenhoffer and Hilgard 1962). Each subject had successfully passed the criterion for amnesia within these scales ("passing" not requiring total amnesia) and an item of posthypnotic automatic writing (Form II, Item 9) adapted from the Stanford Profile Scales (Weitzenhoffer and Hilgard 1967). They scored at approximately the upper 10% of the group of students tested. Apart from earning these high scores in the testing procedures, they had no previous experience of hypnosis and the scales included no prior testing of hypnotic analgesia.

Experimental Design

Subjects participated for 1 hour on each of 4 days, 2 practice days and 2 experimental days. The overall plan was as follows:

Day 1: Practice
Practice in pain reporting was conducted on a numerical scale, both verbally and manually on the keys. There were two keys in a box, the right key for digits and the left for tens. This period provided the waking control test of the ice water pain.

A second type of practice was in deepening hypnosis. Because the subjects were to participate in several sessions, the deepening procedures familiarized them with a numerical scale for reporting their own depth of hypnosis and provided practice both in self-deepening and in detecting whatever signs they used to assure themselves of their hypnotic involvement. The exact meaning of hypnotic depth is problematical, but it has subjective reality for highly responsive hypnotic subjects and serves to legitimize the demands made on them. It may be noted that demand characteristics are of the essence in hypnosis and suggestion: A hypnotic subject will find a rabbit in his lap only if he responds to the demand for a rabbit. The presence of demand characteristics as such does not invalidate hypnotic experiments; they serve special critical purposes in the quasi-control group design proposed by Orne (1972). In that design a difference between "instructed simulators" and "hypnotically reals" is used to show that hypnosis produces some behavior beyond that implied either overtly or covertly by the hypnotist.

In this investigation, the usual demands of hypnosis (e.g., that an arm will become painless) are being offered quite openly, with the full consent of the subject. The evidence for the reality of the effects rests largely on the verbal reports of the subjects, with their honesty commonly shown by the extent to which they do not conform to the demands. The reality of hypnotic analgesia has, in fact, been earlier demonstrated in experiments from another laboratory using the simulator control. Subjects simulating hypnosis did indeed conceal the effects of painful shocks, but when questioned afterwards they admitted suffering the pain, whereas the hypnotized subjects reported that they felt no pain (Shor 1959, 1962).

Practice also assumed the form of automatic talking, as a method of temporarily breaking and restoring the amnesic process. This method has been reported in the earlier papers. Essentially, it makes plausible the breaking of the amnesic process by using the metaphor that some "hidden part" of the person knows more of what is going on than the "hypnotized part" that has reported some distortion of reality. The practice session did not involve pain; instead, it involved breaking the hallucination that an arm, actually held high in the air, was in the subject's lap. Insensitivity of the upraised arm (an indication of dissociation without specific suggestion) was tested by touching it several times but without painful stimulation. The signal for breaking the amnesic barrier and getting into communication with the hidden part was for the hypnotist to place his hand on the subject's shoulder, and the amnesia was restored when he removed his hand. This procedure may not be essential in all its details, but it serves conveniently to reveal how genuine the component experiences are to the subject. When the amnesia was ultimately removed, the subject remembered everything that went on and what was said.

Day 2: Practice

The first practice procedure involved automatic keypressing while consciously naming colors. This portion of the practice was based on the availability of equipment and procedures used in a study of interfering tasks, one conscious, the other out of awareness (Knox, Crutchfield, and Hilgard 1975). The key-pressing task consisted of pressing the right and left keys in a standard pattern of three to the right and three to the left, repeating this pattern for a minute. Under hypnosis, the task can be performed by highly responsive subjects without their awareness that the fingers are pressing the keys. To provide a competing task, the subject named colors arranged on a chart before him. This task was fully conscious and served to occupy the time that he was also pressing the keys out of awareness.

Practice in automatic key pressing concurrently with a hypnotically induced dream was also conducted. Because we desired the subjects to acquire as varied an experience as possible of competing activities, with one out of awareness, we followed an earlier suggestion of Wiseman and Reyher (1962) that the hypnotic dream can be used to facilitate hypnotic amnesia. The usual suggestions were given for the key pressing to go on out of awareness. Following the suggested dream (produced while the key pressing continued), the subject was asked to describe "what happened in the last few minutes." Most subjects responded only with the content of their dreams, failing to mention the key pressing.

Days 3 and 4: Experimental Days—Waking and Hypnotic Analgesia

There were two ice water sessions on each day, both either in waking or in hypnosis; half of the subjects had waking on the first day, half on the second. Pain reduction suggestions were given on both days, via tape recordings, in two forms. One was based on the suggestion that the arm was numb and insensitive "as if just a piece of rubber," following as closely as possible the suggestions used by Spanos, Barber, and Lang (1974). The other was an "absent arm" suggestion, based on the frequent observation by early investigators that an arm out of awareness was also anesthetic. The details will be given at another time because the differences in objective results were not sufficiently great to require treating the two methods separately in this report. The data regarding waking analgesia will also be omitted now, except to indicate that there was no evidence, following waking suggestion of analgesia, that there had been any amnesic distortion of the pain experience. Thus, the hidden reports (obtained during a subsequent hypnosis) were just the same as the usual ones.

Day 4 was symmetrical with Day 3, except that those who had waking analgesia on Day 3 had hypnotic analgesia on Day 4, and vice versa. For the present account, only the data from the hypnotic analgesia day are to be presented. For half of the subjects the condition was on Day 3 and for half on Day 4; therefore, the appropriateness of combining the data must be justified. Statistical comparison of the pain reports of the two subgroups, one on each day, showed no difference in their pain reports, whether by the usual verbal reports within suggested analgesia, the reports obtained by key pressing, or the reports subsequently obtained by automatic talking. In all cases, significances of differences by t test yielded $p > .20$.

Each day was followed by an inquiry after amnesia was lifted regarding all aspects of the reported experiences. The inquiry was recorded on tape, transcribed, and made the basis for the discussion to be presented later.[1]

Results

Pain Reduction within Hypnotic Analgesia

It has previously been shown that pain reports, obtained in the waking state in the cold pressor test, are sufficiently stable for an initial test to serve as a baseline for normal responsiveness to pain. That is, there is little adaptation or learning, so that a second day's results correlate .79 with the initial results and there is no significant change in mean reports over the 2 days (Hilgard et al. 1974). Hence, when a significant change from this baseline is reported within suggested analgesia, it can be taken as a satisfactory measure of the effectiveness of the analgesia suggestions. The amount of reduction is commonly found to correlate about .50 with measured hypnotic susceptibility (Evans and Paul 1970, Hilgard 1967, Shor 1959). There is some uncertainty over the relative effectiveness of waking analgesic suggestions versus suggestions given in hypnosis, but this problem need not be considered here.

The results are given in table 48.1, in which the first column shows the normal wakin paing and the second column shows the pain reported in the usual way in hypnotic analgesia. Attention is now directed to these two columns only.

The subjects have been placed in the order of their success in reducing felt pain through hypnotic analgesia (column 2) and divided into two groups for purposes of studying later some of the correlates of this ability. The 20 subjects all experienced pain normally in the usual waking condition, with the maximum pain at 45 s in the ice water, exceeding the critical level of 10 for all but two of the subjects. Those who were better able to reduce pain did not differ significantly from those less able (column 1). The subjects, although selected for high responsiveness to hypnosis, were not universally able to achieve drastic pain reduction, although all but one reported the maximum pain within hypnotic analgesia to be below the critical level of 10. The reduction of pain as a consequence of suggested analgesia was highly significant, $t(19) = 6.47$, $p < .001$, with every subject reporting some pain reduction. The data in the first two columns merely replicate what has been reported in a number of previous experiments from this laboratory (e.g., Hilgard 1967, 1969, 1971).

Evidence for a Hidden Experience of Pain within Analgesia

The evidence presented in columns 3 and 4 distinguishes this study from earlier research by showing that subjects who have given the usual reports of little pain in analgesia (column 2), at some other processing level report pain often approximating that of the normal waking pain. The reports of maximum pain in columns 2, 3, and 4 are averages obtained from two trials within the day. The trials differed in the suggestion according to which analgesia was produced, but otherwise the procedures were identical. The type of suggestion did not yield significant differences between the means of analgesia obtained, and the scores on the two trials were significantly correlated, so there is ample justification for averaging them.

Primary interest centers in the interrelatedness of the data of columns 2, 3, and 4, all being

Table 48.1

Pain reported in normal waking condition and in hypnotic analgesia

| | Maximum pain within 45 seconds in the ice water | | | |
| | | Hypnotic analgesia | | |
Subject	Normal waking pain (Column 1)	Usual verbal report (Column 2)	Report by concurrent automatic key pressing (Column 3)	Report by retrospective automatic talking (Column 4)
Less pain reported in analgesia				
1	13.0	0.0	6.5	14.0
2	12.0	.5	4.8	4.8
3	18.0	.5	.5	.5
4	8.0	1.0	9.0	9.0
5	25.0	1.0	8.5	8.5
6	25.0	1.0	1.0	1.0
7	9.0	3.0	6.2	10.0
8	11.0	3.0	2.5	3.0
9	13.0	3.0	15.5	18.0
10	15.0	3.8	3.0	3.0
Mean of subgroup (n = 10)	14.9	1.68	5.75	7.18
More pain reported in analgesia				
11	10.0	4.0	8.5	8.5
12	10.0	4.0	7.0	7.0
13	25.0	4.8	4.8	4.8
14	10.0	5.5	5.5	5.5
15	10.0	6.0	6.0	6.0
16	12.0	6.2	6.2	6.2
17	25.0	8.5	7.8	7.8
18	10.0	8.5	10.0	10.0
19	10.0	9.0	9.0	9.0
20	13.0	10.0	10.0	10.0
Mean of subgroup (n = 10)	13.5	6.65	7.48	7.48
Mean of total (n = 20)	14.2	4.16	6.62	7.33

Table 48.2
Statistical tests based on total sample of table 1

Hypnotic analgesia report	t	r
Verbal versus key pressing	−2.96*	.37
Verbal versus automatic talking	−2.94*	.15
Key pressing versus automatic talking	−1.70	.90

Note: $F(2, 38) = 8.18$, $p < .01$.
* $p < .01$.

reports obtained within the same experimental period. Hence, the analysis of variance as reported in table 48.2 is confined to these three columns; it proved satisfactorily significant, $p < .01$, so that t tests between the columns were justified. Both automatic key pressing and automatic talking yielded reports of significantly more pain than in the usual reports with hypnotic analgesia, but they did not differ significantly from each other.

Despite the significant mean results, it should be noted that not all subjects followed the typical trend. For example, whereas the pain reported in column 4 is typically below that in column 1 (normal pain), pain in column 4 was not reduced over column 1 for subjects 1, 4, 7, and 9, all of whom had substantial pain reduction as reported in column 2 (pain in analgesia). Similarly, pain in column 4 was not reduced for subjects 11, 18, 19, and 20, who were less successful in pain reduction as reported in column 2. At the other end of the spectrum are those subjects who failed to report more pain in column 4 than their reduced pains in column 2, including subjects 3, 6, 8, and 10 among the more successful pain reducers, and subjects 13–17 among the less successful. These divergent responses will require further discussion.

Because both key pressing and automatic talking yielded pain reports above the usual reports in hypnotic analgesia, they gave evidence of some hidden experience of pain. The hidden pain was somewhat below the normally ex-

perienced pain, but that is not unreasonable in view of the quiescence of the hypnotized subject. The course of the hidden pain, as reported by automatic key pressing, compared with normal waking pain and hypnotically reduced pain, as usually reported, is shown in figure 48.1. The curves are presented separately for the subjects, divided as in table 48.1 between those more and less analgesic according to their usual verbal reports within hypnotic analgesia. The general relationships hold, apart from the attenuation of the results for the less analgesic.

Results of the Final Inquiry

Relevant information was obtained through the automatic talking reports after each hypnotic session and through subsequent questioning. Each subject was asked about his recollection of what he had said within hypnotic analgesia, and what he had reported by way of the keys and in the automatic talking account. He then elaborated on underlying experiences reflected in these reports. After his free report he was asked specifically about his awareness of the cold water and about the suffering associated with the recollected pain. He was also asked whether or not he had at any time been aware of the key pressing. Subjects did not universally conform to the obvious demands of the experiment. For example, a few were not completely oblivious to the fact that they were pressing the keys while giving their verbal reports; some heard the clicking of the keys while being unaware of the source of the sound. When the subject became fully aware of the keys, the difference between the usual verbal report and the keypressing report tended to disappear. Another type of disagreement with the implied demands of the experiment was shown by nine subjects, successful in hypnotic pain reduction, who failed to show any recovery of felt pain within the automatic reporting procedures. These were subjects 3, 6, 8, 10, and 13–17 of table 48.1, as previously noted.

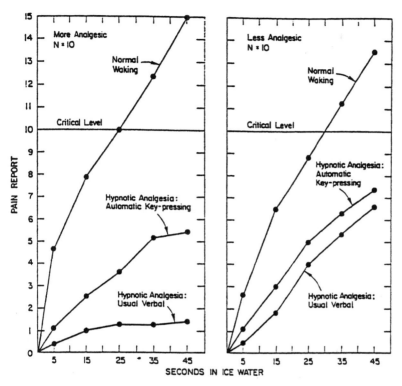

Figure 48.1
Pain reported verbally in the normal waking condition, and in the hypnotic analgesia condition, reported verbally and by automatic key pressing. (Subjects were divided according to the degree of pain reduction as reported verbally on hypnotic analgesia day.)

The final inquiry, when the data had been collected, was conducted after all amnesia was removed and the subject was fully aware of what he had reported at all times. We were particularly interested in his phenomenal account of the nature of the cognitive system responsible for the hidden report that disagreed with his usual or open report within hypnotic analgesia, although other aspects of the experience were also noted.

The Pain–Suffering Dichotomy
In the inquiry regarding the recollection of pain felt in hypnotic analgesia we asked the question

whether the hidden pain was accompanied by suffering. In the case of eight subjects who most clearly sensed a distinction between the usual report of pain in analgesia and that revealed through the automatic methods, all reported that the recollected pain had been felt as a sensory or intellectual experience, and it caused *no distress or suffering*. This is coherent with the results mentioned above for some pilot subjects in an ischemia experiment, although it is at odds with aspects of the findings of Knox et al. (1974). It may very well prove to be the case that hypnotic analgesia relieves suffering more than it relieves sensory pain, but this cannot be considered proven. Were it to be the case, it would be congruent with aspects of the gate-control theory of pain as proposed by Melzack and Wall (1965).

Reactions to the Exposure of the Hidden Experience of Pain

We were interested in how the subjects reacted to their own discovery that, after having reported little or no pain in the usual way in analgesia, they reported more pain through the automatic techniques, thus exposing some felt pain that must either have been denied or in some manner hidden behind a cloak of amnesia. Because this experience was not a clear one for all of the subjects, the more illuminating answers depend on those who had the more vivid experience of change between usual and hidden report. These were 8 of the 20 subjects (subjects 1, 2, 4, 5, 7, 9, 11, and 18 in table 48.1). Of the rest, six (subjects 3, 10, 12, 13, 14, and 17) reported some subjective differences in the roles of the two parts, that is, usual verbal reporting and the automatic reporting systems, but an incomplete separation of one from the other through amnesia. For them, some kind of interpretation in terms of divided attention may prove to be appropriate. The remaining six (subjects 6, 8, 15, 16, 19, and 20) indicated no difference whatever between their usual reports and their automatic ones; either there was no amnesia, or the amnesia that existed was not relieved by the methods used. Obviously, more experimentation is required to produce a completely satisfactory explanation.

The eight who had a sense of separateness between the usual hypnotic analgesia experience and that uncovered by the automatic techniques described the differences in many ways, of which the following verbatim quotes are representative:

I can separate my mind and my head from the rest of my body. The hidden part—reporting on the keys— was controlling my body. My mind was not counting key-pressing. My mind was reporting what it felt, verbally. I've always been aware of the difference between the mind and the body when I've been hypnotized.

It's as though two things were happening simultaneously; I have two separate memories, as if the two things could have happened to different people. The memory of the hidden part is more intellectual, but I can't really comprehend or assimilate the two.

Both parts were concentrating on what you said— not to feel pain. The water bothered the hidden part a little because it felt it a little, but the hypnotized part was not thinking of my arm at all.

Part of me knew that my hand was in the water and it hurt as much as it did the other day [i.e., in the waking control]. The hypnotized part was vaguely aware of the presence of some pain, and that's why I had to concentrate really hard. [Subject reported zero pain.]

When you're hypnotized, there are certain questions that just aren't answered, and you just don't probe them in your mind. I think you're aware that the pain exists, but it's not appropriate to deal with it just then.

I don't think I'm totally unaware that there is some level at which I know exactly what was going on. But when you asked me what I had been doing [i.e., the inquiry within automatic talking], it was really hard to remember. I don't know if I could have. It was like a block.

Today [to the hidden part] the pain was more general, and especially the second time [under the absent arm instruction]. I felt it in my shoulder. That part knew that my arm was there, but part of me knew it wasn't there. The pain was hidden from the hypnotized part.

Part of me knows the pain is there, but I'm not sure I *feel* it. The hypnotized part *doesn't* feel it, but I'm not sure if the hypnotized part may have known it was there but didn't say it. The hypnotized part really makes an effort to not feel it.

Two aspects of the experience run through these comments. One is the activity of the hypnotized subject, a genuine cognitive effort involved in conforming to the demands of the experiment. It is by no means a completely passive experience controlled by the hypnotist. The other is the great difficulty in putting into words the fluctuations that occur within the experience—the fleeting glances at what is going on, even while the events are not fully cognized; separation and fusion; acceptance and denial.

Much of this is familiar in subjective reports of posthypnotic amnesia.

The Amnesic Correlates of the Discrepancies between Pain Reports

It has been repeatedly implied in the foregoing discussion that the concealment of pain that can be recovered through the automatic reporting methods must be amnesic in nature. If that is the case, some of the individual differences in the discrepant reports should correspond to differences in hypnotic amnesia measured in other ways. Two sets of such measures are available: responses within the items concerned with posthypnotic amnesia in the susceptibility tests that were given as part of the subject selection, and indications of amnesia within the training days preparatory to the experiment proper.

All subjects "passed" the amnesia tests according to criteria established in the test standardizations, but the criteria allow the recall of several items so that not all were equally amnesic. Despite the restricted range, it is possible to assign scores to the subjects according to their tested amnesia by making use of both the number of items recalled in the two amnesia tests they had taken and by weighting these scores according to the items recovered when told, "Now you can remember everything."[2] The true hypnotic amnesia is a recoverable one; if items are not recovered, the subject may simply have been inattentive to them or forgotten them for nonhypnotic reasons (Cooper 1972, Kihlstrom and Evans 1973). When subjects were scored for tested amnesia in this way, those who were more analgesic (subjects 1–10 in table 48.1) proved to have higher amnesia scores than those less analgesic (subjects 11–20). The difference, as tested by the Mann–Whitney U test was significant at the .05 level. Of course, a correlation is expected among all tests of hypnotic susceptibility, so this relationship is not surprising, except that it holds within a very restricted range of hypnotic re-

sponsiveness and therefore points to a somewhat specific relation between amnesia and analgesia.

If the rise in pain between the usual report in analgesia and that in automatic talking were a consequence of lifting amnesia, this rise should also be related to amnesia. This did not prove to be the case. Among the more amnesic, 5 of 10 subjects reported substantial gains between the usual and the hidden reports in analgesia, whereas among the less amnesic, 4 of 10 reported corresponding gains. These differences are not significant, so the hypothesis that amnesia would predict the differential pain reports was not supported.

Discussion

The phenomena of pain and suffering are puzzling in themselves and the phenomena of hypnosis are also puzzling, so it not surprising that their combination will yield data difficult to interpret. The data as reported are unequivocal in several respects, and indeterminate in others. It is again demonstrated that the subjective experience of pain and suffering can be reduced by hypnotic analgesia suggestions, especially among those whose hypnotic responsiveness, as measured by hypnotic susceptibility tests, is at a high level. Those who report complete absence of pain are in the minority, even among selected subjects; only 4 of the 20 subjects in this experiment reported complete absence of pain on one of their two test opportunities, although 14 of the 20 reduced their pain by half or more of that reported in the normal waking condition. This pain reduction through suggested analgesia is by now so firmly established that it is unequivocal. Those who are most successful feel neither pain nor suffering.

The second point now established is that for a substantial fraction of those who are able to reduce their pain through hypnotic analgesia, methods can be found to show that information about felt pain of greater magnitude has been processed and can be reported verbally. The methods used here (automatic writing and automatic talking) probably serve to break some sort of amnesic barrier, but the interpretation of how the methods work cannot be considered completely established. The general findings, until recently not confirmed by quantitative experiments, have been occasionally reported in the past, and can be accepted as firm.

A third point, less well established, is that at the hidden level there has been more reduction of suffering than of sensory pain. In the present experiment, all of those with the clearest account of a difference between their absent pain and their recovered pain through the automatic methods reported that there was strongly felt sensory pain but a minimum of suffering. This result might be taken as established, except for the previous findings from our laboratory that under some conditions, although neither pain nor suffering were reported in the usual conditions of hypnotic analgesia, both pain and suffering were reported by the automatic talking procedure (Knox et al. 1974). This uncertainty about the pain–suffering dimension does not reflect, however, on either the demonstration that both pain and suffering are relieved through hypnotic suggestion or that there is processing of the information at some concealed level.

Because of the plausibility that some sort of amnesic process is responsible for the difference between the usual and the hidden analgesic reports, efforts were made to relate measured amnesia in these subjects to their success in the experiments. Unfortunately, the arrangements of the experiments make it difficult to conduct the investigation with subjects who are not capable of demonstrating hypnotic amnesia, so that, pending further experimentation, it was necessary to do the exploratory analyses with a very restricted range of amnesic abilities. Even so, there was a significant relationship between measured amnesia and the amount of hypnotic analgesia shown in the usual way, although there could not be demonstrated any relationship

between measured amnesia and the recovery through the automatic techniques. There appears to be little doubt that an amnesic process of some sort is involved, but because it is an amnesia for something that has not been in awareness previously, it differs from usual posthypnotic amnesia.

If it should be substantiated that the recovery through automatic inquiry methods is of sensory pain, but not of suffering (a result found for a substantial group within this experiment), some interesting problems of interpretation would be involved. The two main problems, reminiscent of the James–Lange theory of emotion, are whether suffering is in reaction to sensory pain or is separately experienced. The separate pathways for pain and suffering that are stressed in the Melzack–Wall gate control theory allow for the second interpretation, although according to the theory there is an interaction between the two systems.

The hypnotic findings (were they to be confirmed) would be that the amnesic effect was only with respect to the sensory pain and there was no amnesic effect on suffering. Thus, recovery of pain but no recovery of suffering would occur. The deeper interpretation could take one of two forms: There might have been some psychophysiological blocking of the suffering mechanism through hypnotic suggestion that operated differently from the blocking of sensory pain, or felt suffering might be in fact only a response to felt pain so that when pain is not felt, no suffering occurs. It is evident in gross observation that the hypnotic subject does not show the usual signs of overt suffering when not experiencing pain; that is, he does not visibly squirm, or sigh, or tense his muscles. If suffering is felt as a reaction to these responses (in the James–Lange spirit), then he does not suffer if the reactions do not occur. There are, of course, some experimental approaches to the clarification of these issues; it is sufficient to point out that they are at present unresolved.

Acknowledgments

This research was supported by Grant MH-03859 from the National Institute of Mental Health to Ernest R. Hilgard in the Laboratory of Hypnosis Research, Department of Psychology, Stanford University.

Notes

1. Verbatim instructions have been reproduced and will be supplied on request.

2. The short form of group test used did not provide data on the recovery of items following amnesia, so the correction could be made for only one of the two amnesia tests.

References

Blum, G. S. Hypnotic programming techniques in psychological experiments. In E. Fromm and R. E. Shor (Eds.), *Hypnosis: Research developments and perspectives.* Chicago: Aldine-Atherton, 1972.

Cooper, L. M. Hypnotic amnesia. In E. Fromm and R. E. Shor (Eds.), *Hypnosis: Research developments and perspectives.* Chicago: Aldine-Atherton, 1972.

Estabrooks, G. H. *Hypnotism* (Rev. ed.). New York: Dutton, 1957.

Evans, M. B., and Paul, G. L. Effects of hypnotically suggested analgesia on physiological and subjective responses to cold stress. *Journal of Consulting and Clinical Psychology*, 1970, *35*, 362–371.

Hilgard, E. R. A quantitative study of pain and its reduction through hypnotic suggestion. *Proceedings of the National Academy of Sciences*, 1967, *57*, 1581–1586.

Hilgard, E. R. Pain as a puzzle for psychology and physiology. *American Psychologist*, 1969, *24*, 103–113.

Hilgard, E. R. Pain: Its reduction and production under hypnosis. *Proceedings of the American Philosophical Society*, 1971, *115*, 470–476.

Hilgard, E. R. A neodissociation interpretation of pain reduction in hypnosis. *Psychological Review*, 1973, *80*, 396–411.

Hilgard, E. R., Morgan, A. H., Lange, A. F., Lenox, J. R., Macdonald, H., Marshall, G. D., and Sachs, L. B. Heart rate changes in pain and hypnosis. *Psychophysiology*, 1974, *11*, 692–702.

Hilgard, E. R., Ruch, J. C., Lange, A. F., Lenox, J. R., Morgan, A. H., and Sachs, L. B. The psychophysics of cold pressor pain and its modification through hypnotic suggestion. *American Journal of Psychology*, 1974, *87*, 17–31.

James, W. Automatic writing. *Proceedings of the American Society for Psychical Research*, 1889, *1*, 584–564.

Kaplan, E. A. Hypnosis and pain. *Archives of General Psychiatry*, 1960, *2*, 657–658.

Kihlstrom, J. F., and Evans, F. J. Recovery of memory after posthypnotic amnesia. *Proceedings of the 81st Annual Convention of the American Psychological Association*, 1973, *8*, 1079–1080.

Knox, V. J., Morgan, A. H., and Hilgard, E. R. Pain and suffering in ischemia: The paradox of hypnotically suggested anesthesia as contradicted by reports from the "hidden observer." *Archives of General Psychiatry*, 1974, *30*, 840–847.

Knox, V. J., Crutchfield, L., and Hilgard, E. R. The nature of task interference in hypnotic dissociation. *International Journal of Clinical and Experimental Hypnosis*, 1975, *23*, 305–323.

Melzack, R., and Wall, P. D. Pain mechanisms: A new theory. *Science*, 1965, *150*, 971–979.

Orne, M. T. On the simulating subject as a quasicontrol group in hypnosis research: What, why, and how. In E. Fromm and R. E. Shor (Eds.), *Hypnosis: Research developments and perspectives.* Chicago: Aldine-Atherton, 1972.

Shor, R. E. Hypnosis and the concept of the generalized reality-orientation. *American Journal of Psychotherapy*, 1959, *13*, 582–602.

Shor, R. E. Three dimensions of hypnotic depth. *International Journal of Clinical and Experimental Hypnosis*, 1962, *10*, 23–38.

Shor, R. E., and Orne, E. C. *The Harvard Group Scale of Hypnotic Susceptibility, Form A.* Palo Alto, Calif.: Consulting Psychologists Press, 1962.

Spanos, N. P., Barber, T. X., and Lang, G. Effects of hypnotic induction, suggestions of analgesia, and demands for honesty on subjective reports of pain. In H. London and R. E. Nisbett (Eds.), *Thought and feeling:*

Cognitive alteration of feeling states. Chicago: Aldine, 1974.

Weitzenhoffer, A. M., and Hilgard, E. R. *The Stanford Scale of Hypnotic Susceptibility, Form C.* Palo Alto, Calif.: Consulting Psychologists Press, 1962.

Weitzenhoffer, A. M., and Hilgard, E. R. *Revised Stanford Profile Scales of Hypnotic Susceptibility, Forms I and II.* Palo Alto, Calif.: Consulting Psychologists Press, 1967.

Wiseman, R. J., and Reyher, J. A procedure utilizing dreams for deepening the hypnotic trance. *American Journal of Clinical Hypnosis*, 1962, 5, 105–110.

V. S. Ramachandran

The social scientists have a long way to go to catch up, but they may be up to the most important scientific business of all, if and when they finally get to the right questions. Our behavior toward each other is the strangest, most unpredictable, and almost entirely unaccountable of all the phenomena with which we are obliged to live.
—Lewis Thomas

Introduction

In 1914, the French neurologist Babinski described an extraordinary neurological syndrome. He noticed that some of his patients, who were completely paralyzed on the left side of the body as a result of a right hemisphere stroke, tended to deny their paralysis and he coined the term "anosognosia" (denial of illness) to describe the condition. Anosognosia can vary in severity from a mere indifference to one's disability to a vehement denial of the paralysis, even when confronted with incontrovertible proof. For example, if the patient is asked to perform a specific task with her paralyzed left hand, she may fail to do so but may continue to insist that she is not paralyzed. In its most extreme form, the patient may even deny that the arm belongs to her and ascribe it to either the examiner or to her spouse! (This disownership phenomenon was called "somatoparaphrenia" by Gerstmann (1942).)

One explanation for anosognosia[1] would be in psychodynamic terms: the patient denies her illness in order to "protect her ego." This interpretation doesn't account for two important aspects of the syndrome. First, the syndrome is seen only when the right parietal lobe is damaged and only rarely when the left parietal lobe is involved (Critchley 1966, Babinski 1914). Second, the denial is often domain specific, for example, the patient will admit she had a severe stroke but denies paralysis or, on occasion, will even admit that her leg is paralyzed but insist

that her arm isn't. For discussions on these topics, the reader is referred to several lucid and insightful recent reviews (Galin 1992; Edelman 1989; Damasio 1994; Heilman 1991; Levine 1990; McGlynn and Schacter 1989; Halligan, Marshall, and Wade 1993) as well as more classic papers in the older neurological literature (Critchley 1962, Juba 1949, Waldenstrom 1939, Ehrenwald 1930, Cutting 1978, Weinstein and Kahn 1950).

Another more "cognitive" interpretation of the syndrome would be in terms of the hemineglect–heminattention that often accompany the denial, that is, one could argue that the patient neglects her paralysis in much the same way that she neglects everything else on the left side. This hypothesis is probably at least partially correct but it doesn't account for why the denial usually persists even when the patient's attention is drawn to the paralysis. Nor does it explain why the patient does not *intellectually correct* her misconception even though she may be quite lucid and intelligent in other respects. Indeed, the reason anosognosia is so puzzling is that we have come to regard the "intellect" as primarily propositional in character and one ordinarily expects propositional logic to be internally consistent. To listen to a patient deny ownership of her arm and yet, in the same breath, admit that it is attached to her shoulder is one of the most perplexing phenomena that one can encounter as a neurologist.

What would happen if the patient is repeatedly asked to perform an action with her left hand? I recently tried this on a patient, Mrs. LR (clinical details for this and other patients are described in a later section). I found that if her failure to perform were pointed out to her, she would usually "rationalize" her failure with statements such as, "My shoulder hurts a lot today; I have arthritis, you know," or "I didn't really want to point that time." After several such trials, however, she eventually admitted she was paralyzed.

Yet, curiously, when questioned again just 10 min. later, she not only reverted to denial—insisting that her left hand was fully functional—but also claimed that she had successfully used that hand during the preceding testing session (Ramachandran 1994a,b)! This was true despite the fact her memory for other details of that session was completely intact. It was almost as though she had "forgotten" or selectively repressed the memory of her failed attempts as well as her verbal acknowledgment of her paralysis. What is especially surprising about this observation is that it implies that her "propositional knowledge" system has no access now to the explicit verbal confession that she had been engaging in just a few minutes earlier (Ramachandran 1994a,b). I realized, therefore, that these patients may provide an opportunity not only for studying denial, but also for studying the mechanism underlying the storage and retrieval of new memories.

Consider another patient BM, a 76-year-old lady who had a recent stroke that left her completely paralyzed on the left side. Although quite lucid when discussing most other topics, she persistently denied her paralysis even when pressed and her answers were not hesitant or lacking in conviction. The following conversation was quite typical:

R: Mrs. M, when were you admitted to the hospital?

M: I was admitted on April 16 because my daughter felt there was something wrong with me.

R: What day is it today and what time?

M: It is sometime late in the afternoon on Tuesday. (This was an accurate response.)

R: Mrs. M, can you use your arms?

M: Yes.

R: Can you use both hands?

M: Yes, of course.

R: Can you use your right hand?

M: Yes.

R: Can you use your left hand?

M: Yes.

R: Are both hands equally strong?

M: Yes, they are equally strong.

R: Mrs. M, point to my student with your right hand.

M: (Patient points.)

R: Mrs. M, point to my student with your left hand.

M: (Patient remains silent.)

R: Mrs. M, why are you not pointing?

M: Because I didn't want to....

The same sequence of questions was repeated the next day with identical answers except that toward the end of the session the patient looked at me and asked:

M: Doctor, whose hand is this (pointing to her own left hand)?

R: Whose hand do you think it is?

M: Well, it certainly isn't yours!

R: Then whose is it?

M: It isn't mine either.

R: Whose hand do you think it is?

M: It is my son's hand, doctor.

One interpretation of this would be that the patient begins with rather simple "denial" of paralysis but when her paralysis becomes increasingly obvious to her with repeated questioning she is pushed into a corner and the only way she can "rationalize" the failure of her arm to perform is to progress into the even more full-blown delusion that the arm belongs to her son! Later in this article, I will consider the hypothesis that what one is seeing here is a replay of the same kinds of delusions and rationalization that all of us engage in some time or the other (Ramachandran 1994a,b). What is puzzling about these cases, however, is the extreme lengths to which they will take the process even though their intelligence, clarity of thought, and mentation is relatively unaffected in every other domain *except* for matters concerning the left hand. The patient I just described, for example, refused a box of candy saying, "I am diabetic, doctor—I can't eat candy. You should know that!" Thus, her anosognosia included her limb but did not extend to her diabetes.

Joseph (1993) has argued that the right parietal patient's statement that her left hand does not belong to her "makes sense" from her point of view since "she," that is, the left hemisphere, no longer has access to either the sensory input or memories of the right hemisphere. (This seems implausible since it is very likely that most memories are bilateraly represented at some level.) In any event it can't be the whole story because it doesn't explain why she doesn't simply plead ignorance instead of engaging in confabulations or why she fails to *intellectually correct* her false belief even in the face of flatly contradictory evidence. For example, in the case of split-brain patients, even though the left hemisphere lacks access to information in the right hemisphere and is sometimes surprised by the actions of the "alien" left hand, the patient certainly doesn't rationalize this by saying, "This isn't my arm," or "This is my brother's arm. It looks big and hairy!" (And I would venture the prediction that if his left arm were to become accidentally paralyzed from a peripheral nerve lesion, he would admit rather than deny the paralysis.) Clearly, something more is involved; something other than just cloudy judgment or dementia, for right parietal patients are often perfectly lucid in other domains.

Mrs. M's excuse for not moving her hand ("Because I didn't want to") is, of course, a classic example of a Freudian rationalization. And, as noted earlier, Ms. LR, who also persistently denied her paralysis, had a whole arsenal of such "defense mechanisms" at her disposal that she used on different occasions. In addition to engaging in rationalizations, she frequently resorted to the use of euphemisms to describe her failure (anything to avoid the dreaded word "paralysis"). For example: "I've never been very ambidextrous, doctor," or "I guess it isn't very fast today, is it?" or, "My arm isn't facilitated." The patient may also use ingenious distraction maneuvers to take the emphasis away from the main thrust of the question. When asked whether she could use her left hand, another patient, Mrs. OS (see below), responded, "Did you know that my father was left-handed? So is my sister.... They were all left-handed—all of them," and so on. And on other occasions, she produced confabulatory responses such as, "Yes, I can use my left hand. In fact, I used it this morning to wash my face," even though her memory for other types of events remained undistorted.

There has been a tendency in the past to regard anosognosia and somatoparaphrenic delusions as a bizarre manifestation of cerebral disease. Contrary to this view, I suggest that what one is really seeing in these patients is an amplified version of Freudian defense mechanisms (Freud 1946, 1895/1961) caught *in flagrante delicto*; mechanisms of precisely the same sort that we all use in our daily lives. However, since the defenses are grotesquely exaggerated, studying them might give us, for the first time, an *experimental handle* on defense mechanisms, that is, we might actually be able to study the rules governing their development by manipulating the stimulus contingencies in individual patients (Ramachandran 1994a,b). For example, it may help us answer an important theoretical question that was never addressed by Freud, namely, what determines which particular defense mechanism is used in a given situation (e.g., rationalization, projection, denial, reaction-formation, intellectualization)? To what extent is the choice determined by the particular environmental *stressor* and to what extent by the patient's premorbid personality?

There are, in fact, two important theoretical issues that we need to deal with. First, why do the Freudian defense mechanisms exist in the first place—even in normal individuals? Do they have a specific biological and/or social role?

Second, why are these mechanisms grossly exaggerated in right parietal patients?

Before I answer these theoretical questions, however, I will describe three sets of experiments that we performed in patients with anosognosia. Although anosognosia has been recognized since the turn of the century, and there have been numerous valuable clinical case studies, there have been remarkably few *experiments* devoted to elucidating the nature and extent of the denial. One of the goals of my experiments will be to conduct formal experiments to determine whether the patient has "tacit" knowledge at some level that she is indeed paralyzed even though she denies it verbally. Additional goals will be to explore memory functions in these patients, for example, if the paralysis is made evident to her, how long does she remember it? Is there a selective amnesia for paralysis? If so, does the amnesia result from "repression" or from failure to acquire the memory in the first place?

The answers to these questions will, in turn, set the stage for developing a new Darwinian theory of defense mechanisms in general and of anosognosia in particular. The rest of this article will, accordingly, consist of two parts. In part 1, I describe the experiments themselves and their immediate implications. In part 2, in keeping with the spirit of this journal, I will use these experiments as a starting point for putting forth a number of highly speculative ideas on such diverse topics as REM sleep, dreams, and laughter. I would emphasize, however, that the two parts are logically independent of each other. Since each part is self-contained, the reader whose main interest is in anosognosia can profitably skip part 2 altogether and just focus on the experiments.

Part 1: Experiments on Anosognosia

Patients

The four patients who participated in our study were elderly women who had recently sustained a right hemisphere stroke causing a left hemiplegia. No formal neuropsychological tests (such as WAIS-R or CVLT) were administered but a routine neurological workup, including a mental status examination, was conducted on each patient. At the time when my experiments were conducted, they did not have any obvious signs of dementia, aphasia, or amnesia and were able to clearly understand our instructions. (LH and BM were sometimes somnolent and/or distractable but I tried to confine our experiments to lucid periods, when they were alert and willing to participate.) Whenever possible a CT scan and/or an MRI was otained.

Case 1

Patient LR, a 78-year-old, right-handed, Caucasian woman with 16 years of schooling and a degree in journalism, was admitted on March 13, 1994, after the sudden onset of loss of strength in her left limbs. The patient was alert, cooperative, and conversed fluently with the experimenters and hospital staff. There were no gross deficits in her memory and orientation (e.g., when I saw her on 2 consecutive days, she clearly recognized me the second time and even remembered the tests that were administered). Touch sensation was partially spared on the left side and clear signs of severe left hemiplegia were present. The patient had left hemispatial neglect, as seen in line cancellation and bisection tasks and also had right head and gaze deviation. She denied any motor or visual impairments, yet admitted she had come to the hospital for treatment of a stroke.

The CT scan performed at admission revealed a right frontoparietal CVA.

Case 2

BM, a 76-year-old, right-handed woman with 3 years of schooling, was admitted April 8, 1994. The patient initially appeared slightly somnolent and easily distractible but was able to successfully communicate through a Spanish/English language interpreter. There were no obvious sign of aphasia or dementia but she did experience difficulty with serial subtraction. Touch and pain sensations were absent on the left side and she showed clear signs of severe left hemiplegia. Extreme left hemispatial neglect was evident from her line cancellations and bisections, and her head, gaze, and trunk were deviated to the right. The patient also denied having any motor or visual deficits and when questioned about the ownership of her left hand, she falsely ascribed it to either the experimenter or to her son, Tony.

An MRI obtained 1 month after admission revealed a large infarct involving much territory of the right middle cerebral artery especially in the right parietooccipital region. There was also an area of hemorrhage in the head of the caudate nucleus.

Case 3

OS, a 65-year-old, right-handed, Caucasian woman, was admitted to the hospital on May 19, 1994. Three days after the stroke she was easily distracted and somnolent, but after a week she became more lucid, mentally alert, and personable. Her memory functions seemed intact but she exhibited some left-right confusion. The patient demonstrated almost complete left hemiplegia with some limited preservation of sensations. Left unilateral neglect and denial of motor or visual impairments were present as well as somatoparaphrenic delusions. When questioned about her left arm, she reported that it belonged to either her son or to her husband.

A CT scan performed 5 days after admission revealed a right temperoparietal infarct.

Case 4

Patient FD was a 77-year-old right-handed female patient who developed a complete left hemiplegia following right hemisphere stroke. At the time when I saw her (8 days after her stroke) she had complete paralysis of left upper and lower limbs, no visual hemineglect (line bisection, line cancellation), and no visual extinction. Touch sensations were partially spared in her left hand, but she showed mild tactile extinction. Visual fields were apparently normal.

Patient FD was very alert and there were no obvious signs of dementia or aphasia; in fact, her intelligence seemed above average. She could do a serial subtraction by twos from 100 without difficulty and was clearly oriented in time and place. When questioned about her family, she provided detailed and accurate descriptions of her son and daughter. She also described the circumstances that led to her hospitalization and was aware she had had a stroke.

Despite the fact that she was mentally lucid, Mrs. D was densely anosognosic and denied her paralysis every time she was questioned. When asked whether she could point she insisted that she could (see under experiment 2 for details). A CT scan performed on the day of admission showed an infarct involving the territory of the right middle cerebral artery and the right cerebellar artery.

Experiment 1: Is There Tacit Knowledge of Paralysis in Anosognosia?

The patients described above repeatedly denied their paralysis, even on those occasions when they were asked to point with their left hand and failed to do so. Is it conceivable, however, that even though they deny their paralysis verbally, they are "aware" at some deeper level that they are in fact paralyzed? And if such tacit knowledge does indeed exist for what types of output is it available?

In my first experiment I confronted the patient with a choice between a unimanual task (e.g., stacking a set of blocks) versus a bimanual task (e.g., tying a shoelace) in a game-like atmosphere. She had to choose only one of these and successfully complete it to obtain a reward (see table 49.1 for a complete list of unimanual/ bimanual task pairs and corresponding prizes). Before each trial, she was first given careful demonstrations of both tasks and told that if she was able to complete one of them, she would be given the corresponding prize. She was also told that if she was unable to accomplish the task successfully, she would be given nothing. The

Table 49.1
Complete list of bimanual and unimanual tasks used in the experiment

Tasks	Prizes
Bimanual	
Tie the laces of a baby shoe	$5.00
Sew yarn around a small card	A ceramic angel
Tie a bow around the large box	A large box of candy
Use scissors to cut a paper circle	
Unimanual	
Screw the nut onto the bolt (mounted on wood to remain perpendicular)	$2.00
Stack five blocks	A bar of scented soap
Pick up objects with a clamp and put them into a bag	A small box of candy
Pick up a toy octopus with a fishing hook and put it into a cup	
Screw a lightbulb onto its holder	

Note: The tasks (left-hand column) were paired randomly with different rewards (right-hand column) on different trials.

combinations of bimanual and unimanual tasks were randomized, along with their prize pairs, but the larger or more valuable prizes were always coupled with the bimanual tasks and the smaller or less valuable prizes with the unimanual tasks.

Since all of the tasks were matched for simplicity, one would expect that nonparalyzed individuals would probably choose the bimanual task, in hopes of receiving the greater reward. (This was validated using two "control" subjects; see below.) Likewise, if the hemiplegic patients were completely unaware of their paralysis then, consistent with their denial, one would expect them also to choose the bimanual task. If, however, they had "tacit" knowledge of their paralysis, they might spontaneously choose the unimanual task.

Results

A total of 19 trials of unimanual versus bimanual choices were administered—8 to Mrs. LR, 6 to Mrs. BM, and 5 to Mrs. OS (Mrs. FD did not participate in this experiment). The experiments were done approximately 2 weeks (LR and BM) or 1 week after the stroke. The tasks (table 49.1) were chosen randomly on different trials and there was usually a 5-min. delay between trials. To Mrs. LR, 4 trials were given on the first day, 2 on the second day, and 2 on the last day and to Mrs. OS all trials were administered during a single testing session. To Mrs. BM the trials were administered on 3 separate days— 2 trials on each day. The tasks, and the corresponding rewards, are described in table 49.1. Two representative trials are described below in some detail.

Patient: LR. Task Choice 1: Tying Bow around Box versus Nut and Bolt The patient was instructed to choose one of two tasks; tying a bow around a large box of candy to receive it as a prize or fastening a nut onto a bolt to win a small box of candy. (The bolt was fixed to a heavy base on the table so that it stood upright and could be easily threaded with one hand.) After hesitating for a few seconds, she decided in favor of the bimanual tying task. The explanation she gave when asked about her choice was that the bigger box "would be easier to work with."

On the second trial with the same tasks and prizes, she immediately chose the unimanual nut and bolt task, but I soon realized that this was because the bow-tying task was located too far in her left visual field, thereby causing her to neglect it. As a result, this trial was not included in the analysis. On all subsequent tasks I took the precaution of presenting the tasks entirely in the right visual field with the exact locations of the objects randomized on different trials.

On the third trial, also with the same task and prize pairs, the patient chose the bimanual option without hesitation. It is interesting to note that her explanation was again, "it seemed easier to work with," yet not even 5 min. had elapsed since she had tried the very same task and failed.

Task Choice 2: Cutting Circle versus Nut and Bolt In this trial the choice was between using scissors to cut out a paper circle (bimanual) for the large box of candy and fastening a nut onto a bolt (unimanual) for the small box. The patient reached for the scissors (bimanual) and attempted unsuccessfully to cut a paper circle (almost 2 min. pass before the first question).

Exp: Why was cutting a circle difficult for you?

Sub: I don't know.

Exp: Try using your other hand.

Sub: Oh, I've never been ambidextrous.

Exp: How many hands does it take to tie a bow?

Sub: Two.

Exp: Can you tie a bow?

Sub: Yes.

Again, it appears that LR has either disregarded or forgotten her previously unsuccessful attempt with the bow-tying task.

Summary of Results from Individual Patients
LR: On 7 of 7 trials, patient LR chose the bimanual task, slowly at first, though it took no more than 2 trials before she was selecting without hesitation. She continued making ineffective attempts to complete the task until interrupted by the experimenter.

BM: On 5 of 6 trials, patient BM chose the bimanual task, sometimes right away and sometimes after a pause. On one occasion (task choice 2 in table 49.1) she immediately chose the unimanual task, reporting that it somehow seemed easier for her.

MS: On 5 of 5 trials, patient MS chose the bimanual task without hesitation. Total for all subjects = 17 of 18 trials bimanual.

Control Condition I also repeated these experiments on two age-matched "control" subjects who had been admitted following an acute right hemisphere stroke producing a left hemiplegia. (The stroke was caused by an infarct in the territory of the right middle cerebral artery.) Both patients had clear signs of left hemineglect, including extinction and right gaze preference but neither of them had any trace of anosognosia. They were thus as close as possible to the experimental group as one could get.

I gave them the unimanual versus bimanual tasks to choose from, as for the experimental group, using identical procedures and instructions. On all 12 trials (8 trials on one subject and 4 on the other) the patients spontaneously chose the unimanual task without any hesitation. At the end of the experiments when I asked them why they had chosen these tasks, they seemed surprised by my question and answered that they had done so because they couldn't use their left hand.

Discussion
We conclude that far from being a mere facade-like condition that leaves room for traces of insight to leak through, anosognosia runs deep. The patients either have no "tacit knowledge" of their paralysis or, even if they do, they cannot access this knowledge when choosing between a unimanual versus bimanual task. It remains to be seen, however, whether other types of tasks might allow the patient to access the knowledge that she is paralyzed. For example, what would happen if the patient were to try to lift a tray full of cocktail glasses? Would her right hand go toward the right side of the tray (as a normal person's might) or would it go straight toward the center of the tray? And what would happen if one were to videotape one of her failed attempts at the bimanual task and play it back to her immediately?[2] Would this enable her to adopt a more abstract attitude toward herself and elicit a confession of paralysis (Ramachandran 1994a,b)

or would it precipitate what Goldstein (1940) has called a "catastrophic reaction?"

It is also important to emphasize, especially, that the patients neither showed obvious signs of *frustration* or distress while trying the bimanual task, nor showed any *learning* despite repeated failures, that is, they seemed to have a selective amnesia for these frustrated attempts even though they recalled other details from the same session quite accurately. For example, during one testing session patient LR remarked that I had been wearing a "tie with pictures of brain scans on it" during the previous session; a fact that many of my students failed to remember. Even on the one occasion when she finally acknowledged her paralysis, she reverted to full denial when questioned again just a few minutes later! I shall return to this point in a later section.

My results also support Babinski's emphasis (1914) on the relatively normal mental status of anosognosics. He described them as being able to remember events and converse lucidly (without confusion, hallucinations, etc.). Like his patient, my three patients also had some subtle abnormalities in judgment and concentration but their denials and delusions were grossly out of proportion to these abnormalities. In any event, such subtle abnormalities of judgment cannot possibly explain why the patient *consistently* chose bimanual task (instead of responding randomly), why they were able to describe the tasks to us clearly, and why they persisted in choosing these tasks despite repeated frustrated attempts.

Experiment 2: The Virtual Reality Box

I will now describe a novel technique that may eventually prove useful in demonstrating "tacit knowledge" of paralysis in patients with anosognosia. The technique is similar to one originally developed for studying intersensory conflict in *normal* subjects (Nielsen 1963), but I realized that it might provide a valuable tool for probing the depth of anosognosia in patients with right parietal lesions (Ramachandran 1994a,b).

The "virtual reality box" was constructed out of cardboard and mirrors. The patient's gloved (paralyzed) left hand is inserted through a window in front of the box and she peeks into the box from a hole in the top to look at what she thinks is her own hand. Unbeknown to the patient, an accomplice inserts his gloved right hand through another opening in the box so that its mirror image is optically superimposed on the patient's left hand and she is "tricked" into thinking that she is looking directly at her own left hand. After being given some practice with the right hand, the patient is instructed to move her (paralyzed) left hand up and down to the rhythm of a metronome. The accomplice then moves his hand to the same rhythm so that the patient is "fooled" into thinking that her hand is indeed obeying her command! The question is would the patient be surprised to see her own left hand come to life even though she doesn't explicitly acknowledge the paralysis? The surprise might manifest itself explicitly (i.e., a verbal exclamation) or at least a change in the patient's expression and/or a galvanic skin response (GSR).

For practical reasons I was able to study only one patient (Mrs. FD) properly, using this procedure. She had sustained a right middle cerebral artery stroke with left hemiplegia and anosognosia (see under Patients for clinical details). Mrs. FD was seen by me on three successive occasions: 8 days, 10 days, and 15 days after her stroke. Even on the first session she spoke slowly but fluently and had no obvious signs of aphasia or dementia; in fact, her clarity of thought and mentation were exceptionally clear. She performed accurately on serial subtraction by twos and was able to give us detailed and accurate information about her family (e.g., her son's job and occupation). Furthermore, she had no hemineglect (line bisection and line cancellation), no visual extinction, and mild tactile extinction. Yet she was densely anosognosic, denying that her left hand was paralyzed. When I grabbed it, raised it toward her nose, and asked her whose hand it was, she said "It is your hand, doctor." (This cannot be ascribed to confusion; when I gripped my student's hand and held it under her nose she said "that is her hand" pointing to my student).

When asked whether she could point to my nose with her left hand she said she could. I then actually asked her to point and asked "Mrs. D, are you now pointing to my nose?" She said, "Yes I am." "Can you clearly see it pointing?" I asked. "Yes I can, it is about 2 inches from your nose," she replied.

Last I asked Mrs. D to clap her hands and she proceeded to do so with gusto, making clapping movements with her right hand alone, as though "clapping" an imaginary left hand! When asked whether she was clapping successfully she said "yes," without hesitation. (Thus, we may, at last, have an answer to the Zen Master's riddle "What is the sound of one hand clapping?" Mrs. D. obviously knew the answer!).

During the following testing session I tried the virtual reality box on Mrs. FD. When she saw her left hand appear to move to the rhythm of the metronome she expressed no surprise whatsoever and when queried specifically, replied "yes I see it moving." I then repeated the experiment with her *normal* hand, asking the stooge to keep her gloved hand absolutely still. Mrs D then started to move her right hand up and down to the metronome, but the view afforded her inside the box was of a perfectly stationary hand (the stooge's). When she looked inside all she could see was a hand that looked perfectly stationary. Yet when questioned again, she maintained that she could clearly see the hand move up and down! This simple experiment demolishes all "neglect" theories of anosognosia since there was certainly no neglect of the right visual (or somatic) field and yet she was producing confabulations about her right hand! Clearly, what is critical is the presence of a *discrepancy* in sensory inputs; it is not critical whether the discrepancy arises from the left or from the right side of the body.[3]

Experiment 3: Repressed Memories: Preliminary Evidence from a Single Case Study

The two experiments that we have discussed so far provided no evidence for "tacit knowledge" of paralysis in these patients. Is it possible, though, that the information is there but simply not accessible? And in the case of the unimanual/bimanual choice experiments, to what extent does the selective anmesia for the failed attempts arise because the relevant memory was never acquired in the first place, given the denial, and to what extent from "repression" causing a failure of retrieval? (This question can be asked of other types of amnesia too, of course, but is especially relevant to the amnesia for paralysis described here.) Certain remarks made by patient LR suggest that the latter explanation might be correct. For example, on one occasion when my student asked her (in my absence) about the previous testing session, she remembered, "That nice Indian doctor ... he asked me to tie shoe laces," and added *without being prompted*, "I did it successfully *using both hands*" (my italics). The vehemence of this assertion is reminiscent of what Freud calls "reaction formation" and it obviously implies tacit knowledge of paralysis. For if she didn't have such knowledge, why would she actually volunteer the information that she used two hands—something that no normal person would do? Mrs. LR's frequent use of euphemisms when directly confronted with her paralysis also strongly suggests that she "knows" about her paralysis at some level (e.g., "I have never been very ambidextrous," "It isn't very fast today, is it?" or "I am unable to *facilitate* my arm").

Would it be possible, however, to demonstrate more *directly* that these patients do indeed repress unpleasant aspects of their experiences? A remarkable piece of evidence for such subconscious knowledge comes from another experiment we did on patient BM. The reader will recall that this patient denied her paralysis even upon repeated questioning and she finally asserted confidently that the arm belonged to her son. Now ordinarily, one thinks of this syndrome as arising from destruction or lesions in the right parietal lobe but, if this is true, how does one explain the fact that parietal lobe syndrome is one of those neurological disorders which show a very high rate of spontaneous remissions within a few weeks? One argument might be that as in the case of phantom limbs (Ramachandran 1993), some other part of the cortex (e.g., the other hemisphere) might "take over" some of these functions but a remarkable discovery made by Bisiach and his co-workers (Bisiach, Rusconi, and Vallar 1992) and by Cappa, Sterzi, Vallar, and Bisiach (1987) suggests an alternative, more exciting possibility. Bisiach et al. studied a patient who had sustained a right hemisphere stroke and was suffering from the delusion that his left arm belonged to someone else. They found, to their surprise, that when they stimulated the vestibular system by irrigating the patient's left ear canal with ice cold water, there was a complete disappearance of symptoms! (Unfortunately, a few hours after the caloric stimulation had worn off, the symptoms returned and the patient once again started denying ownership of his arm.) The important implication of this discovery is that denial and neglect may result from a temporary dysfunction of certain neural circuits in the right hemisphere, rather than from a permanent destruction of neural tissue.

I decided to try a caloric test on patient BM. After she had repeated several times that she was not paralyzed and her arm belonged to her son, I administered 10 cc of ice-cold water into her left ear and waited until nystagmus appeared. My main interest was not only in replicating Bisiach et al.'s observation, but also in specifically asking her questions about her *memory*, an issue that had never been studied directly before on a systematic basis.

E: Do you feel okay?

P: My ear is very cold but other than that I am fine.

E: Can you use your hands?

P: I can use my right arm but not my left arm. I want to move it but it doesn't move.

E: (holding the arm in front of the patient) Whose arm is this?

P: It is my hand, of course.

E: Can you use it?

P: No, it is paralyzed.

E: Mrs. M, how long has your arm been paralyzed? Did it start now or earlier?

P: It has been paralyzed continuously for several days now.

After the caloric effect had worn off completely, I waited for 1/2 h and asked:

E: Mrs. M, can you use your arm?

P: No, my left arm doesn't work.

Finally, the same set of questions was repeated to the patient 8 h later, in my absence, by one of my colleagues.

E: Mrs. M, can you walk?

P: Yes.

E: Can you use both your arms?

P: Yes.

E: Can you use your left arm?

P: Yes.

E: This morning, two doctors did something to you. Do you remember?

P: Yes. They put water in my ear; it was very cold.

E: Do you remember they asked some questions about your arms, and you gave them an answer? Do you remember what you said?

P: No, what did I say?

E: What do you think you said? Try and remember.

P: I said my arms were okay.

These observations have several remarkable implications. First, they confirm Bisiach et al.'s

(1992) observation about remission from anosognosia and delusion following caloric stimulation.[4] Second, they also allow us to draw certain important new inferences about denial and memory repression. Specifically, her admission that she had been paralyzed for several days suggests that even though she had been continuously denying her paralysis, the information about the paralysis was being continuously laid down in her brain, that is, the *denial did not prevent memory consolidation* (Ramachandran 1994a,b). Part of this, of course, could have been simply a confabulatory "filling in" of the gap between her present knowledge of paralysis and the memory of her admission to the hospital but her use of phrases such as "continuously" or "several days" suggests that this was not the case. (And, in any event, the filling-in hypothesis does not explain why she should *confabulate* rather than simply plead ignorance or admit that she had been feeling normal prior to the caloric testing. In this regard, Mrs. BM's apparent lack of surprise at her own admission of paralysis is also noteworthy for it implies that she was now repressing the denial she had been engaging in just 10 min. earlier!). We may tentatively conclude, therefore, that at some deeper level she does indeed have knowledge about the paralysis. Notice also that the insight gained during the caloric stimulation seemed to last at least for 1/2 h after the stimulation had ceased, but that when she was questioned again 8 h later, she not only reverted to denial, but also repressed the admission of paralysis that she had made during her stimulation!

Contrary to the frequently expressed view that memory repression is not a real phenomenon (Holmes 1990), my findings provide compelling experimental/clinical evidence that it is indeed a robust psychological process. Furthermore, these results have important implications for our understanding of how normal memory processes work for they suggest that the separation of memory processes by black-boxologists into "acquisition," "consolidation," "storage," "recognition," "recall," and so on, may be somewhat artificial and misleading. The reason Mrs. BM "forgot" her earlier admission of paralysis may be that it would have been very difficult for her to deny her *present* paralysis and yet admit the insight she had acquired 8 h earlier, while at the same time maintaining an integrated self. Instead of simply retrieving a file from the past, it was almost as though she was completely rewriting the script, for this was the only way she could avoid falling apart completely. We may conclude, therefore, that remembering something even from the recent past entails *a reordering of one's conscious experience to accommodate current demands* (Ramachandran 1994a,b). Right parietal patients provide a valuable opportunity for seeing these phenomena in amplified form but it is probably something we all engage in when trying to remember something.

But when exactly does the "reconceptualization" of experiences and selective repression seen in these patients occur? Does it happen during consolidation or only during subsequent split-second retrieval? Surprising as it might seem, we have to consider the possibility that as soon as the cold water begins to act, the restructuring of experiences occurs almost immediately by altering synaptic weights to accommodate the patient's current ensemble of beliefs. So, in a sense, we are able to create two mutually amnesic conscious beings—the regular Mrs. BM whom we saw in the clinic every morning and the "cold-water Mrs. BM" produced by caloric stimulation.

A Darwinian Theory of Defense Mechanisms

Why do psychological defense mechanisms exist? Freud's suggestion that they serve to defend the ego, although not incorrect, is too vague to be useful since it doesn't tell us why the ego needs to be defended, in the first place. On the face of it holding false beliefs actually seems maladaptive and we must therefore look for a functional or Darwinian explanation to account for their origin.

I suggest that the various defense mechanisms such as rationalization, repression, and so on arise because the brain/mind tries to arrive at the most *probable* and globally consistent interpretation of evidence derived from multiple sources. By way of analogy, consider a military general in a war room trying to make a major strategic decision, for example, whether to invade a particular city at sunrise. He would ordinarily collect evidence from a large number of scouts, weigh the evidence, and arrive at a firm decision. Assume, for the sake of argument, that he has decided to launch the attack at dawn, drawn up his plans accordingly, and directed his soldiers to assume certain strategic positions. Now, if one scout were to show up 15 min. before sunrise and provide information that was somewhat contradictory to the rest (e.g., he might indicate that the enemy had 10,000 soldiers rather than 5000), the general is unlikely to change his strategy. He may ask the scout to shut up and discard the evidence, and, for fear of mutiny, may even ask the scout to "march in tune" with the others and *lie* to the other officers in the army. (The former would be analogous to "denial" and the latter to a "confabulation.") A perpetually indecisive general, on the other hand, would be quite incapable of winning a war.

An analogous process also seems to occur when the visual system tries to combine multiple sources of information about relative depth (e.g., perspective, stereo, occlusion, motion parallax, shading) to yield a vivid coherent impression of depth (Ramachandran 1988, 1989). The rules that the visual system uses to combine multiple cues are poorly understood but may involve:

1. Taking a weighted average. The weighing is important because, statistically speaking, some cues might be inherently more reliable than others and this "wisdom" might be wired into the visual system during ontogeny and phylogeny.

2. Looking for consistency, for example, if six cues yield random values and two yield identical values, then the visual system may "choose" the latter instead of averaging the values. We suggest that the reason for this is that accidental inconsistencies are relatively common in nature (due to noise), whereas accidental consistencies are extraordinarily rare.

Interestingly, once a global interpretation of depth has been reached, the system simply ignores or suppresses the conflicting information. (The purpose of this might be to avoid going into a perpetually indecisive state, i.e., the rule might be that any firm decision is better than none at all.) Now the remarkable thing is that the visual system may, on occasion, even "hallucinate" some of the required evidence in order to preserve consistency, that is, there appears to be a tendency to actually *impose* coherence. It was as though the general had decided not only to ignore the advice of one of his scouts, but also insisted that the scout actually fabricate the evidence required in order to fit the "big picture." Indeed, he may on occasion even employ "yes men" for the specific purpose of cheering him along!

A striking example of this can be observed with the illusory square (Kanizsa 1979) (figure 49.1) which is created by simply aligning four disks from which pie-shaped sectors have been removed. What people usually see when viewing this display is an opaque white square partially occluding four back disks, rather than four disks that have been elaborately prepared and aligned by the experimenter.

Now it should be obvious that when seeing a square in this display, the visual system has to discard the contrary evidence from the homogeneous paper surface about the absence of an edge (for such an edge would usually be associated with a change of luminance). But instead of discarding the perception of a square, the visual system seems to opt for actually hallucinating an illusory edge, which even has an illusory brightness change associated with it. (In a connectionist model, this would be an example of

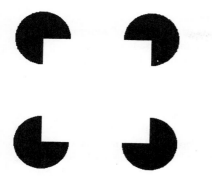

Figure 49.1
An illusory square (Kanizsa 1979). Subjects perceive an illusory white square occluding four black discs in the background rather than four black sectored discs. The illusory perceptual completion seen in these displays may be analogous to the confabulations of right hemisphere patients (see text).

"vector completion.") So here is a clear example of the visual system distorting the evidence in order to impose a coherent interpretation.

Now in my view, the same sort of thing happens in the cognitive/emotional domain. We have a tremendous need to impose a sense of order and coherence in our lives—we need a "story." Of course, when most of the evidence favors one particular interpretation of the available data, we have no difficulty in simply accepting that interpretation. For example, even when a patient's arm is paralyzed, her motor cortex sends messages to her limb and there is a comparator in her brain that ordinarily monitors these feed forward signals and informs her "self" that "I am moving my limb." Therefore, her conscious self tentatively accepts this story. When the evidence is conflicting, however (e.g., if the patient's vision tells her that her arm is not obeying her commands), then instead of wasting time in conflict or oscillating between alternate decisions, her cognitive system simply *picks one story and adheres to it*. Again, in order to do this, it either ignores the conflicting evidence ("denial") or actually fabricates new evidence (ratio-

nalization). The evolutionary purpose of such "defense mechanisms" might be that when limited time is available, *any* decision, however uncertain, is better than an indecisive vacillation—so long as it is the best interpretation of the current data. But to deal with a conflicting source of information that keeps nagging away at the central processor, the latter may actually insert the relevant evidence so that it can go about the rest of its business. What you end up with, therefore, is a "rationalization" or a "denial."[5]

The Anomaly Detector

And that brings me to my last point. The purpose of a "rationalization" we have seen is to eliminate discrepancy by creating fictitious evidence (or false beliefs). But clearly there must be limits to this process, for otherwise defense mechanisms would soon become maladaptive and threaten the individual's survival. It may be a good thing to repress an extremely traumatic memory in order to avoid being paralyzed with fear. This *would* be adaptive. It would be maladaptive, however, to repress every memory that was unpleasant since that would defeat the very purpose of having aversive memories in the first place. I suggest, therefore, that there is a special purpose mechanism—an anomaly detector—in the right parietal lobe whose sole purpose is to serve as a "devil's advocate" that periodically challenges the left hemisphere's "story," detects anomalies or discrepancies, and generates a paradigm shift if the discrepancy is too large. (You can think of this, if you like, as a mechanism for preserving intellectual honesty or integrity.) Hence, I might be willing to engage in some minor rationalization, that is, make some small false assumptions to get on with my life but when the false beliefs become too far removed for reality, my anomaly detector kicks in and makes me reevaluate the situation (e.g., if I was a general about to wage war, it would be quite appropriate, usually, to ignore contrary evidence from a single scout, but if he told me that the enemy was waving a white flag or had nuclear arms, I would be foolish to adhere to my original decision). I suggest, further, that the mechanism for imposing consistency (i.e., the small rationalizations, repressions, etc.) is located in the left hemisphere whereas the "questioning" mechanism that monitors the level of discrepancy, *discovers large-scale anomalies and reacts with the appropriate paradigm shift—including the appropriate emotion—is in the right hemisphere.*[6] This would explain why right hemisphere patients are willing to engage in much more elaborate and fanciful rationalizations than normal individuals or individuls with left hemisphere damage. Conversely, left hemisphere stroke patients may not be able to manage even a minimal amount of denial, rationalization, or confabulatory "gap-filling" and consequently become profoundly depressed. This would be a new interpretation of the common clinical observation that depression is most often associated with left hemisphere (especially left frontal) stroke.

I have not yet adequately dealt with the important question of why anosognosia is apparently *domain specific*; why some patients deny their paralysis and yet admit they had a stroke. One possibility is that this is really a threshold effect, that is, the denial only *appears* to be domain specific but really isn't. The defenses employed by the left hemisphere may be applied selectively only when there is a disturbing discrepancy such as the patient's feeling that she can move her arm versus the verbal and visual feedback she receives informing her that she is paralyzed. The reason patient BM acknowledged her diabetes, however, may simply be because this wasn't quite as threatening to her complacency as being confronted by the immediate reality of her paralysis. A second possibility is there are indeed separate consistency-imposing mechanisms (or even "anomaly detectors") subserving individual domains such as one's body image.[7] The generation of paradigm shifts in response to inconsistencies, on the other hand,

may always require right hemisphere intervention. A more careful study of additional patients might help resolve these issues.

Finally, I emphasize that although the clinical evidence suggests the presence of an anomaly detector in the right hemisphere, the theoretical justification for having a *separate* mechanism for this purpose is unclear. One possibility is that the mechanism prevents the left hemisphere from becoming trapped in local minima by giving it a periodic jolt. The key difference between the two hemispheres, however, may be not that one hemisphere detects anomalies and the other doesn't, but that the way in which they *deal* with anomalies is very different, that is, they have different coping strategies. When a small local anomaly is detected, the left hemisphere tries to *impose consistency by ignoring or suppressing the contrary evidence*, for example, by Freudian defense mechanisms, but when the anomaly reaches threshold, an interaction with the right hemisphere *forces a complete change in one's world view—a paradigm shift*. (And, to that extent, the right hemisphere may be said to be more "sensitive" to anomalies.)[8] Until we have a clearer understanding of the underlying neural mechanisms we must accept these metaphorical explanations as a temporary substitute. Meanwhile, if they suggest interesting new experiments, they will have adequately served their purpose.

Summary and Conclusions

My purpose, in part 1 of this article, has been mainly to present some clinical case studies as well as some novel experimental approaches to the problem of anosognosia. The results of these experiments are still very preliminary, but they have already allowed us to probe this syndrome a little more deeply than in the past. They complement the important work of Bisiach et al. (1992), Galin (1992), Critchley (1966), Heilman (1991), and others and serve to remind us of the important role that this enigmatic disorder is likely to play in any future discussions of consciousness and awareness of self—issues that have traditionally belonged to the province of philosophers.

Part 2: Some Theoretical Speculations

The previous section of this article was concerned mainly with some new empirical findings on patients with anosognosia, together with brief discussions on their theoretical implications. In this section, I would like to use these findings as a starting point to speculate on a wide range of topics such as dreams, humor, REM sleep, and psychoanalysis, topics that are of enduring interest to psychologists studying consciousness and representation of self. I might add that although these ideas are speculative, at least some of them lead to clear, testable predictions.

Humor and Laughter: A Biological Hypothesis

Consider how essentially the same dichotomy between the two hemispheres may help explain another major biological puzzle—the origin of humor and laughter. Theories of humor and laughter go all the way back to Kant (1790) and Schopenhauer (1819), two singularly humorless German philosophers. Typically, humor involves taking someone up along a garden path of expectation so that the left hemisphere (in our scheme) is allowed to construct a story or model and then introducing a sudden unexpected twist at the end. Of course the twist is necessary but certainly not sufficient to generate humor; for example, if my plane were about to land in San Diego and one of the engines failed unexpectedly, I would not regard this as very funny. The key idea here is that the twist has to be novel but *inconsequential*. Thus, we may regard humor as a response to an inconsequential anomaly.

Incongruity theories of humor have a long history (e.g., see Gregory 1991). I would like to take these early ideas a step further by invoking

hemispheric specialization and by proposing a specific explanation for the loud, explosive, stereotyped quality of the sound associated with laughter. I suggest that humor emerges when a dialogue between the consistency imposing tendencies in the left hemisphere and the anomaly detector in the right hemisphere leads to a *premature paradigm shift*. Imagine you are in a dimly lit room late at night and hear some annoying sounds. Ordinarily you interpret this to be the wind or something equally innocuous. If it gets a little louder you continue to ignore it, following the left hemisphere's strategy of ignoring evidence contrary to its preexisting model. But now the sound gets really loud and your right hemisphere forces a paradigm shift; you decide it must be a burglar and orient to the presumed anomaly. Your limbic system is activated so that you are both aroused and angry—preparing to fight or flee. But then you discover that it is in fact your neighbor's cat and so you laugh and harmlessly displace the emotion that has been built up.

But why laughter? Why the particularly loud, explosive, repetitive sound? Freud's view that then you discharge pent-up psychic energy doesn't make much sense without recourse to an elaborate hydaraulic metaphor. I suggest, instead, that laughter evolved specifically to *alert others in the social group that the anomaly is inconsequential*; that is, they need not bother orienting. For example, if someone slips and falls and hurts herself you don't laugh; in fact, you rush to her aid. But if she doesn't get hurt then you do laugh (the basis of all slapstick humor), thereby signaling to others that they need not rush to the fallen person's aid. Thus laughter is nature's "false-alarm" signaling mechanism.

Notice, however, that although this view explains the logical structure of humor, it doesn't explain why humor itself is sometimes used as a psychological defense mechanism. One possibility is that, *jokes are an attempt to trivialize what would otherwise by genuinely disturbing anomalies*. In other words, when an anomaly is detected, it is ordinarily dealt with by orienting or—when appropriate—by denial or repression but if, for some reason, it becomes more conspicuous and starts clamoring for attention, then an alternate strategy would be to *pretend* that it is a trivial anomaly by using a joke (i.e., you set off your own "false alarm" mechanism). Thus, a mechanism that originally evolved specifically as an ethological signal to appease others in the social group, has now become internalized to deal with cognitive anomalies—in the form of a psychological defence mechanism. (Hence the phrase "nervous laughter.")

A Theory of REM Sleep and Dreaming:
Nature's Own Virtual Reality

One of the most curious findings I have considered in this article is the remission of anosognosia and the reactivation of associated memories produced by caloric/vestibular stimulation. Why does vestibular stimulation produce these remarkable effects? I shall suggest three explanations that are not mutually exclusive.

1. The cold water may produce a nonspecific "arousal" of the right hemisphere, and this (in our scheme) allows the anomaly detector in the right hemisphere to become functional again. This hypothesis would be consistent with physiological work on animals that demonstrate a powerful cerebral activation (Fredrickson, Kornhuber, and Schwartz 1974) during vestibular stimulation.

2. The vestibular stimulation may alter the patient's spatial frame of reference by allowing the right hemisphere to "orient" to the left side so as to eliminate the neglect of the left side of the body as. This may make the patient more "aware" of the left side of the body and thus, indirectly, more aware of the paralysis. The fact that we could induce Mrs. D to produce confabulations concerning her *right* hand argues against this interpretation (which is not to say that it doesn't contribute to the anosagnosia at least in some patients).

3. A third, more intriguing possibility is that the vigorous nystagmus itself is somehow causally linked to the chain of events that leads to the remission from anosognosia and the derepression of memories that we observed. This idea is not as farfetched as it sounds. After all, the link between eye movements and reactivation or "derepression" of unconscious memories can also be seen in dreaming associated with REM sleep and it is known that bursts of spontaneous vestibular neuronal activity occur in animals during REM sleep (Pompeiano 1974). One way to test this hypothesis would be to elicit nystagmus in these patients using a rotating striped drum to see if there is any remission from anosognosia. Furthermore, the advent of new imaging techniques such as PET, MEG, and functional MRI might eventually allow us to determine the exact cause-effect sequence that underlies this extraordinary phenomenon.

Developing this theme a little further, I suggest that during ordinary waking life the left hemisphere engages in "on-line" processing of sense data, including the temporal ordering of experiences and the imposition of consistency and coherence. This would necessarily involve the kinds of censoring, repressions, denials, and rationalizations that characterize most of our daily lives. In dream sleep, on the other hand, the mind/brain is allowed to tentatively bring some of the repressed memories out for an "improv" rehearsal on the main stage to see if they can be coherently incorporated into the main script without penalty to the ego. If the rehearsal doesn't lead to a stable organization, however, the material gets repressed again (unless you wake up accidentally, in which case it emerges in disguised form but is not incorporated into your psyche). But if it *does* work, then it gets incorporated seamlessly into the conscious self in the left hemisphere so that you personality becomes progressively more refined and less encumbered by unnecessary defenses. (This might explain why psychoanalysis is so notoriously difficult. What the therapist tries to do during wakefulness is precisely what nature has evolved to *avoid* during wakefulness and allows to occur only during REM sleep.) I suggest, therefore, that the eye movements generated by caloric stimulation in Mrs. BM may have produced their remarkable effects by emulating REM sleep and allowing a temporary "derepression" of her knowledge of paralysis in a manner analogous to what happens normally in dream sleep.

At the risk of pushing the analogy a bit too far, let us return once again to our general in the war room. Recall that during the day, in the heat of battle, he simply had no time to consider the contrary evidence from the single scout and therefore decided to shove it into a drawer marked "Top Secret. Do not open." It is now late at night and while relaxing over a glass of cognac he decides, "maybe I should take a second look at that file, after all, to see if I can incorporate into my battle strategy for the next day." Since he is not, at this time, actively engaged in making more important decisions, he can afford a leisurely contemplation of that file to see if its contents can be incorporated into his plans. And this, in my view, is exactly what happens each time you dream—you open your top-secret files and "psychoanalyze" yourself!

If this hypothesis is correct, one would also expect that in marked contrast to Freud's wish-fulfillment theory, patients with anosognosia should actually *dream that they are paralyzed*, for example, if the patient is woken up during a REM episode, one might expect her to say, "I feel okay now. I can use both hands. But, you know, it's funny—I dreamed that my left hand was paralyzed." This counterintuitive prediction has never been tested directly but the experiment would be easy enough to do. (Recall, also, that in patient BM the effects of caloric stimulation continued for 30 min. after the nystagmus had subsided. Hence, it is not inconceivable that for a short period after the patient is woken up from REM sleep, she might continue to admit her paralysis before eventually reverting once again to denial.)

My hypothesis on dreams is different from—although not inconsistent with—Hobson's (1988) well-known proposal that dreams are essentially an attempt to see meaningful patterns in "noise" generated by PGO activity. It is, however, similar to the ingenious suggestion of Winson (1986), who has postulated that dreaming involves a rehearsal and consolidation of both instinctive and learned patterns of behavior. (It is noteworthy that Winson arrived at his theory starting from a completely different set of initial assumptions based on his physiological work on the hippocampus.) The key difference is that I invoke hemispheric specialization. Furthermore, in my scheme, an important function of dreaming is to allow the vestibular neuronal bursts that occur during REM sleep to selectively *derepress disturbing memories so that you are given the opportunity to unburden yourself of unnecessary or maladaptive defenses.* One can ask, of course, why the same goal cannot be achieved during wakefulness; why can't you simply try out the rehearsals when awake? It makes sense that you can't enact them *literally* since that might actually put you in physical danger, but, as pointed out by Jouvet (1975), this is neatly avoided by using a powerful barrage of inhibitory signals to completely paralyze all your somatic muscles during REM sleep.[9] The reason you can't carry out these rehearsals in your *imagination*, however, is less obvious but three possibilities come to mind. First, during wakefulness the brain may be actively engaged in more important activities like our general in the war room, and daydreaming may simply be too costly an option. Second, for the rehearsals to be effective, they must look and feel like the real thing and this may not be possible when you are awake since you know that the images are internally generated. (As Shakespeare said, "You cannot cloy the hungry edge of appetite with bare imagination of a feast.") Indeed, during wakefulness the system that generates imagery may be temporarily disconnected from your limbic system so that imagery can never actually substitute for the real thing (which would make good evolutionary sense), whereas in dreams there may be limbic activation as well, in order to ensure verisimilitude. Third, and most important in our scheme, unmasking disturbing memories when awake would defeat the very purpose of repressing them in the first place and may have a profound destabilizing effect on the system, whereas unmasking them during REM may permit realistic and emotionally charged simulations (so realistic, in fact, that you may actually have an orgasm with your boss's wife and ejaculate during a dream—the so-called "wet dream"). Dreams may therefore be a way of "having one's cake and eating it too"—of reenacting highly realistic simulations without taking any of the associated emotional risks (in our scheme) or physical risks (in Jouvet's). They are nature's own virtual reality.

A Hypothesis Concerning Classical Anterograde Amnesia

I will consider now how our ideas concerning motivational repression might also help explain bilateral mesial temporal lobe amnesia (Squire 1987), a syndrome characterized by normal immediate memory (e.g., digit span), a profound anterograde amnesia (failure to acquire new "long-term" memories) and intact memories for events that preceded the onset of the disease (i.e., no retrograde amnesia). The currently popular view is that the syndrome results from a failure of consolidation resulting from damage to the hippocampal system, rather than a failure of acquisition or retrieval. The old idea that amnesia (e.g., Korsakoff's amnesia) might result from "motivational repression" fell into disfavor because it fails to explain why even emotionally neutral memories (e.g., a list of words) are quickly forgotten, whereas the patient has no difficulty remembering the emotionally disturbing circumstances (e.g., alcoholism) that led to his hospitalization.

I would like to revive a modified version of the old view in the light of our hypothesis and sug-

gest that the basis of the classical amnesic syndrome is a faulty hippocampal gating system that causes the patient to *indiscriminately repress* all memories rather than just disturbing ones. In other words, the memories are all there but they are locked away in the wrong drawers labeled "don't open." This would explain why the patient has no retrograde amnesia since the older memories were laid down *before* the repression mechanism became faulty.[10] In addition, it would also explain the preservation of "priming" effects and procedures or skills in these patients, since these do not require conscious retrieval and are, therefore, unlikely to be repressed. The "blocked-access" hypothesis makes two simple predictions: (a) That caloric stimulation might help the patient access some of the repressed memories that were apparently forgotten. (b) If woken during REM sleep, the patient might actually report some of the events that occurred during the day, that is, his "day residues" may be just as vivid as that of normal nonamnesic control subjects. Such experiments would be illuminating whether one believed in the particular theory being proposed here.

If my general argument is correct, however, then the derepression of "lost" memories should be seen not only in amnesia but also during routine caloric testing of any neurological patient. One reason such effects have not been reported might be simply that vestibular stimulation only *partially* mimics the unmasking of memories that occur naturally during REM episodes. Consequently, the only memories that would surface would be the ones that were recently repressed, whereas long-lasting traumatic memories that have been strongly censored for many years may not be activated sufficiently to reach threshold.

Summary and Conclusions

The theory of human nature that I have proposed in this article has much more in common with biologically based theories of cognition and perception (Crick 1994, Edelman 1989) than it does with the central tenets of classical AI. As we have pointed out in the past (Ramachandran 1990), classical AI ignores the relevance of the neural machinery in the brain and the evolutionary history of the organism, both of which can provide vital clues to understanding the functional organization of complex biological systems such as the human brain. No engineer in his right mind, for example, could have foreseen a link between the inner ear and cognitive functions such as memory retrieval, dreams, or Freudian psychology.

My purpose, also, has been to provide a new framework for linking several seemingly unrelated phenomena such as anosognosia, REM, amnesia, and laughter. I made two sets of key assumptions (A and B) that are logically independent of each other:

Assumption A

1. The coping strategies of the two hemispheres are fundamentally different.

2. When a small incongruity is detected that doesn't fit the preexisting model or framework, an attempt is made to force a fit. In the cognitive domain this involves denial, rationalization, confabulation, dissociation etc. The purpose of doing this is to ensure consistency and stability of behavior and to avoid indecisive vascillation. (The argument here is that *any* decision, even a partially flawed one, is better than indecision.) Although these psychological defence mechanisms may have originally evolved in a social context they have now become internalized and provide emotional/cognitive stability at the individual level.

3. This particular coping strategy, that is, discarding or distorting the evidence to preserve the status quo, is adopted largely by the left hemisphere (It is important to stress that one is probably dealing with partial rather than exclusive specialization.). I would argue that this is done not just for language but for cognitive consistency in general, although language is the most obvious external manifestation.

4. When the anomaly reaches threshold a "devil's advocate" in the right hemisphere intervenes and forces a paradigm shift, that is, instead of discarding or distorting the evidence an attempt is made to question the status quo and to construct a new model. The paradigm shift also leads to a strong "orienting" and emotional response and to the production of a novel set of behaviors appropriate to the new model.

5. A dialogue between these two opposing tendencies of the two hemispheres may help account for many enigmatic aspects of human nature including the genesis of humor, laughter, and dreams.

Assumption B

1. Vestibular/caloric stimulation eliminates not only anosognosia but also appears to reactivate (or "derepress") the patient's memories of her previous failed attempts.

2. Caloric stimulation may produce its remarkable effects by mimicking the reactivation (or derepression) of memories that is presumed to occur during REM sleep.

These two sets of assumptions (A and B) form the cornerstone of our theory and they lead to several novel predictions. I would emphasize, however, that even if one of these assumptions turns out to be wrong, for example, the view that vestibular stimulation mimics REM sleep, the experimental predictions may still have some heuristic value since they do not depend *critically* on this assumption. For example, the question of whether amnesics remember their "day residues" during REM sleep would be interesting whether or not one believed the particular theory being advanced here. And so, also, would be the outcome of the "virtual reality" experiment[11] or the experiments attempting to elicit tacit knowledge or repressed memories in anosognosia. Indeed, these experiments might have implications for memory research that go well beyond their immediate implications for understanding anosognosia. As well as demonstrating, vividly, that memory is an active, constructive process (as emphasized by Edelman 1989), the study of patients with this disorder may allow us to insert an experimental lever into the mental machinery that merges new memories seamlessly into one's preexisting conceptual categories. Such experiments would be especially easy to conduct in conjunction with the caloric-induced "reversible hyperamnesia"—if that effect is confirmed on additional patients. However, since patients with this syndrome tend to recover spontaneously over a period of several days, the experiments could also in principle be carried out, even without the caloric testing, by simply interviewing the patient repeatedly about her memories as she gradually regained insight.[12] Finally, we would emphasize also that our ideas on the biological function of humor and dreaming depend only on the validity of the assumptions described under (A) rather than (B) and they can be tested directly by a careful study of patients with lateralized focal brain lesions.

Many individual fragments of this puzzle have been around for a long time, for example, Gazzaniga's idea that in split-brain patients the left hemisphere has a language-based "interpreter" that provides a running commentary of events (Gazzaniga 1992), Bogen's novel suggestion (Bogen 1975) that the right hemisphere may be involved in "appositional thinking," that laughter involves a deflation of built-up expectation (Spencer 1860, Kant 1790), or that there may be specialized mechanisms for "reality checks" (Neisser 1967) or "monitoring" (Galin 1992). What I have tried to do, however, is to come up with a unified theory from a Darwinian perspective that can help link a number of seemingly unrelated phenomena, ranging from Freudian defense mechanisms and somatoparaphrenic delusions to REM sleep and laughter. The theory also makes several predictions that would be easy to test; indeed, some of them have already been partially confirmed. For instance, right parietal patients should have a diminished capacity for appreciating humor but paradoxically their remarks should seem funny to the examining physician (e.g., recall Mrs. LR's remark, "I was never very ambidextrous"). Conversely, when the left hemisphere is dysfunctional, there might be a *diminished* toler-

ance for discrepancies or anomalies along with an inability to deploy psychological defense mechanisms.

Anomaly detection may be a prerequisite for seeing the paradoxial nature of certain visual illusions such as Penrose's impossible triangle. (Consistent with this prediction, we found that when one of the original Sperry–Bogen series of split-brain patients, LB, was shown the triangle either in the left or right visual field, he saw the anomaly only in the left visual field, i.e., when the right hemisphere was viewing the display.) Indeed, one could almost argue that our aesthetic appreciation of Escher's engravings arises from a dialogue or "tension" between the oppressing tendencies of the two hemispheres. And in the language domain, right parietal patients should have difficulty in interpreting fables such as the "sour grapes" story that illustrates the fallacy of rationalization. (The fox who couldn't reach the grapes said to himself, "Oh, the grapes are probably sour anyway.") It is known that literal mindedness is a characteristic of right hemisphere disease (Gardner 1993), but to our knowledge no one has specifically tested their interpretation of fables or stories that illustrate Freudian defense mechanisms (as opposed to *any* fable or proverb).

My scheme would explain the curious delusions experienced by patient FD when she failed to see "her" right hand respond to her commands. When confronted with contradictory information from her different sensory systems, her left hemisphere tries to impose consistency by simply inserting the required evidence, that is, the visual appearance of a moving right hand. Since she has a malfunctioning anomaly detector in her right hemisphere, this bizarre delusion goes unchecked and, consequently, she reports that she can actually *see* her hand moving even though this belief is contradicted by the visual appearance of a stationary hand. The result is so surprising, however, that it needs to be repeated carefully on a large number of patients.

Finally, my scheme also provides a way of linking vestibular activation with dreams, REM sleep, and anosognosia. Specifically, I suggest that the *overt* orienting that normally occurs during wakefulness in response to environmental disturbances or anomalies (including vestibular input) becomes replaced with *covert* orienting toward disturbing anomalous, memories that are derepressed in conjunction with eye movements during REM sleep.[13] The involvement of the vestibular system in all this makes perfect evolutionary sense since it is part of a phylogenetically primitive mechanism that generates "orienting" in response to disturbances—either in the environment or in the body—receiving, as it does, information from many sensory systems. As the brain evolved and became increasingly sophisticated, perhaps it also developed a mechanism in the right hemisphere for monitoring *cognitive* anomalies and disturbances. If so, what better way to generate covert orienting in response to such cognitive anomalies than to hook it up to the vestibular orienting system that is already in place?

Freud and the Inner Ear: A Neurological Approach to Psychotherapy

Talking to a patient with anosognosia can be an uncanny experience. Indeed the reason the disorder seems so peculiar to us is because it brings us face to face with some of the most fundamental questions that one can ask as a conscious human being: What is the "self"? What brings about the unity of my conscious experience? What does it mean to will an action? Such questions are often considered to be outside the scope of legitimate scientific enquiry and neuroscientists usually shy away from them. What I have tried to argue in this essay, however, is that patients with anosognosia afford a unique opportunity for experimentally approaching these seemingly intractable problems. As we have seen, they may even help us answer the eternal riddle "What is the sound of one hand clapping?"

Is it conceivable that there are mechanisms in the right hemisphere that are specialized not only for dealing with anomalies involving the corporeal self but also for dealing with other types of anomalies? According to classical psychoanalytical theory, many forms of neuroses arise because the patient's defense mechanisms have become so extreme that they have actually become maladaptive instead of being simply used as a coping strategy. Providing "insight" into these maladaptive defense mechanisms is, therefore, one of the goals of Freudian psychoanalysis and this is usually achieved by several months or years of intensive psychotherapy. But if I am correct in arguing that that "insight" can be enhanced using caloric left ear stimulation in patients with parietal lesions, is it conceivable that such insight could also be induced in neurotic patients who are neurologically intact, in order to eliminate the maladaptive defenses that are said to produce the psychoneuroses? (Notice that the efficacy of this would not necessarily depend on whether the denial is domain specific or not; all we have to assume is that caloric stimulation can also eliminate other types of anosognosia by activation of the right hemisphere—a proposition that can be tested experimentally.)[14] After all, in patient BM, caloric stimulation not only eliminated denial but also allowed the repressed *memory* of the paralysis to be overcome. What I am suggesting then (tongue-in-cheek!) is that the Barany chair may eventually *replace* the analyst's couch as a device for reviving repressed memories and for producing insight.[15] Obviously, these are highly speculative and tentative ideas but at least they are testable and they may not only point to new directions of research but also eventually suggest new ways to treat the numerous psychological ailments to which our species is notoriously prone.

Acknowledgments

I thank L. Levi and D. Rogers-Ramachandran, who collaborated with me in conducting the caloric stimulation experiments; R. McKinney, M.

Stallcup, and A. Schatz, who provided valuable technical assistance in setting up many of the experiments; and L. Stone and G. Arcilla for referring their patients to me. I also thank Patricia and Paul Churchland, F. H. C. Crick, N. Christenfeld, B. Golomb, H. Pashler, W. Rosar, T. Sejnowski, O. Sacks, J. Smythies, and J. Ramachandran for discussions, and the NIMH for support. I also benefited from several stimulating conversations that I had with J. Bogen and D. Galin. Galin (1974) was one of the first to suggest that the activities of the right hemisphere may correspond to the Freudian unconscious. His extensive comments on an early draft of this paper helped improve its clarity, but any errors that remain are entirely my own.

Notes

1. Throughout this paper I restrict the use of the word *anosognosia* to denial of hemiplegia, not to the generic use of the word to indicate denial of other types of deficits.

2. I recently had the opportunity to try some of these experiments on patient FD. When confronted with a tray of cocktail glasses, her right hand went straight for the right side of the tray. For fear of losing the glasses I grabbed the other end of the tray with my right hand and we lifted it together. When asked whether she had raised the tray by herself she seemed surprised by the question and answered "Yes, of course."

I then wheeled her chair up right in front of a full-length wall mirror, so that she could clearly watch her own performance, and asked her to point to her own image in the mirror using her left hand. Seeing her failure to point had no effect whatsoever on her anosognosia; in fact, she insisted that she could clearly see her left hand in the mirror, pointing as it was supposed to. It remains to be seen how general this effect is. (I would emphasise that Mrs. FD had no visual hemineglect, no apraxia, no autotopagnosia, and no radiological evidence of left hemisphere damage).

3. Similar confabulations occurred when the patient was asked to keep her right hand still while the accomplice's hand moved up and down to the rhythm of the metronome. This time the patient insisted that she was *not* seeing her hand move, that it looked perfectly stationary. We are still a long way from understanding the neural basis of such delusions, but the important recent work of Graziano, Yap, and Gross (1994) may be relevant. They found single neurons in monkey supplementary motor area that had visual receptive fields which were "superimposed" on somatosensory fields on the monkey's hand. Curiously, when the monkey moved its hand the visual receptive field moved with the hand, but eye movements had no effect on the receptive field. These hand-centered visual receptive fields ("monkey see, monkey do" cells) may provide a neural substrate for the kinds of somatoparaphrenic delusions I have seen in my patients.

4. On the previous day I had done the control experiment of irrigating Mrs. BM's *right* ear with water. This produced no remission from anosognosia whatsoever. Thus, the remission certainly cannot be attributed to nonspecific "arousal" produced by cold water.

5. Of course, these mechanisms may have evolved originally in a social context, in conjunction with language. But they may have subsequently become internalised to provide cognitive and emotional stability even though they no longer serve an overtly social function. An interesting empirical question is whether anosognosic patients are equally anosognosic when there is no one watching.

A related question concerns the extent to which patients with denial of paralysis are aware of *other people's* deficits. I recently had the opportunity to explore this on another densely anosognosic patient, Mrs. LH, who had left hemiplegia following a right middle cerebral artery stroke. Mrs. LH insisted that she could see her left hand pointing to me, on command. I then asked her to watch another hemiplegic patient, in the adjacent wheelchair, while he attempted to point to my nose with his left hand. When queried, Mrs. LH insisted that she could indeed see him point! Thus, in this one patient at least, the anosognosia seemed to extend to other peoples' equivalent body parts, while at the same time excluding her own dificits in other domains. This result implies that one may need to access one's own body schema even when making judgments about someone elses body parts. (I might add that Mrs. LH had no apraxia or autotopagnosia and no radiological evidence of left parietal damage.)

6. As with most other types of hemispheric specialization, what we are dealing with here almost certainly is

relative rather than absolute specialization. J. Bogen (personal communication) has pointed out the dangers of "dichotomania."

7. Such exquisite domain specificity is, of course, not unique to anosognosia, and it shows up in many areas of neurology. What are we to make of selective loss of vegetable names with sparing of fruits? Or, of loss of inanimate object names but not of animate ones? Such findings pose a serious challenge for any theory of knowledge representation in the brain.

8. This notion is, of course, quite compatible with the traditional view that the right hemisphere sees the "big picture" or gestalt. Seeing the big picture may be a prerequisite for seeing an anomoly.

9. In a disorder called cataplexy, the patient's somatic muscles become suddenly paralyzed in a manner analogous to the paralysis that accompanies in REM sleep, even though the patient is fully awake. Curiously, the attacks are often precipitated by either laughter or surprise, providing yet another link among dreams, REM sleep, and laughter.

10. An alternate formulation of this hypothesis would be that the hippocampal/limbic gating system is needed primarily for attaching a "value" to an object or event and in its absence, the default option is forgetting.

11. Virtual reality may turn out to be a promising technique for studying illusions of body image. We recently used the technique on a patient with a phantom arm to convey the visual illusion that his arm had been resurrected and was obeying his commands. Remarkably, 15 sessions (10 min. each) of this "therapy," distributed over 2 weeks, resulted in a permanent "amputation" of the phantom limb with a disappearance of pain in the phantom elbow (Ramachandran 1994b).

12. Such sequential interviewing of patients with anosognosia—to elicit memories—has rarely been done on a systematic basis. Four months after her repeated denial of paralysis and repeated failure with bimanual tasks (e.g., tying shoelaces), Mrs. OS had recovered completely from anosognosia and she now complained that her left arm was paralyzed. Her memory for various irrelevant details of the early testing sessions were quite vivid but when asked if she had always been paralyzed, she said "yes." When asked whether she remembered denying the paralysis, she said, "Well, if I was, I must have been lying and I don't usually lie."

13. Physiological similarities between brainstem mechanisms that mediate orienting during REM and orienting during wakefulness have also been emphasized by Morrison (1979).

14. For example, would denial of cortical blindness or "Anton's syndrome" be temporarily relieved? And how about the distortions of body image that are said to accompany anorexia nervosa?

15. Soon after I wrote this essay, it was pointed out to me that there is now a fad therapy, popular among some clinical psychologists, that utilizes eye movements to enhance the patients "insight" and to uncover repressed memories. While I would ordinarily be inclined to dismiss this as bizarre, it makes perfect sense from the point of view of my theory!

References

Babinski, M. J. (1914). Contribution a l'etude des troubles mentaux dans l'hemiplegie organique cerebrale. *Revue Neurologique*, 1, 845–848.

Bisiach, E., Rusconi, M. L., and Vallar, G. (1992). Remission of somatophrenic delusion through vestibular stimulation. *Neuropsychologia*, 29, 1029–1031.

Bogen, J. E. (1975). The other side of the brain. *UCLA Education*, 17, 24–32.

Cappa, S., Sterzi, R., Vallar, G., and Bisiach, E. (1987). Remission of hemineglect and anosognosia after vestibular stimulation. *Neuropsychologia*, 25, 755–782.

Critchley, M. (1962). Clinical investigation of disease of the parietal lobes of the brain. *Medical Clinics of North America*, 46, 837–857.

Critchley, M. (1966). *The parietal lobes.* New York: Hafner.

Crick, F. H. C. (1994). *The astonishing hypothesis.* New York: Scribner's.

Cutting, J. (1978). Study of anosagnosia. *Journal of Neurology, Neurosurgery, and Psychiatry*, 41, 548–555.

Damasio, A. (1994). *Descarte's error.* New York: Putnam.

Edelman, G. M. (1989). *The remembered present.* New York: Basic Books.

Ehrenwald, H. (1930). Verandertes erleben des korperbildes mit konsekutiver wahnbildung bie linksseitiger hemiplegie. *Monatsschrift fur Psychiatrie und Neurologie*, 75, 89–97.

Farrah, M. (1991). *Visual agnosia*. Cambridge, MA: MIT Press.

Fredrickson, J., Kornhuber, H., and Schwartz, D. W. (1974). In H. Kornhuber (Ed.), *Handbook of sensory physiology*, (Vol. VI, 1, pp. 565–583). New York: Springer-Verlag.

Freud, A. (1946). *The Ego and the mechanisms of defense*. New York: International Universities Press.

Freud, S. (1961). *The standard edition of the complete works of Sigmund Freud* (Vol. 1–23). London: Hogarth Press. (Original work published 1895)

Galin, D. (1974). Implications for psychiatry of left and right cerebral specialization. *Archives of General Psychiatry*, 31, 572–583.

Galin, D. (1992). Theoretical reflections on awareness, monitoring and self in relation to anosagnosia. *Consciousness and Cognition*, 1, 152–162.

Gardner, H. (1993). In E. Perceman (Ed.), *Cognitive processing in the right hemisphere*. New York: Academic Press.

Gazzaniga, M. (1992). *Nature's mind*. New York: Basic Books.

Gerstmann, J. (1942). Problem of imperception of disease and of impaired body territories with organic lesions: Relation to body scheme and its disorders. *Archives of Neurology and Psychiatry*, 48, 890–913.

Goldstein, K. (1940). *Human nature*. Cambridge, MA: Harvard Univ. Press.

Graziano, M. S. A., Yap, G. S., and Gross, C. (1994). Coding of visual space by premotor neurons. *Science*, 266, 1051–1054.

Gregory, R. L. (1991). *Odd perceptions*. New York: Routledge, Chapman, & Hall.

Haligan, P., Marshall, J., and Wade, D. (1995). Supernumerary phantom limbs. *Journal of Neurology, Neurosurgery, & Psychiatry*, 59, 341–342.

Heilman, J. (1991). In G. Prigatano and D. Schacter (Eds.), *Awareness of deficits after brain injury*. New York/Oxford: Oxford Univ. Press.

Hobson, J. A. (1988). *The dreaming brain*. New York: Basic Books.

Holmes, D. (1990). The evidence for repression: Examination of 60 years of research. In J. L. Singer (Ed.), *Repression and dissociation*. John, D. and Catherine, T.

MacArthur Foundation series on Mental Health and Development. Chicago, IL: Univ. of Chicago Press.

Joseph, R. (1993). *The naked neuron*. New York: Plenum.

Jouvet, M. (1975). The function of dreaming. In M. Gazzaniga and C. Blakemore (Eds.), *Handbook of psychobiology* (pp. 500–524). New York: Academic Press.

Juba, A. (1949). Beitrag zur struktur der ein-und doppelseitigen korperschemastorungen. *Monatsschrift fur Psychiatrie und Neurologie*, 118, 11–29.

Kanizsa, G. (1979). *Organization in vision*. New York: Praeger.

Kant, I. (1790). *Kritik dev*. Berlin: Unteilskraft.

Levine, D. N. (1990). Unawareness of visual and sensorimotor defects: A hypothesis. *Brain and Cognition*, 13, 233–281.

McGlynn, S. M., and Schacter, D. L. (1989). Unawareness of deficits in neuropsychological syndromes. *Journal of Clinical and Experimental Neuropsychology*, 11, 143–205.

Morrison, A. (1979). Brainstem regulation of behavior in sleep and wakefulness. In J. Sprague and A. N. Epstein (Eds.), *Psychobiology and physiological psychology*. New York: Academic Press.

Neisser, V. (1967). *Cognitive psychology*. New York: Appleton–Century–Crofts.

Nielson, T. I. (1963). Volition: A new experimental approach. *Scandinavian Journal of Psychology*, 4, 215–230.

Pompeiano, O. (1974). In H. Kornhuber (Ed.), *Handbook of sensory physiology* (Vol. VI, 1, pp. 583–623).

Ramachandran, V. S. (1988). Perception of depth from shading. *Scientific American*, 269, 76–83.

Ramachandran, V. S. (1989). *The neurobiology of perception*. Presidential Lecture at the Annual meeting of the Society for Neurosciences (USA).

Ramachandran, V. S. (1990). Visual perception in people and machines. In A. Blake and T. Troscianko (Eds.), *AI and the eye*, Bristol: Wiley.

Ramachandran, V. S. (1993). Behavioural and MEG correlates of neural plasticity in the adult human brain. *Proceedings of the National Academy of Science U.S.A.*, 90, 10413–10420.

Ramachandran, V. S. (1994a). How deep is the denial (anosagnosia) of parietal lobe syndrome? *Society for Neuroscience Abstracts*.

Ramachandran, V. S. (1994b). Phanton limbs, somatoparaphrenic delusions, repressed memories and Freudian psychology. In O. Sporns and G. Tononi (Eds.), *Neuronal group selection.* San Diego: Academic Press.

Schopenhauer, A. (1819). *Die Welt als Wille und Vorstellung.* Leipzig.

Spencer, H. (1860). *The physiology of laughter, MacMillan Journals, Ltd.,* 1, 395–402.

Squire, L. (1987). *Memory and the brain.* New York: Oxford Univ. Press.

Waldenstrom, J. (1939). On anosognosia. *Acta Psychiatrica,* 14, 215–220.

Weinstein, E. A., and Kahn, R. L. (1950). The syndrome of anosagnosia. *Archives of Neurology and Psychiatry,* 64, 772–791.

Winson, J. (1986). *Brain and psyche.* New York: Vintage Books, Random House.

50 Implications for Psychiatry of Left and Right Cerebral Specialization: A Neurophysiological Context for Unconscious Processes

David Galin

Students of the brain and behavior recurrently attempt to integrate what is known of neurophysiology and neuroanatomy with what is known of psychodynamic processes. For example, Freud offered an explicit neurological model in the "Project for a Scientific Psychology,"[1] which has been updated by Pribram[2]; and Maclean[3] has proposed that some of the relations between the sexual, aggressive, and oral domains of behavior can be understood in terms of the anatomy and neurophysiology of the limbic system. Such attempts at integration are often resented as reductionism, or dismissed as merely a translation of concepts from one technical language to another. The purpose of this review is not to "neurologize" psychiatric concepts; it is to suggest that our present understanding of the disconnection syndromes and hemispheric specialization can provide a useful framework for developing research and theory.

The two cerebral hemispheres in humans are specialized for different cognitive functions, and when they are surgically disconnected, they each appear conscious; that is, two separate conscious minds in one head. Not only are they separate minds, but because of their specialization they are different, not duplicate minds. This conclusion is the most dramatic and most important to come out of the great volume of studies of commissurotomy patients done in the last decade by R. W. Sperry and his colleagues at the California Institute of Technology; J. E. Bogen, M. Gazzaniga, J. Levy, C. Trevarthen, R. Nebes, and others. These conclusions are extensively documented.[4-11]

Electroencephalogram experiments in our laboratory with normal people have demonstrated lateral specialization in the intact brain.[12-14] It is not an artifact due to the radical surgery or preoperative neurological disorder. Our study of how these two half-brains cooperate or interfere with each other in normal, intact people has just begun. This report briefly reviews experiments and clinical observations that have direct implications for psychiatry, and discusses some questions and opportunities for research that arise from them.

A Neurophysiological Context for Unconscious Processes

Hemispheric Specialization for Different Cognitive Modes

Our understanding of lateral specialization is based on studies of behavioral deficits produced by unilateral lesions and cerebral disconnections, and, most recently, from studies of normal subjects. It is generally agreed that in typical right-handed people, language processes and arithmetic depend primarily on the left hemisphere, and that the right hemisphere is particularly specialized for spatial relations and some musical functions. (The situation with left-handed people is more complex, and has been summarized very well by Hecaen and Ajuriaguerra[15] and others.[16-19]) For example, right temporal lobectomy produces a severe impairment on visual and tactile mazes; left temporal lesions of equal extent produce little deficit on these tasks, but specifically impair verbal memory. In the "split-brain" patients, the left hemisphere is capable of speech, writing, and calculation, but is severely limited in problems involving spatial relationships and novel figures. The right hemisphere can easily carry out tasks involving complex spatial and musical patterns, but can perform simple addition only up to ten, and has the use of relatively few words (very little expressive language, and comprehension of syntax at about the level of a 2-year-old[20,21]; Smith[22] reports on modest recovery or relearning following left hemispherectomy).

This lateralization of cognitive function has been demonstrated in normal subjects with EEG techniques,[12,13,23,24] evoked potentials,[14,25-30] and with studies of left/right visual field differences in perception and reaction time.[31-35]

For example, we have examined the EEGs of normal subjects performing verbal and spatial tasks to determine whether there were differences in activity between the two hemispheres.[12-14] We found relatively higher alpha amplitude (a measure of idling) over the right hemisphere during the verbal tasks, and relatively more alpha over the left hemisphere during the spatial tasks. In other words, the hemisphere expected to be less engaged in the task has more of the idling rhythm. Other investigators have confirmed our observations on changes in alpha asymmetry in studies that contrasted verbal and musical tasks.[23,24] We also found changes in the asymmetry of flash-evoked potentials as subjects switched from verbal to spatial tasks.[14] Other laboratories using the evoked potential method have reported that responses to speech sounds were larger in the left hemisphere than in the right,[28] and that responses to complex visual forms were larger on the right than on the left.[30] Another large group of studies with normal subjects have made use of the different hemispheric projections of the left and right visual fields, and have found, for example, that the left and right hemispheres have opposite superiorities in discriminative reaction times to stimuli such as letters and faces.[34,35]

It is important to emphasize that what most characterizes the hemispheres is not that they are specialized to work with different types of material (the left with words and the right with spatial forms); rather, each hemisphere is specialized for a different cognitive style; the left for an analytical, logical mode for which words are an excellent tool, and the right for a holistic, gestalt mode, which happens to be particularly suitable for spatial relations, as well as music. The difference in cognitive style is explicitly described in

a recent paper by Levy et al.[10] (see also Nebes[11] and Semmes[37]):

Recent commissurotomy studies have shown that the two disconnected hemispheres, working on the same task, may process the same sensory information in distinctly different ways, and that the two modes of mental operation, involving spatial synthesis for the right and temporal analysis for the left, show indications of mutual antagonism.[36] The propensity of the language hemisphere to note analytical details in a way that facilitates their description in language seems to interfere with the perception of an over-all Gestalt, leaving the left hemisphere 'unable to see the wood for the trees.' This interference effect suggested a rationale for the evolution of lateral specialization. . . .

The Hemispheric Disconnection Syndrome

Sperry et al.[4] have summarized the hemispheric disconnection syndrome as follows:

The most remarkable effect of sectioning the cerebral commissures continues to be the apparent lack of change with respect to ordinary behavior. (They) . . . exhibit no gross alterations of personality, intellect or overt behavior two years after operation. Individual mannerisms, conversation and bearing, temperament, strength, vigor and coordination are all largely intact and seem much as before surgery. Despite this outward appearance of general normality in ordinary behavior . . . specific tests indicate functional disengagement of the right and left hemispheres with respect to nearly all cognitive and other psychic activities. Learning and memory are found to proceed quite independently in each separated hemisphere. Each hemisphere seems to have its own conscious sphere for sensation, perception, ideation, and other mental activities and the whole inner realm of gnostic experience of the one is cut off from the corresponding experiences of the other hemisphere—with only a few exceptions as outlined below.

To understand the method of testing and interviewing each half of the brain separately, two points of functional anatomy must be kept in mind. The first is that since language functions (speech, writing) are mediated predominantly by the left hemisphere in most people, the disconnected right hemisphere cannot express itself verbally. Second, the neural pathways carrying information from one side of the body and one half of the visual field cross over and connect only with the opposite side of the brain. This means that sensations in the right hand and images in the right visual space will be projected almost entirely to the *left* hemisphere. Similarly, the major motor output is crossed, and the left hemisphere controls mainly the movements of the right hand. Therefore, patients with the corpus callosum sectioned can describe or answer questions about objects placed in their right hands, or pictures flashed to the right visual field with a tachistoscope, but are unable to give correct verbal reports for test items presented to the left hand or the left visual field. (They will in fact, often confabulate.) However, the mute right hemisphere can indicate its experience through various nonverbal responses, as for example, by manual selection of the proper object from an array. (Ipsilateral motor control is weak and variable; it is minimal for fine movement and distal control. It does improve postoperatively in some cases, confounding interpretations of tests based on lateralized output.)

Dissociation of Experience

The dissociation between the experiences of the two disconnected hemispheres is sometimes very dramatic. Sperry and his associates have photographed some illustrative incidents.

One film segment shows a female patient being tested with a tachistoscope, as described above. In the series of neutral geometrical figures being presented at random to the right and left fields, a nude pin-up was included and flashed to the right (nonverbal) hemisphere. The girl blushes and giggles. Sperry asks "What did you see?" She answers, "Nothing, just a flash of light," and giggles again, covering her mouth with her hand. "Why are you laughing then?" asks Sperry, and

she laughs again and says, "Oh, Dr. Sperry, you have some machine!" The episode is very suggestive; if one did not know her neurosurgical history, one might see this as a clear example of perceptual defense and think that she was "repressing" the perception of the conflictful sexual material—even her final response (a socially acceptable nonsequitur) was convincing (see Sperry[8]).

In another section of the film, a different patient was filmed performing a block design task; he is trying to match a colored geometric design with a set of painted blocks. The film shows the left hand (right hemisphere) quickly carrying out the task. Then the experimenter disarranges the blocks and the right hand (left hemisphere) is given the task; slowly and with great apparent indecision, it arranges the pieces. In trying to match a corner of the design, the right hand corrects one of the blocks, and then shifts it again, apparently not realizing it was correct: the viewer sees the left hand dart out, grab the block to restore it to the correct position—and then the arm of the experimenter reaches over and pulls the intruding left hand off-camera.

Psychiatric Implications

There is a compelling formal similarity between these dissociation phenomena seen in the commissurotomy patients and some phenomena of interest to clinical psychiatry; for example, according to Freud's early "topographical" model of the mind, repressed mental contents functioned in a separate realm that was inaccessible to conscious recall or verbal interrogation, functioning according to its own rules, developing and pursuing its own goals, affecting the viscera, and insinuating itself in the stream of ongoing consciously directed behavior.[38,39]

In later psychoanalytic models, the division of the mental apparatus was based on differences in the formal organization of thought and the control of emotional energy (primary vs secondary processes), rather than primarily on the basis of accessibility to conscious awareness.[39-41] According to Klein,[42] these different formulations have never been adequately synthesized, (Although Arlow and Brenner[40] claim the "structural theory" is in direct conflict with the "topographical theory" and should replace it rather than be reconciled with it, others disagree.[43,44]), and several theorists and experimentalists (Klein,[42] Rapaport,[45] Fischer,[46,47] Shevrin,[48] Piaget,[49] Rubenfine,[50] Deikman,[51] and Horowitz[52]) have continued to explore the interactions between (1) cognitive organization, (2) affective controls, and (3) variations in states of consciousness.

Freud had reluctantly abandoned the attempt to relate the functioning of the parts of the mental apparatus to specific anatomical locations because the neurology of the time was insufficient.[33(pp.107-109)] It may be useful to reconsider these questions now, in the context of our present understanding of the hemispheric disconnection syndromes and the specialization of the two hemispheres for different cognitive modes.

Certain aspects of right hemisphere functioning are congruent with the mode of cognition psychoanalysts have termed primary process, the form of thought that Freud originally assigned to the system Ucs[39(p.119)] (compare particularly Brenner[53(pp.53-55)]).

1. The right hemisphere primarily uses a nonverbal mode of representation, presumably images; visual, tactile, kinesthetic, and auditory.[5,6,10(pp.74-75)]

2. The right hemisphere reasons by a nonlinear mode of association rather than by syllogistic logic; its solutions to problems are based on multiple converging determinants rather than a single causal chain.[5,6,10,11] It is much superior to the left in part-whole relations, for example, grasping the concept of the whole from just a part.

3. The right hemisphere is less involved with perception of time and sequence than the left hemisphere.[54-59]

4. There is considerable evidence that the right hemisphere does possess words, but the words are not organized for use in propositions (see discussion by Bogen[6(pp.146-147)] and Gazzaniga and Hillyard[20]). For example, a patient with a total left hemispherectomy may be able to sing lyrics of a song, but not be able to use the same words in a sentence.[22,60] Therefore, when the right hemisphere did express itself in language, we might expect its use of words to reflect its characteristic holistic style. Because it deals more effectively with complex patterns taken as a whole than with the individual parts taken serially, we might expect metaphors, puns, double-entendre and rebus, that is, *word-pictures*. The elements in these verbal constructions do not have fixed single definitions (are not clearly bounded), but depend on context, and can shift in meaning when seen as parts of a new pattern. This is the sort of language that appears in dreams and slips of the tongue extensively described in *The psychopathology of everyday life*.[61] The right hemisphere is also particularly adept in the recognition of faces,[62,63] which carry much of the meaning in informal and colloquial speech (see Brenner's example,[53(p.55)] "He's a great one." See also Fischer and Mann[64] and Critchley[65] for appearance of poetry following an aphasiogenic left hemisphere lesion).

When the two hemispheres are surgically disconnected, the mental process of each one is inaccessible to deliberate conscious retrieval from the point of view of the other. However, the operation does not affect them so symmetrically with respect to overt behavior; Sperry and his collaborators have found that "in general, the postoperative behavior of [the commissurotomy patients] has been dominated by the major [left] hemisphere ..." except in tasks for which the right hemisphere is particularly specialized.[8,10] In these respects, there seems to be a clear parallel between the functioning of the isolated right hemisphere and mental processes that are repressed, unconscious, and unable to directly control behavior.

Anecdotal observations of the patients suggest that the isolated right hemisphere can sustain emotional responses and goals divergent from the left (e.g., assaulting with one hand and protecting with the other), although how often this occurs is questionable (Gazzaniga[9(p.107)] and Gordon and Sperry.[66]) However, systematic experiments with split-brain monkeys do provide direct support for the possibility of conflicting motivations:

The split hemispheres can experience reinforcing events independently ... at the moment one hemisphere is experiencing a particular stimulus as an effective reinforcer the other hemisphere is either oblivious of this assigned value or free to respond negatively to its own experience[67] ... the probability that a hemisphere will control a response is directly related to its history of obtaining reinforcers. The hemisphere which is most successful in earning reinforcement comes to dominate.[68]

All of the above considerations lead us to examine the hypothesis that in normal, intact people mental events in the right hemisphere can become disconnected functionally from the left hemisphere (by inhibition of neuronal transmission across the corpus callosum and other cerebral commissures), and can continue a life of their own. This hypothesis suggests a neurophysiological mechanism for at least some instances of repression, and an anatomical locus for the unconscious mental contents.

This hypothesis requires that parts of the transmission from one hemisphere to the other can be selectively and reversibly blocked. This does not seem implausible; selective gating has already been demonstrated in the central control of sensory input for all sensory modalities.[69-71] Stimulation of callosal fibers can inhibit as well as excite neuronal discharge in the contralateral cortex[72-74]; noting these reports, Bogen and Bogen[7] proposed "... certain kinds of left hemisphere activity may directly suppress certain kinds of right hemisphere action. Or they may prevent access to the left hemisphere of the products of right hemisphere activity." Presum-

ably there is reciprocity; right hemisphere processes could interfere with or suppress certain left hemisphere activity.

How Integrated Are the Two Hemispheres under Normal Conditions?

We do not know what is the usual relation between the two hemispheres in normal adults, but we can speculate on several arrangements. One possibility is that they operate in alternation, that is, taking turns, depending on situational demands. When one hemisphere is "on" it inhibits the other. A variant of this relationship might be that the dominating hemisphere makes use of one or more of the subsystems of the other hemisphere, inhibiting the rest. The inhibition thus may be only partial, suppressing enough of the subordinate hemisphere as to render it incapable of sustaining its own plan of action. We have some observations of intact people consistent with this view from EEG studies,[12-14] lateral eye movement studies,[75-78] and studies of behavioral interference.[18,19,79-82] (See also Bogen[5(p.102)] for evidence of this kind of inhibition in cases of lesions.) Such a relation of reciprocal inhibition of cognitive systems may be based on the left/right reciprocal inhibition so characteristic of the sensorimotor systems around which the whole brain is built. Another variant is the one hypothesized above; one hemisphere dominates overt behavior, but can only disconnect rather than totally inhibit (disrupt) the other hemisphere, which remains independently conscious. The fourth possible condition, in which the two hemispheres are fully active and integrated with each other, is the condition that Bogen and Bogen associate with creativity, man's highest functioning[7]; unfortunately, this does not seem to occur very often. In fact, they suggest that one of the reasons that the commissurotomy patients appear so normal to casual observation is because the activities of daily life do not demand much integration of holistic and analytic thought.

If the usual condition then is either alternation between the two modes, or parallel but independent consciousness with one of them dominating overt behavior, what factors determine which hemisphere will be "on?" Which will gain control of the shared functions and dominate overt behavior? There are two factors suggested by experiments performed with split-brain monkeys and humans. One could be called "resolution by speed"; the hemisphere that solves the problem first gets to the output channel first. This seems the most likely explanation for the observations in the human patients that "when a hemisphere is intrinsically better equipped to handle some task, it is also easier for that hemisphere to dominate the motor pathways."[10,21]

For example, Sperry and his collaborators have found that while "in general, the postoperative behavior of [the commissurotomy patients] has been dominated by the major [left] hemisphere ..." the right hemisphere dominated behavior in a facial recognition task.[10] Recognition of faces requires a perception of the gestalt, and is relatively resistant to analytical verbal description.[62,83] Therefore, it could be anticipated that the disconnected right hemisphere might be better than the left at recognizing faces. Different photographs were projected simultaneously to the left and right visual fields of commissurotomy patients. When the patients were asked to select the one they had seen from a row of samples, they pointed to the face that had been shown to the right hemisphere.

A second factor determining which hemisphere gets control could be called "resolution by motivation"; the one who cares more about the outcome preempts the output. This is demonstrated in a series of ingenious experiments with split-brain monkeys.[67,68] Each hemisphere was taught a visual discrimination task; two designs were displayed in front of the monkey, and if he pressed the correct one he was rewarded with a drink of fruit juice. Optical apparatus was used so that different cues could be projected to each hemisphere at the same time

from the same apparent location in space. In this way, it could be arranged so that both hemispheres saw the correct cue in the same place (calling for the same response) or in different places (calling for competing responses). After each hemisphere had independently learned the discrimination and was picking the correct cue nearly every time, the monkey was tested in a conflict situation, with each hemisphere seeing the correct cue in a different place. All of the animals showed a clear dominance of one of the hemispheres in this situation, that is, they responded consistently with the correct response for that hemisphere. Then the hemispheres were again trained separately, but with different reward conditions; the cue for the nondominant hemisphere was still rewarded every time it was selected, but the cue for the dominant hemisphere was rewarded only once every six times it was selected. When tested again in the conflict situation, the dominance was changed; the monkey consistently chose the cue that was correct for the previously nondominant hemisphere. Gazzaniga concludes, "Cerebral dominance in monkeys is quite flexible and subject to the effects of reinforcement ... the hemisphere which is most successful in earning reinforcement comes to dominate." I am proposing that this may apply to intact humans as well. As the left hemisphere develops its language capability in the second and third year of life, it gains a great advantage over the right hemisphere in manipulating its environment and securing reinforcements. It seems likely to me that this is the basis for the left hemisphere's suzerainty in overt behavior in situations of conflict with the right hemisphere.

Factors Contributing to a Unity of Consciousness

In spite of their different modes of organization, the two hemispheres are usually not in conflict. There are many unifying factors besides the cerebral commissures, which may also account for the surprisingly ordinary appearance of the commissurotomy patients outside of special laboratory test situations. Sperry et al.[4] describe some of the unifying influences.

Some of these are very obvious ... like the fact that these two separate mental spheres have only one body so they always frequent the same places, meet the same people, see and do the same things all the time and thus are bound to have a great overlap of common, almost identical, experience. The unity of the eyeball as well as the conjugate movements of the eyes causes both hemispheres to automatically center on, focus on, and hence probably attend to, the same items in the visual field all the time.

The sense of personal unity is a compelling subjective experience, and may derive in part from these factors. Sir Charles Sherrington states it elegantly.[84]

This self is a unity ... it regards itself as one, others treat it as one, it is addressed as one, by a name to which it answers. The Law and the State schedule it as one. It and they identify it with a body which is considered by it and them to belong to it integrally. In short, unchallenged and unargued conviction assumes it to be one. The logic of grammar endorses this by a pronoun in the singular. All its diversity is merged in oneness.

But we have good reason to believe that the experience of mental unity is to some extent an illusion, resulting in fact from exactly the conventions of language and law that Sherrington cites. "The strength of this conviction (of unity) is no assurance of its truth."[6(p.156ff)] One of the most striking features of the commissurotomy syndrome is that the patients (at least the hemisphere that can be interviewed) do not experience their obvious duality; they do not notice anything missing after the operation.

These people do not complain spontaneously about a perceptual division or incompleteness in their visual experience.... One can compare the visual experiences of each hemisphere to that of the hemianopic patient who, following accidental destruction of one visual cortex, or even hemispherectomy, may not recognize

the loss of one half of visual space until this is pointed out in formal tests.[4]

There is no indication that the dominant mental system of the left hemisphere is concerned about or even aware of the presence of the minor system under most ordinary conditions except quite indirectly as, for example, through occasional responses triggered from the minor side. As one patient remarked immediately after seeing herself make a left-hand response of this kind, 'Now I know it wasn't me that did that!'[8]

Conditions Favoring the Development of Separate Streams of Consciousness

There are several ways in which the two hemispheres of an ordinary person could begin to function as if they had been surgically disconnected, and decrease their exchange of information.

The first way is by active inhibition of information transfer because of conflict. Imagine the effect on a child when his mother presents one message verbally, but quite another with her facial expression and body language; "I am doing it because I love you, dear," says the words, but "I hate you and will destroy you" says the face. Each hemisphere is exposed to the same sensory input, but because of their relative specializations, they each emphasize only one of the messages. The left will attend to the verbal cues because it cannot extract information from the facial gestalt efficiently; the right will attend to the nonverbal cues because it cannot easily understand the words.[10] Effectively a different input has been delivered to each hemisphere, just as in the laboratory experiments in which a tachistoscope is used to present different pictures to the left and right visual fields. I offer the following conjecture: In this situation, the two hemispheres might decide on opposite courses of action; the left to approach, and the right to flee. Because of the high stakes involved, each hemisphere might be able to maintain its consciousness and resist the inhibitory influence of the other side. The left hemisphere seems to win control of the output channels most of the time,[8] but if the left is not able to "turn off" the right completely, it may settle for disconnecting the transfer of the conflicting information from the other side. The connections between hemispheres are relatively weak compared to the connections within hemispheres,[7] and it seems likely that each hemisphere treats the weak contralateral input in the same way in which people in general treat the odd discrepant observation that does not fit with the mass of their beliefs; first we ignore it, and then, if it is insistent, we actively avoid it.[85]

The mental process in the right hemisphere, cut off in this way from the left hemisphere consciousness that is directing overt behavior, may nevertheless continue a life of its own. The memory of the situation, the emotional concomitants, and the frustrated plan of action all may persist, affecting subsequent perception and forming the basis for expectations and evaluations of future input.

But active inhibition arising from conflicting goals is not the only way to account for a lack of communication between the two hemispheres, and a consequent divergence of consciousness. In the simplest case, because of their special modes of organization and special areas of competence, the knowledge that one hemisphere possesses may not translate well into the language of the other. For example, parts of the experience of attending a symphony concert are not readily expressed in words, and the concept "democracy requires informed participation" is hard to convey in images. What may be transmitted in such cases may be only the conclusion as to action, and not the details on which the evaluation was based.

Opportunities for Research

In the preceding sections I have reviewed some of the literature on hemispheric specialization and the commissurotomy syndrome. I have proposed that in intact people the cognitive specialization of the two hemispheres can lead to the development of separate realms of awareness. I believe that this can provide a useful framework for thinking about the interaction of cognitive structures, defensive maneuvers, and variations in states of consciousness. In the following discussions, I will review reports from several other areas that support this approach, or that provide opportunities for testing its usefulness in clinical and laboratory research.

Hemispheric Specialization and the Expression of Unconscious Processes

After the two hemispheres in man or monkey are surgically disconnected, one side tends to dominate the behavior.[8,10,68] In the human, the left hemisphere usually has preemptive control over the main stream of body activity as well as of propositional speech. If repression in normal intact people is to some extent subserved by a functional disconnection of right hemisphere mental processes, we might expect to see the expression of unconscious ideation through whatever output modes are not preempted by the left hemisphere.

Somatic and Autonomic Expression

One possibility for expression is through somatic representations, psychosomatic disorders, and somatic delusions. We might expect these symptoms to show a predominance on the left side of the body because of the crossing of the sensorimotor pathways. In Ferenczi's paper on hysterical stigmata, he reports just this in a discussion of a case of left hemianesthesia (See also Domhoff[87].):

One half of the body is insensitive in order that it shall be adapted for the representation of unconscious fantasies, and that "the right hand shall not know what the left hand doeth." I derive support for this conception from the consideration of the difference between right and left. It struck me that in general the hemianesthetic stigma occurs more frequently on the left than on the right; this is emphasized too, in a few textbooks. I recalled that the left half of the body is a priori more accessible to unconscious impulses than the right, which, in consequence of the more powerful attention-excitation of this more active and more skillful half of the body, is better protected against influences from the unconscious. It is possible that—in right-handed people—the sensational sphere for the left side shows from the first a certain predisposition for unconscious impulses, so that it is more easily robbed of its normal functions and placed at the service of unconscious libidinal fantasies.[86]

Unfortunately, Ferenczi provides no quantitative documentation for his assertion of the prevalence of left-sided hysterical symptoms, and this report must be considered an opportunity for research rather than support for our hypothesis.

Another channel for somatic expression of right hemisphere attitudes is the autonomic nervous system. In studies of normal humans, Varni et al.[88] concluded, "Asymmetry of autonomic activity is typical rather than atypical." The cerebrum participates extensively in visceral control[89,90] and asymmetrical cerebral activity may be reflected through asymmetrical autonomic activity.[91]

Studies of autonomic activity divide into two classes; those in which the autonomic response is used merely as an indicator of some central nervous system (CNS) process that is the main focus of interest (such as "attention" or "anxiety"), and those in which the autonomic variable itself is the focus of interest, such as blood pressure or heart rate in studies of cardiovascular regulation. In the indicator category, autonomic activity may be even more useful than our EEG alpha asymmetry measure as a sign of lateral cerebral specialization,[12,13,14] because the EEG can sample only those areas on the dorsal convexity of the brain. The autonomic variables probably reflect activity in just those areas of the brain that are not reached by the scalp EEG; the orbital and cingulate cortex, and the deep medial structures of the temporal lobe such as the hippocampus and amygdala.[89,90] If a person is

presented with stimulus material from an area of known conflict, asymmetry in skin conductance responses or digital blood flow might indicate that the two hemispheres had different affective reactions to the material. I am currently pursuing experiments along this line.

Consideration of left/right asymmetry may be useful for the second category of research too, in which the autonomic variable is of interest in itself rather than as an "indicator." There is some evidence of lateral specialization in visceral control just as in the realm of cognition. For example, we know that the right vagus affects primarily the heart rate while the left vagus affects primarily the strength of contraction, and hence systolic pressure.[92] Similar asymmetry has been shown for the sympathetic innervation of the heart.[93,94] (To my knowledge, there are no reports concerning the possibility of functional asymmetries in the abdominal vagus or sympathetic nerves.) If this lateral specialization in visceral control is extensive, it may help in explaining psychosomatic symptom choice, for example, hypertension versus tachycardia or dysrhythmia. Just as there appear to be individual differences in cognitive style, with a predominance of the mode of the left or right hemisphere,[95–98] so there may be a preferred visceral mode. We might expect those psychosomatic symptoms that are the expression of unconscious right hemisphere processes to appear in the right hemisphere visceral mode, as the stigmata of hysteria are alleged to appear in the left side of the body.[86]

Dreams

In periods of inactivity, the right hemisphere might seize the opportunity to express itself, as in daydreams, which occur during pauses in the stream of waking behavior, and in dreams at night. Freud called dreams the "royal road to the unconscious." Is there any link between the right hemisphere and dreams? Is there any evidence that the two hemispheres do not contribute symmetrically to dreams?

The mode of cognition in dreaming is usually of the "primary process" type; mainly nonverbal, image representations, with nonsyllogistic logic, and violations of ordinary temporal sequencing. The parallel between aspects of right hemisphere mentation and primary process thinking has been detailed in the first section of this report.

Humphrey and Zangwill[99] described three patients who spontaneously reported cessation of dreaming following posterior brain injuries. All three had left homonymous hemianopsia, indicating injury to the right hemisphere visual pathways. Impaired visual imagery in the waking state was also found. They cite four other cases in older neurological literature of depression of dreaming and waking visual imagery, usually associated with right parietooccipital lesions. Bogen observed that, following section of the corpus callosum, several patients reported that they no longer had any dreams, in contrast to frequent vivid dreaming before the operation.[6] One interpretation of this observation is that since the report of nondreaming was made by the left (verbal) hemisphere, which no longer had access to the right hemisphere's experience, the right (nonverbal) hemisphere may still be enjoying its dreams.

Austin[100] studied dream reports of people classified as divergent and convergent thinkers: convergent types are those who excel at rational analysis but do relatively poorly on open-ended tests requiring mental fluency and imaginativeness. Convergers tend to specialize in the physical sciences and divergers tend toward the arts. These "types" are consistent with the cognitive specializations of the left and right hemispheres.[6] Austin found that divergers were much more likely to report dreams when awakened in a rapid eye movement (REM) period, and that when convergers did report dreams they were much shorter than the dreams of the divergers. Austin interprets this finding in a manner similar to the interpretation of the reports of loss of dreams by Bogen's "split-brain" patients: the

convergers are having the dreams, but are not able to recall them. In this case, the failure to recall is not because of a lesion but because of what Austin calls their "intellectual bias" against "the emotional and nonrational, which reinforces their capacity for logical construction at the expense of combinatory play."

In our laboratory, we are currently looking for direct evidence on whether or not the right hemisphere is more actively engaged in dream cognition than the left, by studying the EEG asymmetry in REM sleep. In the enormous body of EEG studies on sleep and dreaming, there has been almost no attention given to the question of hemispheric asymmetry in the EEG patterns characterizing the stages of sleep or to the possibility that the two hemispheres make different contributions to the mental activity of sleep. The analysis of the neurological mechanisms relating to sleep have usually been directed toward the vertical organization of the CNS, brainstem mechanisms interacting with cerebral mechanisms. The additional complication of the lateral specialization of the cerebrum for different cognitive modes that is superimposed on this vertical system has not yet been studied.

Hemispheric Differences in Coping Strategies and Affective Reactions

The Denial of Illness

Anosognosia is the term most commonly used to refer to the condition in which a patient with a gross neurological deficit (a hemiplegia, or a hemianopic) is unaware of his disability, or shows an attitude of indifference, or frankly denies it. It is also variously reported as "la douce indifference,"[101] "la belle indifference,"[102] and "anosodiaphoria."[103] Critchley describes the range of this fascinating and frequent symptom as follows:

... hemiplegics may show a diversity of mental attitudes towards their disability. One patient may apparently be unaware of the fact of immobility. Or he may grudgingly admit to some mild degree of disability and then proceed to advance some inadequate excuse ... Or again, a hemiplegic patient may stoutly deny the fact that he is paralysed ... he may declare that he is moving his limbs when he is not. He may deny the ownership of the paralysed limb. Nay, more; he may even proclaim that the limbs belong to some other person, real or imaginary, alive or dead.

Discussion still reigns nevertheless as to the meaning of these facts. Do they, for example, apply particularly to the consequences of disease of the non-dominant hemisphere? ... Are they but arresting instances of a general underlying tendency to avoid looking unpleasant facts in the face—illustrating in this way the "denial syndrome" of Weinstein and Kahn?[104] We must admit that while the problems are not yet wholly settled, we cannot avoid noting the frequency with which such patients display a disability of the non-dominant (right) hemisphere. . . .[103]

These and related symptoms are discussed in detail in his chapter "Disorders of the body image."[105] He presents the indifference reaction as a simple extension of the unilateral spatial neglect, or imperception, which is one of the commonest signs of parietal disease,[105(pp.226ff,340ff,396)] and which is also demonstrable in animals.[106] However, according to Weinstein and Kahn,[104] in human cases, the anosognosia may be due to psychosocial factors, such as social attitudes toward illness or the symbolic significance of the disability, rather than due to a specific brain lesion. In their view, the indifference is a motivated reaction to the deficit, which in its more florid form appears as denial. They interpreted the euphoric reaction as just another variety of the denial reaction, the particular type depending on the defensive character style of the premorbid personality. However, they too agree that anosognosia is much more common following right hemisphere lesions than left (4.5 to 1 in their series). We are thus lead to the conclusion that denial is a characteristic way for the intact left hemisphere to cope with a right hemisphere lesion. This is consistent with the model proposed in the previous sections; the denial could be sustained by an in-

hibition of information transfer across the corpus callosum from the damaged right side.

Is there a coping strategy or emotional reaction that is characteristic following left hemisphere injury? In a recent study, Gainotti[102] reported on 150 cases of unilateral cerebral lesions. He compared the incidence of the indifference reaction and the "catastrophic reaction" described by Kurt Goldstein. The incidence of catastrophic reactions was 62% with left lesions and only 10% with right lesions. In contrast, the incidence of "la belle indifference" was 33% with right lesions and only 11% with left lesions ($P < .01$).

Asymmetry of Affective Reaction to Intracarotid Amobarbital (Amytal)

Another type of evidence suggests that there may be a particular quality of affective reaction associated with injury to each hemisphere. Terzian and Cecotto made this observation in the course of administering the Wada carotid amobarbital test.[107,108] This is a procedure generally used prior to neurosurgery to establish which hemisphere is dominant for language in ambiguous cases, such as when the patient is left-handed, or ambidexterous.[109] A small quantity of the anesthetic is injected into one common carotid artery. This results in anesthetizing only the ipsilateral hemisphere, producing a contralateral hemiplegia and, if it happens to be the side dominant for speech, a complete aphasia. The symptoms last only for a few minutes. Terzian observed that a certain number of his patients had a severe emotional reaction as the anesthetic was wearing off. He describes it as follows:

... Amytal on the left side provokes ... a catastrophic reaction in the sense of Goldstein. The patient ... despairs and expresses a sense of guilt, of nothingness, of indignity, and worries about his own future or that of his relatives, without referring to the language disturbances overcome and to the hemiplegia just resolved and ignored. The injection of the same dose in the contralateral carotid artery of the same subject or in subjects not having received the left injection, produces on the contrary a complete opposite emotional reaction, an euphoric reaction that in some cases may reach the intensity of maniacal reaction. The patient appears without apprehension, smiles and laughs and both with mimicry and words expresses considerable liveliness and sense of well-being.[108]

In a subsequent paper, Alema et al.[110] reported that this specifically lateralized affective response was seen best in patients with no brain damage; in patients with unilateral damage, it was seen only on the intact side, and in cases of diffuse or bilateral damage, it was not seen at all. (The indications for performing the test on the patients with no brain damage were not reported.) These extraordinary observations were confirmed by Rossi and Rosadini[111] and by Hecaen and Ajuriaguerra,[15] but disputed by Milner,[112] who studied the emotional response of 104 patients undergoing the Wada test. She reported only rare depression, and no systematic asymmetry in the euphoria. She related the emotional reaction to the temperament of the patient. Neither Milner nor Rossi was able to account for their divergent results. At this point, we must await further studies to resolve these conflicting reports.

Another provocative study was carried out by Hommes and Panhuysen[113,114] on the effects of unilateral carotid amobarbital in patients hospitalized for depression, with no known brain damage. This report is difficult to evaluate because of many methodological limitations that the authors themselves acknowledge. Nevertheless, because of their implications, their results should be noted.

First, they found much more dysphasia following right hemisphere injections in this depressed population than would be expected in the general population. Second, when they ranked their patients in terms of left hemispheric dominance for speech, they found there was a strong negative correlation with depth of clinical depression (pre-amobarbital); the most depressed had the least left dominance for speech. The authors conclude, "It is therefore possible

that ... the level of functional dominance of the left hemisphere is reduced by the process that leads to depression." They found an elevation of mood with injection on either side, although sometimes much more substantial on one side. They point out that the patients were already depressed, and a further depressive reaction following left hemisphere injection might be inconspicuous.

The interpretation of the affective reaction to unilateral amobarbital injection is especially difficult because it occurs not at the peak of the disability, but as the anesthetic is wearing off, or with doses too small to produce EEG and gross neurological symptoms. Is the affect originating from the injected side, as a reaction to the drug, or from the uninjected side, as the balance of dominance between them is shifted? In other respects, the reported amobarbital emotional asymmetry is similar to that seen following permanent unilateral lesions, described above under "Denial of illness"[104]; depressive catastrophic reactions are more frequent with left lesions, and indifference or euphoria with right lesions.

Unilateral Electroconvulsive Shock Treatment (ECT)

Comparison of Therapeutic Response to Left and Right Hemisphere Treatment
In the past ten years there have been numerous reports that the posttreatment confusion and memory disturbance that commonly follows conventional bitemporal ECT can be minimized by using a unilateral technique; the electrodes are applied only on one side of the head, usually the right. Most authors report no loss in therapeutic effectiveness in relieving the symptoms of depression,[115-121] although some report that unilateral treatment requires more sessions for equivalent results.[122-125] If hemispheric specialization and interaction are related to the organization and integration of personality, then it seems reasonable to expect that which hemi-

sphere gets the shock treatment might effect the therapeutic outcome. What is the evidence for any such differential effect?

Although a substantial literature on unilateral ECT has developed, only a few studies have compared the efficacy of unilateral shock to the left and right hemispheres. Most studies have only compared efficacy of right hemisphere ECT to the conventional bilateral ECT, or have been primarily concerned with the nature and extent of the memory loss and confusion, which are usually held to be unrelated to therapeutic effect.[126] As is usual in clinical outcome studies, gross differences in treatment procedure, patient selection, method and time of evaluation make the comparison of one report with another very difficult. (A summary of methodological problems in ECT studies is given by Costello et al.[117,127].) Nevertheless, a careful reading of this clinical literature does suggest a differential role of the two hemispheres in response to ECT.

Three studies compared the therapeutic effect of left, right, and bilateral ECT in depressives, and included a blind follow-up evaluation at least one month after the last treatment.[115,116,118] Halliday et al. and Cronin et al. both found ECT to the left hemisphere to be significantly less effective in relieving depression than ECT to the right.[115,116] The third study by Fleminger et al., which seems generally comparable, found no difference between the treatments.[118]

Three other studies also compared outcome in left, right, and bilateral ECT and found no difference among the groups,[117,119,128] but they differ substantially in method from those cited above. Two of these mention therapeutic effect only in passing; their patient groups included schizophrenics with depressives, and evaluation was based entirely on the number of treatments given[119] or number of treatments plus the discharge summary.[128] The third[117] rated improvement only to the day following the last treatment, and the authors themselves caution that because of the lack of follow-up, and

because of high variances in the self-report inventories used, their conclusion should be considered exploratory.

The study by Cronin et al.[116] found both right and bilateral treatment were superior to left hemisphere ECT. They emphasized that the difference was not apparent until after the eighth treatment, and had increased further at follow-up one month later.

The study by Halliday et al.[115] tends to show that right hemisphere ECT was more effective than left or bilateral ECT according to overall clinical assessment three months after the end of treatment. Although they point out that a significantly greater number of patients receiving left hemisphere ECT relapsed or dropped out of the study, or both, their overall conclusion was "There was no significant difference in the effect on depression of the three types of ECT." It is worthwhile to consider their results in detail. Five of the patients who dropped out were known to have relapsed under treatment (three with left ECT, one with right ECT, and one with bilateral ECT), but because they were not assessed at the end of the study in the same formal manner as the others, Halliday did not include them in his summary table. With these patients added to the appropriate "worse" groups, the results (as adapted from Halliday et al.[37]) are as follows:

	Left ECT	Right ECT	Bilateral ECT
Recovered	4 (28.5%)	8 (47.0%)	5 (27.8%)
Improved	5 (35.7%)	6 (35.3%)	7 (38.9%)
No change	0 (0%)	2 (11.8%)	0 (0%)
Worse	5 (35.7%)	1 (5.9%)	6 (33.3%)
N =	14	17	18

The effects of left hemisphere ECT and bilateral ECT seem to be similar. The tendency for right ECT to produce superior results (better versus no better) does not reach the .05 level of confidence by the Fischer Exact Probability Test, but the tendency for left ECT to make patients worse (worse vs not worse) is significant at $P < .05$. It would seem important to repeat this study with a larger sample.

Halliday et al. note that the seizure produced by the treatment was wholly or preponderantly unilateral in only one third of the cases. We might hypothesize that the effect in those patients who had bilateral fits was more similar to the effect of bilateral ECT. Therefore, in comparing left and right hemisphere ECT for therapeutic efficacy, the comparison should be restricted to those patients who had unilateral seizures. The difference between the unilateral treatment groups could be diluted by the inadvertent addition of what may be in effect bilateral treatment. If this is correct, then research on methods to confine the seizure to one hemisphere would be very important.

What is reported simply as a "bilateral seizure" may have begun unilaterally and spread to include the other side. Therefore, it may or may not be symmetric in its effects. The EEG could be used to evaluate the extent and duration of the afterdischarge and postictal depression on each side.

Field-Dependence and Lateralization of Brain Function: Effects of Unilateral ECT

A recent study by A. J. Silverman and his colleagues compared the effects of left and right hemisphere ECT in terms of the cognitive style concept, field-dependence.[95,129] Although not explicitly concerned with therapeutic outcome, this suggests a way to understand the clinical empirical results of Cronin et al.[116] and Halliday et al.[115] in terms of changes in balance between the two specialized hemispheres.

Field-dependence is measured by a variety of tests, but most commonly with the rod-and-frame. The subject sits facing a rod surrounded by a tilted frame, and is asked to adjust the rod to a vertical position. People with a strong tendency to be influenced by the frame (the context or "field") and thus to miss the vertical, are called field-dependent. Field-dependence has been related to a great many personality and psychophysiological variables, such as responsiveness to social cues, defensive style (denial vs. intellectualization), and symptom choice in psychosomatic illness.[129] In general, it is the field-dependent who comes out on the pathological, more primitive, less desirable end of the continuum. This may be due to the fact that all the field-dependence tests are set up requiring the subject to be as field-independent as he can. There are none that I know of in which the person is asked to be as responsive to context as possible. In other words, these tests can disclose only an inability to operate in a field-independent mode on demand, not the relative ability to perform in either mode, or the preference for one mode over the other.

In reviewing a series of studies, Silverman and his colleagues concluded that extreme field-dependent subjects had a pattern of deficits that might signify a subclinical cerebral injury; left/right confusion, primitive drawings in the draw-a-person test, poor mirror-tracing and embedded figures performance, and a paradoxical response to amphetamines. In another experiment using a paired associates learning test with word pairs and form pairs, they found that the field-dependent subjects showed relative deficiency on the words section, suggesting a relative deficit in left hemisphere functioning. In order to directly test the relation between left and right cerebral dysfunction and field-dependent performance on the rod-and-frame test, they studied a group of right-handed depressed patients who were undergoing unilateral ECT. They hypothesized that if field-dependence was related to left hemisphere dysfunction, then patients who had ECT on the left hemisphere, rather than on the right, should have increased rod-and-frame error scores. The results were extraordinarily consistent; all 12 patients who had left hemisphere ECT showed more field-dependence on the posttreatment test. But the more startling result was that all 12 patients who had right ECT showed less field-dependence, i.e., fewer errors. In discussing this result, Silverman suggests that it is possible that

... right ECT decreases a subject's ability to respond to a stimulus field such that the more peripheral elements of the field are not attended to. In the case of the Rod-and-Frame task, it is the frame which is both peripheral as well as the major source of interference in performing the task. Thus, with the distracting influence of the frame attenuated the rod can be more accurately brought to true vertical.[129]

Thus, field-dependence is seen to be associated with a relative right hemisphere dominance, rather than a left hemisphere dysfunction per se.

In summary, examination of the literature on unilateral ECT for depression suggests that the two hemispheres differ in the response to treatment, and that it may be useful to consider the effect of this treatment in terms of changing the balance or interaction between the two hemispheres. The results of Halliday et al.,[115] Cronin et al.,[116] Silverman,[129] and Cohen et al.[95] are certainly consistent with the observations discussed in previous sections: the frequency of depressive reaction after amobarbital injection of the left hemisphere, and after lesions of the left hemisphere, and the report of Hommes and Panhuysen[113,114] that their depressed patients showed less than usual left dominance.

Conclusions

In this report, I have proposed that our present knowledge of the two hemispheres' cognitive specialization and potential for independent functioning provides a useful framework for thinking about the interaction of cognitive structures, defensive maneuvers, and variations in states of awareness.

A brief review was presented of the evidence that the left hemisphere is specialized for an analytic, linear mode of information processing, and that the right hemisphere is specialized for a holistic, gestalt mode. The commissurotomy syndrome was described, particularly with respect to observations that indicate that each disconnected hemisphere is independently conscious, and that, in general, the left hemisphere

in these patients seems to dominate their postoperative behavior. A parallel was noted between the functioning of the isolated right hemisphere and mental processes that are repressed, unconscious, and unable to directly control behavior. The congruency between some aspects of the right hemisphere cognitive mode and some aspects of primary process thinking was discussed; both depend mainly on nonverbal, image representations, with nonsyllogistic logic, and are more concerned with multiple simultaneous interactions than with temporal sequencing.

These considerations led to the hypothesis that in normal intact people mental events in the right hemisphere can become disconnected functionally from the left hemisphere (by inhibition of neuronal transmission across the corpus callosum) and can continue a life of their own. This hypothesis suggests a neurophysiological mechanism for at least some instances of repression, and an anatomical locus for the unconscious mental contents.

If repression is to some extent subserved by a functional disconnection of right hemisphere mental processes, we might expect that unconscious ideation would be expressed primarily through channels that are not preempted by the dominant verbal left hemisphere. This notion led me to review several studies that suggest that the right hemisphere plays a special role in dreaming, and that it might be fruitful to look for lateral asymmetries in the autonomic nervous system, and in psychosomatic symptoms.

Another group of studies were reviewed that concern the differences between the two hemispheres in the affective reactions or coping strategies that appear following cerebral injuries or in the course of the intracarotid amobarbital test. Denial of illness or euphoria is seen most often following right lesions, and "catastrophic" or depressive reactions most often following left lesions. At present, the evidence for these differences pertains only to reactions to injury; we do not know whether or to what extent the two hemispheres in the intact brain may each subserve characteristic defensive styles or affective tone.

Finally, the literature on unilateral ECT for the relief of depression was reviewed. It was concluded that the therapeutic effect may depend on which hemisphere gets the treatment. It is suggested that the therapeutic effect can be understood in terms of changing the balance between the specialized hemispheres.

Early attempts to integrate neurology and psychodynamics were not very fruitful, perhaps premature. Since then, the two disciplines have developed extensively, but quite separately, without much cross-fertilization. In this report I have juxtaposed a variety of observations and concepts from neuropsychology and psychiatry. I believe these are complementary rather than competing formulations. The work reviewed here seems to me to indicate a profitable direction for developing research and theory.

Acknowledgments

This investigation was supported in part by National Institute of Mental Health Career Development award MH-28457 and National Institute of Neurological Diseases and Stroke grant NS-10307.

References

1. Freud S: Project for a scientific psychology, in *Origins of Psychoanalysis: Letters to Wilhelm Fliess, Drafts and Notes, 1887–1902.* New York, Basic Books, 1954.

2. Pribram K: The neuropsychology of Sigmund Freud, in Bachrach AJ (ed): *Experimental Foundations for Clinical Psychology.* New York, Basic Books, 1962.

3. Maclean P: New findings relevant to the evolution of psychosexual functions of the brain. *J Nerv Ment Dis* 135:289–301, 1962.

4. Sperry RW, Gazzaniga MS, Bogen JE: Interhemispheric relationships: The neocortical commissures: Syndromes of hemisphere disconnection, in Vinken PJ, Bruyn GW (eds): *Handbook of Clinical Neurology.* Amsterdam, North Holland Publishing Co, 1969, vol 4.

5. Bogen JE: The other side of the brain: I. Dysgraphia and dyscopia following cerebral commissurotomy. *Bull Los Angeles Neurol Soc* 34:73–105, 1969.

6. Bogen JE: The other side of the brain: II. An appositional mind. *Bull Los Angeles Neurol Soc* 34:135–162, 1969.

7. Bogen JE, Bogen GM: The other side of the brain: III. The corpus callosum and creativity. *Bull Los Angeles Neurol Soc* 34:191–220, 1969.

8. Sperry RW: Hemisphere deconnection and unity in conscious awareness. *Am Psychol* 23:723–733, 1968.

9. Gazzaniga MS: *The Bisected Brain.* New York, Appleton-Century-Crofts Inc, 1970.

10. Levy J, Trevarthen C, Sperry RW: Perception of bilateral chimeric figures following hemispheric deconnexion. *Brain* 95:61–78, 1972.

11. Nebes R: Superiority of the minor hemisphere in commissurotomized man for perception of part-whole relations. *Cortex* 7:333–349, 1971.

12. Galin D, Ornstein R: Lateral specialization of cognitive mode: An EEG study. *Psychophysiology* 9:412–418, 1972.

13. Doyle JC, Galin D, Ornstein R: Lateral specialization of cognitive mode: II. EEG frequency analysis. *Psychophysiology,* 11:567–578, 1974.

14. Galin D, Ellis RR: Asymmetry in evoked potentials as an index of lateralized cognitive processes: Relation to EEG alpha asymmetry. *Neuropsychologia,* 13:45–50, 1975.

15. Hécaen H, Ajuriaguerra J: *Lefthandedness.* New York, Grune & Stratton Inc, 1964.

16. Silverman AJ, Adevai G, McGough WE: Some relationships between handedness and perception. *J Psychosom Res* 10:151–158, 1966.

17. James WE, Mefferd RB, Wieland BA: Repetitive psychometric measures: Handedness and performance. *Percept Mot Skills* 25:209–212, 1967.

18. Levy J: Possible basis for the evolution of lateral specialization of the human brain. *Nature* 224:614–615, 1969.

19. Miller E: Handedness and the pattern of human ability. *Br J Psychol* 62:111–112, 1971.

20. Gazzaniga MS, Hillyard SA: Language and speech capacity of the right hemisphere. *Neuropsychologia* 9:273–280, 1971.

21. Levy J, Nebes R, Sperry RW: Expressive language in the surgically separated minor hemisphere. *Cortex* 7:49–58, 1971.

22. Smith A: Speech and other functions after left (dominant) hemispherectomy. *J Neurol Neurosurg Psychiatry* 29:467–471, 1966.

23. McKee G, Humphrey B, McAdam D: Scaled lateralization of alpha activity during linguistic and musical tasks. *Psychophysiology* 10:441–443, 1973.

24. Schwartz G, Davidson RJ, Maer F, et al.: Patterns of hemispheric dominance in musical, emotional, verbal and spatial tasks. Read before the Society for Psychophysiological Research, New Orleans, 1973.

25. Buchsbaum M, Fedio P: Visual information and evoked responses from the left and right hemispheres. *Electroencephalogr Clin Neurophysiol* 26:266–272, 1969.

26. Buchsbaum M, Fedio P: Hemispheric differences in evoked potentials to verbal and non-verbal stimuli in the left and right visual fields. *Physiol Behav* 5:207–210, 1970.

27. McAdam DW, Whitaker HA: Language production: Electro-encephalographic localization in the normal human brain. *Science* 172:499–502, 1971.

28. Morrell LK, Salamy JG: Hemispheric asymmetry of electrocortical responses to speech stimuli. *Science* 174:164–166, 1971.

29. Wood C, Goff WR, Day RS: Auditory evoked potentials during speech perception. *Science* 173:1248–1251, 1971.

30. Vella EJ, Butler SR, Glass A: Electrical correlate of right hemisphere function. *Nature* 236:125–126, 1972.

31. White MJ: Laterality differences in perception: A review. *Psychol Bull* 72:387–405, 1969.

32. Filbey RA, Gazzaniga MS: Splitting the normal brain with reaction time. *Psychol Sci* 17:335, 1969.

33. McKeever WF, Huling M: Left cerebral hemisphere superiority in tachistoscopic word recognition performance. *Percept Mot Skills* 30:763–766, 1970.

34. Rizzolatti G, Umilta C, Berlucchi G: Opposite superiorities of the right and left cerebral hemispheres in discriminative reaction time to physiognomical and alphabetical material. *Brain* 94:431–442, 1971.

35. Berlucchi G, Heron W, Hyman R, et al.: Simple reaction times of ipsilateral and contralateral hand to lateralized visual stimuli. *Brain* 94:419–430, 1971.

36. Levy J: *Information Processing and Higher Psychological Functions in the Disconnected Hemispheres of Human Commissurotomy Patients*, thesis. California Institute of Technology, Pasadena, 1970.

37. Semmes J: Hemispheric specialization: A possible clue to mechanism. *Neuropsychologia* 6:11–26, 1968.

38. Freud S: *Interpretation of Dreams (1900)*. London, Hogarth Press, vols 4 and 5, 1953.

39. Freud S: The unconscious, in *Collected Papers (1915)*. London, Hogarth Press, vol 4, 1948, pp 98–136.

40. Arlow JA, Brenner C: *Psychoanalytic Concepts and the Structural Theory*. New York, International Universities Press, 1964.

41. Freud S: *The Ego and the Id (1923)*. London, Hogarth Press, 1927.

42. Klein GS: Consciousness in psychoanalytic theory: Some implications for current research in perception. *J Am Psychoanal Assoc* 7:5–34, 1959.

43. Gill M: Topography and systems in psychoanalytic theory. *Psychol Issues* 3:10, 1963.

44. Kubie L: *Neurotic Distortion of the Creative Process*. Lawrence, Kan, University of Kansas Press, 1958.

45. Rapaport D: States of consciousness: A psychopathological and psychodynamic view, in Gill MM (ed): *Collected Papers of David Rapaport*. New York, Basic Books, 1967, pp 385–404.

46. Fischer C: Study of the preliminary stages of the construction of dreams and images. *J Am Psychoanal Assoc* 5:5–60, 1957.

47. Fischer C, Paul IH: The effect of subliminal visual stimulation on images and dreams: A validation study. *J Am Psychoanal Assoc* 7:35–83, 1959.

48. Shevrin H: Brain wave correlates of subliminal stimulation, unconscious attention, primary and secondary process thinking, and repressiveness. *Psychol Issues* 8:56–87, 1973.

49. Piaget J: The affective unconscious and the cognitive unconscious. *J Am Psychoanal Assoc* 21:249–261, 1973.

50. Rubenfine DL: Perception, reality testing and symbolism. *Psychoanal Study Child* 16:73–89, 1961.

51. Deikman AJ: Bimodal consciousness. *Arch Gen Psychiatry* 25:481–489, 1971.

52. Horowitz MJ: Modes of representation of thought. *J Am Psychoanal Assoc* 20:793–819, 1972.

53. Brenner C: *An Elementary Textbook of Psychoanalysis*, revised. New York, International Universities Press, 1973.

54. Efron R: Effect of handedness on the perception of simultaneity and temporal order. *Brain* 86:261–284, 1963.

55. Efron R: The effect of stimulus intensity on the perception of simultaneity in right and left-handed subjects. *Brain* 86:285–294, 1963.

56. Efron R: An extension of the Pulfrich stereoscopic effect. *Brain* 86:295–300, 1963.

57. Efron R: Temporal perception, aphasia and deja vu. *Brain* 86:403–424, 1963.

58. Carmon A, Nachshon I: Effect of unilateral brain damage on perception of temporal order. *Cortex* 7:410–418, 1971.

59. Swischer L, Hirsch IJ: Brain damage and the ordering of two temporally successive stimuli. *Neuropsychologia* 10:137–152, 1972.

60. Zangwill OL: Speech and the minor hemisphere. *Acta Neurol Psychiatr Belg* 67:1013–1020, 1967.

61. Freud S: *Psychopathology of Everyday Life*. New York, MacMillan Co, 1926.

62. Hécaen H: Clinical symptomatology in right and left hemispheric lesions, in Mountcastle VB (ed): *Interhemispheric Relations and Cerebral Dominance*. Baltimore, Johns Hopkins Press, 1962.

63. DeRenzi E, Spinnler H: Visual recognition in patients with unilateral cerebral disease. *J Nerv Ment Dis* 142:515–525, 1966.

64. Fischer ED, Mann LB: Shift of writing function to minor hemisphere at the age of 72 years: Report of case with advanced left cerebral atrophy. *Bull Los Angeles Neurol Soc* 17:196–197, 1952.

65. Critchley M: Creative writing by aphasiacs, in Chorobski J (ed): *Neurological Problems*. London, Pergamon Press Inc, 1967, pp 275–286.

66. Gordon H, Sperry RW: Lateralization of olfactory perception in the surgically separated hemispheres of man. *Neuropsychologia* 7:111–120, 1969.

67. Johnson JD, Gazzaniga MS: Reversal behavior in split-brain monkeys. *Physiol Behav* 6:707–709, 1971.

68. Gazzaniga MS: Changing hemisphere dominance by changing reward probability in split-brain monkeys. *Exp Neurol* 33:412–419, 1971.

69. Livingston RB: Central control of receptors and sensory transmission systems, in Magoun HW (ed): *Handbook of Physiology-Neurophysiology, ed 1.* Washington, DC, American Physiological Society, 1959, pp 741–760.

70. Whitfield IC: *The Auditory Pathway*. Baltimore, Williams & Wilkins Co, 1967.

71. Pribram K: *Languages of the Brain*. Englewood Cliffs, NJ, Prentice-Hall Inc, 1971.

72. Asanuma H, Osamu O: Effects of transcallosal volleys on pyramidal tract cell activity of cat. *J Neurophysiol* 25:198–208, 1962.

73. Hossman KA: Untersuchungen über transcallosale Potentiale an der akuten Corpus Callosum-Katze. *Dtsch Z Nervenheilk* 195:79–102, 1969.

74. Eidelberg E: Callosal and non-callosal connections between the sensory motor cortices in cat and monkey. *Electroencephalogr Clin Neurophysiol* 26:557–564, 1969.

75. Galin D, Ornstein R: Individual differences in cognitive style: I. Reflective eye movements. *Neuropsychologia* 12:367–376, 1974.

76. Kocel K, Galin D, Ornstein R, et al.: Lateral eye movement and cognitive mode. *Psychonom Sci* 27:223–224, 1972.

77. Kinsbourne M: Eye and head turning indicates cerebral lateralization. *Science* 176:539–541, 1972.

78. Bakan P: Hypnotizability, laterality of eye-movements and functional brain asymmetry. *Percept Mot Skills* 28:927–932, 1969.

79. Brooks LR: An extension of the conflict between visualization and reading. *Q J Exp Psychol* 22:91–96, 1970.

80. Deutsch D: Tones and numbers: Specificity of interference in immediate memory. *Science* 168:1604–1605, 1970.

81. denHyer K, Barrett B: Selective loss of visual information in STM by means of visual and verbal interpolated tasks. *Psychol Sci* 25:100–102, 1971.

82. Nebes R: Handedness and the perception of the part-whole relationship. *Cortex* 7:350–356, 1971.

83. Rondot P, Tzavaras A: La prosopagnosie après vingt années d'études cliniques et neuropsychologiques. *J Psychol Norm Pathol* 66:133–165, 1969.

84. Sherrington C: *The Integrative Action of the Nervous System*. Cambridge, England, Cambridge University Press, 1947, p xvii.

85. Stent G: Prematurity and uniqueness in scientific discovery. *Sci Am*, 1972, pp 84–93.

86. Ferenczi S: An attempted explanation of some hysterical stigmata, in *Further Contributions to the Theory and Technique of Psychoanalysis.* London, Hogarth Press, 1926.

87. Domhoff GW: But why did they sit on the king's right in the first place? *Psychoanal Rev* 56:586–596, 1969–70.

88. Varni JG, Doerr HO, Franklin JR: Bilateral differences in skin resistance and vasomotor activity. *Psychophysiology* 8:390–400, 1971.

89. Hoff EC, Kell JF, Carroll MN: Effects of cortical stimulation and lesions on cardiovascular function. *Physiol Rev* 43:68–114, 1963.

90. Wang SC: *Neural Control of Sweating.* Madison, University of Wisconsin Press, 1964.

91. Holloway FA, Parsons OA: Unilateral brain damage and bilateral skin conductance levels in humans. *Psychophysiology* 6:138–148, 1969.

92. DeGeest H, Levy MN, Zieske H, et al.: Depression of ventricular contractility by stimulation of the vagus nerves. *Circ Res* 17:222–235, 1965.

93. Randall WC, McNally H, Cowan J, et al.: Functional analysis of cardioaugmentor and cardioaccelerator pathways in the dog. *Am J Physiol* 191:213–217, 1957.

94. Chai CV, Wang SC: Localization of central cardiovascular control mechanisms in the lower brain stem of the cat. *Am J Physiol* 202:25–42, 1962.

95. Cohen BD, Berent S, Silverman AJ: Field-dependence and lateralization of function in the human brain. *Arch Gen Psychiat* 28:165–167, 1973.

96. Cohen RA: Conceptual styles, culture conflict and nonverbal tests of intelligence. *Am Anthropol* 71:828–856, 1969.

97. Bogen JE, DeZure R, Ten Houten WD, et al.: The other side of the brain: IV. The A/P ratio. *Bull Los Angeles Neurol Soc* 37:49–61, 1972.

98. Lee D: Codifications of reality: Lineal and nonlineal. *Psychosom Med* 12:89–97, 1950.

99. Humphrey ME, Zangwill OL: Cessation of dreaming after brain injury. *J Neurol Neurosurg Psychiatry* 14:322–325, 1951.

100. Austin MD: Dream recall and the bias of intellectual ability. *Nature* 231:59, 1971.

101. Alajouanine T, Lhermitte F: Des agnosies electives. *Encephale* 46:505, 1957.

102. Gainotti G: Reactions "catastrophiques" et manifestations d'indifference au cours des atteintes cerebrales. *Neuropsychologia* 7:195–204, 1969.

103. Critchley M: Observations on anosodiaphoria. *Encephale* 46:540–546, 1957.

104. Weinstein EA, Kahn RL: *Denial of Illness: Symbolic and Physiological Aspects.* Springfield, Ill, Charles C Thomas Publisher, 1955.

105. Critchley M: *The Parietal Lobes.* London, Edward Arnold & Co, 1953.

106. Sprague JM: Visual, acoustic, and somesthetic deficits in the cat after cortical and midbrain lesions, in Purpura DP, Yohr M (eds): *The Thalamus.* New York, Columbia University Press, 1966, pp 391–417.

107. Terzian H, Cecotto C: Determinazione e studio della dominanza emisferica mediante iniezione intra carotide di Amytal Sodico nell'uomo (modification cliniche). *Boll Soc Ital Biol Sper* 35:1623–1626, 1959.

108. Terzian H: Behavioural and EEG effects of intracarotid Sodium Amytal injections. *Acta Neurochir (Wien)* 12:230–240, 1964.

109. Wada J, Rasmussen T: Intracarotid injection of Sodium Amytal for the lateralization of cerebral speech dominance. *J Neurosurg* 17:266–282, 1960.

110. Alema G, Rosadini G, Rossi GF: Psychic reactions associated with intracarotid Amytal injection and relation to brain damage. *Excerpta Medica* 37:154–155, 1961.

111. Rossi GF, Rosadini GR: Experimental analysis of cerebral dominance in man, in Millikan DH, Darley FL (eds): *Brain Mechanisms Underlying Speech and Language.* New York, Grune & Stratton Inc, 1967, pp 167–184.

112. Milner B, cited in Rossi GF, Rosadini GR: Experimental analysis of cerebral dominance in man, in Millikan DH, Darley FL (eds): *Brain Mechanisms Underlying Speech and Language.* New York, Grune & Stratton Inc, 1967, p 177ff.

113. Hommes OR, Panhuysen LHHM: Bilateral intracarotid Amytal injection. *Psychiatr Neurol Neurochir* 73:447–459, 1970.

114. Hommes OR, Panhuysen LHHM: Depression and cerebral dominance. *Psychiatr Neurol Neurochir* 74:259–270, 1971.

115. Halliday AM, Davison K, Brown MW, et al.: Comparison of effects on depression and memory of bilateral ECT and unilateral ECT to the dominant and nondominant hemisphere. *Br J Psychiatry* 114:997–1012, 1968.

116. Cronin D, Bodley P, Potts L, et al.: Unilateral and bilateral ECT: A study of memory disturbance and relief from depression. *J Neurol Neurosurg Psychiatry* 3:705–713, 1970.

117. Costello CG, Belton GP, Abra JC, et al.: The amnesic and therapeutic effects of bilateral and unilateral ECT. *Br J Psychiatry* 116:69–78, 1970.

118. Fleminger JJ, Del Horne DJ, Nair NPV, et al.: Differential effect of unilateral and bilateral ECT. *Am J Psychiatry* 127:430–436, 1970.

119. Sutherland EM, Oliver J, Knight D: EEG memory and confusion in dominant and non-dominant and bi-temporal ECT. *Br J Psychiatry* 115:1059–1064, 1969.

120. Zinkin S, Birtchnell J: Unilateral electroconvulsive therapy: Its effects on memory and its therapeutic efficacy. *Br J Psychiatry* 114:973–988, 1968.

121. d'Elia G: Comparison of electroconvulsive therapy with unilateral and bilateral stimulation. *Acta Psychiatr Scand* 215:30–43, 1970.

122. Lancaster NR, Steinert R, Frost I: Unilateral electroconvulsive therapy. *J Ment Sci* 104:221–227, 1958.

123. Impastasto DJ, Karliner W: Control of memory impairment in ECT by unilateral stimulation of the non-dominant hemisphere. *Dis Nerv Syst* 27:182–188, 1966.

124. Bidder TG, Strain JJ, Brunschwig L: Bilateral and unilateral ECT: Follow-up study and critique. *Am J Psychiatry* 127:737–745, 1970.

125. Abrams R, Fink M, Dornbush RL, et al.: Unilateral and bilateral electroconvulsive therapy. *Arch Gen Psychiatry* 27:88–91, 1972.

126. Ottosson JO (ed): Experimental studies of the mode of action of electroconvulsive therapy. *Acta Psychiatr Scand* 35 (suppl 145) 1960.

127. Costello CG, Belton GP: Depression: Treatment, in Costello CG (ed): *Symptoms of Psychopathology.* New York, John Wiley & Sons Inc, 1970, pp 201–215.

128. McAndrew J, Berkey B, Mathews C: Effects of dominant and nondominant unilateral ECT as compared to bilateral ECT. *Am J Psychiatry* 124:483–490, 1967.

128. Silverman AJ: Perception, personality, and brain lateralization. Read before the proceedings of the Fifth World Congress of Psychiatry, Mexico City, 1971.

IX CONSCIOUSNESS AS A STATE: WAKING, DEEP SLEEP, COMA, ANESTHESIA, AND DREAMING

Until fairly recently, the controversial status of consciousness ensured that many researchers carefully avoided using the word *consciousness* in scientific discourse. This prohibition did not extend to clinical neurology, however, where loss of consciousness due to brain-stem damage has always been accepted as a medical commonplace (see Bogen 1995; chap. 53, this section). Such a pathological loss of consciousness has its daily analogue in the hours we all spend in oblivious sleep. Not surprisingly, then, studies of the anatomy and physiology of waking, sleep, and coma have been fundamental to our understanding of the brain basis of consciousness. As this introduction shows, the evidence suggests a useful division between brainstem mechanisms, which appear to control the *state* of consciousness, and cortical activity, which provides the *contents* of consciousness. In this section we focus on state variables.

The Waking Brain

Soon after Moruzzi and Magoun (1949; chap. 51, this volume) announced that damage to the core of the lower brain stem caused coma in experimental animals, a wave of research activity sought to define the nature of this core mechanism, called the *brain stem reticular formation.* Lower brain stem neurons were shown to project to the thalamus, and stimulation of the brain stem reticular formation was shown to trigger waking electrical activity in the cortex of drowsy or sleeping animals. The reticular activating system (RAS) seemed to be the mechanism of wakefulness. Today, introductory textbooks describe the RAS as responsible for transitions from unconscious sleep to waking, and from drowsiness to alertness. In the cortical EEG these changes go from the high-voltage, slow, and regular activity of deep sleep to the low-voltage, fast, and irregular waves of waking and dreaming.

Moruzzi and Magoun's work is widely cited as one of the landmark discoveries of modern brain

science. Yet despite two decades of intensive research, by the 1970s the concept of the RAS had fallen "into desuetude" owing to methodological difficulties in tracing its neurochemical and anatomical relations with the cortex (Steriade 1996). Bogen (1995; chap. 53, this volume) notes that the enthusiasm of early advocates for the reticular-thalamic core as "the indispensable substratum of consciousness" led them to attempt to explain too much. A backlash of sorts ensued among more conservative researchers, as data continued to lag behind conjecture. This led to a return to nineteenth-century conventional wisdom, which holds that all cognitive processes (conscious or otherwise) are the exclusive purview of the cortex. And although evidence has accumulated for a critical role of subcortical areas in episodic memory and attention, most present-day neuroscientists remain circumspect about linking their findings to those of the early pioneers in electroencephalography. Yet EEG remains the most reliable objective marker for distinguishing conscious from unconscious states. Absence of waking EEG is the major criterion for determining "brain death," justifying discontinuation of life support in otherwise viable coma patients.

The chapters in this section provide a broader context for understanding the evidence. As Moruzzi and Magoun predicted, the thalamus has indeed proven to be the critical intermediate link between the reticular formation (RF) and the cortex. Just as its specific nuclei are responsible for relaying all signals to the cortex conveying auditory, somatic, and visual sensations, so the "nonspecific" intralaminar nuclei of the thalamus do so for the midbrain reticular formation. Axonal transport tracing methods developed during the 1970s and 1980s finally confirmed this fact. They also demonstrated some unique anatomical features of the intralaminar neurons extending from thalamus to cortex. Its neurons have thinner, slower conducting axons; their synapses are concentrated outside the middle layers of the cortex (the targets of specific axons); and they are widely distributed in cortex (except in the primary sensory areas). Yet some surprisingly "specific" qualities were discovered as well: projections from discrete intralaminar nuclei generally terminate in circumscribed cortical areas and, as with the sensory cortices, these projections are richly reciprocated. Moreover, both sets of projections employ the excitatory neurotransmitter glutamate. Together they form a vast system of thalamo-cortico-thalamic loops spanning the entire cortex (Macchi and Bentivoglio 1986, Paré and Llinás 1995).

As Bogen's chapter describes, clinical studies lend weight to the hypothesis that the reticular-thalamic core is, in fact, an "indispensable substratum of consciousness." Large areas of the cortex—indeed an entire cerebral hemisphere—can be surgically removed without the loss of consciousness. Bogen cites a study in which, of four patients undergoing a total hemispherectomy, three reported being "acutely aware" *during the course of the operation.* On the other hand, damage to very small parts of the reticular-thalamic core can result in massive coma. For example, in bilateral lesions of the small intralaminar nuclei of the thalamus "unresponsiveness typically ensues.... Sudden onset of coma can occur even when the lesions are only a few cubic centimeters in volume" (Bogen 1995, p. 54; chap. 53, this volume). Of course, circumscribed lesions to the cortex can selectively impair conscious functions like color or object perception, face recognition, perhaps all the major features of sensory consciousness. But as Bogen argues, these cortical lesions have more to do with the *contents* of consciousness, than with consciousness *as a state.* It is the reticular-thalamic core, particularly the intralaminar nuclei, which he believes to be indispensable to generating subjective awareness.

Another closely related element of the thalamus that plays a major role in selective attention and consciousness is the reticular nucleus (nRt, for nucleus reticularis thalami), a thin, shell-like layer covering the egg-shaped thalamus. The nRt had been identified early on by Jasper (1960) and his colleagues as an integral part of the "unspecific" thalamus. Early conjectures that the neurons of this shell were the locus of the "diffuse thalamic projection" were proven to be unfounded by Golgi stain studies by Scheibel and Scheibel (1967). Their research showed that 90% of nucleus reticularis axons projected *back into* the thalamic nuclei they overlay—none to the cortex. Yet, the Scheibels' exquisite detective work also suggested how an array of cells topographically tied to specific thalamic nuclei could exercise global influences as well. For both the specific and nonspecific thalamo-cortical-thalamic loops give off collateral projections to nRt as they pass through it, modulating its inhibitory actions on the underlying thalamus. As Arnold Scheibel argues in his 1980 review of progress on elucidating the RAS (chap. 52, this volume), the accumulated evidence suggested that nucleus reticularis resembles a mosaic of neural "gatelets" sitting astride both the major inputs to the cortex and the outputs from it. Subsequent research has supplemented this picture to include more intricate, looping connectivities from the hippocampus, basal ganglia, and prefrontal cortex to the thalamic extension of the RAS (see Steriade and Llinás 1986 for review). In short, whereas the thalamus may be viewed as the traffic cop governing sensory inflow to the cortex, nRt appears to control the thalamic gates themselves.

Two facts about the reticular nucleus make its gating architecture uniquely suited to the global modulation of cortical processing. First, the gatelets have a topographic structure, allowing them to be activated by particular cortical modules or coalitions of modules. Such excitatory loops, with inhibitory interneurons, constitute a vast bank of oscillating neural amplifiers, capable of mediating a multimodal competition between sensory inputs, RF activation, and cortical feedback upon the thalamus (see Newman, Baars, and Cho 1997; chap. 67, this volume).

Second, the inhibitory dendrites of reticular neurons onto which the excitatory loops synapse, spread out in both directions along the axis of the reticular nucleus, creating a continuous felt-work of dendro-dendritic connections ideally suited to the generation and coherent spreading of neural oscillations, not just across the nucleus itself but over the entire cerebral cortex, by way of thalamocortical loops. Based on this remarkable convergence of connectivities Scheibel (1980; chap. 52, this volume) predicted, "Perhaps here resides the structurofunctional substrate of selective awareness" (p. 55). The viability of this hypothesis has only been strengthened over the years (in this volume, see Newman, Baars, and Cho, chap. 47, and Taylor, chap. 67; Llinás and Paré, chap. 59; also Crick (1984) and LaBerge, chap. 21; Crick and Koch, chap. 3).

Before the discovery of the RAS, it was widely assumed that the sleep-wake cycle was essentially driven by events in the environment. To test this, Moruzzi and Magoun (1949; chap. 51, this volume) went to the extent of not only severing the spinal cord from the brain in some of their cat preparations (*encéphale isolé*), but "full atropinization and curarization" of their bodies. The persistence of desynchronization of the cortical EEG upon reticular-formation stimulation demonstrated that no external stimulus was required to produce central arousal. Conversely, in fully anesthetized but otherwise intact animals—where reticular-formation stimulation produces little effect upon the cortex—stimulating the sensory tracts did evoke a secondary cortical EEG response, but one largely confined to primary cortex.

Such findings demonstrated that the waking state was not a passive response to external stimulation, but an active, endogenous maintenance of an optimal level of cortical arousal for full conscious processing. But what about sleep and dreaming? Were they actively induced, global states as well?

Recent resurgence in interest about EEG rhythms as possible correlates of conscious processes has led some observers to note that most research in this field, until recently, involved fully anesthetized animals, which obviously makes it difficult to study consciousness. But to Moruzzi and Magoun's credit, they tested intact cats under both heavy and light anesthesia, and unanesthetized *encéphale isolé* preparations in spontaneous states ranging from sleep and drowsiness to full alertness. Stimulation of the reticular formation in their drowsy cats (in which alpha "spindles" in the 8–13-Hz range predominate) produced precisely the same "alpha wave blockade" that Berger reported in human subjects in the 1930s: replacing synchronous alpha with fast, asynchronous beta activity (Berger 1969).

Perchance to Dream . . .

The dominant perspective on dreaming today stems from the work of J. Allan Hobson and colleagues at Harvard Medical School, based on the earlier discovery of REM sleep by Dement and Kleitman (1957; chap. 56, this volume). Hobson and McCarley's (1977; chap. 57, this volume) Activation-Synthesis Model of Dream State Generation was largely based on their physiological studies of the brain stem reticular formation in cats. It relied on Dement and Kleitman's earlier demonstration that the dream state has some highly reliable correlates—namely, rapid eye movements (REMs), fast EEG activity virtually indistinguishable from that seen in a fully awake subject, and paralysis of the skeletal muscles. In effect, Dement and Kleitman showed that dreaming was a kind of conscious state. This unexpected finding led researchers to refer to the dream state as "paradoxical sleep," a kind of waking sleep.

As previously noted, the idea of a unified activation system fell "into desuetude" in the 1970s in part because of difficulties in tracing the neurochemical relations of the RAS with the cortex. In particular, the discovery of the major monoaminergic neuromodulators (serotonin, noradrenaline) and their sources in the core of the brain stem did much to undermine such a notion. For although the nuclei that produce these neuromodulators (raphe for serotonin and locus coeruleus for noradrenaline) activate the cortex via widely distributed projections, the bulk of their ascending fibers bypass the thalamus, which suggests not one, but three brain-stem activating systems. And whereas a third cholinergically modulated activating system has been traced from the reticular formation, projecting predominantly to the intralaminar thalamus, the intralaminar projections themselves proved not to be cholinergic. Instead, they utilize the same neurotransmitter as the cortex: glutamate. Now that the central role of the thalamo-cortical-thalamic loops in selectively amplifying cortical activation is known, this makes eminent sense, but it was far from clear when these neurotransmitters were first being traced.

Hobson and McCarley's (1977; chap. 57, this volume) contribution has been to elucidate how these three activation systems interact to produce dreaming and deep sleep. In doing so, they demonstrated the centrality of the cholinergic activating system in both waking and dreaming. They were able to isolate a particular cluster of excitatory neurons in the pontine reticular formation (PRF) whose cyclic activity is maximal during REM sleep. Injecting acetylcholine into the PRF enhanced and prolonged REM activity. Conversely, cells in the nearby locus coeruleus and raphe nuclei showed maximal inhibition during REM. The hyperactivation of PRF has a number of interesting effects. It inhibits nearby motor nuclei (at the same time that it drives REM), producing the characteristic paralysis associated with dream sleep. Brain-stem sensory nuclei for relaying exteroceptive inputs are also markedly attenuated, protecting sleep.

Hobson and McCarley also showed that PRF activation of the midbrain reticular formation

generated EEG activity in the cortex essentially identical to that seen in the waking state. Finally, PRF activates the major thalamic nucleus that relays visual signals to the brain during waking. This nonsensory activation of the nucleus is very likely the mechanism behind the predominance of visual imagery in dreams. Yet despite essentially identical EEG signatures, Hobson and McCarley demonstrated clear physiological differences between the dream state and waking consciousness. Because both the locus coeruleus and serotonergic raphe nuclei have a reciprocally inhibitory relationship with PRF, when they activate upon waking they dampen PRF activity. This appears to allow sensory collaterals given off to the midline reticular formation (as they continue on to the thalamus) to replace PRF activation of the sensory-motor systems. This, as Llinás and Paré (1991; chap. 59, this volume) argue, is the primary difference between dreaming and waking.

The idea that dreaming and waking have much in common, although it may appeal to the artist and psychiatrist, is a rather radical scientific hypothesis. Yet it receives support from an exceptional study in which dreaming subjects were trained to signal when they were consciously aware of a signal *during their dreams*, using an agreed-upon pattern of eye movements (LaBerge, Nagel, Dement, and Zarcone 1981; chap. 58, this volume). Such "lucid dreaming" is now a generally accepted phenomenon. The LaBerge et al. study supports the idea that consciousness—in the sense that subjects can have awareness of, and voluntarily report that they are dreaming—is an intrinsic function of the brain, independent of sense perception.

Two chapters address the still mysterious mechanism of general anesthesia, an artificially induced loss of the conscious state. A range of chemicals induce a loss of consciousness, and much of the scientific challenge is to understand how they do this in seemingly different ways. Flohr's influential hypothesis is that anesthetics have a common mechanism by affecting the functioning of the neurotransmitter NMDA (Flohr 1995; chap. 54, this volume). If this is true, it would explain not only anesthesia but also the nature of neuronal cell assemblies that are widely thought to underlie specific conscious experiences. A different hypothesis is pursued by Alkire, Haier, and Fallon (2000; chap. 55, this volume). These authors present brain imaging evidence for a "thalamocortical switch" triggered by neuronal blockade due to hyperpularization.

Historically, the methods of science have placed the focus almost exclusively on external events as determining reality. And yet our consciousness, which is the very organ by which we observe and report this reality, would seem to depend on a neural substrate more suited to generating personally meaningful, cognitive states than merely reflecting events in the external world. If we think of the brain as a complex system that has evolved over eons to meet the organism's internal needs for planning and self-control, this preoccupation with inner states does not seem so strange. In this context, science's traditional focus on external reality may simply reflect a progression from the study of what is most apparent and tractable to a trained empiricist; today, we may be moving toward an understanding of the mental processes that make such understanding possible.

Returning to our earlier questions about the function of dreaming, as Llinás and Paré note, answers remain "elusive" but certainly the chapters introduced in this section provide vital clues. Hobson and McCarley's classic work argues that what we dream is determined at least as much by the brain's internal physiology as the "residue" of the previous day's events, and that physiology argues against there being a conscious "censor" disguising the latent content of our dreams. In Hobson's model, activation of the cortex by the reticular formation puts its cognitive apparatus in motion and, as in waking, the cortex attempts to synthesize what it is experiencing into a coherent series of episodes. But

because the noradrenergic and serotonergic activation that accompanies cholinergic RAS activity in waking states is inhibited during sleep, cortical processes modulating memory consolidation and focused attention are quiescent. This would appear to cause the cortex to generate bizarre and illogical scenes (sometimes accompanied by vivid emotions). As Hobson and McCarley hypothesize, it may well be that brainstem–generated REM evokes scene shifts as the cortex works to synthesize corollary discharges relayed to it by subcortical sensory and motor nuclei. Alternatively, the "spatial envelope" Scheibel describes in this section as providing a global map of the environment during waking may serve to orient the sleeper in their "dream world" as well.

But to what purpose? After all, the brain functions, ultimately, as a *psychological* not a physiological organ. And to all appearances, it is as cognitively active during REM sleep as waking. Could it be that, despite so little confirmation by science of Freud's particular theories, he was not so far off the mark in calling dreams "the royal road to the unconscious"? Certainly modern cognitive science has demonstrated that many cognitive processes proceed in our brains quite automatically, outside our conscious awareness (see section 7). Indeed, the argument has been made since William James's (1890/ 1983) time that a prime function of consciousness is selecting out what is relevant-in-the-moment from the great "bloom and buzz" of outer events and inner images impinging on our nervous system. Could it be that dreams somehow allow all of this subliminal activity to "have its day" even during sleep? Such a conception is supported not only by the inhibition of noradrenergic activation (increasing noradrenaline facilitates alerting), but Llinás and Paré's observation that, "in contrast to wakefulness, REM sleep was shown to be accompanied by a reduction of inhibitory activity in cortical neurons" (1991, p. 523). Perhaps dreaming is about bringing to completion, or at least quiescence, subliminal thoughts and emotions from preceding days. Given that most of these memories were only half-formed, and unrelated to the day's focus, it would make sense that we seldom remember our dreams. On the other hand, it may be that those dreams we *do* remember have important emotional connotations obscured, not by a "censor," but by the foreignness of dream images to our everyday consciousness. Whatever the case, the papers found in this section leave little doubt that rigorous empirical methods can be fruitfully applied to what many scientists still regard as thoroughly enigmatic phenomena.

References

Berger, H. (1969) On the electroencephalogram of man. Fourth report. *Electroencephalogr Clin Neurophysiol.* 1969:Suppl 28:133.

James, W. (1890/1983) *The principles of psychology.* Revised edition, Cambridge, MA: Harvard University Press.

Jasper, H. H., Proctor, Lorne D., Knighton, R. S., Noshay, W. C., and Costello, R. T., eds. (1958) Reticular formation of the brain. Boston: Little, Brown.

Macchi G., Bentivoglio, M. (1999) Is the "nonspecific" thalamus still "nonspecific"? *Arch Ital Biol.* 137(2–3):201–26.

Paré D., Llinás R. (1995) Conscious and pre-conscious processes as seen from the standpoint of sleep-waking cycle neurophysiology. *Neuropsychologia.* 33(9):1155–68.

Scheibel, M. E., and Scheibel, A. B. (1967) Structural organization of nonspecific thalamic nuclei and their projection toward cortex. *Brain Res.* 6(1):60–94.

Steriade M., and Llinás, R. R. (1988) The functional states of the thalamus and the associated neuronal interplay. *Physiol Rev.* 68(3):649–742.

Steriade, M. (1996) Arousal: revisiting the reticular activating system. *Science,* 272(5259):225–6.

51 Brain Stem Reticular Formation and Activation of the EEG

G. Moruzzi and H. W. Magoun

Transitions from sleep to wakefulness, or from the less extreme states of relaxation and drowsiness to alertness and attention, are all characterized by an apparent breaking up of the synchronization of discharge of elements of the cerebral cortex, an alteration marked in the EEG by the replacement of high-voltage slow waves with low-voltage fast activity. The magnitude of the electrical change parallels the degree of transition, and that most commonly observed in clinical electroencephalography is a minimal one, consisting of an alpha-wave blockade during attention to visual stimulation. Such activation of the EEG may be produced by any type of afferent stimulus that arouses the subject to alertness, or it may be centrally generated, but the basic processes underlying it, like those involved in waking from sleep, have remained obscure.

Recent experimental findings which may contribute to this subject have stemmed from the observation that EEG changes seemingly identical with those in the physiological arousal reactions can be produced by direct stimulation of the reticular formation of the brain stem. The following account describes such features of the response and its excitable substrate as have been determined, provides an analysis of changes in cortical and thalamic activity associated with it, and explores the relations of this reticular activating system to the arousal reaction to natural stimuli. Alterations produced by acute lesions in this system are presented in a succeeding paper. The effects of chronic lesions within it are under investigation.

Methods

The experiments were performed in cats under chloralosane anesthesia (35–50 mgm./K, intraperitoneally) or in the "encéphale isolé" of Bremer, prepared under ether, with exposure margins infiltrated with procaine. Ephedrine was administered intravenously immediately after transection of the cord at C 1. At least an hour elapsed after ether was discontinued before work was begun.

Concentric bipolar electrodes, oriented with the Horsley-Clarke technique, were used for stimulation of, or pickup from, the brain stem. Condenser discharges from a Goodwin stimulator were employed routinely. Lesions were made surgically or electrolytically, and their positions, together with those of electrode placements, were verified histologically.

Potentials were recorded with a Grass model III amplifier and inkwriter. Some cortical records were taken directly from the pial surface, but usually as much of the brain case as possible was left intact, and most cortical pickups were between two screw electrodes, 5–10 mm apart, inserted through burr holes in the calvarium until their tips rested on the dura overlying functional areas. With bipolar leads and by grounding the scalp, stimulus artifacts were negligible. Other technical details are given in the legends.

Results

The response to reticular stimulation consisted of cessation of synchronized discharge in the EEG and its replacement with low-voltage fast activity. The intensity of the alteration varied with the degree of background synchrony present. Conspicuous effects were thus observed against the high-voltage slow waves of chloralosane anesthesia (figures 51.1c,d), while a fully activated EEG was not further affected (figure 51.1a). Responses were seen to best advantage when the unanesthetized brain exhibited some relaxation (figures 51.2b,c) or when light chloralosane

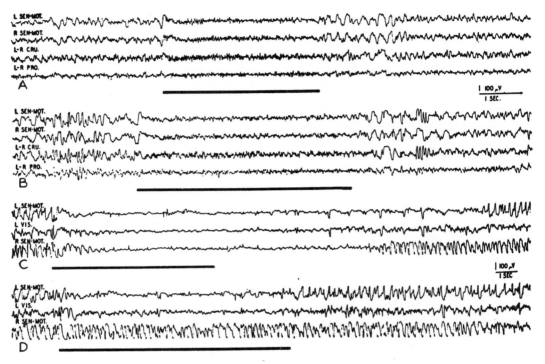

Figure 51.1
Effect of stimulation of the brain stem reticular formation upon electro-cortical activity of chloralosane preparations. (*a*) and (*b*) *Encéphale isolé* with 7 mgm chloralosane/K. Replacement of high-voltage slow waves, present in (*a*) and more pronounced in (*b*), with low-voltage fast activity during left bulbo-reticular stimulation (1.5 V, 300/s). (*c*) Intact cat with 50 mg chloralosane/K. Left bulbo-reticular stimulation (3 V, 300/s) blocks chloralosane waves bilaterally, but more rapidly and for a longer time in the ipsilateral cortex. Note that low-voltage fast activity does not appear. (*d*) like (*c*) but frequency of reticular stimulation reduced to 100/s. Effect limited to ipsilateral cortex and doesn't outlast stimulus. In all records, the origin of activity in different channels is given at the left: L. SEN. MOT. signifies left sensory-motor cortex; L.-R. CRU., left to right cruciate gyrus; L.-R. PRO., left to right gyrus proreus; L. VIS., left visual area; L. AUD., left auditory area; L. THAL., left thalamus. The period of bulbar stimulation is marked by a heavy line beneath the record. Calibration and time are stated.

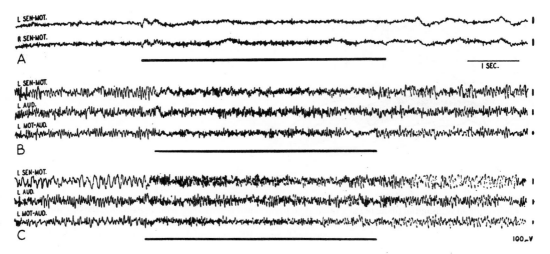

Figure 51.2

Effect of reticular stimulation on electro-cortical activity of the unanesthetized *encéphale isolé*. (*a*)–(*c*) Left bulbo-reticular stimulation (3 V, 300/s) is without effect upon the fully activated cortex (*a*), but evokes characteristic low-voltage fast activity when spontaneous synchrony is present (*b*) and (*c*).

anesthesia had induced synchronization without greatly impairing neural excitability (figures 51.1a,b). With deeper chloralosane, slow waves were blocked, but low-voltage fast activity was not elicited (figures 51.1c,d).

The response was a generalized one, being observed in the sensory-motor cortex (figure 51.1), where it was often most pronounced, and in the visual (figure 51.1c) and auditory (figures 51.2b,c) cortical areas as well. With minimal reticular stimulation, alterations were best obtained in the ipsilateral hemisphere and were sometimes limited to it (figure 51.1d).

The response was readily obtained with low intensities of reticular stimulation; voltages of 1–3 being usually employed. Brief shocks, with a falling phase of 1 ms were used routinely and were as effective as longer lasting ones. Stimulus frequencies of 50/s were the lowest at which definite alterations could be elicited and the response was considerably improved by increasing frequencies up to 300/s, which were regularly

utilized. Thus the EEG response to reticular excitation was best obtained with low voltage, high frequency stimulation.

These responses were not secondary to any peripheral effects of brain stem stimulation. By direct test they were independent of changes in respiration, blood pressure, and heart rate. They occurred in the isolated brain after full atropinization and curarization. As will be seen, they were unquestionably mediated by neural connections between the reticular formation and the cerebral hemisphere.

The distribution of the excitable area is projected upon a reconstruction of the midsagittal plane in figure 51.3 and includes the central core of the brain stem, extending from the bulbar reticular formation forward through the pontile and mesencephalic tegmentum into the caudal diencephalon. At the bulbar level, excitable points were distributed in the ventromedial reticular formation and the area of their distribution coincided with that from which suppression

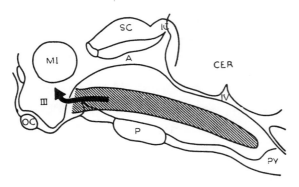

Figure 51.3
Reconstruction of midsagittal plane of cat's brain stem upon which is projected, with cross-lining, the distribution of the ascending reticular activating system. Abbreviations are as follows: A, aqueduct; CER, cerebellum; IC, interior colliculus; MI, massa intermedia; OC, optic chiasma; P, pons; PY, pyramidal crossing; SC, superior colliculus; III, third ventricle; IV, fourth ventricle.

of motor activity (Magoun and Rhines 1946) could be elicited (figure 51.4a). Exploration of the overlying cerebellum has revealed excitable points in its fastigial nuclei, the responses possibly being mediated by connections of the roof nuclei with the brain stem reticular formation (Snider, Magoun, and McCulloch 1949). In the midbrain, responses were obtained from the tegmentum bordering the central grey and extending in a paramedian position beneath it (figure 51.4b). In the caudal diencephalon, effective points were located near the midline in the dorsal hypothalamus and subthalamus (figure 51.4c). From this region, the excitable system is evidently distributed to the overlying thalamus, through which its effects are exerted upon the cortex, and some data bearing on its thalamic mediation will be given later.

The distribution of this ascending system within the midbrain was studied further by observing the effect of lesions here upon the EEG response to bulbo-reticular stimulation. Such responses were unimpaired following sections, of the cerebral peduncles or tectum, but were blocked by injury to the mesencephalic tegmentum (figure 51.4d). Typical cortical responses to

bulbo-reticular stimulation were still obtained after bilateral destruction of all laterally placed mesencephalic structures, including the medial and lateral lemnisci and the spinothalamic tracts (figures 51.4e,f), leaving intact only the paramedian region from which responses were obtained on direct stimulation (figure 51.4b).

A series of ascending reticular relays is presumed to constitute the structural substrate of this brain stem activating system. That responses are not attributable to the antidromic excitation of corticifugal paths, nor to the dromic stimulation of known afferent paths, bordering the reticular area, is indicated by a variety of data.

As regards the pyramidal tract, movements referable to its excitation never accompanied EEG responses to reticular stimulation, and the latter were still obtained from the bulbar level after section of the fibers of this tract in the basis pedunculi (figure 51.4d). Furthermore, single shock stimuli to effective reticular sites did not evoke antidromic potentials in the sensory-motor cortex (figures 51.5c,e) (figure 51.10a), nor did direct stimulation of the bulbar pyramid reproduce the EEG response to reticular stimulation.

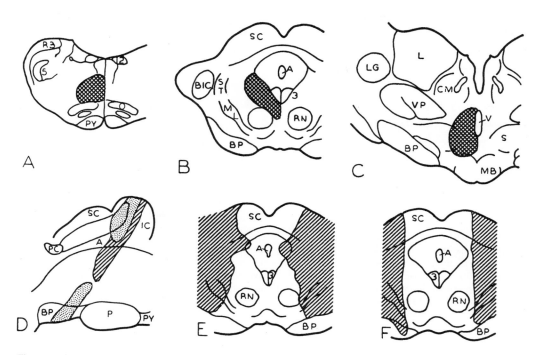

Figure 51.4

(*a*)–(*c*) Transverse sections through bulbar (*a*), mesencephalic (*b*), and caudal diencephalic (*c*) levels, with cross-lining indicating the area from which reticular responses were elicited with lowest voltage and without complications from exciting other ascending or descending neural connections. (*d*) Reconstruction of midsagittal plane of the midbrain upon which is projected, with stipple, the position of tectal and peduncular lesions which failed to block the EEG response to bulbo-reticular stimulation. Cross-lining marks the position of a tegmental lesion which abolished this response to bulbar stimulation. (*e*) and (*f*) Transverse sections through the midbrain of two cats, showing the extent of lesions which interrupted the medial and lateral lemnisci and spinothalamic tracts, but which failed to impair the EEG response to bulbo-reticular stimulation. Abbreviations are as follows: A, aqueduct; BIC, brachium of inferior colliculus; BP, basis penduculi; CM, centre median; IC, inferior colliculus; L, lateral thalamic nucleus; LG, lateral geniculate body; MB, mammillary body; S, subthalamus; SC, superior colliculus; ST, spinothalamic tract; VP, posterior part of ventral thalamic nucleus; 3, oculomotor nucleus; 5, spinal fifth tract and nucleus; 12, hypoglossal nucleus.

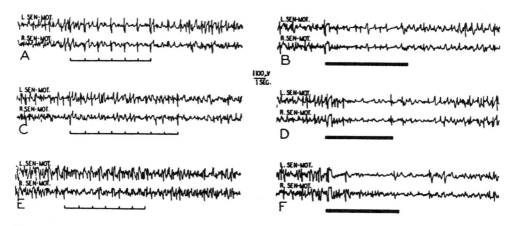

Figure 51.5
Comparison of the effects of stimulating the right posterior column (a, b) and the left reticular activating system at bulbar (c, d) and midbrain (e, f) levels, under full chloralosane anesthesia. Stimulus frequency is 1/s in left records (a, c, e) and 300/s in right records (b, d, f); intensity is 3 V throughout. Single shock stimuli to the posterior column evoke sensory potentials in the cortex (a), not elicited by similar reticular stimulation (c, e). High-frequency stimulation of the posterior column causes some desynchronization of the EEG (b), but more pronounced effects are induced by reticular stimulation (d, f).

A cortico-bulbo-reticular path from area 4-S is distributed to the excitable reticular area of the lower brain stem (figure 51.4a) (McCulloch, Graf, and Magoun 1946), but it is similarly impossible to attribute the EEG responses to its antidromic stimulation. This path accompanies the pyramidal tract in the basis pedunculi (McCulloch, Graf, and Magoun 1946) section of which, as noted, left reticular responses unimpaired. The absence of antidromic potentials in the sensory-motor cortex, on single shock stimuli to the bulbar reticular formation (figure 51.5c, figure 51.10a), might be explained by the small size of the suppressor areas in the cat (Garol 1942), but a more likely possibility is that the unmyelinated terminals of this extrapyramidal path were never excited with the low intensities of reticular stimulation employed in the present experiments. Reticular responses elicited from brain stem levels cephalad to the bulb are, moreover, impossible to explain on the basis of antidromic stimulation of this extrapyramidal pathway.

It is equivalently impossible to ascribe reticular responses to the dromic activation of known afferent pathways ascending to the cortex through the brain stem. The medial lemniscus is adjacent to the excitable reticular area through much of its course, and high frequency stimulation of the lemniscal system, like that of the sciatic nerve (Gellhorn 1947), exerts a desynchronizing influence upon the EEG (figure 51.5b). This influence is not as pronounced as that of the reticular formation and higher voltages of stimulation are required to induce it than those which yield primary and secondary cortical sensory responses.

Three lines of evidence clearly show, however, that the desynchronizing influence of the reticular formation cannot be attributed to activation of the lemniscal system, either through physical spread of stimulating current, or by antidromic excitation of possible lemniscal collaterals to the brain stem reticular formation. First, single shock stimuli to excitable reticular points at bulbar (figure 51.5c) or midbrain (figure 51.5e)

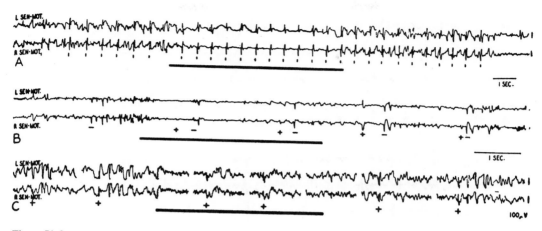

Figure 51.6
Effect of reticular stimulation upon cortical sensory responses. (*a*) Tapping skin of ankle. (*b*) Make and break shocks to the sciatic nerve, under full chloralosane anesthesia as in (*a*). (*c*) Single shocks to the upper end of the posterior column, in *encéphale isolé* with 7 mgm chloralosane/K. In each instance the evoked sensory spike is unaffected, while consequent after-discharge is abolished. Not low-voltage fast activity during reticular stimulation in (*c*), with minimal anesthesia, and its absence in (*a*) and (*b*), with full anesthesia.

levels never evoked potentials in the sensory-motor cortex, as was invariably the case when such shocks were applied to the lemniscal system (figure 51.5a), and this simple control was routinely applied throughout the work. Second, the distribution of the excitable reticular area was distinct from that of the course of the medial lemniscus through the brain stem (figures 51.4a–c). Third and finally, EEG responses to bulbar stimulation were unaffected by mesencephalic lesions which bilaterally interrupted the medial and lateral lemnisci and the spinothalamic tracts (figures 51.4e,f).

Elimination of these possibilities and the distribution of excitable points through the brain stem both indicate that this response is mediated by a paramedian system of ascending reticular connections. Single shock stimuli to effective bulbar sites do not evoke potentials at effective midbrain or diencephalic sites, however, suggesting that a number of relays are present and that the synapses involved are iterative in nature.

Having now described the desynchronization of the EEG induced by brain stem stimulation and presented evidence that this alteration results from exciting a system of reticular relays ascending to the diencephalon, attention may next be directed to the effect of reticular stimulation upon types of evoked activity in the cortex.

Effect upon Evoked Sensory Potentials

In the chloralosane cat, a single afferent volley, initiated either by natural stimuli or by shocks to the sciatic nerve or posterior column, evokes primary and secondary[1] cortical potentials and sensory "after-discharge" succeeding them. The secondary response and after-discharge occur generally in the cortex and are readily observed in the EEG. During stimulation of the brain stem reticular formation, such secondary responses continued to be evoked by afferent volleys, usually without alteration (figure 51.6a), but sometimes with reduction of amplitude and

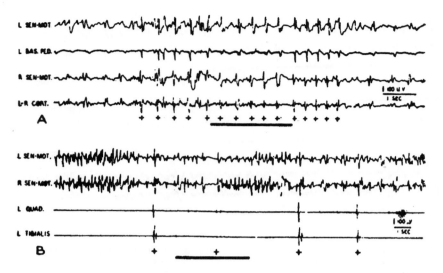

Figure 51.7
Effect of reticular stimulation on pyramidal discharges and chloralosane jerks. (*a*) Break shocks to sciatic nerve cause sensory cortical responses and corresponding pyramidal discharge, recorded from the basis pedunculi (channel 2). The latter and sensory after-discharge are almost abolished by bulbo-reticular stimulation (3 V, 300/s), which leaves cortical sensory spikes unaffected. (*b*) Break shocks to sciatic nerve cause chloralosane jerks, recorded in myograms of the quadriceps and tibialis (channels 3 and 4). Movement was abolished during stimulation of the midbrain tegmentum (3 V, 300/s), although cortical sensory potentials were still elicited. Such midbrain stimulation had no effect on spinal reflexes.

simplification of potential form, particularly in cortical areas outside the sensori-motor region (figure 51.8b). Following conclusion of reticular stimulation, transient enhancement of the secondary response was occasionally observed (figure 51.6b).

The succeeding high-voltage slow waves, called sensory after-discharge, were invariably abolished during reticular stimulation (figures 51.6a–c). In full anesthesia, the cortical record then became flat between secondary responses (figures 51.6a,b), while, if anesthesia was light, low-voltage fast activity was present in these intervals (figure 51.6c). The abolition of sensory after-discharge might thus be simply another manifestation of the desynchronization of the EEG induced by brain stem stimulation. Such

sensory after-discharge was not impaired, however, during cortical desynchronization induced by high frequency stimulation of the sciatic nerve (figure 51.8d).

Effect upon Evoked Pyramidal Discharge

In the chloralosane cat, afferent volleys arriving at the cortex there evoke pyramidal discharges which are responsible for the jerky movements characteristic of this anesthesia (Adrian and Moruzzi 1939). Although afferent volleys continued to reach the cortex during stimulation of the brain stem reticular formation, such pyramidal discharge, recorded from the basis pedunculi, was reduced or abolished (figure 51.7a) and contraction of leg muscles, induced by it, dis-

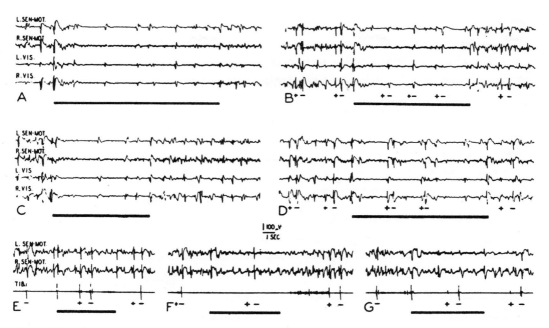

Figure 51.8

Comparison of effect of reticular and sensory stimulation upon spontaneous and evoked electro-cortical activity. (*a*, *c*) Abolition of chloralosane waves during (*a*) bulbo-reticular stimulation (2 V, 300/s) and (*c*) sciatic nerve stimulation (3 V, 300/s). (*b*, *d*) Sensory cortical potentials evoked by make and break shocks to sciatic nerve are reduced by bulbo-reticular stimulation at 2 V, 300/s (*b*), but not by stimulation of the contralateral sciatic nerve at 3 V, 300/s (*d*). (*e*, *f*) Chloralosane jerks evoked by break shocks to the sciatic nerve, and recorded in myograms of the tibialis anticus, were augmented (*e*) by contralateral sciatic nerve stimulation (3 V, 300/s) and abolished (*f*) by stimulation of the midbrain tegmentum (3 V, 300/s). Such midbrain stimulation did not influence tibialis contraction in the ipsilateral flexor reflex (*g*).

appeared (figures 51.7b and 51.8f). This disappearance of movement was not attributable to spinal inhibition, for reflexly induced contraction of the same muscles was not affected by such midbrain stimulation (figure 51.8g). The movements induced by this pyramidal discharge were not reduced during desynchronization of cortical electrical activity by high-frequency sciatic stimulation (figure 51.8e), and the facilitation observed might have been due to spinal alterations. Whether the more pronounced cortical desynchronization resulting from reticular stimulation (figures 51.5b,d,f) opposed simultaneous dis-

charge of a sufficient number of interneurons connecting the sensory with the motor cortex to prevent threshold activation of the cells of origin of the pyramidal tract, or whether these cells were somehow rendered incapable of being excited by afferent cortical volleys, during brain stem stimulation, remains unsettled.

Effect upon Cortical Strychnine Spikes

The recurring spikes produced by local strychnization of the sensori-motor cortex were not prevented by exciting the brain stem reticular

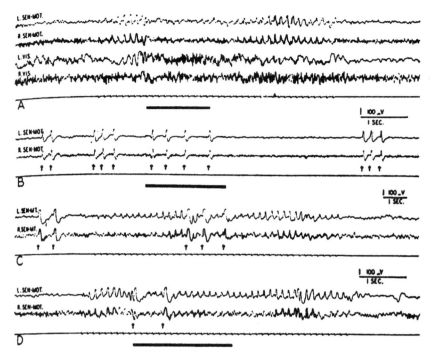

Figure 51.9
Effect of reticular stimulation upon recruiting response and cortical strychnine spikes. (*a*) Recruiting response to left thalamic stimulation (5 V, 7.5/s) in *encéphale isolé*, abolished by left bulbo-reticular stimulation (2 V, 300/s). (*b*) Strychnine spikes in both sensory-motor areas, induced by local application of strychnine to left motor cortex, were not decreased by left bulbo-reticular stimulation (2 V, 300/s). (*c*) Decrease of recruiting response (evoked as in (*a*)), following interspersed strychnine spikes. (*d*) Recruiting response (evoked as in (*a*)) markedly decreased by left bulbo-reticular stimulation (2 V, 300/s), which did not affect strychnine spikes.

formation, nor was conduction of this discharge to the opposite cortex interfered with (figure 51.9b). Synchronized convulsive waves in a cortical fit, induced by supramaximal stimulation of the motor cortex, were similarly unaffected by bulbo-reticular stimulation.

Effect upon Recruiting Response

The cortical response to low frequency stimulation of the diffuse thalamic projection system consists of a series of high-voltage slow waves,

one for each shock, which recruit to a maximum during the initial period of stimulation (figures 51.10–51.13) (Morison and Dempsey 1942, Dempsey and Morison 1942, Jasper and Droogleever-Fortuyn 1946, Jasper 1949). These waves may be confined to the ipsilateral hemisphere, but are usually present, though smaller, contralaterally as well. Depending upon the site of thalamic stimulation, they may be distributed anteriorly, posteriorly, or generally in the cortex.

In the unanesthetized "encéphale isolé", such a recruiting response, in both sensori-motor cor-

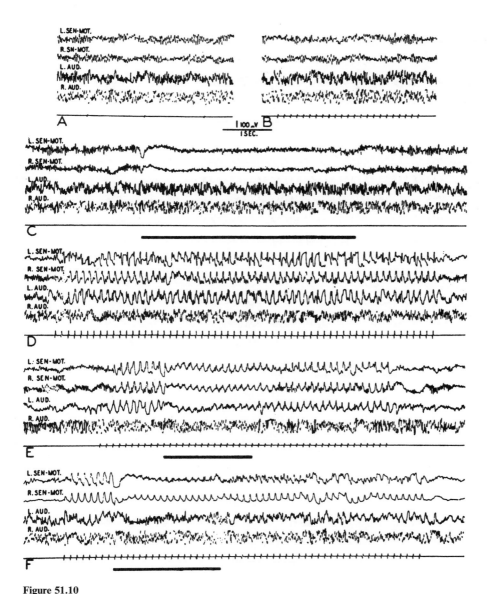

Figure 51.10

Effect of reticular stimulation upon recruiting response. Left bulbo-reticular stimulation at 3 V in *encéphale isolé*. (*a*) Single shocks to bulb do not evoke cortical potentials. (*b*) Bulbar stimulation at 7.5/s does not evoke recruiting response. (*c*) Bulbar stimulation at 300/s activates EEG. (*d*) Recruiting response evoked by left thalamic stimulation (5 V, 7.5/s). (*e*) Recruiting response to left thalamic stimulation reduced or abolished by left bulbar stimulation (3 V, 300/s). (*f*) Recruiting response to right thalamic stimulation reduced or abolished by left bulbar stimulation (3 V, 300/s).

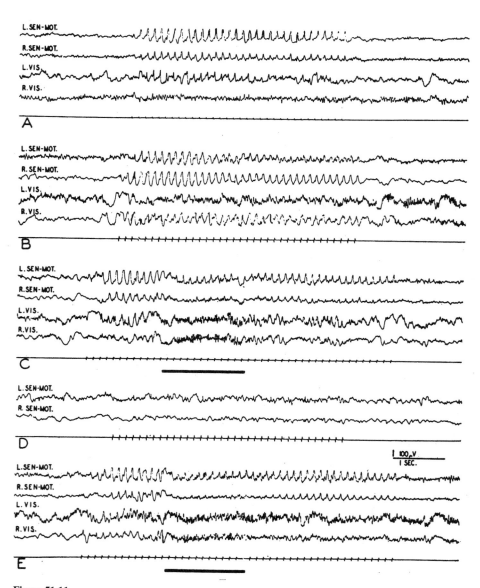

Figure 51.11

Reproduction of reticular response by high-frequency stimulation of diffuse thalamic projection system. (*a*) and (*b*) Recruiting responses induced by left (*a*) and right (*b*) thalamic stimulation (5 V, 7.5/s) in *encéphale isolé*. (*c*) Recruiting response to left thalamic stimulation reduced or abolished by stimulating the same right thalamic site as in (*b*), but with 5 V, 300/s. (*d*) Right electrode lowered into subthalamus, the stimulation of which with 5 V, 7.5/s fails to induce a recruiting response. (*e*) Subthalamic stimulation, with 5 V, 300/s, reduces or abolishes the recruiting response to left thalamic stimulation.

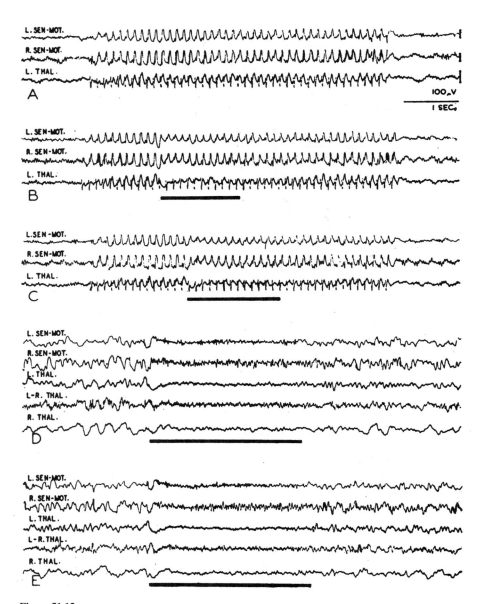

Figure 51.12
Effect of reticular stimulation upon electrothalamogram of diffuse projection system. (*a*)–(*c*) Unanesthetized *encéphale isolé*. (*a*) Recruiting response to right thalamic stimulation (8 V, 7.5/s) is recorded both from cortex and from and between thalamic sites yielding recruiting responses or response on stimulation. (*b*, *c*) Recruiting response in cortex and left thalamus, evoked by right thalamic stimulation as in (*a*), is reduced or abolished during left bulbo-reticular stimulation (3 V, 300/s). (*d*, *e*) Same preparation with 7 mgm chloralosane/K. Chloralosane waves recorded from cortex and from left thalamic site (channel 3), which itself yielded a recruiting stimulation, are abolished in all areas and replaced by low-voltage fast activity during left bulbo-reticular stimulation (2 V, 300/s).

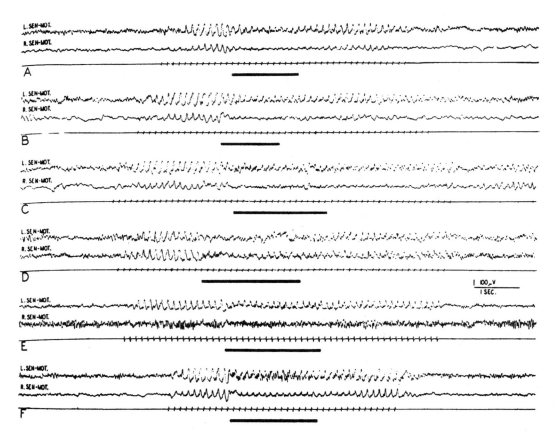

Figure 51.13

Abolition of recruiting responses by sensory and reticular stimulation. Recruiting responses, evoked by left thalamic stimulation (5 V, 300/s) in an *encéphale isolé*. Identically reduced or abolished by loud whistling (*a*), blowing air on head (*b*), rubbing nose (*c*), blowing air on eyes (*d*), stimulating the right posterior column at 2 V, 300/s (*e*), and stimulating the left bulbar reticular formation at 2 V, 300/s (*f*).

tices and the ipsilateral auditory area (figure 51.10d), was either abolished or greatly reduced in all regions during intercurrent bulbo-reticular stimulation and recruited again upon its cessation (figure 51.10e,f). Exciting the rostral end of the reticular system in the subthalamus had a similar effect (figure 51.11e). Another instance is shown in figure 51.9a, in which case, strychnine was then applied locally to the cortex. The recruiting response was transiently abolished following strychnine spikes interspersed in its course, suggesting that identical cortical neurons were involved in these two activities (figure 51.9c). Subsequent repetition of reticular stimulation again opposed the recruiting response without, as noted above, altering the spikes induced by strychnine (figure 51.9d). It should be noted that low frequency stimulation of the ascending reticular system, even in the subthalamus, did not itself induce a recruiting response (figures 51.10b and 51.11d).

Of the different types of evoked cortical activity upon which the effect of reticular stimulation was tested, certain ones, then, secondary sensory responses and strychnine spikes, exhibited little or no alteration, while others, sensory after-discharge and recruiting responses, were abolished. Of the two types of transcortical conduction observed, that from the sensory to the motor cortex, underlying the pyramidal discharge to afferent volleys under chloralosane anesthesia, was blocked, while the other, from a strychninized area of the cortex to the opposite cortex, was unaffected. It is not at present possible to decide whether any common factors underly these similarities and differences.

Thalamic Mediation of Response

The generalized distribution of the alteration in the EEG induced by reticular stimulation has implications for the manner of its mediation by the thalamus. It seems likely that the reticular formation could exert its influence upon all parts of the cortex either by acting generally upon the thalamus or by influencing its diffuse projection system alone. At present, each possibility appears relevant, for there is indication both that the diffuse projection system is involved and that the reticular influence may not operate exclusively through it.

Evidence for the mediation of the reticular effect by the diffuse thalamic projection system is presented in figure 51.12. The low-frequency stimulation of a portion of this system, on one side of the midline, induced recruiting responses not only in both cortices but in a corresponding region of the opposite thalamus as well (figure 51.12a). This evoked intra-thalamic activity was then abolished during intercurrent bulbo-reticular stimulation and returned again upon its cessation (figures 51.12b,c), thus demonstrating a reticular influence upon the diffuse projection system at the thalamic level. It is uncertain whether the corresponding cortical changes were secondary to those in the thalamus in these instances, however, for though cortical recruiting responses were greatly reduced, small cortical waves were still present during reticular stimulation at a time when all synchronized activity was absent from the record of this thalamic sample (figures 51.12b,d: compare left cortical and thalamic channels). This same preparation was next lightly anesthetized with chloralosane, with the development of characteristic high-voltage slow waves both in the cortex and subcortically, within and between components of the diffuse thalamic projection system. Bulbo-reticular stimulation then desynchronized this activity as effectively in the electrothalamogram as in the EEG (figures 51.12d,e).

Further indication that the reticular influence may be mediated by the diffuse thalamic projection system is provided by comparing its effect upon the EEG with that of direct, intrathalamic stimulation of this system. Recruiting responses were obtained by successively stimulating portions of the diffuse system in the left (figure 51.11a) and right (figure 51.11b) sides of the thalamus. The recruiting response to left thalamic stimulation was then repeated and inter-current stimulation of the same right thalamic site at 300/s abolished it as effectively (figure 51.11c) as did subsequent stimulation of the rostral end of the reticular system in the subthalamus (figure 51.11e). As regards the diffuse thalamic projection system, then, reticular stimulation has the same effect upon the electrogram of its thalamic components that it does upon the EEG, and this influence upon the EEG can be reproduced by the direct high-frequency stimulation of this system within the thalamus.

Similar desynchronization, both of spontaneous activity and of the recruiting response has been observed, however, to result from high frequency stimulation of the discretely projecting, posterior part of the ventral thalamic nucleus, and the effect was generalized in the cortex. It remains for further study to determine whether such responses were mediated by direct cortical projections or, as seems more likely, through other subcortical systems.

After ipsilateral destruction of the intra-laminar thalamic region, bulbo-reticular stimulation still desynchronized the EEG bilaterally and as markedly as in initial controls. After extending the lesion until the massa intermedia and intralaminar regions of the thalamus were destroyed bilaterally, bulbar stimulation still seemed to have some effect upon the EEG, but cortical activity was then so reduced that it was difficult to draw conclusions concerning the significance of the results. These findings only serve to introduce the problem of thalamic mediation of the lower brain stem influence upon the EEG, and much added study will be necessary to clarify this subject.

The Reticular Effect and Arousal Reactions

In the acute study of arousal reactions, anesthesia cannot be employed, for its major action is to block them, nor is the unanesthetized "encéphale isolé" suitable, for its EEG is typically activated and only rarely exhibits spontaneous synchrony.

In the latter preparation, however, recruiting responses sometimes provide a background of cortical activity upon which the arousal effect of natural stimuli can be tested. Figure 51.13 shows a series of such instances, in which the high-voltage slow waves of the recruiting response were abolished and replaced by low-voltage fast activity, during loud whistling (a), rubbing the nose (b), and blowing air on the head (c) and eyes (d). Indistinguishable from these changes to natural stimuli, except for somewhat faster low-voltage activity, were those produced by electrical stimulation of the posterior column (e) and bulbar reticular formation (f).

Such abolition of recruiting responses by natural or bulbar stimulation was observed only when the frequency and intensity of thalamic stimulation yielding the recruiting response was just above threshold, and in some cases reticular stimulation could still abolish the recruiting response at a time when natural stimuli were ineffective. Because of these and other difficulties in securing stable testing conditions, attempted repetition of arousing natural stimuli after differential interruption of ascending sensory and reticular paths in the anterior brain stem was abandoned in favor of chronic preparations.

Discussion

The evidence given above points to the presence in the brain stem of a system of ascending reticular relays, whose direct stimulation activates or desynchronizes the EEG, replacing high-voltage slow waves with low-voltage fast activity. This effect is exerted generally upon the cortex and is mediated, in part, at least, by the diffuse thalamic projection system. Portions of this activating system, chiefly its representation in the basal diencephalon, have previously been identified.

In the pioneer studies of Morison and his associates, in which the foundation for so much current work upon the EEG was laid, hypothalamic, subthalamic and medial thalamic excitation was found, in 1943, to suppress intermittent Dial bursts without affecting other types of cortical activity, such as responses to sensory stimulation (Morison, Finley, and Lothrop 1943; Dempsey and Morison 1943). The effect was considered to be inhibitory in nature and was attributed to the excitation of afferent pathways simply passing through this region.

Two years later, Murphy and Gellhorn (1945) found this suppression of Dial bursts, on hypothalamic stimulation, to be accompanied by dispersal of strychnine spikes and by prolonged increase in the frequency and amplitude of low-voltage, background, electro-cortical activity. They pointed out that these latter alterations were excitatory or facilitatory in nature, and attributed the disappearance of bursts to an associated lessened degree of synchrony of firing of cortical neurons, rather than to inhibition. Connections from the hypothalamus to the dorsomedial and intralaminar thalamic region, and thence to cortex, were suggested to provide the channels by way of which these effects were produced and, though the study was undertaken principally to elucidate hypothalamic facilitation of the motor cortex, the generalized distribution of the EEG changes was emphasized.

More recently still, Jasper and his associates (1948) observed a generalized acceleration of spontaneous electrocortical activity, simulating an arousal or waking reaction, from stimulation of the periaqueductal portion of the midbrain, the posterior hypothalamus and the massa intermedia of the thalamus; and Ward (1949) obtained a prolonged generalized increase in both voltage and frequency of the EEG following stimulation of the bulbar reticular formation.

While interpretation of these findings has been varied, their basic similarity can leave little doubt that each of these investigators has dealt with manifestations of the same system as that described above. The present work thus confirms, extends and interrelates these earlier contributions and, from the mass of observations brought to bear upon it, the existence of this brain stem activating system now seems firmly established.

In discussing the general significance of these findings for electroencephalography, attention should certainly be focussed upon the arousal reaction. The breaking up of synchronous cortical discharge by afferent stimulation, first observed by Berger (1930) as alpha blockade on opening the lids, and since found to be a common response to any type of afferent stimulation, is currently attributed to the desynchronizing action of afferent volleys arriving directly at the receiving areas of the cerebral cortex (Adrian and Matthews 1931; Adrian 1947; Bremer 1938, 1944; Walter and Walter 1949). A number of relevant observations are difficult to explain on this basis, however.

More than a decade ago, Ectors (1936) and Rheinberger and Jasper (1932) observed that serially repeated stimulation soon failed to induce activation, though afferent volleys presumably continued to reach the cortex, and it was noted that, in order to be effective in this regard such stimuli must arouse the subject to alertness or attention. In addition, when an activation pattern was so induced, it was by no means confined to the receiving area of the afferent system stimulated (see also Bremer 1943), nor did it appear first in this area and radiate from it. Whether somatic, auditory or, to a lesser extent, visual stimulation was employed, when an arousal reaction was evoked, it appeared simultaneously in all parts of the cortex and often continued for considerable periods in it after afferent stimulation had ceased.

More recently, Monnier's (1949) analysis of the sequence of EEG events induced by visual stimulation in man has shown that alpha blockade is not initiated for a considerable period after the electrocortical changes evoked by the afferent volley are completed, and its prolonged latency might more easily be explained by invoking a subsidiary mechanism than by accounting for it through direct cortical action. Furthermore, the generalized arousal reaction to vestibular stimulation has been shown by Gerebtzoff (1940) to be still elicitable after ablation of the cortical receiving area for this afferent system.

In the present experiments, typical EEG arousal reactions have been reproduced by stimulating the brain stem reticular formation, without exciting classical sensory paths. Crucial evidence that the reticular formation is involved in the arousal reaction to natural stimuli may not yet be obtained but, in addition to being suggested by the data at hand, such a possibility might offer an explanation for the failure of afferent stimuli to evoke arousal from somnolence, lethargy or coma, resulting from injury to the upper brain stem, which left the major sensory paths to the cortex intact (Ingram, Barris, and Ranson 1936; Ranson 1939; Magoun 1948). A conception of the arousal reaction in which collaterals from sensory paths first activated the brain stem reticular formation and exerted their influence upon cortical electrical activity indirectly through it, seems a logical postulate from all these observations, and was, in fact, proposed as long ago as 1940 by Gerebtzoff to account for his observations to which reference was made above.

The proposed participation of the brain stem activating system in the arousal reaction, if established, might represent an aspect of its function concerned with alerting the cortex to abrupt and more or less pronounced alterations in the external environment. It may next be proposed that the presence of a steady background of less intense activity within this cephalically directed brain stem system, contributed to either by liminal inflows from peripheral receptors or preserved intrinsically, may be an important factor contributing to the maintenance of the waking state and that absence of such activity in it may predispose to sleep.

Bremer's fundamental discovery (1935, 1938) that the EEG of the unanesthetized cerebrum, isolated from the rest of the nervous system by mesencephalic transection, resembled that of an intact brain in natural sleep or under barbiturate anesthesia, led him to the conclusion that sleep is the result of deafferentation of the cerebral cortex. Afferent impulses from olfactory and visual receptors are still accessible to such a "cerveau isolé", and more recent work has indicated that sleep changes in the EEG are best produced by basal diencephalic injury (Lindsley, Bowden, and Magoun 1949). But putting these qualifications aside, it should be pointed out that at the time Bremer's discovery was made, classical sensory paths were the only known connections ascending through the midbrain, to the interruption of which the ensuing sleep changes in the "cerveau isolé" could be attributed. The present identification of a second, parallel system of ascending reticular relays, whose direct stimulation induces EEG changes characteristic of wakefulness, now raises a possible alternative interpretation of Bremer's observations, for the obvious question arises: is the production of sleep in the cerebrum, following mesencephalic transection, to be attributed to deafferentation in the strict sense, or to the elimination of the waking influence of the ascending reticular activating system? Two lines of evidence favor this latter possibility.

As regards barbiturate sleep, Forbes et al. (1949) have recently pointed out that the ready conduction of afferent impulses to the cortex under deep barbiturate anesthesia is inconsistent with the view that the sleepinducing properties of these drugs depend upon functional deafferentiation.[2] Conversely, it has been found in the present study that under barbiturate anesthesia, bulbo-reticular stimulation is much less effective in activating the EEG than in a chloralosane or unanesthetized preparation. The fact that hypothalamic stimulation is effective under such anesthesia (Morison, Finley, and Lothrop 1943; Murphy and Gellhorn 1945; Jasper, Hunter, and Knighton 1948) suggests that the blocking of reticular relays within the brain stem may be involved in the production of sleep by barbiturates.

As regards sleep induced by rostral brain stem injury, prolonged somnolence has followed chronic lesions in the basal diencephalon and anterior midbrain which did not involve afferent pathways to the cortex, but which were placed medial and ventral to them in the region of distribution of the ascending reticular activating system (Ingram, Barris, and Ranson 1936; Ranson 1939), and similar results have followed injury to this region from tumors (Fulton and Bailey 1929) or encephalitis (von Economo 1918, Richter and Traut 1940) in man.

Though somnolence was incontestable, EEG studies were not undertaken in the animals or patients to which reference is made, but more recently Ingram, Knott, and Wheatley (1949) have studied alterations in the EEG following chronic, experimental hypothalamic lesions, and the results of acute basal diencephalic and lower brain stem destruction are reported in the succeeding paper (Lindsley, Bowden, and Magoun 1949). In the latter investigation, sleep changes in the EEG, identical with those of barbiturate anesthesia, resulted from basal diencephalic and anterior midbrain lesions which spared sensory pathways to the cortex, but interrupted the rostral distribution of the ascending reticular activating system. Conversely, extensive deafferentiation of the cortex, by section of ascending pathways in the lateral portion of each side of the midbrain, together with bilateral interruption of the optic and olfactory tracts, failed to induce such alterations.

The conception of sleep as a functional deafferentation of the cerebrum is not opposed by this evidence if the term "deafferentation" is broadened to include interruption of the ascending influence of the brain stem reticular activating system, the contribution of which to wakefulness now seems more important than that conducted to the cortex over classical sensory paths.

Summary

1. Stimulation of the reticular formation of the brain stem evokes changes in the EEG, consisting of abolition of synchronized discharge and introduction of low voltage fast activity in its place, which are not mediated by any of the known ascending or descending paths that traverse the brain stem. The alteration is a generalized one but is most pronounced in the ipsilateral hemisphere and, sometimes, in its anterior part.

2. This response can be elicited by stimulating the medial bulbar reticular formation, pontile and midbrain tegmentum, and dorsal hypothalamus and subthalamus. The bulbar effect is due to ascending impulses relayed through these more cephalic structures. The excitable substrate possesses a low threshold and responds best to high frequencies of stimulation.

3. Some background synchrony of electrocortical activity is requisite for manifestation of the response. In the "encephale isolé", reticular stimulation has no additional effect upon the fully activated EEG. With synchrony, in spontaneous drowsiness or light chloralosane anesthesia, the effect of reticular stimulation is strikingly like Berger's alpha wave blockade, or any arousal reaction. In full chloralosane anesthesia, high voltage slow waves are blocked but no increase in lower amplitude, fast activity occurs. With barbiturate anesthesia, the reticular response is difficult to elicit or is abolished.

4. In the chloralosane preparation, the secondary cortical response evoked by a sensory volley is generally unaffected by reticular stimulation. Consequent sensory after-discharge is abolished, however, as is pyramidal tract discharge and jerky movements referable to it. Outside the sensory receiving area, secondary responses themselves may be reduced or prevented.

5. The convulsive spikes produced by local strychnine and those of a fit following supra-

maximal cortical excitation, are not decreased by stimulating the reticular formation.

6. The cortical recruiting response induced by low frequency stimulation of the diffuse thalamic projection system is reduced or abolished by reticular stimulation.

7. There is some indication that the cortical effect of reticular stimulation may be mediated by this diffuse thalamic projection system, for synchronized activity within it is similarly prevented by reticular excitation, and direct high frequency stimulation of this system, within the thalamus, reproduces the reticular response. It is possible, however, that other mechanisms may be involved in its mediation.

8. The reticular response and the arousal reaction to natural stimuli have been compared in the "encéphale isolé", in which EEG synchrony was present during spontaneous relaxation or was produced by recruiting mechanisms, and the two appear identical.

9. The possibility that the cortical arousal reaction to natural stimuli is mediated by collaterals of afferent pathways to the brain stem reticular formation, and thence through the ascending reticular activating system, rather than by intra-cortical spread following the arrival of afferent impulses at the sensory receiving areas of the cortex, is under investigation.

10. The possibility is considered that a background of maintained activity within this ascending brain stem activating system may account for wakefulness, while reduction of its activity either naturally, by barbiturates, or by experimental injury and disease, may respectively precipitate normal sleep, contribute to anesthesia or produce pathological somnolence.

Conclusions

Experiments on cats have identified a cephalically directed brain stem system, the stimulation of which desynchronizes and activates the EEG, replacing high-voltage slow waves with low-voltage fast activity.

This system is distributed through the central core of the brain stem and appears to comprise a series of reticular relays ascending to the basal diencephalon. Its effects are exerted generally upon the cortex and are mediated, in part, at least, by the diffuse thalamic projection system.

Possible implication of this system in the arousal reaction to afferent stimulation and in the maintenance of wakefulness is discussed.

Acknowledgments

The first author was aided by a grant from the National Institute of Mental Health, U.S. Public Health Service. The second author was Visiting Professor of Neurology at Northwestern University Medical School, supported by the Rockefeller Foundation.

Notes

1. These "secondary potentials" resemble those of Forbes and Morison (1939) recorded, in deep barbiturate anesthesia, in and also outside of the somatic receiving area and disappearing when the frequency of afferent stimuli rose above 5/s. Since under chloralosane anesthesia, they are associated with pyramidal discharge they correspond to the "efferent waves" of Adrian (1941).

2. This argument would appear to apply only to the conduction of a single afferent volley. W. H. Marshall (*J. Neurophysiol.*, 1941, 4: 25–43) has observed impairment of conduction of repeated afferent volleys to the cortex under nembutal anesthesia, due to great prolongation of thalamic recovery time.

References

Adrian, E. D. Afferent discharges to the cerebral cortex from peripheral sense organs. *J. Physiol.*, 1941, *100*: 159–191.

Adrian, E. D. The physical background of perception. Oxford, The Clarendon Press, 1947, 95 pp.

Adrian, E. D. and Matthews, B. H. C. The interpretation of potential waves in the cortex. *J. Physiol.*, 1934, *81*: 440–471.

Adrian, E. D. and Matthews, B. H. C. The Berger rhythm: potential changes from the occipital lobes in man. *Brain*, 1934, *57*: 355–385.

Adrian, E. D. and Moruzzi, G. Impulses in the pyramidal tract. *J. Physiol.*, 1939, *97*: 153–199.

Berger, H. Uber das Elektrenkephalogramm des Menschen. II. *J. Physiol. Neurol.*, 1930, *40*: 160–179.

Bremer, F. Cerveau isolé et physiologie du sommeil. *C. R. Soc. Biol., Paris*, 1935, *118*: 1235–1242.

Bremer, F. L'activité cérébrale et le problème physiologique du sommeil. *Boll. Soc. It. Biol. Sp.*, 1938, *13*: 271–290.

Bremer, F. L'activité électrique de l'écorce cérébrale. Paris, Hermann, 1938.

Bremer, F. Etude oscillographique des réponses sensorielles de l'aire acoustique corticale chez le chat. *Arch. Internat. Physiol.*, 1943, *53*: 53–103.

Bremer, F. Aspect théorique de l'électro-encéphalographie. *Arch. Néerl. Physiol.*, 1944–47, *28*: 481–482.

Dempsey, E. W. and Morison, R. S. The production of rhythmically recurrent cortical potentials after localized thalamic stimulation. *Amer. J. Physiol.*, 1942, *135*: 293–300.

Dempsey, E. W. and Morison, R. S. The electrical activity of a thalamocortical relay system. *Amer. J. Physiol.*, 1943, *138*: 283–298.

Economo, C. von. Die Encephalitis Lethargica. Wien, Deuticke, 1918.

Ectors, L. Etude de l'activité électrique du cortex cérébral chez le lapin non narcotisé ni curarisé. *Arch. Internat. Physiol.*, 1936, *43*: 267–298.

Forbes, A., Battista, A. F., Chatfield, P. O. and Garcia, I. P. Refractory phase in cerebral mechanisms. *EEG Clin. Neurophysiol.*, 1949, *1*: 141–193.

Forbes, A. and Morison, B. R. Cortical responses to sensory stimulation under deep barbiturate narcosis. *J. Neurophysiol.*, 1939, *2*: 112–128.

Fulton, J. F. and Bailey, P. Tumors in the region of the third ventricle: their diagnosis and relation to pathological sleep. *J. nerv. ment. Dis.*, 1929, *69*: 1–25, 145–164, 261–272.

Garol, H. W. The functional organization of the sensory cortex of the cat. *J. Neuropath. Exp. Neur.*, 1942, *1*: 320–329.

Gellhorn, E. Effect of afferent impulses on cortical suppressor areas. *J. Neurophysiol.*, 1947, *10*: 125–132.

Gerebtzoff, M. A. Recherches sur la projection corticale du labyrinthe. I. Des effets de la stimulation labyrinthique sur l'activité électrique de l'écorce cérébrale. *Arch. Internat. Physiol.*, 1940, *50*: 59–99.

Hunter, J. and Jasper, H. Reactions of unanesthetized animals to thalamic stimulation. *Trans. Amer. Neur. Ass.*, 1948, *73*: 171–172.

Ingram, W. R., Barris, R. W. and Ranson, S. W. Catalepsy, an experimental study. *Arch. Neurol. Psychiat.*, Chicago, 1936, *35*: 1175–1197.

Ingram, W. R., Knott, J. R. and Wheatley, M. D. Electroencephalograms of cats with hypothalamic lesions III. Meeting Amer. EEG Society, 1949.

Jasper, H. H. and Droogleever-Fortuyn, J. Experimental studies on the functional anatomy of petit mal epilepsy. *Res. Publ. Ass. nerv. ment. Dis.*, 1947, *26*: 272–298.

Jasper, H., Hunter, J. and Knighton, R. Experimental studies of thalamocortical systems. *Trans. Amer. Neur. Ass.*, 1948, *73*: 210–212.

Lindsley, D. B., Bowden, J. and Magoun, H. W. Effect upon the EEG of acute injury to the brain stem activating system. *EEG Clin. Neurophysiol.*, 1949, *1*: 475–486.

Magoun, H. W. Coma following midbrain lesions in the monkey. *Anat. Rec.*, 1948, *100*: 120.

Magoun, H. W. and Rhines, R. An inhibitory mechanism in the bulbar reticular formation. *J. Neurophysiol.*, 1946, *9*: 165–171.

McCulloch, W. S., Graf, C. and Magoun, H. W. A cortico-bulbo-reticular pathway from area 4-S. *J. Neurophysiol.*, 1946, *9*: 127–132.

Monnier, M. Retinal time, retino-cortical time and motor reaction time in man. III. Meeting Amer. EEG Society, 1949.

Morison, R. S. and Dempsey, E. W. A study of thalamocortical relations. *Amer. J. Physiol.*, 1942, *135*: 281–292.

Morison, R. S., Finley, K. H. and Lothrop, G. N. Influence of basal forebrain areas on the electrocorticogram. *Amer. J. Physiol.*, 1943, *139*: 410–416.

Murphy, J. P. and Gellhorn, E. The influence of hypothalamic stimulation on cortically induced movements and on action potentials of the cortex. *J. Neurophysiol.*, 1945, *8*: 339–364.

Ranson, S. W. Somnolence caused by hypothalamic lesions in the monkey. *Arch. Neurol. Psychiat.*, Chicago, 1939, *41*: 1–23.

Rheinberger, M. B. and Jasper, H. H. Electrical activity of the cerebral cortex in the unanesthetized cat. *Amer. J. Physiol.*, 1937, *119*: 186–196.

Richter, R. B. and Traut, E. F. Chronic encephalitis. Pathological report of a case with protracted somnolence. *Arch. Neurol. Psychiat.*, Chicago, 1940, *44*: 848–866.

Snider, R. S., Magoun, H. W. and McCulloch, W. S. A suppressor cerebello-bulbo-reticular pathway from anterior lobe and paramedian lobules. *Fed. Proc.*, 1947, *6*: 207.

Walter, W. G. and Walter, V. J. The electrical activity of the brain. *Ann. Rev. Physiol.*, 1949, *11*: 199–230.

Ward, A. A. The relationship between the bulbar-reticular suppressor region and the EEG. *EEG Clin. Neurophysiol.*, 1949, *1*: 120.

Arnold B. Scheibel

. . . Then felt I like some watcher of the skies
  When a new planet swims into his ken;
Or like stout Cortez, when with eagle eyes
  He stared at the Pacific—and all his men
Look'd at each other with a wild surmise—
  Silent, upon a peak in Darien.
—John Keats

Approximately 25 years have passed since the first great discussion of structure and function of the brain stem reticular core. The proceedings of the Laurentian Symposium (8) are still rewarding reading, laden with ideas and full of the excitement felt by a small group of investigators beguiled by a new neuroscientific concept. A wealth of questions were asked by the participants, many of which seemed unanswerable, perhaps for generations to come. A quarter of a century later, another groundswell of interest in the form and function of the reticular formation, fueled by new techniques, answers many of these questions while raising a host of new ones. This chapter and the five that follow sketch in some of the structural and functional archaeology that must concern us, and provide a sampler of present investigative efforts in these directions.

Nature of the Neurons

Relationships between neuronal form and function have loomed large in the development of the concept of the reticular core. Cajal (37), always a functionalist with a microscope, provided the first substantive notions of reticular cell morphology with his Golgi studies of the neonatal brain stem. The limited number of drawings he provided established the prototypic model of the reticular neuron with its multipolar shape, spreading but sparsely branched dendritic tree, and overlapping dendritic domain structure. The apparently reticulate or diffuse (nonstructured) appearance of the cell ensembles received a

modicum of shaping in his description of three major core zones: (a) the midline or raphe system, (b) the paramedian reticularis alba (or white), and (c) the more laterally lying reticularis grisea (or gray) zones.

Subsequent Golgi-based studies extended these observations up and down the reticular core and into the thalamic medial and intralaminar zones (41, 46, 47, 48, 58). Of particular interest was the idiosyncratic organization of dendrite systems in certain cell groups. The characteristic rostrocaudal compression of dendrite systems in many of the more medial-lying medullopontine reticular neurons stimulated notions about input segregation in an area known for convergence of heterogeneous afferent patterns on individual nerve cells (41, 42, 49). The structural model of this type of cell-dendrite organization, caricatured as a stack of poker chips standing on end, introduced the concept of modular organization into brain form and function (41, 42, 57). Although the module concept suffers obvious deficiencies in terms of appropriate modes for defining modular limits, whether to insist on spatial (and functional) exclusivity, it has provided a means for a more manageable description of neuronal arrays. Functional modularization in cerebral and cerebellar cortices (34, 56, 57) and structural modularization of the neocortical mantle (21, 32, 47, 56, 60) have served to clarify notions regarding information processing at these levels without undue contamination from superficially similar strategies common to contemporary computer technology.

Conceptions about the dendritic surface itself have shown considerable evolution. The classic spine-covered dendrite shafts familiar from Cajal's drawings have proved to be, at best, a special case, time limited to the pre- and early postnatal synaptic periods. With maturation of the organism, spines are progressively lost, leaving shafts appearing remarkably barren (to light microscope viewing), except for occasional irregular excrescences (48). This profound loss of postsynaptic apparatus during the period of maturation is of uncertain significance. It has recently been reported that the same process occurs in the human neonate. Furthermore, in infants dying of crib-death syndrome, the reticular dendrites remain heavily spined (36). The inference follows that postnatal spine loss is a general feature of reticular core maturation and that failure of this involuting process can conceivably result in serious (or fatal) disturbances to cardiorespiratory reflexes.

Despite the obvious strengths of the Golgi method in defining neuronal form and relationships, its limitations are obvious: (a) the partial and largely unpredictable nature of the elements it impregnates, and (b) its inability to identify (as far as we know) any of the biochemical characteristics of the cells visualized. Recently, a number of techniques have become available which enable selective visualization of neurons and some or all of their dendritic (and often axonal) processes, either by uptake at axonal terminals followed by retrograde flow to the cell body of origin (e.g., Horseradish peroxidase [HRP]), or by direct microinjection or iontophoresis of appropriate marker substances into neurons whose electrical activity may have already been monitored intracellularly with fine glass pipettes. Commonly used substances in this category include Alcian blue and HRP. Histofluorescence studies following formalin vapor fixation (7, 12, 62) see also provide another elegant if structurally less revealing group of methods. Even more current and exciting are immunocytochemical methods, whose capacity to delineate the entire soma-dendrite complex of neurons with highly specified chemical signatures promise to overcome both of the primary drawbacks of classic Golgi methodology. Such a technique, in which norepinephrinergic neurons are selectively visualized by staining the enzyme dopamine-beta-hydroxylase (DBH) using specific antibodies to DBH tied to HRP as detector mole-

cules, is described in the chapter by Grzanna and Molliver. The potential significance of extension of this basic method to cell types with other chemical signatures needs no further comment.

Nature of the Input to Individual Neurons and Their Patterns of Response

Kohnstamm and Quesnel (26) were probably the first investigators to conceive of the reticular formation as a central receptive pool (centrum receptorium), basing their conjecture on the apparent presence of fibers entering from the flanking, long-ascending tracts. Cajal (37) made similar assumptions based on the Golgi-demonstrated presence of collaterals seen entering the core from anterolateral, midline, and ventral bundles, He reasoned that these fibers reinforced activity patterns of the third, fourth, and fifth order sensory neurons which he considered constituted the core. Our own Golgi analyses emphasizing transverse, sagittal, and horizontal sections through the brain stem provided further documentation for the enormous convergence of afferent systems, both collateral and terminal, on the substance of the core (40, 41). In addition to both ascending and descending tract systems, the innumerable longitudinal axons of reticular core origin also collateralize richly en route (figure 52.1), thereby adding powerful increments of core-processed information to adjacent or distant levels of the stem. Macroelectrode studies demonstrating such convergence (54) were soon enriched by a group of extracellular microelectrode studies from several laboratories (2, 49). Descriptions of the extensive but not unlimited convergence of central and suprasegmental inputs on most recordable reticular neurons and the apparently unique nature of the input array to each neuron (49) served two immediate functions. Earlier interpretations of the function of the core as a receptive pool were experimentally confirmed; also, abundant hints were supplied as to a degree of specificity of af-

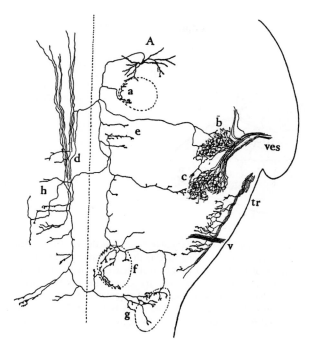

Figure 52.1
Horizontal sagittal section through medullopontine portion of brain stem of young rat showing collateral system generated by descending axon of one neuron in nucleus reticularis pontis caudalis (*a*). Collateral-recipient areas include abducens nucleus (*a*), lateral (*b*), and spinal (*c*) nuclei of vestibular complex, ves; substance of medullary reticular core (*h*), hypoglossal nucleus (*f*), and nucleus gracilis (*g*). Other abbreviations include tract of descending trigeminal nucleus, tr. v., and medial longitudinal fasciculus (*d*). Drawn from Golgi-stained material at 150×.

ferent pattern, and possibly of cell functions not previously suspected. Intracellular studies (4, 29), together with more precise evaluation of points of stimulation in the peripheral receptive field, began to provide a more rigorous mapping of body representation within the core. (Similar data regarding specificities of output organization for these cells are considered elsewhere in this volume.) The technical process of recording these inputs also showed not only the marked attenuation or habituation of response which characterized these cells (22, 43) but also a prominent and previously unsuspected cyclic alteration in afferent receptive properties (44) of

many reticular neurons. Nevertheless, few rigorous statements have been made about the nature of the response of the reticular single unit. The quantitative studies of Freitas de Roche reported below probably represent one of the first attempts to provide the basis for a parametric model for this type of core element activity.

Ascending Systems of the Reticular Core

The organization of the ascending relay system originating in the reticular formation and projecting on diencephalon and telencephalon remains

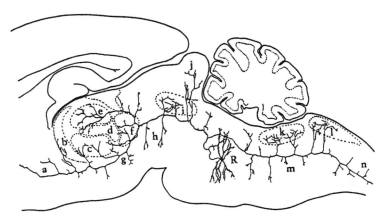

Figure 52.2
Sagittal section showing ascending and descending axon system of single reticular neuron in the nucleus gigantocellularis. Note ascending and descending branches and rich collateral fibers entering the following areas: (*a*) basal forebrain; (*b*) nucleus reticularis thalami; (*c*)–(*e*) complex of medial and intralaminar thalamic nuclei; (*f*) centromedian-parafascicular complex; (*g*) zona incerta; (*h*) mesencephalic tegmentum; (*i*) oculomotor-trochlear nerve nuclear complex; (*j*) inferior complex; (*k*) hypoglossal nucleus; (*l*) nucleus gracilis; (*m*) medullary reticular formation; (*n*) spinal cord. Golgi modification, young rat. (Originally published in Brazier, M.A.B. (1968) *The electrical activity of the nervous system*, 3rd ed. London: Pitman, and Baltimore: Williams & Wilkins. Reprinted by permission of the publisher.)

one of the intriguing problems of core physiology. This system almost certainly serves as substrate for the rest-activity cycle (25), the various levels of sleep and wakefulness, and the enormous range of conscious states which mediate our interactions with the world around us.

The classic conceptions of Cajal (37) and of Moruzzi and Magoun (31) looked toward an interneuronal chain transferring excitation patterns rostrally over multisynaptic links. Electrophysiological studies of Adey et al. (1) provided only partial support for this conception, showing that temporal patterns of evoked ascending waves included a group of short latency responses consonant with a rapid relay. Degeneration studies suggested (6, 33), and Golgi analyses (41, 58) clearly revealed, the characteristic long projection axons from reticular neurons situated in the medial half of the brain stem from medulla through mesencephalon. Many of these ascend-

ing axons originated from parent cells which generated bifurcating axon systems, one branch of which descended to spinal cord levels (figure 52.2).

In our original assessment of this system, we estimated that 10–15% of these ascending axons reached neocortical terminations. The elegant intracellular microelectrode studies of Magni and Willis (29) later confirmed these estimates, but the definitive studies on course, pattern, and terminal stations of chemically identifiable fibers have been left to the histofluorescence techniques pioneered by Falck et al. (12) and applied to the reticular core by Dahlstrom and Fuxe (7). The refinement and extension of this work by Moore's group (62) have added substantially to our understanding of the differential projection pathways and areas of termination of the various monoaminergic systems. In fact, Moore's elegant histochemical dissections may provide, for the first time, some idea of how serotonergic and catecholaminergic systems operate in concert to gate and modulate response patterns of cortical and subcortical neuron ensembles.

Relationship of the Reticular Core to Wakefulness and Sleep

The role of the reticular formation in the mediation of sleeping and waking states and in the selective sampling and response to sensory inputs represents one of the most intriguing areas of brain physiology. The classic studies of Bremer (5) showed that decerebration produced permanent sleep (actually low frequency, high voltage cortical waves) in the experimental animal. These data vigorously reinforced the conception of sleep as a passive state—that is, remove the sensory afferent barrage and the brain lapses into the quiescence of sleep—a conception entirely congruent with the dictates of what Sherrington has called "busy common sense." Hess's data (19, 20), carefully garnered from the first chronically implanted cats indicating that slow repetitive stimulation at a number of brain sites could regularly cause naturally appearing and totally reversible sleep, told a different story. The anti-intuitive qualities of this exotic conception of sleep as an active process, however, determined its destiny to wait 25 years before achieving respectability. Meanwhile, the group of investigators working with Forbes (10, 13) had delimited a central diencephalic core capable of transmitting ascending impulses independently of the classic sensory channels and projecting them widely upon cortex. Later extensions of such studies by Jasper (23) and his colleagues, Penfield (35), and others culminated in the notion of the thalamus as pacemaker for all cortical electrical activity and, in a neo-Jacksonian sense, as the highest hierarchical level of brain function.

The important report of Moruzzi and Magoun (31), together with that of Lindsley et al. (28),

brought into focus the central role of the brain stem reticular formation in modulating levels of cortical activity. Steriade et al. (63) provide, for the first time, cellular level evidence supporting the concept of an ascending reticular mediation of electroencephalogram desynchronization. The studies of Skrebitsky et al. (64) are among the first to show, by intracellular recording, that hyperpolarization is a common membrane accompaniment of the arousal process in cortical neurons.

Since earlier work was linked with, or evocative of, the entire spectrum of sleep and wakeful states independent of the classic sensory paths, the significance of Bremer's findings (5) almost a decade and a half earlier became clear. The conception of sleep as a passive state received added confirmation from these data. It was not until the selective lesion and stimulation studies of Rossi et al. (39) and Jouvet (24) and the electroencephalographic analyses of REM sleep phenomena by Aserinsky, Kleitman, and Dement (3, 9) that the notion of sleep as an active process finally became accepted. Indeed, the intensive study of sleep and dream states during the late 1960s and early 1970s provided the bridge between the epochal yet essentially monolithic concepts of core structure and function of the era we have just briefly considered, and the increasingly rich, mosaic-like notions characterizing the present era.

Substrates of Selective Awareness

One of the most challenging areas for concern within the newer dynamic concepts of conscious behavior is that of selective awareness. How do we turn our attention toward one sensory stream and exclude other inputs? Which core structures are causally involved in the focusing of interest—the all-important "consciousness of what"—now conceptually replacing the more diffuse and probably less meaningful earlier abstraction, "consciousness?"

Anatomical studies already document the profusion of reticular collaterals which invest virtually all sensory (and motor) processing centers. The lucid descriptions of Odutola (65) offer convincing evidence of the complexity of such axon systems. The efficacy of these elements in modulating ongoing activity has been shown in the classic studies of Hernández-Peón (18), Lindsley (27), and Fuster and Uyeda (14), among others. The fact of reticular participation, demonstrated both anatomically and physiologically, in the modulation of all transactions between organism and environment still does not explain the governing principles behind selective awareness. The enormous dispersion of information from individual reticular axon collateral systems argues for the reverse situation —a widespread, diffuse, and nonspecific effect wielded indiscriminately among all neural ensembles receiving presynaptic terminals from the core elements in question. Undoubtedly, processes dedicated to local control, such as presynaptic inhibition (52), are active in selective attenuation of unwanted facilitatory inflows from the core, but there is no hint of supervening intelligence nor pontifical neuronal ensemble determining on which input items our interest shall be focused.

Central to this issue has been the gradual clarification of the connections and functional significance of the nucleus reticularis thalami. Situated like a thin nuclear sheet draped over the lateral and anterior surfaces of the thalamus, it has been likened to the screen grid interposed between cathode and anode in the triode or pentode vacuum tube (45, 46). If its role were modulatory to thalamocorticothalamic interactions, its connections for long seemed too enigmatic to support such a notion. Although Cajal (37) reported that axons of nucleus reticularis neurons in some cases turned caudally toward unknown destinations, many (although not all) anatomists viewed it as a relay in the thalamocortical pathway; Hanbery et al. (17) called it the final common path for nonspecific impulses projecting on cortex.

When more recent Golgi analysis showed that virtually all nucleus reticularis axons played back upon thalamus and mesencephalic tegmentum (45), and these findings were supported by degeneration and axon-tracking techniques (30, 38), more satisfying hypotheses became possible. We suggested that nucleus reticularis thalami ensembles might exert feedback control via tonic and/or phasic inhibition on underlying cell groups of thalamus and mesencephalon (45, 46). In the decade since that suggestion was made, a growing body of data has provided substantial support; today it seems certain that nucleus reticularis neurons, activated by volleys ascending along thalamocortical axons, generate spike bursts which immediately suppress such trains (50, 51, 59, 61, 63). However, a conceptually more panoramic model can now be proposed on the basis of recent physiological studies of mesencephalic units and of thalamofrontal interactions with the nucleus reticularis thalami.

Most reticular core neurons in the mesencephalic tegmentum, especially those constituting nucleus cuneiformis, appear multimodal, responding in particular to visual, somatic, and auditory stimuli, with combinations of the last two stimuli most numerous (4). The common receptive fields of typical bimodal cells in this array show a significant degree of congruence. For instance, a unit responding to stimulation of the hindlimb will usually prove maximally sensitive to auditory stimuli originating well to the rear of the organism. These twin sematic and auditory maps retain approximate register and overlap the visuotopic map laid down in the more peripheral layers of the overlying superior colliculus (11, 15, 55). These data might be interpreted to mean that each deep tectal-tegmental locus maps a point in the three-dimensional spatial envelope surrounding the organism. Further studies suggest the presence of a deep tectal-tegmental motor map closely

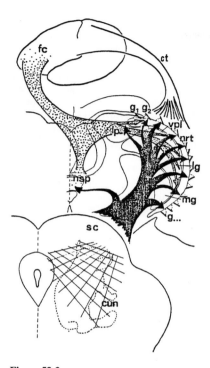

Figure 52.3
Schematic representation of some of the systems operating conjointly upon the gatelets (g_1, g_2, g_3, ...) of the nucleus reticularis thalami (nrt). (*Blackened arrow system*) Projection from the deep layers of superior colliculus (sc) and underlying nucleus cuneiformis (cun) of the mesencephalic tegmentum. Note the shape and position of the animunculus representing the spatial envelope believed to be coded in these tectotegmental cell systems. (*Dotted arrow system*) Projections from frontal granular cortex (fc) and medial nonspecific thalamus (nsp). (*Clear arrow system*) Descending corticothalamic projections (ct). Ascending specific thalamocortical projections are not shown.

matching and in apparent register with the sensory map (16, 19).

Figure 52.3 indicates some general features of this mapped envelope extending three dimensionally through the tectotegmental mesencephalon with caudal portions located caudoventromedially and rostral parts represented rostrodorsolaterally. The axon systems of these cell ensembles sweep forward on a broad front, investing midline thalamus and nucleus reticularis thalami. The investiture is precise in the sense that tectotegmental sites representing specific zones of the spatial envelope (receptive field) project to portions of the nucleus reticularis concerned with similar peripheral fields via projections from both sensory thalamus and sensory-association cortices. Stimulation of the tegmentum produces positive-going slow waves and temporary cessation of nucleus reticularis spike activity along with the disappearance of thalamocortical recruiting phenomena (53, 61). Any external stimulus with alerting value produces the same effect. Conversely, frontal granular cortex, working through the agency of medial thalamic structures, produces negative waves and facilitation of unit response in nucleus reticularis (53, 61).

From these data, the concept emerges of a reticularis complex selectively gating interaction between specific thalamic nuclei and cerebral cortex under the opposed but complementary control of the brain stem reticular core and the frontal granular cortex. In addition, the gate is highly selective; thus, depending on the nature of the alerting stimulus or locus of central excitation, only that portion of nucleus reticularis will open which controls the appropriate subjacent thalamic sensory field. The reticularis gate becomes a mosaic of gatelets, each tied to some specific receptive field zone or species of input. Each is under delicate yet opposed control of (a) the specifically signatured sensory input and its integrated feedback from sensorimotor cortex, (b) the mesencephalic reticular core with its concern more for novelty (danger?) than for specific details of the input experience, and (c) the frontal granular cortex-medial thalamic system more attuned to upper level strategies of the organism, whether based on drive mechanisms (food, sex) or on still more complex derivative phenomena (curiosity, altruism). Perhaps here resides the structurofunctional substrate for selective awareness and in the delicacy and complexity of its connections, our source of knowing, and of knowing that we know.

References

1. Adey, R., Segundo, J., and Livingston, R. (1957): Corticofugal influences on intrinsic brain stem conduction in cat and monkey. *J. Neurophysiol.*, 20:1–17.

2. Amassian, V., and de Vito, R. (1954): Unit activity in reticular formation and nearby structures. *J. Neurophysiol.*, 17:575–603.

3. Aserinsky, E., and Kleitman, N. (1955): A motility cycle in sleeping infants as manifested by ocular and gross bodily activity. *J. Appl. Physiol.*, 8:11–17.

4. Bell, C., Sierra, G., Buendia, N., and Segundo, J. (1964): Sensory properties of neurons in the mesencephalic reticular formation. *J. Neurophysiol.*, 27:961–987.

5. Bremer, F. (1935): Cerveau "isolé" et physiologie du sommeil. *C. R. Soc. Biol.*, 118:1235–1241.

6. Brodal, A., and Rossi, G. (1955): Ascending fibers in brain stem reticular formation of cat. *AMA Arch. Neurol. Psychiatry*, 74:68–87.

7. Dahlstrom, A., and Fuxe, K. (1964): Evidence for the existence of monoamine-containing neurons in the central nervous system. I. Demonstration of monoamines in the cell bodies of brain stem neurons. *Acta Physiol. Scand. [Suppl. 232]*, 63:1–55.

8. Delafresnaye, J. (1954): *Brain Mechanisms and Consciousness*, edited by E. Adrian, F. Bremer, and H. Jasper. pp. xiii–xv. Charles C Thomas, Springfield, Illinois.

9. Dement, W., and Kleitman, N. (1957): Cyclic variations in EEG during sleep and their relation to eye movements, body motility, and dreaming. *Electroenceph. clin. Neurophysiol.*, 9:673–690.

10. Dempsey, E., and Morison, R. (1942): The production of rhythmically recurrent cortical potentials after localized thalamic stimulation. *Am. J. Physiol.*, 135:293–300.

11. Dräger, W., and Huber, D. (1975): Responses to visual stimulation and relationship between visual, auditory, and somatosensory inputs in mouse superior colliculus. *J. Neurophysiol.*, 31:690–713.

12. Falck, B., Hillarp, N., Thraine, G., and Torp, A. (1962): Fluorescence of catecholamines and related compounds condensed with formaldehyde. *J. Histochem. Cytochem.*, 10:348–354.

13. Forbes, A., and Morison, R. (1939): Cortical response to sensory stimulation under deep barbiturate narcosis. *J. Neurophysiol.*, 2:112–128.

14. Fuster, J., and Uyeda, A. (1962): Facilitation of tachistoscopic performance by stimulation at midbrain tegmental points in the monkey. *Exp. Neurol.*, 6:384–406.

15. Gordon, B. (1973): Receptive fields in deep layers of cat superior colliculus. *J. Neurophysiol.*, 36:157–178.

16. Grillner, S., and Shik, M. (1973): On the descending control of the lumbrosacral spinal cord from the "mesencephalic locomotor region." *Acta Physiol. Scand.*, 87:320–333.

17. Hanbery, J., Ajmone-Marsan, C., and Dilworth, M. (1954): Pathways of non-specific thalamocortical projection system. *Electroenceph. clin. Neurophysiol.*, 6:103–118.

18. Hernandez-Peón, R. (1955): Central mechanisms controlling conduction along central sensory pathways. *Acta Neurol. Latinoam.*, 1:256–264.

19. Hess, W. (1931): Le sommeil. *C. R. Soc. Biol. (Paris)*, 107:1333–1364.

20. Hess, W., Burgi, S., and Bucher, V. (1946): Motorische Funktion des Tektal- und Tegmentalgebietes. *Monatsschr. Psychiatr. Neurol.*, 112:1–52.

21. Hubel, D., and Wiesel, T. (1974): Sequence, regularity and geometry of orientation columns in the monkey striate cortex. *J. Comp. Neurol.*, 158:267–294.

22. Huttenlocher, P. (1961): Evoked and spontaneous activity in single units of medial brain stem during natural sleep and waking. *J. Neurophysiol.*, 24:451–468.

23. Jasper, H. (1949): Diffuse projection systems: The integrative action of the thalamic reticular system. *Electroenceph. clin. Neurophysiol.*, 1:405–420.

24. Jouvet, M. (1962): Recherches sur les structures nerveuses et les mécanismes responsables des differentes phases du sommeil physiologique. *Arch. Ital. Biol.*, 100:125–206.

25. Kleitman, N. (1963): The evolutionary theory of sleep and wakefulness. *Perspect. Biol. Med.*, 7:169–178.

26. Kohnstamm, O., and Quesnel, F. (1908): Das Centrum Receptorium (sensorium) der Formatis Reticularis (abstract). *Neurol. Centralb.*, 27:1046–1047.

27. Lindsley, D. (1958): The reticular system and perceptual discrimination. In: *Reticular Formation of the Brain*, edited by H. H. Jasper, L. D. Proctor, R. S. Knighton, W. C. Noshay, and R. T. Costello, pp. 513–534. Little, Brown and Co., Boston.

28. Lindsley, D., Bowden, J., and Magoun, H. (1949): Effects upon the EEG of acute injury to the brain stem activating system. *Electroenceph. clin. Neurophysiol.*, 1:475–486.

29. Magni, F., and Willis, W. (1963): Identification of reticular formation neurons by intracellular recording. *Arch. Ital. Biol.*, 101:681–702.

30. Minderhoud, J. (1971): An anatomical study of the efferent connections of the thalamic reticular nucleus. *Exp. Brain Res.*, 12:435–446.

31. Moruzzi, G., and Magoun, H. (1949): Brain stem reticular formation and activation of the EEG. *Electroenceph. clin. Neurophysiol.*, 1:455–473.

32. Mountcastle, V. (1957): Modality and topographic properties of single neurons of cat's somatic sensory cortex. *J. Neurophysiol.*, 20:408–434.

33. Nauta, W., and Kuypers, H. (1958): Some ascending pathways in the brain stem reticular formation. In: *Reticular Formation of the Brain*, edited by H. H. Jasper, L. D. Proctor, R. S. Knighton, W. C. Noshay, and R. T. Costello, pp. 3–30. Little, Brown and Co., Boston.

34. Palkovitz, M., Magyar, P., and Szentágothai, J. (1971): Quantitative histological analysis of the cerebellar cortex in the cat. I. Number and arrangement in space of the Purkinje cells. *Brain Res.*, 32:1–13.

35. Penfield, W. (1952): Epileptic automatisms and the centrencephalic integrating system. *Res. Publ. Assoc. Res. Nerv. Ment. Dis.*, 30:513–528.

36. Quattrochi, J., Baba, N., and Liss, L. (1978): Sudden infant death syndrome (SIDS): Reticular dendritic spines in infants with SIDS. *Neurosci. Abstr.*, 4:390.

37. Ramón y Cajal, S. (1909–1911): *Histologie du Système Nerveux de l'Homme et des Vertébrés, Vols. I and II*, translated by Azoulay. Maloine, Paris.

38. Rinvik, E. (1972): Organization of thalamic connections from motor and somatosensory cortical areas in the cat. In: *Corticothalamic Projections and Sensorimotor Activities*, edited by T. Frigyesi, E. Rinvik, and M. Yahr, pp. 57–88. Raven Press, New York.

39. Rossi, G., Minobe, K., and Candia, O. (1963): An experimental study of the hypnogenic mechanisms of the brain stem. *Arch. Ital. Biol.*, 101:470–492.

40. Scheibel, A. B. (1955): Axonal afferent patterns in the bulbar reticular formation (abstract). *Anat. Rec.*, 121:361–362.

41. Scheibel, M. E., and Scheibel, A. B. (1958): Structural substrates for integrative patterns in the brain stem reticular cores. In: *Reticular Formation of the Brain*, edited by H. H. Jasper, L. D. Proctor, R. S. Knighton, W. C. Noshay, and R. T. Costello, pp. 31–55. Little, Brown and Co., Boston.

42. Scheibel, M. E., and Scheibel, A. B. (1958): A symposium on dendrites. *Electroenceph. clin. Neurophysiol.*, [*Suppl.*], 10:43–50.

43. Scheibel, M. E., and Scheibel, A. B. (1965): The response of reticular units to repetitive stimuli. *Arch. Ital. Biol.*, 103:279–299.

44. Scheibel, M. E., and Scheibel, A. B. (1965): Periodic sensory nonresponsiveness in reticular neurons. *Arch. Ital. Biol.*, 103:300–316.

45. Scheibel, M. E., and Scheibel, A. B. (1966): The organization of the nucleus reticularis thalami: A Golgi study. *Brain Res.*, 1:43–62.

46. Scheibel, M. E., and Scheibel, A. B. (1967): Structural organization of nonspecific thalamic nuclei and their projection toward cortex. *Brain Res.*, 6:60–94.

47. Scheibel, M. E., and Scheibel, A. B. (1970): Elementary processes in selected thalamic and cortical subsystems. The structural substrates. In: *The Neurosciences—Second Study Program*, edited by F. Schmitt, pp. 443–457. Rockefeller University Press, New York.

48. Scheibel, M. E., Davies, T. L., and Scheibel, A. B. (1973): Maturation of reticular dendrites: Loss of spines and development of bundles. *Exp. Neurol.*, 38:301–310.

49. Scheibel, M., Scheibel, A., Mollica, A., and Moruzzi, G. (1955): Convergence and interaction of afferent impulses on single units of reticular formation. *J. Neurophysiol.*, 18:309–331.

50. Schlag, J., and Waszak, M. (1970): Characteristics of unit responses in nucleus reticularis thalami. *Brain Res.*, 21:286–288.

51. Schlag, J., and Waszak, M. (1971): Electrophysiological properties of units of the thalamic reticular complex. *Exp. Neurol.*, 32:79–97.

52. Singer, W. (1979): Central core control of visual cortex function. In: *The Neurosciences, Fourth Study Program*, edited by F. Schmitt and F. Worden. M.I.T. Press, Cambridge.

53. Skinner, J., and Yingling, C. (1976): Regulation of slow potential shifts in nucleus reticularis thalami by the mesencephalic reticular formation and the frontal granular cortex. *Electroenceph. clin. Neurophysiol.*, 40:280–296.

54. Starzl, T. E., Taylor, C. W., and Magoun, H. W. (1951): Collateral afferent excitation of reticular formation and brain stem. *J. Neurophysiol.*, 14:479–496.

55. Stein, B., Magalhães-Castro, B., and Kruger, L. (1976): Relationship between visual and tactile representation in cat superior colliculus. *J. Neurophysiol.*, 39:401–419.

56. Szentágothai, J. (1971): Some geometrical aspects of the neocortical neuropil. *Acta Biol. Acad. Sci. Hung.*, 22:107–124.

57. Szentágothai, J., and Arbib, M. (1974): Conceptual models of neural organization. *Neurosci. Res. Program Bull.*, 12:370–392.

58. Valverde, F. (1961): Reticular formation of the pons and medulla oblongata. A Golgi study. *J. Comp. Neurol.*, 116:71–99.

59. Waszak, M. (1974): Firing patterns of neurons in the rostral and ventral part of nucleus reticularis thalami during EEG spindles. *Exp. Neurol.*, 43:38–58.

60. Woolsey, T., and Van der Loos, H. (1970): The structural organization of layer IV in the somatosensory region (SI) of mouse cerebral cortex. The description of a cortical field composed of discrete cytoarchitectural units. *Brain Res.*, 17:205–242.

61. Yingling, C., and Skinner, J. (1975): Regulation of unit activity in nucleus reticularis thalami of the mesencephalic reticular formation and the frontal granular cortex. *Electroenceph. clin. Neurophysiol.*, 39:635–642.

62. Moore, R. Y. (1980): The reticular formation: monoamine neuron systems. In: *The Reticular Formation Revisited: Specifying Function for a Nonspecific System*, edited by J. Allan Hobson and Mary A. B. Brazier, pp. 67–81. Raven Press, New York.

63. Steriade, M., Ropert, N., Kitsikis, A., and Oakson, G. (1980): Ascending activating neuronal networks in midbrain reticular core and related rostral systems. In: *The Reticular Formation Revisited: Specifying Function for a Nonspecific System*, edited by J. Allan Hobson and Mary A. B. Brazier, pp. 125–170. Raven Press, New York.

64. Skrebitsky, V. G., Chepkova, A. N., and Sharonova, I. N. (1980): Reticular suppression of cortical inhibitory postsynaptic potentials. In: *The Reticular Formation Revisited: Specifying Function for a Nonspecific System*, edited by J. Allan Hobson and Mary A. B. Brazier, pp. 117–124. Raven Press, New York.

65. Odutola, A. B. (1980): Brain stem reticular projections to rat dorsal column nuclei. In: *The Reticular Formation Revisited: Specifying Function for a Nonspecific System*, edited by J. Allan Hobson and Mary A. B. Brazier, pp. 99–104. Raven Press, New York.

53 On the Neurophysiology of Consciousness: An Overview

Joseph E. Bogen

The main idea in this series of essays is that conscious awareness (more precisely what I call C) is engendered by neuronal activity in and immediately around the intralaminar nuclei (ILN) of each thalamus (Bogen 1993b). Falsification of this proposal is straightforward: find someone with essentially complete, bilateral destruction of ILN whom we would consider conscious. Absolute proof of this claim is unlikely, but I hope to make it plausible. One reason to consider it plausible is that many informed persons have believed it, or something like it, for decades (this includes Wilder Penfield and Herbert Jasper, of whom more later).

There are many facts related to the proposed role of ILN. This chapter indicates the range of materials (including anatomic, physiologic, pathologic, psychologic, philosophic) to be discussed in this series of essays. One way to introduce the series is to enumerate, each with brief exposition, certain assumptions and auxiliary propositions as follows:

1. The crucial, central core of the many, various concepts of consciousness includes subjectivity, the ascription of self or "me-ness" to some percept or affect. Examples include: "It hurts me," "I see red," "I feel thirsty." This central core of conscious awareness is part of what I call C. This proposal means that *whatever else* consciousness involves, without C there is no consciousness. Part 2 of this series discusses in more detail what I exclude from C, including such things as "timebinding" and language.

2. C is provided by some cerebral mechanism (Mc). By "cerebral," I mean to include cerebral cortex, underlying white matter, thalami, and basal ganglia. This view (cerebralism), while explicitly mechanistic, is not necessarily materialistic, fully deterministic, or solely reductionistic. I assume only that Mc necessarily involves neural activity whose nature is discoverable. Part 2 discusses the nonnecessity, for this assumption, of a commitment to materialism.

3. Consciousness involves both a property (C) of varying intensity and a widely varying content. The content (often of cortical origin) is not our main concern here. Rather, we are concerned with Mc which can (serially) endow with C very small fractions of a wide variety of contents. This assumption closely resembles the distinction made between "consciousness *as such*" and "different *contents* of consciousness" by Baars (1993).

By "endowed with C" I mean that some pattern of neuronal activity has acquired two additional attributes: (1) it acquires subjectivity and (2) it has an increased likelihood of influencing other neuronal patterns in the cerebrum by virtue of whatever efferent connections are available to Mc.

4. How Mc momentarily endows with C percepts or affects represented by neuronal patterns situated elsewhere is more likely to be solved when the structures subserving Mc are located. That Mc is localizeable can be argued variously:

a. The usual localizationist argument involves two findings: first, a large deficit in some function (f) is produced by a small lesion in the "center" for that f. (this does *not* imply that the representation of f is wholly contained within some sharp boundary—see Bogen 1976, Bogen and Bogen 1976). Second, a large lesion elsewhere (the right hemisphere in the example of syntactic competence of a right hander) results in a small (or no) loss of f. With respect to C, quite small bithalamic lesions involving both ILN typically impair Mc (see paragraph 5), whereas large bicortical lesions (e.g., bifrontal or bitemporal) typically do not (e.g., Damasio and Damasio 1989).

A striking example of loss of cerebral tissue is "total hemispherectomy" (including cortex, underlying white matter, and basal ganglia). Of the four patients reported by Austin and Grant (1958), one (case 4) was stuporous preoperatively. The other three continued speaking and were "acutely aware" of their surroundings throughout the operation which was done under local anesthesia. All four patients (including case 4) were subsequently able to walk with assistance.

b. Another, less familiar argument analogizes neural circuits with single cells:

A primordial cell has the potentials for a range of activities including multiplication, detoxification, secretion, contraction, conduction, and so on. But cells come to specialize so that skin cells multiply well, liver cells metabolize marvelously, pancreatic islet cells secrete superbly, muscle cells contract best, and the more familiar neurons conduct information better than they secrete, move, multiply, or metabolically adapt.

Analogously, neuronal aggregates form circuits which, early on, have a wide spectrum of potential function. But some come to specialize in the generation of diurnal and other rhythms (e.g., suprachiasmatic nucleus), some in the conversion of short-term memory to long (hippocampus), some in long-term storage (probably including neocortex) and so forth.

Although any sufficiently sizeable aggregate of neurons might early on have a *potential* for Mc, only certain aggregates developmentally organize to subserve Mc (namely, I claim, "nonspecific" thalamus, especially ILN).

5. Support of the proposal that ILN subserve Mc will include, later in this series, detailed discussions of thalamic anatomy, vasculature, and neuropathology. Here it may suffice to note that simultaneous bimedial thalamic infarction can occur because the medial parts of both thalami are occasionally supplied by a single arterial trunk which branches, one branch to each thalamus. If the trunk is occluded before it branches, both thalami will be affected.

When there is simultaneous, partial infarction of the two sets of ILN, unresponsiveness typically ensues (see table 1 in Guberman and Stuss 1983). Sudden onset of coma can occur even when the lesions are only a few cubic centimeters in volume, as in case 4 of Graff-Radford et al. (1990). This is in contrast to retention of responsiveness with very large infarctions elsewhere. Even a quite large lesion involving one (and only one) thalamus rarely if ever causes coma (Plum and Posner 1985).

Emergence from unresponsiveness after bithalamic lesions (not causing death) is commonly accompanied by mental impairments variously described as confusion, dementia, amnesia, and/ or hypersomnia. Which of these impairments dominates depends on precise lesion site as well as size (Castaigne et al. 1981; Gentilini, De Renzi, and Crisi 1987; Guberman and Stuss 1983; Meissner, Sapir, Kokmen, and Stein 1987; Markowitsch, von Cramon, and Schuri 1993).

6. In an intact cerebrum, Mc is double. Whatever the anatomical basis for Mc, the anatomy exists in duplicate. That only one Mc suffices for C is clear from hemispherectomy in humans as well as hemicerebrectomy in cats and monkeys (White et al. 1959, Bogen and Campbell 1960, Bogen 1974).

That with two Mc there can be doubling of C has been inferred from split-brain cats and monkeys (Sperry 1961) as well as humans (Sperry, Gazzaniga, and Bogen 1969). How such a structural duality could be handled by an intact cerebrum is a fascinating and important question (Bogen 1969, 1977, 1990, 1993, 1994), but it is not the issue here. I consider here only how C is engendered in someone with a single cerebral hemisphere.

7. C is *not* produced by cerebral *cortex*. This was considered by Hughlings Jackson before 1900 and, 50 years later, by Penfield and Jasper (1954). Their views derived largely from observations of epilepsy, including that consciousness could be absent during complex behavior (requiring neocortex). Conversely, severe disturbances of function either from cortical removals or cortical hyperactivity need not be accompanied by loss of consciousness. As early as 1937, Penfield noted:

All parts of the brain may well be involved in normal conscious processes but the indispensable substratum of consciousness lies outside of the cerebral cortex, probably in the diencephalon. (p. 241)

To their reasons for this auxiliary conclusion can be added the following: some potential contents of consciousness are quite primitive, that is, unneedful of discrimination, association, or learning. Examples are nausea, fatigue, unelaborated pain (e.g., trigeminal neuralgia), thirst, and the like. Did Mc evolve to give these percepts greater potency, another layer of control over the starting and stopping of ongoing action? Was Mc only subsequently recruited to serve so-called higher functions and more elaborate responses?

We understand that Mc might endow with C instances of complex cortical activity describable as "representations of representations" or "higher order thoughts." But these are special contents, not the crucial core of consciousness. Moreover, such special contents might very well influence other cerebral functions without reaching awareness, as pointed out by Kihlstrom (1987) among others (e.g., Castiello, Paulignan, and Jeannerod 1991; Wexler, Warrenburg, Schwartz, and Janer 1992).

8. Ascending input to ILN can help explain C of primitive percepts. The afference to ILN includes a large fraction of the ascending output of the brainstem reticular formation, which subserves arousal but may well contain information about other bodily states. Other input comes from a phylogenetically old spinothalamic system (conveying temperature and nociceptive information) and from the dentate nuclei in the cerebellum (called by Sherrington the "head ganglion of the proprioceptive system"). There are also ascending inputs to ILN from deep layers of the superior colliculus, substantia nigra, and vestibular nuclei (see figure 53.1 and table 53.1).

9. The existence of connections to ILN from globus pallidus (thought to be collaterals of pallidal projections to VL and VA of thalamus) suggests a monitoring of motor systems, as do the cortical projections to ILN from sensorimotor and premotor cortex. A role in control of motor output is evident in the very substantial projections from ILN to striatum. Is this the pathway for the inhibition (or release from inhibition) supposed by Libet (1983, 1985) to stop (or release) motor plans which have been developing for several hundred milliseconds? Is this the basis for a "volitional" decision?

If it is correct that subjectivity is generated within ILN (and environs), this bears immediately upon the old question of epiphenomenality. This is because the principal output of ILN is to striatum. Hence, awareness of something (i.e., transient subjectivity of a particular content) will necessarily influence motor output.

It is not yet firmly established what the transmitter(s) is for the ILN–striatum projection. Is it glutamate? Can it be inhibitory? Modulatory? Pursuing these and related questions is more likely to lead us to an understanding of Mc (and of C) than equivalent efforts and time spent on other brain parts.

10. It is now widely accepted that the reticular nucleus (nRt) of thalamus affords a physiologic basis for selective attention (Scheibel and Scheibel 1966, Yingling and Skinner 1977, Crick 1984, Mitrofanis and Guillery 1993). Associated with nRt is a plausible theory of C which I consider inadequate for several reasons. It assumes that the thalamocorticothalamic (TCT) activity passing through nRt can grow, in one small locale, so large that it shuts down other TCT activity by a sort of surround inhibition; this would account for the focus of attention. Meanwhile, the level of activity in the small locale could rise above the "threshold for consciousness." Problems with this view include: (1) it does not account for C of primitive content; (2) there may well be focal attention without C (and possibly vice versa); and (3) it makes no provision for an immediate inhibition (or release) of a developing motor plan.

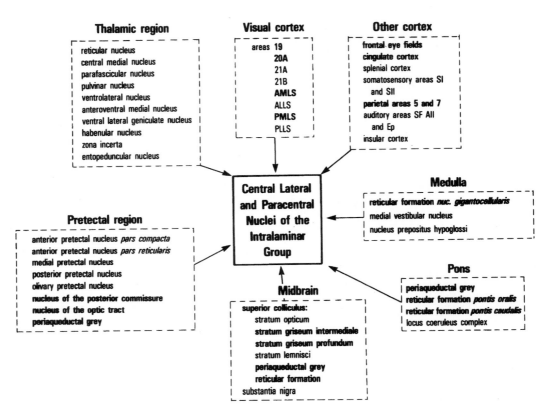

Figure 53.1
Diagram summarizing projections from various brain regions (in cat) to the rostral part of ILN, the central lateral–paracentral complex. Bold type indicates particularly strong connections. Reprinted with permission from Kaufman and Rosenquist 1985.

That focal attention can be influenced by C could have its anatomical basis in collaterals of ILN efferents that terminate in nRt (see figure 53.2).

11. ILN efferents, some of them collaterals of the ILN projection to striatum, are widely and sparsely distributed to most of neocortex. This may provide ongoing cortical computation with immediate notice of the aforementioned "volitional decision." In any case, one can see how ILN could directly influence ideation, insofar as ideation is a function of cortex.

12. Patterns of cortical activity could contact Mc, in some condensed or abstracted form, by virtue of the cortical efferents to ILN. Experiments with small lesions in almost every cortical region provide evidence that these regions project not only to their principal unclei but also to ILN. Interesting is the fact that whereas most TCT projection systems are highly reciprocal, the ILN connections with cortex (relatively diffuse, and sparse, as noted above), are less so, possibly providing for a much less channeled (i.e., less modular) interaction.[1]

Table 53.1

Structures that contain labeled neurons following injections of the centromedian and parafascicular thalamic nuclear complex

Neural structure	HRP	WGA-HRP	RFM
1. Amygdala, central nucleus	+	+	+
2. Entopeduncular nucleus	+	+	+
3. Globus pallidus	+	+	+
4. Thalamus			
(A) Reticular nucleus	+	+	+
(B) Ventral lateral geniculate nucleus	+	+	+
5. Hypothalamus			
(A) Anterior hypothalamic area	0	+	+
(B) Dorsal hypothalamic area	+	+	+
(C) Lateral hypothalamic area	+	+	+
(D) Ventromedial nucleus	+	+	+
(E) Parvocellular nucleus	+	+	+
(F) Posterior hypothalamic area	+	+	+
6. Zona incerta and fields of Forel	+	+	+
7. Substantia nigra			
(A) Pars reticularis	+	+	+
(B) Pars lateralis	+	+	+
(C) Ventral tegmental area	0	+	+
(D) Retrorubral area	+	+	+
8. Pretectum	+	+	+
9. Superior colliculus			
(A) Intermediate layers	+	+	+
(B) Deep layers	+	+	+
10. Periaqueductal gray	+	+	+
11. Dorsal nucleus of the raphe	+	+	+
13. Reticular formation			
(A) Mesencephalic reticular formation	+	+	+
(B) Nucleus reticularis pontis oralis	+	+	+
(C) Nucleus reticularis pontis caudalis	+	+	+
(D) Nucleus reticularis gigantocellularis	+	+	+
(E) Nucleus reticularis ventralis	+	+	+
(F) Nucleus reticularis lateralis	+	+	+
14. Nucleus cuneiformis	+	+	+
15. Marginal nucleus of the brachium conjunctivum	+	+	+
16. Nucleus (locus) coeruleus	+	+	+
17. Trigeminal complex			
(A) Principal sensory nucleus	+	+	+
(B) Spinal nucleus	+	+	+
18. Vestibular complex			
(A) Superior nucleus, medial division	+	+	+
(B) Superior nucleus, lateral division	0	+	+
(C) Medial nucleus	+	+	+

Table 53.1
(continued)

Neural structure	HRP	WGA-HRP	RFM
19. Cerebral nuclei			
(A) Medial cerebellar nucleus	+	+	+
(B) Lateral cerebellar nucleus	+	+	+
(C) Nucleus interpositus	0	+	+
20. Nucleus praepositus hypoglossi	0	+	+
21. Cervical spinal cord	+	+	+

Note: Retrograde labeling of brain regions (in cat) projecting to the caudal part of ILN, the centromedian–parafascicular complex. The three methods used gave similar results: HRP, horseradish peroxidase; WGA-HRP, wheat germ agglutinin-conjugated HRP; and RFM, rhodamine-labeled fluorescent latex microspheres. Reprinted with permission from Royce, Bromley, and Gracco, 1991.

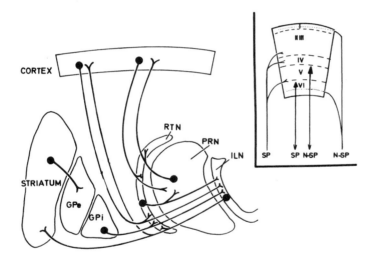

Figure 53.2
Depiction of pathways mentioned in the ext. Reprinted with permission from Jones 1985. Highly schematic outline of the connectivity of the dorsal thalamus and of the associated reticular nucleus (RTN) of the ventral thalamus. Afferent fibers from the cerebral cortex deposit collaterals in the reticular nucleus and continue on to the principal (PRN) of intralaminar (ILN) nuclei. Afferent fibers from the internal segment of the globus pallidus (GPi) also give off collaterals to the reticular nucleus and continue on to the intralaminar nuclei. Efferent fibers from the principal nuclei and from nuclei with nonspecific projections (e.g., the intralaminar nuclei) also give collaterals to the reticular nucleus. The intralaminar nuclei provide the only thalamic input to the striatum, again probably with collaterals to the reticular nucleus. Inset shows laminar pattern of termination of specific and nonspecific afferents in cerebral cortex. Intralaminar nuclei are one of several nuclear groups with nonspecific projections. Corticothalamic fibers to principal thalamic nuclei arise from cells with somata in layer VI. Those reciprocating a nonspecific projection arise from cells with somata in layer V.

13. The foregoing implies that awareness of content requires some as yet unspecified "appropriate interaction" between ILN and the neural representation of that content. It has been suggested (Crick and Koch 1990, Llinás and Ribary 1993) that the "appropriate interaction" involves synchronization of neuronal activity at 40 Hz; problems with this proposal will be discussed in a later part of this series.

As an example of "appropriate interaction" between ILN and cortex, we can consider awareness of the direction of motion of a stimulus. It is now widely understood that motion direction information (MDI) is available in cortex of the superior temporal sulcus, especially area V_5, more commonly called MT (Allman and Kaas 1971; Zeki 1974; Maunsell and Newsome 1987; Boussaoud, Ungerleider, and Desimone 1990; Newsome, Britten, Salzman, and Movshon 1990; Rodman, Gross, and Albright 1990; Murasugi, Salzman, and Newsome 1993; Zeki 1993).

We expect that for the MDI to have a subjective aspect (i.e., to acquire C) there must occur the "appropriate interaction" between ILN and MT (or its targets). We keep in mind that the MDI in MT might well be available for adaptive behavior *whether or not* it acquires C.

In the neurally intact individual, the "appropriate interaction" can be on, or off, or in between, and is quickly adjustable. However, when V_1 (striate cortex) has been ablated, the "appropriate interaction" for vision does not occur. That is, the MDI in MT is not available to verbal output (the individual denies seeing the stimulus). At the same time, the MDI may be available for some other behavior (Stoerig and Cowey 1993). This form of "blindsight" will be enlarged upon in a later essay which will consider several explanations for the effects of V_1 removal. Meanwhile, it appears (when we accept availability to verbal output as the index of awareness) that the "appropriate interaction" between MT and ILN cannot occur in the absence of influences from ipsilateral striate cortex.[2]

14. Some previous objections to ILN being crucial for consciousness have been superseded.

When Penfield and Jasper (1954) advocated the concept of a "centrencephalon," they particularly stressed the role of ILN. Why was this idea eclipsed, to reemerge some 40 years later? At least three reasons can be readily seen:

a. The centrencephalon was supposed to be not only a mechanism for consciousness, but also a source of seizures which were "generalized from the start." The concept of "centrencephalic seizures" has been largely abandoned by epileptologists. However, that Penfield and Jasper combined these two ideas does not require that we do so; arguments for an ILN role in C can be made quite independently of theories about seizure origin and spread.

b. Cerebral commissurotomy (the split-brain) reinforced doubts about the existence of a centrencephalon (Doty 1975). However, the problem of localizing Mc can be approached in terms of a single hemisphere (which we know can have C), postponing to the future the problem of integrating two Mc and how this bears on the "unity of consciousness."

c. Forty (even twenty) years ago, there was considerable doubt of ILN projections to cortex, because unilateral decortication did not produce rapid degeneration in the ILN as it did in most of the ipsilateral thalamus. Another exception to rapid degeneration was nRt which, indeed, we now believe does *not* project to cortex (Scheibel and Scheibel 1966, Jones 1985). However, more recent tracer techniques have shown that ILN *do* project to cortex, and widely.

The "centrencephalon" tried to explain too much. But it contained a germ of truth which now needs to be nourished in terms of ILN as a major constituent of the mechanisms which provide us, and creatures like us, with conscious awareness.

Notes

1. Groenewegen and Berendse (1994) recently reviewed evidence that ILN are more specific than the traditional term "nonspecific" might suggest. They concluded that, "... the major role of the midline-intralaminar nuclei presumably lies in the regulation of the activity and the ultimate functioning of individual basal–ganglia–thalamocortical circuits" (p. 56) and that "the midline-intralaminar nuclei are positioned in the forebrain circuits like a spider in its web" (p. 57).

2. Regarding "blindsight," see also Weiskrantz 1986. The necessity of V_1 for C of MDI has been challenged by Barbur, Watson, Frackowiak, and Zeki 1993.

References

Allman, J. M., and Kaas, J. H. (1971). A representation of the visual field in the caudal third of the middle temporal gyrus of the owl monkey (*Aotus trivirgatus*). *Brain Research*, 31, 85–105.

Austin, G. M., and Grant, F. C. (1958). Physiologic observations following total hemispherectomy in man. *Surgery*, 38, 239–258.

Baars, B. J. (1993). How does a serial, integrated and very limited stream of consciousness emerge from a nervous system that is mostly unconscious, distributed, parallel and of enormous capacity? In G. Broch and J. Marsh (Eds.), *Experimental and theoretical studies of consciousness*. New York: Wiley.

Barbur, J. L., Watson, J. D. G., Frackowiak, R. S. J., and Zeki, S. (1993). Conscious visual perception without V1. *Brain*, 116, 1293–1302.

Bogen, J. E. (1969). The other side of the brain. II: An appositional mind. *Bulletin of the Los Angeles Neurological Society*, 34, 135–162.

Bogen, J. E. (1974). Hemispherectomy and the placing reaction in cats. In M. Kinsbourne and W. L. Smith (Eds.), *Hemispheric disconnection and cerebral function*. Springfield: Thomas.

Bogen, J. E. (1976). Hughlings Jackson's Heterogram. In D. O. Walter, L. Rogers, and J. M. Finzi-Fried (Eds.), *Cerebral dominance*. BIS Conf. Report No. 42. Los Angeles: UCLA, BRI.

Bogen, J. E. (1977). Further discussions on split-brains and hemispheric capabilities. *British Journal of the Philosophy of Science*, 28, 281–286.

Bogen, J. E. (1990). Partial hemispheric independence with the neocommissures intact. In C. Trevarthen (Ed.), *Brain circuits and functions of the mind*. Cambridge, Englang: Cambridge Univ. Press.

Bogen, J. E. (1993a). The callosal syndromes. In K. Heilman and E. Valenstein (Eds.), *Clinical neuropsychology*. (3rd ed., pp. 337–381). New York: Oxford Univ. Press.

Bogen, J. E. (1993b). Intralaminar nuclei and the where of awareness. *Proceedings of the Society for Neuroscience*, 19, 1446.

Bogen, J. E. (1994). Descartes' fundamental mistake: Introspective singularity. *Behavioral and Brain Sciences*, 17, 175–176.

Bogen, J. E. (1995). On the neurophysiology of consciousness: Part II. Constraining the semantic problem. *Consciousness and Cognition*, 4, 137–158.

Bogen, J. E., and Bogen, G. M. (1976). Wernicke's Region—Where is it? *Annals of the New York Academy of Science*, 280, 834–843.

Bogen, J. E., and Campbell, B. (1960). Total hemispherectomy in the cat. *Surgical Forum*, 11, 381–383.

Boussaoud, D., Ungerleider, L. G., and Desimone, R. (1990). Pathways of motion analysis: Cortical connections of the medial superior temporal and fundus of the superior temporal visual areas in the macaque. *Journal of Comparative Neurology*, 296, 462–495.

Campbell, B. (1960). The factor of safety in the nervous system. *Bulletin of the Los Angeles Neurological Society*, 25, 109–117.

Castaigne, P., Lhermitte, F., Buge, A., Escourolle, R., Hauw, J. J., and Lyon-Caen, O. (1981). Paramedian thalamic and midbrain infarcts: Clinical and neuropathological study. *Annals of Neurology*, 10, 127–148.

Castiello, U., Paulignan, Y., and Jeannerod, M. (1991). Temporal dissociation of motor responses and subjective awareness; A study in normal subjects. *Brain*, 114, 2639–2655.

Crick, F. (1984). Function of the thalamic reticular complex: The searchlight hypothesis. *Proceedings of the National Academy of Science, USA*, 81, 4586–4590.

Crick, F., and Koch, C. (1990). Towards a neurobiological theory of consciousness. *Seminars in the Neurosciences*, 2, 263–275.

Damasio, H., and Damasio, A. R. (1989). *Lesion analysis in neuropsychology.* New York: Oxford Univ. Press.

Doty, R. W. (1975). Consciousness from neurons. *Acta Neurobiologiae Experimentalis*, 35, 791–804.

Gentilini, M., De Renzi, E., and Crisi, G. (1987). Bilateral paramedian thalamic artery infarcts: Report of eight cases. *Journal of Neurology, Neurosurgery and Psychiatry*, 50, 900–909.

Graff-Radford, N., Tranel, D., Van Hoesen, G. W., and Brandt, J. P. (1990). Diencephalic amnesia. *Brain*, 113, 1–25.

Groenewegen, J. J., and Berendse, H. W. (1994). The specificity of the "nonspecific" midline and intralaminar thalamic nuclei. *Trends in Neuroscience*, 17, 52–57.

Guberman, A., and Stuss, D. (1983). The syndrome of bilateral paramedian thalamic infarction. *Neurology*, 33, 540–546.

Jones, E. G. (1988). *The thalamus.* New York: Plenum.

Kaufman, E. F. S., and Rosenquist, A. C. (1985). Afferent connections of the thalamic intralaminar nuclei in the cat. *Brain Research*, 335, 281–296.

Kihlstrom, J. D. (1987). The cognitive unconscious. *Science*, 237, 1445–1452.

Kruper, D. C., Patton, R. A., and Koskoff, Y. D. (1961). Delayed object–quality discrimination in hemicerebrectomized monkeys. *Journal of Comparative and Physiological Psychology*, 54, 619–624.

Libet, B. (1985). Unconscious cerebral initiative and the role of conscious will in voluntary action. *Behavioral and Brain Sciences*, 8, 529–566.

Libet, B., Gleason, C. A., Wright, E. W., and Pearl, D. K. (1983). Time of conscious intention to act in relation to onset of cerebral activities (readiness-potential): The unconscious initiation of a freely voluntary act. *Brain*, 106, 623–642.

Llinás, R., and Ribary, U. (1993). Coherent 40-Hz oscillation characterizes dream state in humans. *Proceedings of the National Academy of Science, USA*, 90, 2078–2081.

Markowitsch, H. J., von Cramon, D. Y., and Schuri, U. (1993). Mnestic performance profile of a bilateral diencephalic infarct patient with preserved intelligence and severe amnesic disturbances. *Journal of Clinical and Experimental Neuropsychology*, 15, 627–652.

Maunsell, J. H. R., and Newsome, W. T. (1987). Visual processing in primate extrastriate cortex. *Annual Review of Neuroscience*, 10, 363.

Meissner, I., Sapir, S., Kokmen, E., and Stein, S. D. (1987). The paramedian diencephalic syndrome: A dynamic phenomenon. *Stroke*, 18, 380–385.

Mitrofanis, J., and Guillery, R. W. (1993). New views of the thalamic reticular nucleus in the adult and the developing brain. *Trends in Neuroscience*, 16, 240–245.

Murasugi, C. M., Salzman, C. D., and Newsome, W. T. (1993). Microstimulation in Visual Area MT: Effects of varying pulse amplitude and frequency. *Journal of Neuroscience*, 13, 1719–1729.

Newsome, W. T., Britten, K. H., Salzman, C. D., and Movshon, J. A. (1990). Neuronal mechanisms of motion perception. *Cold Spring Harbor Symp. Quant. Biol.* 55, 697–705.

Penfield, W. (1937). The cerebral cortex and consciousness. In *The Harvey Lectures.* Reprinted (1965) in R. H. Wilkins (Ed.), *Neurosurgical classics.* New York: Johnson Reprint Corp.

Penfield, W., and Jasper, H. H. (1954). *Epilepsy and the functional anatomy of the human brain.* Boston: Little, Brown.

Plum, F., and Posner, J. B. (1985). *The diagnosis of stupor and coma.* Philadelphia: Davis.

Rodman, H. R., Gross, C. G., and Albright, T. D. (1990). Afferent basis of visual response properties in area MT of the macaque. II. Effects of superior colliculus removal. *Journal of Neuroscience*, 10, 1154–1164.

Royce, G. J., Bromley, S., and Gracco, C. (1991). Subcortical projections to the centromedian and parafascicular thalamic nuclei in the cat. *Journal of Comparative Neurology*, 306, 129–155.

Scheibel, M. E., and Scheibel, A. B. (1966). The organization of the nucleus reticularis thalami: A Golgi study: *Brain Research*, 1, 43–62.

Sperry, R. W. (1961). Cerebral organization and behavior. *Science*, 133, 1749–1757.

Sperry, R. W., Gazzaniga, M. S., and Bogen, J. E. (1969). Interhemispheric relationships: The neocortical commissures; syndromes of hemisphere disconnection. *Handbook of Clinical Neurology*, 4, 273–290.

Stoerig, P., and Cowey, A. (1993). Blindsight and perceptual consciousness: Neuropsychological aspects of striate cortical function. In B. Gulyas, D. Ottoson, and P. E. Roland (Eds.), *Functional organisation of the human visual cortex*. Oxford: Pergamon Press.

Weiskrantz, L. (1986). *Blindsight: A case study and implications*. Oxford: Clarendon Press.

Wexler, B. E., Warrenburg, S., Schwartz, G. E., and Janer, L. D. (1992). EEG and EMG responses to emotion-evoking stimuli processed without conscious awareness. *Neuropsychologia*, 30, 1065–1079.

White, R. J., Schreiner, L. H., Hughes, R. A., MacCarty, C. S., and Grindlay, J. H. (1959). Physiologic consequences of total hemispherectomy in the monkey. *Neurology*, 9, 149–159.

Yingling, C. D., and Skinner, J. E. (1977). Gating of thalamic input to cerebral cortex by nucleus reticularis thalami. In J. E. Desmedt (Ed.), *Attention, voluntary contraction and event-related cerebral potentials*. Basel: Karger.

Zeki, S. (1974). Functional organization of a visual area in the superior temporal sulcus of the rhesus monkey. *Journal of Physiology*, 236, 549.

Zeki, S. (1993). *A vision of the brain*. Oxford, England: Blackwell.

Selected Background Sources

Baars, B. J. (1988). *A cognitive theory of consciousness*. Cambridge, England: Cambridge Univ. Press.

Carpenter, M. B., and Sutin, J. (1983). *Human neuroanatomy*. Baltimore: Williams & Wilkins.

Churchland, P. S., and Sejnowski, T. J. (1992). *The computational brain*. Cambridge, MA: MIT Press.

Delafresnaye, J. F. (Ed.) (1954). *Brain mechanisms and consciousness*. Springfield, IL: Thomas.

Gallistel, C. R. (1980). *The organization of action: A new synthesis*. Hillsdale, NJ: Erlbaum.

Jeannerod, M. (1983). *The brain machine: The development of neurophysiological thought* (English trans. by D. Urion, 1985). Cambridge, MA: Harvard Univ. Press.

Marcel, A. J., and Bisiach, E. (Eds.) (1988). *Consciousness in contemporary science*. Oxford: Clarendon Press.

Purves, D., and Lichtman, J. W. (1985). *Principles of neural development*. Sunderland, MA: Sinauer.

Hans Flohr

Introduction

Ideally, general anaesthesia can be defined as the loss of consciousness, that is, the absence of *phenomenal states* or *qualia* [22, 36, 40, 52]. The term "qualia" is badly defined. It is used to denote "sentient states" like perceptions, sensations, memories, emotional states, moods, imagery, thought, intentions, beliefs and the like.

A theory of anaesthesia must explain how these subjective states disappear as the result of the action of anaesthetics on the central nervous system. This means that the theory should not only demonstrate which molecular or cellular effects anaesthetics exert in the central nervous system, but give proof as to whether and why these effects are *relevant* for the disappearance of consciousness. Such a theory should, firstly, contain a hypothesis on those brain states and processes which are *conditional* for the occurrence of consciousness; and, secondly, demonstrate the mode of action of the various anaesthetically active substances in altering these brain states and processes. Previous theories of anaesthesia do not meet these requirements. Their intention was confined to the elucidation of the molecular and cellular effects of anaesthetics. A common mechanism of anaesthetic action has not been found and the "critical changes in brain function that are responsible for the change from 'esthesia' to 'anesthesia'" [40] have not been identified. Actually, this is not at all surprising: one should not expect that the phenomenon of anaesthesia can be explained on the cellular or molecular level.

Identifying the Critical Changes

States of unconsciousness are not always characterized by a global depression of the central nervous system's entire activity. Unconsciousness does neither lead to a complete deprivation of the central nervous system's functions. Depending on the cause of unconsciousness many reflexes *and cognitive performances* remain intact [24, 35]. Consciousness is therefore not a global function of the entire brain, instead, it is obviously bound to a specific subset of brain processes. The main task for a theory of consciousness would consist in identifying this subset of processes and characterizing them physiologically.

As yet such attempts have not only been unsuccessful, indeed we do not even have the faintest idea how such an approach would look like. By no means do we have a *concept* on how physical processes could cause or instantiate states of consciousness [3, 48]. The identification of these brain states does not only present an empirical problem, but, foremost, a theoretical one. The theoretical part of the problem consists in a resumption of the discussion of Du Bois Reymond's [15] famous ignorabimus statement, claiming that a physiological explanation of consciousness could never exist. According to Du Bois Reymond, even a total understanding of all physiological processes going on in the conscious brain would not explain consciousness as a natural phenomenon. Even if we had a detailed description of all the physiological differences between a conscious and an unconscious brain we would not know why the former conditions are bound to the occurrence of phenomenal states, the latter not.

In current discussion this standard objection against *any* attempt to explain consciousness in physiological terms is known as the *absent qualia argument*. It says, briefly, that no physical, functional, or computational description whatsoever gives us the *sufficient conditions* for the occurrence of states of consciousness. The "phenomenal," "subjective" features that characterize these states cannot be captured by *any* physical description, for all of them are logically compatible with the absence of consciousness. It is essential for any theory of consciousness to give proof that this line of argumentation is wrong. It must be shown that some hypotheses on the relationship between physical and psychic phenomena might exist, against which this argumentation does not work.

Information Processing and Phenomenal States

Du Bois Reymond's sceptical position had an enormous impact paralyzing all attempts to search for a theory of consciousness in the following century. This sceptical position is, however, not undisputed. Above all, it is uncertain whether the ignorabimus statement relies on stringent argumentation or whether it is founded on mere intuitions about the nature of conscious states [18–20]. It has been argued that especially the statement that *all* categories of information processing are logically compatible with the absence of consciousness, could be wrong. Contradicting Du Bois Reymond's statement it has been argued that *certain* computational processes necessarily lead to states of consciousness: systems generating and processing *representational states* could, under certain conditions, not only represent external events but also generate representations of their own internal state. They could, whilst representing external events, produce higher-order representations, that is, self-referential representations of their own actual state and representational activity. Such systems can produce states instantiating representations of concepts and beliefs of their own internal state. Under certain conditions they could become what Georges Rey [58, 59] has called recursive believer systems, or, what Daniel Dennett [13] has called an *n*-order intentional system. These systems develop a model of themselves [31, 50], i.e. a mental representation of the self as an agent or experiencer, and are able to bind other mental representations to it. In Nagel's [51] terms, such systems would know "what it is like to be such a system" and have a "subjective perspective."

However, this kind of subjectivity does not comply with our intuitions on the nature of consciousness. According to these intuitions, systems do not already possess consciousness when they have *knowledge* of their own state, but only if they additionally have experiences, sensations, feelings. In other words, the possession of self-referential beliefs is not the same as being in a phenomenal state. Even highly capable *cognitive* systems could be zombies. However, it could be that this distinction between cognitive and sentient systems relies on false intuitions. It has been claimed [18–20] that neither an external observer (like an anaesthetist), nor the system itself could distinguish self-referential cognitive states from "genuine" phenomenal states. Therefore, such a distinction would hardly make any sense. If these assumptions were true, the occurrence of conscious states would be a necessary result of specific computational processes and identical to specific cognitive events. Phenomenal states arise whenever the system's representational activity reaches a certain level: one that is sufficient for the generation of self-referential representations. In this view, consciousness is the product of computational processes.

If the outlined assumptions were true, the questions essential to a theory of anaesthesia could be put more precisely as follows:

1. What are the qualitative or quantitative differences in *information processing* that distinguish conscious from unconscious brains?

2. What cellular or molecular mechanisms are responsible for the action of anaesthetics that, directly or indirectly, cause these differences in information processing in conscious and unconscious brains?

Assemblies, Mental Representations, and the Physiological Conditions of Consciousness

The neurosciences have developed a concept on how mental representations are realized in the nervous system: the idea of cell assemblies as proposed by D. O. Hebb [26, 27]. Cell assemblies are strongly interconnected neurons that exhibit coherent activity. In a randomly interconnected network assemblies will develop automatically, if the neurons of the net are connected by excitatory, activity-dependent Hebb-type synapses. Hebb assumed that the strength of a synapse increases when pre- and postsynaptic activities coincide. Coincident activity at different sites in the network may, for instance, be caused by the various features of an external event. The net detects these coherent properties and represents them as an isomorphic structure, the assembly. An essential modification of Hebb's ideas originates from von der Malsburg [69]. His idea was that the formation of assemblies is not only essential for the *storage* of information but also part of "normal" information processing. He assumed that the formation of assemblies is not only a slow process that leads to permanent changes, but that rapid and transient synaptic changes are also possible allowing the formation of short-lived assemblies within 100–200 ms. Any distributed activity is associated with synaptic changes and a reorganization of the network architecture. The intriguing feature of this idea is that the cortex is conceived as a high-speed generator of rapidly formed, transient representations. Therefore, information processing in the nervous system is not (only) signal transduction and transformation in a rigid net but essentially the self-organization process of representational structures. According to a recently published hypothesis [16, 17] it is this category of information processing that gives rise to conscious states: consciousness will occur, if cortical networks generate complex representational structures.

The essential elements of this hypothesis can be summarized as follows:

1. The occurrence of states of consciousness causally depends on the rapid formation (and disintegration) of complex representational structures. States of consciousness will occur, if and only if cognitive systems develop higher-order, self-referential (meta-) representations, i.e.

states that instantiate concepts and beliefs about their internal states. Phenomenal states are cognitive events.

2. The underlying physiological processes can be identified. In the central nervous system mental representations are instantiated by neural cell assemblies. The occurrence of states of consciousness therefore depends on the formation of complex active assemblies, a process that involves the activation of the NMDA receptor channel complex. This synapse controls different forms of Hebbian plasticity, including rapid changes of the connection strengths. The formation of assemblies can be considered as a self-organizing process in a dynamic system. Representational structures of higher order emerge whenever the plastic changes are accomplished at a specific rate. A high rate of plastic change is the necessary and sufficient condition for the generation of such representational structures. The occurrence of such states is identical with the appearance of conscious states. Awareness is a state of high representational activity. States of consciousness are consequently a function of the activation state of the cortical NMDA synapses.

From these assumptions we can derive a theory of anaesthesia. The various causes of unconsciousness (such as the diverse anaesthetic agents) have a common operative mechanism: They inhibit the formation of neural assemblies. Loss of consciousness will occur, if and only if the rate at which assemblies are formed falls below a critical threshold level. The assembly formation rate is a function of the activation state of the NMDA receptor channel complex which controls fast and slow modifications of connection strengths. Thus, anaesthetics are agents that, directly or indirectly, disturb the activity of the NMDA synapse.

The NMDA Receptor Channel Complex

Numerous reviews have been published on the NMDA synapse. Among others, Collingridge and Lester [8], Lodge [42], Thomson [66], and

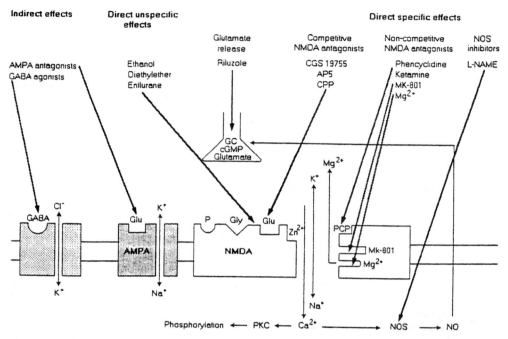

Figure 54.1
The NMDA synapse as a target for anaesthetics. Schematic representation of the NMDA receptor channel complex with its modulatory sites and of neighbouring AMPA and GABA receptors by which the voltage-dependent blockade of the NMDA channel can be influenced. Possible interaction sites for different anaesthetics are indicated by arrows. For details see text.

Yoneda and Ogita [74] have reported on molecular mechanisms and on the pharmacology of the receptor and the receptor-associated channel. The role of the synapse in long-term potentiation and other forms of plasticity were described by Collingridge and Bliss [7], Constantine-Paton et al. [9], Rauschecker [57], Tsumoto [67], Hawkins et al. [25] and Malenka and Nicoll [43]. The important role of nitric oxide as an intracellular messenger in these processes has recently been dealt with by Bruhwyler et al. [6] and Vincent [68]. Relatively few papers, however, have discussed the role of this synapse in "normal" information processing [10, 12, 42]. In the following short overview only those aspects will be

considered which are relevant to the possible role of this synapse in anaesthesia.

The NMDA receptor channel (figure 54.1) has several properties different from all other receptors. It is both ligand-gated and voltage-dependent. The receptor-associated channel opens under two conditions: firstly, the pre-synapse must be active and release the transmitter molecule; secondly, the postsynaptic membrane must be depolarized to about −35 mV. At membrane potentials around the resting potential the channel is closed by a magnesium ion. The blockade is released when the postsynaptic membrane reaches its threshold of depolarization. This mechanism qualifies the

NMDA synapse as a Hebb-synapse: the requirements for an alteration of the transduction properties are met when pre- and postsynaptic activity coincide.

The receptor-associated channel is permeable for Na^+, K^+, Ca^{2+}. Therefore, the channel controls *different* forms of synaptic plasticity, which are either fast and transient or slow and long-lasting:

1. The postsynaptic depolarization required for opening the channel will be achieved only if a sufficient number of neighbouring excitatory synapses are active at the same time. As soon as the activation threshold is reached, the synapse will be switched on and adjoined to the already active connections. In a randomly interconnected network of excitatory NMDA and non-NMDA synapses the activation of NMDA synapses will produce a positive feedback among those neurons reaching the threshold simultaneously. These neurons will be connected preferentially and their activity *coordinated* (which does not necessarily mean that they exhibit an oscillatory activity).

2. Ca^{2+} is an ion that functions as a second messenger and induces a cascade of different reactions in the postsynaptic cell that lead to diverse changes in synaptic efficacy. Firstly, it activates the enzyme nitric oxide synthase (NOS) which is mainly associated with the postsynaptic membrane. This enzyme catalyses the production of nitric oxide (NO) from L-arginine, a reaction that requires the presence of a number of cofactors. NO is a gas that can readily diffuse through the cell membrane. It acts as a retrograde messenger on the transmitter release at the presynaptic terminals, a mechanism, however, which has not yet been entirely elucidated. At first, NO activates soluble guanylyl cyclase in the presynaptic membrane by binding to the heme moiety of the enzyme, thus increasing the presynaptic content of cGMP and succeedingly, the activity of cGMP-dependent protein kinases. The latter control the phosphorylation of proteins involved in transmitter release. These

mechanisms induce a rapid and transient alteration of synaptic efficacy. Secondly, Ca^{2+} triggers a number of biochemical changes inside the postsynaptic terminal that possibly modify *postsynaptic* efficacy. It regulates the activity of various protein kinases that, in turn, modify the activity of various phosphoproteins. As a consequence, either post-translational changes of proteins or changes in protein synthesis may follow. These biochemical reactions probably provide the basis for long-lasting plastic alterations.

This description of the NMDA synapse is decidedly simplified. As yet, probably not all of the functionally relevant properties are known. However, it is essential that this type of synapse realizes the Hebb-rule in various ways, thus controlling the formation of complex patterns of coordinated activity. The activation of the NMDA synapse determines, firstly, the *onset* of Hebbian plastic changes, the *probability of their occurrence* and their *duration*. From this it follows that the activation state of the NMDA synapses determines the rate at which new assemblies are formed, and the complexity that these structures can assume in a given time. Secondly, the ignition of already existing assemblies will be facilitated, if NMDA synapses within these assemblies are switched on. Thirdly, the transient *binding* of pre-existing assemblies to large and complex structures will be promoted as well as their combination with newly formed ones. In short, the activation of the NMDA synapse determines the *representational activity* of the cortex.

The NMDA Synapse as a Target for Anaesthetics

The function of the NMDA synapse can be modulated—physiologically and pharmacologically—in different ways. The synapse is a potential target for a wide range of different chemicals. In this respect, *direct* and *indirect* effects should be distinguished.

In case of direct effects the NMDA receptor channel complex itself is targeted. Direct effects can be either *specific* or *non-specific*. A drug would display specific effects if it reacted selectively with one of those components of the synapse that are essential for its plastic functions. Non-specific agents would also affect one of these components but also have other target sites, for example, by interacting with the lipid or protein fractions of neuronal membranes. The activity of the NMDA synapse is *indirectly* influenced in case the synapses of other cortical neurons are the primary target, which in turn modulate its function. Such indirect effects are mainly exerted by inhibitory or excitatory interneurons of the cortex which have influence on the depolarization of pre- or postsynaptic membranes.

Direct Specific Effects

The NMDA synapse possesses at least four different domains *where a direct and specific* modulation of its function is possible (figure 54.1).

1. The glutamate receptor. A large number of so-called competitive antagonists acting more or less specifically at this site are known.

2. The receptor-associated channel that not only contains the binding site for Mg^{2+} but also other binding sites for so-called non-competitive antagonists.

3. The receptor-associated binding sites for glycine, zinc and polyamines. These ligands modulate the effect of the glutamate molecule on the postsynaptic membrane. Glycine is probably an essential cofactor for the action of glutamate.

4. The NO synthase, which can be inhibited by specific inhibitors.

A number of antagonizing or inhibitory substances are known for each of these interaction sites. The pharmacological spectrum of these substances has been studied more or less extensively (for a recent review, see Rogawski [60]).

All antagonists of these four groups block learning processes. However, the anaesthetic potencies of these substances have not been studied systematically. As yet, only a few occasional observations exist that, taken together, support the assumption that an anaesthetic effect can be obtained by means of any of the above-mentioned direct interventions.

The most thoroughly studied substances in this respect are the non-competitive antagonists to which the dissociative anaesthetics of the arylcyclohexylamine class (like ketamine) and the dioxalan class (like dexoxadrol, etoxadrol) belong. Phencyclidine, ketamine, MK-801, and tiletamine are four representative examples. They bind with high affinity to a receptor inside of the channel, when the receptor is in its ligand-gated open state, thus preventing the influx of Na^+ and Ca^{2+}. Their pharmacological range of actions has been more or less accurately studied. All of the aforementioned channel blockers induce anaesthesia. This form of anaesthesia is different from any other. It is characterized by a relatively *selective* loss of conscious functions and is not accompanied by a general depression of all cortical functions [14]. The anaesthetic potency of the non-competitive antagonists correlates with the affinity to the NMDA receptor [53, 54]. Based on the results known so far, it seems necessary to conclude that all compounds with a high affinity for non-competitive NMDA binding sites inevitably possess anaesthetic properties [61]. Some channel blocking agents, like phencyclidine, also bind to other receptor types, for example, sigma receptors. But there are good reasons to explain the *anaesthetic* effects on account of their action on the NMDA receptor [29, 38, 39, 45, 61, 71].

Anaesthetic potency has also been demonstrated for some competitive antagonists selectively blocking the glutamate recognition site. For instance, AP5 (2-amino-5-phosphonopentanoic acid), CPP {[4-(3-phosphonopropyl)]-2-piperazine carboxylic acid}, CGS 19755 {[cis-4-(phosphonomethyl)]-2-piperidine carboxylic acid} and D-CPP-ene {[D-(−)(E)-4-(3-phos-phonopro-2-enyl)] piperazine-2-carboxylic acid} have been shown to produce anaesthesia in different species [5, 11, 21, 29, 37, 41, 53, 54, 72]. In subanaesthetic doses they potentiate the anaesthetic effects of both volatile and intravenous anaesthetics. Riluzole (2-amino-6-trifluoromethoxybenzothiazole), a novel compound that inhibits glutamate neurotransmission by inhibiting presynaptic glutamate release, and additionally displays some unknown effects on the postsynapse, is also considered as a potent anaesthetic. In subanaesthetic doses it potentiates the effects of ketamine, thiopental, and halothane [44].

It is clear now that the occupation of the glycine recognition site is necessary for the activation of the NMDA receptor [34]. A number of glycine antagonists appear to share, under in vivo conditions, most of the activities which are characteristic for other types of NMDA receptor blockers. Yet, their anaesthetic potencies have not been studied sufficiently. The reason for this may be that most of these compounds, following systemic administration, have little activity in vivo due to their poor penetration of the blood brain barrier. One exception is (+)-HA-966 which interacts stereo-selectively with the glycine recognition site. For this compound *sedative* effects have been observed [63]. The volatile anaesthetic enflurane inhibits glutamate activation of the NMDA receptor. This effect is reversed by glycine [46]. It is therefore possible that enflurane-induced anaesthesia is mediated, at least in part, by an interaction between the anaesthetic and the glycine binding site.

As yet, the potential anaesthetic effects of polyamine antagonists have not been studied either. It is questionable whether such effects are to be expected because their behavioural effects appear to be different from those of other NMDA antagonists.

Three recent publications arriving at contradicting results deal with the potential anaesthetic effects of NOS inhibitors. Johns et al. [30]

found that the specific enzyme inhibitor N^G-*nitro-L-arginine methyl ester (L-NAME)* reduces dose-dependently the minimum alveolar concentration (MAC) for halothane anaesthesia. This effect can be reversed by L-arginine, but not by D-arginine. N^G-nitro-D-arginine had no anaesthetic effect. These findings could not be confirmed by Adachi et al. [1]. L-NAME administered intravenously, intracerebroventricularly or intrathecally did *not* reduce halothane MAC. Adams et al. [2], however, could confirm the anaesthetic effects of NOS inhibitors described by Johns et al. [30] NOS inhibition by L-NAME enhances alcohol-induced narcosis. This effect can be blocked by L-arginine methyl ester (AME), an NOS substrate and by isosorbide dinitrate, an NO donor. Other options of intervention at the site of the NO system have not yet been examined for anaesthetic effects. Blaise et al. [4] discuss a possible direct action of halothane on the NO molecule. Halothane could either shorten the half-time of NO or modify the activated redox form of the molecule. This assumption would be in accordance with the fact that cGMP concentrations in the cortex are considerably reduced in halothane anaesthesia [32].

Direct Non-specific Effects

Anaesthetic substances, reacting with lipids or proteins and thus acting non-specifically, could nevertheless display their anaesthetic effects due to a preferential interaction with the NMDA receptor channel complex. Possible examples are alcohol and diethylether, both depressing the responses of the NMDA receptor [64, 70]. It appears that ethanol interferes with the actions of the co-agonists glutamate and glycine [56, 65], which might explain the relatively high specificity of its action on this receptor subtype. The action of many other anaesthetic compounds could also be due to direct and unspecific effects on the NMDA receptor channel complex. As yet, these actions have not been studied systematically. In particular, it should be examined whether some of those anaesthetics that modulate ion channel kinetics also influence the NMDA channel. This appears to be a highly probable fact for alcanoles [49]. Halothane and isoflurane seem to have a specialized influence on Ca^{2+}-channels [55]. The volatile anaesthetic isoflurane blocks currents gated by NMDA and non-NMDA receptor subtypes of glutamate receptors. It decreases the frequency of the channel opening in low concentrations and causes an additional decrease in mean open time at higher concentrations [73].

Indirect Effects

The activation of the NMDA synapse depends on the degree of depolarization of the postsynaptic membrane. This could explain the actions of *all* anaesthetics that produce their effects by potentiating inhibitory synaptic transmission via $GABA_A$ receptors. To this group belongs a large number of structurally different substances, like barbiturates, benzodiazepines, etomidate, steroids, isoflurane, halothane, and enflurane [23, 33, 62]. It has been assumed, therefore, that the common mechanism for the action of all anaesthetics should be found in a generalized depression of cortical activity resulting from an enhancement of GABA action. As to such hypotheses it must be emphasized that (1) the dissociative anaesthetics do not comply with this mechanism, and (2) a generalized depression of cortical activity is not a necessary condition for anaesthesia.

Antagonists of excitatory synapses that modulate ionic conductances at the NMDA receptor-regulated channel should have similar indirect effects on its function. In fact, it has been shown that NBQX [2.3-dihydroxy-6-nitro-7 sulfamoyl-benzo (f) quinoxaline], a selective antagonist at the glutamatergic AMPA receptor, has anaesthetic properties. It reduces dose-dependently minimum alveolar concentration (MAC) for

halothane and increases sleeping time for pentobarbital anaesthesia [47].

The assumption that a certain depolarization level of the postsynaptic membrane is a necessary condition for the occurrence of conscious states can also explain other forms of unconsciousness [16, 17]. Ever since the classical investigations by Moruzzi and Magoun it is known that lesions of the mesencephalic formatio reticularis lead to the loss of consciousness. A permanent activation of the cortex via unspecific afferents is a necessary condition for the emergence of conscious states. For quite a long time this observation, often confirmed by clinical findings, has not obtained a satisfactory explanation; considering their relevance for consciousness, the *quantitative* or *qualitative* differences between an inactive cortex and a cortex which is activated by the formatio reticularis remained unresolved. According to the hypothesis presented here, the crucial difference consists in the fact that qualitatively different computational processes take place in an activated cortex: processes that are controlled by the NMDA system.

Conclusion

Taken together, there is a considerable number of reliable observations supporting the presented hypothesis. An anaesthetic action has been proven for numerous different chemical substances acting directly and selectively on the NMDA synapse. These substances act physiologically in different ways. Their common mode of action consists in a disturbance of the fast plastic processes controlled by the NMDA synapse. For a number of other, non-specifically acting substances a preferential action on this synapse seems highly probable. Their anaesthetic properties can be explained, at least in part, on account of their action on modulatory sites of the NMDA receptor channel complex. Anaesthetics that enhance neuronal inhibition, like GABA$_A$ agonists, or inhibit excitation pre- or postsynaptically, can exert their effects indirectly by altering the working conditions of the NMDA synapse. It seems to be characteristic for highly effective anaesthetics that they interact with this target in different, functionally synergistic ways. As far as can be seen now, there is no anaesthetic that does not fit into the theoretical framework presented here. Conversely, the anaesthetic potency of the various NMDA antagonists that act directly and specifically, would hardly comply with any other theory of anaesthesia. Beyond this, the presented hypothesis offers the option to explain *other causes* of unconsciousness, such as brain stem lesions, hypoxia or epileptic seizures with the same operative mechanism.

References

1. Adachi, T., Kurata, J., Nakao, S., Murakawa, M., Shichino, T. and Shirakami, G. Nitric oxide synthase inhibitor does not reduce minimum alveolar anesthetic concentration in rats. *Anesth. Analg.* 78, 1154–1157, 1994.

2. Adams, M. L., Meyer, E. R., Sewing, B. N. and Cicero, T. J. Effects of nitric oxide-related agents on alcohol narcosis. *Alcohol clin. exp. Res.* 18, 969–975, 1994.

3. Bieri, P. Was macht Bewußtsein zu einem Rätsel? *Spekt. Wissenschaft* 10, 48–55, 1992.

4. Blaise, G., To, Q., Parent, M., Laguide, B., Asenjo, F. and Sauve, R. Does halothane interfere with the release, action or stability of endothelium-derived releasing factor/nitric oxide? *Anesthesiology* 80, 417–426, 1994.

5. Boast, C. H. and Pastor, G. Characterization of motor activity patterns induced by N-methyl-D-aspartate antagonists in gerbils. *J. Pharmacol. exp. Ther.* 247, 556–561, 1988.

6. Bruhwyler, J., Chleide, E., Liegeois, J. F. and Carreer, F. Nitric oxide: A new messenger in the brain. *Neurosci. Biobehav. Rev.* 17, 373–384, 1993.

7. Collingridge, G. L. and Bliss, T. V. P. NMDA receptors: Their role in long-term potentiation. *Trends Neurosci.* 10, 288–293, 1987.

8. Collingridge, G. L. and Lester, R. J. Excitatory amino acid receptors in the vertebrate central nervous system. *Pharmacol. Rev.* 141, 143–210, 1989.

9. Constantine-Paton, M., Cline, H. T. and Debski, E. Patterned activity, synaptic convergence, and the NMDA receptor in developing visual pathways. *Annu. Rev. Neurosci.* 13, 129–154, 1990.

10. Dale, N. The role of NMDA receptors in synaptic integration and the organization of complex neural patterns. In *The NMDA Receptor*, J. C. Watkins and G. L. Collingridge (Editors), pp. 93–107. Oxford University Press, Oxford, 1989.

11. Daniell, L. C. Effects of CGS 19755, a competitive N-methyl-D-aspartate antagonist, on general anesthetic potency. *Pharmacol. Biochem. Behav.* 40, 767–769, 1991.

12. Daw, N. W., Stein, P. S. G. and Fox, K. The role of NMDA receptors in information processing. *Annu. Rev. Neurosci.* 16, 207–222, 1993.

13. Dennett, D. C. Conditions of personhood. In *Brainstorms*, pp. 267–285. MIT Press, Bradford Books, Cambridge, Mass., 1978.

14. Domino, E. F. and Luby, E. D. Abnormal mental states induced by phencyclidine as a model of schizophrenia. In *PCP (Phencyclidine): Historical and Current Perspectives*, E. F. Domino (Editor), pp. 401–418. NPP Books, Ann Arbor, Mich., 1981.

15. Du Bois Reymond, E. *Über die Grenzen des Naturerkennens*. Veit & Co., Leipzig, 1916.

16. Flohr, H. Brain processes and phenomenal consciousness. A new and specific hypothesis. *Theory Psychol.* 1, 245–262, 1991.

17. Flohr, H. Qualia and brain processes. In *Emergence or Reduction*, A. Beckermann, H. Flohr and J. Kim (Editors), pp. 220–238. de Gruyter, Berlin, 1992.

18. Flohr, H. Denken und Bewußtsein. In *Neuroworlds*, J. Fedrowitz, D. Matejovski and G. Kaiser (Editors), pp. 335–352. Campus, Frankfurt, 1994.

19. Flohr, H. Die physiologischen Bedingungen des Bewußtseins. In *Neue Realitäten—Herausforderung der Philosophie*, H. Lenk und H. Poser (Editors), pp. 222–235. Akademie Verlag, Berlin, 1994.

20. Flohr, H. Sensations and brain processes, *Behav. Brain Res.* 71, pp. 157–161, 1995.

21. France, C. P., Winger, G. D. and Woods, J. H. Analgesic, anesthetic and respiratory effects of the competitive N-methyl-D-aspartate (NMDA) antagonist CGS 19755 in rhesus monkeys. *Brain Res.* 526, 355–358, 1990.

22. Franks, N. P. and Lieb, W. R. Molecular mechanisms of general anaesthesia. *Nature* 300, 487–493, 1982.

23. Gee, K. W. Steroid modulation of the GABA/benzodiazepine receptor-linked chloride ionophore. *Molec. Neurobiol.* 2, 291–317, 1988.

24. Goldmann, L. Cognitive processing and general anesthesia. In *Sleep and Cognition*, R. R. Bertzin, J. F. Kihlstrom and D. L. Schacter (Editors), pp. 127–135. American Psychological Association, Washington, 1990.

25. Hawkins, R. D., Kandel, E. R. and Siegelbaum, S. A. Learning to modulate transmitter release: Themes and variations in synaptic plasticity. *Annu. Rev. Neurosci.* 16, 625–665, 1993.

26. Hebb, D. O. *The Organization of Behavior*. Wiley, New York, 1949.

27. Hebb, D. O. A neuropsychological theory. In *Psychology—A Study of Science*, S. Koch (Editor), Vol. 1, pp. 622–643. McGraw-Hill, New York, 1958.

28. Hoffman, P. L., Rabe, C. S., Grant, K. A., Valverius, P., Hudspith, M. and Tabakoff, B. Ethanol and the NMDA receptor. *Alcohol* 7, 229–231, 1990.

29. Irifune, M., Shimizu, T., Nomoto, M. and Fukuda, T. Ketamine-induced anesthesia involves the N-methyl-D-aspartate receptor-channel complex in mice. *Brain Res.* 596, 1–9, 1992.

30. Johns, R. A., Moscicki, J. C. and Difazio, C. A. Nitric oxide synthase inhibitor dose-dependently and reversibly reduces the threshold for halothane anesthesia. *Anesthesiology* 77, 779–784, 1992.

31. Johnson-Laird, P. N. *The Computer and the Mind*. Harvard University Press, Cambridge, Mass., 1988.

32. Kant, G. J., Muller, T. W., Lenox, R. H. and Meyerhoff, J. L. In vivo effects of pentobarbital and halothane anaesthesia on levels of adenosine $3'$, $5'$-monophosphate and guanosine $3'$, $5'$-monophosphate in rat brain regions and pituitary. *Biochem. Pharmacol.* 29, 1891–1896, 1980.

33. Keane, P. E. and Biziere, K. The effects of general anaesthetics on GABAergic synaptic transmission. *Life Sci.* 41, 1437–1448, 1987.

34. Kemp, J. A. and Leeson, P. D. The glycine site of the NMDA receptor—five years on. *TIPS* 14, 20–25, 1993.

35. Kihlstrom, J. F. The cognitive unconscious. *Science* 237, 1445–1452, 1987.

36. Kihlstrom, J. F. and Schacter, D. L. Anesthesia, amnesia and the cognitive unconscious. In *Memory and Awareness in Anesthesia*, B. Bonke, W. Fitch and K. Miller (Editors), pp. 21–44. Swets & Zeitlinger, Amsterdam, 1990.

37. Koek, W., Woods, J. H. and Ornstein, P. Phencyclidine-like behavioral effects in pigeons induced by systemic administration of the excitatory amino acid antagonist, 2-amino-5-phosphono-valerate. *Life Sci.* 39, 973–978, 1986.

38. Koek, W., Woods, J. H., Mattson, M. V., Jacobson, A. E. and Mudar, P. J. Excitatory amino acid antagonists induce a phencyclidine-like catalepsy in pigeons: structure activity studies. *Neuropharmacology* 26, 1261–1265, 1987.

39. Koek, W., Woods, J. H. and Winger, G. D. MK-801, a proposed non-competitive antagonist of excitatory amino acid neurotransmission, produces phencyclidine-like behavioral effects in pigeons, rats and rhesus monkeys. *J. Pharmacol. exp. Ther.* 245, 969–974, 1988.

40. Krnjević, K. Cellular mechanisms of anesthesia. In *Molecular and Cellular Mechanisms of Alcohol and Anesthetics, Ann. N. Y. Acad. Sci.*, E. Rubin, K. W. Miller and S. H. Roth (Editors), 625, 1–16, 1991.

41. Kuroda, Y., Strebel, S., Rafferty, C. and Bullock, R. Neuroprotective doses of N-methyl-D-aspartate receptor antagonists profoundly reduce the minimum alveolar anaesthetic concentration (MAC) for isoflurane in rats. *Anesth. Analg.* 77, 795–800, 1993.

42. Lodge, D. Modulation of N-methyl-D-aspartate receptor channel complexes. *Drugs Today* 25, 395–411, 1989.

43. Malenka, R. C. and Nicoll, R. A. NMDA receptor-dependent synaptic plasticity: Multiple forms and mechanisms. *Trends Neurosci.* 16, 521–527, 1993.

44. Mantz, J., Cheramy, A., Thierry, A. M., Glowinsky, J. and Desmonts, J.-M. Anesthetic properties of

riluzole (54274 RP) a new inhibitor of glutamate transmission. *Anesthesiology* 76, 844–848, 1992.

45. Martin, D. and Lodge, D. Phencyclidine receptors and N-methyl-D-aspartate antagonism: Electrophysiologic data correlate with known behaviors. *Pharmacol. Biochem. Behav.* 31, 279–286, 1988.

46. Martin, D. C., Abraham, J. E., Plagenhoef, M. and Aronstam, R. S. Volatile anaesthetics and NMDA receptors. Enflurane inhibition of glutamate-stimulated [^{3}H]MK-801 binding and reversal by glycine. *Neurosci. Lett.* 132, 73–76, 1991.

47. McFarlane, C., Warner, D. S., Todd, M. M. and Nordholm, L. AMPA receptor competitive antagonism reduces halothane MAC in rats. *Anesthesiology* 77, 1165–1170, 1992.

48. McGinn, C. *The Problem of Consciousness.* Blackwell, Oxford, 1991.

49. McLarnon, J., Sawyer, D. and Bainbridge, K. Action of intermediate chain-length n-alkanols on single channel NMDA current in rat hippocampal neurons. In *Molecular and Cellular Mechanisms of Alcohol and Anesthetics, Ann. N. Y. Acad. Sci.* E. Rubin, K. W. Miller and S. H. Roth (Editors), 625, 283–286, 1991.

50. Metzinger, T. *Subjekt und Selbstmodell.* Schöningh, Paderborn, 1993.

51. Nagel, T. *The View from Nowhere.* Oxford University Press, Oxford, 1986.

52. Nunn, J. F., Utting, J. E. and Brown, B. R. Jr. (Editors) *General Anaesthesia,* 5th edn. Butterworths, London, 1989.

53. Perkins, W. J. and Morrow, D. R. A dose-dependent reduction in halotane MAC in rats with a competitive N-methyl-D-aspartate (NMDA) receptor antagonist. *Anesth. Analg.* 74, 233, 1992.

54. Perkins, W. J. and Morrow, D. R. Correlation between anesthetic potency and receptor binding constant for non-competitive N-methyl-D-aspartate receptor antagonists. *Anesthesiology* 77, A742 (abstr.), 1992.

55. Puil, E., El-Beheiry, H. and Bainbridge, K. G. Calcium involvement in anesthetic blockade of synaptic transmission. In *Molecular and Cellular Mechanisms of Alcohol and Anesthetics, Ann. N. Y. Acad. Sci.,* E. Rubin, K. W. Miller and S. H. Roth (Editors), 625, 82–90, 1991.

56. Rabe, C. S. and Tabakoff, B. Glycine site-directed agonists reverse the actions of ethanol at the N-methyl-

D-aspartate receptor. *Molec. Pharmacol.* 38, 753–757, 1990.

57. Rauschecker, J. P. Mechanism of visual plasticity: Hebb synapses, NMDA receptors, and beyond. *Physiol. Rev.* 71, 587–615, 1991.

58. Rey, G. A reason for doubting the existence of consciousness. In *Consciousness and Self-regulation, Advances in Research and Theory,* R. J. Davidson, G. E. Schwartz and D. Shapiro (Editors), Vol. 3, pp. 1–39. Plenum Press, New York, 1983.

59. Rey, G. A question about consciousness. In *Perspectives on Mind,* H. R. Otto and J. A. Tuedio (Editors), pp. 5–24. Reidel, Dordrecht, 1988.

60. Rogawski, M. A. The NMDA receptor, NMDA antagonists and epilepsy therapy. A status report. *Drugs* 44, 279–292, 1992.

61. Scheller, M. S., Zornow, M. H., Fleischer, J. E., Shearman, G. T. and Greber, T. F. The noncompetitive NMDA receptor antagonist, MK-801 profoundly reduces volatile anesthetic requirements in rabbits. *Neuropharmacology* 28, 677–681, 1989.

62. Schumacher, M. and McEwen, B. S. Steroid and barbiturate modulation of the GABA receptor. *Molec. Neurobiol.* 3, 275–303, 1989.

63. Singh, L., Donald, A. E., Foster, A. C., Hutson, P. H., Iversen, L. L., Iversen, S. D., Kemp, J. A., Leeson, P. D., Marshall, G. R., Oles, R. J., Priestley, T., Thorn, L., Tricklebank, M. D., Vass, C. A. and Williams, B. J. Enantiomers of HA-966 (3-amino-1-hydroxypyrrolid-2-one) exhibit distinct central nervous system effects: (+)-HA-966 is a selective glycine/N-methyl-D-aspartate receptor antagonist, but (−)-HA-966 is a potent γ-butyrolactone-like sedative. *Proc. natn. Acad. Sci. USA* 87, 347–357, 1990.

64. Snell, L. D., Tabakoff, B. and Hoffman, P. L. Radioligand binding to the N-methyl-D-aspartate receptor/ionophore complex: Alterations by ethanol in vitro and by chronic in vivo ethanol ingestion. *Brain Res.* 602, 91–98, 1993.

65. Tabakoff, B., Rabe, C. S. and Hoffman, P. L. Selective effects of sedative/hypnotic drugs on excitatory amino acid receptors in brain. In *Molecular and Cellular Mechanisms of Alcohol and Anesthetics, Ann. N. Y. Acad. Sci.,* E. Rubin, K. W. Miller and S. H. Roth (Editors), 625, 489–495, 1991.

66. Thomson, A. M. Glycine is a coagonist at the NMDA receptor channel complex. *Progr. Neurobiol.* 35, 53–74, 1990.

67. Tsumoto, T. Long-term potentiation and depression in the cerebral neocortex. *Jpn. J. Physiol.* 40, 573–593, 1990.

68. Vincent, S. R. Nitric oxide: A radical neurotransmitter in the central nervous system. *Progr. Neurobiol.* 42, 129–160, 1994.

69. von der Malsburg, C. The correlation theory of brain function. Internal report 81-2, Department of Neurobiology, Max-Planck-Institute for Biophysical Chemistry, Göttingen, 1981.

70. Weight, F. F., Lovinger, D. M., White, G. and Peoples, R. W. Alcohol and anesthetic actions on excitatory amino acid-activated ion channels. In *Molecular and Cellular Mechanisms of Alcohol and Anesthetics, Ann. N. Y. Acad. Sci.*, E. Rubin, K. W. Miller and S. H. Roth (Editors), 625, 197–207, 1991.

71. Willets, J., Balster, R. L. and Leander, J. D. The behavioral pharmacology of NMDA receptor antagonists. *TIPS* 11, 423–428, 1990.

72. Woods, J. M. Consciousness. *Pharmacol. Biochem. Behav.* 32, 1081, 1989.

73. Yang, J. and Zorumski, C. F. Effects of isoflurane on N-methyl-D-aspartate gated ion channels in cultured rat hippocampal neurons. In *Molecular and Cellular Mechanisms of Alcohol and Anesthetics, Ann. N. Y. Acad. Sci.*, E. Rubin, K. W. Miller and S. H. Roth (Editors), 625, 287–289, 1991.

74. Yoneda, Y. and Ogita, K. Neurochemical aspects of the N-methyl-D-aspartate receptor complex. *Neurosci. Res.* 10, 1–33, 1981.

55

Toward a Unified Theory of Narcosis: Brain Imaging Evidence for a Thalamocortical Switch as the Neurophysiologic Basis of Anesthetic-Induced Unconsciousness

Michael T. Alkire, Richard J. Haier, and James H. Fallon

Introduction

Despite extensive research investigating the cellular mechanisms of general anesthesia (Franks and Lieb 1994), the fundamental question of why anesthesia produces unconsciousness remains unanswered. Findings of animal studies examining anesthetic-induced changes in evoked potential recordings suggest that the primary basis of anesthesia may be the blocking or disruption of sensory information processing through the thalamus (Angel 1991, 1993). This view is consistent with the findings of the effects of anesthetics on evoked potential recordings in humans, as well as some findings from human brain imaging experiments. The magnitude of the drug-induced reduction in thalamic metabolism induced by the benzodiazepine lorazepam correlates with its degree of sleepiness (Volkow et al. 1995). Furthermore, a dose-dependent reduction in thalamic activity accompanies sedative levels of the benzodiazepine midazolam (Veselis et al. 1997). Similarly, regional thalamic functional activity suppression was found during halothane general anesthesia, provided a pixel-based data analysis method (statistical parametric mapping) was used (Alkire et al. 1999). Most recently, a correlational link between a person's level of consciousness and their level of thalamic functioning at various doses of propofol anesthesia has been demonstrated in humans (Fiset et al. 1999).

A number of theories on consciousness propose that a fundamental part of the neural substrate for consciousness is likely to involve thalamocortical-corticothalamic loops (Crick 1994; Joliot, Ribary, and Llinás 1994; Llinás, Ribary, Contreras, and Pedroarena 1998; Lumer, Edelman, and Tononi 1997; Newman 1997). If such loops are involved in generating consciousness, then a change in their functional activity should likely be evident during experimentally induced states of unconsciousness (Llinás and Ribary 1993). Thus, these theories would seem to predict that a specific consequence of anesthetic-induced unconsciousness might be a change in functional thalamocortical activity.

This study, therefore, addressed two issues concerning the role of the thalamus in mediating the anesthetic state in man.

1. Do the regional effects of halothane and isoflurane, when examined with statistical parametric mapping, show commonalities of brain metabolism that offer clues to their mechanism of producing unconsciousness?

2. Will the common effect of these agents, as suggested by findings of animal studies (Angel 1991), be suppression of thalamic activity?

Positron emission tomography (PET) and statistical parametric mapping (SPM) were used to study brain states associated with unconsciousness during general anesthesia in humans. Regional cerebral glucose metabolism using $_{18}$fluorodeoxyglucose (FDG) was recorded as an index of neuronal activity in 11 young, healthy, right-handed male volunteers at baseline and during inhalational anesthesia with either halothane or isoflurane anesthesia titrated to the point of unresponsiveness. The details of the anesthetic administration procedures and the individual anesthetic effects have been reported previously (Alkire, Haier, Shah, and Anderson 1997; Alkire et al. 1999). Presented here are the three-dimensional results of the SPM conjunction analysis between the two different volatile anesthetic agents, which reveals the three-dimensional intersection of those brain regions commonly affected by both inhalational agents.

Further explanation may help clarify the logic of the analysis technique. If, on the one hand, the two agents have completely different neuro-anatomic mechanisms for producing unconsciousness, then the conjunction analysis will not reveal any regionally significant differences between the conscious and unconscious conditions. This would suggest that no overlapping brain areas of effect exist between the two agents. Such a situation could occur, for example, if one anesthetic primarily "turns off" the cerebral cortex, whereas the other agent primarily "turns off" the thalamus. Additionally, such a situation could occur if anesthetic-induced unconsciousness results simply from the global decrease in CNS functioning caused by anesthesia (i.e., subtracting the whole brain from itself would leave nothing). On the other hand, if the two agents have similar neuroanatomic mechanisms for producing unconsciousness, then the conjunction analysis should reveal which key brain regions differ in their functional activity between states of consciousness, irrespective of each agent's particular extemporaneous effects on regional cerebral metabolism.

Materials and Methods

Subject Preparation

All subjects were studied with IRB approval and informed consent. Each of the 11 subjects underwent two separate PET scan procedures, with at least one week between scanning sessions. One scan assessed baseline awake metabolism and the other scan assessed metabolism during the period of unconsciousness induced with either halothane ($n = 5$) or isoflurane ($n = 6$) general inhalational anesthesia. Subjects denied any previous neurological, psychological, or medical problems, and they had a mean ($\pm$sd) age of 22 ± 4 years. All subjects were instructed to avoid caffeine, or any medications, for at least 48 hours prior to each scan. Additionally, subjects fasted at least 8 hours prior to each scan and

they received oral antacid (Sodium Citrate, 30 cc P.O.) before receiving anesthesia. Subject preparation was as similar between sessions and conditions as possible. Each volunteer had two intravenous catheters inserted, one to administer the FDG-PET tracer and one to sample blood for FDG quantification. Monitoring equipment used included a three-lead electrocardiograph, an automated noninvasive blood pressure monitor, a pulse oximeter, end-tidal carbon dioxide monitor, a temperature monitor, and a precordial stethoscope. The experiments took place in a small, darkened, sound-shielded room. One of the subjects participated in both the halothane and isoflurane portions of the study. The baseline-awake scan was obtained while subjects lay quietly on a gurney with their eyes closed. Baseline scans were counterbalanced between subjects and conditions.

Anesthetic Administration

Subjects inhaled the anesthetics (or air, for the baseline condition) through a tight-fitting facemask attached to a semicircle breathing system. The expired end-tidal concentration of each agent was incrementally adjusted upwards in steps of 0.1% every 10–15 min. As the volunteers approached unconsciousness, the eyelash reflex was tested every 3 min., and they were asked to open their eyes until they no longer followed commands. When the volunteers no longer responded to verbal commands, they were stimulated further by mild prodding and shaking. Loss of consciousness was defined as unresponsiveness to both verbal and tactile stimuli (Alkire 1998). Testing for unresponsiveness assured that each subject was actually anesthetized and not just sleeping during the anesthesia scan sessions. Airway instrumentation was not used, and the volunteers maintained spontaneous ventilation throughout each anesthetic. Subjects were thus titrated to a light stage of anesthesia in the 1/2 to 1 minimum alveolar concentration range

(MAC = the minimum alveolar concentration of inhaled anesthetic agent at one atmosphere pressure needed to prevent 50% of patients from moving in response to a surgical skin incision; Eger, Saidman, and Brandstater 1965). The mean $\pm$SD expired isoflurane and halothane concentrations were $0.5 \pm 0.1\%$ and $0.7 \pm 0.2\%$, respectively.

Once unresponsive, 5 mc of FDG were injected intravenously as a bolus and the expired agent concentration remained fixed for the duration of the 32-min. deoxyglucose radiotracer uptake period. Uptake of FDG and metabolic trapping of FDG in the brain as FDG-6-phosphate is 80–90% complete at 32 min. (Phelps et al. 1979). It is primarily the trapped FDG-6-phosphate that reflects regional functional brain activity over time and is the source of the PET scan signal. Thus, following the labeling of brain with the tracer, subjects were allowed to emerge from the anesthetic before being taken to the PET scanner. The resultant PET scan images obtained for the anesthesia condition represent the functional activity of the brain evident during the period of unresponsiveness at the near-steady state level of anesthesia used for each subject and are not representative of the time actually spent in the scanner. The time between the injection of the FDG and the start of the scanning process was standardized across conditions to ensure that it was similar for all subject. Scanning began within 20 min. of the end of each uptake period for each condition. It took approximately 6 min. on average for subjects to open their eyes and become responsive following the discontinuation of the anesthetic agent. In order to standardize cognitive processing during the radiotracer uptake period, the subjects listened to an audiotape of repeated words spoken in normal conversational tone by a pleasant female voice with a frequency of one word every five seconds (Alkire, Haier, Fallon, and Cahill 1998).

PET Imaging

The regional cerebral metabolic rate of glucose utilization (rCMRglu) was measured with a GE2048 head-dedicated scanner. Arterialized venous blood sampling was used, and rCMRglu was calculated (mg/100 gm/min.) using established PET methodology (Huang et al. 1980, Phelps et al. 1979). The scanner has a resolution of 4.5 mm (full-width-half-maximum, FWHM) in plane and 6.0 mm axially. Two sets of 15 image planes, resulting in 30 PET images across the whole brain, were obtained per subject. Subjects were positioned using laser guidance and a thermosetting plastic facemask was used to hold each subject's head stationary during the period of image acquisition for both the awake-baseline and anesthesia conditions. In vivo attenuation correction was obtained by previous transmission scanning using a (^{68}Ge/^{68}Ga)-rod source. PET data were corrected for attenuation and background activity, and reconstructed with a Hanning filter.

Statistical Analysis

Data were processed using the statistical parametric mapping (SPM-96) software from the Wellcome Department of Cognitive Neurology, London, United Kingdom, implemented in Matlab (Mathworks, Sherborn, MA). This process determined regionally significant condition effects for every pixel in standardized space (Friston, Frith, Liddle, and Frackowiak 1991; Friston et al. 1989). This process involved several steps.

1. The data were reconstructed in three-dimensional space.

2. The intercommissural (anterior commissure–posterior commissure) line was identified by an automated routine, and the three-dimensional images were rotated on axis to fit a reference template. A least-squares approach was used to esti-

Table 55.1
Whole brain glucose metabolic rates (mg/100 gm/min)

	Isoflurane			Halothane		
	Awake	Anesthetized	% reduction	Awake	Anesthetized	% reduction
	4.9	3.5	29			
	5.8	4.4	24	4.6	3.3	28
	6.3	3.5	44	5.9	3.9	34
	7.2	3.9	46	6.4	2.9	53
	7.2	3.3	54	7.3	4.3	41
	8.8	3.9	55	7.5	4.2	44
average (SD) =	6.7 (1.4)	3.8 (0.4)	42 (13)	6.3 (1.2)	3.7 (0.6)	40 (10)

mate the six parameters of this rigid body transform (Woods, Cherry, and Mazziotta, 1992).

3. After realignment, all images were transformed into a standardized space (according to the atlas of Talairach and Tournoux 1988).

4. To increase signal-to-noise ratio, and to reduce the effect of variable functional anatomy, the images were smoothed using an isotropic Gaussian kernel (10-mm FWHM).

5. Finally, global differences in glucose metabolic rates were normalized across conditions and volunteers using proportional scaling. This correction ensures that variations in activity caused by differences in global metabolic rates among the volunteers and between the conditions did not obscure the relative regional changes caused by the anesthetics.

Comparisons of regional relative glucose metabolism were performed between conditions on a pixel-by-pixel basis using t statistics. A design matrix was specified such that the locations where a significant conjoint effect of both anesthetics on regional metabolism could be localized. The resulting maps (SPM{t}) were transformed to the unit normal distribution (SPM{z}) and thresholded at $P < 0.05$, corrected for multiple comparisons. The results are dis-

played as a three-dimensional volume of pixels in coronal, transverse and sagittal views of the brain.

Results

General inhalational anesthesia compared to baseline, induced both a global reduction of, and specific regional changes of, brain glucose metabolism. The mean ($\pm$sd) global whole-brain metabolic reduction seen during isoflurane anesthesia was $42 \pm 13\%$, and that seen during halothane was $40 \pm 10\%$ (see table 55.1). For all subjects the anesthetic state was associated with a global decrease in brain metabolism throughout the brain. There were no regions (within the spatial limitations of the scanner) that appeared to increase their absolute metabolic rate under anesthesia to a value greater than that found at baseline. Also, there were no significant differences in relative baseline metabolism between groups, suggesting comparable subjects were sampled between groups.

SPM analysis revealed that the intense and widespread deactivation that occurred during general anesthesia was not uniform; several regions were significantly less active than the rest of the brain. Given that a large decrease in

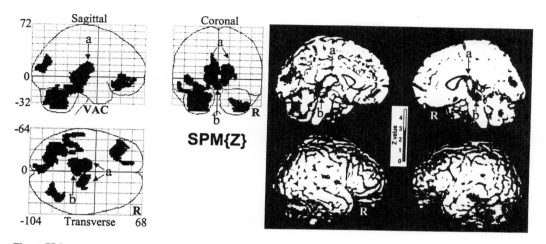

Figure 55.1
SPM projections and MRI renderings show the intersection of effects between halothane ($n = 5$) and isoflurane ($n = 6$) anesthesia. The common brain areas where activity is significantly depressed by the two different inhalational anesthetic agents are shown. Functional PET results are displayed at threshold of $Z = 3.09$ ($P < .05$, corrected), and superimposed, for anatomical reference, upon a T1-weighted magnetic resonance imaging scan normalized to Talairach space (Talairach and Tournoux 1988) (*a*) thalamus; (*b*) midbrain reticular formation.

global metabolism accompanied the anesthetic-induced loss of consciousness seen here, areas with significantly decreased relative metabolism indicate those brain regions which were most affected by the anesthetic agents. The intersection of the relative functional regional neuro-anatomic effects common to both agents are shown in figure 55.1 and listed in table 55.2.

The results show a significant conjoint effect between the two different anesthetic agents such that both agents caused specific relative reductions of regional cerebral glucose metabolism primarily in the thalamus, and also in the midbrain reticular formation, basal forebrain, cerebellum, and occipital cortex. These results provide the first comprehensive description of the three-dimensional regional distribution of cerebral activity evident during unconsciousness induced with different inhalational anesthetic agents in human subjects.

Discussion

As the conjunction analysis between the two different anesthetics clearly centers primarily on the thalamus, and our subjects were anesthetized to a loss of consciousness endpoint, our data support the idea that a reduction of thalamocortical output may underlie the loss of consciousness associated with the anesthetic state in humans. The mechanism of anesthetic-induced thalamic processing disruption appears from animal work to be dependent on how anesthetics interact with a few specific brain sites including: the thalamus, the cerebral cortex (especially layer V) and the thalamic reticular nucleus (Angel 1991). An anesthetic-induced decrease in cortico-thalamic and cortico-reticulo-thalamic signaling is thought to increase inhibition on excitatory thalamic neurons, thereby decreasing their output to the cortex (Angel 1991).

Table 55.2
Areas of significant relative glucose metabolic decreases during anesthesia

Region	Brod-mann's Area	Coordinates X	Y	Z	Cluster size (voxels)	Corrected P value of Cluster size	Voxel z-Score	Corrected P value of Z-score
Cuneus (L)	**18**	**−4**	**−78**	**20**	**338**	**0.003**	**5.50**	**0.001**
Cuneus	18	−6	−92	12			3.62	ns
Medial Frontal gyrus (L)	**47**	**−36**	**32**	**−10**	**552**	**0.003**	**5.13**	**0.005**
Inferior Frontal gyrus (L)	47	−46	38	−2			4.42	ns
Inferior Frontal gyrus (L)	47	−26	28	−14			4.42	ns
Thalamus—anterior nucleus (R)		**10**	**−12**	**18**	**1800**	**<0.001**	**4.98**	**0.009**
Thalamus—VLN (R)		14	−16	10			4.81	0.02
Midbrain (L)		−2	−32	−12			4.73	0.03
Inferior Temporal gyrus (L)		**−58**	**−34**	**−16**	**2319**	**<0.001**	**4.71**	**0.03**
Temporal lobe (L)		−40	−60	−44			4.52	ns
Fusiform gyrus (L)	36	−42	−34	20			4.40	ns
Cerebellum (R)		**32**	**−66**	**−42**	**454**	**0.007**	**3.81**	**ns**
Cerebellum (R)		40	−58	−48			3.78	ns
Cerebellum posterior lobe (R)		26	−64	−36			3.50	ns

Only areas with a z-score >3.09 (P < 0.05, corrected) and an extent threshold >223 voxels (P < 0.01, corrected) are listed. The coordinates are given (in millimeters) for the maximally significant pixel in each cluster (BOLD), and the next highest maxima within each cluster (plain text) according to a standard stereotactic space (Talairach and Tournoux, 1988). x = lateral displacement from the midline (+ for the right hemisphere), y = anteroposterior displacement relative to the anterior comm (+ for positions anterior to the latter), z = vertical postition relative to the AC-PC line (+ if above this line); R = right, L = left, VLN = Ventral lateral nucleus.

Toward a Unified Theory of Anesthetic-Induced Unconsciousness

Thalamocortical cells have two primary modes of firing—tonic and burst. Onset of physiologic sleep switches these cells from a predominately tonic-firing pattern to a predominately burst-firing pattern (Steriade, McCormick, and Sejnowski 1993). The change in firing pattern occurs coincident with changes in the EEG pattern from one of behavioral arousal (i.e., low voltage, fast activity) to one of slow-wave sleep (i.e., spindle and delta wave oscillations, high voltage, slow activity) (Steriade 1992). Animal physiology studies show that the switch in thalamocortical cell firing and the change in the EEG oscillation pattern happens because the thalamocortical cells become hyperpolarized. This hyperpolarization establishes a block to the transmission of sensory information through the thalamus, which results in the cortex being functionally disconnected from outside sensory experience with the onset of sleep-induced unconsciousness (Steriade 1994). During sleep this hyperpolarization block develops because of a decrease in tonic excitation from brainstem arousal centers (Steriade 1994). During anesthesia a hyperpolarization block likely develops not only from anesthetic effects on brainstem arousal centers, but also from direct effects of certain anesthetics themselves.

Based on direct in vitro demonstration of halothane's ability to hyperpolarize thalamic parafascicular nucleus neurons, Sugiyami and colleagues (Sugiyama, Muteki, and Shimoji 1992) proposed that a hyperpolarization block of thalamocortical neurons may be mechanistically related to the loss of consciousness seen during halothane anesthesia. Our previous in vivo human results with halothane did reveal that a relative decrease of thalamic activity accompanies halothane anesthesia, but a number of other areas, such as the basal forebrain and cerebellum, were also noted to be affected by halothane (Alkire et al. 1999). Thus, a clear relationship between thalamic suppression and "unconsciousness" was not obvious in the single-agent halothane study. However, the present intersection analysis clearly focuses attention to a relatively limited number of brain regions that are commonly affected by both halothane and isoflurane. Here, the fact that isoflurane appears to have mechanisms in common with halothane for affecting thalamic activity strengthens the idea that a hyperpolarization block of thalamocortical neurons has general import for understanding the loss of consciousness induced by anesthesia. Studies are underway to determine whether hyperpolarization of thalamocortical neurons is a general underlying principle of all anesthetics.

Our findings suggest that hyperpolarization of thalamocortical neurons and the transition of thalamocortical activity from tonic to burst firing is likely to be a general principle of anesthesia which can occur through different mechanisms with different anesthetic agents (see figure 55.2).

Anesthetics can affect the activity within thalamocortical-corticothalamic loops and cause thalamocortical hyperpolarization, coincident with the loss of consciousness, by at least four possible mechanisms including: direct cellular hyperpolarization, inhibition of excitement, enhancement of inhibition, or any combination of these. These points are elaborated below.

1. The inhalational agents are known to have direct hyperpolarizing effects on thalamic and cortical neuronal membrane potentials (Berg-Johnsen and Langmoen 1987; Nicoll and Madison 1982; Sugiyama, Muteki, and Shimoji 1992). How much this direct effect contributes to the solidity of the hypothesized hyperpolarization block of anesthetic-induced unconsciousness remains to be determined. However, this factor does predict that those agents with more potent hyperpolarization ability should induce unconsciousness easier than those agents that have limited hyperpolarization ability.

2. Consciousness is an energy-requiring active brain state. Keeping the brain awake requires arousing inputs to the corticothalamic-thalamocortico-reticulothalamic loops from central core structures (brainstem, diencephalon, and basal forebrain) and cortex (Steriade 1993a; Steriade, McCormick, and Sejnowski 1993). The central core structures impinge on the thalamus and thalamic reticular nucleus with tonic excitation from cholinergic, glutamatergic, and aminergic cellular inputs (Steriade 1993b). Our imaging data show that inhalational anesthesia has, as one of its effects, an ability to specifically suppress the functional activity in midbrain/pontine areas involved with regulating arousal. Thus, for the inhalational agents, anesthetic-induced suppression of normal tonic excitatory activity from lower brain structures will directly contribute to hyperpolarization of thalamocortical neurons and a functional decrease in thalamic metabolism. Therefore, just as with natural sleep, removal of excitatory arousal circuitry inputs to the thalamocortical-corticothalamic loops will contribute to thalamocortical hyper-

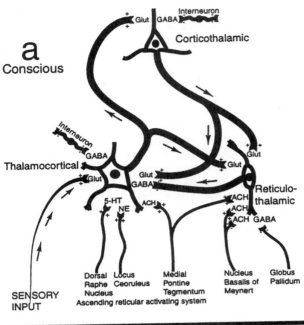

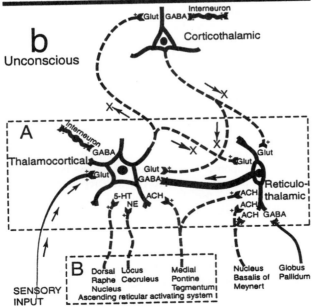

polarization. Anesthetics will accomplish this removal of excitatory inputs primarily through inhibition of glutamatergic and cholinergic synaptic neurotransmission (Dildy-Mayfield, Eger, and Harris 1996; Durieux 1996; Violet et al. 1997).

3. Enhancement of inhibitory circuitry functioning within the thalamocortical loops, primarily through enhancement of GABAergic synaptic neurotransmission is one of the primary mechanisms of sleep regulation (Juhasz, Emri, Kekesi, and Pungor 1989; Steriade, Dossi, and Nunez 1991). Enhancement of GABAergic synaptic neurotransmission has often been proposed as a possible mechanism of anesthesia (Cheng and Brunner 1987, Juhasz et al. 1989). The present empirical results provide a functional neuroanatomic bridge for understanding the link between endogenous sleep mechanisms, GABAergic signaling, and anesthetic-induced unconsciousness.

4. Any individual anesthetic agent might need to use only one of these proposed mechanisms, such as barbiturate enhancement of GABAergic activity. Alternatively some agents (like the inhalationals) might use various proportions of nearly all of these different mechanisms (Franks and Lieb 1994). In essence, any substance or event that pushes thalamocortical cells towards hyperpolarization, through whatever mechanism, will drive the brain towards unconsciousness. Unconsciousness will result when the thalamocortical switch is "pushed" far enough

and the thalamocortical cells change from tonic to burst firing.

Halothane and isoflurane are in the same general class of general anesthetic agents. Thus, after the fact, it seems not at all surprising that their global and regional effects on functional cerebral metabolism would be found to be somewhat similar. Nonetheless, prior to this study, a number of physiologic/functional differences were known to exist between these two agents, which made predicting a loci for a common effect between them a speculative proposition, at best. On an equal MAC basis, the agents differ in their ability to suppress cerebral metabolism, isoflurane is the most potent inhalational agent at suppressing cerebral metabolism, halothane is one of the least potent (Todd and Drummond 1984). Halothane is the most potent at increasing cerebral blood flow; isoflurane is one of the least potent. Halothane induces EEG "sleep" spindle activity that is morphologically nearly identical to the spindles found with natural sleep (Keifer, Baghdoyan, and Lydic 1996). Isoflurane also induces EEG spindle activity, but the spindles of isoflurane have a morphology more reminiscent of those found with the barbiturates and burst suppression patterns. Numerous functional differences between agents also exist on the cellular level (Chan and Durieux 1997, Nietgen et al. 1998, Schotten et al. 1998). Thus, though one could argue that the main theoretical hypothesis of this paper would have been better tested if different classes of general

Figure 55.2

A neuroanatomic/neurophysiologic model of anesthetic-induced unconsciousness. The key cellular players are the thalamocortical, corticothalamic, and reticulothalamic cells. (*a*) The system during consciousness, when sensory information can be processed through the thalamus. (*b*) The system during anesthetic-induced unconsciousness. Sensory information processing is blocked at the level of the thalamus secondary to thalamocortical hyperpolarization, which switches the thalamocortical cells from tonic to burst firing mode. The thalamus/thalamic reticular area (A) and the midbrain region (B) specifically suppressed by inhalational anesthesia in humans (from figure 55.1) are outlined. Anesthetics affect numerous interaction points within the thalamocortical-corticothalamic-reticulothalamic loops, and cause thalamocortical hyperpolarization through many mechanisms including, direct hyperpolarization, GABA agonism, glutamate antagonism, and cholinergic antagonism. ACH = acetylcholine, 5-HT = 5-hydroxy-tryptamine, GABA = gamma amino butyric acid, Glut = glutamate, NE = norepinephrine.

anesthetic agents were studied (intravenous versus inhalational, for example), the agents that were studied were, nonetheless, functionally divergent in a number of important respects.

Strong support for the theoretical framework proposed here has recently emerged from the report by Fiset and colleagues (Fiset et al. 1999). They studied the effects of the intravenous anesthetic agent propofol on regional cerebral blood flow during different depths of sedation/anesthesia in humans. Using a correlational approach between propofol blood levels and PET blood flow images, they found a strong relationship exists between a person's level of "consciousness" and the amount of activity in the thalamus, basal forebrain, and occipital lobe. The regional results from that study and the regional results presented here are remarkably similar. The regions identified in both studies qualitatively appear to differ only in the magnitude of how much each region is identified. Their occipital and frontal findings are larger than ours, and our thalamic finding is larger than theirs. By visual inspection, an intersection analysis between the three agents (i.e., halothane, isoflurane, and now propofol) would reveal the thalamus as the primary focus of the intersection. This overlap in findings is made even more striking when one considers that this completely different group of investigators used a different type of imaging technique (blood flow versus glucose metabolism), with a different type of analysis technique (correlational versus subtractive) to find similar regional effects on consciousness with a different class of anesthetic (intravenous versus inhalational). Thus, the regional results found by Fiset and colleagues integrate extremely well with the theoretical framework proposed here.

Neural Correlates of Consciousness: Where or How?

Do these data help us answer the questions: Does the neural substrate of conscious awareness depend upon activation of a particular set of neurons, or does it depend upon the resonant or regenerative patterns of activity across select groups of neurons? What do the present findings say about thalamocortical functioning as the basis of waking consciousness? These broader issues may come into focus with more discussion on how the present findings can be interpreted.

The overall logic of the experimental approach used here is rather straightforward. Subjects are studied in two conditions: conscious and unconscious. A subtraction image between these two conditions should reveal something about the functional neuroanatomy of "consciousness." A number of possible results could be expected from such a subtraction analysis. At best, those brain areas that generate consciousness will be identified. In other words, the subset of brain regions whose functional activity results in a subjective experience of consciousness will be visualized (i.e., a neural correlate of consciousness). Alternatively, those brain areas whose functional activity is required for consciousness to occur will be identified. In other words, rather than identifying those neurons which directly contain consciousness itself, the subtraction analysis may reflect primarily those neurons required to be active in order to allow consciousness to occur (i.e., the power switch). Another possibility, is that no regions would be identified. This could happen if consciousness is a widely diffuse phenomenon that depends on the global functioning of the brain (i.e., the Dennett explanation; Dennett 1991). Or, this could happen if the neurons that mediate consciousness are clustered in groups smaller than the spatial resolution of the PET technique. The regions identified may have nothing to do with consciousness, per se, or the regulation of consciousness, but may simply reflect those areas most affected by the agents causing the unconsciousness. For example, Cohen and Hood showed that radio-labeled halothane had a particular affinity for the granular layer of the cerebellum (Cohen and Hood 1969). Therefore, it is conceivable that the regional cerebellar metabolic decrease found in this report may be related to some unique ability of the inhalational anesthetics to specifically suppress metabolism in the cerebellum. Recently, Eckenhoff and colleagues showed that radio-labeled halothane has affinity for regions with high synaptic density (Eckenhoff and Eckenhoff 1998). Similar regional affinities may exist in other brain areas, perhaps the basal forebrain and thalamus are specifically sensitive to the effects of inhalational anesthesia because of a relatively higher synaptic density. Finally, a combination of any of these results could occur.

What did happen? We propose our results are best interpreted as a mixture of the above possibilities. Using neuroanatomy and neurophysiology as guides, we hypothesize that the thalamic and midbrain reticular formation findings are probably related to the suppression of a specific set of consciousness requiring neurons (i.e., the thalamocortical hyperpolarization hypothesis). Prior to these empirical results, these regions were often proposed as important by a number of authors expounding a number of theories about the functional neuroanatomy of consciousness (for review, see Smythies 1997). Furthermore, since the pioneering work of Moruzzi and Magoun (1949), the connection between the need for functional activity in these brain regions and the regulation of levels of consciousness is well established. In some sense then, these specific regional findings demonstrate and confirm in vivo what is to be expected from years of research related to regulation of levels of consciousness. As such, these results focus attention back to the old reticular formation hypothesis of anesthetic action. However, these results and our theoretical framework build on that older hypothesis by placing the most important region of anesthetic action not in the reticular formation itself, but rather in the thalamically gated regions regulated by the arousal centers located within the reticular formation. Given all of that, it would appear that these empirically demonstrated regional findings fit remarkably well with the extended reticular-thalamic activating system (ERTAS) theory of consciousness proposed by Newman and Baars (Newman and Baars 1993). Furthermore, these results fit well with the idea that the activity within some small subcortical structures may be required for the state of waking consciousness, whereas cortical projection areas may provide the perceptual content of consciousness (Baars 1995).

The findings of the left dorso-lateral prefrontal cortex and the left temporal gyrus are probably related to the fact that the subjects were listening to an audiotape during both awake and anesthetized conditions. During the awake scans the subjects would likely have been internally rehearsing the words on the audiotape. Yet, during the anesthetized scans such rehearsal was probably not possible. Hence, this region shows up in a subtraction analysis. However, a more intriguing possibility for why this region shows up is to suggest that the dorso-lateral prefrontal cortex finding might represent a neural correlate of consciousness, itself. For many people the internal perception of being conscious is having the ability to think to oneself and follow a "stream of consciousness" that is primarily a running verbal commentary. Putting the thalamic findings with the dorso-lateral prefrontal cortex findings and realizing that the subject's attention was likely focused on the auditory input, raises the possibility that a functional "consciousness circuit" may have been directly visualized for the first time in the human brain. Such a functional circuit would fit well with the ERTAS model of consciousness. Of course, many more controlled brain imaging experiments, such as replicating the procedures done here without the auditory input, need to be performed to follow up on this speculative idea.

The cerebellar and occipital lobe changes seen here may be related to the decreased sensory state the subjects were in while unconscious. Or, as previously suggested, they might simply represent some regional selectivity of the anesthetic agents themselves. If the cerebellum was involved with mediating waking consciousness then it would likely have shown up in the propofol study of Fiset and colleagues (1999). Likewise, the large occipital lobe effect seen by Fiset and colleagues (1999), which was not seen here (with the study of the inhalational agents), is likely related to a specific effect of propofol. As one can see by this example, separating the regional functional brain changes associated with consciousness itself from the extemporaneous effects agents can have on regional brain metabolism can be significantly helped by utilizing an intersection analysis approach.

Were subjects conscious while "unconscious"? The word anesthesia literally means to be without sensation (an + aisth• sis). On emergence from the anesthetic experience all subjects reported a sensation of complete oblivion during the anesthetic. No subject could remember anything about the time they were unconscious, even after repeated questioning. Many offered the statement that their mind was a complete blank for the period of anesthesia, and many had a sensation that time had stopped while they were unconscious. Thus, in the proposed model, with the thalamic "consciousness" switch thrown, sensory information would have been prevented from reaching each subject's cortex and the subjects were likely rendered in a cognitive state of sensory deprivation. Nevertheless, even though no new sensory information was coming into each subject's cortex, perhaps some subjects were in some sort of "dreamlike" state and still able to ruminate about thoughts already within their brains.

The idea that these subjects may have retained some level of consciousness during anesthesia should be considered to be highly unlikely. Most anesthetics, including alpha-chloralose and urethane cause a significant decrease in global brain metabolism (Dudley, Nelson, and Samson 1982; Ito, Miyaoka, and Ishii 1984), even though functional brain reactivity may remain somewhat intact (Dudley, Nelson, and Samson 1982).

Remember that the appearance of the thalamic switch, in the present report, is really superimposed on the back of a large global reduction in brain functioning for both of these inhalational agents (see table 55.1). Such a large global decrease in brain functioning means that cortical brain functioning is dramatically reduced during the anesthetic exposure. If one presupposes that cortical projection areas may contain the content of consciousness (Baars 1995), then a direct anesthetic effect on the cortex should directly suppress consciousness.

Did consciousness go away in our subjects because of neuronal suppression or discharge disruption? In other words, it may not be which neurons are firing that determines the presence or absence of consciousness; rather it may be how select groups of neurons fire that generates consciousness. This distinction underlies a number of theories on consciousness related to oscillatory neuronal firing patterns. Given that the imaging technique used has a relatively long temporal resolution and can only really measure suppression (or activation) of activity, it is not really possible to address this question with these data. Nonetheless, to speculate on this issue and as a prelude to future experiments, only a few anesthetics might fit into the disruption rather than the suppression category. These agents include ketamine, nitrous oxide, and xenon. Interestingly, these agents may have their primary anesthetic affects mediated primarily through the NMDA receptor (Franks et al. 1998).

Although it is common usage to state that a patient under anesthesia has been "put to sleep," our data suggest that this statement may not be far from the truth. Our findings reveal that the physiology of the unconsciousness induced by anesthesia likely shares a common mechanism with that of the unconsciousness caused by non-REM sleep (Lydic and Biebuyck 1994). This is not to say that anesthesia is a form of sleep. Anesthesia fundamentally differs from sleep in a number of important respects, such as the inability to be aroused from anesthesia and anesthetic-induced inhibition of thermoregulation and vasomotor tone. Another primary difference between the two states of awareness is that anesthetics inhibit those systems that allow cortical arousal and REM functioning to occur (e.g., primarily basal forebrain and reticular formation cholinergic activation) (Keifer, Baghdoyan, and Lydic 1996), and thus anesthesia can be likened to a form of slow-wave sleep from which one can not be aroused. Therefore, it might be more precise to state that anesthetics do not "put one to sleep"; rather, they "prevent one from being awake." In any event, the novel idea here is that the underlying neurophysiology that produces the "unconsciousness" of both slow-wave sleep and anesthesia is likely to be the same.

Conclusion

Functional brain imaging data of two different commonly used inhalational anesthetic agents obtained from volunteers rendered unconscious with anesthesia revealed the thalamus and midbrain reticular formation to be at the intersection of the anesthetic effect on human consciousness. These data offer strong support for theories attempting to relate the neuronal basis of consciousness to the functional activity in thalamocortical-corticothalamic loops. Moreover, these data lead to the proposal of a new unifying neurophysiologic model of anesthetic-induced unconsciousness. The essence of the model explains the multiple different pathways through which various anesthetic agents may act to produce unconsciousness by all ultimately causing the development of a hyperpolarization block in thalamocortical neurons.

Acknowledgments

The authors thank James L. McGaugh, Ph.D. and Larry Cahill, Ph.D. for helpful discussion of the manuscript.

References

Alkire, M. T. (1998). Quantitative EEG correlations with brain glucose metabolic rate during anesthesia in volunteers. *Anesthesiology*, 89, 323–333.

Alkire, M. T., Haier, R. J., Fallon, J. H., and Cahill, L. (1998). Hippocampal, but not amygdala, activity at encoding correlates with long-term, free recall of nonemotional information. *Proceedings of the National Academy of Sciences of the United States of America*, 95, 14506–14510.

Alkire, M. T., Haier, R. J., Shah, N. K., and Anderson, C. T. (1997). Positron emission tomography study of regional cerebral metabolism in humans during isoflurane anesthesia. *Anesthesiology*, 86, 549–557.

Alkire, M. T., Pomfrett, C. J., Haier, R. J., Gianzero, M. V., Chan, C. M., Jacobsen, B. P., and Fallon, J. H. (1999). Functional brain imaging during anesthesia in humans: Effects of halothane on global and regional cerebral glucose metabolism. *Anesthesiology*, 90, 701–709.

Angel, A. (1991). The G. L. Brown lecture: Adventures in anaesthesia. *Experimental Physiology*, 76, 1–38.

Angel, A. (1993). Central neuronal pathways and the process of anaesthesia. *British Journal of Anaesthesia*, 71, 148–163.

Baars, B. J. (1995). Tutorial commentary: Surprisingly small subcortical structures are needed for the state of waking consciousness, while cortical projection areas seem to provide perceptual contents of consciousness [comment]. *Consciousness and Cognition*, 4, 159–162.

Berg-Johnsen, J., and Langmoen, I. A. (1987). Isoflurane hyperpolarizes neurones in rat and human cerebral cortex. *Acta Physiologica Scandinavica*, 130, 679–685.

Chan, C. K., and Durieux, M. E. (1997). Differential inhibition of lysophosphatidate signaling by volatile anesthetics. *Anesthesiology*, 86, 660–669.

Cheng, S. C., and Brunner, E. A. (1987). A hypothetical model on the mechanism of anesthesia. *Medical Hypotheses*, 23, 1–9.

Cohen, E. N., and Hood, N. (1969). Application of low-temperature autoradiography to studies of the uptake and metabolism of volitile anesthetics in the mouse. 3. Halothane. *Anesthesiology*, 31, 553–559.

Crick, F. (1994). *The astonishing hypothesis.* New York: Scribner.

Dennett, D. C. (1991). *Consciousness explained.* Boston: Little, Brown.

Dildy-Mayfield, J. E., Eger, II, E. I., and Harris, R. A. (1996). Anesthetics produce subunit-selective actions on glutamate receptors. *Journal of Pharmacology and Experimental Therapeutics*, 276, 1058–1065.

Dudley, R. E., Nelson, S. R., and Samson, F. (1982). Influence of chloralose on brain regional glucose utilization. *Brain Research*, 233, 173–180.

Durieux, M. E. (1996). Muscarinic signaling in the central nervous system: Recent developments and anesthetic implications. *Anesthesiology*, 84, 173–189.

Eckenhoff, M. F., and Eckenhoff, R. G. (1998). Quantitative autoradiography of halothane binding in rat brain. *Journal of Pharmacology and Experimental Therapeutics*, 285, 371–376.

Eger, II, E. I., Saidman, L. J., and Brandstater, B. (1965). Minimum alveolar anesthetic concentration: A standard of anesthetic potency. *Anesthesiology*, 26, 756–763.

Fiset, P., Paus, T., Daloze, T., Plourde, G., Meuret, P., Bonhomme, V., Hajj-Ali, N., Backman, S. B., and Evans, A. C. (1999). Brain mechanisms of propofol-induced loss of consciousness in humans: A positron emission tomographic study. *Journal of Neuroscience*, 19, 5506–5513.

Franks, N. P., Dickinson, R., de Sousa, S. L., Hall, A. C., and Lieb, W. R. (1998). How does xenon produce anaesthesia? [letter]. *Nature*, 396, 324.

Franks, N. P., and Lieb, W. R. (1994). Molecular and cellular mechanisms of general anaesthesia. *Nature*, 367, 607–614.

Friston, K. J., Frith, C. D., Liddle, P. F., and Frackowiak, R. S. (1991). Comparing functional (PET) images: The assessment of significant change. *Journal of Cerebral Blood Flow and Metabolism*, 11, 690–699.

Friston, K. J., Passingham, R. E., Nutt, J. G., Heather, J. D., Sawle, G. V., and Frackowiak, R. S. (1989). Localisation in PET images: Direct fitting of the intercommissural (AC-PC) line. *Journal of Cerebral Blood Flow and Metabolism*, 9, 690–695.

Huang, S. C., Phelps, M. E., Hoffman, E. J., Sideris, K., Selin, C. J., and Kuhl, D. E. (1980). Noninvasive determination of local cerebral metabolic rate of glucose in man. *American Journal of Physiology*, 238, E69–82.

Ito, M., Miyaoka, M., and Ishii, S. (1984). [Alterations in local cerebral glucose utilization during various anesthesia: The effect of urethane and a review]. *No To Shinkei*, 36, 1191–1199.

Joliot, M., Ribary, U., and Llinás, R. (1994). Human oscillatory brain activity near 40 Hz coexists with cognitive temporal binding. *Proceedings of the National Academy of Sciences USA*, 91, 11748–11751.

Juhasz, G., Emri, Z., Kekesi, K., and Pungor, K. (1989). Local perfusion of the thalamus with GABA increases sleep and induces long-lasting inhibition of somatosensory event-related potentials in cats. *Neurosci Lett*, 103, 229–233.

Keifer, J. C., Baghdoyan, H. A., and Lydic, R. (1996). Pontine cholinergic mechanisms modulate the cortical electroencephalographic spindles of halothane anesthesia. *Anesthesiology*, 84, 945–954.

Llinás, R., and Ribary, U. (1993). Coherent 40-Hz oscillation characterizes dream state in humans. *Proceedings of the National Academy of Sciences USA*, 90, 2078–2081.

Llinás, R., Ribary, U., Contreras, D., and Pedroarena, C. (1998). The neuronal basis for consciousness. *Philosophical Transactions of the Royal Society of London B*, 353, 1841–1849.

Lumer, E. D., Edelman, G. M., and Tononi, G. (1997). Neural dynamics in a model of the thalamocortical system. I. Layers, loops, and the emergence of fast synchronous rhythms. *Cerebral Cortex*, 7, 207–227.

Lydic, R., and Biebuyck, J. F. (1994). Sleep neurobiology: Relevance for mechanistic studies of anaesthesia [editorial]. *British Journal of Anaesthesia*, 72, 506–508.

Moruzzi, G., and Magoun, H. W. (1949). Brain stem reticular formation and activation of the EEG. *Electroencephalography and Clinical Neurophysiology*, 1, 455–473.

Newman, J. (1997). Putting the puzzle together. Part 1: Towards a general theory of the neural correlates of consciousness. *Journal of Consciousness Studies*, 4, 46–66.

Newman, J., and Baars, B. J. (1993). A neural attentional model for access to consciousness: A global workspace perspective. *Concepts in Neuroscience*, 4, 255–290.

Nicoll, R. A., and Madison, D. V. (1982). General anesthetics hyperpolarize neurons in the vertebrate central nervous system. *Science*, 217, 1055–1057.

Nietgen, G. W., Honemann, C. W., Chan, C. K., Kamatchi, G. L., and Durieux, M. E. (1998). Volatile anaesthetics have differential effects on recombinant m1 and m3 muscarinic acetylcholine receptor function. *British Journal of Anaesthesia*, 81, 569–577.

Phelps, M. E., Huang, S. C., Hoffman, E. J., Selin, C., Sokoloff, L., and Kuhl, D. E. (1979). Tomographic measurement of local cerebral glucose metabolic rate in humans with (F-18)2-fluoro-2-deoxy-D-glucose: Validation of method. *Annals of Neurology*, 6, 371–388.

Schotten, U., Schumacher, C., Sigmund, M., Karlein, C., Rose, H., Kammermeier, H., Sivarajan, M., and Hanrath, P. (1998). Halothane, but not isoflurane, impairs the beta-adrenergic responsiveness in rat myocardium. *Anesthesiology*, 88, 1330–1339.

Smythies, J. (1997). The functional neuroanatomy of awareness: With focus on the role of various anatomical systems in the control of intermodal attention. *Consciousness and Cognition*, 6, 455–481.

Steriade, M. (1992). Basic mechanisms of sleep generation. *Neurology*, 42, 9–17; discussion 18.

Steriade, M. (1993a). Central core modulation of spontaneous oscillations and sensory transmission in thalamocortical systems. *Current Opinion in Neurobiology*, 3, 619–625.

Steriade, M. (1993b). Cholinergic blockage of network- and intrinsically generated slow oscillations promotes waking and REM sleep activity patterns in thalamic and cortical neurons. *Progress in Brain Research*, 98, 345–355.

Steriade, M. (1994). Sleep oscillations and their blockage by activating systems. *Journal of Psychiatry and Neuroscience*, 19, 354–358.

Steriade, M., Dossi, R. C., and Nunez, A. (1991). Network modulation of a slow intrinsic oscillation of cat thalamocortical neurons implicated in sleep delta waves: Cortically induced synchronization and brainstem cholinergic suppression. *Journal of Neuroscience*, 11, 3200–3217.

Steriade, M., McCormick, D. A., and Sejnowski, T. J. (1993). Thalamocortical oscillations in the sleeping and aroused brain. *Science*, 262, 679–685.

Sugiyama, K., Muteki, T., and Shimoji, K. (1992). Halothane-induced hyperpolarization and depression of postsynaptic potentials of guinea pig thalamic neurons in vitro. *Brain Research*, 576, 97–103.

Talairach, J., and Tournoux, P. (1988). *Co-planar stereotaxic atlas of the human brain, a 3-dimensional proportional system: an approach to cerebral imaging* (Mark Rayport, Trans.). New York: Thieme Medical Publishers.

Todd, M. M., and Drummond, J. C. (1984). A comparison of the cerebrovascular and metabolic effects of halothane and isoflurane in the cat. *Anesthesiology*, 60, 276–282.

Veselis, R. A., Reinsel, R. A., Beattie, B. J., Mawlawi, O. R., Feshchenko, V. A., DiResta, G. R., Larson, S. M., and Blasberg, R. G. (1997). Midazolam changes cerebral blood flow in discrete brain regions: an H2(15)O positron emission tomography study. *Anesthesiology*, 87, 1106–1117.

Violet, J. M., Downie, D. L., Nakisa, R. C., Lieb, W. R., and Franks, N. P. (1997). Differential sensitivities of mammalian neuronal and muscle nicotinic acetylcholine receptors to general anesthetics [see comments]. *Anesthesiology*, 86, 866–874.

Volkow, N. D., Wang, G. J., Hitzemann, R., Fowler, J. S., Pappas, N., Lowrimore, P., Burr, G., Pascani, K., Overall, J., and Wolf, A. P. (1995). Depression of thalamic metabolism by lorazepam is associated with sleepiness. *Neuropsychopharmacology*, 12, 123–132.

56 The Relation of Eye Movements During Sleep to Dream Activity: An Objective Method for the Study of Dreaming

William Dement and Nathaniel Kleitman

The study of dream activity and its relation to physiological variables during sleep necessitates a reliable method of determining with precision when dreaming occurs. This knowledge, in the final analysis, always depends upon the subjective report of the dreamer, but becomes relatively objective if such reports can be significantly related to some physiological phenomena which in turn can be measured by physical techniques.

Such a relationship was reported by Aserinsky and Kleitman (1), who observed periods of rapid, conjugate eye movements during sleep and found a high incidence of dream recall in Ss awakened during these periods and a low incidence when awakened at other times. The occurrence of these characteristic eye movements and their relation to dreaming were confirmed in both normal Ss and schizophrenics (4), and they were shown to appear at regular intervals in relation to a cyclic change in the depth of sleep during the night as measured by the EEG (5).

This paper represents the results of a rigorous testing of the relation between eye movements and dreaming. Three approaches were used:

1. Dream recall during rapid eye movement or quiescent periods was elicited without direct contact between E and S, thus eliminating the possibility of unintentional cuing by E.

2. The subjective estimate of the duration of dreams was compared with the length of eye movement periods before awakening, reasoning that there should be a positive correlation if dreaming and eye movements were concurrent.

3. The pattern of the eye movements was related to the dream content to test whether they represented a specific expression of the visual experience of dreaming or merely a random motor discharge of a more active central nervous system.

Method

The Ss for the experiments were seven adult males and two adult females. Five were studied intensively while the data gathered from the other four were minimal with the main intent of confirming the results on the first five.

In a typical experiment, S reported to the laboratory a little before his usual bedtime. He was instructed to eat normally but to abstain from alcoholic or caffeine-containing beverages on the day of the experiment. Two or more electrodes were attached near the eyes for registering changes in the corneoretinal potential fields as the eyes moved. Two or three electrodes were affixed to the scalp for recording brain waves as a criterion of depth of sleep. The S then went to bed in a quiet, dark room. All electrode lead wires were further attached to the top of the head and from there to the lead box at the head of the bed in a single cord to minimize the possibility of entanglement and allow S a free range of movement. The potentials were amplified by a Model III Grass Electroencephalograph in an adjoining room. The electroencephalograph was run continuously throughout the sleep period at a paper speed of 3 or 6 mm/s, which allowed easy recognition of eye-movement potentials. A faster speed (3 cm/s) was used for detailed examination of the brain waves although the slower speed permitted at least an approximate estimation of the gross pattern. The criteria of eye-movement potentials and their differentiation from brain wave artifacts have been discussed at length elsewhere (1, 4).

At various times during the night Ss were awakened to test their dream recall. The return to sleep after such an awakening invariably took less than 5 min. Table 56.1 is a summary of the experiments showing the number of nights each S slept and the number of awakenings. In all,

Table 56.1
Summary of experiments

Ss	Nights slept	Awaken-ings	Average nightly awaken-ings	Average sleeping time
DN	6	50	8.3	7:50
IR	12	65	5.4	4:20
KC	17	74	4.4	6:00
WD	11	77	7.0	6:30
PM	9	55	6.1	6:20
KK	2	10	5.0	6:00
SM	1	6	6.0	6:40
DM	1	4	4.0	7:00
MG	2	10	5.0	6:10
Totals	61	351	5.7	6:00

21% of the awakenings fell in the first 2 hr. of sleep, 29% in the second two, 28% in the third two, and 22% in the fourth two.

Results

The Occurrence of Rapid Eye Movements

Discrete periods during which their eyes exhibited rapid movements were observed in all nine Ss every night they slept. These periods were characterized by a low-voltage, relatively fast pattern in the EEG. The interspersed periods in which rapid eye movements were absent showed EEG patterns indicative of deeper sleep, either a predominance of high-voltage, slow activity, or frequent, well-defined sleep spindles with a low-voltage background. No REMs were ever observed during the initial onset of sleep although the EEG always passed through a stage similar to that accompanying the rapid eye movement periods occurring later in the night. These findings concerning associated EEG patterns were identical with previous observations on uninterrupted sleep (5).

An accurate appraisal of the mean duration of the REM periods was impossible since most were terminated artificially by an awakening. However, those that were not so terminated varied between 3 and 50 min. in duration with a mean of about 20 min., and they tended to be longer the later in the night they occurred. The eyes were not constantly in motion during such periods; rather, the activity occurred in bursts of 1 or 2, up to 50 or 100 movements. A single movement was generally accomplished in 0.1–0.2 s and was followed by a fixational pause of varying duration. The amount, pattern, and size of the movements varied irregularly from period to period.

The REM periods occurred at fairly regular intervals throughout the night. The frequency of occurrence seemed to be relatively constant and characteristic for the individual. DM and WD averaged one eye-movement period every 70 min. and every 75 min., respectively. KC averaged one eye-movement period every 104 min. The other Ss fell between these two extremes. The average for the whole group was one REM period every 92 min.

Despite the considerable disturbance of being awakened a number of times, the frequency and regularity with which REM periods occurred was almost exactly comparable to that seen previously in a study of uninterrupted sleep (5). If the awakening occurred during a NREM period, the return to sleep was never associated with REM's, nor was the time of onset of the next REM period markedly changed from that which would have been expected in the absence of an awakening. An awakening during an REM period generally terminated the REMs until the next period, and the sequence of EEG changes, excluding the brief period of wakefulness, was the same as that following an REM period that ended spontaneously. Exceptions occurred when S was awakened during an REM period in the final hours of sleep when the period was likely to be quite long if uninterrupted. On these occasions, the REMs sometimes started up again when S fell asleep. It seemed as though a period of heightened CNS activity had not run its normal course and, although S was able to fall asleep, he continued to dream.

Eye Movement Periods and Dream Recall

For all awakenings to elicit dream recall, the arousing stimulus was the ringing of an ordinary doorbell placed near the bed and sufficiently loud to ensure immediate awakening in all levels of sleep. The Ss then spoke into a recording device near the bed. They were instructed to first state whether or not they had been dreaming and then, if they could, to relate the content of the dream. When S had finished speaking E, who could hear their voices, occasionally entered the room to further question them on some particular point of the dream. There was no communication between S and E in any instance, it must be emphasized, until S had definitely commited himself. The Ss were considered to have been dreaming only if they could relate a coherent, fairly detailed description of dream content. Assertions that they had dreamed without recall of content, or vague, fragmentary impressions of content, were considered negative.

The awakenings were done either during REM periods or at varying increments of time after the cessation of eye movements during the interspersed periods of NREMs. The Ss, of course, were never informed when awakened whether or not their eyes had been moving.

Table 56.2 shows the results of the attempts to recall dreams after the various awakenings. The REM or NREM awakenings for PM and KC were chosen according to a table of random numbers to eliminate any possibility of an unintentional pattern. For DN, a pattern was followed: first three REM awakenings, then three NREM awakenings, and so on. WD was told he would be awakened *only* when the recording indicated that he was dreaming, but REM and NREM awakenings were then interspersed

Table 56.2

Instances of dream recall after awakenings during periods of rapid eye movements or periods of no rapid eye movements

S	Rapid eye movements		No rapid eye movements	
	Dream recall	No recall	Dream recall	No recall
DN	17	9	3	21
IR	26	8	2	29
KC	36	4	3	31
WD	37	5	1	34
PM	24	6	2	23
KK	4	1	0	5
SM	2	2	0	2
DM	2	1	0	1
MG	4	3	0	3
Totals	152	39	11	149

randomly. The type of awakenings for IR was chosen according to the whim of E.

The Ss uniformly showed a high incidence of dream recall following REM awakenings and a very low incidence of recall following awakenings during periods of NREMs regardless of how the awakenings were chosen. In particular, DN was not more accurate than the others although there was a pattern he might have learned, and WD was not less accurate although he was deliberately misled to expect to have been dreaming every time he was awakened. Over a narrow range, some Ss appeared better able to recall dreams than others.

Table 56.3 compares the results of the first half of the series of REM awakenings with the last half. Practice was certainly not a significant factor as only one S showed any degree of improvement of recall on later nights as compared with the early ones.

The incidence of dream recall dropped precipitously almost immediately upon cessation of

Table 56.3

Comparison of first half of series of rapid eye movement awakenings with second half

S	First half		Second half	
	Dream recall	No recall	Dream recall	No recall
DN	12	1	5	8
IR	12	5	14	3
KC	18	2	18	2
WD	19	2	18	3
PM	12	3	12	3
Total	73	13	67	19

REMs. In 17 NREM awakenings that were done within 8 min. after the end of a REM period, five dreams were recalled. Although small, this was a much higher incidence of dream recall than occurred when the NREM awakenings followed the end of REM periods by *more* than 8 min. In the latter category only six dreams were recalled in 132 awakenings.

In general, *S*s were best able to make an emphatic statement that they had not been dreaming when the NREM awakenings were done during an intermediate stage of sleep as indicated by a brain-wave pattern of spindling with a low-voltage background. When aroused during a deep stage of sleep characterized by high-voltage, slow waves in the EEG, *S*s often awoke somewhat bewildered. In this state they frequently felt that they must have been dreaming although they could not remember the dream or, on the other hand, that they had not been asleep at all. They sometimes had a great variety of feelings to describe—such as pleasantness, anxiety, detachment, and so on, but these could not be related to any specific dream content.

Most of the instances of inability to recall dreaming after awakenings during REM periods occurred in the early part of the night. Of 39 negative reports in the entire study, 19 occurred after awakenings during REM periods falling in

the first 2 hr. of sleep, 11 after REM awakenings during the second 2 hr., 5 in the third 2 hr., and 4 in the last 2 hr. There was no such variation relating to awakenings during the interspersed periods of ocular quiescence, the incidence of dream recall being uniformly low, regardless of whether the early or late part of the night was being considered.

Length of Rapid Eye Movement Periods and Subjective Dream-Duration Estimates

If the length of the REM periods were proportional to the subjectively estimated duration of the dreams, it would further help to establish the relatedness of the two and would give some information about the rate at which dreaming progresses.

At first, *S*s were awakened at various increments of time after the REMs had begun and were requested to estimate to the nearest minute the amount of time they had been dreaming. This proved to be too difficult, although the estimates were always of the same order of magnitude as the lengths of the REM periods, and were occasionally exactly right.

A series was then done in which *S*s were awakened either 5 or 15 min. after the onset of REMs and were required on the basis of their recall of the dream to decide which was the correct duration. The 5- or 15-min. periods were chosen on the basis of a random series. Table 56.4 shows the results of these awakenings. All *S*s were able to choose the correct dream duration with high accuracy except DN. This *S*, however, made most of his incorrect choices by estimating 15 min. to be 5 min. This is consistent with the interpretation that the dream was longer, but he was only able to recall the latter fraction and thus thought it was shorter than it actually was.

In addition to depending on the amount of actual dreaming, the lengths of the dream narratives were undoubtedly influenced by many other factors as, for example, the loquacity or

Table 56.4

Results of dream-duration estimates after 5 or 15 min. of rapid eye movements

	5 minutes		15 minutes	
S	Right	Wrong	Right	Wrong
DN	8	2	5	5
IR	11	1	7	3
KC	7	0	12	1
WD	13	1	15	1
PM	6	2	8	3
Total	45	6	47	13

Table 56.5

Correlation between duration of REM periods in minutes and number of words in dream narratives

Subjects	Number of dreams	r	P
DN	15	.60	<.02
IR	25	.68	<.001
KC	31	.40	<.05
WD	35	.71	<.001
PM	20	.53	<.02

taciturnity of *S*. However, the lengths of the dream narratives still showed a significant relationship to the duration of REM periods before awakening. Table 56.5 shows the correlations between minutes of REMs and lengths of dream narratives for each *S*. The number of words in the narrative was the measurement of length. Of the 152 dreams recalled, 26 were not included because poor recording did not allow complete transcription. Dream narratives recalled after 30 or as much as 50 min. of REMs were not a great deal longer than those after 15 min. although *S*s had the impression that they had been dreaming for an unusually long time. This was perhaps due to inability to remember all the details of very long dreams.

Specific Eye-Movement Patterns and Visual Imagery of the Dream

The quality and quantity of the REMs themselves showed endless variation. There was much or little movement, big or small movements, and so on. As has been stated, the movements occurred in bursts of activity separated by periods of relative inactivity. However, the brain-wave stage during the whole period remained the same whether there was much or little movement at any given moment of the period.

It was hypothesized that the movements represented the visual imagery of the dream, that is, that they corresponded to where and at what the dreamer was looking. An attempt to account for every movement by having *S* state chronologically in what directions he had gazed in the dream proved futile. The *S*s could not recall the dream with such a high order of detail and precision.

In a slightly different approach, *S*s were awakened as soon as one of four predominant patterns of movement had persisted for at least 1 min. and were asked to describe in detail the dream content just before awakening. The four patterns were: (a) mainly vertical eye movements, (b) mainly horizontal movements, (c) both vertical and horizontal movements, and (d) very little or no movement. The prevalence of the horizontal or vertical components was determined by placing leads both vertically and horizontally around the eyes.

A total of 35 awakenings was accumulated from the nine *S*s. Periods of either pure vertical or horizontal movements were extremely rare. Three such periods of vertical movements were seen. After each of these the dream content involved a predominance of action in the vertical plane One *S* dreamed of standing at the bottom of a tall cliff operating some sort of hoist and looking up at climbers at various levels and down at the hoist machinery. Another *S* dreamed of climbing up a series of ladders looking up and down as he climbed. In the third instance the dreamer was throwing basketballs at a net, first shooting and looking up at the net, and then looking down to pick another ball off the floor. Only one instance of pure horizontal movement was seen. In the associated dream S was watching two people throwing tomatoes at each other. On 10 occasions Ss were awakened after 1 min. of little or no eye movement. In these, the dreams all had the common property that the dreamer was watching something at a distance or just staring fixedly at some object. In two of these awakenings in different Ss the patterns were the same, as follows: about a minute of ocular inactivity followed by several large movements to the left just a second or two before the awakening. Both instances, interestingly enough, were virtually identical as regards dream content. In one case S was driving a car and staring at the road ahead. He approached an intersection and was startled by the sudden appearance of a car speeding at him from the left as the bell rang. In the other, the dreamer was also driving a car and staring at the road ahead. Just before the awakening he saw a man standing on the left side of the road and hailed him as he drove past.

In the 21 awakenings after a mixture of movements Ss were always looking at things close to them, objects or people. Typical reports were of talking to a group of people, looking for something, fighting with someone, and so forth. There was no recall of distant or vertical activity.

In order to confirm the meaningfulness of these relationships, 20 naive Ss as well as 5 of the experimental Ss were asked to observe distant and close-up activity while awake. Horizontal and vertical electrodes were attached. The eye-movement potentials in all cases were comparable in both amplitude and pattern to those occurring during dreaming. Furthermore, there was virtually no movement, as indicated by the eye potentials, when viewing distant activity, and much movement while viewing close-up activity. Vertical eye-movement potentials were always at a minimum except for the upward movements accompanying blinking, and in a few cases when E tossed a ball in the air for them to watch.

Discussion

The results of these experiments indicate that dreaming accompanied by REMs and a low-voltage electroencephalogram occurred periodically in discrete episodes during the course of a night's sleep. It cannot be stated with complete certainty that some sort of dream activity did not occur at other times. However, the lack of recall and also the fact that the brain waves were at the lightest level of sleep only during REM periods and at deeper levels at all other times, makes this unlikely. The few instances of dream recall during NREM periods are best accounted for by assuming that the memory of the preceding dream persisted for an unusually long time. This is borne out by the fact that most of these instances occurred very close, within 8 min., after the end of REM periods.

Other workers have attempted to relate dreaming to physiological phenomena during sleep. Wada (12) felt that dreaming and gastric contractions occurred simultaneously. However, this conclusion was based on only seven awakenings in two Ss. One was unable to recall dream content although he felt he had been dreaming and the other remembered dream content in three of four awakenings. Scantlebury, Frick, and Patterson (11) also studied gastric activity and dreaming. They felt, on the basis of three instances of dream recall out of seven awakenings, that the two were probably related, but judiciously stated that "the exact time during which a dream occurs is elusive of record." The occurrence of dreaming during a series of foot twitches occurring immediately after the onset of sleep was postulated by McGlade (9). However, he based this conclusion mainly on dreams recalled on the morning after the experiments which is highly unreliable, and only 3 out of the 25 Ss studied exhibited foot twitches.

Incidental observations have been made on the occurrence of dreaming by investigators studying brain waves during sleep (2, 3, 6, 7, 8). All stages of brain waves were related to dreaming in these five papers, but no mention was made of whether or not actual dream content was recalled, and the number of reports by sleepers was generally very small.

In other studies of dreaming, excellently reviewed by Ramsey (10), attempts were made to localize dream activity by simply awakening Ss at various times during the night. In general it was found that dreams might be recalled at any time during the night, but that most were recalled in the later hours of sleep. This would correspond to the statistical incidence of REMs as previously reported (1, 4), and is also consistent with the finding in this study that, even when the awakenings occurred during REM periods, recall was still more difficult earlier in the night.

It was stated herein that all Ss showed periods of REMs *every* night they slept. This was also the case in another briefly reported series of experiments involving 16 Ss who were observed a total of 43 nights (5). It is felt on the basis of these and other studies which are unreported that periods of REMs and dreaming and the regularity with which they occur are an intrinsic part of normal sleep. In view of this, the failure to observe REMs in occasional Ss reported in earlier work (1, 4) deserves some consideration. One explanation is that the recording was done by sampling rather than continuously. If the REM periods were shorter than usual, they may have occurred in the intervals between the samples, thus escaping observation. Another explanation is that a lower amplification of the REM potentials was employed which, although usually adequate, did not clearly record very small movements. A third possibility is that the dreams of these Ss happened to be the sort, such as watching distant activity, in which eye movement was at a minimum. Since the association

of the characteristic low-voltage, non-spindling EEG was not realized at the time and thus could not aid in identifying this sort of period, they very likely would have been overlooked.

There was nothing in the experiments reported in this paper to indicate that the dreams occurred instantaneously, or with great rapidity, as some have suposed. Rather, they seemed to progress at a rate comparable to a real experience of the same sort. An increment in the length of REM periods was almost invariably associated with a proportional increase in the length of the dream. This could not have occurred if dreaming were instantaneous, since any length of REM periods would then easily accommodate a virtually infinite amount of dream activity.

It seems reasonable to conclude that an objective measurement of dreaming may be accomplished by recording REMs during sleep. This stands in marked contrast to the forgetting, distortion, and other factors that are involved in the raliance on the subjective recall of dreams. It thus becomes possible to objectively study the effect on dreaming of environmental changes, psychological stress, drug administration, and a variety of other factors and influences.

Summary

Regularly occurring periods of REMs were observed during every night of experimental sleep in nine adult Ss. A high incidence of dream recall was obtained from Ss when awakened during REM periods and a very low incidence when they were awakened at other times. A series of awakenings was done either 5 or 15 min. after the REMs (dreaming) had begun and Ss judged the correct dream duration with high accuracy. The pattern of the REMs was related to the visual imagery of the dream, and the eye movements recorded in analogous situations while awake corresponded closely in amplitude and pattern to those observed during dreaming.

Acknowledgments

Aided by a grant from the Wallace C. and Clara A. Abbott Memorial Fund of the University of Chicago.

References

1. Aserinsky, E., and Kleitman, N. Two types of ocular motility occurring in sleep. *J. appl. Physiol.*, 1955, 8, 1–10.

2. Blake, H., Gerard, R., and Kleitman, N. Factors influencing brain potentials during sleep. *J. Neurophysiol.*, 1939, 2, 48–60.

3. Davis, H., Davis, P., Loomis, A. L., Harvey, E. N., and Hobart, G. A. Human brain potentials during the onset of sleep. *J. Neurophysiol.*, 1938, 1, 24–38.

4. Dement, W. Dream recall and eye movements during sleep in schizophrenics and normals. *J. nerv. ment. Dis.*, 1955, 122, 263–269.

5. Dement, W., and Kleitman, N. Incidence of eye motility during sleep in relation to varying EEG pattern. *Fed. Proc.*, 1955, 14, 216.

6. Henry, C. E. Electroencephalographic individual differences and their constancy. I. During sleep. *J. exp. Psychol.*, 1941, 29, 117–132.

7. Knott, J. R., Henry, C. E., and Hadley, J. M. Brain potentials during sleep; a comparative study of the dominant and non-dominant alpha groups. *J. exp. Psychol.*, 1939, 24, 157–168.

8. Loomis, A. L., Harvey, E. N., and Hobart, G. A. Cerebral states during sleep as studied by human brain potentials. *J. exp. Psychol.*, 1937, 21, 127–144.

9. McGlade, H. B. The relationship between gastric motility, muscular twitching during sleep and dreaming. *Amer. J. digest. Dis.*, 1942, 9, 137–140.

10. Ramsey, G. Studies of dreaming. *Psychol. Bull.*, 1953, 50, 432–455.

11. Scantlebury, R. E., Frick, H. L., and Patterson, T. L. The effect of normal and hypnotically induced dreams on the gastric hunger movements of man. *J. appl. Psychol.*, 1942, 26, 682–691.

12. Wada, T. An experimental study of hunger and its relation to activity. *Arch. Psychol.*, N. Y., 1922, 8, No. 57.

57 The Brain as a Dream State Generator: An Activation-Synthesis Hypothesis of the Dream Process

J. Allan Hobson and Robert W. McCarley

Since the turn of the century, dream theory has been dominated by the psychoanalytic hypothesis that dreaming is a reactive process designed to protect consciousness and sleep from the disruptive effect of unconscious wishes that are released in sleep (1). Thus dreaming has been viewed as a psychodynamically determined state, and the distinctive formal features of dream content have been interpreted as manifestations of a defensive transformation of the unconscious wishes found unacceptable to consciousness by a hypothetical censor. A critical tenet of this wish fulfillment-disguise theory is that the transformation of the unconscious wish by the censor disguises or degrades the ideational information in forming the dream imagery. We were surprised to discover the origins of the major tenets of psychoanalytic dream theory in the neurophysiology of 1890 and have specified the transformations made by Freud in an earlier, related article (2). In detailing the neurophysiological origins of psychoanalytic dream theory, the concept of mind-body isomorphism, denoting similarity of form between psychological and physiological events, was seen as an explicit premise of Freud's thought.

Sharing Freud's conviction that mind-body isomorphism is a valid approach, we will now review modern neurophysiological evidence that we believe permits and necessitates important revisions in psychoanalytic dream theory. The activation-synthesis hypothesis that we will begin to develop in this paper asserts that many formal aspects of the dream experience may be the obligatory and relatively undistorted psychological concomitant of the regularly recurring and physiologically determined brain state called "dreaming sleep." It ascribes particular formal features of the dream experience to the particular organizational features of the brain during that state of sleep. More specifically, the theory details the mechanisms by which the brain becomes periodically activated during sleep and specifies the means by which both sensory input and motor output are simultaneously blocked, so as to account for the maintenance of sleep in the face of strong central activation of the brain. The occurrence and character of dreaming are seen as both determined and shaped by these physiological processes.

The most important tenet of the activation-synthesis hypothesis is that during dreaming the activated brain generates its own information by a pontine brain stem neuronal mechanism, which will be described in detail. We hypothesize that this internally generated sensorimotor information, which is partially random and partially specific, is then compared with stored sensorimotor data in the synthesis of dream content. The functional significance of the brain activation and the synthesis of endogenous information in dreaming sleep is not known, but we suggest that state-dependent learning is at least as likely a result of dreaming as is tension reduction or sleep maintenance.

While we believe that the two processes emphasized in this paper—activation and synthesis—are major and important advances in dream theory, we wish to state explicitly and comment on some of the things that our theory does not attempt to do. The activation-synthesis hypothesis does not exclude possible defensive distortions of the value-free sensorimotor dream stimuli, but it does deny the primacy of any such process in attempting to explain *formal* aspects of dream content or the fundamental impetus to dreaming itself. The idea that dreams reveal wishes is also beyond the direct reach of our new theory, but some specific alternatives to this interpretation of several classic dream situations can be advanced.

The new theory cannot yet account for the emotional aspects of the dream experience, but we assume that they are produced by the activation of brain regions subserving affect in parallel with the activation of the better known sensorimotor pathways. Finally, the new theory does not deny meaning to dreams, but it does suggest (1) a more direct route to their acquisition than anamnesis via free association, since dream origins are in basic physiological processes and not in disguised wishes, (2) a less complex approach to their interpretation than conversion from manifest to latent content, since unusual aspects of dreams are not seen as disguises but as results of the way the brain and mind function during sleep, and (3) a broader view of their use in therapy than that provided by the transference frame of reference, since dreams are not to be interpreted as the product of disguised unconscious (transference) wishes. Dreams offer a royal road to the mind and brain in a behavioral state, with different operating rules and principles than during waking and with the possibility of clinically useful insights from the product of these differences. These points are discussed in the last section of this paper and elsewhere (3).

What Is a Dream?

A dream may be defined as a mental experience, occurring in sleep, which is characterized by hallucinoid imagery, predominantly visual and often vivid; by bizarre elements due to such spatiotemporal distortions as condensation, discontinuity, and acceleration; and by a delusional acceptance of these phenomena as "real" at the time that they occur. Strong emotion may or may not be associated with these distinctive formal properties of the dream, and subsequent recall of these mental events is almost invariably poor unless an immediate arousal from sleep occurs.

That this technical jargon describes a universal human experience seems certain, since the five key points in this definition are easily elicited from both naive and sophisticated individuals when they are asked to characterize their dreams. We leave aside the question of whether other less vivid and nonperceptual forms of mental activity during sleep should also be called "dreams" and confine ourselves here to the psychophysiology of the hallucinoid type of dream. In doing so, we not only simplify the immediate task at hand but may also gain insight into the mechanisms underlying the most florid symptoms of psychopathology. We mean, of course, the hallucinations and delusions of the psychotic experience, which have so often invited comparison with the dream as we have defined it here.

What Is the State of the Brain during Dreaming Sleep?

The physiological substrate of the dream experience is the CNS in one of its three principal operating states: waking (W), synchronized sleep (S), and desynchronized sleep (D). These states can be reliably and objectively differentiated by recording the EEG, the electromyogram (EMG), and the electrooculogram (see table 57.1). Hal-

Table 57.1
Electrographic criteria for behavioral state determination

State	Electro-myogram	EEG	Electro-oculogram
Waking	+	Low voltage, fast	+
Sleep Synchronized	−	High voltage, slow	−
Desynchronized	−	Low voltage, fast	+

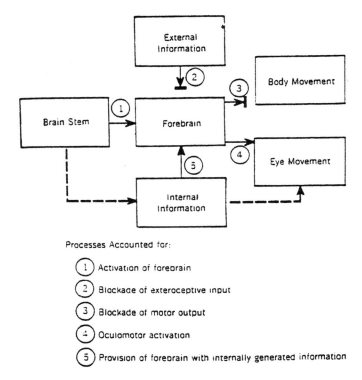

Figure 57.1
Systems model of dream state generation.

lucinoid dreaming in man occurs predominantly during the periodically recurrent phase of sleep characterized by EEG desynchronization. EMG suppression, and REMs (4). We call this kind of sleep "D" (meaning desynchronized, but also conveniently denoting dreaming).

In the systems analysis terms used in figure 57.1, this D brain state is characterized by the following "sensorimotor" properties: activation of the brain; relative exclusion of external input; generation of some internal input, which the activated forebrain then processes as information; and blocking of motor output, except for the oculomotor pathway. In this model the sub-

strate of emotion is considered to be a part of the forebrain; it will not be further distinguished here because we have no specific physiological evidence as to how this part of the system might work in any brain state. Memory is not shown but is considered to be a differentiated function of the brain that operates during the D state, such that output from long-term storage is facilitated but input to long-term storage is blocked. A highly specific hypothesis about dream amnesia has previously been derived (5) from the same evidence that we will now review in our attempt to account for the general sensorimotor aspects of the dream process.

Electrophysiology of the Brain during the Dream State

The three major electrographic features of the D state are of obvious relevance to our attempt to answer the following three questions about the organization of the brain in the dream state.

How Is the Forebrain Activated in the D State?

Since EEG desynchronization also characterizes waking, similar mechanisms of "activation" may be involved in both instances. Physiological evidence suggests that this is so: the reticular formation of the anterior brain stem is at least as active in D sleep as it is in the waking state (see figure 57.2).

How Is Motor Output Blocked in the D State?

Physiological evidence clearly shows that the profound EMG suppression of D sleep is a consequence of the direct inhibition of spinal cord motoneurons (6). As a consequence, any organized motor patterns that might be generated

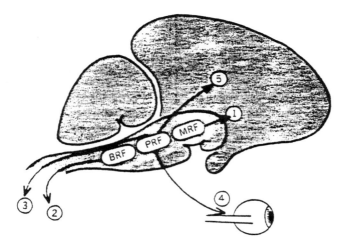

Processes Accounted for:

① Activation of forebrain

② Blockade of exteroceptive input

③ Blockade of motor output

④ Oculomotor activation

⑤ Provision of forebrain with internally generated information

Figure 57.2
Physiological model of dream state generation using the sagittal section of the cat brain and showing the bulbar (BRF), pontine (PRF), and midbrain (MRF) divisions of the reticular formation.

during the intense brain activation of D sleep cannot be expressed.

That organized movement patterns are in fact generated, but not expressed, in normal D sleep is dramatically demonstrated by cats with lesions of the anterodorsal pontine brain stem (7). The animals show all of the major manifestations of D sleep except the atonia; instead of the fine twitches of the digits and the limb jerks that are normally present in D, these cats display complex motor behaviors including repetitive paw movements and well-coordinated attack and defense sequences that have no apparent relationship to the environment.

How Is Sensory Imagery Generated in the D State?

In waking, a corollary discharge of the oculomotor system has been shown to suppress visual transmission during saccadic eye movements, possibly contributing to the stability of the visual field during that state (8). The same mechanisms might underlie the hallucinoid dream imagery by inhibiting and exciting neurons of the lateral geniculate body (9) and the visual cortex (10) during D sleep, when retinal input is reduced and unformed.

The possibility that oculomotor impulses trigger visual imagery is particularly intriguing in view of the demonstrated quantitative correlation between eye movement intensity and dream intensity (11). More specific correlations have also been reported to relate eye movement direction to orientation of the hallucinated gaze in dreams (12). This finding has been interpreted as indicative of "scanning" the visual field— implying cortical control of the eye movements in dreaming sleep. An alternative, although not exclusive, hypothesis is that the oculomotor activity is generated at the brain stem level and that the cortex is then provided with feed-forward information about the eye movements. According to this view, we are not so much scanning dream imagery with our D sleep eye movements as we are synthesizing the visual imagery appropriate to them. We will return to the implications of this intriguing possibility in discussing the generation of eye movements in dreaming sleep, but we wish to stress here the general significance of this clue to the identity of an "internal information generator" operating at the brain stem level in the dreaming sleep state.

The eye-movement-related inhibition of sensory relays (13), as well as the possible occlusion of exogenous inputs by internally generated excitation, may also contribute to the maintenance of sleep in the face of strong central activation of the brain. In this sense the dream process is seen as having a sleep maintenance mechanism built into its physiological substrate rather than a sleep guardian function operating at the psychological level.

A firm general conclusion can be reached at this point: the desynchronized phase of sleep is the physiological substrate of hallucinoid dreaming, as defined. This conclusion is of profound significance to psychophysiology, since we can now reliably and objectively characterize and measure many aspects of the brain when it is in the dream state. For example, one feature that emerges from the psychophysiological study of dreaming and one that was not at all evident from introspective, psychoanalytically oriented research, is that the brain enters the dream state at regular intervals during sleep and stays in that state for appreciable and predictable lengths of time. One clear implication of this finding is that dreaming is an automatically preprogrammed brain event and not a response to exogenous (day residue) or endogenous (visceral) stimuli. A second implication is that the dream state generator mechanism is periodic, that is, the dream state generator is a neurobiological clock (14). Since the length of the sleep cycle and, by inference, the frequency of dreaming, is a function of body size within and across mammalian species (15), the system controlling the length of the period must have a structural substrate. Thus we must account for size-related periodicity with our model of the dream state generator.

An Animal Model of the Brain during the Dream State

We said that the length of the sleep cycle varies "across species." Does that mean that nonhuman animals dream? Unfortunately we cannot know, but we are willing to assert that if they do so, it is when their brains are in the D sleep state. Because we have no direct evidence of any significant difference between the brain state of man and the brain state of other mammals in D sleep, we therefore feel justified in asserting that the brain state of our experimental animal, the cat, constitutes a reasonable subject for our study of the brain as a dream process generator, whether or not cats dream. This assertion seems justified since we are restricting our attention here to formal aspects of the dream experience; our experimental model need not dream or even possess "consciousness" to be useful as a source of physiological information. If we accept this argument and use the definition of dreaming offered above, then the presence of D sleep in cats (16) offers nothing less than an animal model in which to study the neurophysiological basis of a hallucinoid mental process in man. Such a model is as important in experimental psychiatry as it is rare. Let us now turn to the biological data upon which our sketches of the brain as a dream state generator are based.

Localization of the Power Supply or Trigger Zone of the Dream State Generator

Lesion, stimulation, and recording studies pioneered by Jouvet (17) have strongly implicated the pontine brain stem as critical to the generation of the desynchronized sleep phase (see figure 57.3 for a summary of the neuroanatomy of this region). Important findings supporting this hypothesis include the following.

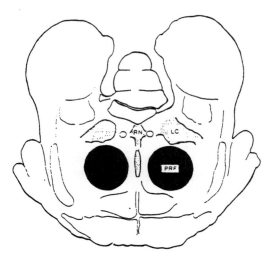

Figure 57.3
The anatomy of the pontine brain stem. On this frontal section of the cat brain stem, the cells that are selectively activated are in the paramedian reticular formation. On this frontal section of the cat brain stem, the cells that are selectively activated are in the paramedian reticular formation (PRF) (giganto cellular tegmental field), while the cells that are selectively inactivated lie more dorsally (in the region of the locus coeruleus [LC]) and medially (in the region of the raphe nuclei [RN]). Compare this with figure 57.5, which summarizes the neurophysiology and shows the anatomy in a sagittal section.

Large lesions of the pontine reticular formation prevent the occurrence of desynchronized sleep for several weeks in cats (17). This suggests that the pontine reticular formation may be the site of an executive or triggering mechanism for desynchronized sleep. Prepontine transections and forebrain ablation have no effect upon periodicity or duration of the skeletal, muscular, and oculomotor manifestations of D sleep (17). The data indicate that the trigger, the power supply, and the clock are pontine.

The pontine brain stem is thus implicated as the site of both the trigger and the clock. The periodicity of the D sleep clock in poikilothermic pontine cats lengthens as temperature declines, indicating orthodox metabolic mediation of the cycle, in contrast to the temperature independence of circadian rhythms. If we assume that the physiological substrate of consciousness is in the forebrain, these facts completely eliminate any possible contribution of ideas (or their neural substrate) to the primary driving force of the dream process.

Small lesions of the dorsal pontine brain stem, in the region of the locus coeruleus (LC), may eliminate the atonia but no other aspects of desynchronized sleep (7). This suggests that inhibition of muscle tone is somehow dependent upon the integrity of the LC. The elaborate motor behavior that characterizes the D sleep of cats with LC lesions has been described as "pseudo-hallucinatory" (7). Whether or not one accepts the sensory implications of that designation, the importance of motor inhibition in quelling the effects of central excitation during the dream state is clear.

This finding has an important bearing on mechanisms of dream paralysis and suggests that in the classic chase dream, the dreamer who has trouble fleeing from a pursuer is as much accurately reading the activated state of his motor pattern generator and the paralyzed state of his spinal neurons as he is "wishing" to be caught. This dream experience is so universal and the feeling of constrained motor action so impressive as to make its physiological basis in the descending inhibition of motoneurons seem to us inescapable. Conversely, this reasonable and adequate explanation of the paradox of the chase dream makes its interpretation as wish fulfillment less compelling. Other implications of the D sleep activation of various motor system pattern generators for movements and dream plots have been discussed elsewhere (3).

The vestibular system, as classically established, integrates head position and movement with eye position and posture. Pompeiano and Morrison (18) showed that lesions of the vestibular nuclei interfered with the bursts of REM but not with the isolated eye movements of D. This finding suggested that the vestibular system contributed to the elaboration and rhythmicity of the eye movements but that the eye movement generator was extravestibular. Magherini and associates (19) found that systemic injections of the anticholinesterase agent physostigmine produced rhythmic eye movements in decerebrate cats, suggesting that the eye movement generator may be cholinergic. Thus the central, automatic activation during sleep of the vestibular system may provide a substrate for endogenously generated, specific information about body position and movement. Flying dreams may thus be a logical, direct, and unsymbolic way of synthesizing information generated endogenously by the vestibular system in D sleep. In view of this reasonable and direct explanation, it seems gratuitous to "interpret" the sensual flying dream as sexual.

In accord with the isomorphism principle, the degree of neuronal activation in brain systems should parallel the frequency and intensity of dreams to these systems (3), and the predominance of visual sensorimotor activity in both brain and mind supports this notion. Symbol formation and the often bizarre juxtaposition of sensations in the dream may be a reflection of the heightened degree of simultaneous activation of multiple sensory channels in dreaming as compared with waking (3).

Long-term electrical stimulation of the pontine brain stem results in the earlier appearance of sleep episodes and in increases in the absolute amounts of desynchronized sleep, but it does not affect the periodicity of its occurrence (20). By implication, the delivery of electrical energy accomplishes what most psychological and behavioral treatments fail to achieve: an increase in the duration of dreaming sleep. Testing the assumption that the generator neurons are cholinoceptive, our laboratory team has recently established that injection of the cholinergic agent carbachol into the pontine reticular formation produces prolonged enhancement of D-like sleep behavior

(21). In man the parenteral injection of the anti-cholinesterase agent physostigmine potentiates D sleep, and the pharmacologically induced episodes are associated with hallucinoid dreaming (22). The time of occurrence and duration of dreams may thus be chemically determined.

In summary, these results support the hypothesis that the pontine brain stem is the generator zone for the D sleep state. The trigger mechanism for the whole system, including the eye movement generator, may be cholinoceptive and the executive zones are probably in the reticular formation. The LC is involved, possibly in a permissive or reciprocal way, and is especially important in mediating spinal reflex inhibition. Together, these two regions may constitute the clock. We will have more to say about the hypothesis of reciprocal interaction between them later in this paper.

Although the brain stem mechanisms mediating atonia remain obscure, it is clear from the work of Pompeiano (6) that both monosynaptic and polysynaptic spinal reflexes are tonically inhibited during D sleep (see figure 57.4). In addition, during the bursts of REM, there is a descending presynaptic inhibition of the most rapidly conducting (group Ia) spinal afferent endings. Both presynaptic and postsynaptic inhibition appear to be of brain stem origin. Phasic presynaptic inhibition has also been shown to occur in sensory relays elsewhere in the brain during D sleep (6). Thus motor output is tonically damped throughout D and sensory input is phasically damped in concert with the REM bursts. In other words, we are not only paralyzed during our dreams, but the degree to which we are paralyzed fluctuates in concert with the intensity of the internally generated information and the degree to which we suppress exogenous input.

On the basis of this evidence, the systems terminology used earlier (see figure 57.1) can be tentatively translated into the anatomical and physiological terms of figure 57.2; and the activation-synthesis hypothesis of dreaming can be

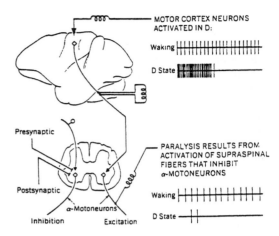

Figure 57.4
Mechanisms of sleep paralysis. The upper part of the figure illustrates the intense activation in D sleep of antidromically identified pyramidal tract neurons of the motor cortex. Note the relatively regular discharge in waking (W) and the clustering of discharges in D sleep in these models of 3-s epochs of microelectrode recordings (vertical lines indicate discharges). The lower portion of the figure shows the inhibitory events of D at the spinal cord level that largely prevent alpha motoneuron discharge and consequent muscle excitation, despite the activation of excitatory (arrow) pyramidal tract fibers. Both presynaptic and postsynaptic inhibition (bars) are present in D (sketched on the left side of the cord section). Absence of this inhibition in W allows alpha motoneuron discharge in response to excitation from pyramidal tract fibers (17).

stated as follows: during D sleep, a cholinergic mechanism in the reticular formation of the pontine brain stem is periodically activated. The consequences of this activation are as follows:

1. The forebrain is tonically activated, probably via the midbrain reticular formation that is also responsible for its activation during waking. Thus the forebrain is made ready to process information.

2. The spinal reflexes are tonically inhibited, possibly via the bulbar reticular formation and LC; thus motor outflow is blocked despite high

levels of activity in the brain, including the motor cortex.

3. The oculomotor and vestibular systems are phasically activated by the pontine reticular formation so as to produce eye movements. This circuitry, in its entirety, is an internal information source or generator that provides the forebrain with spatially specific but temporally disorganized information about eye velocity, relative position, and direction of movement. Information may similarly be derived from the brain stem generators of patterned motor activity.

4. At the same time that internal information feedback is being generated by the activation of various motor systems, exteroceptive input to sensory systems is phasically blocked. This may intensify the relative impact of the endogenous inputs to the brain, accounting for the intensity of dream imagery and preventing sleep disruption by the externally generated excitation.

This working sketch of the dream state generator, based on the classical localizing methods of experimental neurology, is intriguing but unsatisfying in that it fails to specify the mechanisms by which the pontine generator is turned on, kept active for a time, and then shut off. Further, it does not say anything about the mechanism of periodicity. To provide details about the anatomy and physiology of the periodic trigger mechanisms of the generator process, we will now turn our attention to the neuronal level of analysis. In doing so, we also come full circle in our reaffirmation of isomorphism since it was the neuron that Freud recognized as the physical unit of the nervous system on which he based his dream theory (2).

Histological Features of Relevance to the Periodic Triggering of the Dreaming Sleep State Generator

Several structural details of the pontine brain stem are notable as possible elements of a D

sleep control device with rhythmic properties (see figure 57.3 for an illustration of the anatomy discussed).

In his discussion of the histology of the potine brain stem. Cajal (23) emphasized three points:

1. The paramedian reticular giant cells, with their rostral and caudal axonal projections, are admirably suited to serve as output elements of the generator; when excited they could influence many other cells. The work of Brodal (24) and the Scheibels (25) shows that the spinal cord and thalamus receive projections from these elements. Although they are relatively few in number, conservative estimates of their postsynaptic domain indicate that each directly projects to nine million (9×10^6) postsynaptic neurons. Thus the 3,000 pontine reticular giant cells in the cat might make many billions of synapses (2.9×10^{10}). Since the giant cells also project to other brain stem nuclei and have recurrent axons to themselves, mutual interaction with raphe-type elements (see below) and self-reexcitation are both possible. These two features could be used to create excitability variability, with powerful consequences for the whole nervous system.

2. The raphe neurons of the midline are ideally situated and connected to regulate excitability of paramedian elements, and they also have extensive projections to other brain regions. The discovery that these cells concentrate the biogenic amine serotonin (26) gives this regulatory hypothesis an attractive corollary: these cells might regulate excitability of their postsynaptic neurons via specific transmitter substances. Another brain stem cell group, in the locus coeruleus, has been shown to concentrate the amine norepinephrine (26). There are thus at least two neuronal candidates for a level setting role, and both are probably inhibitory. Since the giant cells are excitatory (and probably cholinergic; see below), a substrate for reciprocal interaction is established.

3. Cajal (23) suggested that input to the central reticular core might be via small stellate cells in the lateral zone. This input channel, which we

now know to be more diffuse than was originally suspected, could be used to abort or damp the core oscillator at critical ambient stimulus levels. This is an important feature, since adaptation depends on the capacity to interrupt the cycle and not to incorporate all exogenous stimuli into the dream plot.

Cellular Activity in the Pontine Brain Stem during the Sleep Cycle

A direct experimental approach to the question of D state control has been made with cats by recording from individual neurons in many parts of the brain as the sleep cycle normally evolved. In this experimental paradigm, the frequency and pattern of extracellular action potentials, which are the signal units of nerve cells, are taken as indices of a cell's excitability; the influence of a recorded neuron upon other cells and that neuron's own control mechanism may also be inferred from the data. This method has the advantage of being relatively physiological since it does little to alter or damage the properties of the system under study. When cats are kept active at night, they will sleep under the necessary conditions of restraint during the daytime. The microelectrodes can then be stereotaxically directed at the brain stem and individual cell activity recorded for as long as 20 hours, allowing many successive sleep cycles to be studied (see figure 57.5).

The pontine brain stem control hypothesis has been tested in three ways at the level of single cells.

Selectivity Criterion: Which Cells Change Rate Most in D?

We assumed that cells which showed pronounced alterations in discharge rate over the sleep cycle were more likely to be playing a controlling role than those showing minimal change. We further assumed that those cells having peaks of activity in phase with the D phase of the cycle

were more likely to be specifically and actively involved in dreaming sleep state control than those with multiple peaks. We found that the giant cells of the pontine tegmentum concentrated their discharge in the D phase of sleep to a greater extent than any other group of neurons (27). They became our prime candidate for a generator function.

Tonic Latency Criterion: Which Cells Change Rate First in D Onset?

If the cells with positive discharge selectivity were driving the dreaming sleep phase of the sleep cycle, then their rates would be expected to increase in advance of the behavioral state change. Such phase leads might well be longer than those of the follower neurons under the control of the giant cells. The giant cells, when recorded over entire sleep cycles and through repeated sleep cycles, were found to change rate continuously (28). Significant rate increases occurred *as long as 5 min.* before a desynchronized sleep phase. When the 2 min. just prior to desynchronized sleep onset were studied, a rate increase in a pool of giant cells was observed 10 s before a similar increase in a pool of cerebral cortical neurons.

The rapidly accelerating limb of the giant cell activity curves at D sleep phase onset indicated that this was a time of maximal excitability change in this pool of neurons. The goodness of fit of the data by an exponential curve indicated that reexcitation within the pool might be superimposed upon disinhibition from without. The positive tonic latency indicated that the activation of the forebrain might be a consequence of activation of the brain stem but that the converse could not be the case.

Phasic Latency Criterion: Which Cells Fire before Eye Movements of D?

Because of the proximity and direct projections to oculomotor neurons from giant cells, we tested the possibility that they might be generat-

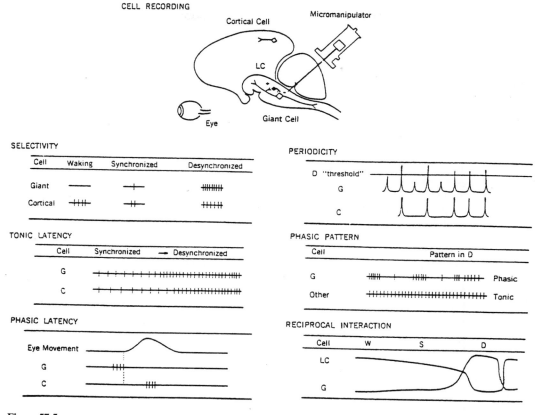

Figure 57.5

Cellular neurophysiology of dream state generation. The cell recordings are made from hydraulically driven microelectrodes that can be stereotaxically directed at neurons in the cat brain during natural sleep. Two classes of brain stem neurons are represented by the reticular giant cell (G in the physiological models) and the LC cell; the synaptic interactions suggested are detailed in figure 57.8. A cortical cell is also shown. The results of the cell recording experiments are shown in six models representing the criteria used to quantify discharge properties: selectivity—giant cells concentrate their discharge in D to a greater extent than cerebral cortical or other brain stem neurons; tonic latency—giant cells show rate increases that precede those of cortical neurons during the S and D transition; phasic latency—giant cells fire before the REMs of D, while cortical neurons fire after them; periodicity—peaks in the giant cell activation curves are periodic and the higher peaks are associated with D sleep episodes and peaks of cortical activity; phasic pattern—giant cells show a higher degree of clustered firing in D than do other neurons; and reciprocal interaction—the rate curves of giant cells and LC cells are reciprocal over the sleep cycle.

ing the REMs so characteristic of the desynchronized phase of sleep by determining the time
of occurrence of short-term rate increases by
the giant cells in relation to eye movement onset.
On the average, such rate increases were more
prominent and anticipated eye movement by
longer intervals than other brain stem neurons
(29). Rate increases by presumed follower elements (in the posterolateral cerebral cortex) *followed* the eye movements by many milliseconds.
It could therefore be concluded that the eye
movements might be initiated by giant cells but
could not be generated by cortical neurons.
This finding practically wrecks the scanning hypothesis and strongly favors the idea that visual
cortical events are determined by events in the
oculomotor brain stem.

At this point we felt justified in concluding
that the giant cells of the pontine tegmentum
were critical output elements in a sleep cycle
control mechanism. More particularly, we proposed that they might be generator elements for
some of the tonic and phasic excitatory events in
the desynchronized sleep phase of the cycles:
most important to the activation-synthesis hypothesis of dreaming are the determination of
EEG desynchronization (activation of the forebrain) and REMs (provision of forebrain with
internally generated information). At the very
least, we felt that we had found an important
avenue to understanding sleep cycle control,
since we could now examine the properties and
possible mechanisms of giant cell excitability
regulation. In this regard there are three additional points worthy of emphasis.

Periodicity Criterion

Long-term recordings of giant cells revealed
peaks of activity in phase with each full-blown
desynchronized sleep episode (30) (see figure
57.6). Less prominent peaks were associated with
abortive episodes and were rarely seen with no
electrographic evidence of desynchronized sleep.
Spectral analysis of these long-term data confirmed the impression of powerful periodicity in
the discharge peaks, indicting that sleep cycles
are periodic, underlying cell activity is probably
even more so, and by definition, cell excitability
is under the control of a neurobiological clock.
The possible mechanisms of excitability control
are thus of great interest.

Phasic Pattern Criterion

The pattern of giant cell discharge within each D
sleep episode indicated that classical pacemaker
mechanisms are *not* involved in giant cell excitability regulation (31). Regular interspike intervals were exceptional, indicating that the rate
increases were not caused by endogenous membrane depolarizations. The tendency, rather, was
for giant cells to discharge in intermittent, prolonged clusters of irregularly distributed spikes
as if the cells were responding to excitatory
postsynaptic potentials from other neurons (see
figure 57.7). In our view, a likely source of much
of this input, especially as the longer clusters
developed, was other giant cells. Once other
neurons were excited, feedback from them is to
be expected. It also seemed likely that the clusters of giant cell discharge were causally related
to the eye movement bursts of the D sleep phase.

Reciprocal Interaction Criterion

If giant cell excitability change is not an intrinsic
property of the giant cells, what other cell group
might regulate it and in what way might that
regulation be effected? Since all indices showed
giant cells to discharge first in relation to both
the tonic and phasic events of desynchronized
sleep, we considered the possible contribution of
inhibitory neurons. Since interneurons do not
appear to exist in the giant cell fields, such cells
should be discrete from but proximal to the giant
cell. To be effective, projections should be abundant and should have inhibitory transmitter
action upon the giant cells. Reciprocal rate
changes during the sleep cycle are to be expected

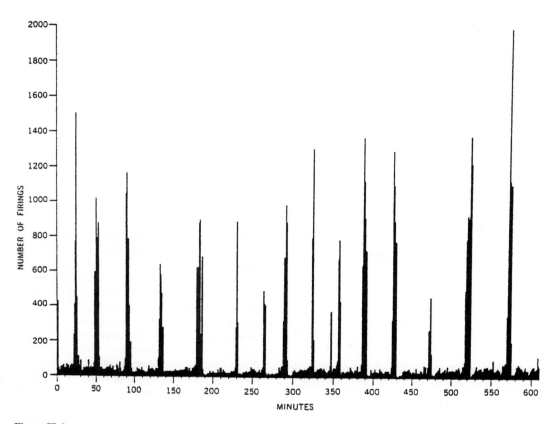

Figure 57.6
Discharge activity of a giant cell neuron recorded over multiple sleep-waking cycles. Each peak corresponds to a desynchronized sleep episode, and a regular trend of discharge activity over a cycle is observable: a peak in desynchronized sleep; a rapid decline at the end of the desynchronized sleep episode; a trough, often associated with waking; a slow rise (in synchronized sleep and preceding all electrographic signs of desynchronized sleep); and an explosive acceleration at the onset of desynchronized sleep. Note also the extreme modulation of activity and the periodicity (30). Reprinted by permission from *Science*, 189, 58–60, July 4, 1975. Copyright 1975 by the American Association for the Advancement of Science.

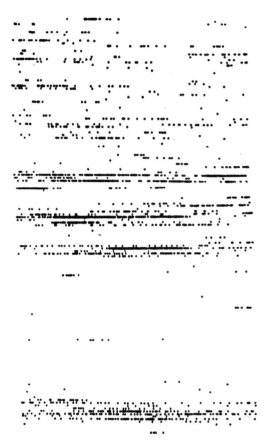

Figure 57.7
Temporal clustering of extracellularly recorded discharges of cat giant cell neurons during D sleep. Each discharge is represented by a dot; the time sequence runs left to right and top to bottom, with each line 1 s in duration. The figure encompasses about 200 s of D sleep activity. Clustering is visible as closely spaced dots and, over longer durations, as "bands" of activity, some of which appear to occur rhythmically. Note the various durations of clusters and the presence of shorter duration clusters of activity within longer duration clusters. Clusters are delimited by periods of relative inactivity. Such sequences of giant cell neuronal activity are temporally associated with runs of eye movements and ponto-geniculo-occipital waves, and

if such cells exist. We have discovered just such changes in a small number of unidentified cells in the region of the posterior locus coeruleus and the nucleus subcoeruleus (32). Not only is discharge concentration of these elements quantitatively inverse to those of the giant cells in the phases of the cycle, but their decelerating rate curve is the approximate mirror image of that of the giant cells at desynchronized sleep onset as seen in part C. We called such cells "D-off" cells to contrast their activity curves with those of the giant cells, prototypes of the "D-on" species of neurons. We do not know if the "D-off" cells are catecholaminergic but their location and discharge properties make this possible.

McGinty and associates (33) have found similar reciprocal rate changes in the dorsal raphe nucleus (DRN) neurons and we have recently confirmed this finding. The low regular rates of discharge by these cells in waking suggest a level-setting or pacemaker function. Their location and discharge properties are the same as those cells thought to be serotonergic on the basis of pharmacological experiments (34). Since both the LC and DRN are adjacent to and project to giant cells, and since giant cells receive abundant serotonergic and catecholaminergic endings, we thought that the mutual interconnections of these D-on and D-off cells could form a substrate for reciprocal interaction which regulated sleep cycle oscillation (30).

A Model for a Brain Stem Sleep Cycle Oscillator

Restricting attention to within-sleep changes, we constructed a physiological model that bears a striking resemblance to the a priori schema derived from Cajal (see figure 57.8, top portion).

similar sequences of executive neuron discharges may represent the neuronal substrate of dream sequences in man (Hobson and McCarley, unpublished data).

a.

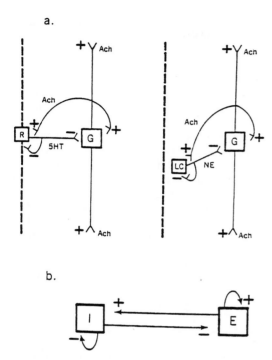

b.

Figure 57.8
Reciprocal interaction model of generator process. Physiological models used to organize and interpret results of pharmacological experiments on desynchronized sleep. The G cells are seen as executive elements; they excite with and are excited by acetylcholine (Ach). They interact reciprocally with two aminergic cell groups, the LC and raphe (R), which utilize norepinephrine (NE) and serotonin (5HT), respectively. Both amines are hypothesized to be inhibitory to the G cells. D sleep will therefore be enhanced by increasing G cell excitability, and this can occur by either adding cholinergic drive or subtracting aminergic inhibition. Conversely, D sleep will be suppressed by subtracting cholinergic drive or by adding aminergic inhibition. Formal reduction of the elements in the top portion of the figure yields the general model of reciprocal interaction, of inhibitory (I.-) and excitatory (E.-) populations, each of which contains a self-loop as well as a projection to the other set. The resulting oscillation of activity in the two sets can be mathematically described by the Lotka-Volterra equations.

Most of the connections have been demonstrated but many of the synaptic assumptions are as yet unproven physiologically. In addition to being explanatory, the model suggests experiments, particularly those employing pharmacological methods, the results of which will lead to its future modification. Since the LC, DRN, and giant cell groups are chemically differentiated, we deduced that their action and interaction may involve specific neurotransmitters.

In preliminary tests of the model, we have found that microinjection of the cholinomimetic substance carbachol into the giant cell zone not only gives more potent desynchronized sleep phase enhancement than injections into the adjacent tegmental fields but simultaneously activates giant cells. The results also indicate that an opposite effect is obtained at locus coeruleus sites (as if an inhibitory cell group were being activated). We have not yet tested this last hypothesis directly, but the LC cells do resume firing before the end of D sleep. We assume that as FTG excitation declines and LC inhibition grows, the cycle ends. In the decerebrate cat, physostigmine-induced D episodes are associated with activation of neurons in the giant cell and suppression of firing by cells in the LC and DRN (35).

The physiological model can be reduced to a simple unit susceptible to mathematical analysis (see figure 57.8, bottom portion). Cell group E (giant cell) and cell group I (raphe and/or LC) are assumed to be mutually interconnected; cell group E is excitatory to itself and to group I, which inhibits itself and group E. Growth of activity in one group occurs at the expense of growth in the other, and vice versa. As such the cell groups are analogous to two populations, prey and predator, whose interaction can be described by a set of nonlinear differential equations, the Lotka-Volterra equations (30). As shown in figure 57.9, the time course of activity of cell group E closely resembles that predicted by these equations. It is now possible to plot the activity curves of cell group I and compare

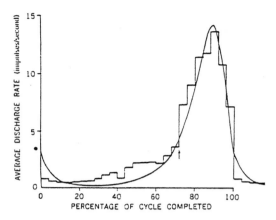

Figure 57.9
Time course of giant cell activity over the sleep cycle. The histogram shows the average discharge level (impulses/second) of a giant cell neuron over 12 sleep-waking cycles, each normalized to constant duration. The cycle begins and ends with the end of a desynchronized sleep period. The arrow indicates the average time of D sleep onset. The smooth curve is derived from a mathematical model of sleep cycle control and shows a good fit to the experimental data. The probability of obtaining dream-like mentation reports might be expected to show the same trajectory as these curves (30). Reprinted by permission from *Science*, 189, 58–60, July 4, 1975. Copyright 1975 by the American Association for the Advancement of Science.

the actual data with the curves predicted by the model. The phase lag between the reciprocal cycles remains to be explained and the previously noted fact that cycle length is proportional to brain size suggests that a distance factor may be at work. The distance between the two cell fields could be such a factor through its determination of protein transport time. Assuming an average LC-FTG internuclear distance of 2.5 mm and a fast protein transport time of 96 mm/day, a period length of about 35 min. is predicted for the cat. This figure is within limits normal for that species. Another possible substrate for the long, size-dependent time constant of the cycle is the

recently discovered class of long-duration postsynaptic transmitter actions (36) that may be mediated by second messengers such as cyclic AMP (37). Since the cyclic nucleotides activate protein kinases, the metabolic activity of the neuron, including the synthesis of neurotransmitters, can be linked to and entrained by membrane events.

An important point is that the mathematical model parallels, but is not identical to, the physiological model. This means that even if the specific assumptions about physiological interaction are incorrect, the mathematical model may be viable and useful in another system—for example, the coupling of the circadian and ultradian oscillators (14) or, at another level of analysis, in a molecular system. This is particularly important to keep in mind since it is also at the molecular level that time constant elements necessary to explain the long periodicity of the sleep-dream cycle may be found.

Psychological Implications of the Cellular Neurophysiology of Dream Sleep Generation

Hallucinoid dreaming is regarded as the psychological concomitant of D sleep. Brain activity in the D state has been analyzed to account for activation of the forebrain, occlusion of sensory input, blockade of motor output at the spinal cord level, and the generation of information within the system. The evidence that the pontine brain stem contains a clock-trigger mechanism that contributes to activation of the forebrain, occlusion of sensory input, and the generation of internal information has been reviewed. The periodicity of the triggering mechanism is hypothesized to be a function of reciprocal interaction of reciprocally connected, chemically coded cell groups in the pontine brain stem.

The psychological implications of this model, which we call the activation-synthesis hypothesis of the dream process (schematically represented in figure 57.10), contrast sharply with many

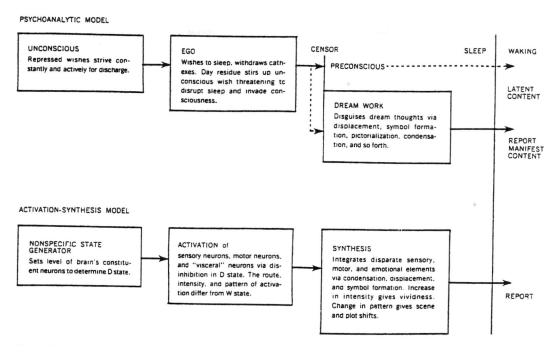

PSYCHOANALYTIC MODEL

Figure 57.10

Two models of the dream process. In the psychoanalytic model the motive force of the process is the dynamically repressed unconscious wish that is released from control in sleep. The dream thoughts that emerge threaten consciousness and sleep; they are deterred by the censor. The "dream work" transforms the unconscious wish by the processes that are listed. The product, or manifest content, that becomes conscious thus contains only disguised elements of the original (latent) dream thoughts. The activation-synthesis model is designed to contrast activation-synthesis theory with the guardian-censorship theory illustrated in the top portion of this figure. The motive force of the process is seen to be nonspecific neural energy or excitation hypothesized to arise from a nonspecific generator. This excitation affects the component systems of the forebrain represented in the upper box: sensory systems generate scene frames, structural fragments, and qualitative features: cognitive systems generate ideas that may be conscious (day residue thoughts) or unconscious (instinctually determined); emotion is also generated at the first stage. The dream report, easily obtainable if a state change to waking occurs, is seen as an accurate reflection of the integrated product of disparate, internally generated elements.

tenets of the dream theory provided by psycho-analysis (also represented in figure 57.10) in the following ways:

1. The primary motivating force for dreaming is not psychological but physiological since the time of occurrence and duration of dreaming sleep are quite constant, suggesting a prepro-grammed, neurally determined genesis. In fact, the neural mechanisms involved can now be precisely specified. This conclusion does not, of course, mean that dreams are not also psycho-logical events; nor does it imply that they are without psychological meaning or function. But it does imply that the process is much more basic than the psychodynamically determined, evanes-cent, "guardian of sleep" process that Freud had imagined it to be; and it casts serious doubt upon the exclusively psychological significance attached to both the occurrence and quality of dreams.

2. Specific stimuli for the dream imagery ap-pear to arise intracerebrally but from the pontine brain stem and not in cognitive areas of the ce-rebrum. These stimuli, whose generation appears to depend upon a largely random or reflex pro-cess, may provide spatially specific information which can be used in constructing dream imag-ery; but the unusual intensity, intermittency, and velocity of the eye movements may also contrib-ute to features of the dream experience which are formally bizarre and have been interpreted as defensive by psychoanalysis. Thus such features as scene shifts, time compression, personal con-densations, splitting, and symbol formation may be directly isomorphic with the state of the ner-vous system during dreaming sleep. In other words, the forebrain may be making the best of a bad job in producing even partially coherent dream imagery from the relatively noisy signals sent up to it from the brain stem.

The dream process is thus seen as having its origin in sensorimotor systems, with little or no primary ideational, volitional, or emotional con-tent. This concept is markedly different from that

of the "dream thoughts" or wishes seen by Freud as the primary stimulus for the dream. The sen-sorimotor stimuli are viewed as possibly provid-ing a frame into which ideational, volitional, or emotional content may be projected to form the integrated dream image, but this frame is itself conflict free. Thus both the major energetic drive for the dream process and the specific primary stimulus of the dream content are genotypically determined and therefore conflict free in the spe-cifically psychodynamic sense of the term.

3. The elaboration of the brain stem stimulus by the perceptual, conceptual, and emotional structures of the forebrain is viewed as primarily a synthetic constructive process, rather than a distorting one as Freud presumed. Best fits to the relative inchoate and incomplete data provided by the primary stimuli are called up from mem-ory, the access to which is facilitated during dreaming sleep. The brain, in the dreaming sleep state, is thus likened to a computer searching its addresses for key words. Rather than indicating a need for disguise, this fitting of phenotypic experiential data to genotypic stimuli is seen as the major basis of the "bizarre" formal qual-ities of dream mentation. There is, therefore, no need to postulate either a censor or an informa-tion degrading process working at the censor's behest. The dream content elaborated by the forebrain may include conflictually charged memories, but even this aspect of dream con-struction is seen as synthetic and transparent rather than degradative and opaque.

4. With respect to the forgetting of dreams, the normally poor recall is seen principally to reflect a state-dependent amnesia, since a care-fully effected state change, to waking, may pro-duce abundant recall even of highly charged dream material. There is thus no need to in-voke repression to account for the forgetting of dreams. This hypothesis is appealingly economi-cal, and in the light of the reciprocal interaction hypothesis dream amnesia can now be modeled in a testable way as the result of a different bal-

ance between cholinergic and aminergic neuronal activity and the resulting effects on second messengers and macromolecules (5). Among its other surprising gifts to psychophysiology, dreaming sleep may thus also provide a biological model for the study of memory, and a functional role for dreaming sleep in promoting some aspect of the learning process is suggested.

Summary and Conclusions

Assuming that isomorphism, or identity of form, must characterize the simultaneous physiological and psychological events during dreaming, we have reviewed the general and cellular neurophysiology of dreaming sleep in search of new ways of accounting for some of the formal aspects of dream psychology. We have noted that the occurrence of dreaming depends upon the periodic activation of the forebrain during sleep. We have hypothesized that the activated forebrain synthesizes the dreams by fitting experiential data to information endogenously and automatically generated by reticular, vestibular, and oculomotor neurons in the pontine brain stem. A specific physiological and mathematical model of the pontine generator, based upon single cell recording studies in cats, is described: the model posits reciprocal interaction between inhibitory aminergic (level-setting) and excitatory cholinergic (generator) neurons.

Some of the "bizarre" formal features of the dream may directly reflect the properties of the brain stem neuronal generator mechanism. The physiological features of the generator mechanisms and their corresponding psychological implications include the following: the automaticity and periodicity of activation indicate a metabolically determined, conflict-free energetics of the dream process; the random but specific nature of the generator signals could provide abnormally sequenced and shaped, but spatiotemporally specific, frames for dream imagery; and the clustering of runs of generator signals

might constitute time-marks for dream subplots and scene changes. Further, the activation by generator neurons of diffuse postsynaptic forebrain elements in multiple parallel channels might account for the disparate sensory, motor, and emotional elements that contribute to the "bizarreness" of dreams; the suppression of motor output and sensory input simultaneous with central activation of both sensory and motor patterns could assure the maintenance of sleep in the face of massive central excitation of the brain; and the change in the ratio of neurotransmitters affecting forebrain neurons might account for dream amnesia and indicate a state-dependent alteration of neural plasticity, with implications for the learning process.

Acknowledgments

Based on the text of the Sandoz Lecture presented by Dr. Hobson at the University of Edinburgh, April 23, 1975.

The research described herein was supported by Alcohol, Drug Abuse, and Mental Health Administration grant MH-13923 from the National Institute of Mental Health and by the Milton Fund of Harvard University.

The authors wish to express their appreciation to Drs. John Nemiah and John Nelson for their helpful comments on the manuscript.

References

1. Freud S: The interpretation of dreams (1900), in The Complete Psychological Works, standard ed, vols 4 and 5. Translated and edited by Strachey J. London, Hogarth Press, 1966

2. McCarley RW, Hobson JA: The neurobiological origins of psychoanalytic dream theory. Am J Psychiatry 134:1211–1221, 1977

3. McCarley RW: Mind-body isomorphism and the study of dreams, in Advances in Sleep Research, vol 6. Edited by Fishbein W. New York, Spectrum, 1981

4. Dement W, Kleitman N: The relation of eye movements during sleep to dream activity: an objective method for the study of dreaming. J Exp Psychol 53:89–97, 1957

5. Hobson JA: The reciprocal interaction model of sleep cycle control: implication for PGO wave generation and dream amnesia, in Sleep and Memory. Edited by Drucker-Colin R, McGaugh J. New York, Academic Press, 1977, pp 159–183

6. Pompeiano O: The neurophysiological mechanisms of the postural and motor events during desynchronized sleep. Res Publ Assoc Res Nerv Ment Dis 45:351–423, 1967

7. Jouvet M, Delorme F: Locus coeruleus et sommeil paradoxol. Soc Biol 159:895, 1965

8. Volkman F: Vision during voluntary saccadic eye movements. J Opt Soc Am 52:571–578, 1962

9. Bizzi E: Discharge pattern of single geniculate neurons during the rapid eye movements of sleep. J Neurophysiol 29:1087–1095, 1966

10. Evarts EV: Activity of individual cerebral neurons during sleep and arousal. Res Publ Assoc Res Nerv Ment Dis 45:319–337, 1967

11. Hobson JA, Goldfrank F, Snyder F: Sleep and respiration. J Psychiatr Res 3:79–90, 1965

12. Roffwarg HP, Dement WC, Muzio JN, et al: Dream imagery: relationship to rapid eye movements of sleep. Arch Gen Psychiatry 7:235–258, 1962

13. Pompeiano O: Sensory inhibition during motor activity in sleep, in Neurophysiological Basis of Normal and Abnormal Motor Activities. Edited by Yahr MD, Purpura DP. New York, Raven Press, 1967, pp 323–375

14. Hobson JA: The sleep-dream cycle, a neurobiological rhythm, in Pathobiology Annual. Edited by Ioachim H. New York, Appleton-Century-Crofts, 1975, pp 369–403

15. Zepelin H, Rechtschaffen A: Mammalian sleep, longevity and energy metabolism. Brain Behav Evol 10:425–470, 1974

16. Dement W: The occurrence of low-voltage fast electroencephalogram patterns during behavioral sleep in the cat. Electroencephalogr Clin Neurophysiol 10:291–296, 1958

17. Jouvet M: Recherches sur les structures nerveuses et les mecanismes responsables des differentes phases du sommeil physiologique. Arch Ital Biol 100:125–206, 1962

18. Pompeiano O, Morrison AR: Vestibular influences during sleep. I. Abolition of the rapid eye movements of desynchronized sleep following vestibular lesions. Arch Ital Biol 103:569–595, 1965

19. Magherini PC, Pompeiano O, Thoden U: Cholinergic mechanisms related to REM sleep. I. Rhythmic activity of the vestibulo-oculomotor system induced by an anticholinesterase in the decerebrate cat. Arch Ital Biol 110:234–259, 1972

20. Frederickson CJ, Hobson JA: Electrical stimulation of the brain stem and subsequent sleep. Arch Ital Biol 108:564–576, 1970

21. Amatruda TT, Black DA, McKenna TM, et al: Sleep cycle control and cholinergic mechanisms: differential effects of carbachol at pontine brain stem sites. Brain Res 98:501–515, 1975

22. Sitaram N, Wyatt RJ, Dawson S, et al: REM sleep induction by physostigmine infusion during sleep. Science 191:1281–1283, 1976

23. Cajal R: Histologie du System Nerveux, vol 1. Madrid, Consejo Superior de Investigaciones Cientificas, 1952

24. Brodal A: The Reticular Formation of the Brain Stem. Anatomical Aspects and Functional Correlations. Edinburgh, Oliver and Boyd, 1957

25. Scheibel ME, Scheibel AB: Anatomical basis of attention mechanisms in vertebrate brains, in The Neurosciences: A Study Program. Edited by Quarton GC, Melnechuk T, Schmitt FO. New York, Rockefeller University Press, 1967, pp 577–602

26. Dahlstrom A, Fuxe K: Evidence for the existence of monoamine-containing neurons in the central nervous system. I. Demonstration of monoamines in the cell bodies of brain stem neurons. Acta Physiol Scand 62:1–55, 1964

27. Hobson JA, McCarley RW, Pivik RT, et al: Selective firing by cat pontine brain stem neurons in desynchronized sleep. J Neurophysiol 37:497–511, 1974

28. Hobson JA, McCarley RW, Freedman R, et al: Time course of discharge rate changes by cat pontine brain stem neurons during the sleep cycle. J Neurophysiol 37:1297–1309, 1974

29. Pivik RT, McCarley RW, Hobson JA: Eye movement-associated discharge in brain stem neurons

during desynchronized sleep. Brain Res 121:59–76, 1977

30. McCarley RW, Hobson JA: Neuronal excitability modulation over the sleep cycle: a structural and mathematical model. Science 189:58–60, 1975

31. McCarley RW, Hobson JA: Discharge patterns of cat pontine brain stem neurons during desynchronized sleep. J Neurophysiol 38:751–766, 1975

32. Hobson JA, McCarley RW, Wyzinski PW: Sleep cycle oscillation: reciprocal discharge by two brainstem neuronal groups. Science 189:55–58, 1975

33. McGinty DJ, Harper RM, Fairbanks MK: 5 HT-containing neurons: unit activity in behaving cats, in Serotonin and Behavior. Edited by Barchas J, Usdin E. New York, Academic Press, 1973, pp 267–279

34. Aghajanian GK, Foote WE, and Sheard MH: Action of psychogenic drugs on single midbrain raphe neurons. J Pharmacol Exp Ther 171:178–187, 1970

35. Pompeiano O, Hoshino K: Central control of posture: reciprocal discharge by two pontine neuronal groups leading to suppression of decerebrate rigidity. Brain Res 116:131–138, 1976

36. Libet B: Generation of slow inhibitory and excitatory postsynaptic potentials. Fed Proc 29:1945–1955, 1970

37. Bloom FE: Role of cyclic nucleotides in central synaptic function. Rev Physiol Biochem Pharmacol 74:1–103, 1975

58

Stephen P. LaBerge, Lynn E. Nagel, William C. Dement, and Vincent P. Zarcone, Jr.

That we sometimes dream while knowing that we are dreaming was first noted by Aristotle. According to accounts of conscious or "lucid" dreaming, as this phenomenon is commonly termed, the dreamer can possess a consciousness fully comparable in coherence, clarity, and cognitive complexity to that of the waking state, while continuing to dream vividly (Van Eeden 1913, Brown 1936, Green 1968, Tart 1979, LaBerge 1980b). As a result of theoretical assumptions about the nature of dreaming, contemporary dream researchers have questioned whether these experiences take place during sleep or during brief periods of hallucinatory wakefulness. The purpose of the present study was to give an empirical answer to this question by determining the physiological conditions in which lucid dreaming occurs.

Our experimental approach was suggested by previous investigations (Antrobus, et al. 1965, Salamy 1970, Brown and Cartwright 1978), showing that sleeping subjects are sometimes able to produce behavioral responses highly correlated with dreaming. Since these subjects have not, according to Cartwright (1978), been conscious of making the responses, these earlier studies do not provide evidence for voluntary action (and thus, reflective consciousness) during sleep. However, we reasoned that what could be done unconsciously could also be done consciously.

The experience of one of us (S.P.L.) indicated that, if subjects became aware they were dreaming, they could also remember to perform previously intended dream actions. Because dreamed gaze and limb actions have sometimes shown very good correlations with polygraphically recorded eye movements and muscle activation (Rechtschaffen 1973), it seemed plausible that lucid dreamers could signal that they knew they were dreaming by means of intentional dream actions having observable physiological correlates.

Method and Results

Five subjects, trained in the method of lucid dream induction (MILD) described by LaBerge (1980c), were selected on the basis of their claimed ability to have lucid dreams on demand, and studied for 2–20 nonconsecutive nights (see table 58.1). Standard polysomnograms (Rechtschaffen and Kales 1968), that is, electroencephalogram (EEG), electro-oculogram (EOG), and chin electromyogram (EMG), were recorded, as well as left and right wrist EMG (for signaling). The subjects attempted to follow a predetermined procedure of signaling whenever they became aware that they were dreaming. A variety of signals were specified, generally consisting of a combination of dreamed eye movements and a pattern of left and right dream-fist clenches. The subjects demonstrated the signals during pre-recording calibrations but were asked not to practice further while awake.

In the course of the study, 35 lucid dreams were reported subsequent to spontaneous awakening from various stages of sleep as follows: rapid-eye-movement (REM) sleep in 32 cases, non-REM (NREM) stage 1 twice, and during the transition from NREM stage 2 to REM once.

The subjects reported signaling during 30 of these lucid dreams. After each recording, the reports mentioning signals were submitted along with the respective polysomnogram to a judge uninformed of the times of the reports. The judge was asked to determine whether one (or none) of the polysomnographic epochs corresponded with the reported lucid dream signal. In 24 cases, the judge was able to select the ap-

Table 58.1
Summary of lucid dream signaling experiments

Subject (age, sex)	Nights recorded	Lucid dreams reported (sleep stage)	Lucid dream signals verified*/reported
S.L. (32 yr., M)	20	17 (REM)	14/15
R.K. (28 yr., M)	4	5 (REM)	3/5
L.L. (34 yr., F)	2	1 (REM)	0/0
		2 (NREM-1)	0†/1
B.K. (27 yr., F)	6	6 (REM)	5/6
		1 (NREM-2/REM)††	0/0
S.P. (26 yr., M)	2	2 (REM)	2/2

* Blindly matched for correspondence between reported and observed signals.
† On awakening from NREM Stage 1 sleep (2 min. after having awakened from REM), the subject reported performing the agreed-upon signal during a vivid and lengthy lucid dream. However, neither her EOG nor wrist EMG showed any sign of the reported signals, as might be expected from the normal lack of correspondence between dream gaze and eye movements during descending Stage 1 sleep (Rechtschaffen, 1973).
†† The subject awoke, in this case, during the transition from NREM Stage 2 to REM.

propriate 30-s epochs (out of about 1000 per polysomnogram) on the basis of correspondence between reported and observed signals (table 58.1). The probability that the selections were correct by chance alone is astronomically small. All signals associated with lucid dream reports occurred during epochs of unambiguous REM sleep scored according to the standard criteria (Rechtschaffen and Kales 1968). The lucid dream signals were followed by an average of 1 min. (range: 5–450 s) of uninterrupted REM sleep.

Inspection of the polysomnographic epochs preceding the lucid dream signal reports suggested the failures with blind matching (the "false negatives") were due to high baseline EOG and wrist EMG activity, resulting in an unfavorable signal-to-noise ratio. However, no clear instances of signals were observed except where reported, that is, there were no "false positives." On the other hand, in many cases, the reported signals were unequivocal (see figures 58.1 and 58.2). The most reliable signal was a series of extreme horizontal eye movements (left, right, left, right.)

The most complicated signal (shown in figure 58.1) consisted of a single upward dream-eye movement followed by a series of left (L) and right (R) dream-fist clenches in the order "LLL LRLL." This sequence is equivalent to the subject's initials in Morse code (LLL = $\cdots$ = S; LRLL = $\cdot - \cdot\cdot$ = L). The complexity of this signal argues against the possibility that the EMG discharges might be spontaneous.

That all cases of lucid dream signaling occurred during epochs scored as REM sleep specifies, to a certain extent, the physiology of lucid dreaming as "a relatively low voltage, mixed frequency EEG in conjunction with episodic REMs and low amplitude electromyogram (EMG)" (Rechtschaffen and Kales 1968). This definition allows variation in the three parameters, the details of which will be reported elsewhere. In brief, the variations in the EEG patterns of the lucid dream polysomnograms were typical of REM sleep, that is, sporadic "saw-tooth" waves as well as alpha and theta rhythm, and not wakefulness. The occasional, but normal, appearance of alpha rhythm (a brain wave usually associated with wakefulness), in the

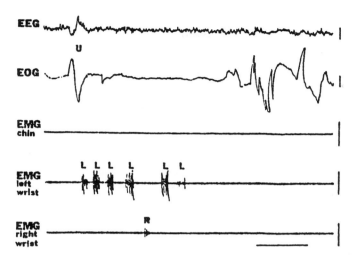

Figure 58.1
Polygraph record of a subject signaling that he knows he is dreaming. The subject awoke approximately 20 s after this excerpt and reported recognizing that he was dreaming and performing the agreed upon signal in the dream, that is, he directed his dream gaze upwards momentarily (U) and then executed a sequence of dreamed left (L) and right (R) fist clenches, Morse code for S. L., the subject's initials. Note that unlike the predominantly horizontal eye movements (above right), the extreme upward eye movement (U) produces characteristic artifact in the EEG channel. All three of the scoring criteria for REM sleep are met: low amplitude chin EMG, episodic REMs, and low-voltage, mixed-frequency EEG (Rechtschaffen and Kales 1968). The EEG shows occasional 10-Hz (alpha) activity as is normal during REM sleep (Rechtschaffen 1973); integration of the alpha band-pass filtered EEG showed the amount of alpha activity during the lucid dream did not significantly differ from that during the preceding nonlucid portion of the REM period. (Calibrations: 50 μV; 5 s)

EEG during REM periods raises the possibility that lucid dreaming could occur during momentary partial arousals or "micro-awakenings" (Schwartz and Lefebvre 1973). However, alpha rhythm need not be present during lucid dream signaling, as is shown by figure 58.2. Furthermore, some of the lucid dreams were several minutes long, ruling out any explanation based on the notion of brief intrusions of wakefulness.

Discussion

How do we know that the subjects were "really asleep" when they communicated the signals? If we allow perception of the external world as a criterion of being awake, we can conclude the subjects were indeed asleep: Although they knew they were in the laboratory, this knowledge was a matter of memory, not perception; upon awakening, they reported having been totally in the dream world and not in sensory contact with the external world. Neither were the subjects merely not attending to the environment, for example, as when absorbed in reading or daydreaming; according to their reports, they were specifically aware of the *absence* of sensory input from the external world. If subjects were to claim to have been awake while showing physiological signs of sleep, or vice versa, we might doubt their subjective reports. However, in the present case, the subjective accounts and physiological mea-

(A) AWAKE

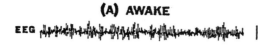

EEG

(B) LUCID DREAM

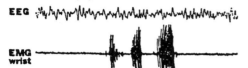

EEG

EMG
wrist

Figure 58.2
Comparison of EEG (C3/A2) during lucid dream signaling (*b*) and immediately after awakening (*a*). The continuous waking alpha (10 Hz) activity for this subject is clearly distinct from the mixed frequency patterns during REM sleep. Although other EEG patterns are compatible with wakefulness, the tracing illustrated is the pattern normally exhibited when subjects awaken from sleep. The 2- and 4-Hz EEG activity prominent in the lucid dream sample (*b*) is highly characteristic of REM sleep. (Calibrations: 50 µV; 1 s)

sures are in clear agreement, and it would be extremely unparsimonious to suppose that subjects who believed themselves to be asleep while showing physiological indications of sleep were actually awake.

The two principal conclusions of this study are that lucid dreaming can occur during REM sleep and that it is possible for lucid dreamers to signal intentionally to the environment while continuing to dream. These findings have both theoretical and practical consequences. The first result shows that under certain circumstances, dream cognition during REM sleep can be much more reflective and rational than has been commonly assumed. Evidence indicating that lucid dreaming is a learnable skill (LaBerge 1979, 1980a,b,c), taken with the second result, suggests the feasibility of a new approach to dream research: lucidly dreaming subjects could carry out diverse experiments marking the exact time of occurrence of particular dream events,

which would allow the derivation of precise psychophysiological correlations and methodical testing of hypotheses.

Acknowledgments

The writing of this manuscript was supported, in part, by the Holmes Center for Research in Holistic Healing. We are grateful to Drs. J. van den Hoed and R. Coleman for helpful comments and Mr. R. Baldwin, Ms. S. Bornstein, and Mr. S. Coburn for expert technical assistance.

References

Antrobus, J. S., Antrobus, J. S., and Fisher, C. Discrimination of dreaming and nondreaming sleep. *Archives of General Psychiatry*, 1965, 12, 395–401.

Brown, A. E. Dreams in which the dreamer knows he is asleep. *Journal of Abnormal and Social Psychology*, 1936, 31, 59–66.

Brown, J. N., and Cartwright, R. Locating NREM dreaming through instrumental responses. *Psychophysiology*, 1978, 15, 35–39.

Cartwright, R. [Response to review of Brown and Cartwright (1978).] *Sleep Reviews*, 1978, 166, 30.

Green, C. *Lucid dreams*. London: Hamilton, 1968.

LaBerge, S. Lucid dreaming: some personal observations. *Sleep Research*, 1979, 8, 153.

LaBerge, S. P. Induction of lucid dreams. *Sleep Research*, 1980, 9, 138. (a)

LaBerge, S. P. Lucid dreaming: an exploratory study of consciousness during sleep. Ph.D. dissertation, Stanford Univer., 1980. (University Microfilms International, 80-24, 691) (b)

LaBerge, S. P. Lucid dreaming as a learnable skill: a case study. *Perceptual and Motor Skills*, 1980, 51, 1039–1042. (c)

Rechtschaffen, A. The psychophysiology of mental activity during sleep. In F. J. McGuigan and R. A. Schoonover (Eds.), *The psychophysiology of thinking*. New York: Academic Press, 1973. Pp. 153–200.

Rechtschaffen, A., and Kales, A. (Eds.), *A manual of standardized terminology, techniques and scoring system for sleep stages of human subjects.* Washington, D.C.: United States Government Printing Office, 1968. (National Institute of Health Publication No. 204)

Salamy, J. Instrumental responding to internal cues associated with REM sleep. *Psychonomic Science*, 1970, 18, 342–343.

Schwartz, B. A., and Lefebvre, A. Contacts veille/ P.M.O. II: Les P.M.O. morcelees. *Revue d'Electroencephalographie et de Neurophysiologie Clinique*, 1973, 3, 165–176.

Tart, C. S. From spontaneous event to lucidity: a review of attempts to control nocturnal dreaming. In B. B. Wolman (Ed.), *Handbook of dreams*. New York: Van Nostrand Reinhold, 1979. Pp. 226–268.

VanEeden, F. A. A study of dreams. *Proceedings of the Society for Psychical Research*, 1913, 26, 431–461. [Reprinted in C. T. Tart (Ed.), *Altered states of consciousness*. New York: Wiley, 1969. Pp. 145–158]

59

Commentary: Of Dreaming and Wakefulness

Rodolfo Llinás and Denis Paré

Introduction

Some of the truly important issues in neuroscience relate to the ability of the brain to generate global functional states that may significantly alter the relationship of the organism to its environment. Among these, the differences between the wakefulness and sleep states are perhaps the best known to everyone. Nevertheless, and in spite of considerable advances toward an understanding of the physiological and behavioral characterization of these states,[40] their functional meaning remains elusive.[106]

A point that we consider fundamental to understanding CNS function lies in the similarities and differences between wakefulness and paradoxical sleep. In fact, at the end of this essay, we will conclude that, from the standpoint of the thalamocortical system, *the overall functional states present during paradoxical sleep and wakefulness are fundamentally equivalent* although the handling of sensory information and cortical inhibition is different in the two states. The implications of this conclusion are far reaching since wakefulness may then be considered as nothing other than a highly coherent intrinsic functional state strongly modulated by sensory input. That is, paradoxical sleep and wakefulness are seen as almost identical intrinsic functional states in which subjective awareness is generated.[60]

Paradoxical Sleep

Four major sleep stages (stages I–IV) have been distinguished on the basis of behavioral and physiological criteria and most of the functional variables examined fluctuate according to the stages. For example, the electrorhythmicity [electroencephalogram (EEG), electromyogram, electrooculogram][6,22] autonomic responsiveness[83] and sensory thresholds for awaken-

ing[89,117] vary in a well-defined manner with the sleep stages.

Aserinsky and Kleitman[6] and Dement and Kleitman[22] were the first to describe the cyclic variations of the human EEG during sleep. About every 90–100 min, the EEG cycles between the low-amplitude, high-frequency waves typical of stage I and the high-amplitude, low-frequency waves of stage IV. As sleep proceeds, the amount of time spent in the deeply synchronized stages (stages III and IV) progressively decreases while that spent in desynchronized sleep increases.[6,22] Finally, it was soon recognized by those authors that the EEG-desynchronization occurring during sleep (called paradoxical sleep) was, in fact, quite similar to the desynchronized activity that characterizes wakefulness.

Perhaps the most salient differences between wakefulness and rapid eye movement (REM) sleep are: (i) paradoxical sleep is characterized by the repeated occurrence of REMs,[7] from which the alternative designation "REM sleep" was derived: (ii) sensory input does not generate the expected cognitive consequences it does in the awake state; and (iii) from a motor point of view, complete muscular atonia is present during REM sleep.

With respect to other sleep states, REM sleep differs in that (i) sensory thresholds for awakening are the highest in REM sleep, except for stage IV[89,117] and (ii) subjects awakened during REM sleep often report having been dreaming.[6]

Studies in other mammalian forms extended these findings in several important respects. For instance, it was found by Jouvet and collaborators that REM sleep in felines is characterized by generalized muscular atonia,[49] which upon further investigation was found to be accompanied by a marked depression of motor reflexes.[87] These phenomena are probably due to the increased activity of the inhibitory medullary reticulospinal neurons.[30,77] A detailed study of the REMs that accompany REM sleep demonstrated that concurrent with their appearance were bursts of electrical activity in the pons, lateral geniculate nucleus (LGN), oculomotor nuclei, and occipital cortex. These transients were called ponto-geniculooccipital (PGO) waves and occur just before[110] and during REM sleep.[50,74,80] More modern research has pinpointed the actual site of generation of this activity.[65,66]

Rapid Eye Movement Sleep and Wakefulness Are Fundamentally Equivalent Functional States

Physiological Comparison of the Two States

Sensory Evoked Potentials and Unit Activities Elicited by Central Electrical Stimulation

Sensory Stimuli In general, the averaged evoked potentials (AEPs) recorded from the scalp in response to sensory stimulation during waking and REM sleep are very similar, but differ strikingly from those recorded during non-REM sleep. We will consider auditory and somatosensory human studies as well as animal studies in which the excitability of thalamic and cortical neurons was tested by means of direct electrical stimulation.

The Auditory System The auditory evoked potential comprises several components. In humans, the early components (<10 ms, thought to reflect the responses of various brainstem and possibly thalamic nuclei)[76] do not display state-dependent fluctuations during the sleep-waking cycle[15,29,86] apart from small-latency variations related to changes in body temperature.[8] However, some middle-latency components (10–80 ms, thought to reflect early thalamocortical activity) decreased in amplitude from waking to stage IV but, returned to normal[16] or surpassed waking values in REM sleep.[20,72,73]

Few studies have dealt with the state-dependent fluctuations of the long-latency components which are relatively insensitive to the properties of the stimulus, but do change with attention level and task requirements.[76] In a study by Wesensten and Badia,[112] subjects learned to differentiate between target and non-target stimuli and auditory evoked responses were recorded for each type of stimulus during various stages of sleep. Although the evoked responses to targeted and non-targeted stimuli were most clearly distinguished when the subjects were awake, a slight difference between these two types of response was also seen during REM sleep. This indicates that the presence of a weak sensory specification may occur during REM sleep. In agreement with this finding is the common observation that occasionally sensory stimuli may be embedded into an ongoing dream or trigger a specific dream sequence, in which such stimulus is a nucleating point. Alternatively, these stimuli may be integrated into cognitive constructs in which their significance may be quite different from that in the waking stage.

The Somatosensory System Short-, middle- and long-latency components are also distinguished in somatosensory evoked potentials. Although the latencies and anatomical correlations are the subject of some controversy, the early components (<19 ms) are thought to reflect activity in the peripheral nerve (9 ms), spinal cord (11 ms), dorsal column nuclei and brainstem (12 ms), as well as in the cerebellum and thalamus (14–18 ms). The earliest activity in the cerebral cortex (19–20 ms) is followed by middle- and long-latency components which are highly dependent on task requirements and attentional level.[25]

Among the early components, only the positivity at 15 ms (P15) did not display state-dependent fluctuations.[119] The amplitude of the other components decreased markedly from waking to stage IV but partially recovered in REM sleep[119] (figure 59.1). The latency of the

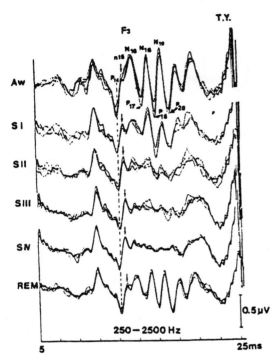

Figure 59.1
State-dependent fluctuations of short-latency somatosensory evoked potentials in humans. Digitally filtered (250–2500 Hz) traces showing the potentials evoked by median nerve stimulation during different sleep stages (indicated on the left). Note that most components are attenuated during stages I–IV but recover in REM sleep. (Reproduced with permission from Yamada et al.[119])

P20 component (which presumably reflects the primary cortical response) increased from waking to stage IV, but returned close to waking values in REM sleep.[119] However, the late components (P100, P200, P300) were abolished in REM sleep.[32,111]

Electrical Stimuli

The Visual System The excitability of the visual pathways during REM sleep cannot be tested

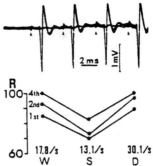

Figure 59.2
Antidromic responsiveness of a corticothalamic neuron during the sleep-waking cycle. Area 5 neuron backfired from the nucleus centrum medianum of a cat. A four-shock train was applied periodically during a complete sleep cycle and the probability of antidromic invasion (R, bottom part) to the first, second, and fourth shocks was computed in waking (W), slow-wave sleep (S), and REM sleep (D). Note that the responsiveness decreased from waking to slow-wave sleep but returned to waking levels in REM sleep. (Reproduced with permission from Steriade et al.[104])

with photic stimulation due to miosis.[10] We must therefore turn our attention to experiments performed in chronically implanted, naturally sleeping animals. In this case the spontaneous and evoked activity of thalamocortical and corticofugal neurons were tested with central electrical stimulation. Single-unit recordings showed that the discharge rate of thalamocortical and corticofugal neurons is generally higher in REM sleep than in the waking state.[cf.105] In addition, the ortho- and/or antidromic excitability of these cells was the same or higher in REM sleep than in awake animals[13,31,82,102,104] (figure 59.2). In particular, the probability of orthodromic activation of dorsal LGN neurons by optic tract stimulation increased above waking levels during REM sleep.[13]

At the cortical level, evoked potential studies of thalamic and cortical regions devoted to motor control suggest that their synaptic excit-

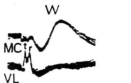
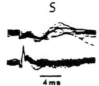
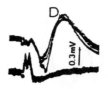

Figure 59.3
Simultaneously recorded field potentials in the ventral lateral thalamic nucleus (VL) and motor cortex (MC) followed stimulation of the superior cerebellar peduncle during waking (W), slow-wave sleep (S), and REM sleep (D). t, Presynaptic (tract) components; r, monosynaptic response. Note the almost complete abolition of thalamic and cortical responses in slow-wave sleep and their recovery above waking values in REM sleep. (Reproduced with permission from Steriade et al.[102])

ability diminishes from waking (W) to slow-wave sleep (S) but surpasses waking values in REM sleep[99,102] (figure 59.3). Finally, in contrast to wakefulness, REM sleep was shown to be accompanied by a reduction of inhibitory activity in cortical neurons.[95]

Significance of the High Sensory Thresholds for Awakening During Rapid Eye Movement Sleep

Since the brain's response to sensory stimulation is very similar during REM sleep and wakefulness, the threshold for awakening should be lowest in REM sleep. Animal and human studies indicate that this in fact is not the case. In cats, Jouvet and collaborators[50] found that the auditory threshold for awakening was clearly higher in REM sleep than in deep slow-wave sleep while Dement[21] found that the auditory threshold was comparable or slightly lower in REM sleep than in deep slow-wave sleep.

Similarly, studies in humans found that the percentage of awakenings evoked by auditory stimuli decreased from stage I to stage IV with REM sleep displaying intermediate values between stages III and IV.[89,117]

These studies draw our attention to the central paradox of REM sleep. Namely, that stimuli which are perceived in the waking state do not awaken subjects in REM sleep, even though the amplitude of the primary evoked cortical responses is generally similar to, or higher than, in the waking state (see section "Physiological Comparison of the Two Gates"). In other words, although the thalamocortical network appears to be at least as excitable during REM sleep as in the waking state, the input is mostly ignored.

Does the lack of behavioral response to suprathreshold sensory stimuli reflect the somatic paralysis characterizing REM sleep, or rather, a difference in the way the brain processes sensory input? The latter explanation seems to be more likely.

The first line of evidence comes from studies of the sensory responsiveness of sleeping cats in which the muscular atonia of REM sleep was suppressed by a small pontine lesion.[48] Although these animals can execute complex sequences of species-specific behavior during REM sleep, they were unresponsive to peripheral stimulation.[48] Similar events occur in humans with pontine lesions due to the lack of motor paralysis which normally accompanies REM sleep. These patients act their dreams out, endangering their lives and that of their bed-fellows.[90]

The second line of evidence is found in cases of sleep disturbances such as the cataplexy of narcoleptic patients,[51] or the postdormatory paralysis displayed by otherwise normal patients.[1] Indeed, about 70% of narcoleptics report cataplexy and are otherwise fully awake and conscious of their environment but cannot move.[51] Following the period of cataplexy, these subjects can provide a detailed description of events occurring during such periods.[1] Similarly, although subjects experiencing postdormatory paralysis are fully awake and oriented, they lack muscle tone and cannot make voluntary movements. These paralytic attacks generally occur at the end of a night of sleep and can be terminated by a slight stimulation such as a light touch.[1]

Therefore, if the high sensory thresholds to awakening do not reflect somatic paralysis during REM sleep, the resolution of the paradox probably lies in the nature of brain function, in a most fundamental sense. In particular, that the late potentials (P100, P200, P300) following sensory stimuli are abolished in REM sleep[32,111] suggests that the ongoing activity that generates cognition during dreaming prevents the early thalamocortical activation from being incorporated into the intrinsic cognitive world. Perhaps then, an altered state of attention is the most likely origin for the high awakening from REM sleep. This issue will be discussed further later on.

Wakefulness as an Intrinsic State Fundamentally Similar to Rapid Eye Movement Sleep, but Specified by Sensory Inputs

The only tool available to study the functional state of the brain during REM sleep is a comparison of the dreams of control subjects with those of patients suffering from various central and peripheral dysfunctions.

Developmental studies by cognitive psychologists have led to the conclusion that dreaming is subjected to the constraints of general cognitive maturation.[28]

Moreover, the decline of higher cognitive abilities following circumscribed lesions of the temporal and parietal associative areas is also reflected in dream contents.[89a] For instance,

patients afflicted with unilateral neglect resulting from right parietal lobe damage in which the opposite half of the visual field is not perceived, report a similar lack of perception in their dreams (M. Mesulam, personal communication). Similarly, people inhabiting the dreams of prosopagnosic subjects are faceless (A. Damasio, personal communication). Interestingly, when awake these patients perceive facial features but they cannot use such features to recognize individual faces. This fact suggests that dreaming operates on integrated symbolic structures and that sensory inputs which are not integrated in these structures during the waking state cannot be reproduced in the dreaming process. Furthermore, these observations indicate that mentation during dreaming operates on the same anatomical substrate as does perception during the waking state.

This view is supported by the analysis of the dream content of patients who acquire peripheral sensory neuropathologies late in life. In these patients, the dream scenes contain vivid sensations that incorporate the affected sensory modalities. For example, one subject who suffered total blindness due to bilateral retinal detachment in his adult life reported totally detailed visual imagery during dreaming but "returns to blindness" upon waking up.[41]

Thus, the evidence reviewed so far indicates that waking and REM sleep are similar in a number of respects. As far as we can tell from the studies on the state-dependent changes in sensory evoked potentials, the excitability of the thalamocortical system is essentially equivalent in the two states. Moreover, neuropsychological investigations indicate that even if dreams may seem irrational by waking standards, they still reflect the cognitive abilities present in the waking state.

Following upon what has been discussed, we may conclude that a possible approach to understanding the nature of wakefulness is to consider it as one element in a category of intrinsic brain functions, in which REM sleep is another element. The difference between these two states would be that in REM sleep, the sensory specification of the functionalities carried out by the brain is fundamentally altered. That is, *REM sleep can be considered as a modified attentive state in which attention is turned away from the sensory input, toward memories.* This hypothesis could, in principle, explain the total rejection of or, otherwise, the alteration of sensory input into our dreaming.[37,89]

Let us formally propose then *that wakefulness is nothing other than a dreamlike state modulated by the constraints produced by specific sensory inputs.*[60] Findings in support of this rather outrageous statement come from morphological and electrophysiological studies.

Morphological Evidence

Survey of Quantitative Studies of Thalamocortical Connectivity and Its Functional Implications

Quantitative morphological evidence suggests that only a minor part of the thalamocortical connectivity is devoted to the transfer of sensory input. Rather, the thalamocortical network appears to be a complex machine largely devoted to generating an internal representation of reality that may operate in the presence or absence of sensory input.

The thalamus is considered to be the functional and morphological gate to the forebrain.[103] Indeed, with the exception of the olfactory system, all sensory messages reach the cerebral cortex through the thalamus.[47] Yet, synapses established by specific thalamocortical fibers comprise a minority of cortical contacts. For example, in the primary somatosensory and visual cortices, the axons of ventroposterior thalamic and dorsal LGN neurons account for, respectively, 28% and 20% of the synapses in layer IV and adjacent parts of layer III[55,113] (where most thalamocortical axons project). Even in primary sensory cortical areas, most of the connectivity does not represent sensory

input transmitted by the thalamus, but input from cortical and non-thalamic CNS nuclei. Indeed, corticostriatal, corticocortical and corticothalamic pyramidal neurons receive, respectively, 0.3–0.9, 1.5–6.8 and 6.7–20% of their synapses from specific thalamocortical fibers, while less than 4% of the synaptic contacts on multipolar aspiny neurons in layer IV originate in the thalamus.[113–116]

Equally important is the fact that the connectivity between the thalamus and the cortex is bidirectional. Indeed, layer VI pyramidal cells project back to that area of the thalamus where their specific input arises.[46] The number of corticothalamic fibers is about one order of magnitude larger than the number of thalamocortical axons.[118] Moreover, the number of optic nerve axons projecting to the LGN is smaller than the number of corticothalamic axons projecting to the same nucleus.[118]

Clearly, the sensory input arising from the thalamus is necessary for perception as in the absence of specific inputs, there is no externally guided sensory function. However, the specific thalamocortical input accounts for a minority of the synaptic contacts in the cortex.

What are the implications of these morphological data for brain function? Specifically, what is the function of the majority of inputs to the cortex and how is their activity related to sensory input? One conclusion seems inescapable. The ability to see, that is, to place sensory input into the context of consciousness or a state resembling consciousness, requires an enormous computational machine. This is not surprising since the essence of brain function seems, to us, to be that of generating the functional scaffolding required to create an internal image consistent with external reality. And more importantly, such a consistent image of reality, requires that inputs from different sensory modalities coalesce into a singular perceptual event. Interestingly, most of the connectivity necessary for this amalgamation is present at birth,[38] that is, the connectivity allows a cognitive capacity that is truly a priori. By this, we do not mean, however, that the total content of consciousness is innate. Even though the mechanisms necessary for its generation are present at birth, the emergence of consciousness arises out of interactions between the brain and its environment. Yet, the internalization of sensory events and the elaboration of memories require an intrinsic mechanism different from that which is primarily responsible for the acquisition and central conduction of sensory inputs.

The Relation between Brain States and External Reality

Let us briefly discuss the nature of the interaction between this set of innate mechanisms and the sensory world. At the outset, it must be recognized that sensory events are nothing other than simplifications determined by the physical properties of our sensory organs. Similarly, the internal representation derived from the sensory specification is constrained by the computational capabilities of the brain. In our opinion, the model of the world emerging during ontogeny is governed by innate predispositions of the brain to categorize and integrate the sensory world in certain ways. Although the particular computational world model derived by a given individual is a function of the sensory exposure he is subjected to, the resulting functional accommodation is genetically determined. As a result, sensory inputs presented during adult life would only convey the parameters required to specify the dimensions relevant to the cognitive templates which stemmed from this accommodative process. Finally, these cognitive templates could be used to recreate world-analogs during dreaming or, once specified by sensory inputs, to generate an adaptive representation of the environment.

Thus, we may consider a closely related problem, that of the open (extrinsic) or closed (intrinsic) nature of nervous system function. One view stipulates that the brain states which repre-sent the external world are nothing other than point-to-point representations having as the basic coinage for functioning the elaboration of reflexes. This view may be traced back, in modern times, to William James,[44] who suggested that as sensory inputs proceed through the nervous system they generate functional states which serve as representations of external reality. James referred to this flow of activity as a "stream of consciousness." His assumption that consciousness is generated solely as a by-product of sensory input was for many years a most pervasive view of how the brain works. Indeed, most physiological thinking in the first two-thirds of this century was dominated by the idea that the nervous system is essentially organized as an extrinsic, open device.

An opposite point of view is that the nervous system is basically a closed device. Support for this proposal comes from electrophysiological studies indicating that the intrinsic membrane properties of neurons allow them to oscillate or resonate at different frequencies and that such intrinsic activity may play a fundamental role in CNS function.[61] We will argue that the insertion of such elements into complex synaptic networks allows the brain to generate dynamic oscillatory states which deeply influence the brain activity evoked by sensory stimuli.

Graham Brown[12] was among the first to propose that physiological states, such as locomotion, are products of oscillatory events intrinsic to the spinal cord. These oscillatory states are synaptically transferred to motor neurons, into a well-defined set of muscle movements, resulting in locomotion. Recent evidence indicates that intrinsic neuronal activity in the spinal cord is at the foundation of locomotion.[36] In this context, the function of sensory input in locomotion is to modulate the intrinsic oscillatory properties of the spinal cord network in order to adapt it to the irregularities of the terrain on which the animal moves. This view of spinal cord function may be extended to the brainstem and forebrain.

Intrinsic Oscillations in the Brainstem and the Forebrain

Inferior Olive In structures such as the inferior olive (IO), electrophysiological studies have shown that the function of a neuronal system is not determined only by its connectivity, but is also directly related to the intrinsic membrane properties of the constitutive elements. Conductances which endow nerve cells with the ability to act as single-cell oscillators were first described in the IO.[58,59] Recent studies have demonstrated the importance of oscillations of IO neuronal ensembles in the accurate timing of motor neuron activity that is required to generate co-ordinated movements.[63]

Thalamus Similar experiments in the thalamus were performed both under in vitro and in vivo conditions. The in vitro experiments characterized the electroresponsiveness and intrinsic membrane properties of thalamic cells.[42,43] The in vivo studies explored the functional consequences of the incorporation of these cells into complex synaptic circuits.[24,98–101]

A new view of thalamic operations emerged from these studies. Indeed, the thalamus appeared to be capable not only of controlling the transfer of sensory input to the cerebral cortex, but of expressing its own electrical activity, these two aspects of thalamic functions being intimately related.[103]

Other Brain Areas Other systems capable of demonstrating autorhythmicity are discovered daily in studies of the mammalian nervous system. Examples of the richness of the intrinsic electrical activity of central neurons are found in the neocortex,[56] hypothalamus,[3] entorhinal cortex[4] and brainstem.[54]

The Brain as a Closed System

Several factors suggest that the brain is essentially a closed system. In addition, this system is capable of self-generated oscillatory activity which determines the functional events specified by the sensory stimuli. First, as stated above, only a minor part of the thalamocortical connectivity is devoted to the reception and transfer of sensory input (see section "Survey of Quantitative Studies of Thalamocortical Connectivity and Its Functional Implications"). Second, the number of cortical fibers projecting to the specific thalamic nuclei is larger than the number of fibers conveying the sensory information to the thalamus.[118] Thus, a large part of the thalamocortical connectivity is devoted to re-entrant[27] or to reverberating activity.[64] Third, the insertion of neurons with intrinsic oscillatory capabilities into this complex synaptic network allows the brain to generate global oscillatory states which shape the computational events evoked by sensory stimuli. In this context, functional states such as wakefulness (or REM sleep and other sleep stages) appear to be particular examples of the multiple variations provided by the self-generated brain activity.

The neuropsychological evidence discussed in section "Significance of the High Sensory Thresholds for Awakening During Rapid Eye Movement Sleep" also supports this view of the brain as a closed system in which sensory input plays an extraordinarily important but, nevertheless, a mainly modulatory role. The cases of prosopagnosic patients dreaming of faceless characters indicate that the significance of sensory cues is largely dependent on their incorporation into larger cognitive entities and upon the functional state of the brain. In other words, sensory cues gain their significance by virtue of triggering a pre-existing disposition of the brain to be active in a particular way.

Spatial and Temporal Mapping

A discussion of how the brain might use space and time to elaborate cognitive and perceptual constructs will be used in formulating a hypothesis to account for the difference between waking and REM sleep.

That general connectivities present at birth in humans are not fundamentally modified during normal maturation has been known from the inception of neurological research.[14,38] The localization of function in the brain began with the identification of a cortical speech center by Broca in 1861[11] and was followed by the discovery of point-to-point somatotopic maps in the motor and sensory cortices[85] in the thalamus[78,79] and more recently in the superior colliculus.[33,52,91]

A totally different type of functional geometry[84] has emerged in which that of temporal mapping, in addition to its spatial counterpart, are important variables. Temporal mapping has been far more difficult to understand and to study than spatial mapping since its study requires an understanding of natural computation and the importance of simultaneity in brain function.

Synchronous Activation in the Face of Spatial Disparity

The question of temporal simultaneity with spatial disparity had been addressed in studies of the discharge of electrical organs in teleosts. Maximal current density is achieved when the electroplaques at different distances from the command nucleus are activated synchronously.[9] The solution to the problem is elegant. The conductance time from the command nucleus to the individual electroplaques is uniform because the conduction velocity of the motor axons varies directly with the distance of the individual electroplaques from the motoneurons; axons of the closest electroplaques have the slowest conduction velocity.

Recent studies of the olivocerebellar system have shown that a similar mechanism is used to achieve isochronic activation of Purkinje cells following direct IO activation.[109] Similarly, the volley entering the optic nerve following activation of the entire ganglion cell population is close to synchronous.[94] Thus, activity from peripheral and centrally located ganglion cells reaches the optic nerve at the same time.[94]

40-Hz Activity and Cognitive Conjunction

Synchronous activation has recently been seen in the mammalian cerebral cortex. Visual stimulation with light bars of optimal dimensions, orientation and velocity may synchronously activate cells in a given column of the visual cortex.[26,34,35] Moreover, the components of a visual stimulus which relate to a singular cognitive object (such as a line in a visual field) produce coherent 40-Hz oscillations in regions of the cortex that may be separated by as much as 7 mm.[34,35] Also a high correlation coefficient has been found for 40-Hz oscillatory activity between related cortical columns.

These findings have inspired a number of theoretical papers with the view that temporal mapping is very important in nervous system function (e.g., references 26, 92). The central tenet can be summarized simply. Spatial mapping allows a limited number of possible representations. However, the addition of a second component (serving to form transient functional states by means of simultaneity) generates an indefinitely large number of functional states, as the categorization is accomplished by the conjunction of spatial and temporal mapping.

Magnetoencephalographic recordings performed in awake humans[57] have revealed the presence of continuous 40-Hz oscillations over the entire cortical mantle. The presentation of auditory stimuli having random frequency components produced a clear synchronization of this 40-Hz activity (figure 59.4). Phase comparison between the oscillatory activity recorded from different cortical regions revealed the presence of a close to 12-ms phase shift between the rostral and caudal pole of the brain (figure 59.5). What could be the mechanisms underlying this well-organized 40-Hz activity and what function might it serve?

The high level of organization displayed by this 40-Hz oscillation suggests that the candidate mechanisms must: (i) be able to produce and maintain a synchronized pattern of activity in very distant groups of neurons; and (ii) have ex-

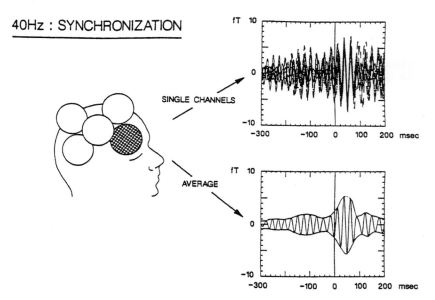

Figure 59.4
Synchronization of human magnetic 40-Hz oscillatory activity during auditory processing within seven single channels of one probe placed over lower frontal areas. The graph on the top right indicates a superimposition of 40-Hz activities, time locked to the stimulus onset, recorded from the seven channels. The graph on the lower right indicates an average of the seven individual channels, demonstrating synchronization over a large area (around 25 cm²). (Reproduced from Llinás and Ribary.[57])

tensive projections to the cerebral cortex. Furthermore, if this oscillatory activity were to play a significant role in providing a context for sensory events transmitted by specific thalamocortical systems, return projections from the cerebral cortex would be necessary.

Few prosencephalic structures have extensive reciprocal connections with the cerebral cortex: the thalamus[47] and the amygdala[5] probably constitute the best-known examples. It has already been hypothesized that the thalamus is involved in 40-Hz activity.[62] Specifically, it was proposed that sparsely spiny layer IV neurons which are able to generate intrinsic 40-Hz oscillations[56] would produce an inhibition-rebound sequence (probably sodium dependent) in thalamically projecting pyramidal neurons. These cells would then generate a 40-Hz inhibitory rebound oscillation in cells of the reticular thalamic nucleus (RE), a group of GABAergic neurons projecting to most relay nuclei of the thalamus.[45,108] More recently, it has been demonstrated that thalamic neurons in vivo can also oscillate intrinsically at the same frequency using a similar ionic mechanism.[96] Consequently, cortico-thalamo-cortical pathways could be led to resonant oscillation at 40 Hz (figure 59.6). According to this hypothesis, RE cells would be responsible for the synchronization of the 40-Hz oscillations in distant thalamic and cortical territories. Indeed, it has been shown that neighboring RE cells are linked by dendrodendritic and intranuclear axon collaterals.[23,120]

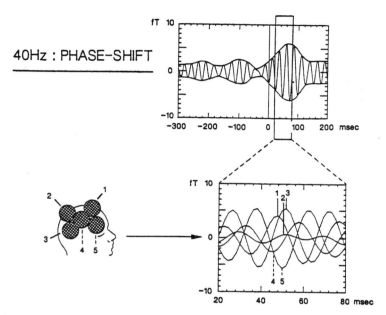

Figure 59.5
Phase shift of human magnetic 40-Hz oscillatory activity during auditory processing. The time period between 20 and 80 ms after the onset of the auditor stimuli is enlarged in the lower panel. The lowest panel shows the superposition of averaged responses from all sensors in each of the five probe positions (hatched and numbered at left). Note the large, consistent phase shifts from region to region, indicating a continuous rostrocaudal phase shift over the hemisphere. (Reproduced from Llinás and Ribary.[57])

The amygdala may also play an important role in the generation of 40-Hz activity. Golgi and immunohistochemical studies indicate that, like the thalamus, most amygdaloid nuclei contain two populations of cells: projection cells and GABAergic interneurons.[71,81] In addition, the amygdala is endowed with a group of GABAergic cells,[81] the intercalated cells, which appear to play a role analogous to the RE nucleus in the thalamus: they are contacted by projection cell axon collaterals and seem to project within the amygdaloid nuclei.[75] However, in contrast with the thalamus, the projection cells have intranuclear recurrent collaterals which probably contact neighboring projection and local-circuit cells.[71] In addition, there is an important system of connections linking various amygdaloid nuclei.[2] Because projection cells are believed to use glutamate as a neurotransmitter,[17] these intra- and internuclear links could constitute a means to synchronize projection cells rapidly through excitatory connections. Such a mechanism seems more potent than the subtler influence produced by the aforementioned inhibitory rebound mechanism.[56]

Another reason to favor the amygdala as a candidate for the synchronization of the 40-Hz oscillations lies in the role it is believed to play in memory.[5,93] If we assume that a function of this 40-Hz activity is to maintain a general, continuous neuronal humming against which intra- or externally generated "irregularities" can stand

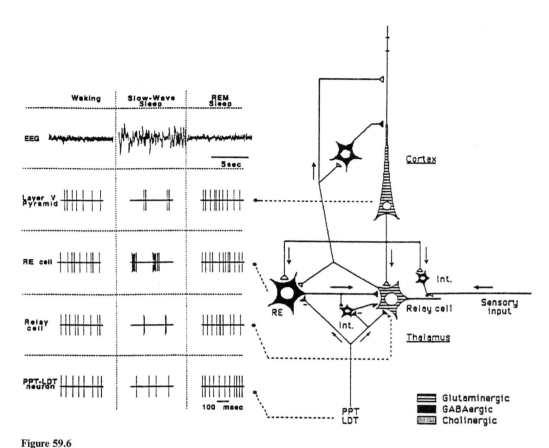

Figure 59.6
Schematic diagram showing the interconnections of the basic cellular components of the thalamocortical system (right). The left panel illustrates simulated spike trains of these various cell types in waking, slow-wave sleep, and REM sleep (first to third column, respectively). Note the sharp contrast between the activity of thalamic and cortical cells in slow-wave sleep and EEG-desynchronized states. The spike trains were derived from publications by Steriade et al.[97, 103]

out, the importance of a structure which could communicate this "irregularity" to other neuronal groups becomes self-evident. Indeed, through preferential intra-amygdaloid connections reinforced by previous experiences, neuronal groups which are relevant to the computations required by the irregularity in question could be led to oscillate in phase with each other, thereby maximizing the effectiveness of synaptic interactions between them.

However, a variety of neuronal types are endowed with intrinsic membrane properties which allow them to generate voltage-dependent 40-Hz oscillations, as in the cerebral cortex,[56] and thalamus.[96] These observations suggest that it might be a mistake to search for a single site for the generation and synchronization of this oscillation.

The Nature of the Differences between Wakefulness and Rapid Eye Movement Sleep: a Hypothesis

Electrophysiological Properties of the Thalamocortical Cells and Circuit

It is well known that the thalamus has two basic operating modes: a relay mode characterizing EEG-desynchronized states, such as waking and REM sleep; and an oscillatory mode characterizing EEG-synchronized states such as drowsiness and slow-wave sleep.[98] In the relay mode, thalamocortical cells show an increased synaptic responsiveness, tonic discharge and short periods of inhibition. In contrast, the oscillatory mode is characterized by a decreased ability to transfer incoming sensory inputs and by long-lasting periods of inhibition interrupted by burst discharges.

These two functional states arise from interactions between the intrinsic membrane properties of thalamocortical cells and the properties of the complex synaptic network in which they are embedded. Indeed, the firing mode of

thalamocortical cells varies with their membrane potential.[42,43] From a depolarized level, a suprathreshold depolarizing pulse evokes a tonic discharge during the pulse, whereas from a hyperpolarized level it evokes a brief (30 ms), high-frequency (250–400 Hz) burst of fast sodium-dependent action potentials riding on a slow calcium-mediated spike.[42,43] Single-unit recordings throughout the dorsal thalamus in naturally sleeping cats[104] have shown that thalamocortical cells display a burst discharge in slow-wave sleep (when their membrane potential is relatively hyperpolarized), and a tonic discharge during EEG-desynchronization (when their membrane potential is relatively depolarized[39]).

Brainstem Influence on Thalamic Firing Mode

While the firing mode of thalamocortical cells is related to the expression of intrinsic membrane properties, the state-dependent fluctuations in membrane potential result from extrinsic synaptic influences. Morphological and electrophysiological data suggest that cholinergic cells of the pedunculopontine and laterodorsal tegmental nuclei are largely responsible for modulating the operating mode of thalamocortical cells during the transition from EEG-synchronized to EEG-desynchronized states.[105] In vitro studies in the dorsal LGN suggest that the cholinergic effects result from: (i) the hyperpolarization of somata of thalamic interneurons[67] and reticularis thalamic cells,[68] and (ii) the increased input resistance of thalamocortical cells[69,70] (by closing various types of potassium channels), thereby increasing their sensitivity to incoming synaptic volleys. These findings are consistent with the results of in vivo intracellular studies performed in a variety of thalamic nuclei.[18,19]

During REM sleep, the tonic discharge rate of most thalamically projecting pedunculopontine (PPT) and laterodorsal tegmental (LDT) neurons increases above waking levels (on average from 24 to 34 Hz[97]), thereby activating thalamocortical neurons. A large proportion of PPT and LDT neurons increase phasically their discharge rate before and during PGO waves.[107] These tonic and phasic increases in the discharge rate of PPT and LDT neurons during REM sleep could be largely responsible for the corresponding tonic and PGO-related phasic augmentations in firing displayed by thalamocortical cells during REM sleep.[103] Since most humans sleep in a relatively stimulation-free environment, the activity of thalamocortical neurons has no immediate external meaning. Therefore, although the ongoing neuronal events reflect normal thalamocortical interactions, the activity generated has a totally different nature than the same activity would have during the waking state.

Hypothesis

We propose that wakefulness and REM sleep are fundamentally the same type of functional state and that the main difference between them lies in what particular input is most prevalent. But both are most probably related to coherent thalamocortical activity. As mentioned above, recent results from EEG and magneto-encephalography studies suggest that during the waking state, there are organized 40-Hz oscillations throughout the cortex.[57] Sensory stimuli in this case will reset this intrinsic rhythmicity in a way similar to that described in single cells.[26,34,35] During REM sleep, the brain would be turned away from the sensory world because sensory stimuli would not be able to take hold of the consciousness-generating apparatus, that is, the thalamocortical system.

Thus, during REM sleep, temporal associations which generate subjectivity do not coincide with the temporal maps, and only strong sensory inputs are capable of resetting such temporal conditions. In short, if the sensory input coming to the brain is not put in the context of thalamocortical reality by being correlated temporally with ongoing activity, the stimulus does not exist as a functionally meaningful event.

Consciousness and Subjectivity Are Intrinsic Properties of the Brain

The most fundamental conclusion to be drawn from the states described above is that consciousness is an intrinsic property arising from the expression of existing dispositions of the brain to be active in certain ways. It is a close kin to dreaming, where sensory input by constraining the intrinsic functional states specifies, rather than informs, the brain of those properties of external reality that are important for survival.

If this is the case, we may conclude that the perception of external reality is an a priori cognitive ability of the CNS developed and honed by the same evolutionary pressures that generated other biological specializations. Moreover, this implies that secondary qualities of our senses such as colors, identified smells, tastes and sounds, are inventions of our CNS which allow the brain to interact with the external world in a predictive manner.[60] The degree to which our perception of reality and "actual" reality overlap is inconsequential as long as the predictive properties of the computational states generated by the brain meet the requirements of successful interaction with the external world.

Indeed, that one person sees red as having the same subjective quality as another person is unimportant. The important variable is that of distinguishing red from green or blue, as colors are intrinsic functional events that do not necessarily correspond to any reality in the external world. Rather, they are a means for the brain to distinguish between rather small differences in surface spectral reflectances.

That consciousness is generated intrinsically is not difficult to understand when one considers the completeness of the sensory representations in our dreams or in the hallucinations of the mentally impaired or the pharmacologically challenged.

Rapid Eye Movement Sleep, Hallucinations, and Daydreaming

The possible intrinsic nature of consciousness has serious implications for our understanding of psychiatric conditions characterized by illusional states in which the intrinsic view of reality and the emotional states generated by them are in discord with the perception of other individuals in the same social setting.

What would happen if the differences between intrinsically generated REM sleep and extrinsically modulated dream imagery were to go awry? According to the views expressed above, the thalamocortical system is ultimately responsible for the generation of consciousness. Thus, individuals who experience certain forms of hallucinatory states may be convinced that their hallucination indeed corresponds to events in the external world.

Finally, when one considers that attentiveness is selective, that is, paying attention to certain external events while not paying attention to others, the lack of responsiveness of a person dreaming, hallucinating or deep in thought (daydreaming) becomes clear. In all three cases, intrinsically generated activity similar to that observed in REM is rampant and does not necessarily heed the vicissitudes of external reality.

The above statement addresses the two important issues of the nature of consciousness and the nature of attention. Of interest here is the fact that electrophysiological studies indicate that REM responsiveness resembles non-attentive responsiveness rather than responsiveness to attended stimuli (see section "Physiological Comparison of the Two States"). Thus the possibility arises, as proposed above, that dreaming is basically a hyperattentive state in many ways similar to full wakefulness. If we assume this is the case, what follows?

Consciousness as a Thalamocortical Temporally Dependent Conjunctive State

As stated in the previous section, those aspects of brain function which form part of our consciousness must occur at the same time, most probably with 40-Hz activity recently described in animals and humans (see section "40-Hz Activity and Cognitive Conjunction). This may be taken to indicate that attentive states are those that fall within neuronal circuits displaying 40 Hz at any particular time. Indeed, recent experiments indicate the existence of coherent 40-Hz activity in the human brain which demonstrates a phase shift in the rostrocaudal direction with a conductance time near 12 ms (figures 59.4 and 59.5). This rostral-to-caudal 12-ms phase shift of 40-Hz activity suggests that synchronous events may be occurring within our head with a frequency close to 80 Hz.[57]

If we assume that the phase shift observed in these preliminary studies is related to the presence of simultaneity waves which scan our brain at 80 Hz, we can conclude that consciousness is not a continuous event. Rather, it is determined by the simultaneity of activity in the thalamocortical system, modulated by the brainstem, and fed when one is awake by sensory input, and when one is asleep by circuits that support memories.

Thalamocortical Activity as the Functional Basis for Consciousness

From the above, it follows that the major development in the evolution of the brain of higher primates, including man, is the enrichment of the corticothalamic system. This is supported by evolutionary studies if one considers the increase in corticalization in mammals. The increase in the surface area of the neocortex in man is approximately three times that of higher apes.[53]

How can this thalamo-cortico-thalamic functional state generate the unique experience we all recognize as existence of self or existence of the here and now? In principle, the activity generated via thalamocortical interactions may mimic the responsiveness generated during the waking state (i.e. reality-emulating states, such as hallucinations, may be generated). The implications of this proposal are of some consequence, for this means that if consciousness is a product of thalamocortical activity, *it is the dialogue between the thalamus and the cortex that generates subjectivity.*

Acknowledgments

This work was supported by NIH grant NS 13742. D. Paré is an MRC postdoctoral fellow.

References

1. Adams R. D. and Victor M. (1985) *Principles of Neurology.* McGraw-Hill, New York.

2. Aggleton J. P. (1985) A description of intra-amygdaloid connections in old world monkeys. *Expl Brain Res.* 57, 390–399.

3. Alonso A. and Llinás R. (1988) Voltage-dependent calcium conductances and mammillary body neurons autorhythmicity an in vitro study. *Soc. Neurosci. Abstr.* 14, 900.

4. Alonso A. and Llinás R. R. (1989) Subthreshold theta-like rhythmicity in stellate cells of entorhinal cortex layer II. *Nature* 342, 175–177.

5. Amaral D. G. (1987) Memory: anatomical organization of candidate brain regions. In *Handbook of Physiology* (eds Mountcastle V. B. and Plum F.), pp. 211–294. American Physiological Society, Bethesda.

6. Aserinsky E. and Kleitman N. (1953) Regularly occurring periods of eye motility and concurrent phenomena during sleep. *Science* 118, 273–274.

7. Aserinsky E. and Kleitman N. (1955) Two types of ocular motility occurring in sleep. *J. appl. Physiol.* 8, 1–10.

8. Bastuji H., Larrea L. G., Bertrand O. and Mauguière F. (1988) PAEP latency changes during nocturnal sleep are not correlated with sleep stages but with body temperature variations. *Electroenceph. clin. Neurophysiol.* 70, 9–15.

9. Bennet M. V. L. (1971) Electric organs. In *Fish Physiology* (eds Hoar W. S. and Randall D. J.), pp. 347–391. Academic Press, New York.

10. Berlucchi G., Moruzzi G., Salvi G. and Strata P. (1964) Pupil behavior and ocular movements during synchronized and desynchronized sleep. *Archs. ital. Biol.* 102, 230–244.

11. Broca P. (1888) *Mémoire sur le Cerveau de l'Homme.* Reinwald, Paris.

12. Brown T. G. (1981) The intrinsic factors in the act of progression in the mammal. *Proc. R. Soc. Biol. Sci. Ser. B. Lond.* 84, 308–319.

13. Burke W. and Cole A. M. (1978) Extraretinal influences on the lateral geniculate nucleus. *Rev. Physiol. Biochem. Pharmac.* 80, 105–166.

14. Cajal S. R. (1929) *Etude sur la Neurogénèse de quelques Vertébrés.* Thomas, Springfield.

15. Campbell K. B. and Bartoli E. A. (1986) Human auditory evoked potentials during natural sleep: the early components. *Electroenceph. clin. Neurophysiol.* 65, 142–149.

16. Chen B. M. and Buchwald J. S. (1986) Midlatency auditory evoked responses: differential effects of sleep in the cat. *Electroenceph. clin. Neurophysiol.* 65, 373–382.

17. Christie M. J., Summers R. J., Stephenson J. A., Cook C. J. and Beart P. M. (1987) Excitatory amino acid projections to the nucleus accumbens septi in the rat: a retrograde transport study utilizing D[^{3}H]aspartate and [^{3}H]GABA. *Neuroscience* 22, 425–439.

18. CurróDossi R., Paré D. and Steriade M. (1991) Short-lasting nicotinic and long-lasting muscarinic depolarizing responses of thalamocortical neurons to stimulation of mesopontine cholinergic nuclei. *J. Neurophysiol.* 65, 393–406.

19. CurróDossi R., Paré D. and Steriade M. (1991) Various types of inhibitory post-synaptic potentials

in anterior thalamic cells are differentially altered by stimulation of laterodorsal tegmental cholinergic nucleus. *Neuroscience* (submitted).

20. Deiber M. P., Bastuji H., Fischer M. D. and Maugière F. (1989) Changes of middle latency auditory evoked potentials during natural sleep in humans. *Neurology* 39, 806–813.

21. Dement W. (1958) The occurrence of low voltage, fast, electroencephalogram patterns during behavioral sleep in the cat. *Electroenceph. clin. Neurophysiol.* 10, 291–296.

22. Dement W. and Kleitman N. (1957) Cyclic variations in EEG during sleep and their relation to eye movements, body motility, and dreaming. *Electroenceph. clin. Neurophysiol.* 9, 673–690.

23. Deschênes M., Madariaga-Domich A. and Steriade M. (1985) Dendrodendritic synapses in the cat reticularis thalami nucleus: a structural basis for thalamic spindle synchronization. *Brain Res.* 334, 165–168.

24. Deschênes M., Paradis M., Roy J. P. and Steriade M. (1984) Electrophysiology of neurons of lateral thalamic nuclei in cat: resting properties and burst discharges. *J. Neurophysiol.* 51, 1196–1219.

25. Desmedt J. E. (1981) Scalp-recorded cerebral event-related potentials in man as point of entry into the analysis of cognitive processing. In *The Organization of the Cerebral Cortex* (eds Schmitt F. O., Worden F. G., Adelman G. and Dennis S. G.), pp. 441–473. MIT Press, Cambridge.

26. Eckhorn R., Bauer R., Jordan W., Brosch M., Kruse W., Munk M. and Reitbock H. J. (1988) Coherent oscillations: a mechanism of feature linking in the visual cortex? *Biol. Cybern.* 60, 121–130.

27. Edelman G. M. (1987) *Neuronal Darwinism: The Theory of Neuronal Group Selection.* Basic Books, New York.

28. Foulkes D. (1983) Dream ontogeny and dream psychophysiology. In *Sleep Disorders: Basic and Clinical Research* (eds Chase M. H. and Weitzman E. D.), pp. 347–362. Spectrum, New York.

29. Giard M. H., Perrin F., Pernier J. and Perronnet F. (1988) Several attention related waveforms in auditory areas: a topographic study. *Electroenceph. clin. Neurophysiol.* 69, 371–384.

30. Glenn L. L. (1985) Brainstem and spinal control of lower limb motoneurons with special reference to phasic events and startle reflexes. In *Brain Mechanisms of Sleep* (eds McGinty D., Drucker-Colin R. R., Morrison A. and Parmeggiani P. L.), pp. 81–95, Raven Press, New York.

31. Glenn L. L. and Steriade M. (1982) Discharge rate and excitability of cortically projecting intralaminar thalamic neurons during waking and sleep states. *J. Neurosci.* 2, 1387–1404.

32. Goff W. R., Allison T., Shapiro A. and Rosner B. S. (1966) Cerebral somatosensory responses evoked during sleep in man. *Electroenceph. clin. Neurophysiol.* 21, 1–9.

33. Grantyn R. (1988) Gaze control through superior colliculus: structure and function. In *Neuroanatomy of the Oculomotor System* (ed. Buttner-Ennever J. A.), pp. 273–333. Elsevier, New York.

34. Gray C. M., Konig P., Engel A. K. and Singer W. (1989) Oscillatory responses in cat visual cortex exhibit inter-columnar synchronization which reflects global stimulus properties. *Nature* 338, 334–337.

35. Gray C. M. and Singer W. (1989) Stimulus-specific neuronal oscillations in orientation columns of cat visual cortex. *Proc. natn. Acad. Sci. U.S.A.* 86, 1698–1702.

36. Grillner S. (1981) Control of locomotion in bipeds, tetrapods and fish. In *Handbook of Physiology* (ed. Brooks V. B.), pp. 1179–1236. American Physiological Society, Bethesda.

37. Gross M. M. (1963) Discussion of the paper by Williams (1963). *Ann. N.Y. Acad. Sci.* 112, 172–181.

38. Harris W. A. (1987) Neurogenetics. In *Encyclopedia of Neuroscience* (ed. Adelman G.), pp. 791–793. Birkhäuser, Basel.

39. Hirsch J. C., Fourment A. and Marc M. E. (1983) Sleep-related variations of membrane potential in the lateral geniculate body relay neurons of the cat. *Brain Res.* 259, 308–312.

40. Hobson J. A. and Steriade M. (1986) Neuronal basis of behavioural state control. In *Intrinsic Regulatory Systems of the Brain* (ed. Bloom F. E.), pp. 701–823. American Physiological Society, Bethesda.

41. Hull J. M. (1990) *Touching the Rock: an Experience of being Blind.* S.P.C.K., London.

42. Jahnsen H. and Llinás R. (1984) Electrophysiological properties of guinea-pig thalamic neurones: an in vitro study. *J. Physiol., Lond.* 349, 205–226.

43. Jahnsen H. and Llinás R. (1984) Ionic basis for the electro-responsiveness and oscillatory properties of

guinea-pig thalamic neurons in vitro. *J. Physiol., Lond.* 349, 227–248.

44. James W. (1890) *The Principles of Psychology.* Henry Holt, London.

45. Jones E. G. (1975) Some aspects of the organization of the thalamic reticular complex. *J. comp. Neurol.* 162, 285–308.

46. Jones E. G. (1984) Laminar distribution of cortical efferent cells. In *Cerebral Cortex: Cellular Components of the Cerebral Cortex* (eds Peters A. and Jones E. G.), pp. 521–552. Plenum Press, New York.

47. Jones E. G. (1985) *The Thalamus.* Plenum Press, New York.

48. Jouvet M. and Delorme F. (1965) Locus coeruleus et sommeil paradoxal. *C. R. Soc. Biol. Paris* 159, 895–899.

49. Jouvet M. and Michel F. (1959) Corrélations électromyographiques du sommeil chez le chat décortiqué et mésencéphalique chronique. *C. R. Soc. Biol., Paris* 153, 422–425.

50. Jouvet M., Michel F. and Courjon J. (1959) Sur un stade d'activité électrique cérébrale rapide au cours du sommeil physiologique. *Compt. Rend. Soc. Biol., Paris* 153, 1024–1028.

51. Karacan I. and Howell J. W. (1988) Narcolepsy. In *Sleep Disorders: Diagnosis and Treatment* (eds Williams R. L., Karacen I. and Moore C. A.), pp. 87–105. John Wiley, New York.

52. Knudsen E. I., du Lac S. and Esterly S. D. (1987) Computational maps in the brain. *A. Rev. Neurosci.* 10, 41–65.

53. Lande R. (1979) Quantitative genetic analysis of multivariate evolution, applied to brain-body size allometry. *Evolution* 33, 400–416.

54. Leonard C. S. and Llinás R. R. (1990) Electrophysiology of mammalian pedunculopontine and laterodorsal tegmental neurons in vitro: implications for the control of REM sleep. In *Brain Cholinergic Systems* (eds Steriade M. and Biesold D.), pp. 205–223. Oxford University Press, New York.

55. LeVay S. and Gilbert C. D. (1976) Laminar patterns of geniculocortical projection in the cat. *Brain Res.* 113, 1–19.

56. Llinás R. R. and Grace A. A. (1989) Intrinsic 40 Hz oscillatory properties of layer IV neurons in guinea pig cerebral cortex in vitro. *Soc. Neurosci. Abstr.* 15, 660.

57. Llinás R. R. and Ribary U. (1991) Rostrocaudal scan in human brain: a global characteristic of the 40 Hz response during sensory input. In *Induced Rhythms in the Brain* (eds Basar E. and Bullock T.). Birkhäuser, Boston (in press.)

58. Llinás R. R. and Yarom Y. (1981) Electrophysiology of mammalian inferior olivary neurones in vitro. Different types of voltage-dependent ionic conductances. *J. Physiol., Lond.* 315, 549–567.

59. Llinás R. R. and Yarom Y. (1981) Properties and distribution of ionic conductances generating electroresponsiveness of mammalian inferior olivary neurones in vitro. *J. Physiol., London.* 315, 569–584.

60. Llinás R. R. (1988) "Mindness" as a functional state of the brain. In *Mind Waves* (eds Blakemore C. and Greenfield S. A.), pp. 339–358. Blackwell, Oxford.

61. Llinás R. R. (1988) The intrinsic electrophysiological properties of mammalian neurons: insights into central nervous system function. *Science* 242, 1654–1664.

62. Llinás R. R. (1990) Intrinsic electrical properties of mammalian neurons and CNS function. In *Fidia Research Foundation Neuroscience Award Lectures*, pp. 175–194. Raven Press, New York.

63. Llinás R. R. and Sasaki K. (1989) The functional organization of the olivo-cerebellar system as examined by multiple Purkinje cell recordings. *Eur. J. Neurosci.* 1, 587–602.

64. Lorente de Nó R. (1932) Studies on the structure of the cerebral cortex. *J. F. Psychol. und Neurol.* 45, 381–438.

65. McCarley R. W. and Ito K. (1983) Intracellular evidence linking medial pontine reticular formation neurons to PGO generation. *Brain Res.* 280, 343–348.

66. McCarley R. W. and Ito K. (1985) Desynchronized sleep-specific changes in membrane potential and excitability in medial pontine reticular formation neurons: implications for concepts and mechanisms of behavioral state control. In *Brain Mechanisms of Sleep* (eds McGinty D., Drucker-Colin R., Morrison A. and Parmeggiani P. L.), pp. 63–80. Raven Press, New York.

67. McCormick D. A. and Pape H. C. (1988) Acetylcholine inhibits identified interneurones in the cat lateral geniculate nucleus. *Nature* 334, 246–248.

68. McCormick D. A. and Prince D. A. (1986) ACh induces burst firing in thalamic reticular neurones

by activating a K^+ conductance. *Nature* 319, 402–405.

69. McCormick D. A. and Prince D. A. (1988) Actions of acetylcholine in the guinea pig and cat medial and lateral geniculate nuclei, in vitro. *J. Physiol., Lond.* 392, 147–165.

70. McCormick D. A. and Prince D. A. (1987) Neurotransmitter modulation of thalamic neuronal firing pattern. *J. Mind Behav.* 8, 573–590.

71. McDonald A. J. (1982) Neurons of the lateral and basolateral amygdaloid nuclei: a Golgi study in the rat. *J. comp. Neurol.* 212, 293–312.

72. Mendel M. I. and Goldstein R. (1971) Early components of the averaged electroencephalographic response to constant level clicks during all-night sleep. *J. Speech. Hear. Res.* 14, 829–840.

73. Mendel M. I. and Kuperman G. L. (1974) Early components of the averaged electroencephalographic response to constant level clicks during rapid eye movement sleep. *Audiology* 13, 23–32.

74. Mikiten T., Niebyl P. and Hendley C. (1961) EEG-desynchronization during behavioural sleep associated with spike discharges from the thalamus of the cat. *Fedn Proc.* 20, 327.

75. Millhouse O. E. (1986) The intercalated cells of the amygdala. *J. comp. Neurol.* 247, 246–271.

76. Moller A. R. and Burgess J. (1986) Neural generators of the brain-stem auditory evoked potentials (BAEPs) in the rhesus monkey. *Electroenceph. clin. Neurophysiol.* 65, 361–372.

77. Morales F. and Chase M. H. (1981) Post-synaptic control of lumbar motoneuron excitability during active sleep in the chronic cat. *Brain Res.* 225, 279–295.

78. Mountcastle V. B. and Hennemann E. (1949) Pattern of tactile representation in thalamus of cat. *J. Neurophysiol.* 12, 85–100.

79. Mountcastle V. B. and Hennemann E. (1952) The representation of tactile sensibility in the thalamus of the monkey. *J. comp. Neurol.* 97, 409–440.

80. Mouret J. R., Jeannerod M. and Jouvet M. (1963) L'activité électrique du système visuel au cours de la phase paradoxale du sommeil chez le chat. *J. Physiol., Paris* 55, 305–306.

81. Nitecka L. and Ben-Ari Y. (1987) Distribution of GABA-like immunoreactivity in the rat amygdaloid complex. *J. comp. Neurol.* 266, 45–55.

82. Paré D., Bouhassira D., Oakson G. and Datta S. (1990) Spontaneous and evoked activities of anterior thalamic neurons during waking and sleep states. *Expl Brain Res.* 80, 54–62.

83. Parmeggiani P. L., Morrison A., Drucker-Colin R. R. and McGinty D. (1985) Brain mechanisms of sleep: an overview of methodological issues. In *Brain Mechanisms of Sleep* (eds McGinty D., Drucker-Colin R. R., Morrison A. and Parmeggiani P. L.), pp. 1–33. Raven Press, New York.

84. Pellionisz A. and Llinás R. R. (1982) Space-time representation in the brain. The cerebellum as a predictive space-time metric tensor. *Neuroscience* 7, 2949–2970.

85. Penfield W. and Rasmussen T. (1950) *The Cerebral Cortex of Man.* MacMillan, New York.

86. Picton T. W. and Hillyard S. A. (1974) Human AEPs. II. Effect of attention. *Electroenceph. clin. Neurophysiol.* 36, 191–199.

87. Pompeiano O. (1967) The neurophysiological mechanisms of the postural and motor events during desynchronized sleep. *Proc. assoc. Nerv. Ment. Dis.* 45, 351–423.

88. Price J. L. and Amaral D. G. (1981) An autoradiographic study of the projections of the central nucleus of the monkey amygdala. *J. Neurosci.* 1, 1242–1259.

89. Rechtschaffen A., Hauri P. and Zeitlin M. (1966) Auditory awakening thresholds in REM and NREM sleep stages. *Percept. Mot. Skills* 22, 927–942.

89a. Sacks O. (1991) Neurological dreams. *Medical Doctor* 35, 29–32.

90. Schenck C. H., Bundlie S. R., Ettinger M. G. and Mahowald M. W. (1986) Chronic behavioral disorders of human REM sleep: a new category of parasomnia. *Sleep* 9, 293–308.

91. Sparks D. L. (1986) Translation of sensory signals into commands for control of saccadic eye movements: role of primate superior colliculus. *Physiol. Rev.* 66, 118–171.

92. Sporns O., Gally J. A., Reeke G. N. and Edelman G. M. (1989) Reentrant signaling among simulated neuronal groups leads to coherency in their oscillatory activity. *Proc. natn. Acad. Sci. U.S.A.* 86, 7265–7269.

93. Squire L. R. (1987) Memory: neural organization and behavior. In *Handbook of Physiology* (eds Mount-

castle V. B. and Plum F.), pp. 295–370. American Physiological Society, Bethesda.

94. Stanford L. R. (1987) Conduction velocity variations minimize conduction time differences among retinal ganglion cell axons. *Science* 238, 358–360.

95. Steriade M. (1976) Cortical inhibition during sleep and waking. In *Mechanisms in Transmission of Signal for Conscious Behavior* (ed. Desiraju T.), pp. 209–248. Elsevier, Amsterdam.

96. Steriade M., CurróDossi R., Paré D. and Oakson G. (1991) Fast oscillations (20–40 Hz) in thalamocortical systems and their potentiation by mesopontine cholinergic nuclei in the cat. *Proc. natn. Acad. Sci. U.S.A.* 88, 4396–4400.

97. Steriade M., Datta S., Paré D., Oakson G. and Curró-Dossi R. (1990) Neuronal activities in brainstem cholinergic nuclei related to tonic activation processes in thalamocortical systems. *J. Neurosci.* 10, 2527–2545.

98. Steriade M., Deschênes M., Domich L. and Mulle C. (1985) Abolition of spindle oscillations in thalamic neurons disconnected from nucleus reticularis thalami. *J. Neurophysiol.* 54, 1473–1497.

99. Steriade M., Deschênes M., Wyzinski P. and Hallé J. Y. (1974) Input-output organization of the motor cortex during sleep and waking. In *Basic Sleep Mechanisms* (eds Petre-Quadens O. and Schlag J.), pp. 144–200. Academic Press, New York.

100. Steriade M., Domich L. and Oakson G. (1986) Reticularis thalamic neurons revisited: activity changes during shifts in states of vigilance. *J. Neurosci.* 6, 68–81.

101. Steriade M., Domich L., Oakson G. and Deschênes M. (1987) The deafferented reticular thalamic nucleus generates spindle rhythmicity. *J. Neurophysiol.* 57, 260–273.

102. Steriade M., Iosif G. and Apostol V. (1969) Responsiveness of thalamic and cortical motor relays during arousal and various stages of sleep. *J. Neurophysiol.* 32, 251–265.

103. Steriade M., Jones E. G. and Llinás R. R. (1990) *Thalamic Oscillations and Signalling*. John Wiley, New York.

104. Steriade M., Kitsikis A. and Oakson G. (1979) Excitatory-inhibitory processes in parietal association neurons during reticular activation and sleep-waking cycle. *Sleep* 1, 339–355.

105. Steriade M. and Llinás R. R. (1988) The functional states of the thalamus and the associated neuronal interplay. *Physiol. Rev.* 68, 649–742.

106. Steriade M. and McCarley R. W. (1990) *Brainstem Control of Wakefulness and Sleep*. Plenum Press, New York.

107. Steriade M., Paré D., Oakson G. and Curró-Dossi R. (1990) Different cellular types in mesopontine cholinergic nuclei related to ponto-geniculo-occipital waves. *J. Neurosci.* 10, 2560–2579.

108. Steriade M., Parent A. and Hada J. (1984) Thalamic projections of nucleus reticularis thalami of cat: a study using retrograde transport of horseradish peroxidase and double fluorescent tracers. *J. comp. Neurol.* 229, 531–547.

109. Sugihara I., Lang E. and Llinás R. (1990) Uniform conduction times of climbing fibers determined at different folial depths using a multiple electrode recording paradigm. *Soc. Neurosci. Abstr.* 16, 637.

110. Thomas J. and Benoit O. (1967) Individualisation d'un sommeil à ondes lentes et activités phasiques. *Brain Res.* 5, 221–235.

111. Velasco F., Velasco M., Cepeda C. and Munoz H. (1980) Wakefulness-sleep modulation of cortical and subcortical somatic evoked potentials in man. *Electroenceph. clin. Neurophysiol.* 48, 64–72.

112. Wesensten N. J. and Badia P. (1988) The P300 component in sleep. *Physiol. Behav.* 44, 215–220.

113. White E. L. (1978) Identified neurons in mouse Sm1 cortex which are postsynaptic to thalamocortical axon terminals: a combined Golgi-electron microscopic and degeneration study. *J. comp. Neurol.* 181, 627–662.

114. White E. L. and Hersch S. M. (1982) A quantitative study of thalamocortical and other synapses involving the apical dendrites of corticothalamic projection cells in mouse Sm1 cortex. *J. Neurocytol.* 11, 137–157.

115. White E. L. and Hersch S. M. (1981) Thalamocortical synapses of pyramidal cells which project Sm1 to Ms1 cortex in the mouse. *J. comp. Neurol.* 198, 167–181.

116. White E. L. and Rock M. P. (1981) A comparison of thalamocortical and other synaptic circuits to dendrites of two non-spiny neurons in a single barrel of mouse Sm1 cortex. *J. comp. Neurol.* 195, 265–277.

117. Williams H. L., Hammack J. T., Daly R. L., Dement W. C. and Lubin A. (1964) Responses to au-

ditory stimulation, sleep loss and the EEG stages of sleep. *Electroenceph. clin. Neurophysiol.* 16, 269–279.

118. Wilson J. R., Friedlander M. J. and Sherman S. M. (1984) Ultrastructural morphology of identified X- and Y-cells in the cat's lateral geniculate nucleus. *Proc. R. Soc.* B221, 411–436.

119. Yamada T., Kameyama S., Fuchigami Z., Nakazumi Y., Dickins Q. S. and Kimura J. (1988) Changes of short latency somatosensory evoked potential in sleep. *Electroenceph. clin. Neurophysiol.* 70, 126–136.

120. Yen C. T., Conley M., Hendry S. H. C. and Jones E. G. (1985) The morphology of physiologically identified GABAergic neurons in the somatic sensory part of the thalamic reticular nucleus in the cat. *J. Neurosci.* 5, 2254–2268.

X THEORY

A surprisingly rich theoretical field has emerged in the last decade, attempting to deal with aspects of consciousness. Although there is clearly still a gap between theory and evidence, that gap seems to be narrowing. Three overlapping types of theories can be distinguished. First, there are theories that emphasize resonant neuronal assemblies, with roots in Hebbian theory, neuronal net models, and biological group-selection theory. A second set particularly emphasizes temporal coordination of large populations of neurons. Finally, emerging from the literature on cognitive architectures, Global Workspace theory combines a small, central domain related to working memory with a vast distributed set of specialized unconscious processors.

Reentry, Adaptive Resonance, and Neural Nets

Tononi and Edelman (1998; chap. 60, this volume) provide the first example of resonance theories. Gerald Edelman has long advocated the view that brain states emerge both embryologically and in environmental adaptation from a kind of Darwinian neuronal group selection, in which neurons that sustain each other by way of feedback survive and create additional connections, whereas less "fit" neurons and connections tend to die out. Tononi and Edelman extend that conception to the issue of consciousness, making use of formulae derived from the mathematical theory of information. They propose a "dynamic core hypothesis," in which consciousness corresponds to a reentrantly activated population of neurons in the thalamocortical system. Although this is a widely held view, Tononi and Edelman connect their hypothesis by way of precise mathematical definitions to testable evidence (see Tononi, Srinivasan, Russell, and Edelman 1998; chap. 7, this volume) and to fundamental concepts of mutual information and the emergence of organized patterns in massive parallel and distributed populations of neurons.

Grossberg (1999; chap. 61, this volume) provides a second example of a resonance theory, based on many years of modeling of specific structures in the brain. Grossberg's Adaptive Resonance Theory (ART) has been developed over two decades and has been applied to a sizable set of psychological and brain phenomena. The same basic principles appear to cast light on perception, recognition, attention, reinforcement, recall, and memory search. Grossberg suggests that all conscious states are resonant states. According to ART the important resonant states for consciousness are those that connect top-down and bottom-up processes (cognitive and sensory processes) in the process of reaching attentive consensus between expectations and sensory data.

Taylor (1992; chap. 62, this volume) also believes that conscious contents are determined by the intermingling of past and present. The reticular nucleus of the thalamus (nRt) appears to control the major sensory highways to cortex, and Taylor has provided a model for intersensory competition based on this evidence. Rather than a simple winner-take-all competition, he suggests that consciousness corresponds to a wave of activity of the coupled thalamic-nRt-cortical system, a multidimensional "bubble" of neuronal firing patterns. Such a winning wave will have many spatial regions over cortex that have nonzero activity.

Although there are distinct pros and cons to each theoretical perspective, the general impression is of a surprising degree of consensus on a set of fundamental ideas. The next two proposals add the dimension of temporal coordination to these basic ideas.

Temporal Correlation and Binding

Antonio Damasio's (1989; chap. 63, this volume) proposal specifically aims to understand recognition and recall from long-term memory. Like previous authors, Damasio advances a theory involving looping feedforward and feedback circuits of neurons—a kind of massive, resonant assembly of cells. To this fundamental mechanism he adds a specific role for sensory projection areas of the cortex (local convergence zones) and their neighboring higher-order association areas (nonlocal convergence zones). The notion of temporal synchrony is proposed to account for retrieval of information from memory, when neuron ensembles are activated in a time-locked fashion in the local and nonlocal convergence zones of the cortex. Memories are stored as large sets of fragmentary features in large populations of neurons, and are retrieved by means of synchronous activation of related firing patterns in a subset of the same cell population.

Wolf Singer's research group at the Max Planck Institute in Frankfurt has been pursuing the matter of temporal correlation longer and more systematically than any comparable group (see Engel et al., chap. 8, this volume). Singer and Gray (1995; chap. 64, this volume) present an excellent summary of the case for temporal synchrony as a way to coordinate and "bind" large populations of neurons. Temporal correlations have been observed between and within columns of cells in the cortex, between cortical regions and hemispheres, and between cortex, thalamus, and other areas of the brain. Time-correlated activity may be directly related to perceptual consciousness by way of the Gestalt laws, which determine how novel sensory elements go together to create whole conscious perceptual ensembles.

These two papers are variations on a theme. Global Workspace theory employs a different vocabulary, but one that is broadly compatible with resonance and temporal correlation theories.

Cognitive Architectures: Global Workspace Theory

Global Workspace (GW) theory emerges from a different tradition, but it is broadly consistent with resonance theories and with the idea of temporal synchrony. Early work on GW theory is stated in an artificial intelligence vocabulary, but Baars (1998; chap. 65, this volume) presents the theory in terms of a widely used analogy, which can broadly be called the "theater metaphor." Such heuristic analogies are common in the history of science, from the notion of "current flow" in electrical theory to the "lock and key" analogy of neurotransmitters to receptor sites. Ranging from Plato and the Upanishads to Francis Crick (1984; chap. 18, this volume), thinkers have talked about consciousness by analogy to a theater filled with unconscious spectators. The contents of consciousness correspond to the actors declaiming in a bright spot on the stage of the theater, cast by a spotlight under executive direction; and what happens in the bright spot is widely distributed to the audience, which includes large arrays of neurons in and outside of cortex.

GW theory was initially worked out as a cognitive architecture in the tradition of Allan Newell, Herbert A. Simon, and John R. Anderson (see Baars 1983, 1988, 1998). Specific mechanisms were proposed to deal with a vast array of psychological processes, from perceptual analysis to spontaneous problem solving, memory retrieval, language production, and the like. GW theory therefore appears to be the most broadly worked out explicit theory of conscious processes today, at a high level of description.

The evidentiary basis for GW theory is a set of some 30–40 contrastive cases in which comparable conscious and unconscious events appear to take place (see Introduction). The most prominent of these contrasts involves the limited capacity of conscious contents at any given moment, compared to the vastness and complexity of unconscious neuronal circuits. Thus consciousness is associated with limited capacity, seriality, and integration, whereas comparable unconscious processes are of much greater capacity, parallelism, and distributed autonomy.

Consciousness in such a massively parallel nervous system appears to represent a biological trade-off. The survival cost of limited capacity becomes apparent when we consider that prey animals are often caught when they are distracted—in ambush at a watering hole, for example. It is not possible for a giraffe to simultaneously bend down to drink, watch for predators, protect its young, and maintain its competitive dominance in the herd. Vertebrate brains were not designed to handle all those tasks simultaneously, at least not with full attention. The reality of "distraction" as a threat to survival is of course another way of talking about limited capacity. Predators, from their perspective, pay similar costs: they may die when they fail to catch a prey when it zigs or zags in a way they cannot track attentively. Limited capacity thus seems to exact a high biological cost, and this in turn suggests that it must have significant countervailing advantages (Baars 1993; chap. 66, this volume).

The answer suggested by GW theory is that in a large "society of mind" there are numerous autonomous brain functions that must be coordinated by a global distribution capacity, comparable to a newspaper or broadcasting station in a human society. Such a global workspace serves the needs of integration, coordination, and control. But such functioning also implies that the global coordinating system must be able to concentrate its resources on only one system-wide topic at any given moment. The limited capacity that is associated with consciousness thus has an indispensible advantage for any large nervous system, to make up for its apparent biological cost.

Newman, Baars, and Cho (1997; chap. 67, this volume) aim to cast the global workspace framework in a more neurally realistic form, giving special regard to thalamocortical mechanisms. Their work represents an effort to integrate GW theory with the neuronal resonance theories discussed before. They propose that, to a first approximation, the neural circuitry can be described in terms of repeating, parallel loops of thalamocortical neurons that pass through a thin sheet of neurons known as the nucleus reticularis thalami (nRt). The overall framework suggests a neurocognitive model in which consciousness is viewed as a global integration and dissemination system, nested in a large-scale, distributed array of specialized bioprocessors, which controls the allocation of processing resources in the central nervous system.

In an ambitious research effort, Franklin and Graesser (1999; chap. 68, this volume) are implementing the general claims of GW theory in applied contexts. If consciousness is functional, and if GW theory captures some of that functionality, then it should be possible to show how computer implementations of the theory can actually do useful things in the real world. The first project along these lines is called CMattie (for "Conscious" Mattie), an autonomous agent for sending and receiving email messages for organizing seminars at a university. Where GW theory postulates a collection of specialized unconscious processors in the brain, CMattie has a collection of specialized "codelets," each able to implement a single function, such as searching for related emails, decoding natural language expressions, and generating templates for answering e-mails. When CMattie encounters difficulties in assigning single codelets to a task, it can perform a global broadcast to recruit a coalition of codelets, which together may be able to solve the problem. This is the single most important function of a global workspace—to bring together multiple sources of knowledge in order to solve problems in ways that cannot be anticipated ahead of time (Baars 1988, 1997). Franklin and Graesser's effort is important to test whether the qualitative claims made about the theory are actually implementable, and whether they carry out the functions that are claimed. Franklin and Graesser are optimistic about these issues and suggest that computer simulations of GW theory meet a number of other empirical constraints that characterize conscious processes in the brain.

Although consciousness has only recently returned as a central focus of the brain and behavioral sciences, current theoretical proposals capture a good deal of the evidence, in a broad way. A critical mass of scientists appears to be succeeding in collecting relevant evidence and developing reasonable theory. Science is always a matter of confronting the unknown, and predictions about science are inherently risky. Nevertheless, it seems that we are better prepared today than ever before to try to understand human consciousness.

References

Baars, B. J. (1998) A cognitive theory of consciousness. Cambridge University Press.

Baars, B. J. (1997) In the theater of consciousness: The workspace of the mind. NY: Oxford University Press.

Giulio Tononi and Gerald M. Edelman

What is the neural substrate of conscious experience? While William James concluded that it was the entire brain (1), recent approaches have attempted to narrow the focus: are there neurons endowed with a special location or intrinsic property that are necessary and sufficient for conscious experience? Does primary visual cortex contribute to conscious experience? Are brain areas that project directly to prefrontal cortex more relevant than those that do not (2)? Although heuristically useful, these approaches leave a fundamental problem unresolved: How could the possession of some particular anatomical location or biochemical feature render some neurons so privileged that their activity gives rise to subjective experience? Conferring this property on neurons seems to constitute a category error, in the sense of ascribing to things properties they cannot have (3).

Here, we pursue a different approach. Instead of arguing whether a particular brain area or group of neurons contributes to consciousness or not, our strategy is to characterize the kinds of neural processes that might account for key properties of conscious experience. We emphasize two properties: conscious experience is integrated (each conscious scene is unified) and at the same time it is highly differentiated (within a short time, one can experience any of a huge number of different conscious states). We first consider neurobiological data indicating that neural processes associated with conscious experience are highly integrated and highly differentiated. We then provide tools for measuring integration (called functional clustering) and differentiation (called neural complexity) that are applicable to actual neural processes. This leads us to formulate operational criteria for determining whether the activity of a group of neurons contributes to conscious experience. These criteria are incorporated into the dynamic core

hypothesis, a testable proposal concerning the neural substrate of conscious experience (4).

General Properties of Conscious Experience

Consciousness, as William James pointed out, is not a thing, but a process or stream that is changing on a time scale of fractions of seconds (1). As he emphasized, a fundamental aspect of the stream of consciousness is that it is highly unified or integrated.

Integration

Integration is a property shared by every conscious experience irrespective of its specific content: Each conscious state comprises a single "scene" that cannot be decomposed into independent components (5). Integration is best appreciated by considering the impossibility of conceiving of a conscious scene that is not integrated, that is, one which is not experienced from a single point of view. A striking demonstration is given by split-brain patients performing a spatial memory task in which two independent sequences of visuospatial positions were presented, one to the left and one to the right hemisphere (6). In these patients, each hemisphere perceived a separate, simple visual problem and the subjects were able to solve the double task well. Normal subjects could not treat the two independent visual sequences as independent, parallel tasks. Instead, they combined the visual information into a single conscious scene and into a single, large problem that was much more difficult to solve.

The unity of conscious experience is also evidenced by our inability to perform multiple tasks, unless some tasks are highly automatic and impinge less on consciousness. Moreover, we cannot make more than a single conscious decision within an interval of a few hundreds of milliseconds, the so-called psychological refractory period (7). Furthermore, we cannot be aware of two incongruent scenes at the same time, as indicated by the bistability of ambiguous figures and the phenomenon of perceptual rivalry (8). Unity also entails that conscious experience is private, that is, it is always experienced from a particular point of view and cannot fully be shared (1).

Differentiation

While each conscious state is an integrated whole, perhaps the most remarkable property of conscious experience is its extraordinary differentiation or complexity. The number of different conscious states that can be accessed over a short time is exceedingly large. For example, even if we just consider visual images, we can easily discriminate among innumerable scenes within a fraction of a second (9). More generally, the occurrence of a given conscious state implies an extremely rapid selection among a repertoire of possible conscious states that is, in fact, as large as one's experience and imagination. Differentiation among a repertoire of possibilities constitutes information, in the specific sense of reduction of uncertainty (10). Although this is often taken for granted, the occurrence of one particular conscious state over billions of others therefore constitutes a correspondingly large amount of information. Furthermore, it is information that makes a difference, in that it may lead to different consequences in terms of either thought or action.

The informativeness of consciousness helps dispose of many of the paradoxes raised about conscious experience. Consider a photodiode that can differentiate between light and dark and then provide an audible output, and a conscious human performing the same task and giving a verbal report. Why should the differentiation between light and dark performed by the human be associated with conscious experience, while presumably that performed by the photodiode is not? The paradox disappears if one considers the information generated by such discriminations. To the photodiode, the discrimination between darkness and light is the only one available, and is therefore minimally informative. To a conscious human, by contrast, an experience of complete darkness and an experience of complete light are two specific conscious experiences selected out of an enormous repertoire, and their selection implies the availability of a correspondingly large amount of information. To understand consciousness, it is important to identify underlying neural processes that are both integrated and capable of such exceptionally informative differentiations.

General Properties of Neural Processes Underlying Conscious Experience

Distributed neural activity, particularly in the thalamocortical system, is almost certainly essential for determining the contents of conscious experience (4, 11). We suggested previously that a key neural mechanism underlying conscious experience are the reentrant interactions between posterior thalamocortical areas involved in perceptual categorization and anterior areas related to memory, value, and planning for action. Such interactions among neuronal groups in distributed brain areas may be necessary in order to generate a unified neural process corresponding to a multimodal conscious scene (4). Recent experimental findings are consistent with this hypothesis and suggest some generalizations about the neural processes that underlie conscious experience.

Activation and Deactivation of Distributed Neuronal Populations

Changes in specific aspects of conscious experience correlate with changes in activity in specific brain areas, whether the experience is driven by external stimuli, by memory, or by imagery and dreams (12). Conscious experience as such, however, involves the activation or deactivation of widely distributed brain areas (13), although what should count as the appropriate reference state for comparison is not clear. In subjects who are comatose or deeply anesthetized, unconsciousness is associated with a profound depression of neural activity in both the cerebral cortex and thalamus (13). During slow-wave sleep, in which consciousness is severely reduced or lost, cerebral blood flow is globally reduced as compared to both waking and REM (rapid eye movement) sleep, two brain states associated with vivid conscious reports (14). A more specific reference state would be the response to a simple sensory input when a subject is unaware of it versus when the subject is aware of it. We have used magnetoencephalography to measure brain responses to flickering visual stimuli under conditions of binocular rivalry (15). A vertical grating flickering at one frequency was presented to one eye and a horizontal grating, flickering at a different frequency, was presented to the other eye. Although the stimuli were presented together, the subjects perceived either the vertical grating or the horizontal grating, with an alternation every few seconds. It was found that the power of steady-state neuromagnetic responses at the frequency of the flickering stimulus (its frequency tag) was higher by 30–60% in many sensor locations when the subject was conscious of that stimulus. The sensors with frequency tags that correlated with conscious experience were widely distributed over both posterior (occipital and temporal) and anterior (frontal) areas. Furthermore, there were considerable variations among different subjects (figure 60.1).

A change in the degree to which neural activity is distributed within the brain may accompany the transition between conscious, controlled performance and unconscious, automated performance. When tasks are novel, brain activation related to the task is widely distributed;

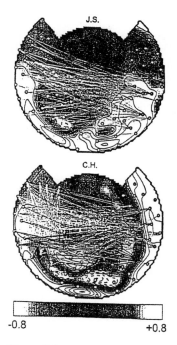

Figure 60.1
Amplitude and coherence differences between the steady-state neuromagnetic responses during binocular rivalry when subjects were conscious of a stimulus and when they were not. The differences are taken between amplitude and coherence values at 7.41 Hz when the subjects were conscious of a vertical grating flickered at 7.41 Hz and when they were not (that is, when they were conscious of a horizontal grating flickered at 9.5 Hz). Amplitude differences are topographically displayed for two subjects. Color scale is in picotesla. Significant positive differences in coherence at 7.41 Hz between pairs of distant sensors are indicated by superimposed cyan lines. Blue lines indicate negative differences in coherence. Filled green circles indicate channels with signal-to-noise ratio > 5 that have coherence values > 0.3 with at least one other channel. See (15) for details.

when the task has become automatic, activation is more localized and may shift to a different set of areas (16). In animal studies, neural activity related to sensory stimuli can be recorded in many brain regions before habituation. After habituation sets in (a time when humans report that stimuli tend to fade from consciousness), the same stimuli evoke neural activity exclusively along their specific sensory pathways (17). These observations suggest that when tasks are automatic and require little or no conscious control, the spread of signals that influence the performance of a task involves a more restricted and dedicated set of circuits that become "functionally insulated." This produces a gain in speed and precision, but a loss in context-sensitivity, accessibility, and flexibility (18).

Integration through Strong and Rapid Reentrant Interactions

Activation and deactivation of distributed neural populations in the thalamocortical system are not sufficient bases for conscious experience unless the activity of the neuronal groups involved is integrated rapidly and effectively. We have suggested that such rapid integration is achieved through the process of reentry—the ongoing, recursive, highly parallel signaling within and among brain areas. Large-scale computer simulations have shown that reentry can achieve the rapid integration or "binding" of distributed, functionally specialized neuronal groups dynamically, that is, in a unified neural process rather than in a single place (19, 20).

Substantial evidence indicates that the integration of distributed neuronal populations through reentrant interactions is required for conscious experience. An indication comes from the study of patients with disconnection syndromes, in which one or more brain areas are anatomically or functionally disconnected from the rest of the brain due to some pathological process (21). In the paradigmatic disconnection syndrome (the split brain), visual or somato-

sensory stimuli can activate the nondominant hemisphere and lead to behavioral responses, but the dominant, verbal hemisphere is not aware of them (22). Although the two hemispheres can still communicate through indirect, subcortical routes, rapid and effective neural interactions mediated by direct reentrant connections are abolished by the lesion of the corpus callosum. Modeling studies suggest that a telltale sign of effective reentrant interactions is the occurrence of short-term temporal correlations between the neuronal groups involved (19). Experiments on cats show that short-term temporal correlations between the activity of neuronal groups responding to the same stimulus, but located in different hemispheres, are abolished by callosal transections (23). Other studies indicate that various kinds of cognitive tasks are accompanied by the occurrence of short-term temporal correlations among distributed populations of neurons in the thalamocortical system (24). The magnetoencephalographic study of binocular rivalry mentioned above (15) also indicates that awareness of a stimulus is associated with increased coherence among distant brain regions (figure 60.1).

The requirement for fast, strong, and distributed neural interactions may explain why stimuli that are feeble, degraded, or short-lasting, often fail to be consciously perceived. Although such stimuli may produce a behavioral response [perception without awareness (25, 26)], they are unlikely to ignite neural activity of sufficient strength or duration to support fast distributed interactions. Conversely, attention may increase the conscious salience of certain stimuli by boosting the corresponding neural responses as well as the strength of neural interactions (27). Neural activity is also more likely to contribute effectively to distributed neural interactions if it is sustained for hundreds of milliseconds. This would lead to the functional closure of longer reentrant loops and thereby support reentrant interactions among more distant regions (19, 20). Experimental findings are consistent with this idea. High-frequency somatosensory stimuli delivered to the thalamus require about 500 ms for the production of a conscious sensory experience, while less than 150 ms are sufficient for sensory detection without awareness (28). The sustained evoked potentials associated with a conscious somatosensory sensation are apparently generated by the excitation of pyramidal neurons of primary somatosensory cortex through reentrant interactions with higher cortical areas (29).

Evidence for a correlation between conscious experience and sustained neural activity also comes from tasks involving visuospatial working memory—the ability to rehearse or "keep in mind" a spatial location. Working memory is used to bring or keep some item in consciousness or close to conscious access (30). In working memory tasks, sustained neural activity is found in prefrontal cortex of monkeys, and it is apparently maintained by reentrant interactions between frontal and parietal regions (31). Sustained neural activity may facilitate the integration of the activity of spatially segregated brain regions into a coherent, multimodal neural process that is stable enough to permit decision-making and planning (32).

Differentiated Patterns of Activity

Although strong and fast reentrant interactions among distributed groups of neurons are necessary for conscious experience, in themselves, they are still not sufficient. This is strikingly demonstrated by the unconsciousness accompanying generalized seizures and slow-wave sleep. During generalized seizures, the brain is not only extremely active, but most neurons fire in a highly synchronous manner. For example, the electroencephalogram (EEG) during petit mal absences indicates that groups of neurons over the whole brain are either all firing together or all silent together, with these two neural states alternating every third of a second. Although such hypersynchronous firing is indicative of strong and distributed interactions, a subject who is prey to such a seizure is unconscious. Similarly, during slow-wave sleep, neurons in the thalamocortical system are active as well as remarkably interactive, as shown by their synchronous firing in a stereotyped, burst-pause pattern. During this stage of sleep, however, it is rare to obtain vivid and extensive conscious reports (33). By contrast, during REM sleep, when neural activity is not globally synchronous but resembles the rapid and complex patterns of waking, subjects typically report vivid dreams if awakened. We suggest that the low-voltage, fast-activity EEG characteristic of waking and REM sleep reflects the availability of a rich and diverse repertoire of neural activity patterns. If the repertoire of differentiated neural states is large, consciousness is possible. Conversely, if this repertoire is reduced, as when most groups of neurons in the cortex discharge synchronously and functional discriminations among them are obliterated, consciousness is curtailed or lost (34).

Theoretical Concepts and Measures

This brief review of neurological and neurophysiological data indicates that the distributed neural process underlying conscious experience must be functionally integrated and at the same time highly differentiated. As mentioned above, two key properties of conscious experience are that it is integrated, in the sense that it cannot be subdivided into independent components, and that it is extremely differentiated, in the sense that it is possible, within a short time, to select among an enormous number of different conscious states. It is a central claim of this article that analyzing the convergence between these phenomenological and neural properties can yield valuable insights into the kinds of neural processes that can account for the corresponding properties of conscious experience. Such an analysis requires the availability of satisfactory measures of integration and differentiation that can be applied to actual neural processes, as well as an understanding of the neural mechanisms of integration.

Functional Clustering: How to Identify an Integrated Process

How can one determine whether a neural process is unified or simply a collection of independent or nearly independent subprocesses? We have suggested that a subset of distributed elements within a system gives rise to a single, integrated process if, at a given time scale, these elements interact much more strongly among themselves than with the rest of the system—for example, if they form a functional cluster. This criterion has been formalized by introducing a direct measure of functional clustering (35) which we summarize here.

Consider a jth subset of k elements (X_j^k) taken from an isolated neural system X, and its complement $(X - X_j^k)$. Interactions between the subset and the rest of the system introduce statistical dependence between the two. This is measured most generally by their mutual information $\mathrm{MI}(X_j^k; X - X_j^k) = \mathrm{H}(X_j^k) + \mathrm{H}(X - X_j^k) - \mathrm{H}(X)$, which captures the extent to which the entropy of X_j^k is accounted for by the entropy of $X - X_j^k$ and vice versa (H indicates statistical entropy (36)). The statistical dependence within a subset can be measured by a generalization of mutual information, which is called integration and is given by $\mathrm{I}(X_j^k) = \Sigma \mathrm{H}(x_i) - \mathrm{H}(X_j^k)$, where $\mathrm{H}(x_i)$ is the entropy of each element x_i considered independently. We then define the functional cluster index $\mathrm{CI}(X_j^k) = \mathrm{I}(X_j^k)/\mathrm{MI}(X_j^k; X - X_j^k)$ as a ratio of the statistical dependence within the subset and the statistical dependence between that subset and the rest of the system. Based on this definition, a subset of neural elements that has a CI value much higher than 1 and does not itself contain any smaller subset with a higher CI value constitutes a functional cluster. This is a single, integrated neural process that cannot be

decomposed into independent or nearly independent components.

We have applied these measures of functional clustering both to simulated datasets and to positron emission tomography data obtained from schizophrenic subjects performing cognitive tasks (35). Theoretically sound measures that can detect the occurrence of functional clustering at the time scale (fractions of a second) crucial for conscious experience may require additional assumptions. Nevertheless, it would appear that the rapid establishment of synchronous firing among cortical regions and between cortex and thalamus should be considered as an indirect indicator of functional clustering, since it implies strong and fast neural interactions among the neural populations involved (19, 20). The mechanisms of rapid functional clustering among distributed populations of neurons in the thalamocortical system have been studied with the help of large-scale simulations (19, 20). These have shown that the emergence of high-frequency synchronous firing in the thalamocortical system depends critically on the dynamics of corticothalamic and corticocortical reentrant circuits and on the opening of voltage-dependent channels in the horizontal corticocortical connections (37).

Neural Complexity: Measuring the Differences That Make a Difference

Once an integrated neural process is identified, we need to determine to what degree that process is differentiated. Does it give rise to a large repertoire of different activity patterns or neural states? It is essential to consider only those differences between activity patterns that make a difference to the system itself. A TV screen may, for example, go through a large number of "activity patterns" that look different to an external observer, but that make no difference to the TV.

A possible approach to measuring differences that make a difference within an integrated neural system is to consider it as its own "observer." This can be achieved by dividing the system (which, we assume, constitutes a functional cluster) into two subsets and then measuring their mutual information (38). The value of $MI(X_j^k; X - X_j^k)$ between a jth subset X_j^k of the isolated system X and its complement $X - X_j^k$ will be high if two conditions are met. Both X_j^k and $X - X_j^k$ must have many states (their entropy must be relatively high (10)), and the states of X_j^k and of $X - X_j^k$ must be statistically dependent (the entropy of X_j^k must be largely accounted for by the interactions with $X - X_j^k$, and vice versa). The expression $MI(X_j^k; X - X_j^k)$ reflects how much, on average, changes in the state of $X - X_j^k$ make a difference to the state of X_j^k, and vice versa.

To obtain an overall measure to how differentiated a system is, one can consider not just a single subset of its constituent elements, but all its possible subsets. The corresponding measure, called neural complexity, is given by $C_N(X) = 1/2\Sigma\langle MI(X_j^k; X - X_j^k)\rangle$, where the sum is taken over all k subset sizes and the average is taken over all jth combinations of k elements. Complexity is thus a function of the average mutual information between each subset and the rest of the system, and it reflects the number of states of a system that result from interactions among its elements (39).

It can be shown that high values of complexity reflect the coexistence of a high degree of functional specialization and functional integration within a system, as appears to be the case for systems such as the brain. For example, the dynamic behavior of a simulated cortical area containing thousands of spontaneously active neuronal groups (38) resembled the low-voltage fast-activity EEG of waking states and had high complexity. Such a system, whose connections were organized according to the rules found in the cortex, visited a large repertoire of different activity patterns that were the result of interactions among its elements. If the density of the connections was reduced, the dynamic behavior of the model resembled that of a noisy TV screen and had minimal complexity. A large number of activity patterns were visited, but they were merely the result of the independent fluctuations of its elements. If the connections within the cortical area were instead distributed at random, the system yielded a hypersynchronous EEG that resembled the high-voltage waves of slow-wave sleep or of generalized epilepsy. The system visited a very limited repertoire of activity patterns, and its complexity was low.

Measures of complexity, like measures of functional clustering, can also be applied to neurophysiological data to evaluate the degree to which a neural process is both integrated and differentiated (40). This opens the way to comparisons of the values of neural complexity in different cognitive and arousal states and to empirical tests of the relationships between brain complexity and conscious experience.

The Dynamic Core Hypothesis

A final issue we should consider is whether the neural process underlying conscious experience extends to most of the brain, as was concluded by William James, or is restricted to varying subsets of neuronal groups. Several observations support the latter possibility.

1. Classical lesion and stimulation studies suggest that many brain structures outside the thalamocortical system have no direct influence on conscious experience. Even within the thalamocortical system, many regions can be lesioned or stimulated without producing direct effects on conscious experience (41).

2. Neurophysiological studies indicate a possible dissociation between conscious experience and ongoing neural activity within portions of the thalamocortical system. During binocular rivalry in monkeys, a large proportion of neurons in early visual areas, such as V1, V4, and MT, continued to fire to their preferred stimulus even

when it was not consciously perceived (42). The activity of only a subset of the neurons recorded in these areas was correlated with the percept, although in higher areas such as IT and STS, the percentage reached 95%. In our magneto-encephalographic study of binocular rivalry in humans (figure 60.1) (15), we found that the responses of only a subset of occipital, temporal, and frontal areas was correlated with the conscious perception of a stimulus, although several other regions showed widespread responses to stimuli that were not consciously perceived.

3. The firing of neurons dealing with rapidly varying local details of a sensory input or a motor output does not seem to map to conscious experience. The latter deals with invariant properties of objects that are highly informative as well as more stable and easily manipulated. For example, patterns of neural activity in the retina and other early visual structures correspond faithfully to spatial and temporal details of the visual input and are in constant flux. During each visual fixation, however, humans extract the meaning of a scene and are not conscious of considerable changes in its local details (43). Groups of neurons responding in a stable way to invariant properties of objects are therefore more likely to contribute to conscious experience.

4. Many neural processes devoted to carrying out highly automated routines that make it possible to talk, listen, read, write, and so forth, in a fast and effortless way do not appear to contribute directly to conscious experience, although they are essential in determining its content (44). As mentioned above, neural circuits carrying out such highly practiced neural routines may become functionally insulated except at the input or output stages. There is also some evidence that cortical regions that are part of a fast system for controlling action, such as the dorsal visual stream, may not contribute significantly to conscious experience (45).

5. Although the sheer anatomical connectivity of the brain may hint that, over a sufficiently long time scale, everything can interact with everything else, modeling studies indicate that only certain interactions within the thalamocortical system are fast and strong enough to lead to the formation of a large functional cluster within a few hundred milliseconds (46).

These observations suggest that changes in the firing of only certain distributed subsets of the neuronal groups that are activated or deactivated in response to a given task are associated with conscious experience. What is special about these subsets of neuronal groups, and how can they be identified? We suggest the following:

1. A group of neurons can contribute directly to conscious experience only if it is part of a distributed functional cluster that achieves high integration in hundreds of milliseconds.

2. To sustain conscious experience, it is essential that this functional cluster be highly differentiated, as indicated by high values of complexity.

We propose that a large cluster of neuronal groups that together constitute, on a time scale of hundreds of milliseconds, a unified neural process of high complexity be termed the "dynamic core," in order to emphasize both its integration and its constantly changing activity patterns. The dynamic core is a functional cluster: its participating neuronal groups are much more strongly interactive among themselves than with the rest of the brain. The dynamic core must also have high complexity: its global activity patterns must be selected within less than a second out of a very large repertoire.

The dynamic core would typically include posterior corticothalamic regions involved in perceptual categorization interacting reentrantly with anterior regions involved in concept formation, value-related memory, and planning (4), although it would not necessarily be restricted to the thalamocortical system. The term "dynamic core" deliberately does not refer to a unique, invariant set of brain areas (be they prefrontal, extrastriate, or striate cortex), and the core may change in composition over time (47). Because our hypothesis highlights the role of the functional interactions among distributed groups of neurons rather than their local properties (2), the same group of neurons may at times be part of the dynamic core and underlie conscious experience, while at other times it may not be part of it and thus be involved in unconscious processes. Furthermore, since participation in the dynamic core depends on the rapidly shifting functional connectivity among groups of neurons rather than on anatomical proximity, the composition of the core can transcend traditional anatomical boundaries (48). Finally, as suggested by imaging studies (15), the exact composition of the core related to particular conscious states is expected to vary significantly across individuals.

The dynamic core hypothesis avoids the category error of assuming that certain local, intrinsic properties of neurons have, in some mysterious way, a privileged correlation with consciousness. Instead, this hypothesis accounts for fundamental properties of conscious experience by linking them to global properties of particular neural processes. We have seen that conscious experience is a process that is unified and private, that is extremely differentiated, and that evolves on a time scale of hundreds of milliseconds. The dynamic core is a process, since it is characterized in terms of time-varying neural interactions, not as a thing or a location. It is unified and private, because its integration must be high at the same time as its mutual information with what surrounds is low, thus creating a functional boundary between what is part of it and what is not. The requirement for high complexity means that the dynamic core must be highly differentiated—it must be able to select, based on its intrinsic interactions, among a large repertoire of different activity patterns. Finally, the selection among integrated states must be achieved within hundreds of milliseconds, thus reflecting the time course of conscious experience (49).

A number of experimental questions and associated predictions are generated by this hypothesis. A central prediction is that, during cognitive activities involving consciousness, there should be evidence for a large but distinct set of distributed neuronal groups that interact over fractions of a second much more strongly among themselves than with the rest of the brain. This prediction could, in principle, be tested by recording, in parallel, multiple neurons whose activity is correlated with conscious experience. Multielectrode recordings have already indicated that rapid changes in the functional connectivity among distributed populations of neurons can occur independently of firing rate (50). Recent studies in monkey frontal cortex also show abrupt and simultaneous shifts among stationary activity states involving several, but not all recorded neurons (51). A convincing demonstration of rapid functional clustering among distributed neuronal groups requires, however, that these studies be extended to larger populations of neurons in several brain areas. Another possibility would be to examine whether the effects of direct cortical microstimulation spread more widely in the brain if they are associated with conscious experience than if they are not. In humans, the extent and boundaries of neural populations exchanging coherent signals can be evaluated through methods of frequency tagging (15). Techniques offering both wide spatial coverage and high temporal resolution could also help establish how large a dynamic core normally is, how its composition changes, and whether certain brain regions are always included or always exlcuded. It is also significant to ask whether the dynamic core can split, and thus whether multiple dynamic cores can coexist in a normal subject. A reasonable prediction would be that certain disorders of consciousness, notably dissociative disorders and schizophrenia, should be reflected in abnormalities of the dynamic core and possibly result in the formation of multiple cores.

A strong prediction based on our hypothesis is that the complexity of the dynamic core should correlate with the conscious state of the subject.

For example, we predict that neural complexity should be much higher during waking and REM sleep than during the deep stages of slow-wave sleep, and that it should be extremely low during epileptic seizures despite the overall increase in brain activity. We also predict that neural processes underlying automatic behaviors, no matter how sophisticated, should have lower complexity than neural processes underlying consciously controlled behaviors. Finally, a systematic increase in the complexity of coherent neural processes is expected to accompany cognitive development.

The outcome of such tests should indicate whether conscious phenomenology can indeed be related, as we suggest, to a distributed neural process that is both highly integrated and highly differentiated. The evidence available so far supports the belief that a scientific explanation of consciousness is becoming increasingly feasible (52).

References and Notes

1. W. James, *The Principles of Psychology* (Holt, New York, 1890).

2. F. Crick and C. Koch, *Cold Spring Harbor Symp. Quant. Biol.* 55, 953 (1990); *Nature* 375, 121 (1995); S. Zeki and A. Bartels, *Proc. R. Soc. London Ser. B* 265, 1583 (1998).

3. G. Ryle, *The Concept of Mind* (Hutchinson, London, 1949).

4. G. M. Edelman, *The Remembered Present* (Basic Books, New York, 1989); G. M. Edelman and G. Tononi, *Consciousness: How Matter Becomes Imagination* (Basic Books, New York, in press); see also G. Tononi and G. M. Edelman, in *Consciousness*, H. Jasper et al., Eds. (Plenum, New York, 1998), pp. 245–280.

5. A "conscious state" is meant here as an idealization, exemplified by viewing a rapid succession of slides.

6. J. D. Holtzman and M. S. Gazzaniga, *Neuropsychologia* 23, 315 (1985).

7. H. Pashler, *Psychol. Bull.* 116, 220 (1994). The duration of this interval is comparable with the duration

8. F. Sengpiel, *Curr. Biol.* 7, R447 (1997).

9. H. Intraub, *J. Exp. Psychol. Hum. Percept. Perform.* 7, 604 (1981); I. Biederman, *Science* 177, 77 (1972).

10. C. E. Shannon and W. Weaver, *The Mathematical Theory of Communication* (Univ. of Illinois Press, Urbana, IL, 1963). Note that the Informativeness of consciousness also helps us to understand its evolutionary value (4).

11. V. B. Mountcastle, in *The Mindful Brain*, G. M. Edelman and V. B. Mountcastle, Eds. (MIT Press, Cambridge, MA, 1978), p. 7; A. Damasio, *Cognition* 33, 25 (1989); R. Llinas, U. Ribary, M. Joliot, X.-J. Wang, in *Temporal Coding in the Brain*, G. Buzsaki, R. Llinás, W. Singer, Eds. (Springer-Verlag, Berlin, 1994); J. Newman, *Consciousness Cognit.* 4, 172 (1995); T. W. Picton and D. T. Stuss, *Curr. Biol.* 4, 256 (1994).

12. R. S. J. Frackowiak, *Human Brain Function* (Academic Press, San Diego, CA, 1997); P. E. Roland, *Brain Activation* (Wiley-Liss, New York, 1993); M. I. Posner and M. E. Raichle, *Images of Mind* (Scientific American Library, New York, 1994). These imaging studies confirm and extend previous lesion and stimulation studies.

13. Lesion studies indicate that consciousness is abolished by widely distributed damage but not by localized cortical damage. The only localized brain lesions resulting in loss of consciousness typically affect the reticular core in the upper brainstem and hypothalamus or its rostral extensions in the reticular and intralaminar thalamic nuclei [F. Plum, in *Normal and Altered States of Function*, A. Peters and E. G. Jones, Eds. (Plenum, New York, 1991), vol. 9, p. 359]. Although it has been suggested that the reticular core may have a privileged connection to conscious experience [J. E. Bogen, *Consciousness Cognit.* 4, 52 (1995)], its activity may simply be required to sustain distributed activity patterns in the cortex.

14. A. R. Braun et al., *Science* 279, 91 (1998); P. Maquet et al., *Nature* 383, 163 (1996). Neural activity in slow-wave sleep is reduced in both anterior neocortical regions (most of the prefrontal cortex), as well as in posterior cortical regions (especially parietal association areas), in paralimbic structures (anterior cingulate cortex and anterior insula), and in centrencephalic structures (reticular activating system,

of conscious states [A. L. Blumenthal, *The Process of Cognition* (Prentice-Hall, Englewood Cliffs, NJ, 1977)].

thalamus, and basal ganglia); in contrast, it is not depressed in unimodal sensory areas (primary visual, auditory, and somatosensory cortex).

15. G. Tononi, R. Srinivasan, D. P. Russell, G. M. Edelman, *Proc. Natl. Acad. Sci. U.S.A.* 95, 3198 (1998); R. Srinivasan, D. P. Russell, G. M. Edelman, G. Tononi, *Soc. Neurosci. Abstr.* 24, 433 (1998).

16. S. E. Petersen, H. vanMier, J. A. Fiez, M. E. Raichle, *Proc. Natl. Acad. Sci. U.S.A.* 95, 853 (1998); R. J. Haier et al., *Brain Res.* 570, 134 (1992).

17. J. A. Horel et al., *Science* 158, 394 (1967).

18. B. J. Baars, *A Cognitive Theory of Consciousness* (Cambridge Univ. Press, New York, 1988).

19. O. Sporns, G. Tononi, G. M. Edelman, *Proc. Natl. Acad. Sci. U.S.A.* 88, 129 (1991); G. Tononi, O. Sporns, G. M. Edelman, *Cereb. Cortex* 2, 310 (1992).

20. E. D. Lumer, G. M. Edelman, G. Tononi, *Cereb. Cortex* 7, 207 (1997); ibid., p. 228. For example, in a large-scale model of the visual system, reentrant interactions between groups of neurons in perceptual or "posterior" areas and in executive or "anterior" areas rapidly led to their synchronous firing and to a correct behavioral discrimination. This discrimination was based on the dynamic binding of multiple visual attributes (position, movement, color, form) and of different levels of stimulus generalization (local features, invariant aspects of stimuli).

21. B. Kolb and I. Q. Whishaw, *Fundamentals of Human Neuropsychology* (Freeman, New York, 1996). Psychiatric dissociation syndromes and conversion disorders may originate from a similar alteration of reentrant interactions, although in these cases, the disconnection would be functional rather than anatomical [J. F. Kihlstrom, *Consciousness Cognit.* 1, 47 (1992)]. Some explicit-implicit dissociations, such as amnesia, may also be due to a partial disconnection of a lesioned area from the more global pattern of neural activity that is associated with consciousness [D. L. Schacter, *Proc. Natl. Acad. Sci. U.S.A.* 89, 11113 (1992)].

22. M. S. Gazzaniga, *Neuron* 14, 217 (1995).

23. A. K. Engel, P. König, A. K. Kreiter, W. Singer, *Science* 252, 1177 (1991).

24. S. L. Bressler, *Brain Res. Rev.* 20, 288 (1995); W. Singer and C. M. Gray, *Annu. Rev. Neurosci.* 18, 555 (1995); M. Joliot, U. Ribary, R. Llinas, *Proc. Natl. Acad. Sci. U.S.A.* 91, 11748 (1994); A. Gevins et al., *Electroencephalogr. Clin. Neurophysiol.* 98, 327 (1996).

25. A. J. Marcel, *Cognit. Psychol.* 15, 238 (1983); ibid., p. 197; P. M. Merikle, *Am. Psychol.* 47, 792 (1992). In some cases, perception without awareness has been shown to occur with stimuli that are not short-lasting or weak [F. C. Kolb and J. Braun, *Nature* 377, 336 (1995); S. He, H. S. Smallman, D. I. A. Macleod, *Invest. Ophthalmol. Visual Sci.* 36, S438 (1995)].

26. S. He, P. Cavanagh, J. Intriligator, *Nature* 383, 334 (1996).

27. J. H. Maunsell, *Science* 270, 764 (1995); K. J. Friston, *Proc. Natl. Acad. Sci. U.S.A.* 95, 796 (1998).

28. B. Libet, *Ciba Found. Symp.* 174, 123 (1993).

29. L. Cauller, *Behav. Brain Res.* 71, 163 (1995).

30. A. Baddeley, *Proc. Natl. Acad. Sci. U.S.A.* 93, 13468 (1996).

31. J. M. Fuster, R. H. Bauer, J. P. Jervey, *Brain Res.* 330, 299 (1985); P. S. Goldman-Rakic and M. Chafee, *Soc. Neurosci. Abstr.* 20, 808 (1994).

32. The idea that neural activity must persist for a minimum period of time in order to contribute to conscious experience is also suggested by the phenomenon of masking [J. L. Taylor and D. I. McCloskey, *Exp. Brain Res.* 110, 62 (1996); K. J. Meador et al., *Neurology* 51, 721 (1998)].

33. M. Steriade, *Cereb. Cortex* 7, 583 (1997); D. Kahn, E. F. Pace-Schott, J. A. Hobson, *Neuroscience* 78, 13 (1997).

34. Neural activity must also exhibit sufficient variance in time to support conscious perception. For example, if images on the retina are stabilized, perception fades rapidly, and a similar effect is seen in Ganzfeld stimulation. Short-lasting visual stimuli become invisible if the transient neuronal responses associated with their onset and offset are suppressed by masking stimuli [S. L. Macknik and M. S. Livingstone, *Nature Neurosci.* 1, 144 (1998)].

35. G. Tononi, A. R. McIntosh, D. P. Russell, G. M. Edelman, *Neuroimage* 7, 133 (1998).

36. As a measure of statistical dependence, mutual information has the virtue of being highly general, because it is multivariate and sensitive to high-order moments of statistical dependence [A. Papoulis, *Probability, Random Variables, and Stochastic Processes* (McGraw-Hill, New York, 1991)]. Note that mutual information reflects a statistical dependence among subsets of a system, irrespective of its source. The presence and direction of causal interactions between

two subsets of a system can be evaluated, at least in principle, by measuring the change in mutual information obtained by perturbing or deefferenting each subset in turn.

37. These observations are of interest in view of the well-known action of certain so-called dissociative anesthetics, such as ketamine and phencyclidine, that act as noncompetitive antagonists of the *N*-methyl-D-aspartate receptor [H. Flohr, *Behav. Brain Res.* 71, 157 (1995)].

38. G. Tononi, O. Sporns, G. M. Edelman, *Proc. Natl. Acad. Sci. U.S.A.* 91, 5033 (1994). A complexity measure that does not involve the calculation of average values of integration and mutual information can also be defined as the amount of the entropy of a system that is accounted for by the interactions among its elements and is given by $\Sigma MI(X_j^1; X - X_j^1) - I(X)$. Note that complexity measures should be applied to a single system (a functional cluster) and not to a collection of independent or nearly independent subsystems.

39. Changes in complexity can be obtained without modifying the anatomical connectivity of the model by simulating the transition between the burst-pause pattern of firing typical of slow-wave sleep and the tonic mode of firing typical of waking and REM sleep (G. Tononi, unpublished material). It should be noted that high complexity is not easy to achieve. A system of elements that are randomly interconnected, for instance, may look very complicated, but it has low values of complexity. On the other hand, systems that undergo selective processes so as to match the statistical structure of a rich environment will gradually increase their complexity [G. Tononi, O. Sporns, G. M. Edelman, *Proc. Natl. Acad. Sci. U.S.A.* 93, 3422 (1996)].

40. K. J. Friston, G. Tononi, O. Sporns, G. M. Edelman, *Hum. Brain Mapp.* 3, 302 (1995).

41. W. Penfield, *The Excitable Cortex in Conscious Man* (Thomas, Springfield, IL, 1958).

42. D. A. Leopold and N. K. Logothetis, *Nature* 379, 549 (1996); D. L. Shenberg and N. K. Logothetis, *Proc. Natl. Acad. Sci. U.S.A.* 94, 3408 (1997). For other instances of dissociation, see (26); M. Gur and D. M. Snodderly, *Vision Res.* 37, 377 (1997); I. N. Pigarev, H. C. Nothdurft, S, Kastner, *Neuroreport* 8, 2557 (1997); D. C. Bradley, G. C. Chang, R. A. Andersen, *Nature* 392, 714 (1998).

43. D. J. Simons and D. T. Levin, *Trends Cogn. Sci.* 1, 261 (1997). The neurological evidence is in agreement with these psychological observations. In the adult, lesions of the retina produce blindness, but they do not eliminate visual imagery, visual memories, and visual dreams, while the latter are eliminated by lesions of certain visual cortical areas [M. Solms, *The Neuropsychology of Dreams* (Erlbaum, Mahwah, NJ, 1997)]. V1 may be important, however, to provide visual consciousness with a certain degree of detail. See also R. Jackendoff [*Consciousness and the Computational Mind* (MIT Press, Cambridge, MA, 1987)].

44. R. M. Shiffrin, in *Scientific Approaches to Consciousness*, J. D. Cohen and J. W. Schooler, Eds. (Erlbaum, Mahwah, NJ, 1997), p. 49; L. L. Jacoby, D. Ste-Marie, J. P. Toth, in *Attention: Selection, Awareness, and Control*, A. D. Baddeley and L. Weiskrantz, Eds. (Clarendon, Oxford, 1993), p. 261; W. Schneider, M. Pimm-Smith, M. Worden, *Curr. Opin. Neurobiol.* 4, 177 (1994).

45. A. D. Milner, *Neuropsychologia* 33, 1117 (1995); A. D. Milner and M. A. Goodale, *The Visual Brain in Action* (Oxford Univ. Press, New York, 1995).

46. The organization of the anatomical connectivity of certain brain regions, such as the thalamocortical system, is much more effective in generating coherent dynamic states than that of other regions, such as the cerebellum or the basal ganglia (G. Tononi, unpublished material). Consistent with this, although in cortical and thalamic areas 20–50% of all pairs of neurons recorded are broadly synchronized, neurons in the internal segment of the globus pallidus, the output station of the basal ganglia, are almost completely uncorrelated [H. Bergman et al., *Trends Neurosci.* 21, 32 (1998)].

47. If the fast integration of neural activity comes at a premium in terms of number of connections and energetic requirements, neuronal groups in "higher" areas should be privileged members of the dynamic core underlying consciousness. Everything else being equal, their firing is more informative, in the sense that it rules out a larger number of possibilities. For example, the firing of face-selective neurons in area IT considerably reduces uncertainty about a visual scene (seeing a face rules out countless other visual scenes), while the firing of retinal neurons reduces uncertainty by much less (a bright spot in a certain position of the visual field is consistent with countless visual scenes). The results of studies of binocular rivalry in monkeys and humans mentioned above are consistent with this view.

48. We emphasize that the dynamic core, the highly complex, rapidly established functional cluster pro-

posed to underlie conscious experience, is in no way the only integrated but distributed neural process that is relevant to brain function. We have hypothesized that distributed but integrated neural processes called global mappings, encompassing portions of the thalamocortical system, as well as parallel loops through cortical appendages such as the basal ganglia, the hippocampus, and the cerebellum, underlie the unity of behavioral sequences (4). The functional integration of global mappings is envisioned to occur at longer time scales than the dynamic core (seconds as opposed to fractions of a second). However, these two kinds of dynamic processes are expected to partially overlap for short periods of time.

49. Qualia—the seemingly inexplicable phenomenological manifestations of conscious experience—are conceived within this framework as rapid, highly informative discriminations within a repertoire of billions of neural states available to a unified neural process of great complexity. They correspond to the generation of a large amount of information in a short period of time. In this view, each quale—even a seemingly simple quale like a feeling of "redness"—corresponds to a discriminable state of the dynamic core in its entirety, and not merely to the state of a specific group of neurons in a certain brain area. The subjective meaning or quale of "redness," for example, would be defined by the (increased) activity of red-selective neurons as much as by the (reduced or unmodified) activity of neuronal groups selective for green or blue, for visual motion or shape, for auditory or somatosensory events, and for proprioceptive inputs, body schemas, emotions, intentions, and so forth, that jointly constitute the dynamic core. This view is antithetical to modular or atomistic approaches to consciousness (2).

50. E. Vaadia et al., *Nature* 373, 515 (1995).

51. E. Seidemann, I. Meilijson, M. Abeles, H. Bergman, E. Vaadia, *J. Neurosci.* 16, 752 (1996).

52. It is perhaps worth pointing out that our analysis predicts the possibility of constructing a conscious artifact and outlines some key principles that should constrain its construction. This work was carried out as part of the theoretical neurobiology program at The Neurosciences Institute, which is supported by Neurosciences Research Foundation. The Foundation receives major support for this program from Novartis Pharmaceuticals Corporation and the W. M. Keck Foundation.

61   Brain Learning, Attention, and Consciousness

Stephen Grossberg

How Do We Continue to Learn Throughout Life?

We experience the world as a whole. Although myriad signals relentlessly bombard our senses, we somehow integrate them into unified moments of conscious experience that cohere together despite their diversity. Because of the apparent unity and coherence of our awareness, we can develop a sense of self that can gradually mature with our experiences of the world. This capacity lies at the heart of our ability to function as intelligent beings.

The apparent unity and coherence of our experiences is all the more remarkable when we consider several properties of how the brain copes with the environmental events that it processes. First and foremost, these events are highly context-sensitive. When we look at a complex picture or scene as a whole, we can often recognize its objects and its meaning at a glance, as in the picture of a familiar face. However, if we process the face piece-by-piece, as through a small aperture, then its significance may be greatly degraded. To cope with this context-sensitivity, the brain typically processes pictures and other sense data in parallel, as *patterns* of activation across a large number of feature-sensitive nerve cells, or neurons. The same is true for senses other than vision, such as audition. If the sound of the word GO is altered by clipping off the vowel O, then the consonant G may sound like a chirp, quite unlike its sound as part of GO.

During vision, all the signals from a scene typically reach the photosensitive retinas of the eyes at essentially the same time, so parallel processing of all the scene's parts begins at the retina itself. During audition, each successive sound reaches the ear at a later time. Before an entire pattern of sounds, such as the word GO, can be processed as a whole, it needs to be re-coded, at a later processing stage, into a simultaneously available spatial pattern of activation. Such a processing stage is often called a working memory, and the activations that it stores are often called short-term memory (STM) traces. For example, when you hear an unfamiliar telephone number, you can temporarily store it in working memory while you walk over to the telephone and dial the number.

In order to determine which of these patterns represents familiar events and which do not, the brain matches these patterns against stored representations of previous experiences that have been acquired through learning. Unlike the STM traces that are stored in a working memory, the learned experiences are stored in long-term memory (LTM) traces. One difference between STM and LTM traces concerns how they react to distractions. For example, if you are distracted by a loud noise before you dial a new telephone number, its STM representation can be rapidly reset so that you forget it. On the other hand, if you are distracted by a loud noise, you (hopefully) will not forget the LTM representation of your own name.

The problem of learning makes the unity of conscious experience particularly hard to understand, if only because we are able to rapidly learn such enormous amounts of new information, on our own, throughout life. For example, after seeing an exciting movie, we can tell our friends many details about it later on, even though the individual scenes flashed by very quickly. More generally, we can quickly learn about new environments, even if no one tells us how the rules of each environment differ. To a surprising degree, we can rapidly learn new facts without being forced to just as rapidly forget what we already know. As a result, we do not need to avoid going out into the world for fear that, in learning to recognize a new friend's face, we will suddenly forget our parents' faces.

I have called the problem whereby the brain learns quickly and stably without catastrophically forgetting its past knowledge the *stability-plasticity dilemma*. The stability-plasticity dilemma must be solved by every brain system that needs to rapidly and adaptively respond to the flood of signals that subserves even the most ordinary experiences. If the brain's design is parsimonious, then we should expect to find similar design principles operating in all the brain systems that can stably learn an accumulating knowledge base in response to changing conditions throughout life. The discovery of such principles should clarify how the brain unifies diverse sources of information into coherent moments of conscious experience.

This article reviews evidence that the brain does operate in this way. It summarizes several recent brain modeling studies that illustrate, and further develop, a theory called Adaptive Resonance Theory, or ART, that I introduced in 1976 (Grossberg 1976a,b, 1978, 1980, 1982). In the present chapter, I will briefly summarize results selected from four areas where ART principles have been used to explain challenging behavioral and brain data. These areas are visual perception, visual object recognition, auditory source identification, and variable-rate speech recognition. On first inspection, the behavioral properties of these visual and auditory phenomena may seem to be entirely unrelated. On a deeper computational level, their governing neural circuits are proposed to incorporate a similar set of computational principles.

I should also say right away, however, that ART principles do not seem to be used in all brain learning systems. Whereas ART learning designs help to explain sensory and cognitive processes such as perception, recognition, attention, reinforcement, recall, working memory, and memory search, other types of learning seem to govern spatial and motor processes. In these latter task domains, it *is* adaptive to forget old coordinate transformations as the brain's control systems adjust to a growing body and to other changes in the body's sensory-motor endowment throughout life.

Sensory and cognitive processes are often associated with the What cortical processing stream that passes from visual cortex through inferotemporal cortex, whereas spatial and motor processes are associated with the Where (or How) cortical processing stream that passes from visual cortex through parietal cortex (Goodale and Milner 1992; Mishkin, Ungerleider, and Macko 1983; Ungerleider and Mishkin 1982). Our research over the years has concluded that many processes in the two distinct streams, notably their matching and learning processes, obey different, and even complementary, laws. This fact bears heavily on questions of consciousness, and helps to explain why procedural memories are not conscious (Cohen and Squire 1980, Mishkin 1982, Scoville and Milner 1957, Squire and Cohen 1984). Indeed, a central hypothesis of ART since its inception is:

ART Hypothesis: All conscious states are resonant states.

As noted in greater detail below, many spatial and motor processes involve a form of inhibitory matching and mismatch-based learning that does not support resonant states. Hence, by the ART Hypothesis, they cannot support a conscious state. Although ART predicts that all conscious states are resonant states, the converse statement, that all resonant states are conscious states, is not yet asserted.

Various other models of cognitive learning and recognition, such as the popular back-propagation model (Parker 1982; Rumelhart, Hinton, and Williams 1986; Werbos 1974), are based on a form of mismatch-based learning. They cannot, therefore, generate resonant states and, in fact, are well known to experience catastrophic forgetting under real-time learning conditions. A comparative survey of ART versus backpropagation computational properties is provided in Grossberg (1988).

How Do We Perceive Illusory Contours and Brightness?

Let me start by providing several examples of the diverse phenomena that ART clarifies. Consider the images in figure 61.1. Figure 61.1a shows an image called an Ehrenstein figure in which some radial black lines are drawn on a uniformly white paper. Remarkably, our minds construct a circular illusory contour that touches each line end at a perpendicular orientation. This illusory contour is a collective, emergent property of all the lines that only occurs when their positions relative to each other are suitable. For example, no illusory contour forms at the line ends in figure 61.1b even though they end at the same positions as the lines in figure 61.1a. Note also that the illusory contour in figure 61.1a surrounds a disk that seems uniformly brighter than its surround. Where does the brightness enhancement come from? It certainly does not always happen when illusory contours form, as can be seen by inspecting figure 61.1c. Here a vertical illusory contour can be recognized as interpolating the two sets of offset horizontal lines, even though neither side of the contour seems brighter than the other. How we can con-

sciously *recognize* something that we cannot *see*, and is thus perceptually invisible, is a fascinating aspect of our conscious awareness about which quite a bit is now known. Such percepts are known as *amodal* percepts (Michotte, Thines, and Crabbe 1964) in order to distinguish them from modal, or visible, percepts. Amodal percepts are experienced in response to many naturalistic scenes, notably in response to scenes in which some objects are partially occluded by other objects. How both modal and amodal percepts can occur is modeled in Grossberg (1994, 1997). Of particular interest from the viewpoint of ART processing is why the Ehrenstein disk looks bright, despite the fact that there are no local contrasts within the image itself that describe a disk-like object. Gove, Grossberg, and Mingolla (1995) provide an explanation of this illusion using ART mechanisms that are described below.

How Do We Learn to Recognize Visually Perceived Objects?

The Ehrenstein example concerns the process of visual perception. The next example concerns a process that goes on at a higher level of the visual system. It is the process whereby we visually recognize objects. A key part of this process concerns how we learn to categorize specific instances of an object, or set of objects, into a more general concept. For example, how do we learn that many different printed or script letter fonts can all represent the same letter A? Or how do we learn that several different combinations of patient symptoms are all due to the same disease? Moreover, how do we control how general our categories will become? For some purposes, like recognizing a particular face, we need highly specific categories. For others, like knowing that every person has a face, the categories are much more general. Finally, how does our learning and memory break down when something goes wrong in our brain? For example, it is known

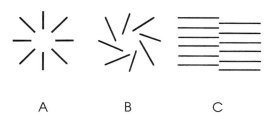

A   B   C

Figure 61.1
(*a*) The Ehrenstein pattern generates a circular illusory contour that encloses a circular disk of enhanced illusory brightness. (*b*) If the endpoints of the Ehrenstein pattern remain fixed while their orientations are tilted, then both the illusory contour and brightness vanish. (*c*) The offset pattern generates a vertical boundary that can be recognized even though it cannot be seen.

that lesions to the human hippocampal system can cause a form of amnesia whereby, among other properties, patients find it very hard to learn new information and hard to remember recently learned information, but previously learned information about which their memory has "consolidated" can readily be retrieved. Thus, an amnesic patient can typically carry out a perfectly intelligent conversation about experiences that occurred a significant time before the lesion that caused the amnesia occurred.

What computational properties do the phenomena of bright illusory disks and amnesic memory have in common? I will suggest below that their apparent differences conceal the workings of a general unifying principle.

How Do We Solve the Cocktail Party Problem?

To continue with our list, let us now consider a different modality entirely; namely, audition. When we talk to a friend in a crowded noisy room, we can usually keep track of our conversation above the hubbub, even though the sounds emitted by the friendly voice may substantially overlap the sounds emitted by other speakers. How do we separate this jumbled mixture of sounds into distinct voices? This is often called the cocktail party problem. The same problem is solved whenever we listen to a symphony or other music wherein overlapping harmonic components are emitted by several instruments. If we could not separate the instruments or voices into distinct sources, or auditory streams, then we could not hear the music as music, or intelligently recognize a speaker's sounds. A striking and ubiquitous property of such percepts, and one which has not yet been understand by alternative modeling approaches, is how future events can alter our conscious percepts of past events in a context-sensitive manner.

A simple version of this competence is illustrated by the auditory continuity illusion (Bregman 1990). Suppose that a steady tone shuts off

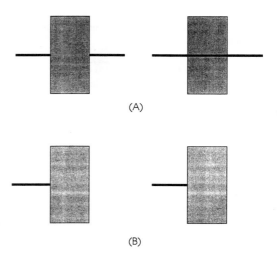

(A)

(B)

Figure 61.2
(*a*) Auditory continuity illusion. When a steady tone occurs both before and after a burst of noise, then under appropriate temporal and amplitude conditions, the tone is perceived to continue through the noise. (*b*) This does not occur if the noise is not followed by a tone.

just as a broadband noise turns on. Suppose, moreover, that the noise shuts off just as the tone turns on once again; see figure 61.2a. When this happens under appropriate conditions, the tone seems to continue right through the noise, which seems to occur in a separate auditory "stream." This example shows that the auditory system can actively extract those components of the noise that are consistent with the tone and use them to track the "voice" of the tone right through the hubbub of the noise.

In order to appreciate how remarkable this property is, let us compare it with what happens when the tone does not turn on again for a second time, as in figure 61.2b. Then the first tone does not seem to continue through the noise. It is perceived to stop before the noise. How does the brain know that the second tone will turn on after the noise shuts off, so that it can continue the tone through the noise, yet not continue the tone through the noise if the second tone does not eventually occur? Does this not seem to require that the brain can operate "backwards in time" to alter its decision as to whether or not to continue a past tone through the noise based on future events?

Many philosophers and scientists have puzzled about this sort of problem. I will argue that the process whereby we consciously hear the first tone takes some time to unfold, so that by the time we hear it, the second tone has already begun. To make this argument, we need to ask why does conscious audition take so long to occur after the actual sound energy reaches our brain? Just as important, why can the second tone influence the conscious percept so quickly, given that the first tone could not? Finally, I will indicate what these auditory phenomena have to do with bright Ehrenstein disks and amnesia.

How Do We Consciously Perceive Speech?

The final examples also involve the auditory system but at a higher level of processing. They concern how we understand speech. In these examples, too, the process whereby conscious awareness occurs takes a long time, on the order of 100 ms or more. An analysis of these percepts will also give us more clues about the nature of the underlying process. The first example is called phonemic restoration. Suppose that a listener hears a noise followed immediately by the words "eel is on the ...". If this string of words is followed by the word "orange," then "noise-eel" sounds like "peel." If the word "wagon" completes the sentence, then "noise-eel" sounds like "wheel." If the final word is "shoe," then "noise-eel" sounds like "heel."

This marvelous example, which was developed by Richard Warren and his colleagues more than 20 years ago (Warren 1984, Warren and Sherman 1974), vividly shows that the bottom-up occurrence of the noise is not sufficient for us to hear it. Somehow the sound that we *expect* to hear based upon our previous language experi-

ences influences what we do hear, at least if the sentence is said quickly enough. As in the auditory continuity illusion, it would appear that the brain is working "backwards in time" to allow the meaning imparted by a later word to alter the sounds that we consciously perceive in an earlier word.

I suggest that this happens because, as the individual words occur, they are stored temporarily via STM traces in a working memory. As the words are stored, they activate LTM traces which attempt to categorize the stored sound stream into familiar language units like words at a higher processing level. These list categories, in turn, activate learned top-down expectations that are *matched* against the contents of working memory to verify that the information expected from previous learning experiences is really there. This concept of bottom-up activation of learned categories by a working memory, followed by read-out of learned top-down expectations, is illustrated in figure 61.3a.

What is the nature of this matching, or verification, process? Its properties have been clarified by experiments of Arthur Samuel (1981a,b) and others in which the spectral content of the noise was varied. If the noise includes all the formants of the expected sound, then that is what the subject hears, and other spectral components of the noise are suppressed. If some formants of the expected sound are missing from the noise, then only a partial reconstruction is heard. If silence replaces the noise, then only silence is heard. The matching process thus cannot "create something out of nothing." It can, however, selectively amplify the expected features in the bottom-up signal and suppress the rest, as in figure 61.3b.

The process whereby the top-down expectation selectively amplifies some features while suppressing others helps to "focus attention" upon information that matches our momentary expectations. This focusing process helps to filter out the flood of sensory signals that would otherwise overwhelm us, and to prevent them from destabilizing our previously learned memories. Learned top-down expectations hereby help to

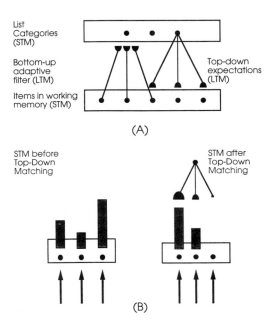

List
Categories
(STM)

Bottom-up
adaptive
filter (LTM)

Top-down
expectations
(LTM)

Items in working
memory (STM)

(A)

STM before
Top-Down
Matching

STM after
Top-Down
Matching

(B)

Figure 61.3
(*a*) Auditory items activate STM traces in a working memory, which send bottom-up signals toward a level at which list categories, or chunks, are activated in STM. These bottom-up signals are multiplied by learned LTM traces which influence the selection of the list categories that are stored in STM. The list categories, in turn, activate LTM-modulated top-down expectation signals that are matched against the active STM pattern in working memory. (*b*) This matching process confirms and amplifies STM activations that are supported by contiguous LTM traces, and suppresses those that are not.

solve the stability-plasticity dilemma by focusing attention and preventing spurious signals from accidentally eroding our previously learned memories. In fact, Gail Carpenter and I proved mathematically in 1987 that such an ART matching rule assures stable learning of an ART model in response to rapidly changing environments wherein learning becomes unstable if the matching rule is removed (Carpenter and Grossberg 1987a).

What does all this have to do with our conscious percepts of speech? This can be seen by asking: If top-down expectations can select consistent bottom-up signals, then what keeps the selected bottom-up signals from reactivating their top-down expectations in a continuing cycle of bottom-up and top-down feedback? Nothing does! In fact, this reciprocal feedback process takes awhile to equilibrate, and when it does, the bottom-up and top-down signals lock the STM activity patterns of the interacting levels into a resonant state that lasts much longer and is more energetic than any individual activation. ART hereby, suggests how only resonant states of the brain can achieve consciousness, and that the time needed for a bottom-up/top-down resonance to develop helps to explain why a conscious percept of an event takes so long to occur after its bottom-up input is delivered.

The example of phonemic restoration also clarifies another key point about the conscious perception of speech. If noise precedes "eel is on the shoe," we hear and understand the meaning of the sentence "heel is on the shoe." If, however, noise is replaced by silence, we hear and understand the meaning of the sentence "eel is on the shoe," which has a quite different, and rather disgusting, meaning. This example shows that the process of resonance binds together information about both meaning and phonetics. Meaning is not some higher-order process that is processed independently from the process of conscious phonetic hearing. Meaning and phonetics are bound together via resonant feedback into a global emergent state in which the phonetics that we hear are linked to the meaning that we understand.

ART Matching and Resonance: The Link between Attention, Intention, and Consciousness

Adaptive resonance theory claims that, in order to solve the stability-plasticity dilemma, only resonant states can drive new learning. That is why the theory is called *adaptive* resonance theory. I will explain how this works more completely below. Before doing so, let me emphasize some implications of the previous discussion that are worth reflecting about. The first implication provides a novel answer to why, as philosophers have asked for many years, humans are "intentional" beings who are always anticipating or planning their next behaviors and their expected consequences. ART suggests that "stability implies intentionality." That is, stable learning requires that we have expectations about the world that are continually matched against world data. Otherwise expressed, without stable learning, we could learn very little about the world. Having an active top-down matching mechanism greatly amplifies the amount of information that we can stably learn about the world. Thus the mechanisms that enable us to know a changing external world, through the use of learned expectations, set the stage for achieving internal self-awareness.

It should be noted here that the word "intentionality" is being used, at once, in two different senses. One sense concerns the role of expectations in the anticipation of events that may or may not occur. The second sense concerns the ability of expectations to read out planned sequences of behaviors aimed at achieving definite behavioral goals. The former sense will be emphasized first; the latter towards the end of the article. My main point in lumping them together is that ART provides a unified mechanistic perspective with which to understand both uses of the word.

The second implication is that "intention implies attention and consciousness." That is, expectations start to focus attention on data worthy of learning, and these attentional foci are confirmed when the system as a whole incorporates them into resonant states that include (I claim) conscious states of mind.

Implicit in the concept of intentionality is the idea that we can get *ready* to experience an expected event so that, when it finally occurs, we can react to it more quickly and vigorously, and until it occurs, we are able to ignore other, less desired, events. This property is called *priming*. It implies that, when a top-down expectation is read-out in the absence of a bottom-up input, it can subliminally sensitize the cells that would ordinarily respond to the bottom-up input, but not actually fire them, whereas it suppresses cells whose activity is not expected. Correspondingly, the ART matching rule computationally realizes the following properties at any processing level where bottom-up and top-down signals are matched:

- *Bottom-up automatic activation:* A cell, or node, can become active enough to generate output signals if it receives a large enough bottom-up input, other things being equal.

- *Top-down priming:* A cell can become sensitized, or subliminally active, and thus cannot generate output signals, if it receives only a large top-down expectation input. Such a top-down priming signal prepares a cell to react more quickly and vigorously to subsequent bottom-up input that matches the top-down prime.

- *Match:* A cell can become active if it receives large convergent bottom-up and top-down inputs. Such a matching process can generate enhanced activation as resonance takes hold.

- *Mismatch:* A cell is suppressed even if it receives a large bottom-up input if it also receives only a small, or zero, top-down expectation input.

I claim that this ART matching rule and the resonance rule that it implies operate in all the examples that I have previously sketched, and do so to solve the stability-plasticity dilemma. All the examples are proposed to illustrate how we can continue to learn rapidly and stably about new experiences throughout life by matching bottom-up signal patterns from more peripheral to more central brain processing stages against top-down signal patterns from more central to more peripheral processing stages. These top-down signals represent the brain's learned expectations of what the bottom-up signal patterns should be based on past experience. The matching process is designed to reinforce and amplify those combinations of features in the bottom-up pattern that are consistent with the top-down expectations and to suppress those features that are inconsistent. This top-down matching step initiates the process whereby the brain selectively pays attention to experiences that it expects, binds them into coherent internal representations through resonant states, and incorporates them through learning into its knowledge about the world.

Given that such a resonant matching process occurs in the brain, how does the brain react when there is a mismatch situation? The ART matching rule suggests that a big enough mismatch between a bottom-up input and a top-down expectation can rapidly attenuate activity at the matching level. This collapse of bottom-up activation can initiate a rapid *reset* of activity at both the matching level itself and at the subsequent levels that it feeds, thereby initiating a memory search for a more appropriate recognition category or creating a new one.

Resonant Dynamics during Speech Categorization

Many examples of such a reset event occur during variable-rate speech perception. As one example, consider how people hear combinations of vowels (V) and consonants (C) in VC–CV sequences. Bruno Repp at Haskins Laboratories has studied perception of the sequences [ib]–[ga] and [ib]–[ba] when the silence interval between the initial VC syllable and the terminal CV syllable is varied (Repp 1980). If the silence interval is short enough, then [ib]–[ga] sounds like [iga] and [ib]–[ba] sounds like [iba]. Repp ran a number of conditions, leading to the several data curves displayed in figure 61.4. The main point

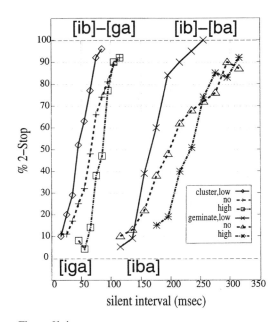

Figure 61.4
The left-hand curves represent the probability, under several experimental conditions, that the subject will hear [ib]–[ga] rather than [iga]. The right-hand curves do the same for [ib]–[ba] rather than the fused percept [iba]. Note that the perception of [iba] can occur at a silence interval between [ib] and [ba] that is up to 150 ms longer than the one that leads to the percept [iga] instead of [ib]–[ga]. (Data are reprinted with permission from B. H. Repp (1980), Haskins Laboratories Status Report on Speech Research, SR-61, 151–165.)

for present purposes is that the transition from a percept of [iba] to one of [ib]–[ba] occurs after 100–150 ms more silence than the transition from [iga] to [ib]–[ga]. One hundred milliseconds is a very long time relative to the time scale at which individual neurons can be activated. Why is this shift so large?

My colleagues Ian Boardman and Michael Cohen and I have quantitatively simulated these data using a model, called the ARTPHONE model, of how a resonant wave develops due to

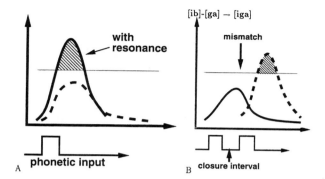

Figure 61.5
(*a*) Response to a single stop, such as [b] or [g], with a without resonance. Suprathreshold activation is shaded. (*b*) Rest due to phonologic mismatch between [ib] and [ga].

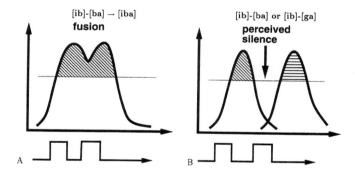

Figure 61.6
(*a*) Fusion in response to proximal similar phones. (*b*) Perceptual silence allows a two-stop percept.

bottom-up and top-down signal exchanges between a working memory that represents the individual speech items and a list categorization network that groups them together into learned language units, or chunks (Grossberg, Boardman, and Cohen 1997). We have shown how a mismatch between [g] and [b] rapidly resets the working memory if the silence between them is short enough, thereby preventing the [b] sound from reaching resonance and consciousness, as in figure 61.5. We have also shown how the development of a previous resonance involving [b]

can resonantly fuse with a subsequent [b] sound to greatly extend the perceived duration of [iba] across a silence interval between [ib] and [ba]. Figure 61.6a illustrates this property by suggesting how the second presentation of [b] can quickly reactivate the resonance in response to the first presentation of [b] before the resonance stops. This phenomenon uses the property that it takes longer for the first presentation of [b] to reach resonance than it does for the second presentation of [b] to influence the maintenance of this resonance.

If, however, [ib] can fuse across time with [ba], then how do we ever hear distinct [ib]–[ba] sounds when the silence gets long enough? Much evidence suggests that after a resonance fully develops, it spontaneously collapses after awhile owing to a habituative process that goes on in the pathways that maintain the resonance via bottom-up and top-down signals. Thus, if the silence is long enough for resonant collapse of [ib] to occur, then a distinguishable [ba] resonance can subsequently develop and be heard, as in figure 61.6b.

Such a habituative process has also been used to explain many other data about perception, learning, and recognition, notably data about the reset of visual, cognitive, or motor representations in response to rapidly changing events. Relevant visual data include properties of light adaptation, visual persistence, aftereffects, residual traces, and apparent motion (Carpenter and Grossberg 1981; Francis and Grossberg 1996a,b; Francis, Grossberg, and Mingolla 1994). Abbott, Varela, Sen, and Nelson (1997) have recently reported data from visual cortex that they modeled using the same habituative law that was used in all of these applications. At bottom, such a habituative law is predicted to be found so ubiquitously across brain systems because it helps to rapidly reset and rebalance neural circuits in response to rapidly changing input conditions, notably as part of an opponent process (Grossberg 1980).

The Repp (1980) data illustrate the important fact that the duration of a consciously perceived interval of silence is sensitive to the phonetic context into which the silence is placed. These data show that the phonetic context can generate a conscious percept of continuous sound across 150 ms of silence—that can be heard as silence in a different phonetic context. Our explanation of these data in terms of the maintenance of resonance in one case, but its rapid reset in another, is consistent with a simple, but revolutionary, definition of silence: Silence is a temporal discontinuity in the rate with which the auditory resonance evolves in time. Various other models of speech perception, having no concept like resonance on which to build, cannot begin to explain data of this type. Several such models are reviewed by Grossberg, Boardman, and Cohen (1997).

Resonant Dynamics during Auditory Streaming

A similar type of resonant processing helps to explain cocktail party separation of distinct voices into auditory streams, as in the auditory continuity illusion of figure 61.2. This process goes on, however, at earlier stages of auditory processing than speech categorization. My colleagues Krishna Govindarajan, Lonce Wyse, and Michael Cohen and I have developed a model, called the ARTSTREAM model, of how distinguishable auditory streams are resonantly formed and separated (Grossberg 1998b; Govindarajan, Grossberg, Wyse, and Cohen 1995). Here the two main processing levels (figure 61.7) are a spectral stream level at which the frequencies of the sound spectrum are represented across a spatial map, and a pitch stream level at which pitch nodes respond to the harmonics at the spectral stream level that comprise a given pitch. After the auditory signal is preprocessed, its spectral, or frequency, components are redundantly represented in multiple spectral streams; that is, the sound's preprocessed frequency components are represented in multiple spatial maps, each one of which can subserve the percept of a particular auditory stream.

Each of these spectral streams is filtered by bottom-up signals that activate its own pitch stream representation at the pitch stream level; that is, there are multiple pitch streams, one corresponding to every spectral stream. This multiple representation of a sound's spectral components and pitch interact to break up the entire sound stream that is entering the system into distinct acoustic sources or voices. This happens as follows. A given sound spectrum is

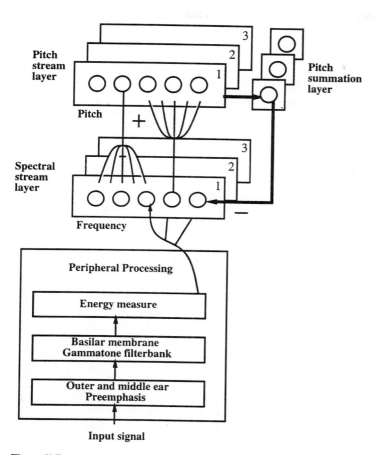

Figure 61.7
Block diagrams of the ARTSTREAM auditory streaming model. Note the nonspecific top-down inhibitory signals from the pitch level to the spectral level that realize ART matching within the network.

multiply represented at all the spectral streams and then redundantly activates all of the pitch nodes that are consistent with these sounds. These pitch representations compete to select a winner, which inhibits the representations of the same pitch across streams while also sending top-down matching signals back to the spectral stream level. By the ART matching rule, the frequency components that are consistent with the winning pitch node are amplified, and all others are suppressed, thereby leading to a spectral-pitch resonance within the stream of the winning pitch node. In this way, the pitch layer coherently binds together the harmonically related frequency components that correspond to a prescribed auditory source. All the frequency components that are suppressed by ART matching in this stream are freed to activate and resonate with a different pitch in a different stream. The net result is multiple resonances, each selectively grouping together into pitches those frequencies that correspond to distinct auditory sources.

Using the ARTSTREAM model, we have simulated many of basic streaming percepts, including the auditory continuity illusion of figure 61.2. It occurs, I contend, because the spectral-stream resonance takes a time to develop that is commensurate to the duration of the subsequent noise. Once the tone resonance develops, the second tone can quickly act to support and maintain it throughout the duration of the noise, much as [ba] fuses with [ib] during perception of [iba]. Of course, for this to make sense, one needs to accept the fact that the tone resonance does not start to get consciously heard until just about when the second tone occurs.

A Circuit for ART Matching

Figure 61.7 incorporates one of the possible ways that Gail Carpenter and I proposed in the mid 1980s for how the ART matching rule can be realized (Carpenter and Grossberg 1987a).

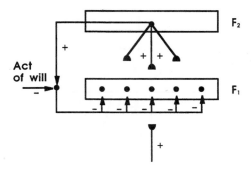

Figure 61.8
One way to realize the ART matching rule using top-down activation of nonspecific inhibitory interneurons. Several mathematically possible alternative ways are suggested in the Appendix of G. A. Carpenter and S. Grossberg 1987a.

This matching circuit is redrawn in figure 61.8 for clarity. It is perhaps the simplest such circuit, and I have found it in subsequent studies to be the one that is implicated by data time and time again.

In this circuit, bottom-up signals to the spectral stream level can excite their target nodes if top-down signals are not active. Top-down signals try to excite those spectral, or frequency component, nodes that are consistent with the pitch node that activates them. By themselves, top-down signals fail to activate spectral nodes because the pitch node also activates a pitch summation layer that nonspecifically inhibits all spectral nodes in its stream. The nonspecific top-down inhibition hereby prevents the specific top-down excitation from supraliminally activating any spectral nodes. On the other hand, when excitatory bottom-up and top-down signals occur together, then those spectral nodes that receive both types of signals can be fully activated. All other nodes in that stream are inhibited, including spectral nodes that were previously activated by bottom-up signals but received no subsequent top-down pitch support. Attention hereby selectively activates consistent nodes while nonselectively inhibiting all other nodes in a stream.

How Early Does Attention Act in the Brain?

It has classically been thought that attention first acts at higher levels of cortical organization. In vision, for example, it was thought that attention occurred no earlier than the extrastriate visual cortex (McAdams and Maunsell 1997; Motter 1994a,b; Reynolds, Nicholas, Chelazzi, and Desimone 1995). However, recent experiments have suggested that attentional modulation can occur in primary visual cortex (V1), and even at the earlier Lateral Geniculate Nucleus via top-down cortico-geniculate pathways (Hupé, James, Girard, and Bullier 1997; Ito, Westheimer, and Gilbert 1997; Johnson and Burkhalter 1997; Lamme, Zipser, and Spekreijse 1997; Press and van Essen 1997). Is there a contradiction here? The answer depends upon how you define attention. If attention refers only to processes that can be controlled voluntarily, then corticogeniculate feedback, being automatic, may not qualify. On the other hand, such top-down feedback does appear to have the selective properties of an "automatic" attention process, even at the earliest stages of sensory processing.

Is there direct experimental evidence for the prediction that corticogeniculate feedback supports ART matching and resonance? In a remarkable 1994 *Nature* article, Sillito and his colleagues (Sillito, Jones, Gerstein, and West 1994) published neurophysiological data that strikingly support this prediction. They wrote in particular that:

cortically induced correlation of relay cell activity produces coherent firing in those groups of relay cells with receptive field alignments appropriate to signal the particular orientation of the moving contour to the cortex ... this increases the gain of the input for feature-linked events detected by the cortex ... the cortico-thalamic input is only strong enough to exert

an effect on those dLGN cells that are additionally polarized by their retinal input ... the feedback circuit searches for correlations that support the "hypothesis" represented by a particular pattern of cortical activity.

In short, Sillito verified all the properties of the ART matching rule.

Attention at All Stages of Sensory and Cognitive Neocortex?

It has, in fact, been suggested how similar automatic attentional processes are integrated within the laminar circuits of visual cortex, notably the circuits of cortical areas V1 and V2 that are used to generate perceptual groupings, such as the illusory contours in figure 61.1 (Grossberg 1998a). In this proposal, the ART matching rule is realized as follows. Top-down attentional feedback from cortical area V2 to V1 is predicted to be mediated by signals from layer 6 of cortical area V2. These top-down signals attentionally prime layer 4 of cortical area V1 via an on-center off-surround network within V1 from layer 6 to layer 4. In this conception, layer 6 of V2 activates layer 6 of V1, possibly via a multisynaptic pathway via layers 1 and 5. Layer 6 then activates layer 4 of V1 via an on-center off-surround network from layer 6-to-4. This analysis predicts that the layer 6-to-4 on-center circuit can *prime*, or *modulate*, layer 4 cells, but cannot fully activate them because the top-down attentional prime, acting by itself, is subliminal. Such a modulatory effect is achieved by appropriately balancing the strength of the on-center and off-surround signals within the layer 6-to-4 network.

Related modeling work has shown how such balanced on-center off-surround signals can lead to self-stabilizing development of the horizontal connections within layers 2/3 of V1 and V2 that subserve perceptual grouping (Grossberg and Williamson 1997, 1998). It has also been shown how the top-down on-center off-surround circuit from area V1 to LGN can self-stabilize the development of disparity-sensitive complex cells in area V1 (Grunewald and Grossberg 1998). Other modeling work has suggested how a similar top-down on-center off-surround automatical attentional circuit from cortical area MST to MT can be used to generate coherent representations of the direction and speed with which objects move (Chey, Grossberg, and Mingolla 1997). Taken together, these studies show how the ART matching rule may be realized in known cortical circuits, and how it can self-stabilize development of these circuits as a precursor to its role in self-stabilizing learning throughout life. Grossberg (1998a) has predicted that the same ART matching circuit exists within the laminar organization that is found universally in all sensory and cognitive neocortex, including the various examples of auditory processing that are reviewed above. This prediction does not, of course, deny that these various circuits may be specialized in various ways to process the different types of information with which they are confronted.

Given that the cortical organization of top-down on-center off-surround attentional priming circuits seem to be ubiquitous in visual cortex, and by extension in other types of cortex, it is important to ask: What more does the brain need to add in order to generate a more flexible, task-dependent type of attention switching? This question leads us to consider visual object recognition, and how it breaks down during medial temporal amnesia. Various other models of object recognition, and their conceptual and explanatory weaknesses relative to ART, are reviewed by Grossberg and Merrill (1996).

Self-Organizing Feature Maps for Learned Object Recognition

Let us begin with a two-level network that illustrates some of the main ideas in the simplest possible way. Level $\mathscr{F}_1$ in figure 61.9 contains a network of nodes, or cell populations, each of which is activated by a particular combination of

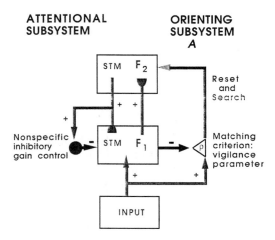

Figure 61.9
An example of a model ART circuit in which attentional and orienting circuits interact. Level $\mathscr{F}_1$ encodes a distributed representation of an event by a short-term memory (STM) activation pattern across a network of feature detectors. Level $\mathscr{F}_2$ encodes the event using a compressed STM representation of the $\mathscr{F}_1$ pattern. Learning of these recognition codes occurs at the long-term memory (LTM) traces within the bottom-up and top-down pathways between levels $\mathscr{F}_1$ and $\mathscr{F}_2$. The top-down pathways read out learned expectations whose prototypes are matched against bottom-up input patterns at $\mathscr{F}_1$. The size of mismatches in response to novel events are evaluated relative to the vigilance parameter p of the orienting subsystem $\mathscr{A}$. A large enough mismatch resets the recognition code that is active in STM at $\mathscr{F}_2$ and initiates a memory search for a more appropriate recognition code. Output from subsystem A can also trigger an orienting response. (*a*) Block diagram of circuit. (*b*) Individual pathways of circuit, including the input level F_0 that generates inputs to level $\mathscr{F}_1$. The gain control input g_1 to level $\mathscr{F}_1$ helps to instantiate the matching rule (see text). Gain control g_2 to level $\mathscr{F}_2$ is needed to instate a category in STM.

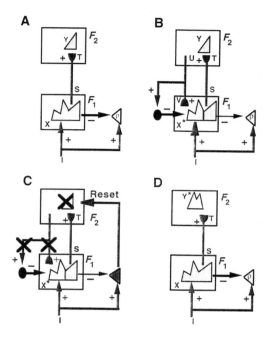

Figure 61.10
ART search for a recognition code. (a) The input pattern **I** is instated across the feature detectors at level $\mathscr{F}_1$ as a short-term memory (STM) activity pattern **X**. Input **I** also nonspecifically activates the orienting subsystem $\mathscr{A}$; see figure 61.1. STM pattern **X** is represented by the hatched pattern across $\mathscr{F}_1$. Pattern **X** both inhibits A and generates the output of pattern **S**. Pattern **S** is multiplied by long-term memory (LTM) traces and added at $\mathscr{F}_2$ nodes to form the input pattern **T**, which activates the STM pattern **Y** across the recognition categories coded at level $\mathscr{F}_2$. (b) Pattern **Y** generates the top-down output pattern **U**, which is multiplied by top-down LTM traces and added at $\mathscr{F}_1$ nodes to form the prototype pattern **V** that encodes the learned expectation of the active $\mathscr{F}_2$ nodes. If **V** mismatches **I** at $\mathscr{F}_1$, then a new STM activity pattern **X*** is generated at $\mathscr{F}_1$. **X*** is represented by the hatched pattern. It includes the features of **I** that are confirmed by **V**. Inactivated nodes corresponding to unconfirmed features of **X** are unhatched. The reduction in total STM activity that occurs when **X** is transformed into **X*** causes a decrease in the total inhibition from $\mathscr{F}_1$ to $\mathscr{A}$. (c) If inhibition decreases sufficiently, $\mathscr{A}$ releases a

sensory features via inputs. Level $\mathscr{F}_2$ contains a network of nodes that represent recognition codes, or categories, which are selectively activated by the activation patterns across $\mathscr{F}_1$. Each $\mathscr{F}_1$ node sends output signals to a subset of $\mathscr{F}_2$ nodes. Each $\mathscr{F}_2$ node thus receives inputs from many $\mathscr{F}_1$ nodes. The thick bottom-up pathway from $\mathscr{F}_1$ to $\mathscr{F}_2$ in figure 61.9 represents in a concise way an array of diverging and converging pathways. Let learning take place at the synapses denoted by semicircular endings in the $\mathscr{F}_1 \rightarrow \mathscr{F}_2$ pathways. Pathways that end in arrowheads do not undergo learning. This bottom-up learning enables $\mathscr{F}_2$ category nodes to become selectively tuned to particular combinations of activation patterns across $\mathscr{F}_1$ feature detectors by changing their LTM traces.

Why is not bottom-up learning sufficient in a system that can autonomously solve the stability-plasticity dilemma? Why are learned top-down expectations also needed? To understand this, we consider a type of model that is often called a self-organizing feature map, competitive learning, or learned vector quantization. This type of model shows how to combine associative learning and lateral inhibition for purposes of learned categorization.

In such a model, as shown in figure 61.10a, an input pattern registers itself as a pattern of activity, or STM, across the feature detectors of level $\mathscr{F}_1$. Each $\mathscr{F}_1$ output signal is multiplied or gated, by the adaptive weight, or LTM trace, in its respective pathway. All these LTM-gated

nonspecific arousal wave to $\mathscr{F}_2$, which resets the STM pattern **Y** to $\mathscr{F}_2$. (d) After **Y** is inhibited, its top-down prototype signal is eliminated, and **X** can be reinstated at $\mathscr{F}_1$. Enduring traces of prior reset lead **X** to activate a different STM pattern **Y*** at $\mathscr{F}_2$. If the top-down prototype due to **Y*** also mismatch **I** at $\mathscr{F}_1$, then the search for an appropriate $\mathscr{F}_2$ code continues until a more appropriate $\mathscr{F}_2$ representation is selected. Then an attentive resonance develops and learning of attended data is initiated. (Reprinted with permission from Carpenter and Grossberg 1993.)

Table 61.1

The state of node x_j as a function of the state of connection S_i and the weight w_{ij}

		Case 1	Case 2	Case 3	Case 4
State of S_i		+	−	+	−
State of x_j		+	+	−	−
State of w_{ij}		↑	↓	↔	↔

Note: + = active; − = inactive; ↑ = increase; ↓ = decrease; ↔ = no change.

inputs are added up at their target $\mathcal{F}_2$ nodes. The LTM traces hereby *filter* the STM signal pattern and generate larger inputs to those $\mathcal{F}_2$ nodes whose LTM patterns are most similar to the STM pattern. Lateral inhibitory, or competitive, interactions within $\mathcal{F}_2$ contrast-enhance this input pattern. Whereas many $\mathcal{F}_2$ nodes may receive inputs from $\mathcal{F}_1$, lateral inhibition allows a much smaller set of $\mathcal{F}_2$ nodes to store their activation in STM. These are the $\mathcal{F}_2$ nodes whose LTM patterns are most similar to the STM pattern. These inhibitory interactions also tend to conserve the total activity that is stored in STM (Grossberg 1982), thereby realizing an interference-based capacity limitation in STM.

Only the $\mathcal{F}_2$ nodes that win the competition and store their activity in STM can influence the learning process. STM activity opens a learning gate at the LTM traces that abut the winning nodes. These LTM traces can then approach, or track, the input signals in their pathways, a process called steepest descent. This learning law is thus often called gated steepest descent, or instar learning. This type of learning tunes the winning LTM patterns to become even more similar to the STM pattern, and to thereby enable the STM pattern to more effectively activate the corresponding $\mathcal{F}_2$ nodes. I introduced this learning law into neural network models in the 1960s (e.g., Grossberg 1969), and into ART models in the 1970s (Grossberg 1976a,b, 1978, 1980). Such

an LTM trace can either increase (Hebbian) or decrease (anti-Hebbian) to track the signals in its pathway (table 61.1). It has been used to model neurophysiological data about learning in the hippocampus (also called long term potentiation and long term depression) and about adaptive tuning of cortical feature detectors during early visual development (Artola and Singer 1993, Levy 1985, Levy and Desmond 1985, Rauschecker and Singer 1979, Singer 1983), thereby lending support to ART predictions that these systems would employ this type of leaning.

Self-organizing feature map models were introduced and computationally characterized by Christoph von der Malsburg and myself during the 1970s (Grossberg 1972, 1976a, 1978; von der Malsburg 1973; Willshaw and Malsburg 1976). These models were subsequently applied and further developed by many authors, notably Teuvo Kohonen (Kohonen 1984). They exhibit many useful properties, especially if not too many input patterns, or clusters of input patterns, perturb level $\mathcal{F}_1$ relative to the number of categorizing nodes in level $\mathcal{F}_2$. I proved that, under these sparse environmental conditions, category learning is stable in the sense that its LTM traces converge to fixed values as learning trials proceed. Additionally, the LTM traces track the statistics of the environment, are self-normalizing, and oscillate a minimum number of times (Grossberg 1976a). Also, the category selection rule, like a Bayesian classifier, tends to minimize error. I also proved, however, that under *arbitrary* environmental conditions, learning becomes unstable (Grossberg 1976b). Such a model could forget your parents' faces when it learns a new face. Although a gradual switching off of plasticity can partially overcome this problem, such a mechanism cannot work in a learning system whose plasticity is maintained throughout adulthood.

This memory instability is due to basic properties of associative learning and lateral inhibition, which are two processes that occur ubiquitously in the brain. An analysis of this instability, together with data about human and animal categorization, conditioning, and attention, led me to introduce ART models to stabilize the memory of self-organizing feature maps in response to an arbitrary stream of input patterns.

How Does ART Stabilize Learning of a Self-Organizing Feature Map?

How does an ART model prevent such instabilities from developing? As previously noted, in an ART model, learning does not occur when some winning $\mathscr{F}_2$ activities are stored in STM. Instead, activation of $\mathscr{F}_2$ nodes may be interpreted as "making a hypothesis" about an input at $\mathscr{F}_1$. When $\mathscr{F}_2$ is activated, it quickly generates an output pattern that is transmitted along the top-down adaptive pathways from $\mathscr{F}_2$ to $\mathscr{F}_1$. These top-down signals are multiplied in their respective pathways by LTM traces at the semicircular synaptic knobs of figure 61.10b. The LTM-gated signals from all the active $\mathscr{F}_2$ nodes are added to generate the total top-down feedback pattern from $\mathscr{F}_2$ to $\mathscr{F}_1$. It is this pattern that plays the role of a learned expectation. Activation of this expectation may be interpreted as "testing the hypothesis," or "reading out the prototype," of the active $\mathscr{F}_2$ category. As shown in figure 61.10b, ART networks are designed to match the "expected prototype" of the category against the bottom-up input pattern, or exemplar, to $\mathscr{F}_1$. Nodes that are activated by this exemplar are suppressed if they do not correspond to large LTM traces in the top-down prototype pattern. The resultant $\mathscr{F}_1$ pattern encodes the cluster of input features that the network deems relevant to the hypothesis based upon its past experience. This resultant activity pattern, called $\mathbf{X}^*$ in figure 61.10b, encodes the pattern of features to which the network "pays attention."

If the expectation is close enough to the input exemplar, then a state of resonance develops as the attentional focus takes hold. The pattern $\mathbf{X}^*$ of attended features reactivates the $\mathscr{F}_2$ category $\mathbf{Y}$ which, in turn, reactivates $\mathbf{X}^*$. The network locks into a resonant state through a positive feedback loop that dynamically links, or binds, $\mathbf{X}^*$ with $\mathbf{Y}$. The resonance binds spatially distributed features into either a stable equilibrium or a synchronous oscillation, much like the synchronous feature binding in visual cortex that has recently attracted so much interest after the experiments of Reinhard Eckhorn, Wolf Singer, and their colleagues (Eckhorn et al. 1988; Gray and Singer 1989; also see Grossberg and Grunewald 1997).

In ART, the resonant state, rather than bottom-up activation, is predicted to drive the learning process. The resonant state persists long enough, at a high enough activity level, to activate the slower learning processes in the LTM traces. This helps to explain how the LTM traces can regulate the brain's fast information processing without necessarily learning about the signals that they process. Through resonance as a mediating event, the combination of top-down matching and attentional focusing helps to stabilize ART learning and memory in response to an arbitrary input environment. The stabilizing properties of top-down matching may be one reason for the ubiquitous occurrence of reciprocal bottom-up and top-down cortico-cortical and cortico-thalamic interactions in the brain.

How is the Generality of Knowledge Controlled?

A key problem about consciousness concerns what combinations of features or other information are bound together into object or event representations. ART provides a new answer to this question that overcomes problems faced by earlier models. In particular, ART systems learn prototypes, rather than exemplars, because the attended feature vector $\mathbf{X}^*$, rather than the input exemplar itself, is learned. Both the bottom-up LTM traces that tune the category nodes and the top-down LTM traces that filter the learned expectation learn to correlate activation of $\mathscr{F}_2$ nodes with the set of all *attended* $\mathbf{X}^*$ vectors that they have ever experienced. These attended STM vectors assign less STM activity to features in the input vector $\mathbf{I}$ that mismatch the learned top-down prototype $\mathbf{V}$ than to features that match $\mathbf{V}$.

Given that ART systems learn prototypes, how can they also learn to recognize unique experiences, such as a particular view of a friend's face? The prototypes learned by ART systems accomplish this by realizing a qualitatively different concept of prototype than that offered by previous models. In particular, Gail Carpenter and I have shown with our students how ART prototypes form in a way that is designed to conjointly maximize category generalization while minimizing predictive error (Bradski and Grossberg 1995; Carpenter and Grossberg 1987a,b; Carpenter, Grossberg, and Reynolds 1991; Carpenter et al. 1992). As a result, ART prototypes can automatically learn individual exemplars when environmental conditions require highly selective discriminations to be made. How the matching process achieves this is discussed below.

Before describing how this is achieved, let me note what happens if the mismatch between bottom-up and top-down information is too great for a resonance to develop. Then the $\mathscr{F}_2$ category is quickly reset and a memory search for a better category is initiated. This combination of top-down matching, attention focusing, and memory search is what stabilizes ART learning and memory in an arbitrary input environment. The attentional focusing by top-down matching prevents inputs that represent irrelevant features at $\mathscr{F}_1$ from eroding the memory of previously learned LTM prototypes. Additionally, the memory search resets $\mathscr{F}_2$ categories so quickly when their prototype $\mathbf{V}$ mismatches the input vector $\mathbf{I}$ that the more slowly varying LTM traces do not have an opportunity to correlate the attended $\mathscr{F}_1$ activity vector $\mathbf{X}^*$ with them. Conversely, the resonant event, when it does oc-

cur, maintains and amplifies the matched STM activities for long enough and at high enough amplitudes for learning to occur in the LTM traces.

Whether or not a resonance occurs depends upon the level of mismatch, or novelty, that the network is prepared to tolerate. Novelty is measured by how well a given exemplar matches the prototype that its presentation evokes. The criterion of an acceptable match is defined by an internally controlled parameter that Carpenter and I have called vigilance (Carpenter and Grossberg 1987a). The vigilance parameter is computed in the orienting subsystem $\mathscr{A}$; see figure 61.9. Vigilance weighs how similar an input exemplar $\mathbf{I}$ must be to a top-down prototype $\mathbf{V}$ in order for resonance to occur. Resonance occurs if $\rho|\mathbf{I}| - |\mathbf{X}^*| \leq 0$. This inequality says that the $\mathscr{F}_1$ attentional focus $\mathbf{X}^*$ inhibits $\mathscr{A}$ more than the input $\mathbf{I}$ excites it. If $\mathscr{A}$ remains quiet, then an $\mathscr{F}_1 \leftrightarrow \mathscr{F}_2$ resonance can develop.

Either a larger value of ρ or a smaller match ratio $|\mathbf{X}^*||\mathbf{I}|^{-1}$ makes it harder to satisfy the resonance inequality. When ρ grows so large or $|\mathbf{X}^*||\mathbf{I}|^{-1}$ is so small that $\rho|\mathbf{I}| - |\mathbf{X}^*| > 0$, then $\mathscr{A}$ generates an arousal burst, or novelty wave, that resets the STM pattern across $\mathscr{F}_2$ and initiates a bout of hypothesis testing, or memory search. During search, the orienting subsystem interacts with the attentional subsystem (figures 61.10c,d) to rapidly reset mismatched categories and to select better $\mathscr{F}_2$ representations with which to categorize novel events at $\mathscr{F}_1$, without risking unselective forgetting of previous knowledge. Search may select a familiar category if its prototype is similar enough to the input to satisfy the resonance criterion. The prototype may then be refined by attentional focusing. If the input is too different from any previously learned prototype, then an uncommitted population of $\mathscr{F}_2$ cells is selected and learning of a new category is initiated.

Because vigilance can vary across learning trials, recognition categories capable of encoding widely differing degrees of generalization or abstraction can be learned by a single ART system. Low vigilance leads to broad generalization and abstract prototypes. High vigilance leads to narrow generalization and to prototypes that represent fewer input exemplars, even a single exemplar. Thus a single ART system may be used, say, to learn abstract prototypes with which to recognize abstract categories of faces and dogs, as well as "exemplar prototypes" with which to recognize individual faces and dogs. A single system can learn both, as the need arises, by increasing vigilance just enough to activate $\mathscr{A}$ if a previous categorization leads to a predictive error. Thus the contents of a conscious percept can be modified by environmentally sensitive vigilance control.

Vigilance control hereby allows ART to overcome some fundamental difficulties that have been faced by classical exemplar and prototype theories of learning and recognition. Classical exemplar models face a serious combinatorial explosion, since they need to suppose that all experienced exemplars are somehow stored in memory and searched during performance. Classical prototype theories face the problem that they find it hard to explain how individual exemplars are learned, such as a particular view of a familiar face. Vigilance control enables ART to achieve the best of both types of model, by selecting the most general category that is consistent with environmental feedback. If that category is an exemplar, then a "very vigilant" ART model can learn it. If the category is at an intermediate level of generalization, then the ART model can learn it by having the vigilance value track the level of match between the current exemplar and the prototype that it activates. In every instance, the model tries to learn the most general category that is consistent with the data. This tendency can, for example, lead to the type of overgeneralization that is seen in young children until further learning leads to category refinement (Chapman, Leonard, and Mervis 1986; Clark 1973; Smith, Carey, and Wiser 1985; Smith and Kemler 1978; Ward

1983). Many benchmark studies of how ART uses vigilance control to classify complex data bases have shown that the number of ART categories that is learned scales well with the complexity of the input data; see Carpenter and Grossberg 1994 for a list of illustrative benchmark studies.

Corticohippocampal Interactions and Medial Temporal Amnesia

As sequences of inputs are practiced over learning trials, the search process eventually converges upon stable categories. Carpenter and I mathematically proved (Carpenter and Grossberg 1987a) that familiar inputs directly access the category whose prototype provides the globally best match, while unfamiliar inputs engage the orienting subsystem to trigger memory searches for better categories until they become familiar. This process continues until the memory capacity, which can be chosen arbitrarily large, is fully utilized. The process whereby search is automatically disengaged is a form of memory consolidation that emerges from network interactions. Emergent consolidation does not preclude structural consolidation at individual cells, since the amplified and prolonged activities that subserve a resonance may be a trigger for learning-dependent cellular processes, such as protein synthesis and transmitter production. It has also been shown that the adaptive weights which are learned by an ART model at any stage of learning can be translated into if-then rules (e.g., Carpenter et al. 1992). Thus the ART model is a self-organizing rule-discovering production system as well as a neural network.

The attentional subsystem of ART has been used to model aspects of inferotemporal (IT) cortex, and the orienting subsystem models part of the hippocampal system. The interpretation of ART dynamics in terms of IT cortex led Miller, Li, and Desimone (1991) to successfully test the prediction that cells in monkey IT cortex are reset after each trial in a working memory task. To illustrate the implications of an ART interpretation of IT-hippocampal interactions, I will review how a lesion of the ART model's orienting subsystem creates a formal memory disorder with symptoms much like the medial temporal amnesia that is caused in animals and human patients after hippocampal system lesions (Carpenter and Grossberg 1994, Grossberg and Merrill 1996). In particular, such a lesion in vivo causes unlimited anterograde amnesia; limited retrograde amnesia; failure of consolidation; tendency to learn the first event in a series; abnormal reactions to novelty, including perseverative reactions; normal priming; and normal information processing of familiar events (Cohen 1984; Graf, Squire, and Mandler 1984; Lynch, McGaugh, and Weinberger 1984; Squire and Butters 1984; Squire and Cohen 1984; Warrington and Weiskrantz 1974; Zola-Morgan and Squire 1990).

Unlimited anterograde amnesia occurs because the network cannot carry out the memory search to learn a new recognition code. Limited retrograde amnesia occurs because familiar events can directly access correct recognition codes. Before events become familiar, memory consolidation occurs which utilizes the orienting subsystem (figure 61.10c). This failure of consolidation does not necessarily prevent learning per se. Instead, learning influences the first recognition category activated by bottom-up processing, much as amnesics are particularly strongly wedded to the first response they learn. Perseverative reactions can occur because the orienting subsystem cannot reset sensory representations or top-down expectations that may be persistently mismatched by bottom-up cues. The inability to search memory prevents ART from discovering more appropriate stimulus combinations to attend. Normal priming occurs because it is mediated by the attentional subsystem.

Similar behavioral problems have been identified in hippocampectomized monkeys. Gaffan (1985) noted that fornix transection "impairs ability to change an established habit ... in a different set of circumstances that is similar to the first and therefore liable to be confused with it." In ART, a defective orienting subsystem prevents the memory search whereby different representations could be learned for similar events. Pribram (1986) called such a process a "competence for recombinant context-sensitive processing." These ART mechanisms illustrate how, as Zola-Morgan and Squire (1990) have reported, memory consolidation and novelty detection may be mediated by the same neural structures. Why hippocampectomized rats have difficulty orienting to novel cues and why there is a progressive reduction in novelty-related hippocampal potentials as learning proceeds in normal rats is also clarified (Deadwyler, West, and Lynch 1979; Deadwyler, West, and Robinson 1981). In ART, the orienting system is automatically disengaged as events become familiar during the memory consolidation process. The ART model of normal and abnormal recognition learning and memory is compared with several other recent models of these phenomena by Grossberg and Merrill (1996).

At this point, it might also be useful to note that the processes of automatic and task-selective attention may not be independent in vivo. This is because higher-order attentional constraints, that may be under task-selective control, can in principle propagate downwards through successive cortical levels via layer 6-to-layer 6 linkages. For example, recent modeling work has suggested how prestriate cortical areas may separate visual objects from one another and from their backgrounds during the process of figure-ground separation (Grossberg 1994, 1997; Grossberg and McLoughlin 1997). Such constraints may propagate top-down toward earlier cortical levels, possibly even area V1, to modulate the cells that get active there to be consistent with these figure-ground constraints. Still higher cortical processes, such as those involved in learned categorization, may also propagate their modulatory constraints to lower levels. How the strength of such top-down modulatory influences depends upon the source cortical area and on the number of synaptic steps to the target cortical area is a topic that has yet to be systematically studied.

How Universal are ART Processes in the Brain?

In all the examples discussed above—from early vision, visual object recognition, auditory streaming, and speech recognition—ART matching and resonance have played a central role in models that help to explain how the brain stabilizes its learned adaptations in response to changing environmental conditions. This type of matching can be achieved using a top-down nonspecific inhibitory gain control that down-regulates all target cells except those that also receive top-down specific excitatory signals, as in figure 61.8. Are there yet other brain processes that utilize these mechanisms?

With my colleagues Mario Aguilar, Dan Bullock, and Karen Roberts, a neural model has been developed to explain how the superior colliculus learns to use visual, auditory, somatosensory, and planned movement signals to control saccadic eye movements (Grossberg, Roberts, Aguilar, and Bullock 1997). This model uses ART matching and resonance to help explain behavioral and neural data about multimodal eye movement control. The model clarifies how visual, auditory, and planned movement signals use learning to form a mutually consistent movement map, and how attention gets focused on a movement target location after all these signals compete to determine where the eyes will move.

Nobuo Suga and his colleagues (Gao and Suga 1998, Yan and Suga 1998) have recently reported neurophysiological data showing how ART-like top-down matching signals can modulate learning in the auditory system.

Recent experiments from Marcus Raichle's lab at Washington University using positron emission tomography (PET) support the idea that ART top-down priming also occurs in human somatosensory cortex (Drevets, Burton, and Raichle 1995). In their experiments, attending to an impending stimulus to the fingers caused inhibition of nearly cortical cells that code for the face, but not cells that code the fingers. Likewise, priming of the toes produced inhibition of nearby cells that code for the fingers and face, but not cells that code for the toes.

ART models have also been used to explain a great deal of data about cognitive-emotional interactions, notably about classical and instrumental conditioning (Grossberg 1987b) and about human decision making under risk (Grossberg and Gutowski 1987). In these examples, the resonances are between cognitive and emotional circuits, and help to focus attention upon, and release actions towards, valued events in the world.

Thus all levels of vision, visual object recognition, auditory preprocessing and streaming, speech recognition, attentive selection of eye movement targets, somatosensory representation, and cognitive-emotional interactions may all incorporate variants of the circuit depicted in figure 61.8. These results suggest that a type of "automatic" attention operates even at early levels of brain processing, such as the lateral geniculate, but that higher processing levels benefit from an orienting subsystem that can be used to flexibly reset attention and to facilitate voluntary control of top-down expectations.

Internal Fantasy, Planned Movement, and Volitional Gating

Given this type of circuit, how could top-down priming be released from inhibition to enable us to voluntarily experience internal thinking and fantasies? This can be achieved through an "act of will" that activates inhibitory cells which inhibit the nonspecific inhibitory interneurons in the top-down on-center off-surround network of figure 61.8. This operation disinhibits the cells receiving the excitatory top-down signals in the on-center of the network. These cells are then free to generate supraliminal resonances. Such self-initiated resonances can, for example, be initiated by the read-out of top-down expectations from higher-order planning nodes into temporally organized working memories, say in the prefrontal cortex (Fuster 1996). It is, for example, well known that the basal ganglia can use such a disinhibitory action to gate the release of individual movements, sequences of movements, and even cognitive processes (Hikosaka 1994, Middleton and Strick 1994, Sakai et al. 1998).

These examples also help to understand how top-down expectations can be used for the control of planned (viz., intentional) behavioral sequences. For example, once such planning nodes read out their top-down expectations into working memory, the contents of working memory can be read out and modified by on-line changes in "acts of will." These volitional signals enable invariant representations of an intentional behavior to rapidly adapt themselves to changing environmental conditions. For example, Bullock, Grossberg, and Mannes (1993) have modeled how such a working memory can control the intentional performance of handwriting whose size and speed can be modified by acts of will, without a change of handwritten form. Bullock, Grossberg, and Guenther (1993) have shown how a visual target that is stored in working memory can be reached with a novel tool that has never been used before. The latter study shows how a such a model can learn its own parameters through a type of Piagetian perform-and-test developmental cycle.

Thus we arrive at an emerging picture of how the adaptive brain works wherein the core issue of how a brain can learn quickly and stably about a changing world throughout life leads towards a mechanistic understanding of attention, intention, thinking, fantasy, and consciousness. The mediating events are adaptive resonances that effect a dynamic balance between the complementary demands of stability and plasticity, and of expectation and novelty, and which are a necessary condition for consciousness.

What versus Where: Why Are Procedural Memories Not Conscious?

Although the type of ART matching, learning, and resonance that have been reviewed above seem to occur in many sensory and cognitive processes, they are not the only types of matching and learning to occur in the brain. In fact, there seems to be a major difference between the types of learning that occur in sensory and cognitive processes versus those that occur in spatial and motor processes. In particular, sensory and cognitive processes are carried out in the What processing stream that passes through the inferotemporal cortex, whereas spatial and motor processes are carried out in the Where processing stream that passes through the parietal cortex. What processing includes object recognition and event prediction. Where processing includes spatial navigation and motor control. I suggest that the types of matching and learning that go on in the What and Where streams are different, indeed complementary, and that this difference is appropriate to their different roles. First consider how we use a sensory expectation. Suppose, for example, that I ask you to "Look for the yellow ball, and if you find it within 300 ms, I will give you $1,000,000." If you believed me, you could activate a sensory expectation of "yellow balls" that would make you much more sensitive to yellow and round objects in your environment. As in ART matching, once you detected a yellow ball, you could then react to it much more quickly and with a much more energetic response than if you were not looking for it. In other words, sensory and cognitive expectations lead to a type of excitatory matching.

Now consider how we use a motor expectation. Such an expectation represents where we want to more (Bullock and Grossberg 1988). For example, it could represent a desired position for the hand to pick up an object. Such a motor expectation is matched against where the hand is now. After the hand actually moves to the desired position, no further movement is required to satisfy the motor expectation. In this sense, motor expectations lead to a type of inhibitory matching. In summary, although the sensory and cognitive matching process is excitatory, the spatial and motor matching process is inhibitory. These are complementary properties. Models such as ART quantify how excitatory matching is accomplished. A different type of model, called a Vector Associative Map, or VAM, model, suggests how inhibitory matching is accomplished (Gaudiano and Grossberg 1991; Grossberg, Guenther, Bullock, and Greve 1993; Guenther, Bullock, Greve, and Grossberg 1994).

As shown in the discussions of ART above, learning within the sensory and cognitive domain is often a type of *match* learning. It takes place only if there is a good enough match of top-down expectations with bottom-up data to risk altering previously stored knowledge within the system, or it can trigger learning of a new representation if a good enough match is not available. In contrast, learning within spatial and motor processes, such as VAM processes, is *mismatch* learning that is used to either learn new sensory-motor maps (e.g., Grossberg et al. 1993) or to adjust the gains of sensory-motor commands (e.g., Fiala, Grossberg, and Bullock 1996). These types of learning are also complementary.

Why are the types of learning that go into spatial and motor processes complementary to those that are used for sensory and cognitive processing? My answer is that ART-like learning allows the brain to solve the stability-plasticity dilemma. It enables us to continue learning more about the world in a stable fashion throughout life without forcing catastrophic forgetting of our previous memories. On the other hand, catastrophic forgetting is a good property when it takes place during spatial and motor learning. We have no need to remember all the spatial and motor maps that we used when we were infants or children. In fact, those maps would cause us a lot of trouble if they were used to control our adult limbs. We want our spatial and motor processes to continuously adapt to changes in our motor apparatus. These complementary types of learning allow our sensory and cognitive systems to stably learn about the world and to thereby be able to effectively control spatial and motor processes that continually update themselves to deal with changing conditions in our limbs.

Why, then, are procedural memories unconscious? The difference between cognitive memories and procedural, or motor, memories has gone by a number of different names, including the distinction between declarative memory and procedural memory, knowing that and knowing how, memory and habit, or memory with record and memory without record (Bruner 1969; Mishkin 1982, 1993; Ryle, 1949; Squire and Cohen 1984). The amnesic patient H. M. dramatically illustrated this distinction by learning and remembering motor skills like assembly of the Tower of Hanoi without being able to recall ever having done so (Bruner 1969, Scoville and Milner 1957, Squire and Cohen 1984). We can now give a very short answer to the question of why procedural memories are unconscious: The matching that takes place during spatial and motor processing is often inhibitory matching. Such a matching process cannot support an excitatory resonance. Hence, it cannot support consciousness.

In this regard, Goodale and Milner (1992) have described a patient whose brain lesion has prevented accurate visual discrimination of object orientation, yet whose visually guided reaching behaviors towards objects are oriented and sized correctly. We have shown, in a series of articles, how head-centered and body-centered representations of an object's spatial location and orientation may be learned and used to control reaches of the hand-arm system that can continuously adapt themselves to changes in the sensory and motor apparatus that is used to plan and execute reaching behaviors (Bullock, Grossberg, and Guenther 1993; Carpenter, Grossberg, and Lesher 1998; Gaudiano and Grossberg 1991; Grossberg et al. 1993; Guenther et al. 1994). None of these model circuits has resonant loops; hence, they do not support consciousness.

When these models are combined into a more comprehensive system architecture for intelligent behavior, the sensory and cognitive match-based networks in the What processing stream through the inferotemporal cortex provide self-stabilizing representations with which to continually learn more about the world without undergoing catastrophic forgetting, whereas the Where/How processing stream's spatial and motor mismatch-based maps and gains can continually forget their old parameters in order to instate the new parameters that are needed to control our bodies in their present form. This larger architecture illustrates how circuits in the self-stabilizing match-based sensory and cognitive parts of the brain can resonate into consciousness, even while they are helping to direct the contextually appropriate activation of spatial and motor circuits that cannot.

Acknowledgments

Supported in part by the Defense Advanced Research Projects Agency and the Office of Naval Research (ONR N00014-95-1-0409), National Science Foundation (IRI-97-20333), and the Office of Naval Research (ONR N00014-95-1-0657).

The author wishes to thank Cynthia E. Bradford, Diana Meyers, and Robin Amos for their valuable assistance in the preparation of this manuscript.

References

Abbott, L. F., Varela, K., Sen, K., and Nelson, S. B. (1997). Synaptic depression and cortical gain control. *Science*, 275, 220–223.

Artola, A. and Singer, W. (1993). Long-term depression of excitatory synaptic transmission and its relationship to long-term potentiation. *Trends in Neurosciences*, 16, 480–487.

Bradski, G. and Grossberg, G. (1995). Fast learning VIEWNET architectures for recognizing 3-D objects from multiple 2-D views. *Neural Networks* 8, 1053–1080.

Bregman, A. S. (1990). Auditory scene analysis: The perceptual organization of sound. Cambridge, MA: MIT Press.

Bruner, J. S. (1969). In G. A. Talland and N. C. Waugh (Eds.), *The pathology of memory*. New York: Academic Press.

Bullock, D. and Grossberg, S. (1988). Neural dynamics of planned arm movements: Emergent invariants and speed-accuracy properties during trajectory formation. *Psychological Review*, 95, 49–90.

Bullock, D., Grossberg, S. and Guenther, F. H. (1993). A self-organizing neural model of motor equivalent reaching and tool use by a multijoint arm. *Journal of Cognitive Neuroscience*, 5, 408–435.

Bullock, D., Grossberg, S. and Mannes, C. (1993). A neural network model for cursive script production. *Biological Cybernetics*, 70, 15–28.

Carpenter, G. A. and Grossberg, S. (1981). Adaptation and transmitter gating in vertebrate photoreceptors. *Journal of Theoretical Neurobiology*, 1, 1–42. Reprinted in S. Grossberg (Ed.), *The adaptive brain*, II. Amsterdam: Elsevier Publishing, 1987, 271–310.

Carpenter, G. A. and Grossberg, S. (1987a). A massively parallel architecture for a self-organizing neural pattern recognition machine. *Computer Vision, Graphics, and Image Processing*, 37, 54–115.

Carpenter, G. A. and Grossberg, S. (1987b). ART 2: Self-organization of stable category recognition codes for analog input patterns. *Applied Optics*, 26, 4919–4930.

Carpenter, G. A. and Grossberg, S. (1993). Normal and amnesic learning, recognition, and memory by a neural model of cortico-hippocampal interactions. *Trends in Neurosciences*, 116, 131–137.

Carpenter, G. A. and Grossberg, S. (1994). Integrating symbolic and neural processing in a self-organizing architecture for pattern recognition and prediction. In V. Honavar and L. Uhr (Eds.), *Artificial intelligence and neural networks: Steps towards principled prediction.* San Diego: Academic Press, 387–421.

Carpenter, G. A., Grossberg, S. and Lesher, G. W. (1998). The What-and-Where filter: A spatial mapping neural network for object recognition and image understanding. *Computer Vision and Image Understanding*, 69, 1–22.

Carpenter, G. A., Grossberg, S. Markuzon, N., Reynolds, J. H., and Rosen, D. B. (1992). Fuzzy ART-MAP: A neural network architecture for incremental supervised learning of analog multidimensional maps. *IEEE Transactions on Neural Networks*, 3, 698–713.

Carpenter, G. A., Grossberg, S. and Reynolds, J. H. (1991). ARTMAP: Supervised real-time learning and classification of nonstationary data by a self-organizing neural network. *Neural Networks*, 4, 565–588.

Chapman, K. L., Leonard, L. B., and Mervis, C. G. (1986). The effect of feedback on young children's inappropriate word usage. *Journal of Child Language*, 13, 101–107.

Chey, J., Grossberg, S. and Mingolla, E. (1997). Neural dynamics of motion grouping: From aperture ambiguity to object speed and direction. *Journal of the Optical Society of America*, 14, 2570–2594.

Clark, E. V. (1973). What's in a word? On the child's acquisition of semantics in his first language. In T. E. Morre (Ed.), *Cognitive development and the acquisition of language.* New York: Academic Press, 65–110.

Cohen, N. J. (1984). Preserved learning capacity in amnesia: Evidence for multiple memory systems. In L. Squire and N. Butters (Eds.), *The neuropsychology of memory.* New York: Guilford Press, pp. 83–103.

Cohen, N. J. and Squire, L. R. (1980). Preserved learning and retention of a pattern-analyzing skill in amnesia: Dissociation of knowing how and knowing that. *Science*, 210, 207–210.

Deadwyler, S. A., West, M. O., and Lynch, G. (1979). Activity of dentate granule cells during learning: Differentiation of perforant path inputs. *Brain Research*, 169, 29–43.

Deadwyler, S. A., West, M. O., and Robinson, J. H. (1981). Entorhinal and septal inputs differentially control sensory-evoked responses in the rat dentate gyrus. *Science*, 211, 1181–1183.

Drevets, W. C., Burton, H., and Raichle, M. E. (1995). Blood flow changes in human somatosensory cortex during anticipated stimulation. *Nature*, 373, 249.

Eckhorn, R., Bauer, R., Jordan, W., Brosch, M., Kruse, W., Munk, M., and Reitboeck, H. J. (1988). Coherent oscillations: A mechanism of feature linking in the visual cortex? *Biological Cybernetics*, 60, 121–130.

Fiala, J. C., Grossberg, S., and Bullock, D. (1996). Metabotropic glutamate receptor activation in cerebellar Purkinje cells as substrate for adaptive timing of the classically conditioned eye-blink response. *Journal of Neuroscience*, 16, 3760–3774.

Francis, G. and Grossberg, S. (1996a). Cortical dynamics of boundary segmentation and reset: Persistence, afterimages, and residual traces. *Perception*, 35, 543–567.

Francis, G. and Grossberg, S. (1996b). Cortical dynamics of form and motion integration: Persistence, apparent motion, and illusory contours. *Vision Research*, 36, 149–173.

Francis, G., Grossberg, S., and Mingolla, E. (1994). Cortical dynamics of feature binding and reset: Control of visual persistence. *Vision Research*, 34, 1089–1104.

Fuster, J. M. (1996). Frontal lobe and the cognitive foundation of behavioral action. In A. R. Damasio, H. Damasio, and Y. Christen (Eds.), *The neurobiology of decision-making.* New York: Springer, 47–61.

Gaffan, D. (1985). Hippocampus: Memory, habit, and voluntary movement. *Philosophical Transactions of the Royal Society of London*, B308, 87–99.

Gao, E. and Suga, N. (1998). Experience-dependent corticofugal adjustment of midbrain frequency map in bat auditory system. *Proceedings of the National Academy of Sciences USA* 95, 12663–12670.

Gaudiano, P. and Grossberg, S. (1991). Vector associative maps: Unsupervised real-time error-based learning and control of movement trajectories. *Neural Networks*, 4, 147–183.

Goodale, M. A. and Milner, D. (1992). Separate visual pathways for perception and action. *Trends in Neurosciences*, 15, 20–25.

Gove, A., Grossberg, S., and Mingolla, E. (1995). Brightness perception, illusory contours, and corticogeniculate feedback. *Visual Neuroscience*, 12, 1027–1052.

Govindarajan, K. K., Grossberg, S., Wyse, L. L., and Cohen, M. A. (1995). A neural network model of auditory scene analysis and source segregation. Technical Report: CAS/CNS-TR-94-039. Boston, MA: Boston University.

Graf, P., Squire, L. R., and Mandler, G. (1984). The information that amnesic patients do not forget. *Journal of Experimental Psychology: Learning, Memory, and Cognition*, 10, 164–178–183.

Gray, C. M. and Singer, W. (1989). Stimulus-specific neuronal oscillations in orientation columns of cat visual cortex. *Proceedings of the National Academy of Sciences USA*, 86, 1698–1702.

Grossberg, S. (1969). On learning and energy-entropy dependence in recurrent and nonrecurrent signed networks. *Journal of Statistical Physics*, 1, 319–350.

Grossberg, S. (1972). Neural expectation: Cerebellar and retinal analogs of cells fired by learnable or unlearned pattern classes. *Kybernetik*, 10, 49–57.

Grossberg, S. (1976a). Adaptive pattern classification and universal recoding, I: Parallel development and coding of neural feature detectors. *Biological Cybernetics*, 1976, 23, 121–134.

Grossberg, S. (1976b). Adaptive pattern classification and universal recoding, II: Feedback, expectation, olfaction, and illusions. *Biological Cybernetics*, 1976, 23, 187–202.

Grossberg, S. (1978). A theory of human memory: Self-organization and performance of sensory-motor codes, maps, and plans. In R. Rosen and F. Snell (Eds.), *Progress in theoretical biology*, Vol. 5. New York: Academic Press, 1978.

Grossberg, S. (1980). How does a brain build a cognitive code? *Psychological Review*, 1, 1–51. How does a brain build a cognitive code? *Psychological Review*, 1980, 1, 1–51.

Grossberg, S. (1982). *Studies of mind and brain: Neural principles of learning, perception, development, cognition, and motor control.* Dordrecht: Kluwer.

Grossberg, S. (1987b). *The adaptive brain*, I. Amsterdam: North-Holland.

Grossberg, S. (1988). Nonlinear neural networks: Principles, mechanisms, and architectures. *Neural Networks*, 1, 17–61.

Grossberg, S. (1994). 3-D vision and figure-ground separation by visual cortex. *Perception and Psychophysics*, 1994, 55, 48–120.

Grossberg, S. (1997). Cortical dynamics of three-dimensional figure-ground perception of two-dimensional figures. *Psychological Review*, 1997, 104, 618–658.

Grossberg, S. (1999). How does the cerebral cortex work? Learning, attention, and grouping by the laminar circuits of visual cortex. Technical report CAS/CNS TR-97-023. Boston, MA: Boston University. *Spatial Vision*, 12, 163–185.

Grossberg, S. (1998). Pitch based streaming in auditory perception. In N. Griffith and P. Todd (Eds.), *Musical networks: Parallel distributed perception and performance.* Cambridge, MA: MIT Press.

Grossberg, S., Boardman, I., and Cohen, M. A. (1997). Neural dynamics of variable-rate speech categorization. *Journal of Experimental Psychology: Human Perception and Performance*, 23, 481–503.

Grossberg, S. and Grunewald, A. (1997). Cortical synchronization and perceptual framing. *Journal of Cognitive Neuroscience*, 9, 117–132.

Grossberg, S., Guenther, F., Bullock, D., and Greve, D. (1993). Neural representations for sensory-motor control, II: Learning a head-centered visuomotor representation of 3-D target position. *Neural Networks*, 1993, 6, 43–67.

Grossberg, S. and Gutowski, W. (1987). Neural dynamics of decision making under risk: Affective balance and cognitive-emotional interactions. *Psychological Review*, 1987, 94, 300–318.

Grossberg, S. and McLoughlin, N. P. (1997). Cortical dynamics of three-dimensional surface perception: Binocular and half-occluded scenic images. *Neural Networks*, 10, 1583–1605.

Grossberg, S. and Merrill, J. W. L. (1996). The hippocampus and cerebellum in adaptively timed learning, recognition, and movement. *Journal of Cognitive Neuroscience*, 3, 257–277.

Grossberg, S., Roberts, K., Aguilar, M., and Bullock, D. (1997). A neural model of multimodal adaptive saccadic eye movement control by superior colliculus. *Journal of Neuroscience*, 17, 9706–9725.

Grossberg, S. and Williamson, J. R. (1997). Linking cortical development to visual perception. *Society for Neuroscience Abstract*, 23, 568, Number 227.9.

Grossberg, S. and Williamson, J. R. (1998). A neural model of how visual cortex develops a laminar architecture capable of adult perceptual grouping. Technical Report CAS/CNS-TR-98-022. Boston, MA: Boston University.

Grunewald, A. and Grossberg, S. (1998). Self-Organization of binocular disparity tuning by reciprocal corticogeniculate interactions. *Journal of Cognitive Neuroscience*, 10, 199–215.

Guenther, F. H., Bullock, D., Greve, D. and Grossberg, S. (1994). Neural representations for sensory-motor control, III: Learning a body-centered representation of 3-D target position. *Journal of Cognitive Neuroscience*, 6, 341–358.

Hikosaka, O. (1994). Role of basal ganglia in control of innate movements, learned behavior and cognition—a hypothesis. In G. Percheron, J. S. McKenzie, and J. Feger (Eds.), *The basal ganglia*, IV. New York: Plenum Press, 589–595.

Hupé, J. M., James, A. C., Girard, P. and Bullier, J. (1997). Feedback connections from V2 modulate intrinsic connectivity within. *Society for Neuroscience Abstracts*, 406.15, 1031.

Ito, M., Westheimer, G., and Gilbert, D. C. (1997). Attention modulates the influence of context on spatial integration in V1 of alert monkeys. *Society for Neuroscience Abstracts* 603.2, 1031.

Johnson, R. R. and Burkhalter, A. (1997). A circuit for amplification of excitatory feedback input from rat extrastriate cortex to primary visual cortex. *Society for Neuroscience Abstracts*, 651.7, 1669.

Kohonen, T. (1984). *Self-organization and associative memory*. New York: Springer-Verlag.

Lamme, V. A. F., Zipser, K., and Spekreijse, H. (1997). Figure-ground signals in V1 depend on consciousness and feedback from extra-striate areas. *Society for Neuroscience Abstracts*, 603.1, 1543.

Levy, W. B. (1985). Associative changes at the synapse: LTP in the hippocampus. In W. B. Levy, J. Anderson, and S. Lehmkuhle (Eds.), *Synaptic modification, neu-ron selectivity, and nervous system organization*. Hillsdale, NJ: Erlbaum, 5–33.

Levy, W. B. and Desmond, N. L. (1985). The rules of elemental synaptic plasticity. In W. B. Levy, J. Anderson, and S. Lehmkuhle (Eds.), *Synaptic modification, neuron selectivity, and nervous system organization*. Hillsdale, NJ: Erlbaum Associates, 105–121.

Lynch, G., McGaugh, J. L., and Weinberger, N. M. (Eds.) (1984). *Neurobiology of learning and memory*. New York: Guilford Press.

McAdams, C. J. and Maunsell, J. H. R. (1997). Spatial attention and feature-directed attention can both modulate neuronal responses in macaque area V4. *Society for Neuroscience Abstracts*, 802.5, 2062.

Michotte, A., Thines, G., and Crabbe, G. (1964). *Les complements amodaux des structures perceptives*. Louvain: Publications Universitaires de Louvain.

Middleton, F. A. and Strick, P. L. (1994). Anatomical evidence for cerebellar and basal ganglia involvement in higher cognitive function. *Science*, 166, 458–461.

Miller, E. K., Li, L., and Desimone, R. (1991). A neural mechanism for working and recognition memory in inferior temporal cortex. *Science*, 254, 1377–1379.

Mishkin, M. (1982). A memory system in the monkey. *Philosophical Transactions Royal Society of London*, B, 298, 85–95.

Mishkin, M. (1993). Cerebral memory circuits. In T. A. Poggio and D. A. Glaser (Eds.), *Exploring brain functions: Models in neuroscience*. New York: Wiley and Sons, 113–125.

Mishkin, M., Ungerleider, L. G., and Macko, K. A. (1983). Object vision and spatial vision: Two cortical pathways. *Trends in Neurosciences*, 6, 414–417.

Motter, B. C. (1994a). Neural correlates of attentive selection for color or luminance in extrastriate area V4. *Journal of Neuroscience*, 14, 2178–2189.

Motter, B. C. (1994b). Neural correlates of feature selective memory and pop-out in extrastriate area V4. *Journal of Neuroscience*, 14, 2190–2199.

Murphy, P. C. and Sillito, A. M. (1987). Corticofugal feedback influences the generation of length tuning in the visual pathway. *Nature*, 329, 727–729.

Parker, D. B. (1982, October). Learning-logic (Invention Report 581-64, File 1). Office of Technology Licensing. Stanford University, Stanford, CA.

Press, W. A. and van Essen, D. C. (1997). Attentional modulation of neuronal responses in macaque area V1. *Society for Neuroscience Abstracts*, 405.3, 1026.

Pribram, K. H. (1986). The hippocampal system and recombinant processing. In R. L. Isaacson and K. H. Pribram (Eds.), *The hippocampus*, Vol. 4, New York: Plenum Press, 329–370.

Rauschecker, J. P. and Singer, W. (1979). Changes in the circuitry of the kitten's visual cortex are gated by postsynaptic activity. *Nature*, 280, 58–60.

Repp, B. H. 1980. A range-frequency effect on perception of silence in speech. *Haskins Laboratories Status Report on Speech Research*, SR-61, 151–165.

Reynolds, J., Nicholas, J., Chelazzi, L., and Desimone, R. (1995). Spatial attention protects macaque V2 and V4 cells from the influence of non-attended stimuli. *Society for Neuroscience Abstracts*, 21.3, 1759.

Rumelhart, D. E., Hinton, G. E. and Williams, R. J. (1986). Learning internal representations by error propagation. In D. E. Rumelhard and J. L. McClelland (Eds.), *Parallel distributed processing*. Cambridge, MA: MIT Press.

Ryle, G. (1949). *The concept of mind*. New York: Hutchinson Press.

Sakai, K., Hikosaka, O., Miyauchi, S., Takino, R., Sasaki, Y., and Putz, B. (1998). Transition of brain activation from frontal to parietal areas in visuomotor sequence learning. *Journal of Neuroscience*, 18, 1827–1840.

Samuel, A. G. (1981a). The role of bottom-up confirmation in the phonemic restoration illusion. *Journal of Experimental Psychology: Human Perception and Performance*, 7, 1124–1131.

Samuel, A. G. (1981b). Phonemic restoration: Insights from a new methodology. *Journal of Experimental Psychology: General*, 110, 474–494.

Scoville, W. B. and Milner, B. (1957). Loss of recent memory after bilateral hippocampal lesion. *Journal of Neurology, Neurosurgery, and Psychiatry*, 20, 11–21.

Sillito, A. M., Jones, H. E., Gerstein, G. L., and West, D. C. (1994). Feature-linked synchronization of thalamic relay cell firing induced by feedback from the visual cortex. *Nature*, 369, 479–482.

Singer, W. (1983). Neuronal activity as a shaping factor in the self-organization of neuron assemblies. In E. Basar, H. Flohr, H. Haken, and A. J. Mandell (Eds.), *Synergetics of the brain*. New York: Springer-Verlag.

Smith, C., Carey, S., and Wiser, M. (1985). On differentiation: A case study of the development of the concept of size, weight, and density. *Cognition*, 21, 177–237.

Smith, L. B. and Kemler, D. G. (1978). Levels of experienced dimensionality in children and adults. *Cognitive Psychology*, 10, 502–532.

Squire, L. R. and Butters, N. (Eds.) (1984). *Neuropsychology of memory*. New York: Guilford Press.

Squire, L. R. and Cohen, N. J. (1984). Human memory and amnesia. In G. Lunch, J. McGaugh, and N. M. Weinberger (Eds.), *Neurobiology of learning and memory*. New York: Guilford Press, 3–64.

Ungerleider, L. G. and Mishkin, M. (1982). Two cortical visual systems: Separation of appearance and location of objects. In D. L. Ingle, M. A. Goodale, and R. J. W. Mansfield (Eds.), *Analysis of visual behavior*. Cambridge, MA: MIT Press, 549–586.

von der Malsburg, C. (1973). Self-organization of orientation sensitive cells in the striate cortex. *Kybernetik*, 14, 85–100.

Ward, T. B. (1983). Response temp and separable-integral responding: Evidence for an integral-to-separable processing sequencing in visual perception. *Journal of Experimental Psychology: Human Perception and Performance*, 9, 1029–1051.

Warren, R. M. (1984). Perceptual restoration of obliterated sounds. *Psychological Bulletin*, 96, 371–383.

Warren, R. M. and Sherman, G. L. (1974). Phonemic restorations based on subsequent context. *Perception and Psychophysics*, 16, 150–156.

Warrington, E. K. and Weiskrantz, L. (1974). The effect of prior learning on subsequent retention in amnesic patients. *Neuropsychology*, 12, 419–428.

Werbos, P. (1974). Beyond regression: New tools for prediction and analysis in the behavioral sciences. Unpublished doctoral thesis, Harvard University, Cambridge, MA.

Willshaw, D. J. and Malsburg, C. von der. (1976). How patterned neural connections can be set up by self-organization. *Proceedings of the Royal Society of London*, B, 194, 431–445.

Yan, W. and Suga, N. (1998). Corticofugal modulation of the midbrain frequency map in the bat auditory system. *Nature Neuroscience*, 1, 54–58.

Zola-Morgan, S. M. and Squire, L. R. (1990). The primate hippocampal formation: Evidence for a time-limited role in memory storage. *Science*, 250, 288–290.

A Global Competitive Network for Attention

J. G. Taylor and F. N. Alavi

Introduction

There is developing interest in creating neural network models of attention. Various attempts have been made to approach this by means of competitive networks [15], [38] and more recently by more complicated nets which describe the psychological or global level of response effectively. However, none of these references, and the many more using competitive nets to explain other aspects of neurobiological processing, appear to have any strong foundation in neurobiological fact. A non-trivial proportion of neurons, suggested at about 25%, are inhibitory, but long-range connections between cortical areas appear to be excitatory [8], although with feedback inhibition coming from local lateral inhibition. There is good evidence for inhibitory effects in orientation sensitivity in early cortex [20] but this has at most been suggested as arising from half a hypercolumn distance, or about 0.5 mm, and giving fine-tuning of earlier sensitivity [39].

It appears, therefore, that the absence of any long-range inhibitory connections leading to the production of competition between activity in the numerous areas (occipital parietal, temporal and frontal lobe) involved in guiding the various aspects of attention [26] requires that one search elsewhere than in the cortex. A particularly desirable feature of the competitive mechanism would be that it leads not only to efficient competition but also to *global guidance*. By this we mean the ability of a winning input to a portion of cortex to control activity in other parts of cortex at the same (or in very closely subsequent) time. This latter activity which loses the competition is not destroyed, but is allowed to exist only in certain forms, guided by the winning input.

Global guidance is not a standard property of winner-take-all (WTA) type networks.[2] Indeed it appears to be very different and not compatible with any known WTA architecture. One possible class of neural networks able to implement global guidance to some degree is that of nets with spatial instability. Such nets have been known since the time of the work on visual hallucinations [9] and from the wealth of examples of instability and pattern formation in reaction-diffusion equations [22]. We present here results on a particular brain network, the nucleus reticularis thalami (NRT), which we propose functions by means of its special lateral inhibitory connectivity so as to achieve global guidance as well as a more local competitive form of action. The manner in which such global guidance can be used in attentive processing is still to be analysed. However we briefly explore this possibility, and the even more conjectural manner in which this system may contribute to consciousness, at the end of the paper. This follows the earlier sections on the basis of the model, its theoretical analysis, and simulation results.

The Model

We start by describing the crucial feature of the model, the nucleus reticularis thalami (NRT).

Nucleus Reticularis of the Thalamus

The NRT, present in all mammals, is a thin, curved sheet of cells so situated between thalamic relay cells and their cortical target sites as to be highly suggestive of its possible controlling influence on cortical input and activity. It is pierced by thalamo-cortical and returning cortico-thalamic fibres in a roughly topographic fashion, especially for inputs to and from primary sensory cortical areas. The main organisational principle [14] is that the NRT can be considered as a series of overlapping sectors, each related to a particular dorsal thalamic nucleus (or nuclei). The axons penetrating NRT give off excitatory collaterals to it, whilst NRT cells themselves only feed back inhibitorily in a roughly topographic fashion to the thalamic relay cells from which they have received their collaterals. The main NRT cell neurotransmitter is GABA, which is a well-known inhibitor. The NRT structure eminently qualifies it to be some sort of integrative filter modulating thalamic and cortical activity, the filter itself controlled by cortical, mid-brain, and some brain stem structures (which also have inputs to NRT). That NRT performs a control function has been remarked on briefly in numerous papers. For example, as noted by Schiebel [27]: "Situated like a thin nuclear sheet draped over the lateral and anterior surfaces of the thalamus, it has been likened to the screen grid interposed between cathode and anode in the triode or pentode vacuum tube." This was also stated by [40], with a wealth of neurophysiological support: "The possibility that NRT may function as a topographically specific feedback circuit makes it a prime candidate for selective regulation of thalamo-cortical activities."

There are various features of the detailed circuitry and functionality which must be properly accounted for in any serious modeling:

1. Firstly, the nature of the inter-connectivity on the NRT sheet is itself species specific. Thus in the rat, fine structure analysis shows only axo-dendritic synapses of presumed excitatory or inhibitory type [23], but that of the cat and monkey have very clear dendro-dendritic synapses [24], some of these even being reciprocal [7]. It should be added that these dendro-dendritic synapses occur near cell bodies, and not on their distal dendrites.

2. Secondly, the exact nature of the inhibitory effect of the GABAergic NRT cells is unclear. Thus evidence has been presented [21], [28] that local application of GABA to NRT neurons causes depolarisation of cell membrane rather than hyperpolarisation. Direct evidence of lat-

eral inhibition of NRT neurons on each other was earlier provided by [1]. Moreover, the equilibrium potential E_{Cl} of the chloride conductance (the ion channel by which GABA influences the membrane potential) is about -65 mV [21] whilst the average membrane potential is about -56 mV [3]. Thus the effect of GABA on neurons at or above their resting potential will be expected to be inhibitory. It is interesting to note that this effect will become excitatory if the membrane potential goes below E_{Cl}. This may be a useful control mechanism to prevent NRT neurons becoming so hyperpolarised as to be in their bursting state. Throughout this paper we will assume the action of GABA on NRT is inhibitory, and that the neurons have membrane potentials always above E_{Cl} (although this latter will not be explicitly discussed in the modelling). The effect of GABAergic feedback in thalamic relay cells and interneurons will be considered later.

3. Thirdly, the continuous nature of the NRT sheet is reasonably well supported by anatomical and cytoarchitectonic evidence, except for that part of it adjacent to the visual input (through the lateral geniculate nucleus, LGN) termed the perigeniculate nucleus (PGN). Presently, the weight of opinion is in favour of complete connectivity between PGN and NRT.

4. Fourthly, there are at least two modes of action of thalamic relay and NRT neurons:

(i) relay-like behaviour, defined by tonic firing in response to inputs.

(ii) a phasic bursting discharge behaviour, with the ability to maintain rhythmic burst discharges at about 6–8 Hz.

There is great relevance of mode (ii) in thalamic and cerebral spindling (sequences of rhythmic bursting) activity in sleep and in the sleep-wake transition [3]. Since we are mainly interested here in the waking state, only mode (i) of the NRT (and thalamic) neurons will be considered explicitly.

5. Fifthly, there is an important species-specific difference in the NRT feedback to thalamus. In the rat, only LGN has inhibitory interneurons, but other thalamic nuclei with output to NRT are known to possess very few nonrelay cells [4], [11]. In the cat and monkey, however, such interneurons are apparently widespread. Inhibitory NRT feedback on these latter interneurons was used as an important part of the model of [31] and later by [16]. This model assumed disinhibition of interneuronal input control by inhibitory NRT feedback. However, in rat, without such interneurons, one might expect NRT inhibition to feed back directly on to input thalamic relay cells, so having just the opposite effect on thalamic inputs. We will discuss this problem when we turn to the details of our model, and in particular consider it in the context of stability.

6. Sixthly, there are also interesting features of the global wiring diagram in which NRT is concerned. Thus NRT is claimed not to be connected at all to the anterior thalamic nuclei in cats [14], [25], but there is apparently such connectivity in rats [23]. The question of how important NRT inputs are to conscious processing will be discussed later in the paper.

7. Seventhly, there is [29] a clear change of cellular type in NRT from cells with round dendritic fields (termed R-type), of about 200 μm across, at the anterior pole to more elongated large fusiform cells (F-type) moving posteriorly, to even more elongated small fusiform cells (f-type) on the medial and lateral borders of the sheet. F and f-type cells have dendrites running either vertically or horizontally in the plane of the NRT sheet (the elongated dendritic fields of f-type usually being horizontal), the f-type extending up to 300–400 μm in length from the cell body. The f-cells seem to be located especially in the region of the NRT related to sensory thalamic nuclei, and receive afferents from sensory cortex. The most important aspects of these features of NRT are summarised in table 62.1, for future reference.

Table 62.1

Species differences between various structural properties of NRT

Property of NRT	Rat	Cat, primate
1. Dendro-dendritic synapses	No	Yes
2. Inhibitory interneurons in non-sensory thalamic nuclei	No	Yes
3. Inhibitory interneurons in LGN	Yes	Yes
4. NRT connected to anterior thalamic nuclei	Yes	No

Neural Modelling

In order to deduce properties of neural models it is usual to do so either by general arguments or, alternatively and more precisely, to simulate them using simplified models of the neurons which they contain. The latter approach becomes difficult if there are many neurons and/or many coupled nets. Since we wish to attempt to consider both of these latter cases we appear to be forced to attempt to use the more general method. We will try to be more precise, however, be using the techniques of dynamical systems theory to allow us to deduce qualitative results for a class of models. This is a method which has now become well established and for which there are numerous texts and reviews. The main concepts are attractors (fixed points, cycles, strange attractors) and stability (bifurcations of various types). These have been discussed in the cortical context in a general fashion in [9], and many more discussions are now appearing, which are too numerous to mention. In specific cases quantitative results are being obtained which permit even more precise descriptions of various biological neural processes.

The main model of the neuron we will use is the leaky integrator neuron, with output describing its mean firing rate, given by a suitable sigmoidal function of the membrane potential. The input is a linear sum of the outputs of other neurons. This is now standard in the field of artificial neural networks, and has proved increasingly effective in many industrial applications. The model is obviously an enormous simplification of any biologically realistic neuron. However, we argue in support of simplicity on two grounds. Firstly, general features of simulations of nets of highly complex neurons have been duplicated by using the simple neurons we are advocating [18]. Secondly, if it is possible to achieve insight into basic principles for new paradigms of information processing that might be used by the brain in terms of such simple model neurons, then it could give a valuable guidance to further research. One would then have to ascertain if the use of biologically more realistic neurons would make such processing as, if not more than, effective. It also might help in developing further new paradigms for ever more global information processing, again with the purpose of guiding understanding of additional styles of brain processing. These new paradigms could occur on using more global wiring diagrams to understand the functionality of an even larger range of brain regions than those under the initial detailed scrutiny, but involved with these latter in an important manner. We will describe such extensions later.

Part of the important advances being made by artificial neural networks is in their ability to learn any suitably smooth function with simple sigmoidally responding neurons and with a one hidden layer feedforward architecture [12]. This aspect of neural networks allows an adaptive feedforward net to be arbitrarily flexible. On the face of it such powers would seem to make easier the problem of modelling attention and consciousness for one might think of trying to train a neural net to become conscious. However, such a method appears difficult to make effective. That is because the criteria for an attentional net are not simple to specify. One might claim that a single competitive net will achieve effective results [15]. However, it is well known [26] that attention has several stages, containing at least

the steps of disengagement, movement, and re-engagement. There is also the difference between exogenous and endogenous attention. Several nets therefore must be involved in the overall action of attending. This makes the desired input-output transforms of each net less obvious. Moreover, it is likely that not until after being attended to does recognition and memory storage of an object occur. Thus the on-going net learning should not take place until after attention. Adaptive processes may be necessary to develop suitable feature detectors for preprocessing [19] but that need not be regarded as part of the activity we must consider most specifically during actual attentional processing. Nor has the study of the development of feature detectors led to any perceptible insight into attention.

In the face of these difficulties we will use the hints which can be gleaned from lesion studies and gross circuit diagrams [26] amd from the details of the microneuroanatomy we have presented above, and the neurophysiology of the appropriate neural circuits, as contained, for example, in [31] and [32].

The Analytic Model

We now turn to the detail of the equations used to describe the C-NRT-TH interacting system, whose general structure is shown in figure 62.1. Excitatory neurons are assumed to be at co-ordinate position $\mathbf{r}$ (using the same coordinate frame for NRT, C and TH) on the thalamic and cortical sheets and to have membrane potentials labelled $u_1(\mathbf{r})$ and $u_3(\mathbf{r})$, and outputs $f_i(u_i)$, ($i = 1$ and 3 respectively), where $f_i(x) = \left[1 + \exp\left(\frac{x - S_i}{T_i}\right)\right]^{-1}$, with threshold S_i and temperature T_i. Inhibitory neurons in thalamus and on NRT (with the same co-ordinate positions) have membrane potentials denoted $v_1(\mathbf{r})$, $v_2(\mathbf{r})$ with similar sigmoidal outputs g_1, g_2 to the other neurons. Connection weights from the j'th excitatory (inhibitory) neuron at $\mathbf{r}'$ to the i'th

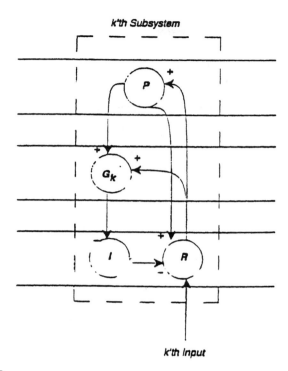

k'th Subsystem

k'th Input

cm

Figure 62.1
(a) Schematic of a typical k'th subsystem. (b) Schematic of connected subsystems. Symbols: I—inhibitory inter-neuron; R—relay cell; G_k—k'th gating neuron; P—pyaimidal cell.

excitatory (inhibitory) neuron at $\mathbf{r}$ are denoted $a_{ij}(\mathbf{r}, \mathbf{r}')(e - e)$, $b_{ij}(\mathbf{r}, \mathbf{r}')(e - i)$, $c_{ij}(\mathbf{r}, \mathbf{r}')(i - e)$ and $d_{ij}(\mathbf{r}, \mathbf{r}')(i - i)$. The resulting leaky integrator neurons (LIN) satisfy

$$\dot{u}_3(\mathbf{r}) = -\frac{1}{\tau_3} u_3(\mathbf{r}) + \frac{1}{\tau_3} \sum_{\mathbf{r}'} a_{31}(\mathbf{r}, \mathbf{r}') f_1(u_1(\mathbf{r}')), \quad (1)$$

$$\dot{v}_2(\mathbf{r}) = -\frac{1}{\tau_2} v_2(\mathbf{r}) + \frac{1}{\tau_2} \sum_{\mathbf{r}'} [c_{23}(\mathbf{r}, \mathbf{r}') f_3(u_3(\mathbf{r}'))$$

$$+ c_{21}(\mathbf{r}, \mathbf{r}') f_1(u_1(\mathbf{r}')) + d_{22}(\mathbf{r}, \mathbf{r}') g_2(v_2(\mathbf{r}'))]$$

$$+ \text{dendro-dendritic terms}, \quad (2)$$

$$\dot{v}_1(\mathbf{r}) = -\frac{1}{\tau_1'} v_1(\mathbf{r}) + \frac{1}{\tau_1'} \sum_{\mathbf{r}'} d_{12}(\mathbf{r}, \mathbf{r}') g_2(v_2(\mathbf{r}')), \quad (3)$$

$$\dot{u}_1(\mathbf{r}) = -\frac{1}{\tau_1} u_1(\mathbf{r}) + \frac{1}{\tau_1} \sum_{\mathbf{r}'} [a_{13}(\mathbf{r}, \mathbf{r}') f_3(u_3(\mathbf{r}'))$$

$$+ b_{11}(\mathbf{r}, \mathbf{r}') g_1(v_1(\mathbf{r}'))] + \frac{1}{\tau_1} I(\mathbf{r}) \quad (4)$$

(where we are using the notation $\dot{u} = \partial u / \partial t$). We have rescaled all the connection weights, and the input on TH cells, so that the decay constants τ_i, τ_1' drop out for stationary activity. Moreover the dendrodenritic contribution has yet to be included in (2).

This dendro-dendritic term can be following the analysis of [33], in which the capacitative current $C\dot{v}_2$ for the NRT cell plus the current injected by the cell into the NRT net by the dendrodendritic synapse (taken to be on or near to the cell body) is equal to the excitatory input currents from the TH and C cells (already incorporated in the right-hand side of (2)). The dendro-dendritic synaptic current is equal to $\sum_{\mathbf{r}'} F(v_2(\mathbf{r}) - v_2(\mathbf{r}'))$, where the summation is over the N nearest neighbours at $\mathbf{r}'$ to $\mathbf{r}$, and F is the (in general) non-linear voltage-current relation at the synapse. F is understood to be a sigmoidal function of the negative of its variable, being saturated for large values of that variable. Let us assume that the synaptic transfer function is linear (the non-linear case will be investigated in section "Softer Gating Model"). If G_2 is the dendro-dendritic conductance in this linear case (taken to be negative), this leads to the extra dendro-dendritic term in (2) equal to

$$-G_2(Nv_2(\mathbf{r}) - \sum v_2(\mathbf{r}')). \tag{5a}$$

Taking a purely rectangular net with four neighbours at horizontal and vertical distances $a_\pm$, $b_\pm$ (so $\mathbf{r}' = (\mathbf{r} + (a_\pm, b_\pm))$) gives, in the continuum limits [33],

$$+G_2(\mathbf{v} \cdot \nabla v_2 + \frac{1}{2}\lambda^2 \cdot \nabla^2 v_2) + \text{(higher order terms)}, \tag{5b}$$

where $\mathbf{v} = (a_+ - a_-, b_+ - b_-)^T$, $\lambda^2 = (a_+^2 + a_-^2, b_+^2 + b_-^2)^T$, $\nabla^2 = (\partial_x^2, \partial_y^2)^T$. The equation (2) thus reduces to a negative Laplacian net, with a linear derivative term proportional to $\mathbf{v}$. The inputs to the net depend, however, in a non-linear manner on v_2 as given by (1), (3), (4).

Analysis of the Model

The simplest model preserving the Laplacian net structure has no other lateral connections, so that in the continuum limit all connection weights are two-dimensional δ-functions. Only the symmetrical net is considered, with $a_+ = a_-$,

$b_+ = b_-$. Moreover, cortical activity can be dropped if the purely gating activity of the NRT-TH system is being explored. Finally, only the hard-limiting (zero temperature) outputs equal to step functions $Y(x)$ are taken (with $Y(x) = 0$ for $x < 0$; $Y(x) = 1$ for $x > 0$). Then (2), (3), (4) in the static limit, reduce to:

$$v_2(\mathbf{r}) + a^2\nabla^2 v_2 = \bar{c}_{21} Y(u_1(\mathbf{r}) - \bar{s}_1), \tag{6}$$

$$v_1(\mathbf{r}) = -\bar{d}_{12} Y(v_2(\mathbf{r}) - s_2), \tag{7}$$

$$u_1(\mathbf{r}) = I(\mathbf{r}) - \bar{b}_{11} Y(v_1(\mathbf{r}) - s_1), \tag{8}$$

where the constants $\bar{b}_{11}$, $\bar{c}_{21}$, $\bar{d}_{12}$ are all positive and a is a real constant. We note that for suitable choices of the connection strengths and thresholds on the right-hand sides of (6), (7) and (8), these latter behave as the simple model of NRT-TH feedback discussed in the text requires. Thus strong enough input I brings $u_1(\mathbf{r})$ positive enough (above $\bar{s}_1$) to give a source term in (6). Neglecting the Laplacian term in (6), v_2 becomes large enough (above s_2) to make $v_1 = -\bar{d}_{12}$ from (7). This activity effectively switches off the thalamic interneuron if $\bar{d}_{12} + s_1 < 0$, so leaving the thalamic relay cell potential u_1, large enough so that relay activity continues (provided $I_1 > \bar{s}_1$). If I is reduced, or v_2 is reduced by lateral inhibition, then u_1 goes below $\bar{s}_1$ to make $v_2 < s_2$, and the inhibitory interneuron is no longer inhibited. Assuming $s_1 < 0$, this neuron is active, and inhibits the thalamic relay cell sufficiently to leave $u_1 < \bar{s}_1$; there is no relay cell output.

It can be seen that the effect of the Laplacian term in (6) is important: it brings about global correlation of activity on NRT. This arises because (6), for given u_1, is the well-known Schrödinger equation in quantum mechanics for the wave function v_2. The extra term on the right-hand side of (6) leads to regions in which its value is zero, and to other regions where it takes the value $\bar{c}_{21}$. Let us denote these regions I and II respectively. Then (6) is analogous, (but not identical), to a Schrödinger equation in a piecewise constant potential. In order that (6) be satisfied everywhere it is necessary, following similar arguments to those used in the analogous situation, that across the boundaries B between I and II (assuming these exist), v_2 and ∂v_2 (the derivative of v_2 along the normal to B) be continuous. Otherwise δ-function terms arise on differentiation of v_2 which destroy the possibility of (6) being satisfied (these will be more discontinuous than that arising from the step-function in (6), so we need not be more precise about the latter). It is these boundary conditions which "sew together" the values of v_2 in I and II and give global control.

An important feature of (2) and (5b) is that they correspond to a negative diffusion term. Thus the continuity argument just given does not exclude a trivial constant response to a constant input for positive diffusion, as is well known. However, negative diffusion, together with further stabilising terms, can lead to non-trivial pattern formation [22]. It is clear that the stability analysis of the full non-linear system is important. This will be discussed later.

It is possible to solve (6), (7), (8) explicitly in the one-dimensional situation, where these equations reduce to

$$v_2 + a^2 v_2'' = \begin{cases} 0 & \text{(in region I)} \\ c & \text{(in region II).} \end{cases} \tag{9}$$

Let I be the set of intervals $(x^{(1)}, x^{(2)})$, $(x^{(3)}, x^{(4)}), \ldots, (x^{(2r-1)}, x^{(2r)}), \ldots, (x^{(2N-1)}, x^{(2N)})$ and II the intervals $(0, x^{(1)}), (x^{(2)}, x^{(3)}), \ldots, (x^{(2r)}, x^{(2r+1)}), \ldots, (x^{(2N)}, x^{(2N+1)})$; there are three other choices with I having lowest or highest intervals, but similar results obtain. The solution in the intervals $(x^{(2r-1)}, x^{(2r)})$ and $(x^{(2r)}, x^{(2r+1)})$ have the form, respectively,

I: $A_1^{(r)} \cos\left(\dfrac{x - \theta_1^{(r)}}{a}\right)$

$(r = 1, 3, 5, \ldots, 2N - 1)$,

$$\tag{10}$$

II: $A_2^{(r)} \cos\left(\dfrac{x - \theta_2^{(r)}}{a}\right) + c$

$(r = 0, 2, \ldots, 2N)$.

There are N intervals in I, $(N + 1)$ in II, so that there are $2(2N + 1)$ constants $\{A_i^{(r)}, \theta_i^{(r)}\}$, $(i = 1, 2)$ and a further $2N$ unknowns $x^{(1)}, \ldots, x^{(2N)}$, assuming $x^{(2N+1)} = h$ is fixed by the size of NRT. There are the boundary conditions on the continuity of v_2, v_2' at each $x^{(r)}$, $r = 1, 2, \ldots, 2N$, giving $4N$ conditions. There are also the conditions on the sign of v_2 in order that it fit correctly in I or II according to the collapse of (6), (7), (8) to (9). For suitable choices of weights and thresholds this reduces to the conditions:

$$v_2 \leq 0 \text{ in I}, \quad v_2 \geq 0 \text{ in II.} \tag{11}$$

But then the continuity conditions on v_2 at the I/II boundaries B require $v_2 = 0$ at each point $x^{(r)}$, $(r = 1, 2, \ldots, 2N)$. There are thus a further $2N$ constraints. The solutions (10) will thus be a two-parameter family, depending, say, on v_2 and v_2' at $x = 0$. It can be shown by more detailed analysis that each interval of I can fit one half-wave of $\cos a^{-1}x$, whilst each interval of II can fit about a full wavelength. This leads to the rough estimate

$$N \sim \frac{L}{3\pi a} \tag{12}$$

for the number of 'bunches' of activity which can be fitted into the interval $[0, L]$. Thus for $L \sim 1$ cm, $a \sim 200$ μm, there will be about 10 such bunches of activity. It is interesting to note the recent discovery of a repeated lattice of columnar encoding of complex features in temporal cortex [10], similar to that in striate cortex for orientation sensitivity, but now with about half the distance between columns (0.5 mm as compared to 1 mm separation). One might conjecture that there may be some relation between the spatial NRT pattern and the columnar cortical patterns; this will be investigated elsewhere.

Softer Gating Model

The possible solutions (10) seem to have a limited flexibility, only depending on the values of v_2 and v_2' at one point. But (6), (7) and (8) are idealisations of the underlying non-linear system (1)–(5). In the static and continuum limits of these equations, with no lateral coupling in TH or cortical contribution, and again for the symmetric Laplacian, they reduce to

$$v_2 + a^2 \mathbf{V}^2 v_2 = \bar{c}_{21} f_1(u_1(\mathbf{r}))$$

$$- \bar{d}_{22} \int K(\mathbf{r}, \mathbf{r}') g_2(v_2(\mathbf{r}')) d^2 \mathbf{r}', \quad (13)$$

$$v_1 = -\bar{d}_{12} g_2(v_2(\mathbf{r})), \quad (14)$$

$$u_1 = I - \bar{b}_{11} g_1(v_1(\mathbf{r})), \quad (15)$$

These equations are identical to (6), (7), (8), but with the replacement of the thresholded step functions by the appropriate sigmoidal output functions, and with the extra lateral inhibitory term on NRT. The kernel $K(\mathbf{r}, \mathbf{r}')$ could, for example, be $\exp(-|\mathbf{r} - \mathbf{r}'|/d)$, for some d. This system, except for the Laplacian term, is somewhat like the class of neuronal equations already discussed over a decade ago [9]. They showed that the existence of localised regions of activity could persist if the inhibitory connections in a net were longer ranged than the excitatory ones, and suitable relations occurred between the coupling strengths. We also wish to consider the possible existence of localised states with and without the presence of the Laplacian term. We consider the extreme case when the lateral inhibitory NRT term is set to zero, giving rise to the single equation

$$v_2 + a^2 \mathbf{V}^2 v_2 = \bar{c}_{21} f_1(I(\mathbf{r}) - \bar{b}_{11} g_1(-\bar{d}_{12} g_2(v_2(\mathbf{r})))), \quad (16)$$

This can also be written as

$$v_2 + a^2 \mathbf{V}^2 v_2 = F(I(\mathbf{r}), v_2(\mathbf{r})), \quad (17)$$

where F is sigmoidal in both its variables. For suitably smooth F, we suppose we can approximate (17) by its linearised expansion about $v_2 = 0$, which we take to be of the form $F_0(I(\mathbf{r})) + v_2(\mathbf{r})F_1(I(\mathbf{r}))$ for certain non-linear functions F_0, F_1, which are both sigmoidal in I. Then there is an input-dependent modification of

the wavelength determined by a in (17) to a value $\bar{a}$, given by

$$\bar{a}^2 = \frac{a^2}{1 - F_1(I(\mathbf{r}))}. \quad (18)$$

This will allow more flexibility in that the number and spacing of pockets of activity and adjacent inactivity on NRT will be modified as the input changes. Since $F_1(x) = \bar{b}_{11}\bar{d}_{12} g_2'(0) g_1'(-\bar{d}_{12} g_2(0)) \cdot f_1'(x - \bar{b}_{11} g_1(-\bar{d}_{12} g_2(0)))$ then F_1 is positive and varying proportionally to $(1 - f_1(x)) f_1(x)$ for large x. This has a maximum value of $\frac{1}{4}$ at $x = \bar{b}_{11} g_1(-\bar{d}_{12} g_2(0))$. The maximum value of a at this input value gives rise to the largest number of packets of activity, as determined by (12) with a replaced by $\bar{a}$. However, solutions are still expected to be controlled by boundary values of v_2 at the edge of the NRT sheet.

Local Control Models

In the rat there are no dendro-dendritic synapses, so that the model of the previous part (equations (13), (14), (15)) without the Laplacian term reduces to

$$v_2(\mathbf{r}) = F_2(v_2(\mathbf{r}), I) - \bar{d}_{22} \int K(\mathbf{r}, \mathbf{r}') g_2(v_2(\mathbf{r}')) d^2 r', \quad (19)$$

where $F_2(x, I) = \bar{c}_{21} f_1(I - \bar{b}_{11} g_1(-\bar{d}_{12} g_2(x)))$, being sigmoidal in both x and I. We may use the method of [9] to conclude that for suitably large current there can be localised states of activity for v_2, so of input to the cortex. The existence of such localised solutions depends on the form of K, chosen in the case referred as having exponential fall-off. As these authors point out, the net can act as a localised flip-flop. This indicates that there may not be the same level of global control as is possible with the presence of the Laplacian term.

Control Possibilities

The limited global control of activity obtained either with the hard limiter model (i) or the softer output functions used in (ii) does not correspond to what would be required of a top-down control system. That would have global control of NRT (and of TH output and cortical activity) by activity over a wider range of C, NRT or TH than at the NRT boundary. Neither cortical activity, fan-in and fan-out of C, NRT or TH activity to the other sheets, nor time dependence have yet been analysed in detail, although they are all inherently present in the basic equations (1)–(4). Firstly, both cortical activity and time dependence may be added to the models (i) or (ii) above. The former adds new non-linear terms in v_2 on the right hand sides of (6), (7), (8) or (13), (14), (15), but does not change the control nature of the solution for v_2 in terms of values given at the boundary of NRT. The latter adds to the left-hand side of (6), upon taking more careful account of the NRT structure as in (5), the terms

$$-\frac{1}{\tau_1}\dot{v}_2 + \frac{1}{\tau_1}(v_x\partial_x v_2 + v_y\partial_y v_2). \qquad (20)$$

Assuming u_1 and v_1 follow v_2 with no time lag then (20) will lead to travelling waves depending on $v_2((\mathbf{v}\cdot\mathbf{r})/|\mathbf{v}|^2 - t)$, with $\mathbf{v} = (v_x, v_y)^T$ and v_2 satisfies the time-independent equations (9) or (13) (for hard- and soft-limiting outputs respectively). Thus neither extension modifies the nature of the control problem for v_2.

The second approach is to include more realistic fan-in and fan-out on the various sheets C, TH, NRT. This corresponds to using, say, Gaussian lateral connections for the connection matrices $a_{ij}(\mathbf{r},\mathbf{r}')$, $b_{ij}(\mathbf{r},\mathbf{r}')$, $c_{ij}(\mathbf{r},\mathbf{r}')$ and $d_{ij}(\mathbf{r},\mathbf{r}')$ which enter in (1). In general this changes the boundary value problem, but only marginally. This can be seen from the addition of the fan-in term on the right-hand side of (13). In the linearised limit, with $K(\mathbf{r},\mathbf{r}') = K(|\mathbf{r}-\mathbf{r}'|)$, (13) becomes in Fourier space (with Fourier variables capped by tildes)

$$(1 - a^2\mathbf{k}^2 - \tilde{K})\tilde{v}_2 = d\tilde{I}, \qquad (21)$$

where $\tilde{K}$ is expected to be monotone decreasing in $\mathbf{k}^2$. The operator on the left in (21) remains elliptic on NRT for a suitable set of small enough kernels K, so that the boundary values of v_2 and NRT for later times, plus the critical values v_2 over NRT at $t = 0$, are expected to specify the unique solution of (21).

Use of External Control

It was indicated in the text that the subicular complex (including the entorhinal cortex) exerts an important influence on the mediodorsal thalamus (MD) and anterior pole of NRT in a unidirectional fashion. Thus such anterior input must be added to the right-hand side of (2) and (4) to allow the control system to become effective. However, we must consider temporal delays more carefully than so far, since cortical input to the subicular complex and its hippocampal and Papez circuit transforms, must be incorporated into the model. This cortical transformation will involve time delays, so that the subicular inputs to be added to (2) and (4) would be some unknown, but time delayed, transforms of the NRT-processed neo-cortical association area outputs as part of (1). These transforms would also involve sub-cortical information flowing into the Papez circuit and other circuits in which the subicular output (and that from other sources) would go to MD. Thus the addition to the right-hand sides of (2) and (4) will be time-delayed transforms $T_1(u_3(t - \delta), g(t))$, $(i = 1, 2)$, where δ is an appropriate time delay and $g(t)$ denotes non-cortical influences which do not activate NRT directly but only through the projection to MD. The static or asymptotic limit (in time) of this effect gives rise to control by the inputs g alone, for suitably behaved T_1, T_2.

The Triadic Synapse

The thalamic triadic synapse can be modelled by assuming linearity at each part of the synapse, and that the effect of the serial dendro-dendritic channel (from optic nerve axon to interneuron dendrite to relay cell dendrite) is simply multiplicative. In terms of the variable used in equations (1)–(4) the effect will therefore be an additional term

$$-c_{12}v_1(\mathbf{r})I(\mathbf{r}) \tag{22}$$

to be added to the right-hand side of (4), where c_{12} is a positive constant. This term can be seen to make the feedback control system more efficient. Thus in the simplified model of (6), (7), (8) the term (22) replaces the input I on the right-hand side of (8) by the term

$$I[1 + \bar{d}_{12}c_{12} Y(v_2 - s_2)]. \tag{23}$$

When v_2 is enhanced, the factor $[\cdots]$ in (23) enhances the input; for small enough v_2 the extra factor is set to unity.

Stability and Extensions of the Laplacian Net

The Laplacian term (5b) in the dispersion relation for (2) contributes the value $-G_2a^2k^2$. This brings about instability for large enough k^2 (as mentioned earlier), and indicates a limitation of the approximation of taking the Laplacian approximation to (5a) for high wave numbers. Thus the results of the analysis associated with (9) are only valid for small values of v_2, thus for short times after initiation of NRT activity. Returning to (5a), and working only in one dimension, the contribution to the dispersion relation is now $-G_2\left(2 \sin \frac{1}{2}ka\right)^2$, where the neighbours to r are at $r \pm a$. This is bounded in k, so that there is now stability for all k for a small enough value for $-G_2$. On increasing this quantity the energy will first change sign at the value (π/a), giving the number of wavelengths of the resulting spatial wave bifurcating from the constant solution as $L/2a$. A somewhat similar result holds also for the case when there is a continuous distribution of inhibited neighbours, with decrease of the neighbouring density function to occur at a distance a. For these variations

of the original negative Laplacian net, the same global control is expected to occur, and a large enough spatially constant input will generate a spatial oscillatory response in the NRT net (and so in cortex). This will not be the case for (13), (14), (15) with $a = 0$, as noted above. There are other sources of stability in the system:

1. addition of the shunting-inhibition term, so that (6) (and the later equations in which $\mathbf{V}^2$ appears) has the Laplacian term replaced by

$$a^2(v_2 - E)\mathbf{V}^2v_2, \tag{24}$$

where $E < 0$. The factor $(v_2 - E)$ stabilises the unbounded Laplacian contribution for $v_2 < E$, although it does not do so for $v_2 > E$.

2. the range of values of v_2 are limited above, since if v_2 exceeds the threshold then the cell generates a nerve impulse, resetting v_2 to the resting value, and a refractory period ensues.

3. there is an upper bound on the range of spatial momenta due to the finite lattice spacing of the net, so that $|\mathbf{k}| \lesssim \pi/a$.

4. It may be that the NRT system works in an unstable manner, to produce patterns of activity as suggested by [9] and reviewed in [22]. This instability, however, can be more controlled by considering the next higher order term in (5a), of value $(a_+^4 + a_-^4)\partial_x^4 + (b_+^4 + b_-^4)\partial_y^4$. This gives the further term $G_2a^4k^4$ in the dispersion relation for (2). For $v_2 \sim \exp\{\lambda t + ikx\}$, this dispersion relation will have the form

$$\lambda = -C + Ak^2 - Bk^4, \quad A = |G_2|a^4 \tag{25}$$

where $A, B, C > 0$. The homogenous solution is unstable for $|G_2| > C$, so that there is an interval on the k-axis for which $\lambda > 0$ (this being $\frac{1}{2}[1 - \sqrt{1 - 4/|G_2|}] < k < \frac{1}{2}[1 + \sqrt{1 + 4/|G_2|}]$). As in the discussion of the formation of heterogeneous patterns for hallucinations and monocularity. [9], [22] it is necessary to simulate the full non-linear system to observe the resulting stable activity; this is expected to depend crucially on the initial conditions.

5. Inclusion of the non-linear synaptic response function F defined at the beginning of the appendix. Since for large values of v_2, F becomes constant, it is to be expected that stabilisation of the state oscillatory solutions discussed in (i) will occur. It is to be noted that the analogy with the OPL of the retina breaks down here, since the OPL has gap junctions which are assumed to give a more linear transfer function than for the chemically transmitting dendro-dendritic synapses of NRT.

6. There is known inhibitory feedback from NRT to TH relay cells [6]. This might be effective to turn off the output of such cells above a certain threshold for NRT activity, and hence reduce it.

Towards a Mathematics of Attention

We must now briefly make explicit the crucial mathematical features of our approach, and delineate the outstanding questions. It is that the system (1)–(4) is supposed to function as a global controller of the inputs. We may regard these equations as giving a transformation from the input I to the cortical activity u_3 (and hence to cortical output) which enables global control to be achieved. By this we mean that the TH output $f_1(u_1)$ and I are suitably similar (say to within ε in distance). Only for a certain class of inputs, which we call 'allowed inputs', does such similarity occur. Thus we have the definition:

Allowed Inputs: Such an input I is one for which

$$\|f_1(u_1) - I\| < \varepsilon \qquad (26)$$

over some interval of time, where $\| \circ \|$ is an L_2-type of norm on the spatial and temporal dependence of the function involved (so $\|u_1\|^2 = \int_{NRT} d^2\mathbf{r}|u_1(r)|^2$ in the purely spatial case). An asymptotically allowed input is one for which (26) is valid for a constant input I and the asymptotic values of the TH output.

The mathematical problem we have to explore is the detailed nature of the set of allowed inputs

for (1)–(4), with variants of the dendro-dendritic synapse and the triadic synapse contributions as described in earlier parts of this appendix. From (4) above, we know that for certain values of the parameters a suitable large constant input is unstable and will develop asymptotically into a heterogeneous pattern for v_2. We assume that an input I formed of such a heterogeneous pattern may be asymptotically stable. The problem we are faced with is to delineate the space of such allowed inputs. In particular we wish to determine how much impressed activity on a subset of NRT, such as that coming from the limbic circuit onto the anterior pole of NRT, can determine allowed inputs elsewhere. Thus the emphasis here is on the input dependence of pattern formation as compared to initial value dependence of such structure, as reviewed, for example, in [22].

Computer Simulation Results

In this section, we present the results of a series of computer simulations that were carried out to verify some of the predictions of the mathematical analysis we have carried out above.

The Simulation Model

The simplified model we investigated is illustrated in figure 62.1. It is essentially one-dimensional, which corresponds to a line of TH, NRT and C neurons. In future work, it is intended to extend the simulation work to the more realistic case of two-dimensional sheets of TH, NRT and C neurons.

Consider first the boxed subsystem in figure 62.1. The entire neuro-physical system under investigation is obtained by replicating this subsystems in a geometrically linear fashion, with inhibitory lateral coupling occuring between the NRT units of each subsystem. Within each particular subsystem, we have inter-unit "signal flow" as specified by the arrow-tipped curves;

Table 62.2

Subsystem units and their differential equations

Unit name	Unit ID	Location	Unit Differential Equation
Inhibitory interneuron	I	Thalamus	(27)
Relay cell	R	Thalamus	(28)
Gating neuron	G_k	Nucleus	(29)
Pyramidal cell	P	Cortex	(30)

every such tip labelled with a "+" signifies an excitatory incoming signal, while every "−" label corresponds to an inhibitory signal.

Each unit in every subsystem solves its own unique non-linear differential equation, which determines its output voltage evolution. We had occasion to write down these differential equations in (1)–(4). In table 62.2, we identify explicitly every unit's differential equation, from the list in (27)–(30); the coefficients W_{AB} identify the connection weight for the signal from a source with Unit ID A to a target with Unit ID B. The subscript k refers to the k'th subsystem. Note that (29) is incomplete; it lacks terms on the RHS that corresponds to the lateral dendro-dendritic interaction with the $(k \pm 1)$'th subsystems. These will be discussed later. I_k in (28) corresponds to the input to the k'th subsystem.

$$\dot{v}_1 = -\frac{1}{\tau_1'} v_1 + \frac{1}{\tau_1'} W_{G_k I} f(v_2), \qquad (27)$$

$$\dot{u}_1 = -\frac{1}{\tau_1} u_1 + \frac{1}{\tau_1} W_{IR} f(v_1) + \frac{1}{\tau_1} W_{PR} f(u_3) + I_k, \qquad (28)$$

$$\dot{v}_2 = -\frac{1}{\tau_2} v_2 + \frac{1}{\tau_2} W_{RG_k} f(u_1) + \frac{1}{\tau_2} W_{PG_k} f(u_3)$$

$$+ \text{dendro-dendritic terms}, \qquad (29)$$

$$\dot{u}_3 = -\frac{1}{\tau_3} u_3 + \frac{1}{\tau_3} W_{RP} f(u_1). \qquad (30)$$

In these equations, the non-linear gain function $f(x_A)$, where A is the unit ID, is defined by

$$f(x_A) = h_A Y(x_A - \theta_A)[1 - \exp\{-\beta_A(x_A - \theta_A)\}], \qquad (31)$$

where h_A is a scaling parameter, θ_A is the threshold for unit A and β_A is its inverse temperature. This particular choice is identical to that used by [17], and is particularly suitable in a simulation environment since it restricts $f(x_A)$ to a smooth and pseudo-linear gain function, where saturation is less likely.

In order to proceed with the simulations, it was found necessary to obtain limits on the ranges of the large number of parameters involved. To obtain an idea of what constitutes 'good' parameter ranges, consider the equations (27)–(31) in the static limit (obtained by setting $du_i/dt = dv_i/dt = 0$, or, equivalently, by allowing the τ_i's, $i = 1, \ldots, 3$ to go to zero):

$$v_1 = W_{G_k I} Y(v_2 - \theta_2), \qquad (27')$$

$$u_1 = I_k + W_{IR} Y(v_1 - \theta_1') + W_{PR} Y(u_3 - \theta_3), \qquad (28')$$

$$v_2 = W_{RG_k} Y(u_1 - \theta_1) + W_{PG_k} Y(u_3 - \theta_3), \qquad (29')$$

$$u_3 = W_{RP} Y(u_1 - \theta_1), \qquad (30')$$

Note that in these equations, we have taken the full non-linearity $Y(\circ)$ for the function in (31). To distinguish between zero and finite external inputs, we define further $I_k^- = I_k = 0$ and $I_k^+ = I_k \neq 0$. In order to set up the subsystem so that we can achieve global control, we require that units R, G_k and P be switched "off" whenever unit I is "on" in the case of zero external input, and *vice versa* in the case of finite external input.[1] Looking at (28') separately for the case when $I_k = I_K^-$ and $I_k = I_k^+$, it is easy to show that the thresholds of each of the units have to lie in the ranges

$$I_k^- - W_{IR} < \theta_1 < I_k^+ + W_{PR}, \quad -W_{G_k I} < \theta_1' < 0, \qquad (32)$$

$$0 < \theta_2 < W_{RG_k} + W_{PG_k}, \quad 0 < \theta_3 < W_{RP}.$$

In the following sections, we detail the results of our actual simulation runs, where the param-

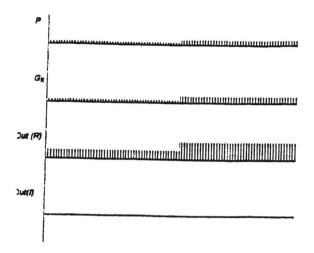

Figure 62.2
Simulation results for non-constant input to thalamic cells, with 100 noninteracting subsystems. The inputs are 50 neighbouring neurons with an activity of 10 units, and the remaining neurons have an input activity of 20 units. In figures 62.2–62.13, cells P and G_k (the symbols described in figure 62.1), the membrane potentials are plotted, whilst the outputs are shown for R and I.

eter ranges were subject to the constraints in the set (32). These constraints are completely analogous to those arising out of the analysis in section "Analysis of the Model."

Simulation Results

The series of simulations we carried out reflect in part the major aim of establishing the existence of the global control model for the NRT.

As a first exercise, the very simplest setup one can begin to experiment with is simply a series of N non-interacting subsystems, such that $k = 1, \ldots, N$, linearly arranged. Applying the Runge-Kutta fourth order integration routines (with fixed step size)[2] to the differential equations (27)–(30), we obtained first the set of outputs in figure 62.2. In this figure (and all subsequent plots), note that the abcissa represents the spatial position of the N units ($N = 100$

in these simulations), linearly arranged. The ordinates represent OUT(R) and OUT(I) in the case of the thalamic units, and the actual raw voltages generated from the Runge-Kutta integrator in the case of the gating neuron G_k and the pyramidal cell P. Time delays for the signals to propagate from one unit to another were set to zero (although the simulation code is quite capable of accomodating these) for the sake of simplicity. It is seen that with no lateral interaction between the N units, all output coming into every subsystem effectively travels up and generates an output voltage at a cortical unit.

In figure 62.3, we introduce the lateral connectivity between the N subsystems. This initially takes the form of a difference of Gaussian interaction (DOG), given by adding the following term to the RHS of (29):

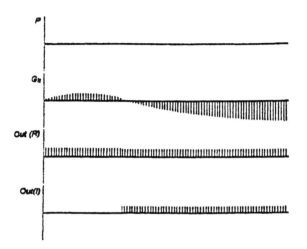

Figure 62.3
Simulation results for non-constant input to thalamic cells, with DOG lateral connectivity. The inputs is identical to that for figure 62.2.

$$\frac{1}{\tau_2} \sum_{l=-s_1}^{+s_1} A_1 \left(\exp\left[\frac{-|\mathbf{r}_j - \mathbf{r}_l|^2}{d_1^2} \right] \right.$$
$$\left. - \exp\left[\frac{-|\mathbf{r}_j - \mathbf{r}_l|^2}{d_2^2} \right] \right) f(v_2), \qquad (33)$$

where s_1 is a lateral spread count, A_1 is a scaling parameter and d_1 and d_2 are widths of the respective Gaussian terms. The "vectors" $\mathbf{r}_j$ and $\mathbf{r}_l$ are, in this simple one-dimensional case, simply the values of k times typical interneuronal distances (about 10^{-4} m). As can be seen, the addition of this term leads to interesting activity being generated on the NRT; the first sign of a distributed spatial wave is now evident.

In figure 62.4, we replace (33) by the proposed dendro-dendritic term,

$$\frac{1}{\tau_2} \sum_{l=-s_2}^{+s_2} \exp\left(\frac{-|\mathbf{r}_j - \mathbf{r}_l|}{\lambda} \right)$$
$$\times A_2 \left(\frac{1}{1 + \exp[-\beta_2(v_2 - \theta_2)]} - \frac{1}{1 + \exp[\beta_2\theta_2]} \right), \qquad (34)$$

with s_2 another lateral spread count, A_2 a scaling parameter and λ determines the sharpness of this term. Looking at figure 62.4, we see that this term has a much more significant effect upon the lateral connections than (33), and also brings about strong effects on the relay cell and cortical cell outputs.

In figure 62.5, we combine the effects of both (33) and (34). Here we see very strong control over the allowed cortical response. Effectively, the larger part of the two inputs completely dominates the smaller and destroys it.

In figure 62.6, the wave pattern in all layers' response to a constant input is clearly seen. The control enacted by this wave pattern over thalamic inputs depends sensitively on the nature of the inputs, as is demonstrated in figures 62.7–62.9. In particular, the cortical activity persisting in these cases does not reflect the inputs I to the thalamic relay cell R, as especially seen in figures 62.7 and 62.8; even in figure 62.9, only half of each of the main input activities gets through to the cortex.

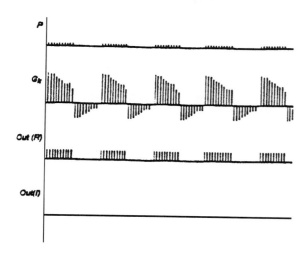

Figure 62.4
Simulation results for non-constant input to thalamic cells, with dendro-dendritic lateral connectivity (eq. 34). The inputs are five peaks and five troughs, with activities of 20 and 10 units, respectively.

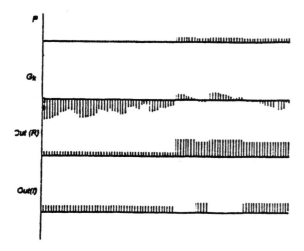

Figure 62.5
Simulation results for non-constant input to thalamic cells, with a combination of DOB and dendro-dendritic connectivity. Same inputs as for figure 62.4.

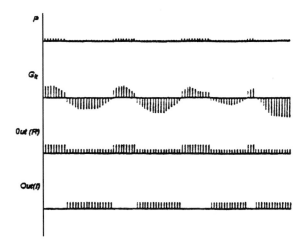

Figure 62.6
Simulation results for a constant input to thalamic cells, with both DOG and dendro-dendritic connectivity. Same inputs as for figure 62.4.

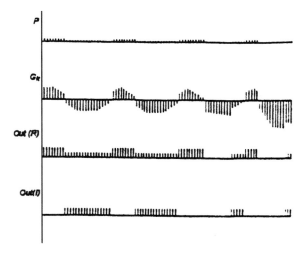

Figure 62.7
Simulation results for non-constant input to thalamic cells, with both DOG and dendro-dendritic connectivity. Same inputs as for figure 62.4.

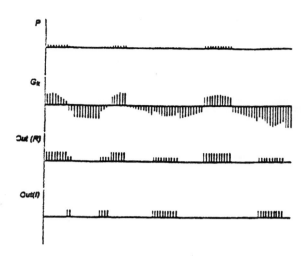

Figure 62.8
As for figure 62.7, but with stronger connectionist weights.

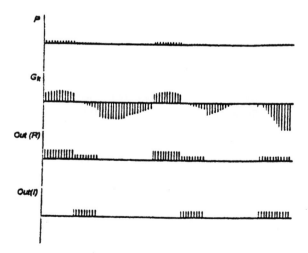

Figure 62.9
As for figure 62.7, but with another non-constant input, having fewer than five peaks and troughs.

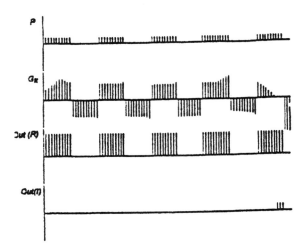

Figure 62.10
Simulation result for constant input to thalamic cells, with strong DOG and dendro-dendritic connectivity. The inputs are three peaks and three troughs, with activities of 20 and 10 units, respectively.

The extent of the lateral control exerted by the NRT is the next topic to be discussed. The manner this can be achieved is seen is figure 62.1b, where three connected TH-NRT-C regions are affecting each other. The NRT activity may develop a non-linear structure, for large A_1 or A_2, as seen in figure 62.10, with dependence on the structure of inputs being non-trivial, as seen in figure 62.11.

The complexity of the activities on the different layers is seen in figure 62.12, where a constant input produces oscillatory activity in NRT and the inhibitory interneuron I, but constant activities in the right thalamus and the cortex. Dependence on the feedback strengths in (33) is seen by NRT activity in figure 62.13.

We can conclude from the above that the TH-NRT-C complex of (27)–(34), with 60 free parameters, can achieve a variety of control mechanisms. In particular, figure 62.5 indicates how global control across the left-most 50 neurons can be achieved from the right-most 50; in other words the larger input wins! This is also seen in figures 62.6–62.9.

We recognise from these figures two separate principles for global competition:

• *completely global:* by a global wave of activity on NRT, so confining inputs to agree with the oscillatory character on NRT; for example, in figure 62.8 the wave in NRT gets cut off—this is therefore a wavelength-dependent control, but one with global character

• *partially global:* Amplitude competition, determined by spread. In figure 62.5, for example, with wavelengths ≪ size of competition, the spread determines size of the competitive region. This may not be so global as in the previous case.

Discussion

In the previous two sections we showed, firstly by mathematical analysis, and secondly by simulation, that the NRT can act in a manner so as to achieve effective control over the thalamic inputs to the cortex. This control depends (as

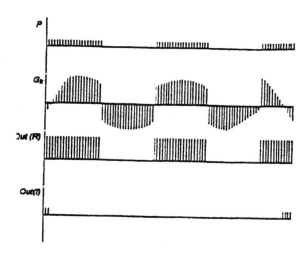

Figure 62.11
As for figure 62.10, with even stronger connectivity.

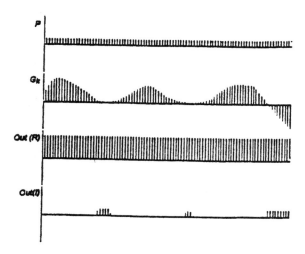

Figure 62.12
Simulation results for constant input to thalamic cells, showing oscillatory behaviour in NRT layer.

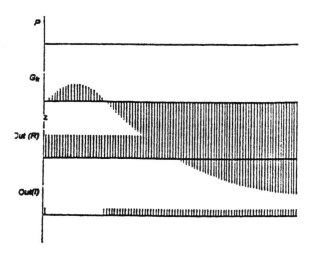

Figure 62.13
As for figure 62.12, but with stronger feedback weights.

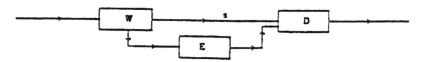

Figure 62.14
Schematic of the connectivity of a neural net with meaning. The net *W* is the preprocessing net, while *E* is the episodic net. The final net *D* is the decision net.

does the whole of the TH-NRT-C activity) critically on the 60 parameters entering the model. In spite of this difficult problem of searching through a high-dimensional space, and especially guided by the mathematical analysis, the simulation showed two types of control that the NRT can exert:

1. Global, by means of wave activity set up on the NRT.

2. Extensive, but non-global, given by lateral inhibitory effects of input-driven non wave-like NRT activity.

It is clear that the global control of type 1 is of more interest than that of type 2, although both may be occuring as part of ongoing activity. We claim that our results are in strong support of the ideas on consciousness presented elsewhere [34], and developed further in [35], [36], [37], which we summarise here:

• The Relational Theory of the Mind, in which semantically coded input and its related episodic memories are compared in some decision unit, as shown in figure 62.14, and

• The "Conscious I" NRT, in which global competition is carried out through activity on

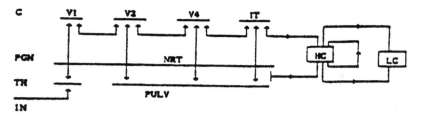

Figure 62.15
Schematic of the flow diagram for information in the global NRT control model. Only visual input is considered explicitly. The arrows denote direction of flow of information. Top-down control by the limbic system is shown by the output from HC to MD, with collaterals to anterior NRT. Abbreviations: IN, input; TH, thalamus; MD, mediodorsal thalamus; C, cortex; IT, inferotemporal lobe; HC, hippocampus; LC, limbic circuit (which includes hippocampus); V1, striate cortex; V2, etc., extra striate areas; PGN, pergeniculate nucleus.

NRT, and more specifically by means of the feedback control system, so that the features of figure 62.15 arise.

Our results so far justify the competitive response of the TNC complex carried out on thalamic inputs. We now have to try to combine the above features (1) and (2) to obtain consciousness. More specifically, we have to attempt to understand how the TNC system of figure 62.15, which produces the comparator/decision unit of figure 62.14, leads to consciousness as experienced by the "private" or subjective world. To do that, we turn to the manner in which feedback connections from the episodic memory store need to be involved.

There are two crucial features to be considered here. One is the manner in which the episodic memories are stored and re-excited. It is clear that the re-excitation has to be of a whole host of earlier memories, which can give the consciousness "colour" to experience. That could not be achieved by a pattern completion or attractor network, since only a single pattern would result. The most suitable memory structure is a matrix memory for a one-layer feedforward net in which the connection weight matrix A_{ij} has the form $A_{ij} = \sum a_i^{(m)} a_j^{(m)}$. The response $\mathbf{y} = \mathbf{A}\mathbf{x}$ will then have the form

$$\mathbf{y} = \sum \mathbf{a}^{(m)} (\mathbf{a}^{(m)} \cdot \mathbf{x}) \tag{35}$$

being a weighted sum of projections of $\mathbf{x}$ along the various memories. Assuming that attention has been caught by $\mathbf{x}$, it would seem reasonable to assume further that memories $\mathbf{a}^{(m)}$ suitable close to $\mathbf{x}$ would therefore be allowed to be reactivated in earlier cortex by the TNC complex. The details of how close such memories should be to $\mathbf{x}$ (the "metric" of the comparator) depend of the nature of the TNC complex, and are indicated by the simulation presented earlier. Thus the "Conscious I" leads to a specific class of comparators in the Relational Mind theory of figure 62.14.

The second important feature is that feedback to associative and even primary cortex must be present to allow re-excitation of features of the appropriate episodic memories $\mathbf{a}^{(m)}$ of (35). This is necessary in order that the detailed content of these memories be "unscrambled" from the high level coding they have been represented as in medial temporal lobe areas. Indeed, the important feedback connections in cortex, and also those through the TNC complex, may have exactly the form required to achieve this amplification of the memories. In this approach, consciousness arises from the imagery arising from feedback of excited memories allowed to persist with the input $\mathbf{x}^{(m)}$ in (35) by the action of the TNC competitive complex. In order for such feedback to be effective, some form of priming of inputs would seem essential for these inputs to be re-accessed, so explaining how consciousness can exist in people with temporal lobe loss (who have a normal short-term memory (STM) and normal priming). It would seem that either STM and/or priming is essential for consciousness; as is said in [5], "no case of a person who is conscious but has lost all forms of STM has been reported."

The preceding ideas lead to the following sequence of predictions, in increasing order of importance:

1. No STM or priming implies no consciousness.

2. No cortical feedback implies no consciousness.

3. No NRT implies no single consciousness.

4. NRT activity structure and anterior-posterior sweep speed is determined by the detailed parameters of the NRT activity.

5. The detailed NRT activity corresponds to a spatial wave during attentive processing.

6. Exogenous attention arises from BRF reset of the NRT wave.

7. The detailed form of TNC feedback depends of the content of LTM.

8. A matrix memory, not a pattern completer, must be used in LTM.

It is hoped that these predictions can be experimentally tested to ascertain the viability and more detailed features of the model.

There are many other predictions which will be made as more specific features of the model are implemented. The seemingly most accessible area of investigation seems to be that involving priming, short term memory and imagery. Indeed, the model can be expressed succintly as

Consciousness = controlled imagery of
short term memory

Of course, the terms on the right hand side of (2) are not themselves very well defined, in spite of extensive investigations on imagery and STM. There is strong impetus to investigate both of these features from the proposed identification (36), as is that for significance and self memory from the identity

Self-consciousness = controlled imagery of
self-memory

It is hoped to consider these questions more fully elsewhere.

Acknowledgments

One of us (F. A.) would like to thank the Science and Engineering Research Council of the U. K. for financial support whilst this work was being performed.

Notes

1. The "on" state corresponds to OUT (unit) = 1, while the "off" state is OUT (unit) = 0, with OUT having its usual artificial neural network meaning.

2. We found it unnecessary to use adaptive step sizes, since the fixed step size algorithm generated very good results.

References

1. Ahlsén G., Lindstöm S.: Mutual inhibition between perigeniculate neurons. Brain Res., 236, 1982, 482–486.

2. an der Heiden: Analysis of neural networks. Lecture Notes in Biomathematics, No. 35, Springer-Verlag, 1980.

3. Avanzini G., de Curtis M., Ferruccio P., Spreafico, R.: Intrinsic properties of nucleus reticularis thalami neurons of the rat studied (in vitro). J. Physiol., 416, 1989, 111–122.

4. Barbaresi P., Spreafico R., Frassoni C., Rustioni, A.: GABA-ergic neurons are present in the dorsal col-

umn nuclei but not in the ventroposterior complex of rats. Brain Res., 382, 1986, 305–326.

5. Crick F.H.C., Koch C.: Seminars in Neuroscience, 2, 1990, 237–249.

6. Crunelli V., Leresche N.: A role for GABA$_B$ receptors in excitation and inhibition of thalamo-cortical cells. Trends in Neurosci., 14, 1991, 16–21.

7. Deschénes M., Madariage-Domich A., Steriade M.: Dendro-dendritic synapses in the cat reticularis thalami nucleus: A structural basis for thalamic spindle synchronisation. Brain Res., 334, 1989, 165–168.

8. Douglas R.J., Martin K.A.: A functional microcircuit for cat visual cortex. J. Physiol., 440, 1991, 735–769.

9. Ermentrout G.B., Cowan J.D.: Some aspects of the "eigenbehaviour of neural nets." Studies in Mathematics: The Mathematical Assoc. of America, 15, 1978, 67–117.

10. Fujita I., Tanaka K., Ito M., Cheng K.: Columns for visual features of objects in monkey inferotemporal cortex. Nature, 360, 1992, 343–346.

11. Harris R.M., Hendrickson A.E.: Local circuit neurons in the rat ventrobasal thalamus—A GABA immunocytochemical study. Neurosci., 21, 1987, 229–236.

12. Hornik K., Stinchcombe M., White H.: Multilayer feedforward networks are universal approximators. Neural Networks, 2, 1989, 359–368.

13. Humphreys G.W., Muller H.J.: SEarch via Recursive Rejection: A connectionist model of visual search. Cog. Psych., 25, 1993, 43–110.

14. Jones E.G.: Some aspects of the organisation of the thalamic reticular complex. J. Comp. Neurobiol., 162, 1975, 285–308.

15. Koch C., Ullman S.: Shifts in selective visual attention: Towards the underlying circuitry. Human Neurobiol., 4, 1985, 219–227.

16. La Berge D.: Thalamic and cortical mechanisms of attention suggested by recent positron emission tomographic experiments. J. Cog. Neurosci., 2, 1990, 358–373.

17. La Berge D., Carter M., Brown V.: A network simulation of thalamic circuit operations in selective attention. Neural Computation, 4, 1992, 318–331.

18. Lijenström H.: Modelling the dynamics of olfactory cortex using simplified network units and realistic architectures. Int. J. Neurosci., 1–2, (to appear), 1991.

19. Linsker R.: Self-organisation in a perceptual network. Computer, 21, 1988, 105–117.

20. Martin K.A.: From single cells to single circuits in the cerebral cortex. Quart. J. Exp. Physiol., 73, 1988, 637–702.

21. McCormick D.A., Prince D.A.: Acetylcholine induces burst firing in thalamic reticular neurons by activating a potassium conductance. Nature, 319, 1986, 402–405.

22. Murray J.M.: Mathematical Biology, Springer-Verlag, 1989.

23. Ohara P.T., Lieberman A.R.: The thalamic reticular nucleus of the adult rat: experimental anatomical studies. J. Neurocyt., 14, 1985, 365–411.

24. Ohara P.T.: Synaptic organisation of the thalamic reticular neclus. J. Elect. Mic. Tech., 10, 1988, 283–292.

25. Paré D., Steriade M., Deschénes M., Oakson G.: Physiological characteristics of anterior thalamic nuclei, a group devoid of inputs from reticular thalamic nucleus. J. Neurophysiol., 57, 1987, 1669–1685.

26. Posner M.I., Petersen S.E.: The attention system of the human being. Ann. Rev. Neurosci., 13, 1990, 25–42.

27. Schiebel A.B.: in Reticular Formation Revisited, eds. J.A. Hobson and B.A. Brazier, Raven Press, New York, 1990.

28. Spreafico F., De Curtis M., Frassoni C., Avanzini G.: Electrophysiological characteristics of morphologically identified reticular thalamic neurons from rat slices. Neurosci., 27, 1988, 629–638.

29. Spreafico F., Battaglia G., Frassoni C.: The reticular thalamic nucleus (RTN) of the rat: Cytoarchitectural, golgi, immunocytochemical and horseradish peroxidase study. J. Comp. Neuro., 304, 1991, 478–490.

30. Squire L.R.: Memory and Brain, Oxford Univ. Press, 1987.

31. Steriade M., Domich L., Oakson G.: Reticularis thalami neurons revisited: Activity changes during shifts in states of vigilance. J. Neurosci., 6, 1986, 68–81.

32. Steriade M., Curro-Dossi R., Oakson G.: Fast oscillations (20–40 Hz), in thalamocortical systems and their potentiation by mesopontine cholinergic nuclei in the cat. Proc. Nat. Acad. Sci., 88, 1991, 4396–4400.

33. Taylor J.G.: A silicon model of vertebrate retinal processing. Neural Networks, 3, 1990, 171–178.

34. Taylor J.G.: Can neural networks ever be made to think? Neural Network World, 1, 1991, 4–12.

35. Taylor J.G.: From single neuron to cognition. In: Advances in Neural Networks II, eds. I. Aleksander and J.G. Taylor, Elsevier, 1992a.

36. Taylor J.G.: Temporal processing in brain activity. In: Complex Neurodynamics, Proc. 1991 Vietri Conference, eds. J.G. Taylor et al., Springer-Verlag, 1992b.

37. Taylor J.G.: Towards a neural network model of the mind. Neural Network World, 2, 1992c, 797–812.

38. van der Malsburg Ch., Schneider W.: A neural cocktail-party processor. Biol. Cyb., 54, 1986, 29–40.

39. Wörgötter F., Niebur E., Koch C.: Isotropic connections generate functional asymmetrical behaviour in visual cortical cells. J. Neurophysiol., (in press), 1991.

40. Yingling C.D., Skinner J.E.: Gating of thalamic inputs to cerebral cortex by nuclear reticularis thalami. Prog. Clin. Neurophysiol., 1, 1977, 70–96.

63 Time-Locked Multiregional Retroactivation: A Systems-Level Proposal for the Neural Substrates of Recall and Recognition

Antonio R. Damasio

Introduction

This proposal describes a neural architecture capable of supporting the experiences that are conjured up in recall and are used for recognition, at the level of systems that integrate macroscopic functional regions. It arose out of dissatisfaction with available accounts of the neural basis of higher behaviors, especially those implicit in center localizationism, behaviorism, functional equipotentiality, and disconnection syndrome theory.

The title captures the two principal notions in the proposal. First, perceptual experience depends on neural activity in multiple regions activated simultaneously, rather than in a single region where experiential integration would occur. Second, during free recall or recall generated by perception in a recognition task, the multiple region activity necessary for experience occurs near the sensory portals and motor output sites of the system rather than at the end of an integrative processing cascade removed from inputs and outputs. Hence the term retroactivation to indicate that recall of experiences depends on reactivation close to input and output sites rather than away from them.

The two critical structures in the proposed architecture are the fragment record of feature-based sensory or motor activity, and the convergence zone, an amodal record of the combinatorial arrangements that bound the fragment records as they occurred in experience. There are convergence zones of different orders; for example, those that bind features into entities, and those that bind entities into events or sets of events, but all register combinations of components in terms of coincidence or sequence, in space and time. Convergence zones are an attempt to provide an answer to the binding problem, which I see as a central issue in cognitive processing, at all taxonomic levels and scales of operation.

The adult organization described here operates on the basis of neurobiological and reality constraints. During interactions between the perceiver's brain and its surround, those constraints lead to a process of feature, entity, and event grouping based on physical structure similarity, spatial placement, temporal sequence, and temporal coincidence. The records of those perceptuomotor interactions, both at fragment level and at combinatorial level, are inscribed in superimposed and overlapped fashion; yet, because of the different conditions according to which they are grouped, they become committed to separate neural regions. In cognitive terms I will refer to these processes as domain formation (a creation of relatively separable areas of knowledge for faces, man-made objects, music, numbers, words, social events, disease states, and so on), and recording of contextual complexity (a recording of the temporal and spatial interaction of entities within sets of concurrent events). In neural terms I will refer to these grouping processes as regionalization.

The same type of neuron ensembles, operating on the same principles, constitutes the substrate for different cognitive operations, depending on the location of the ensemble within they system and the connections that feed into the ensemble and that feed back out of it. Location and communication lines determine the topic of the neuron ensemble. The connectivity of functional regions defines the systems-level code for cognitive processes.

The neuroanatomical substrates for this organization are:

1. primary and early association cortices, both sensory and motor, which constitute the substrate for feature-based records;

2. association cortices of different orders, both sensory and motor, some limbic structures (entorhinal cortex, hippocampus, amygdala, cingulate cortices), and the neostriatum/cerebellum, which constitute the substrate for convergence zones;

3. feed-forward and feedback connectivity interrelating (1) and (2), at multiple hierarchical levels, with reciprocal patterns;

4. non-specific thalamic nuclei, hypothalamus, basal forebrain, and brainstem nuclei.

The cognitive/neural architecture outlined above can perform: (1) perceptuomotor interactions with the brain's surround; (2) learning of those interactions at the representational level defined above; (3) internal activation of experience-replicative representations in a recall (perception-independent) mode; (4) problem solving, decision making, planning, and creativity; and (5) communication with the evironment. All those functions are predicated on a key operation: the attempted reconstitution of learned perceptuomotor interactions in the form of internal recall and motor performance. Attempted perceptuomotor reconstitution is achieved by time-locked retroactivation of fragmentary records, in mutiple cortical regions as a result of feedback activity from convergence zones. The success of this operation depends on attention, which is defined as a critical level of activity in each of the activated regions, below which consciousness cannot occur.

According to this proposal, there is no single site for the integration of sensory and motor processes. The experience of spatial integration is brought about by time-locked multiple occurrences. I thus propose a recursive, iterative design to substitute for the traditional unidirectional processing cascades.

Although the notion of representation covers all the inscriptions related to an entity or event, that is, both fragment and binding code records,

the proposal posits that only the multiregional retroactivations of the fragment components become a content of consciousness. The perceptuomotor reconstitutions that form the substrate of consciousness thus occur in an anatomically restricted sector of the cerebrum, albeit in a distributed, multiple-site manner.

In this proposal, and unlike traditional neurological models, there is no localizable single store for the meaning of a given entity within a cortical region. Rather, meaning is reached by widespread multiregional activation of fragmentary records pertinent to a stimulus, wherever such records may be stored within a large array of sensory and motor structures, according to a combinatorial arrangement specific to the entity. A display of the meaning of an entity does not exist in permanent fashion. It is recreated for each new instantiation. The same stimulus does not produce the same evocations at every instantiation, though many of the same or similar sets of records will be evoked in relation to the same or comparable stimuli. The records that pertain to a given entity are distributed in the telencephalon both in the sense that they are inscribed over sizable synaptic populations and in the sense that they are to be found in multiple loci of cerebral cortex and subcortical nuclei.

The proposal permits the reinterpretation of the main types of higher cognitive disorder—the agnosias, the amnesias, and the aphasias—and prompts testable hypotheses for further investigation of those disorders. It also provides a basis for neural hypotheses regarding psychiatric conditions such as sociopathy, phobias and schizophrenia. Several predictions based on this proposal are now being tested in humans, with or without focal brain lesions, using advanced imaging methods and cognitive probes. Some anatomical and physiological aspects of the proposal can be investigated in experimental animals. The concept of convergence zone can be explored with computational techniques.

The Need for Temporo-Spatial Integration and Its Traditional Solution

Current knowledge from neuroanatomy and neurophysiology of the primate nervous system indicates unequivocally that any entity or event that we normally perceive through multiple sensory modalities must engage geographically separate sensory modality structures of the central nervous system. Since virtually every conceivable perception of an entity or event also calls for a motor interaction on the part of the perceiver and must include the concomitant perception of the perceiver's somatic state, it is obvious that perception of external reality and the attempt to record it are a multiple-site neurophysiological affair. This notion is reinforced by the discovery, over the past decade, of a multiplicity of subsidiary functional regions that show some relative dedication not just to a global sensory modality or motor performance but also to featural and dimensional aspects of stimuli (see Damasio 1985a, Van Essen and Maunsell 1983, Livingstone and Hubel 1988, for a pertinent review). The evidence from psychological studies in humans is equally compelling in suggesting featural fragmentation of perceptual processes (see Barlow 1981, Julesz 1971, Posner 1980, Triesman and Gelade 1980). Early geographic parcellation of stimulus properties has thus grown rather than receded, and the condition faced by sensory and motor representations of the brain's surround is a fragmentation of the inscription of the physical structures that constitute reality, at virtually every scale. The physical structure of an entity (external, such as an object, or internal, such as a specific somatic state) must be recorded in terms of separate constituent ingredients, each of which is a result of secondary mappings at a lower physical scale. And the fragmentation that obtains for concrete entities is even more marked for abstract entities and events, considering that abstract entities correspond to criterion-governed conjunctions of dimensions and features present in concrete entities, and that events are an interplay of entities.

The experience of reality, however, both in ongoing perception as well as in recall, is not parcellated at all. The normal experience we have of entities and events is coherent and "in-register," both spatially and temporally. Features are bound in entities, and entities are bound in events. How the brain achieves such a remarkable integration starting with the fragments that it has to work with is a critical question. I call it the *binding problem* (I use the term "binding" in a broader sense than it has been used by Treisman and others, to denote the requisite integration of components at all levels and scales, not only in perception but also in recall). The brain must have devices capable of promoting the integration of fragmentary components of neural activity, in some sort of ensemble pattern that matches the structures of entities, events, and relationships thereof. The solution, implicitly or overtly, has been, for decades, that the components provided by different sensory portals are projected together in so-called multimodal cortices in which, presumably, a representation of integrated reality is achieved. According to this intuitively reasonable view, perception operates on the basis of a unidirectional cascade of processors, which provides, step by step, a refinement of the extraction of signals, first in unimodal streams and later in a sort of multimedia and multitrack apparatus where integration occurs. The general direction of the cascade is caudo-rostral, in cortical terms, and the integrative cortices are presumed to be in the anterior temporal and anterior frontal regions. Penfield's findings in epileptics undergoing electrical stimulation of temporal cortex seemed to support this traditional view (Penfield and Jasper 1954), as did influential models of the neural substrates of cognition in the postwar period, such as Geschwind's (1965) and Luria's (1966). The major discoveries of neurophysiology and neuroanatomy over the past two decades have also seemed compatible with it. On the face of it, anatomical projections do radiate from primary sensory cortices and do create multiple-stage sequences toward structures in the hippocampus and prefrontal cortices (Jones and Powell 1970, Nauta 1971, Pandya and Kuypers 1969, Van Hoesen 1982). Moreover, without a doubt, single-cell neurophysiology does suggest that, the farther away neurons are from the primary sensory cortices, the more they have progressively larger receptive fields and less unimodal responsivity (see Desimone and Ungerleider 1988 for a review and restatement of the traditional view). Until recently, the exception to this dominant view of anterior cerebral structures as the culmination of the processing cascade was to be found in Crick's (1984) hypothesis for a neural mechanism underlying attention.

The purpose of this text is to question the validity of the conventional solution. I doubt that there is a unidirectional cascade. I also question the information-processing metaphor implicit in the solution, that is, the notion that finer representations emerge by progressive extraction of features, and that they flow caudo-rostrally. Specifically, we believe that by using this view of brain organization and function the experimental neuropsychological findings in patients with agnosia and amnesia become unmanageably paradoxical. I also suggest that there is a lack of neuroanatomical support for some requirements of the traditional view, and that there are neuroanatomical findings to support an alternative model. Finally, I believe that available neurophysiological data can be interpreted to support the alternative theory I propose.

Paradoxes and Contradictions of the Traditional Solution

Objections from Human Studies with the Lesion Method

If temporal and frontal integrative cortices were to be the substrate for the integration of neural activity on the basis of which perceptual experience and its attempted recall unfold, the following should be found:

1. That the bilateral destruction of those cortices should preclude the perception of reality as a coherent multimodal experience and reduce experience to disjointed, modality-specific tracks of sensory or motor processing to the extent permitted by the single modality association cortices;

2. That the bilateral destruction of the integrative cortices should reduce the quality of even such modality-specific processing, that is, reduce the richness and detail of perception and recall commensurate with the quality obtainable by the level of non-integrative stations left intact;

3. That the bilateral damage to the rostral integrative cortices should disable memory for any form of past integrated experience and interfere with all levels and types of memory, including memory for specific entities and events, even those that constitute the perceiver's autobiography, memory for non-unique entities and events, and memory for relationships among features, entities, and events.

The results of bilateral destruction of the anterior temporal lobes, either in the medial sector alone or the entire anterior temporal region, as well as bilateral destruction of prefrontal cortices, either in separate sectors or in combination, deny all but a fraction of one of these predictions.

Evidence from Anterior Temporal Cortex Damage

It is *not* true that coherent, multimodal, perceptual experience is disturbed by bilateral lesions of the temporal integrative units, and it is *not* true that those lesions cause the perceptual quality of experience to diminish. On the contrary, all available evidence indicates that at both consciously reportable and non-conscious covert levels, the quality of perceptual experience of subjects who have sustained major selective damage to anterior temporal cortices is comparable to controls (see Corkin 1984; Damasio et al. 1985a,b, 1987). Such subjects can report on what they see, hear, and touch, in ways that observers cannot distinguish from what they themselves see, hear, and touch. A variety of covert knowledge paradigms (e.g., forced recognition and passive skin conductance) indicates that they can also discriminate stimuli, probably on the basis of non-conscious activation of detailed knowledge about the items under scrutiny (Bauer 1984; Tranel and Damasio 1985, 1987, 1988). More importantly, the knowledge that such subjects can evoke consciously, at a non-autobiographical level, indicates that ample memory stores of "integrated experience" remain intact after damage to the alleged integrative units. These facts support the contentions: (1) that a considerable amount of integration must take place early on in the system well before higher-order cortices are reached; (2) that integrated information can be recorded there without the agency of rostral integrative units; and (3) that it can be re-evoked there too, without the intervention of rostral integrative structures.

The only accurate prediction regarding the role of alleged integrative units applies to anterior temporal cortices and concerns the loss of the ability to recall unique combinations of representations that were conjoined in experience within a specific time lapse and space unit. That ability is indeed lost, along with the possibility of creating records for new and unique experiences. This is exemplified by the neuropsychological profile of the patient Boswell, whose cerebral damage entirely destroyed, bilaterally, both hippocampal systems (including the entorhinal cortex, the hippocampal formation, and the amygdala), the cortices in anterolateral and anteroinferior temporal lobes (including areas 38, 20, 21, anterior sector of 22, and part of 37), the entire basal forebrain region bilaterally

(including the septal nuclei, the nucleus accumbens and the substantia innominata, which contains a large sector of the nucleus basalis of Meynert), and the most posterior part of the orbitofrontal cortices. Boswell's perception in all modalities but the olfactory is flawless and the descriptions he produces of complex visual or auditory entities and events are indistinguishable from those of his examiners. All aspects of his motor performance are perfect. His use of grammar, his phonemic and phonetic processing, and his prosody are intact. His memory for most entities is preserved, and at generic/categorical levels his defect only becomes evident when subordinate specificity is required for the recognition of uniqueness or for the disambiguation of extremely similar exemplars. For instance, he recognizes virtually any man-made object such as a vehicle, tool, utensil, article of furniture or clothing, but cannot decide whether he has previously encountered the specific exemplar, or whether or not it is his. Although he can recognize the face of a friend as a human face, or his house as a house, and provide detailed descriptions of the features that compose them, he is unable to conjure up any event of which the unique face or house was a part, and which belong to his autobiography. In short, his essential perceptuomotor interaction with the environment remains normal provided uniqueness of recognition, recall, or action are not required. Recognition, recall, and imagery operate as they should for large sectors of knowledge at the generic/categorical level.

Evidence from Anterior Frontal Lobe Damage

Damage to bilateral prefrontal cortices, especially those in the orbitofrontal sector, is compatible with normal perceptual processes and even with normal memory for entities and events, except when they pertain to complex domains such as social knowledge (Damasio and Tranel 1988, Eslinger and Damasio 1985). Bilateral lesions in superior mesial and in dorsolateral cortices cause defects in drive for action, attention, and problem solving, that may secondarily influence perceptual tasks. However, even extensive ablation of virtually the entire prefrontal cortices is compatible with normal perception. The study of Brickner's patient A, of Hebb's and Ackerly and Benton's patients (see Damasio 1985b for a review), and of our subject EVR (see Eslinger and Damasio 1985) provides powerful evidence in this regard. Frontal lobe structures, with their multiple loci for the anchoring of processing cascades (Goldman-Rakic 1988), are even less likely candidates to be the single, global site of integration than their temporal counterparts.

Evidence from Damage in Single-Modality Cortices

Perhaps the most paradoxical aspect of these data, when interpreted in light of the traditional view, is that damage in certain sectors of sensory association cortices does affect the quality of some aspects of perception within the sensory modality of those cortices. For instance, damage in early visual association cortices can disrupt perception of color, texture, stereopsis, and spatial placement of the physical components of a stimulus. The range of loss depends on which precise region of visual cortex is most affected (Damasio 1985a).

The perceptual defect is accompanied by an impairment of recall and recognition. For instance, achromatopsia (loss of color perception) also precludes imaging color in recall (Damasio 1985; Farah 1989 and unpublished observations), that is, no other cortices, and certainly no other higher-order, integrative cortices, are capable of supporting the recall of the perceptually impaired feature. The coupling of perceptual and recall impairments is strong evidence that the same cortices support perception and recall. This finding, based on lesion method studies, is in line with evidence from normal human experiments (Kosslyn 1980). It also suggests an economical

approach to brain mapping of knowledge that might obviate the problem of combinatorial explosion faced by the traditional view. In my proposal, the brain would not re-inscribe features downstream from where it perceives them. Furthermore, damage within some sectors of modal association cortices can disturb recall and recognition of stimuli presented through that modality, even when basic perceptual processing is not compromised. The domain of stimuli, and the taxonomic level of the disturbance, depend on the specification of the lesion in terms of site, size, and uni- or bilaterality (Damasio and Tranel 1989; see also work on category-related recognition defects reviewed in Damasio 1989 and McCarthy and Warrington 1988). Lesions within visual association cortices may impair the recognition of the unique identity of faces, while allowing for the recognition of facial expressions, non-unique objects, and visuo-verbal material. Or lesions may compromise object recognition and leave face recognition untouched (Feinberg, Rothi, and Heilman 1986; Newcombe and Ratcliff 1974), or compromise reading but not object or face recognition (Damasio and Damasio 1983, Geschwind and Fusillo 1966). The key point is that damage in a caudal and modal association cortex *can disrupt recall and recognition at even the most subordinate taxonomic level*. It can preclude the kind of integrated experience usually attributed to the rostral cortices, that is, an evocation made up of multiple featural components, based on different modalities, constituting entities and events. This can happen without disrupting perception within the affected modality and without compromising recall or recognition in other modalities. Damage in modal cortices also disrupts learning of new entities and events presented through the modality (Damasio et al. 1989a).

These findings indicate that a substantial amount of perceptual integration takes place within single-modality cortices, and that knowledge recalled at categoric levels (also known as semantic, or generic)[1] is largely dependent on records and interactions among posterior sensory cortices and the interconnected motor cortices.

It also indicates that recall and recognition of knowledge at the level of unique entities or events (also known as episodic)[1] requires *both* anterior *and* posterior sensory cortices, an indication that a more complex network is needed for intricate subordinate-level mappings and that anterior integrative structures alone are not sufficient to record and reconstruct knowledge at such levels.

The implications are:

1. that the posterior sensory cortices are sites where fragment records are inscribed and reactivated, according to appropriate combinatorial arrangements (by fragments I mean "parts of entities," at a multiplicity of scales, most notably at the feature level, for example color, movement, texture, and shape); such cortices are also capable of binding features into entities and thus re-enact the perceptual experience of entities and their operations ("local" or "entity" binding). But posterior cortices cannot map non-local contextual complexity at event level, which is to say they cannot map the spatial and temporal relationships assumed by entities within the multiple concurrent events that usually characterize complex interactions with the environment.

2. the inscription of contextual complexity, that is, the complexity of the combinatorial arrangement exhibited by many concurrent events (non-local or event binding), requires anterior cortices, although its re-enactment also depends on posterior cortices.

The posterior cortices contain all the fragments with which experiences can potentially be reconstituted, given the appropriate combinatorial arrangement (binding). But as far as combinatorial arrangements are concerned, the posterior cortices contain primarily the records for "local" entity or simple event binding. They do not contain records for "non-local" concurrent event

binding and are thus unable to reconstitute experiences based on the contextually complex, multi-event situations that characterize one's autobiography.

The anterior cortices do contain such non-local, concurrent event binding records. The critical point is that since posterior cortices contain *both* fragment and local binding records, they are essential for *all* experience-replicative operations. Anterior cortices are only required to assist experiences that depend on high-level contextual complexity.

I would predict, based on the above hypotheses, that simultaneous damage in strategic regions of *several* single-modality cortices, for example visual, auditory, somatosensory, in spite of intactness of the so-called rostral integrative cortices, would preclude recognition and recall of a sweeping range of stimuli defined by features and dimensions from those modalities, *both* at generic and episodic levels. The central premise behind my proposal, then, is that extensive damage in "early" sensory cortices is the only way of producing the effect normally posited for destruction of the anterior units, namely the suspension of multimodal recognition and recall, from which would follow the abolition of experiences.

A testable hypothesis drawn from this premise is that damage in intermediate cortices (cortices in parts of areas 37, 36, 35, and 39 that constitute virtual "choke points" for the feed-forward-feedback projections that interlock earlier and higher-order cortices) should have a comparable disrupting effect. There is preliminary evidence that this is so from findings on patients with lesions in these areas (Horenstein, Chamberlin, and Conomy 1967), and a study is currently under way to analyze additional evidence.

Neuroanatomical and Neurophysiological Evidence

Leaving aside the fact that no bilateral lesion in a presumed "anterior integrative cortex" is capable of precluding coherent perception of any entity or event, or categorical recall, one might turn around and pose a purely neuroanatomical question: which area or set of areas could possibly function as a fully encompassing and single convergence region, based on what is currently known about neural connectivity? The simple answer is: none. The entorhinal cortex and the adjacent hippocampal system (hippocampal formation and amygdala) do receive connections from all sensory cortices, and come closest to the mark. Prefrontal cortices, inasmuch as one can envisage their connectivity from neuroanatomical studies in non-human primates, do not fit the bill either. They have no single point of anatomical convergence equivalent to the entorhinal cortex, only separate convergence points with different and narrower admixtures of innervation. The hypothesis suggested by these facts is that the integration of sensory and motor activity necessary for coherent perception and recall must occur in multiple sites and at multiple levels. A single convergence site is nowhere to be found.

In fact, developments in neuroanatomy and neurophysiology have emphasized the notion of segregation while beginning to reveal different possibilities for integration. For instance, Hubel and Livingstone (1987) and Livingstone and Hubel (1984) have demonstrated that separate cellular channels within area 17 are differently dedicated to the processing of color, form and motion. Beyond area 17 the evidence shows:

1. Early channel separation and divergence into several functional regions revealed by neurophysiological studies (Allman, Miezin, and McGuinness 1985; Hubel and Livingstone 1987; Livingstone and Hubel 1984; Van Essen and Maunsell 1983), and characterized in part by studies of connectivity (Gilbert 1983; Livingstone and Hubel 1987a; Lund, Hendrickson, Ogren, and Tobin 1981; Rockland and Pandya 1979, 1981). This form of organization is describable by the attributes divergent, one-to-many, parallel, and sequential.

2. The existence of back-projections to the feeding cortical origin, capable of affecting processing in a retroactive manner, and capable of cross-projecting to regions of the same level (Van Essen 1985; Zeki 1987, personal communication). This anatomical pattern opens the possibility for various forms of local integration.

3. Existence of convergence into functional regions downstream (projections from visual, auditory, and somatosensory cortices) can be encountered in combinations from two and three modalities, in progressively more rostral brain regions such as areas 37, 36, 35, 38, 20 and 21 (Jones and Powell 1970; Seltzer and Pandya 1976, 1978; Pandya and Yeterian 1985),[2] a design feature describable by the attributes convergent, many-to-few, parallel, and sequential. In humans, judging from evidence in non-human primates, trimodal combinations are likely to occur in functional regions within Brodmann's areas 37, 36, 35, 38, 39; bimodal combinations are likely in areas 40, 20 and 21.

4. Existence of further feedback from the latter cortices, that is, "convergence regions", have the power to back-project divergently to the feeding cortices.

The pattern of forward convergence and retro-divergence is repeated in the rostral cortices of the entorhinal and prefrontal regions. For instance, neuron ensembles in higher-order cortices project into the circumscribed clusters found in layer II and superficial parts of layer III of the entorhinal cortex (Van Hoesen 1982; Van Hoesen and Pandya 1975a,b; Van Hoesen, Pandya, and Butters 1975). I describe this design feature as convergent, and few-to-fewer. Convergence continues into the hippocampal formation proper, by means of perforant pathway projections to the dentate gyrus and of projections from there into CA3 and CA1. Convergence is again followed by divergent feedbacks via several anatomical routes:

1. a direct route, using the subiculum and layer IV of the entorhinal cortex, diverges into the cortices that provide the last station of input into the hippocampus (Kosel, Van Hoesen, and Rosene 1982; Rosene and Van Hoesen 1977); as noted above, those cortices project back to the previous feeding station;

2. an indirect route, so far only revealed in rodents but possibly present in primates, which feeds back into virtually all previous stations, divergently and in saltatory fashion, rather than in recapitulatory manner (Swanson and Kohler 1986);

3. an even less direct and specific route, which uses pathways in the fornix and exerts influence over thalamic, hypothalamic, basal forebrain, and frontal structures, all of which in turn, directly and indirectly, can influence the operation of the cerebral cortices in widespread fashion. The latter route provides the cortex with regionally selective or widespread neurochemical influence (e.g., acetylcholine, norepinephrine, dopamine, and serotonin) based on the activity of neurotransmitter nuclei in basal forebrain and brainstem (Lewis et al. 1986; Mesulam, Mufson, Levey, and Wainer 1983).

The findings clearly indicate that the hippocampus-bound projection systems point as much forward as backward. Furthermore, the convergence noted anteriorly is always partial, never encompassing the full range of sensory and motor processes that may be involved in complex experiences. Precisely the same argument could be presented for the multiplicity of prefrontal cortices that serve as end-points for projections from parietal and temporal regions. The feed-forward projections remain segregated among parallel streams and are reciprocated by powerful feedbacks to their originating cortices or their vicinity (Goldman-Rakic 1988).

The fact that the receptive fields of neurons increase dramatically in a caudal-rostral direction has implicitly supported the notion of ros-

tral integration. A look at this issue in the visual system reveals that the size of the receptive field of neurons in area 17 (V_1) is extremely small; it enlarges by as much as one hundred times at the level of V_4, and at the level of the higher-order cortices of areas 20 and 21 virtually encompasses the entire visual scene (Desimone, Schein, Moran, and Ungerleider 1985). This gradual enlargement of receptive fields, all the way from small and lateralized to large and bilateral, has been viewed as an indication that anteriorly placed neurons not only see more of the world but represent a finer picture of it (Desimone and Ungerleider 1989, Perrett et al. 1987). However, nothing in those data indicates that the fewer and fewer neurons that are linked to larger and larger receptive fields contain any concrete representation whatsoever of the perceptual detail upstream or that those neurons are committed and the end-point of multiple-channel processing. Those data are certainly compatible with the proposal I present below: (a) that fewer and fewer neurons placed anteriorly in the system are projected on by structures upstream and thus subtend a broader compass of feed-forwarding regions; (b) that they serve as pivots for reciprocating feedback projections rather than as the recipients and accumulators of all the knowledge inscribed at earlier levels; and (c) that in such a capacity they are intermediaries in a continuous process that systematically returns to early cortices.

The unavoidable conclusion is that, while it is possible to conceive of the integration of sensory processes within a few neuronal regions necessary to define a single entity, it is apparent that no single area in the human brain receives projections from all the regions involved in the processing of an event. More importantly, it is inconceivable that any single region of the brain might integrate spatially all the fragments of sensory and motor activity necessary to define a set of unique events. An answer to this puzzle, namely the ability to generate an integrated experience in the absence of any means to bring the experience's components together in a single spatial meeting ground, might be a trick of timing. It would allow the perceiver or recaller to experience spatial integration and continuity in relation to sets of activity that are spatially discontinuous but do occur in the same time window, an illusory intuition.

A Different Solution

Following on the evidence and reflections outlined above and incorporating additional neuropsychological and neuroanatomical data, I propose the following solution:

1. The neural activity that embodies physical structure representations entity occurs in *fragmented fashion and in geographically separate cortices* located in modal sensory cortices. The so-called integrative, rostral cortices of the anterior temporal and prefrontal regions cannot possibly contain such fragmentary inscriptions.

2. The integration of multiple aspects of reality, external as well as internal, in perceptual or recalled experiences, both within each modality and across modalities, depends on the time-locked co-activation of geographically separate sites of neural activity within sensory and motor cortices, rather than on a neural transfer and integration of different representations towards rostral integration sites. The conscious experience of those co-activations depends on their simultaneous, but temporary, enhancement (here called co-attention), against the background activity on which other activations are being played back.

3. The representations of physical structure components of entities are recorded in precisely the same neural ensembles in which corresponding activity occurred during perception, but the combinatorial arrangements (binding codes) which describe their pertinent linkages in entities and events (their spatial and temporal coincidences) are stored in separate neural ensembles called *convergence zones*. The former

and the latter neuron ensembles are interlocked by reciprocal projections.

4. The concerted reactivation of physical structure fragments, on which recall of experiences depends, requires the firing of convergence zones and the concomitant firing of the feedback projections arising from them.

5. Convergence zones bind neural activity patterns corresponding to topographically organized fragment descriptions of physical structure, which were pertinently associated in previous experience on the basis of similarity, spatial placement, temporal sequence, temporal coincidence, or any combination of the above. Convergence zones are located throughout the telencephalon, at multiple neural levels, in association cortices of different orders, limbic cortices, subcortical limbic nuclei, and non-limbic subcortical nuclei such as the basal ganglia.

6. The geographic location of convergence zones varies among individuals but is not random. It is constrained by the subject matter of the recorded material (its domain), by degree of contextual complexitiy in events (the number of component entities that interact in an event and the relations they adopt), and by the anatomical design of the system.

7. The representations inscribed in the above architecture, both those that preserve topographic/topologic relationships, and those that code for temporal coincidences, are committed to populations of neuron ensembles and their synapses, in distributed form.

8. The co-occurrence of activities at multiple sites, which is necessary for temporary conjunctions, is achieved by iteration across time phases.

Thus I propose not a single direction of processing, along single or multiple channels, but rather a recursive and iterative form of processing. Such processing is parallel and, because of the many time phases involved in multiple steps, it is also sequential. Convergence zones provide integration, and, although the convergence zones that realize the more encompassing integration are more rostrally placed, the activities that all levels of convergence zone end up promoting, and on the basis of which representations are reconstituted and evoked, actually take place in caudal rather than rostral cortices. And because convergence zones return the chain of processing to earlier cortices where the chain can start again towards another convergence zone, there is no need to postulate an ultimate integration area. In other words, this model can accommodate the astonishing segregation of processing streams that the work of Livingstone and Hubel has revealed so dramatically.

The sensory and motor cortices are thus seen as the distributed and yet restricted sector of the brain on which both perception and recall play themselves out, and on which self-consciousness must necessarily be based. Perception and self-consciousness are assigned the same brain spaces at the border between the world within and the world without.

In the following section I present a framework based on these views and discuss its structures, systems, organization, and operation.

Timelocked Multiregional Retroactivation: Framework, Structures, Systems Organization, and Operation

Framework

Because of its origin in mutually constraining sets of cognitive and neural data, the theory developed here is both cognitive and neural. The cognitive architecture implicit in the theory assumes representations that can be described as psychological phenomena and interrelated according to combinatorial semantics and syntax. The proposed neural organization, however, is not a mere hardware implementation apparatus for any potential type of cognitive processes, in that its specifications severely restrict the range of representations and algorithms that it can implement; that is, it is not likely to implement representations other than the ones its anatomy

and physiology embody and are destined to operate. The key level of neural architecture is that of systems of macroscopic functional regions in cerebral cortex and gray matter nuclei.

The theory describes an adult neural/cognitive organization presumed to be relatively stable and yet modifiable by experience, to produce temporary or long-lasting partial reorganizations. The issues of neural and cognitive development are not addressed, nor does the theory deal with microneural specifications at synaptic and molecular levels. However, it does assume that any inscription of perceptuomotor activity is based on a distributed transformation of physiological parameters, occurring over ensembles of neurons at the level of their synapses, according to some variant of Hebbian principles. The theory operates on the basis of neurobiological and reality constraints.

Neurobiological Constraints

These correspond to the structural design of the nervous system prior to interactions with the environment: the basic circuitry of cellular structures and their interconnectivity, which can be changed by epigenetic interactions. The design includes neuroanatomically embodied values of the organism (e.g., goals and drives of the species), external and internal spatial reference maps, and a variety of processing biases that are likely to guide, in part, the mapping of interactions with the environment, that is, the domains of knowledge that the brain prefers to acquire and the choice of neural sites to support such knowledge. The effect of these constraints is to provide a certain degree of innate modularization of "faculties" upon exposure to the reality constraints discussed below.

Reality Constraints: The World Without and the World Within

The description of the characteristics of the universe surrounding the brain, both inside and outside the organism, can be made at the multiple levels that current knowledge of philosophy, psychology, physics, chemistry, and biology permit. From my point of view, however, it is sensible to focus the description on the levels from which we derive psychological meaning: (1) a broad range of objects to which I will refer to as entities and which encompass both natural and man-made kinds; (2) the features and dimensions that compose those entities; and (3) the interplay of entities in unique events or episodes occurring in temporal and spatial units. Thus, the set of reality constraints corresponds to:

1. The existence of concrete entities external to both brain and organism, and external to the brain but internal to the organism (somatic). External entities are themselves composed of various aggregated features and dimensions in an entity-intrinsic space (the space defined by the physical limits of the entity) and are, in turn, placed within an entity-extrinsic space (the coordinate space where the entity and other entities lie or more). Internal entities consist of: (a) motor interactions of the organism with external entities by means of movements in hands, head, eyes, and whole body; (b) baseline somatic states of internal milieu and of smooth and striated musculature during interaction with external entities; and (c) modification of somatic states triggered by and occurring during interaction with external entities.

2. The existence of abstract entities are criterion-governed conjunctions of features and dimensions present in the concrete entities outlined above.

3. The fact that entities necessarily occur in unique interactive combinations called events, and that events often take place concurrently, in complex sets.

Entities are definable by the number of components, the modality range of those components (e.g., single or multiple modality), the mode of assembly, the size of the class formed on the ba-sis of physical structure similarity, their operation and function, their frequency of occurrence, and their value to the perceiver.

As is the case with entities, events can be both external and internal, and both concrete and abstract. The concurrence of many events which characterize regular life episodes generates "contextual complexity," which can be defined by the number of entities and by the relational links they assume as they interplay in such complex sets of events. Naturally, during the unfolding of events, other entities and events are recalled from autobiographical records. The records co-activated in that process add further to the contextual complexity of the experiences that occur within a given time unit. It is thus contextual complexity which sets entities and events apart and which confers greater or lesser uniqueness to those entities and events. In other words, contextual complexity sets the taxonomic level of events and entities along a continuum that ranges from unique (most subordinate) to non-unique (less subordinate and more supraordinate).

Domain Formation and Recording of Contextual Complexity

During interactions between the perceiver's brain and its surround, the two sets of constraints lead to some critical operations that can be described as follows from a psychological standpoint:

1. domain formation, which is a process of feature, entity, and event grouping based on physical structure similarity, spatial placement, temporal sequence, and temporal coincidence;

2. the creation of records of contextual complexity that register the temporal coincidence of entities and their interrelationships within sets of events.

It is on the basis of this psychological-level description and on the evidence that category-related recognition defects can be associated to damage in specific brain loci that we hypothesize neural substrates for different knowledge domains and levels of knowledge processing. It must be noted that for the purposes of modeling we are here inverting the natural order of things: domains exist *because* of neurobiological and reality constraints, not the other way around.

Functional Regionalization

The process of regionalization occurs for both fragments of perceptuomotor activity and convergence zones. I conceive it as a way of recruiting a neuron population for a limited range of cortical inputs (and, by extension, to the domain or level defined by the feed-forwarding neuronal populations). In other words, certain topics (at feature, entity, or event level) are assigned to a circumscribed neuronal population. Within that polulation, however, different synaptic patterns define individual features, or entities, or events. In simple terms one might say that generally similar material stacks up together within the same regions and systems.

As I will discuss further on, the superimposed, overlapped nature of the records poses problems for their appropriate separation during recall. The solution I envisage, and that may appear counterintuitive at first glance, resides with the wealth and complexity of the record at the synaptic level. The greater the number of defining sub-components and distinctive links, the greater the chance of establishing uniqueness at the time of recording and at the time of reactivation.

The key to regionalization is the detection, by populations of neurons, of coincident or sequential spatial and temporal patterns of activity in the input neuron populations. Precisely the same type of neuron ensembles, operating on precisely the same principles, will constitute the substrate for different cognitive operations depending on the location of the ensemble within the system and the connections that feed into the ensemble and that feed back out of it. In other words, location and communication lines determine the topic of the synaptic patterns within a given neuron ensemble (the domain of a convergence zone), without there being a need to posit special neuron types or special physiological codes in order for convergence zones to serve different domains or cognitive operations.

The Nature of Representations

Human experiences as they occur ephemerally in *perception* are the result of multiple sensory and motor processing of a collection of features and dimensions in external and internal entities. Specifically they are based on the cerebral representation of concrete external entities, internal entities, abstract entities, and events.

Such representations are interrelated by combinatorial arrangements so that their internal activation in recall and the order with which they are attended, permits them to unfold in a "sentential" manner. Such "sentences" embody semantic and syntactic principles.

In my view, the words of any language are also concrete external entities. The combinatorial semantics and syntax of thought and language might be embodied in the relationships that describe the constitution of entities and events (although the universal grammar behind language may be based on additional language-specific principles and rules).

This cognitive/neural architecture implies a high degree of sharing and embedding of representations. Both the representation of abstract entities and of events are derived from the representation of concrete entities and are thus individualized on the basis of combinatorial arrangement rather than remapping of constituents. The representation of concrete entities themselves share subrepresentations of component features so that individuality is again conferred by combinatorial formulas.

Human experiences, as they occur ephemerally in *recall*, are based on records of the multiple-site and multiple-level neural activities previously engaged by perception. Recalled experiences constitute an attempted reconstruction of perceptual experience based on activity in a set of pertinent sensory and motor cortices, controlled by a reactivation mechanism specified below.

The Components of Representations

Feature-Based Fragments
I propose that the experienceable (conscious) component of representations results from an attempt at reconstituting feature-based, topographic or topologically organized fragments of sensory and motor activity; that is, only the feature-based components of a representation assembled in a specific pattern can become a content of consciousness. The maximal size of the feature-based fragment is a critical issue. Stimuli such as human faces, verbal lexical entities, and body parts of the self, must be permanently represented by large-scale fragments on the basis of which rapid reconstitution can occur. It is unlikely that such stimuli would depend on a reconstruction from the smallest-scale level of neural activity (equivalent, for the visual system, to Bela Julesz' textons, 1981). But many fragments are small-scale and can be shared by numerous entities and used interchangeably in the reconstitution attempt.

Convergence Zones

The Structure and Role of Convergence Zones
Because feature-based fragments are recorded and reactivated in sensory and motor cortices, the reconstitution of an entity or event so that it resembles the original experience depends on the recording of the combinatorial arrangement that conjoined the fragments in perceptual or recalled experience. The record of each unique combinatorial arrangement is the binding code, and it is based on a device I call the convergence zone.

Convergence zones exist as synaptic patterns within multi-layered neuron ensembles in association cortices, and satisfy the following conditions: (1) they have been convergently projected upon by multiple cortical regions according to a connectional principle that might be described as many-to-one; (2) they can reciprocate feed-forward projections with feedback projection (one-to-many); (3) they have additional, interlocking feed-forward/feedback relations with other cortical and subcortical neuron ensembles. The signals brought to convergence zones by cortico-cortical feed-forward projections, represent temporal coincidences (co-occurrence) or temporal sequences of activation in the feeding cortices (rather than re-representations of inscriptions contained in the feeding cortices). I envision the binding code as a synaptic pattern of activity such that when one of the projections which feedforward to it is reactivated, firing in the convergence zone leads to simultaneous firing in all or most of the feed-back projections which reciprocated the feed-forward from the original set. By means of those reciprocating feedback lines, convergence zones can trigger simultaneous activity in all or part of the originally feeding cortices, in a retroactive and divergent manner, according to certain principles of operation specified below. The proposal does not address the issue of the number or size of convergence zones, although it assumes that the zone's size is defined during development as a result of input-output connection patterns, and the patterns of lateral interaction that help structure the ensemble as a unit.

Convergence zones are *a*modal, in that they receive signals from the same or different modalities but do *not* map sensory or motor activity in a way that preserves feature-based, topographic and topological relations of the external environment as they appear in psychological experience. Convergence zones do not embody a refined representation, in the sense that would be assumed in an information-processing model, although they do route information in the sense of information theory. They know "about" neural activity in the feeding cortices and can promote further cortical activity by feedback/retroactivation. In themselves, however, they are uninformed as to the content of the representations they assist in attempting to reconstruct. The role of convergence zones is to enact formulas for the reconstitution of fragment-based momentary representations of entities or events in sensory and motor cortices—the experiences we remember.[3]

Operating Principles

Convergence zones signal the related binding of the similarity, spatial placement, temporal sequence, or temporal coincidence of feature-based fragments highlighted in the perceiver's experience. Convergence zones prompt sensory and motor co-activation by means of back-projections into cortices located upstream. In the extreme view (a mere caricature), all that would be required of a convergence zone would be to function as a pivot, that is, to cause retroactivation in sites that it fed back to, after a threshold defined by concurrent inputs had been reached. The general operating principle would be stated as: (a) reactivate itself when fired upon; (b) reactivation promotes firing toward any site to which there are back-projections, reciprocating feed-forward inputs that generated the synaptic pattern that defines the zone. But because of superimposition and overlapping of convergence zones within the same neuron population, and of the ensuing high number of synaptic interactions, the range of back-firing of each convergence zone is modulated rather than rigid. It depends on the momentary number and nature of cortical feed-foward inputs (relative to the total number of possible feedback outputs that the zone can have), and on the momentary inputs from other areas of cortex and from limbic system, thalamus, basal forebrain, and so froth.

As a consequence, convergence zones can produce different ranges of retroactivation in the cortex, depending on the concurrent balances of inputs they receive. Also, convergence zones can blend responses, that is, produce retroactivation of fragments that did not originally belong to the same experiential set, because of under-specification of cortical feed-forward inputs, or higher-order cortical feedbacks, or subcortical feedbacks. When pathological combinations of input are reached, the zone malfunctions, for example, it may generate "fantastic" or "psychotic" responses, or not operate at all.

It is important to note that the lines activated by feedback from convergence zones are not rigid. They should be seen as facilitated paths that may or may not be travelled depending on the ensemble pattern of synaptic interactions within a population.

Types of Convergence Zones

I envisage permanent convergence zones in the cortex and temporary convergent zones in limbic structures and basal ganglia/cerebellum, based on current findings regarding the profile of retrograde amnesia following hippocampal damage. The domain of the convergence zone is determined by its immediate and remote feed-forward inputs which are co-extensive with its back-projection targets.

I propose two types of convergence zones. In type 1, the zone fires back simultaneously and produces concomitant activations. Type 1 zones inscribe temporal coincidences and aim at replicating them. Type 2 convergence zones fire back in sequence, producing closely ordered activations in the target cortices. Such zones have inscribed temporal sequences and aim at replicating them. The time scale for firing from Types 1 and 2 convergence zones would be different.

Type 1 convergence zones are located in sensory association cortices of low and high order, and are assisted in learning by the hippocampal system. Type 2 convergence zones are the hallmark of motor-related cortices, and are assisted in learning by basal ganglia and cerebellum.

In the normal condition, the two types of convergence zone interlock at multiple levels so that learning relative to an entity or event recruits both types of convergence zones. Likewise normal recall and recognition involve operations in both types of convergence zone, even when the triggering stimulus only activates one type of convergence zone at the outset of the process.

The Development of Convergence Zones

The placement of convergence zones is partly the result of the genetically expressed neuroanatomical design and partly the result of the sculpting process introduced by learning. Convergence zones develop in association cortices that: (a) receive projections in a convergent manner from a wider array of cortices located upstream; (b) can reciprocate projections to the feeding cortices; (c) can project downstream to other cortices and subcortical structures; and (d) can receive a wide array of projections from several subcortical and motor structures.

It is the genetic pattern of neuroanatomical connections that first constrains the potential domain of convergence zones. For example, a convergence zone in early visual association cortices cannot possibly bind anything but visually related activity at the level of component features, whereas a convergence zone in anterior temporal cortices can be told about activity related to numerous simultaneous events and bind their coincidence. But the ultimate anatomical location and functional destiny of convergence zones is determined by learning, as neuron ensembles become differentially dedicated to certain types of occurrence in feeding cortices.

Convergence zones are created during learning as a result of concurrent activations in neuron ensembles within association cortices of different order, hippocampus, amygdala, basal ganglia, and cerebellum. The concurrent activations come from convergent feed-forward signals generated by neural activity in: (a) sensory and motor cortices (as caused by perception or recall of external or internal entities); (b) feedback projections from other convergence zones in association cortices; (c) direct and indirect feedback projections from convergence zones in limbic cortices and from limbic related nuclei: (d)

direct and indirect feedback projections from basal ganglia, non-motor thalamus, and cerebellum; and (e) local microcircuitry interactions.

As noted above, convergence zones have thresholds and levels of response. The activation of a convergence zone depends on its internal constitution, the size, locus, number, and location of sensory and motor representation sites that it subtends. It also depends on the momentary concurrent combination of potential trigger weights, from neural activity related to externally generated representations, internally recalled representations, and back-projection from all the neuronal sites listed previously.

Superposition of Signals

Convergence zones contain overlapping binding codes for many entities and events. Such rich binding is the source of the widening retroactivation that permits recognition and thought processes, and yet its wealth, if unchecked, would eventually result in co-activations bearing only minimal relationships to previous specific experiences and on inability to reconstitute unique events. Ultimately, fantastic and cognitively catastrophic combinations would occur, as they do in fact occur in a variety of neuropsychological disorders caused by the neuropathological processes at several levels of the system. In the normal brain, the constraints that impose specificity of co-evocations depend on concurrent inputs from the following systems: (a) other convergence zones, at multiple neural levels, whose subtended retroactivation provides neural context and thereby helps constrain co-activation; and (b) non-specific limbic nuclei (basal forebrain and brain stem) activated by antero-temporal limbic units (amygdala, hippocampus).

Attention

In a system that produces multiple-site activations incessantly, it is necessary to enhance pertinently linked sites in order to permit binding by salient coincidences. I use the term attention to designate the "spotlighting" process that generates simultaneous and multiple-site salience and thus permits the emergence of evocations. Consciousness occurs when multiple sites of activation are simultaneously enhanced in keeping or not with real past experiences. (Some psychotic and demential states are possibly examples of simultaneous enhancement of activations whose combination does not conform to reality; in non-pathological states the same applies to day-dreams). As defined here, attention depends on numerous factors and mechanisms. First, there is a code for enhancement of activations that is part of the record of the activation pattern it enhances. Type 2 convergence zones are especially suited to this role. Secondly, the state of the perceiver and the context of the process play important roles in determining the level of activations. The reticular activating system, the reticular complex of the thalamus, and the limbic system mediate such roles under partial control of the cerebral cortex.

The evocations that constitute experienced recall occur in specified sensory and motor cortices, albeit in parcellated fashion. Experienced recall thus occurs where physical structures of external entities or body states were mapped in feature fragment manner, notwithstanding the fact that a complex neural machinery made up of numerous other areas of cortex and subcortical nuclei cooperates to reconstruct the co-activation patterns and enhance them.

The Placement of Convergence Zones

Convergence zones have different placements within association cortices and other gray matter regions, and varied activation thresholds. There are numerous levels of convergence zone depending on knowledge domain and contextual complexity (taxonomic level). The functional regionalization of a domain corresponds to the neural inscription of separate sensory and motor activities related to features and dimensions of different exemplars. The inscriptions are naturally superimposed to the extent that the respec-

tive features and dimensions overlap, or coincide in time. The inscriptions are naturally contiguous when the respective features or acts they represent occurred in temporal sequence. As superimpositions accrue, categories emerge from the blends and mergings of separate exemplars. It is important to note that for each separate exemplar to be recalled as an individual entity, it is necessary to add contextual complexity to its representation. This is accomplished by connecting its inscription to the inscription of other entities and events so that an entirely unique set can be defined. When additional inscriptions are not linked to create unique or nearly unique sets, the superimposition of exemplars remains categorical or generic, and recall can reconstitute any one previously learned exemplar or else a blend of exemplars. The creation of records of contextual complexity, which code for the temporal entities and events, is thus critical for recall or recognition at unique (episodic) level.

It is important to note that in this perspective the building of categories occurs while inscribing episodes. The system operates so that it always attempts to inscribe as much as possible of the entire context. Even if the system fails to inscribe the whole episode—or if it does inscribe it, but recall cannot fully reconstitute it—the operation preserves enough of the core inscription of an entity (or event) for categorization to develop from this and other related inscriptions. The inscription of categories precedes episode inscription; that is, it is neuroanatomically and neurophysiologically more caudal. This disposition explains the impairment of episodic memory and preservation of generic memory following damage to anterior temporal cortices.

Knowledge of objects, faces, numbers, among many others, created by perceptuomotor interactions, is anatomically and functionally regionalized in a manner different from classic localizationism of function, but that does admit a notable degree of anatomical specialization. This form of specialization does not follow traditional anatomical boundaries such as are known for sensory modalities, or cytoarchitectonic brain areas. Nor does it conform to the functional centers of traditional neurology. The fragment representations that comprehensively describe an entity are dispersed by multiple functional regions which are, in turn, located in different cytoarchitectonic areas. The many convergence zones necessary to bind the fragments relationally are located in yet other neural sites. The region thus formed obeys anatomical criteria dictated by the nature of the entity represented, and by the interaction between perceiver and entity, and is secondarily constrained by the potential offerings of the anatomy. The comprehensive representation of a specific entity or category is distributed not only within a population of neurons but is also distributed in diverse types of neural structure, cortically and subcortically. In this proposal, the term localization can only refer to an imaginary space defined by neural sites likely to contain convergent zones necessary for the retroactivation of a given set of entities or events. The borders of such a space are not only fuzzy but changeable, in the sense that for different instantiations of retroactivation of a given entity the set of necessary convergence zones varies considerably.

Applications of the Framework

In the following two sections I discuss briefly the application of this proposal to learning and memory and language.

Learning and Memory

The Relative Segregation of Memory Domains

The fact that different neural regions support memory for different domains is the reason why striking performance dissociations can occur in human amnesia. For instance, after lesions in the hippocampal system, patients retain previously learned perceptuomotor skills (so-called procedural knowledge) or even learn new ones, while memory and learning for new faces or objects is no longer possible (Cohen and Squire 1980; Damasio et al. 1985a,b, 1987; Eslinger and Damasio 1986; Milner, Corkin, and Teuber 1968). This dissociation occurs because the representations of motor entities rely on structures that remain intact in those patients: somatosensory and motor cortices, neo-striatum and cerebellum. As noted above, the functional essence behind the system formed by those structures is the recording and re-encactment of temporal sequences and relies on type 2 convergence zones.

Participation of the hippocampal system is not at all necessary for the acquisition and maintenance of procedural memories, provided they are used only at a covert level, and the subject is not required to recollect the factual information related to the acquisition of the skill or to the circumstances in which the skill has been previously exercised. Conscious recall of the source of knowledge requires patency of at least one hippocampal region.

By contrast, the weight of recording factual knowledge, in spite of its diverse base on sensory and motor activities, relies most importantly on sensory cortices and necessitates hippocampal activity. The functional essence in this system is the recording of neural activity related to physical structure (of features, entities, and events), spatial contiguity (of features and entities), and temporal coincidence (of entities and events). Type 1 convergence zones in the hippocampal-bound association cortices are required. Perhaps the most dramatic lesion-related dissociation within factual knowledge is the one that compromises memory for complex social events but spares general knowledge of entities and events outside of a social context (Damasio and Tranel 1988, Eslinger and Damasio 1985). Other striking dissociations abound, however, for different categories of objects, for verbal and non-verbal knowledge, and for different types of verbal knowledge (Damasio et al. 1989b).

Different Levels of Memory Processing

In essence, the distinction between generic and episodic memories is a distinction of processing levels during recall or recognition. We can recall at generic levels, with little contextual complexity attached to an entity, no definition of uniqueness, and no connection to our autobiography. Or we can recall at progressively richer episodic levels, with the evocation of greater contextual complexity and the experience of autobiographic events in which entities play more specific roles. I believe the brain normally attempts to capture the maximal complexity of every event, although the stability of the recording of such complexity varies with the value of the event and with the anticipated need to recall it.

The Mapping of Uniqueness and of Entity-Centered Knowledge

The critical distinction between generic and episodic knowledge, from the standpoint of learning, resides with the ability to record temporal coincidence (co-occurrence) of entities within a wide and complex context. It is a matter of magnitude that distinguishes generic from episodic levels of processing, somewhat artificially, along a continuum.

When a perceiver interacts with a novel entity, learning consists of recording any additional patterns of physical structure, somatic state, or relational binding that transpired during the interaction but were *not previously recorded*. The same applies to learning of new events.

In virtually all instances of learning beyond the early acquisition periods of infancy and childhood, any new pattern of activity related to perception of new entities and events also evokes multiple and previously stored patterns that are thus co-experienced with the novel stimuli. Learning does not entail the recording of all the information contained in a new event. Rather, it calls for the co-evocation of many physical structures and relations previously recorded for related events, the recording of any novel features that had not been recorded before, and the linking of novel records with the pre-existing records so that a new specific set is defined and the code for its potential reconstitution committed to a convergence zone.

There is a large sharing of memory records such that the same neural patterns can be applied to many entities and events by superimposition and overlap whenever and wherever their physical structure or relational bindings are shared. The inscription of a specific entity or event can be made unique only by means of connecting a particular component to others. Such an organization is extremely economical and promotes a large memory capacity. However, it is also prone to ambiguity and an easily disordered operation if one of its many supporting devices malfunctions. Confusional states and some amnesic syndromes caused by subcortical lesions are an expression of such malfunctions. At a milder level, fatigue, sleep deprivation, or distraction can cause the same.

Neural Substrates for Learning and Memory at Systems Level

The critical neural substrate for learning and memory comprises two major subsystems: one that interconnects sensory cortices assigned to mapping physical structure and temporal coincidence with the hippocampus; and a second that interconnects sensory and motor cortices assigned to mapping temporal sequence with the basal ganglia/cerebellum and the dorsolateral frontal cortices. Normal operation of these subsystems is cooperative rather than independent.

The neuroanatomical design of the entorhinal cortex and of the sequence of cellular regions in the hippocampus to which it projects deserves special mention. This subsystem provides a set of auto-interacting convergence zones of great complexity. It is the only brain region in which signals originally triggered by neural activity in all sensory cortices and in centers for autonomic control can actually co-occur over the same neuron ensembles. As such, this is the appropiate substrate for a detector of temporal coincidences, the function that I have previously proposed for this system and that I believe to be lost in amnesia following hippocampal damage (see Damasio et al. 1985a). Such a function is compatible, in essence, with the type of physiological basis for learning proposed by Hebb, a presynaptic/postsynaptic coincidence mechanism. It is also compatible with a variety of recent cellular and molecular evidence regarding the phenomenon of long-term potentiation (LTP) and the role of NMDA-gated calcium channels as detectors of coincidence (see Gustafsson and Wigstrom 1988 for a review).

Once detection of co-occurrence takes place, the region acts via its powerful feedback system into cortical and subcortical neural stations, to assist in the creation or modification of convergence zones located in the cortices that originally projected into the entorhinal cortex. It is also apparent that such a structure, especially the autocorrelation matrix of CA_3, could store within itself binding codes of the kind I envisage for convergence zones, capable of content-addressed completion. It appears unlikely, however, that the hippocampal complex remains as a storage site for long periods, not only because of what that would mean in terms of capacity limits and risk of malfunction, but also because bilateral damage confined to the entorhinal cortex/hippocampus appears to cause only limited impairments of retrograde memory (Corkin 1984), and the same appears to be true of bilateral damage to the hippocampus alone (Zola-Morgan, Squire, and Amaral 1986). The definitive account on this issue is not available yet. In humans, the left and right hippocampi appear to be dedicated to different operations and may also operate differently in terms of their long-term role in retrieval.

Consciousness and Self-Consciousness

As previously noted, consciousness emerges when retroactivations attain a level of activity that confers salience. Coincident salient sites of activity define a set that separates itself from background activity and emerges, in psychological terms, as a conscious content on evocation as opposed to non-salient retroactivations that remain covert.

Conscious contents are all contents about which one can give testimony, in verbal narrative form, but I wish to distinguish them from the subset of conscious content we call self-conscious contents. The difference resides with the notion of self and autobiography. In my view, self-consciousness only emerges when conscious contents relative to an ongoing stimulus are experienced in the context of pertinent autobiographical data. The distinction is not specious. Patient Boswell is conscious of his environment and properly recognizes the stimuli around him but not in relation to his autobiography. Whether the stimulus is something that he ought to have recognized as unique, or something truly new to him, his ability to put it in the perspective of his life experience is restricted. His self-consciousness is thus limited and unlike that of perceivers in whom evocations generated by novel percepts are co-attended simultaneously with autobiographical evocations.

Language

The representations related to language, that is, the representations of lexical entries and grammatical operations, including syntactic rules or principles, phonology, morphology, and semantics which constitute the internalized or mental grammar, are perceived, acquired, and co-activated according to the principles articulated for non-verbal entities. As noted above, the framework does not address the issue of innate versus acquired aspects of language, although from a perspective of biological evolution as well as from the investigation of universal properties of the world's diverse languages it is likely that the substrates for combinatorial semantics and syntactical principles are partly innate.

The lexicon and language-specific aspects of the grammar, as cultural artifacts, are a subset of reality characterized by certain physical structures (the physical phonetic articulatory gestures and resultant acoustic correlates of linguistic units and structures, that is, phones, phonemes, morphemes, words, phrases, sentences, etc.) and logical relationships (grammatical functions) at multiple levels. Those external physical structures and relations constitute a corpus of signals capable of symbolizing, in sentential terms, most non-language aspects of reality at any level. By means of both feature-based physical fragment representations and binding convergence zones, the brain stores the potential for reconstituting any lexical entry or relational arrangement that it has learned, as well as the implicit rules by which novel utterances are produced and comprehended. This would not deny the possibility that highly frequent lexical entries would be recorded at large-scale fragment level, for instance, the level of an entire word stem, a condition that would be highly adaptive.

The brain not only inscribes language constituents but also provides direct and dynamic neural links between verbal representations and the representation of non-language entities or events that are signified by language. In other words, the brain embodies (materializes) in neural hardware the combined biological and cultural bond that culture has assigned between a language representation (a signifier) and a segment of non-verbal reality (a signified), to borrow Saussure's suggestive terminology. It is that neural bond that permits the two-way, uninhibitable translation process that can automatically convert non-verbal co-activation into a verbal narrative (and vice versa), at every level of neural representation and operation.

Testing the Framework

There are fundamentally four approaches to test the validity of the hypotheses expressed here.

One relies on the lesion method, the approach on which most of these ideas are based. Small focal and stable lesions in humans with neurological disease can be used to probe neuropsychological predictions based on the hypotheses expressed here. Another approach involves the use of positron emission tomography in both normals and patients with focal brain damage, to explore temporal correlations among different cortical regions activated by controlled stimuli. Another approach would involve computational modeling and testing of the concept of convergence zone. Finally, it will be possible in experiments using multiple recording from different cortical sites to test the notion of time-locked activations. For instance, in an experiment where one would record simultaneously from multiple cortical sites encompassing two sensory modalities, the following should be observed:

1. After a delay compatible with feedback firing, electrical stimulation of convergence zones would produce synchronous activity in separate cortical sites presumed to contain feature-fragments related to the convergence zone.

The regions chosen for stimulation would be guided by knowledge of neurons in association cortex that respond constantly to specific stimuli, for example, faces. Likewise, the choice of areas to guide the search for time-locked activity in early cortices would come from knowledge of areas known to be activated by the perception of a specific stimulus, for example, a face.

2. The lack of finding of time-locked activity across a vast array of cortical regions theoretically presumed to be necessary for the reconstitution of a perceptual set would constitute evidence against the notion of convergence zones proposed here.

Situating the Proposal

I see the following features of the theory as distinctive:

1. The notion that there is a major distinction between records of physical structure fragments, and records of combinatorial arrangements among those records.

2. The notion that the experience of entities or events in recall always depends on the time-locked retroactivation of fragmentary records contained in multiple sensory and motor regions and thus on momentary attempted reconstitutions of the once perceived components of reality.

3. The notion that while evocations only exist momentarily, they are the only directly inspectable aspect of brain activity. Their fleeting existence makes them no less real. Furthermore, although their existence depends on a complex machinery distributed by multiple brain sites and levels, the proposal specifies that the attempted reconstitutions occur in an anatomically restricted sector of the cerebrum.

4. The notion that certain aspects of the interaction between perceiver and reality generate domains of knowledge, which become regionalized according to neural constraints rather than conceptual-lexical labels.

5. The notion that the anatomical placement and connectional definition of a convergence zone, that is, the specification of its inputs and outputs at the point in the system that is located, also defines the knowledge domain the convergence zone embodies.

6. The role attributed to feedback projections, especially cortico-cortical, in the mechanisms of reconstitution of experiences. Feedback is distinguished from re-entry as used in the automata of Edelman and Reeke (1982). Feedback and feed-forward carry signals about activity in interconnected units but they do not transport a movable representation being entered or re-entered. Feed-forward signals mark the presence of activity upstream in the network, and indicate the whereabouts of records of activity. Feedback reactivates such upstream records. The convergence zones record those relationships and operate to route activity. No representations of

reality as we experience it are ever transferred in the system; that is, no concrete contents and no psychological information move about in the system.

7. The value accorded to representations of internal somatic states in all their aspects and levels. Somatic states are generally relegated to a subsidiary position, a matter of non-specific influence on the general workings of a network concerned with representations of external reality. In this proposal somatic states are memorized in feature-based fragment records (linked by binding convergence zones), just as external stimuli are. The source for this notion was our studies of humans with focal lesions, especially those with conditions such as anosognosia and acquired disorders of conduct (Damasio and Anderson 1989).

It is perhaps useful to compare this proposal to other recent proposals that deal with cognitive processes and the organization of their putative neural substrates. In order to do this we will choose two reference points: the classical model of cognitive architecture, as presented, for instance, by Fodor and Pylyshyn (1988), and a range of models known under the designations "parallel distributed processing" or "connectionism" (see Rumelhart and McClelland 1986).

We believe that the structures and operations described in this theory occupy an intermediate position and are compatible with the proposals in these reference points. The neural organization we propose is at the level of systems formed by macroscopic functional regions. It embodies and can implement some predicates of a classical cognitive architecture. On the other hand, it is conceivable that connectionist nets and alogrithms may realize some of the microscopic levels underlying the organization proposed here. By the same token our theory is also compatible with neuronal group selection theory (Edelman and Finkel 1984). Although the specification of neuron units in those theories is designed in "brain-style," the overall networks are not yet "brain-like." The principles of structure and operation of the machines so designed are not aimed at the superstructure organization necessary for cognitive processes such as thought, language, or consciousness; that is, to our knowledge they do not yet compel separate units to hook themselves up in a particular way capable of making a system thoughtful and self-conscious. By contrast, this theory seeks to propose precisely some of those higher organization principles. Cognitive architecture proposals refer to psychological phenomena that our framework aims at capturing. Connectionist models refer to microstructure and function situated below the levels at which our description concentrates, but that might conceivably carry on some of the necessary implementations, at least in certain sectors of the neural structure.

Acknowledgments

This work was supported by NINCDS grant PO1 NS19632. I thank my associates Hanna Damasio, Gary Van Hoesen, and Daniel Tranel for helping me shape many of the ideas summarized here, over the past decade. I also thank other colleagues who read previous versions of this manuscript over the past few years and made numerous helpful suggestions: Patricia Churchland, Victoria Fromkin, Jack Fromkin, Edward Klima, Francis Crick, Terry Sejnowski, Jaques Paillard, Marge Livingstone, David Hubel, Freda Newcombe, Ursula Bellugi, Arthur Benton, Peter Eimas and Albert Galaburda.

Notes

1. The terms "semantic" and "episodic" were proposed by Tulving (1972). Our term "generic" is largely equivalent to semantic and categorical. Elsewhere in the text I refer generic or categorical knowledge as "supraordinate" or "basic object level" knowledge, and to episodic knowledge as "subordinate level" knowledge. The latter terms are drawn from Rosch's nomenclature for taxonomic levels (Rosch et al. 1976).

2. The human areas 37 (mesially), 36, and 35 largely correspond to fields TF and TH in the monkey, and to fields TF and TH of von Economo and Koskinas in the human. They are extremely developed in the human, especially area 37. Area 38 corresponds to TG; areas 20 and 21 to TE. Area 39 (the angular gyrus) also represents a major human development and may correspond to expansion of cortices in both posterior superior temporal sulcus and inferior parietal lobule. Area 40 (the supramarginal gyrus) is largely a new human area.

3. The notion of separating storage of fragments of experience, from storage of a catalogue for their reconstitution, was inspired by our study of patient Boswell, along with the notion that a unidirectional caudal-rostral processing cascade was less likely than a multidirectional, recursive organization. The idea of convergence zones came from reflection on patterns of cortico-limbic projections, especially the multiplicity of parallel and converging channels, and the progressive size reduction of the neural convergence sites along a caudal-rostral axis. The pattern of disruption of cortico-limbic and cortico-cortical feed-forward and feedback projections in patients with Alzheimer's disease (see Van Hoesen and Damasio 1987 for a review) provided the blueprint for the construct.

References

Allman, J., Miezin, F., and McGuinness, E. (1985). Stimulus specific responses from beyond the classical receptive field: Neurophysiological mechanisms for local-global comparisons in visual neurons. *Annual Review of Neuroscience, 8,* 407–430.

Barlow, H. B. (1981). Critical limiting factors in the design of the eye and visual cortex. (The Ferrier Lecture, 1980). *Proceedings of the Royal Society London, (Biology), 212,* 1–34.

Bauer, R. M. (1984). Autonomic recognition of names and faces in prosopagnosia: A neurophysiological application of the Guilty Knowledge Test. *Neuropsychologia, 22,* 457–469.

Bruce, C. J., Desimone, R., and Gross, C. G. (1981). Visual properties of neurons in a polysensory area in superior temporal sulcus of the macaque. *Journal of Neurophysiology, 46*, 369–384.

Chavis, D. A., and Pandya, D. N. (1976). Further observations on corticofrontal connections in the rhesus monkey. *Brain Research, 117*, 369–386.

Cohen, N. J., and Squire, L. R. (1980). Preserved learning and retention of pattern-analyzing skill in amnesia: Dissociation of knowing how and knowing that. *Science, 210*, 207–210.

Corkin, S. (1984). Lasting consequences of bilateral medial temporal lobectomy: Clinical course and experimental findings in HM. *Seminars in Neurology, 4*, 249–259.

Crick, F. (1984). Function of the thalamic reticular complex: The searchlight hypothesis. *Proceedings of the National Academy of Science USA, 81*, 4586–4590.

Damasio, A. R. (1979). The frontal lobes. In K. Heilman and E. Valenstein (Eds.), *Clinical neuropsychology*. New York: Oxford University Press.

Damasio, A. R. (1985a). Disorders of complex visual processing. In M. M. Mesulam (Ed.), *Principles of behavioral neurology*. Philadelphia: Davis.

Damasio, A. R. (1985b). The frontal lobes. In K. Heilman and E. Valenstein (Eds.), *Clinical neuropsychology* (2nd edition). New York: Oxford University Press.

Damasio, A. R., and Anderson, S. (1989). Anosognosia as a domain-specific memory defect. *Journal of Clinical and Experimental Neuropsychology, 11*, 17.

Damasio, A. R., and Damasio, H. (1983). The anatomic basis of pure alexia. *Neurology, 33*, 1573–1583.

Damasio, A., Damasio, H., and Tranel, D. (1989a). Impairments of visual recognition as clues to the processes of memory. In G. M. Edelman, W. E. Gall, and W. M. Cowan (Eds.), *Signal and sense: Local and global order in perceptual maps*. In press.

Damasio, A. R., Damasio, H., and Tranel, D. (1989b). New evidence in amnesic patient Boswell: Implications for the understanding of memory. *Journal of Clinical and Experimental Neuropsychology, 11*, 61.

Damasio, A., Damasio, H., Tranel, D., Welsh, K., and Brandt, J. (1987). Additional neural and cognitive evidence in patient DRB. *Society for Neuroscience, 13*, 1452.

Damasio, A., Damasio, H., and Van Hoesen, G. W. (1982). Prosopagnosia: Anatomic basis and behavioral mechanisms. *Neurology, 32*, 331–341.

Damasio, A., Eslinger, P., Damasio H., Van Hoesen, G. W., and Cornell, S. (1985a). Multimodal amnesic syndrome following bilateral temporal and basal forebrain damage. *Archives of Neurology, 42*, 252–259.

Damasio, A., Graff-Radford, N., Eslinger, P., Damasio, H. and Kassell, N. (1985b). Amnesia following basal forebrain lesions. *Archives of Neurology, 42*, 263–271.

Damasio, A. R., and Tranel, D. (1988). Domain-specific amnesia for social knowledge. *Society for Neuroscience, 14*, 1289.

Desimone, R., Albright, T. D., Gross, C. G., and Bruce, C. (1984). Stimulus-selective responses of inferior temporal neurons in the macaque. *Journal of Neuroscience, 4*, 2051–2062.

Desimone, R., Schein, S. J., Moran, J., and Ungerleider, L. G. (1985). Contour, color and shape analysis beyond the striate cortex. *Vision Research, 25*, 441–452.

Desimone, R., and Ungerleider, L. (1989). Neural mechanisms of visual processing in monkeys. In A. Damasio (Ed.), *Handbook of neuropsychology: Disorders of visual processing* (Vol. II, pp. 267–299). Amsterdam: Elsevier.

Edelman, G. M., and Finkel, L. H. (1984). Neuronal group selection in the cerebral cortex. In G. M. Edelman, W. E. Gall, and W. M. Cowan (Eds.), *Dynamic aspects of neocortical function*. New York: Wiley.

Edelman, G. M., and Reeke, G. N. (1982). Selective networks capable of representative transformations, limited generalizations, and associative memory. *Proceedings of the National Academy of Science USA, 79*, 2091–2095.

Eslinger, P. J., and Damasio, A. R. (1985). Severe disturbance of higher cognition after bilateral frontal lobe ablation. *Neurology, 35*, 1731–1741.

Eslinger, P. J., and Damasio, A. R. (1986). Preserved motor learning in Alzheimer's disease. *Journal of Neuroscience, 6*, 3006–3009.

Farah, M. (1989). The neuropsychology of mental imagery. In A. Damasio (Ed.), *Handbook of neuropsychology: Disorders of visual processing*. (Vol. II, pp. 395–413). Amsterdam: Elsevier.

Feinberg, T., Rothi, L., and Heilman, K. (1986). Multimodal agnosia after unilateral left hemisphere lesion. *Neurology, 36*, 864–867.

Fodor, J. A., and Pylyshyn, Z. W. (1988). Connectionism and cognitive architecture: A critical analysis. *Cognition, 28,* 3–71.

Geschwind, N. (1965). Disconnexion syndromes in animals and man. *Brain, 88,* 237–294.

Geschwind, N., and Fusillo, M. (1966). Color-naming defects in association with alexia. *Archives of Neurology, 15,* 137–146.

Gilbert, C. D. (1983). Microcircuitry of the visual cortex. *Annual Review of Neuroscience, 6,* 217–247.

Goldman-Rakic, P. S. (1984). The frontal lobes: Uncharted provinces of the brain. *Trends in Neurosciences, 7,* 425–429.

Goldman-Rakic, P. S. (1988). Topography of cognition: Parallel distributed networks in primate association cortex. In: *Annual Review of Neuroscience, 2,* 137–156.

Gustafsson, B., and Wigstrom, H. (1988). Physiological mechanisms underlying long-term potentiation. *Trends in Neurosciences, 11,* 156–162.

Horenstein, S., Chamberlin, W., and Conomy, J. (1967). Infarction of the fusiform and calcarine regions: Agitated delirium and hemianopia. *Transactions of the American Neurological Association, 92,* 85–89.

Hubel, D. H., and Livingstone, M. S. (1987). Segregation of form, color, and stereopsis in primate area 18. *Journal of Neuroscience, 7,* 3378–3415.

Hubel, D. H., and Wiesel, T. N. (1977). Functional architecture of macaque monkey visual cortex. *Proceedings of the Royal Society London Series B, 198,* 1–59.

Jones, E. G., and Powell, T. P. S. (1970). An anatomical study of converging sensory pathways within the cerebral cortex of the monkey. *Brain, 93,* 793–820.

Julesz, B. (1971). *Foundation of cyclopean perception.* Chicago: University of Chicago Press.

Julesz, B. (1981). Textons, the elements of texture perception and their interaction. *Nature, 290,* 91–97.

Kosel, K. C., Van Hoesen, G. W., and Rosene, D. L. (1982) Nonhippocampal cortical projections from the entorhinal cortex in the rat and rhesus monkey. *Brain Research, 244,* 202–214.

Kosslyn S. M. (1980). *Image and mind.* Cambridge, MA: Harvard University Press.

Lettvin, J. Y., Maturana, H. R., McCulloch, W. S., and Pitts, W. H. (1959). What the frog's eye tells the frog's brain. *Proceedings of the IRE, 47,* 1940–1949.

Lewis, D. A., Campbell, M. J., Foote, S. L., and Morrison, J. H. (1986). The monoaminergic innervation of primate neocortex. *Human Neurobiology, 5,* 181–188.

Livingstone, M. S., and Hubel, D. H. (1984). Anatomy and physiology of a color system in the primate visual cortex. *Journal of Neuroscience, 4,* 309–356.

Livingstone, M. S., and Hubel, D. H. (1987a). Connections between layer 4B of area 17 and thick cytochrome oxidase stripes of area 18 in the squirrel monkey. *Journal of Neuroscience, 7,* 3371–3377.

Livingstone, M. S., and Hubel, D. H. (1987b). Psychological evidence for separate channels for the perception of form, color, movement, and depth. *Journal of Neuroscience, 7,* 3416–3468.

Livingstone, M. S., and Hubel, D. H. (1988). Segregation of form, color, movement, and depth: Anatomy, physiology, and perception. *Science, 240,* 740–749.

Lund, J. S., Hendrickson, A. E., Ogren, M. P., and Tobin, E. A. (1981). Anatomical organization of primate visual cortex area VII. *Journal of Comparative Neurology, 202,* 19–45.

Luria, A. R. (1966). *Higher cortical functions in man.* New York: Basic Books.

McCarthy, R. A., and Warrington, E. K. (1988). Evidence for modality-specific meaning systems in the brain. *Nature, 334,* 428–430.

Mesulam, M. M., Mufson, E. J., Levey, A. I., and Wainer, B. H. (1983). Cholinergic innervation of the cortex by basal forebrain: Cytochemistry and cortical connections of the septal area, diagnosal band nuclei, nucleus basalis (substantia innominata) and hypothalamus in the rhesus monkey. *Journal of Comparative Neurology, 214,* 170–197.

Milner, B., Corkin, S., and Teuber, H. L. (1968). Further analyses of the hippocampal amnesic syndrome: 14 year follow-up study of H. M. *Neuropsychologia, 6,* 215–234.

Mishkin, M., Malamut, B., and Bachevalier, J. (1984). Memories and habits: Two neural systems. In G. Lynch, J. L. McGaugh, and N. M. Weinberger (Eds.), *Neurobiology of learning and memory* (pp. 65–77). New York: Guilford Press.

Mountcastle, V. B., Lynch, J. C., and Georgopoulous, A. (1975). Posterior parietal association cortex of the monkey: Command functions for operations within extra-personal space. *Journal of Neurophysiology, 38,* 871–908.

Nauta, W. J. H. (1971). The problem of the frontal lobe: A reinterpretation. *Journal of Psychiatric Research, 8,* 167–187.

Newcombe, F., and Ratcliff, G. (1974). Agnosia: A disorder of object recognition. In F. Michel and B. Schott (Eds.), *Les syndromes de disconnexion calleuse chez l'homme.* Lyon: Colloque international de Lyon.

Paillard, J. (1971). Les determinants moteurs de l'organization de l'espace. *Cahiere de Psychologie, 14,* 261–316.

Pandya, D. N., and Kuypers, H. G. J. M. (1969). Cortico-cortical connections in the rhesus monkey. *Brain Research, 13,* 13–36.

Pandya, D. N., and Yeterian, E. H. (1985). Architecture and connections of cortical association areas. In A. Peters and E. G. Jones (Eds.), *Cerebral cortex, (Vol. 4).* New York: Plenum Press.

Penfield, W., and Jasper, W. (1954). *Epilepsy and the functional anatomy of the human brain.* Boston: Little, Brown.

Perrett, D. I., Mistlin, A. J., and Chitty, A. J. (1987). Visual neurons responsive to faces. *Trends in Neurosciences, 10,* 358–364.

Perrett, D. I., Rolls, E. T., and Caan, W. (1982). Visual neurons responsive to faces in the monkey temporal cortex. *Experimental Brain Research, 47,* 329–342.

Posner, M. I. (1980). Orienting of attention. *Quarterly Journal of Experimental Psychology, 32,* 3–25.

Rockland, K. S., and Pandya, D. N. (1979). Laminar origins and terminations of cortical connections of the occipital lobe in the rhesus monkey. *Brain Research, 179,* 3–20.

Rockland, K. S., and Pandya, D. N. (1981). Cortical connections of the occipital lobe in rhesus monkey: Interconnections between areas 17, 18, 19 and the superior temporal gyrus. *Brain Research, 212,* 249–270.

Rosch, E., Mervis, C., Gray, W., Johnson, D., and Boyes-Braem, P. (1976). Basic objects in natural categories. *Cognitive Psychology, 8,* 382–439.

Rosene, D. L., and Van Hoesen, G. W. (1977). Hippocampal efferents reach widespread areas of the cerebral cortex in the monkey. *Science, 198,* 315–317.

Rumelhart, D. E., and McClelland, J. L. (1986). *Parallel distributed processing (Vol. 1).* Cambridge, MA: MIT Press.

Sejnowski, T. J. (1986). Open questions about computation in cerebral cortex. In J. L. McClelland and D.

R. Rumelhart (Eds.), *Parallel distributed processing* (pp. 372–389). Cambridge, MA: MIT Press.

Seltzer, B., and Pandya, D. N. (1976). Some cortical projections to the parahippocampal area in the rhesus monkey. *Experimental Neurology, 50,* 146–160.

Seltzer, B., and Pandya, D. N. (1978). Afferent cortical connections and architectonics of the superior temporal sulcus and surrounding cortex in the rhesus monkey. *Brain Research, 149,* 1–24.

Squire, L. R. (1987). *Memory and brain,* New York: Oxford University Press.

Swanson, L. W., and Kohler, C. (1986). Anatomical evidence for direct projections from the entorhinal area to the cortical mantle in the rat. *Journal of Neuroscience, 6,* 3010–3023.

Tranel, D., and Damasio, A. (1985). Knowledge without awareness: An autonomic index of facial recognition by prosopagnosics. *Science, 228,* 1453–1454.

Tranel, D., and Damasio, A. (1987). Autonomic (covert) discrimination of familiar stimuli in patients with visual agnosia. *Neurology, 37,* 129; *Society for Neuroscience, 13,* 1453.

Tranel, D., and Damasio, A. (1988). Nonconscious face recognition in patients with face agnosia. *Behavioral Brain Research, 30,* 235–249.

Treisman, A., and Gelade, G. (1980). A feature-integration theory of attention. *Cognitive Psychology, 12,* 97–136.

Tulving, E. (1972). Episodic and semantic memory. In E. Tulving and W. Donaldson (Eds.), *Organization of memory.* New York: Academic Press.

Ungerleider, L. G., and Mishkin, M. (1982). Two cortical visual systems. In D. J. Ingle, R. J. W. Mansfield, and M. A. Goodale (Eds.), *The analysis of visual behavior.* Cambridge, MA: MIT Press.

Van Essen, D. C. (1985). In A. Peters and E. G. Jones (Eds.), *Functional organization of primate visual cortex.* New York: Plenum Publishing.

Van Essen, D. C., and Maunsell, J. H. R. (1983). Hierarchical organization and functional streams in the visual cortex. *Trends in Neurosciences, 6,* 370–375.

Van Hoesen, G. W., and Damasio, A. R. (1987). Neural correlates of the cognitive impairment in Alzhermer's disease. In F. Plum (Ed.), *Higher functions of the nervous system: The handbook of physiology* (pp. 871–898).

Van Hoesen, G. W., and Pandya, D. N. (1975a). Some connections of the entorhinal (area 28) and perirhinal (area 35) cortices in the rhesus monkey. I. Temporal lobe afferents. *Brain Research*, *95*, 1–24.

Van Hoesen, G. W., and Pandya, D. N. (1975b). Some connections of the entorhinal (area 28) and perirhinal (area 35) cortices in the rhesus monkey. III. Entorhinal cortex efferents. *Brain Research*, *95*, 39–59.

Van Hoesen, G. W., Pandya, D. N., and Butters, N. (1975). Some connections of the entorhinal (area 28) and perirhinal (area 35) cortices in the rhesus monkey. II. Frontal lobe afferents. *Brain Research*, *95*, 25–38.

Van Hoesen, G. W. (1982). The primate parahippocampal gyrus: New insights regarding its cortical connections. *Trends in Neurosciences*, *5*, 345–350.

Zeki, S. M. (1987). Personal communication.

Zola-Morgan, S., Squire, L. R., and Amaral, D. (1986). Human amnesia and the medical temporal region: Enduring memory impairment following a bilateral lesion limited to the CAI field of the hippocampus. *Journal of Neuroscience*, *6*, 2950–2967.

64 Visual Feature Integration and the Temporal Correlation Hypothesis

Wolf Singer and Charles M. Gray

Introduction

The Combinatorial Problem

The mammalian visual system is endowed with a nearly infinite capacity for the recognition of patterns and objects. To have acquired this capability the visual system must have solved what is a fundamentally combinatorial problem. Any given image consists of a collection of features, consisting of local contrast borders of luminance and wavelength, distributed across the visual field. For one to detect and recognize an object within a scene, the features comprising the object must be identified and segregated from those comprising other objects. This problem is inherently difficult to solve because of the combinatorial nature of visual images. To appreciate this point, consider a simple local feature such as a small vertically oriented line segment placed within a fixed location of the visual field. When combined with other line segments, this feature can form a nearly infinite number of geometrical objects. Any one of these objects may coexist with an equally large number of other possible objects. The problem becomes daunting when we expand this scenario to account for the wide array of possible local features and the fact that objects may appear in different spatial locations and orientations. The possible combinations that confront the visual system are virtually unlimited. Yet when faced with any new scene, the visual system usually has no problem in segmenting the image into its component objects within a fraction of a second. This observation suggests that the visual system has adapted a very efficient mechanism for the flexible integration of featural information.

Population Coding and the Binding Problem

Considering what is presently known about the anatomical and functional organization of the mammalian visual system, we can clearly see that the requirement for flexible integration presents a fundamental problem to our understanding. The mammalian visual cortex consists of numerous interconnected areas (Rosenquist 1985, Felleman and van Essen 1991, Sereno and Allman 1991, Payne 1993). These different regions possess numerous feedforward, feedback, and intrinsic connections and are thought to be devoted to the analysis of different but often overlapping attributes of visual images (DeYoe and Van Essen 1988, Livingstone and Hubel 1988, Merigan and Maunsell 1993). At early stages of processing, cortical areas are retinotopically organized; neurons have relatively simple receptive field properties; and cells with similar functional properties are grouped together into functional streams (DeYoe and Van Essen 1988, Livingstone and Hubel 1988). This organization gradually gives way to a largely nonretinotopic mapping at higher levels in the hierarchy, and the receptive field properties of cortical neurons concurrently increase in size and complexity owing to convergence and divergence of connections from cells in lower areas. Although the functional streams are preserved, in the sense that separate areas tend to have distinct functional properties, extensive cross-talk occurs among areas at every processing stage.

It is apparent from this organization that the representation of a perceptual object, and its attributes such as location in space or direction of motion, are not likely to be processed at a single location but rather involve a large population of cells distributed over several different cortical areas. This raises the question as to how relations are established among the spatially distributed responses occurring within and between different levels of processing. Similar binding problems are also likely to arise at lower levels. A common assumption is that the representation of a particular local feature is achieved by the graded responses of a population of neurons.

This notion is attractive because the relatively broad tuning of neuronal receptive fields suggests that single contours evoke simultaneous responses in many neurons. For the same reason, the response amplitude of any individual cell is an ambiguous descriptor of a particular feature because response vigor is equally influenced by the location of a contour and its orientation, contrast, and extent. Representation of a feature by a population of cells raises binding problems when nearby contours evoke graded responses in overlapping groups of neurons. Of the many simultaneous responses, those evoked by the same contour need to be distinguished and evaluated together to avoid interference with the responses elicited by neighboring contours. A similar need for response selection and binding arises in the context of perceptual grouping. Once the elementary features of a scene have been represented, some grouping operation must be performed to identify those neurons responding to the features of a particular object and to segregate the activity of neurons responding to the features of other objects or to the background. The implementation of units that receive converging inputs from cells whose responses require integration may allow this type of binding. The activity of such cells would then represent either elementary features or, at higher levels of processing, a particular constellation of elementary features. Finally, by iteration of this operation, units could be created that respond with high selectivity to single perceptual objects.

The analysis of single-cell receptive fields at different levels of visual processing suggests that the visual system does exploit the option of binding by convergence. Cells at higher levels of processing tend to have larger receptive fields and to respond selectively to rather complex constellations of elementary features, such as stereotypes of faces or patterns (Gross et al. 1972, Baylis et al. 1985, Desimone et al. 1985, Perrett et al. 1987, Sakai and Miyashita 1991, Fujita et al. 1992, Gallant et al. 1993). However, several observations indicate that binding is probably not achieved solely by the convergence of distributed signals onto specialized cells. Although such a mechanism could enable the rapid and unambiguous association of a limited set of key features, the number of units required to implement it as a universal mechanism scales very unfavorably with the number of possible patterns to be represented. Essentially, one cell would be required for every distinguishable feature, for each higher-order feature combination, and ultimately for every distinguishable perceptual object. Moreover, because of its inherent lack of flexibility, such a mechanism cannot easily cope with the representation of new or modified patterns. Experimental data also suggest that binding by convergence is probably not the only strategy for the association of distributed neuronal responses. The pattern-specific cells in the inferotemporal cortex are not selective for individual perceptual objects but for characteristic components of patterns (Fujita et al. 1992). Hence, these cells respond to a whole family of related patterns, and conversely, a particular pattern is likely to activate many neurons simultaneously (Young and Yamane 1992).

The representation of features and objects by the joint activity of neuronal populations has several undisputed advantages (Hebb 1949; Braitenberg 1978; Ballard et al. 1983; Singer 1985, 1990; von der Malsburg 1985; Edelman 1987; Gerstein et al. 1989; Grossberg 1980; Palm 1990; Abeles 1991). One essential feature of such assembly coding is that individual cells can participate at different times in the representation of different patterns. This strategy substantially reduces the number of cells required for the representation of different patterns and allows for greater flexibility in the generation of new representations. The assumption is that just as a particular feature can be present in many different patterns, the group of cells coding for this feature can be shared by many different representations in that they participate at different times in different assemblies of coactive neurons. The code is thus relational and the significance of an individual response depends entirely on the context set by the other members of the assembly.

To exploit the advantages of population coding, however, mechanisms are required that enable the flexible association of neuronal activity. Those active cells participating in a particular representation must be unambiguously identified as belonging together. One way to distinguish a given subset of cells is to enhance their saliency by increasing their relative firing rates (Olshausen et al. 1993). The output of these cells then has a greater impact because of temporal summation. However, selecting neurons solely on the basis of enhanced discharge rates has two potential disadvantages: First, it limits the option of encoding information about stimulus properties by the graded activity of neuronal groups. Second, it limits the number of populations that can be enhanced simultaneously without becoming confounded. Only those populations that are clearly defined by a place code would remain segregated. However, although place codes can in principle reduce ambiguity, they are again expensive in terms of neuron numbers, and most importantly, they sacrifice flexibility. To maintain the position code, interactions between assemblies in different areas must be forbidden, because they would reintroduce the ambiguity that one wants to overcome. It has been proposed, therefore, that response selection could be achieved by the synchronization of activity among a distributed population of neurons rather than by solely increasing their discharge rate (Milner 1974; von der Malsburg 1981, 1985; von der Malsburg and Schneider 1986).

Two features of cortical connectivity suggest that synchronization may be a particularly effective way of enhancing response saliency. First, cortical cells contact each other with only a few synapses whose efficiency is usually low (Komatsu et al. 1988, Mason et al. 1991, Braitenberg and Schüz 1991, Nicoll and Blakemore 1993, Thomson and West 1993). Second, synaptic transmission among cortical neurons is characterized by pronounced frequency attenua-

tion (Thomson and West 1993). Hence, increasing the summation of activity by synchronizing inputs may more effectively enhance transmission than raising discharge rates (see Abeles 1991). Another (and in this context) crucial advantage of synchronization is that it expresses unambiguous relations among neurons because it enhances selectively only the saliency of synchronous responses. Simulation studies by Softky and Koch (1993) suggest that the interval for effective summation of converging inputs is only a few milliseconds in cortical neurons. Thus, if synchronization of discharges can be achieved with a precision in the millisecond range, it can define relationships among neurons with very high precision. Moreover, if synchrony is established rapidly and maintained only over brief intervals, different assemblies can be organized in rapid temporal succession. In principle, a particular assembly can be defined by a single barrage of synchronous action potentials whereby each individual cell needs to contribute only a few spikes (Buzsaki et al. 1992). Such synchronous events are likely to be very effective in eliciting responses in target populations, and because they are statistically improbable, their information content is high.

In summary, the hypothesis predicts that the discharges of neurons undergo a temporal patterning and become synchronous if they participate in the encoding of related information. This synchronization is thought to be based on a self-organizing process that is mediated by a selective network of corticocortical and corticothalamic connections. Thus, distributed groups of coactive neurons that code for a particular feature, or at higher levels, for constellations of features corresponding to a perceptual object, would be identifiable as members of an assembly because their responses would contain episodes during which their discharges are synchronous. These theoretical considerations yield several predictions regarding the organization of neuronal assemblies in cortical networks. In the following paragraphs we enumerate these predictions and review the experimental evidence for their validation.

Predictions

The first requirement of the temporal correlation hypothesis, and the one with the most supporting evidence, predicts that cells recorded simultaneously should, under appropriate conditions, exhibit synchronous firing on a millisecond time scale. Specifically, correlated firing should occur between cells recorded in (a) the same cortical column of a given area to enable the coding of local features, (b) different columns within an area to enable the linking of spatially disparate but related features, (c) different cortical areas to provide for the binding of information across different feature categories and different locations in space, (d) the two cerebral hemispheres to link information present in the two visual hemifields, and (e) different sensory and motor modalities to contribute to the processes of sensorimotor integration. Second, the probability for intra- and interareal response synchronization should reflect some of the Gestalt criteria for perceptual grouping (Koffka 1935). Third, individual cells should be able to rapidly change the partners with which they synchronize their responses if stimulus configurations change and require new associations. Fourth, if more than one object is present in a scene, several distinct assemblies should form. Cells belonging to the same assembly should exhibit synchronous response episodes, whereas no consistent temporal relationships should exist between the discharges of neurons belonging to different assemblies. This prediction, however, may apply differently to different levels in the cortical hierarchy. In retinotopically organized areas synchronous assemblies of active cells can be spatially separated. In nonretinotopic areas, such as inferotemporal cortex, spatial segregation is less likely. Thus, few assemblies or even a single assembly of synchronously active neurons may be present at any given time. This could contribute to the serial nature of visual attention (Crick and Koch 1990). Fifth, the connections determining synchronization probability should be specific and yet modifiable according to a correlation rule whereby synaptic connections should strengthen if pre- and postsynaptic activity is often correlated, and they should weaken when there is no correlation. This is required to enhance grouping of cells that code for features that often occur in consistent relations, as is the case for features constituting a particular object. Finally, the patterns of synchronized activity should bear some specific relation to visual discrimination behavior.

Experimental Testing of Predictions

Intracolumnar Interactions

Multielectrode recording experiments have revealed neuronal response synchronization over each of the predicted spatial scales. The bulk of these studies have focused on the occurrence and properties of local (<1 mm) intra- and intercolumnar interactions. The literature contains many examples of temporal synchrony between cells recorded within the same cortical column (<200 μm separation) in different areas of the cat or monkey visual cortex (Toyama et al. 1981a,b; Michalski et al. 1983; Ts'o et al. 1986; Ts'o and Gilbert 1988; Aiple and Kruger 1988; Hata et al. 1988, 1991; Gochin et al. 1991; Schwarz and Bolz 1991; Gawne and Richmond 1993). These synchronous interactions occur among various cell types in different layers of cortex and are most often characterized by central peaks in cross-correlation histograms, which indicates a common excitatory or inhibitory input (Perkel et al. 1967). Occasionally, the correlograms exhibit peaks or troughs at specific latencies indicative of direct excitatory or inhibitory synaptic interactions.

In our own studies, the systematic search for dynamic, stimulus-dependent interactions between cortical neurons was initiated by the finding that adjacent neurons in area 17 of the cat visual cortex often transiently engage in highly synchronous discharges when presented with their preferred stimulus (Gray and Singer 1987, 1989). Groups of neurons recorded simultaneously with a single electrode discharge synchronously at intervals of 15–30 ms. These sequences of synchronous rhythmic firing occur preferentially when cells are activated with slowly moving contours of optimal orientation. They typically last a few hundred milliseconds and may occur several times during a single passage of a moving stimulus (figure 64.1). Accordingly, autocorrelation histograms computed from such response epochs often exhibit a periodic modulation (Gray and Singer 1987, 1989; Eckhorn et al. 1988; Gray et al. 1990; Schwarz and Bolz 1991). During such episodes of synchronous firing, an oscillatory field potential can be recorded by the same electrode; here, the negative phase of the signal coincides with the cells' discharges (figure 64.1). The occurrence of the local field response indicates that many cells in the vicinity of the electrode synchronize their discharges (Gray and Singer 1989). This conjecture is supported by recent multiple single-unit recordings employing new spike extraction techniques (figure 64.2) (Gray and Viana Di Prisco 1993).

The locally synchronous firing has since been observed in recordings of multiple units and local field potentials (LFP) in several areas of the visual cortex of anesthetized cats (areas 17–19 and Posteromedial Lateral Suprasylvian (PMLS)) (Eckhorn et al. 1988, 1992; Gray and Singer 1989; Gray et al. 1990; Engel et al. 1991c; Schwarz and Bolz 1991), in striate cortex of awake, behaving cats (figure 64.2) (Raether et al. 1989, Gray and Viana Di Prisco 1993) and monkeys (Eckhorn et al. 1993), in the optic tectum of awake pigeons (Neuenschwander and Varela 1993), and in area 17 (Livingstone 1991)

and area MT (Kreiter and Singer 1992, Engel et al. 1992) of anesthetized and awake, behaving monkeys, respectively. In each instance the activity is characterized by properties similar to those observed in the cat striate cortex:

1. The spike trains consist of repetitive burst discharges at semiregular 15- to 30-ms intervals.

2. Neither the onset latency nor the phase of the synchronous episodes are precisely related to the position of the stimulus within the neuron's receptive field. When cross-correlation functions are computed between responses to identical stimuli, these shift predictors reveal no correlation (Gray and Singer 1989, Gray et al. 1990, Jagadeesh et al. 1992). This finding rules out the possibility that the synchronous firing is related to some fine spatial structure in the receptive fields of cortical neurons.

3. The locally synchronous firing often, but not always, results in the appearance of a correlated field potential signal at the same frequency (Eckhorn et al. 1988, 1993; Gray and Singer 1989; Engel et al. 1991c; Livingstone 1991; Kreiter and Singer 1992).

Although these properties appear to be general, several studies have found little or no evidence for rhythmic firing in single- and multiple-unit recordings from areas V1, MT, and the inferotemporal cortex of the macaque (Bair et al. 1992, Tovee and Rolls 1992, Young et al. 1992). The reasons for these conflicting results are not readily apparent. One possibility is suggested by data from the olfactory bulb (Freeman 1975, Gray and Skinner 1988) and the hippocampus (Alonso and Garcia-Austt 1987, Buzsaki et al. 1992) where rhythmic activity is prominent at the level of field potentials but often not apparent in the autocorrelograms computed from single-unit activity. In these systems, however, the timing of spike discharges are often well correlated with the phase of the LFP. Thus, even though little evidence supports rhythmicity in the discharge of single units, the cells do participate

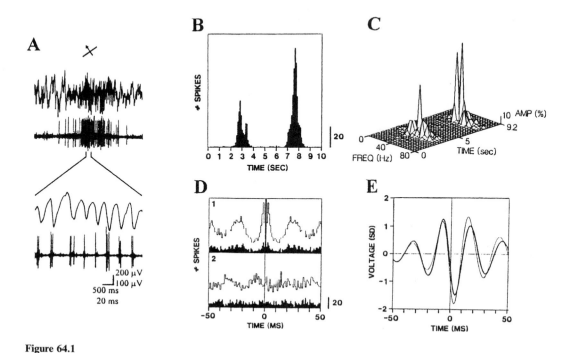

Figure 64.1

Multiunit and local field-potential responses to the presentation of an optimally oriented light bar recorded from a single electrode in area 17 of an adult cat. Oscilloscope records show the response to the preferred direction of movement on a single trial. In the upper two traces, at a slow time scale, the onset of the response is associated with an increase in high-frequency activity in the local field potential. The lower two traces display the activity at an expanded time scale. Note the presence of oscillations in the local field potential correlated with the occurrence of the unit discharges. (*b*)–(*e*) Quantitative properties of multiunit and local field potential activity recorded on a single electrode in the striate cortex of a 6-week-old kitten in response to a moving light bar of optimal orientation. (*b*) Post-stimulus-time histogram (PSTH) of the multiunit activity. The light bar was first moved over the receptive field in one direction (1–4 s) and then in the opposite direction (6–9 s). (*c*) Compressed spectral array of the LFP recorded on a single trial illustrating the time course and frequency content of the oscillatory response. The signal was bandpass filtered between 20 and 100 Hz. (*d*) Autocorrelation histograms and associated shift predictor histograms computed from the multiunit activity. The unfilled bars are for the second direction of stimulus movement (4–9 s). The shift predictors are flat, indicating that the oscillatory signals are not time locked to the visual stimulus. (*e*) Spike-triggered average of the LFP demonstrating that spike activity occurs with the highest probability during the negative phase of the field potential oscillations. The thick line represents the second direction.

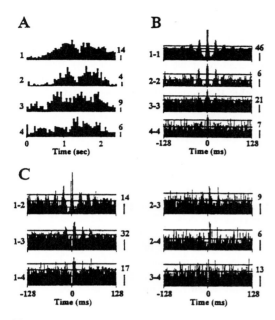

as members of a population that exhibits oscillatory behavior. The lack of rhythmicity in the spike trains is thought to be a consequence of the low firing rates of the cells, the frequency variability of the rhythmic population events, and the variation of phase differences between the single-unit discharges and the population oscillations. These sources of variance combine to produce a spike train that appears Poisson when analyzed using relatively short epochs of data.

Figure 64.2 shows an example of this effect. The sampling problem is alleviated with multi-unit recordings if several of the recorded cells are synchronized to the same rhythm. But variations in the frequency of the rhythm may yield autocorrelograms lacking any oscillatory modulation. Because the detectability of oscillatory activity in the gamma frequency range has become a major issue in the context of the correlation hypothesis, we emphasize that no conclusions regarding the formation of assemblies can be drawn from the presence or absence of oscillatory firing patterns in single-unit activity. First, oscillatory firing is in itself not thought to convey significant information regarding the stimulus. It is too variable in frequency and magnitude (Gray and Singer 1989; Engel et al. 1990; Gray et al. 1990, 1992; Ghose and Freeman 1992). Second, evidence for or against assembly formation can only be obtained with simultaneous recordings from two or more units or field-potential signals because the relevant parameter is the temporal correlation among the discharges of groups of neurons. Oscillations may provide an important mechanism for establishing synchrony, especially over large distances (König et al. 1994), but the nervous system contains many examples of nonrhythmic synchronous firing.

Figure 64.2
Rhythmic firing in area 17 of the alert cat is locally synchronous. Multiunit activity was recorded from a single electrode in area 17 while the cat maintained its gaze on a central fixation spot for a period of 2.4 s. Four single units were extracted from the multiunit recording using principal components analysis to identify separate spike waveforms. (*a*) PSTHs computed from each of the four spike trains (1–4). (*b*) Auto-correlation histograms computed from the activity of each single unit during the response to the visual stimulus. Note that oscillatory firing is readily apparent in the activity of units 1 and 2, less so for unit 3, and not at all for unit 4. (*c*) Cross-correlation histograms computed for each cell pair. Note that the discharges of cells 1 and 2 are in phase while cells 3 and 4 display a 4- to 5-ms lag relative to these cells. Also note that correlograms 1–4 and 2–4 exhibit a significant peak even though cell 4 shows little or no evidence of rhythmicitiy. The thick and thin horizontal lines passing through the histograms in (*b*) and (*c*) represent the mean and the 99% confidence interval computed from the shift predictors. (From Gray and Viana Di Prisco 1993.)

Intercolumnar Interactions

Measurements of intercolumnar correlations are fewer in number but have revealed similar patterns of synchronous firing. The majority of these studies have been performed in area 17 and have sought to determine the relationship between receptive field properties and the occurrence of synchronous firing. Two general findings have emerged. First, the probability and strength of correlated firing falls off with distance in cortex (Michalski et al. 1983, Ts'o et al. 1986, Aiple and Kruger 1988, Ts'o and Gilbert 1988, Gray et al. 1989, Engel et al. 1990, Kruger 1990, Hata et al. 1991, Schwarz and Bolz 1991). Cells that have overlapping receptive fields and that are separated by less than 2 mm are far more likely to exhibit synchronous firing than cells with nonoverlapping fields that have a separation greater than 2 mm. Nevertheless, numerous examples of long-range synchronous firing have been observed over distances spanning several hypercolumns in area 17 (Ts'o et al. 1986, Ts'o and Gilbert 1988, Gray et al. 1989, Engel et al. 1990, Schwarz and Bolz 1991).

The second general finding obtained from these studies is that intercolumnar correlated firing occurs with greater probability for cells that have similar receptive field properties. Correlations tend to occur most often between cells with similar orientation preferences (Ts'o et al. 1986, Ts'o and Gilbert 1988, Gray et al. 1989, Hata et al. 1991, Schwarz and Bolz 1991), similar ocular dominances (Ts'o et al. 1986, Ts'o and Gilbert 1988), and similar color selectivities (Ts'o and Gilbert 1988). Moreover, cells with specific types of complex and simple receptive fields tend to interact with other cells of the same type (Ts'o et al. 1986, Schwarz and Bolz 1991), although there are exceptions to this, as yet, poorly defined rule (Schwarz and Bolz 1991). These long-range correlations have generally been thought to reflect the specificity of intra-cortical horizontal axonal connections that preferentially link functional columns with similar feature specificities (Ts'o et al. 1986; Ts'o and Gilbert 1988; Martin and Whitteridge 1984; Gilbert and Wiesel 1983, 1989; but see Matsubara et al. 1987). In most instances, however, inter-

columnar correlation measurements have been performed using two stimuli, one optimal for each of the two recorded cells. Cells that have different receptive field properties are thus activated by stimuli that have different features. Within the context of the theory presented here, such a featural difference in the stimuli introduces a potential cue for the segregation of assemblies and the consequent absence of correlated firing. This point is discussed in detail below.

When interactions occur over larger tangential distances in the cortex, the cross-correlograms exhibit two other prominent features. First, the peak in the histograms is usually centered around zero delay. The half width at half height of this peak is often on the order of 2–3 ms, indicating that most of the action potentials occur nearly simultaneously (Ts'o and Gilbert 1986, Gray et al. 1989, Schwarz and Bolz 1991). Second, when cells engage in long-distance synchronization, the firing patterns of the local groups often exhibit synchronous repetitive discharges as described above. The central peak in the correlogram is thus often flanked on either side by troughs that result from refractory periods between the synchronous bursts. When the duration of these pauses is sufficiently constant throughout the episode of synchronization, the cross-correlograms show a periodic modulation with additional side peaks and troughs (Eckhorn et al. 1988, Gray et al. 1989, Engel et al. 1990, Schwarz and Bolz 1991, Livingstone 1991). Synchronous oscillations are readily apparent if the LFP is also recorded from each electrode (figure 64.3) (Engel et al. 1990, Gray et al. 1992). This pattern of rhythmic synchronization rarely, if ever, occurs in the absence of visual stimulation. Such intercolumnar synchronization has been observed over distances of up to 7 mm in the cat (Gray et al. 1989) and up to 5 mm in area V1 of the squirrel monkey (M. Livingstone, personal communication). In the cat, cells separated by more than 2 mm that have nonoverlapping receptive fields are more likely to exhibit synchronous firing if they have similar orientation preferences (Gray et al. 1989, Engel et al. 1990, Schwarz and Bolz 1991). If the cells are separated by less than 2 mm and have overlapping receptive fields, the synchronous firing occurs largely irrespective of the preferred orientation of the cells (Gray et al. 1989, Engel et al. 1990), provided that they can be activated with a single stimulus.

Interareal and Interhemispheric Interactions

In agreement with the predictions of the temporal correlation hypothesis, response synchronization has also been found between groups of cells located in different cortical areas. In the cat, stimulus-evoked synchronous firing has been observed between cells in areas 17 and 18 (Eckhorn et al. 1988, 1992; Nelson et al. 1992b); between cells in areas 17 and 19, and 18 and 19 (Eckhorn et al. 1992); between cells in area 17 and area PLMS, an area specialized for motion processing (figure 64.4) (Engel et al. 1991c); and between cells in area 17 of the two hemispheres (Engel et al. 1991a, Eckhorn et al. 1992, Nelson et al. 1992a). In the macaque, synchronous firing has been observed among neurons in areas V1 and V2 (Bullier et al. 1992, Roe and Ts'o 1992, Nowak et al. 1994).

In the studies of Nelson et al. (1992b) interareal synchronous firing in cats occurs spontaneously and during the presentation of visual stimuli. The interactions span a wide tripartite range of temporal scales, which produces correlograms with central peaks of narrow, medium, and broad width. The narrow coupling is most often seen between cells that have overlapping receptive fields with similar properties. The broader coupling encompasses a much wider range of receptive-field separations and orientation-preference differences (Nelson et al. 1992b). Synchronous interactions between cells in V1 and V2 in the monkey show similar broad peaks. Synchrony occurs between cells that have both overlapping and nonoverlapping receptive fields (Bullier et al. 1992, Nowak et al. 1994) and

is most frequent between cells of similar color selectivity in the two areas (Roe and Ts'o 1992).

In the studies of Eckhorn et al. (1988, 1992) and Engel et al. (1991a,c), interareal and interhemispheric synchronous firing occurred primarily, if not exclusively, during coactivation of the cells by visual stimuli, and was particularly pronounced during periods of oscillatory firing. These data reveal several additional similarities to the intra- and intercolumnar oscillatory interactions. The occurrence of synchronous firing depends on, but is not locked to, the visual stimulus. The probability of occurrence and the magnitude of interareal temporal correlations are somewhat greater for cells that have overlapping receptive fields and similar orientation preferences. When receptive fields are nonoverlapping and cells are activated with two stimuli, synchronization probability is greatest when the stimuli move at the same speed in the same direction (Engel et al. 1991a,c). Interhemispheric synchrony also requires the integrity of the corpus callosum. Surgical sectioning of this structure markedly reduces the probability of synchronous firing between the two hemispheres (Engel et al. 1991a, Nelson et al. 1992a). These studies provide the first results demonstrating that corticocortical connections are critical for the establishment of synchronous firing.

Evidence for Synchrony in Nonvisual Structures

In the preceding discussion, we have reviewed the evidence for synchronous activity revealed by multielectrode recordings from visual cortical areas. Comparable multicell recordings are still rare in nonvisual structures, but considerable data are available from field-potential studies. The data indicate that synchronous rhythmic activity occurs over a range of spatial scales in several different cortical and subcortical systems throughout the brains of mammals (Basar and Bullock 1992, Gray 1993, Singer 1993).

In the mammalian olfactory system, for example, 40- to 80-Hz oscillatory activity is evoked

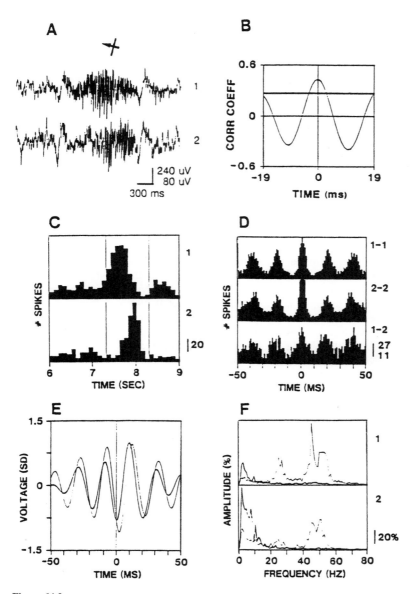

Figure 64.3
The local field potential and multiunit activity recorded at two sites in area 17 separated by 7 mm show similar temporal properties and correlated interactions. (*A*) Plot of the LFP responses (1–100 Hz bandpass) recorded on a single trial to the presentation of two optimally oriented light bars passing over the receptive fields of the recorded

during inspiration in both the olfactory bulb and piriform cortex (Adrian 1950; Freeman 1975, 1978; Bressler 1984). This activity is synchronous over a scale of several millimeters both within and between the two structures (Bressler 1984, 1987; Freeman 1987). The patterns of activity that emerge during these coherent states correspond to specific odors, the animal's past experience with the odors, and their behavioral significance (Freeman 1987). The oscillatory activity by itself is not thought to convey any specific information; instead, it is viewed as a mechanism for establishing synchrony among large populations of coactive cells (Freeman 1987).

Similar rhythmic activities have been discovered in both the somatosensory and motor cortices of cats and monkeys. In the studies of Bouyer and colleagues, field potential oscillations in the beta and gamma ranges occur in the somatosensory cortex when animals are in a state of focused attention (Bouyer et al. 1981). These rhythmic activities are synchronous over relatively large areas of cortex (Bouyer et al. 1987), occur in phase with similar activity in the ventrobasal thalamus (Bouyer et al. 1981), and are regulated by dopaminergic input from the ventral tegmentum (Montaron et al. 1982). Oscillatory field potential and unit activities in the range of 20–40 Hz have also been observed in

the motor cortex of alert monkeys (Murthy and Fetz 1992, Sanes and Donoghue 1993). These signals are synchronous over widespread areas of the motor cortical map within and between the two cerebral hemispheres, between the visual and motor cortices (E. Fetz, personal communication), and between the motor and somatosensory cortices. They are also enhanced in amplitude when the animals are performing new and complicated motor acts (Murthy and Fetz 1992). The rhythms are suppressed, however, during the execution of trained movements (Sanes and Donoghue 1993).

The hippocampus exhibits several forms of synchronous rhythmic activity that are associated with particular behavioral states. Foremost among these is the theta rhythm, a 4- to 10-Hz oscillation of neuronal activity that occurs during active movement and alert immobility. Theta field potentials are often synchronous between the two hemispheres and over distances extending up to 8 mm along the longitudinal axis of the hippocampus (Bland et al. 1975). Local populations of cells also exhibit a high degree of synchronous firing during theta activity (Kuperstein et al. 1986). Furthermore, two other hippocampal neuronal rhythms have been discovered. One has a frequency of 30–90 Hz, occurs during a variety of behavioral states (Buzsaki et al. 1983, Leung 1992, Bragin et al.

neurons at each site. The peaks of the responses overlap in time but are not in precise register. (*B*) The average cross-correlogram computed between the two LFP signals (20–100 Hz bandpass) at a latency corresponding to the peak of the oscillatory responses. The thick horizontal line represents the 95% confidence limit for significant deviation from random correlation. (*C*) PSTHs of the multiunit activity recorded over 10 trials at the same two cortical sites as shown in panel *A*. Again the responses overlap but are not in precise register. (*D*) Auto- (1–1, 2–2) and cross- (1–2) correlograms of the multiunit activity recorded at each site. Note the presence of clear periodicity in each correlogram, which indicates that the responses are oscillatory and that they show a consistent phase relationship. (*E*) Plots of the spike-triggered averages of the LFP signals at each site computed over all 10 trials. The thick and thin lines correspond to electrodes 1 and 2 respectively. Note that the peak negativity of the waveform is correlated with the occurrence of neuronal spikes at 0-ms latency. (*F*) Normalized average power spectrum of the LFP signals computed from periods of spontaneous (*thick line*) and stimulus-evoked (*thin line*) activity. The frequency of the activity is similar in both the autocorrelograms of the multiunit activity (MUA) and the power spectra of the LFPs. (From Gray et al. 1992.)

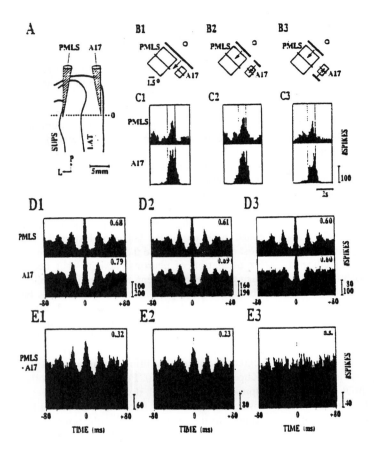

Figure 64.4
Interareal synchronization is sensitive to global stimulus features. (*a*) Position of the recording electrodes. A17, area 17; LAT, lateral sulcus; SUPS, suprasylvian sulcus; P, posterior; L, lateral. (*b1–3*) Plots of the receptive fields of the PMLS and area 17 cells. The diagrams depict the three stimulus conditions tested. The circle indicated the visual field center. (*c1–3*) PSTHs for the three stimulus conditions. The vertical lines indicate 1-s windows for which auto- and cross-correlation histograms were computed. (*d1–3*) Comparison of the autocorrelation histograms computed for the three stimulus paradigms. (*e1–3*) Cross-correlation histograms computed for the three stimulus conditions. Note that the response amplitudes are minimally affected by changes of stimulus configuration, whereas the synchronization of activity is largely absent for stimuli moving in opposite directions. (From Engel et al. 1991c.)

1994), and is both locally and bilaterally synchronous. Another more recently discovered signal with a frequency around 200 Hz is associated with alert immobility and the presence of sharp waves in the hippocampal EEG (Buszaki et al. 1992, Ylinen et al. 1994). These events have been termed population oscillations because single cells do not exhibit high-frequency periodic firing. Rather they fire at low rates in synchrony with the surrounding population of cells, which in the composite yields a periodic signal that is synchronous over distances up to 2.1 mm (Buzsaki et al. 1992, Ylinen et al. 1994).

Oscillatory components in the beta- and gamma-frequency ranges have also been documented in humans. In several early studies, depth recordings of the local EEG from several cortical and subcortical sites revealed episodes of synchronous rhythmic activity during particular behavioral states (Sem-Jacobsen et al. 1956, Chatrian et al. 1960, Perez-Borja 1961). Surface EEG and MEG recordings have revealed gamma-frequency components in the auditory evoked potential (Galambos et al. 1981, Basar 1988, Sheer 1989, Pantev et al. 1991, Tiitinen et al. 1993), the somatomotor cortex (Murphy et al. 1994), and a broad distribution over the entire cerebral mantle (Ribary et al. 1991). Recently, however, direct surface recordings of the EEG over the somatosensory cortex in humans have revealed that gamma-band activity does not predominate over activity in other frequency ranges (Menon et al. 1994). In spite of this there is ample evidence from animals and humans that brain structures other than the visual cortex engage in synchronous rhythmic activity in the beta- and gamma-frequency ranges.

Stimulus Dependence of Response Synchronization

Another important prediction of the temporal correlation hypothesis is that the probability for distributed cells to join an assembly should reflect the Gestalt criteria, according to which, features in images tend to be grouped together into objects. Described early this century (see Koffka 1935), these criteria include the categories of proximity, similarity, continuity, and common fate, reflecting the fact that objects typically consist of features that exist in close proximity; that have common properties such as form, color, and depth; that are spatially contiguous; and that, when they move, tend to do so with a common or linked direction of motion. Evidence reviewed in the previous section supports the notion that response synchronization satisfies the criteria of proximity and similarity.

Additional evidence suggests that response synchronization fulfills the criteria of continuity and common fate. In one study, Gray et al. (1989) recorded multiunit activity from two locations separated by 7 mm in striate cortex. The receptive fields of the cells were nonoverlapping, had nearly identical orientation preferences, and were spatially displaced along the axis of preferred orientation. This arrangement enabled stimulation of the cells with bars of the same orientation under three different conditions: two bars moving in opposite directions, two bars moving in the same direction, and one long bar moving across both fields coherently. Under these conditions, no significant correlation was found in the first case; a weak correlation was seen in the second; and a robust synchronization was found in the third case. This effect occurred in spite of the fact that the firing rates of the two cells and the oscillatory patterning of the responses were similar in the three conditions (Gray et al. 1989). Further support for the notion that response synchronization is influenced by stimulus continuity was obtained in a study by Schwarz and Bolz (1991). They demonstrated that the probability of detecting intercolumnar synchronization between standard complex cells in layer 5 and simple or complex cells in layer 6 is highest not only when the cells have the same orientation preferences but when their receptive fields are aligned colinearly.

In a related experiment, Engel et al. (1991c) obtained evidence that the criteria of continuity and common fate are also satisfied by interareal interactions. They made simultaneous recordings from cells in areas 17 and PMLS (a motion-sensitive area in the lateral suprasylvian sulcus of the cat) that had nonoverlapping receptive fields with similar orientation preference and colinear alignment. This technique allowed them to examine the effects of continuity and coherent motion on response synchronization using the paradigm described above. They found little or no correlation when the cells were activated by oppositely moving contours, a weak but significant correlation in response to two bars moving in the same direction, and a robust synchronization when the cells were coactivated by a single long bar moving over both fields (figure 64.4) (Engel et al. 1991c). Recently, Sillito et al. (1994) demonstrated an analogous influence of stimulus continuity and coherent motion on the synchronization of activity in the lateral geniculate nucleus (LGN). They showed that cells having nonoverlapping receptive fields displayed little or no evidence of synchronization when activated by a pair of stationary spots. If, however, the cells were driven by a single long bar or an extended grating drifting over both receptive fields, the cells often engaged in synchronous firing. This effect was abolished by removal of the overlying visual cortex, suggesting that the thalamic synchronization is controlled by feedback from the visual cortex.

These findings, combined with the earlier results, suggest that the global properties of visual stimuli can influence the magnitude of synchronization between widely separated cells located within and between different cortical areas and thalamus. Single contours, but also spatially separate contours, which move coherently and therefore appear as parts of a single figure, are more efficient in inducing synchrony among the responding cell groups than oppositely moving contours that appear as parts of independent figures. This finding demonstrates that synchro-nization probability and magnitude depends not only on the spatial separation of cells and on their feature preferences, but also on the configuration of the stimuli.

A central prediction of the correlation hypothesis posits that individual cells must be able to change the partners with which they become synchronized in order to join different assemblies at different times. Thus, as the features in an image change, the relationships among the activity patterns of the cells responding to those features should change in a way that reflects the Gestalt properties of the image.

Tests of this prediction have been conducted by Engel et al. (1991b) in cat area 17 and by Kreiter and colleagues in area MT of the anesthetized monkey (Kreiter et al. 1992). In the cat, multiunit activity was recorded from up to four electrodes that had a spacing of approximately 0.5 mm. The proximity of the electrodes yielded recordings in which all the cells had overlapping receptive fields and covered a broad range of orientation preferences. This configuration enabled these investigators to compare the correlation of activity among cells coactivated by either one or two moving bars. In the majority of cases, cells with different orientation preferences fired synchronously when coactivated by a single bar of intermediate orientation. But when the same cells were activated by two independent bars of differing orientation, moving in different directions, the responses were not synchronized (Engel et al. 1991b).

Kreiter and Singer (1994) recently demonstrated that this process is a general property of the visual cortex and is not confined to the visual cortex of anesthetized cats. Recordings of multiunit activity were made from two electrodes in area MT of an alert macaque. The electrode separation was less than 0.5 mm, which yielded cells with nearly completely overlapping receptive fields but often differing directional preferences. This setup enabled them to repeat the earlier experiment conducted in the cat (Engel et al. 1991b) by coactivating the cells with one bar and then with two independently moving bars. The firing of the cells was synchronized when responses were evoked by a single bar moving over both fields but not when the responses were evoked by two independent bars (figure 64.5) (Kreiter and Singer 1994). Repeated measurements of the responses from the same cells under identical conditions revealed that the effect was stable.

Taken together, these data (Engel et al. 1991b, Kreiter and Singer 1994) demonstrate that two overlapping, but independent, stimuli evoke simultaneous responses in a large array of spatially interleaved neurons. The active neuronal populations can become organized into two assemblies that are distinguished by the temporal coherence of activity within and the lack of coherence between the cell groups responding to the two different stimuli. Cells representing the same stimulus exhibit synchronized response epochs, while no consistent correlations occur between the responses of cells that are activated by different stimuli. This observation suggests that the pattern of temporal correlation among the responses of individual cells provides additional information to signal that two objects are present in nearby or overlapping regions of the visual field. More generally, these examples demonstrate that under appropriate conditions visual stimulus properties can influence the synchronization of activity of two or more groups of neurons, thus supporting the hypothesis that response synchrony can serve to establish relations between spatially distributed features in a visual image. It must be pointed out, however, that there do exist examples in which the correlated firing of neurons in visual cortex is not influenced by changes in the pattern of visual stimulation (Schwarz and Bolz 1991). Thus, further experiments are required to rigorously determine the conditions under which this type of dynamic correlation occurs.

The theoretical arguments put forth here with respect to visual processing also apply to tactile and auditory processing, motor control, and higher cognitive functions. Hence, transient synchronization of distributed neuronal responses should also occur within and across other regions of cortex. Moreover, these temporal correlations of neuronal firing should be flexible. Single cells or populations of cells should be able to participate in different assemblies at different times depending on stimulus properties or the context of a particular behavioral task. Supporting this prediction are recent studies in the alert monkey that were based on multineuron activities in the auditory and frontal cortex (Ahissar et al. 1992, Vaadia and Aertsen 1992) and on field potential signals in sensory, motor, parietal, and frontal cortices (Bressler et al. 1993). These investigators found instances in which changes in either stimulus properties or behavioral-task conditions led to marked changes in the correlated firing of two neurons without an appreciable change in their firing rate (Ahissar et al. 1992, Vaadia and Aertsen 1992) or a change in the pattern of multiregional coherence of activity between different cortical areas (Bressler et al. 1993). These findings suggest that dynamic, stimulus- and context-dependent modulations of response synchronization are a general property of cortical networks.

Experience-Dependent Influences on Intraareal Synchronization

The temporal correlation hypothesis implies that assemblies based on synchronous firing patterns form as a result of the synaptic interactions among the constituent cells. The experiments on interhemispheric synchronization have confirmed this supposition by identifying corticocortical connections as the anatomical substrate for synchrony. Therefore, the criteria by which particular features are grouped together must be built into the functional architecture of the corticocortical connections. If this architecture is specified entirely by genetic instructions, perceptual grouping criteria will have to be regarded

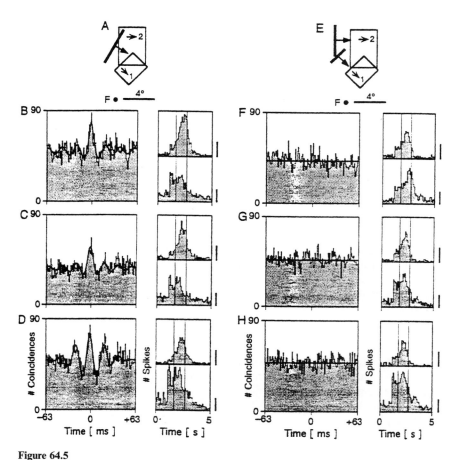

Figure 64.5
Stimulus-dependent synchronization in area MT of an awake macaque. (*a, e*) Plots of the receptive fields and the stimulus configurations. Panels (*a*)–(*d*) illustrate the single-bar configuration, while panels (*e*)–(*h*) show the results when two bars are moved simultaneously but in different directions over the two receptive fields. Both stimulus conditions were applied in six alternating blocks, each containing 10 trials. Cross-correlation histograms and PSTHs computed for the single-bar condition appear in panels (*b*), (*c*), and (*d*) and those for the dual bar condition in panels (*f*), (*g*), and (*h*). The thin vertical lines in the PSTHs mark the time window in which the cross-correlation histograms were computed. The scale bars correspond to 40 spikes. Note that the single-bar stimulus results in a clear synchronization, as shown by the pronounced peaks in the cross-correlograms, while no synchronization occurs with the two-bar stimulus. (From Kreiter and Singer 1994.)

as genetically determined. If the architecture is modifiable by activity and hence experience, some of these criteria could be acquired by learning. The numerous similarities in the layout of cortical connections indicate that some of the basic principles of cortical organization are determined genetically. But extensive evidence also supports epigenetic modifications. In mammals, corticocortical connections develop mainly postnatally (Innocenti and Frost 1979, Price and Blakemore 1985, Luhmann et al. 1986, Callaway and Katz 1990) and attain their final specificity through an activity-dependent selection process (Innocenti and Frost 1979, Luhmann et al. 1990, Callaway and Katz 1991).

Direct evidence for experience-dependent modifications of synchronizing connections comes from experiments with strabismic kittens (Löwel and Singer 1992). The primary visual cortex of kittens raised with artificially induced strabismus is split into two subpopulations of cells of about equal size, each responding rather selectively to stimulation of one eye only (Hubel and Wiesel 1965b). The changes in the thalamocortical connections elicited by squint suggest that input to cells driven by different eyes is only rarely correlated. A recent study showed that horizontal intercolumnar connections were reorganized in strabismic kittens, and unlike in normal animals, no longer connected neurons receiving input from different eyes (Löwel and Singer 1992). This finding suggests that experience-dependent selection of cortical connections occurs according to a correlation rule in a manner similar to other levels of the visual system (for review, see Stryker 1990). Moreover, in strabismic cats response synchronization does not occur between cell groups connected to different eyes, whereas the incidence and magnitude of synchronization appears normal between cell groups connected to the same eye (König et al. 1993). Because strabismic subjects are unable to bind signals conveyed by different eyes into coherent percepts (von Noorden 1990), this result also supports the hypothesis that response synchronization serves binding.

Further indications for a relation between response synchrony and visual function come from a recent study of strabismic cats that had developed amblyopia, a condition in which the spatial resolution and perception of patterns through one of the eyes is impaired. The identification of neuronal correlates of these deficits in animal models of amblyopia has remained inconclusive because the contrast sensitivity and spatial acuity of neurons in the retina and in the lateral geniculate nucleus were found to be normal, and evidence for correlates of the perceptual deficits in the visual cortex has remained controversial (see Crewther and Crewther 1990, Blakemore and Vital Durand 1992). However, multielectrode recordings from the striate cortex of cats exhibiting behaviorally verified amblyopia have revealed significant differences in the synchronization behavior of cells driven by the normal and the amblyopic eye. The synchronization of activity among cells connected to the amblyopic eye was much less than that observed between cells responsive to the normal eye (figure 64.6) (Roelfsema et al. 1994). This difference was even more pronounced for responses elicited by gratings of high spatial frequency. Apart from these differences, the response properties of the cells appeared normal. Thus, cells connected to the amblyopic eye continued to respond vigorously to gratings whose spatial frequency had been too high to be discriminated with the amblyopic eye in the preceding behavioral tests. These results suggest that disturbed temporal coordination of responses may be one of the neuronal correlates of the amblyopic deficit.

Mechanisms Controlling Oscillations and Their Functional Importance

As reviewed above, synchronous activity is often associated with oscillatory firing patterns. This common finding raises the question of how oscillatory processes are generated and whether

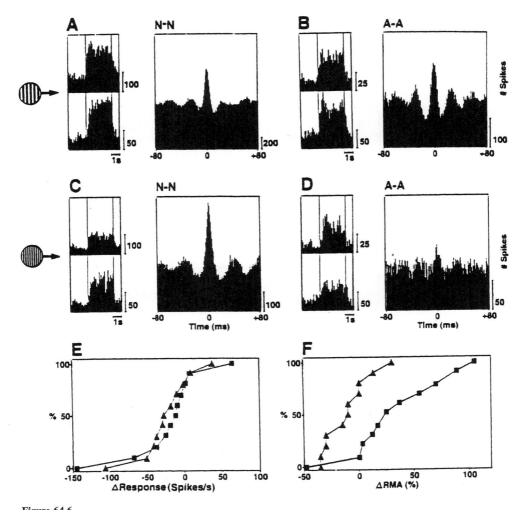

Figure 64.6

PSTHs (left panels) and associated cross-correlograms (right panels) computed from the activity recorded in response to the presentation of gratings of different spatial frequencies in cats with strabismic amblyopia. (*a*)–(*d*) Neuronal responses to low (*a*, *b*) and high (*c*, *d*) spatial frequencies gratings, recorded simultaneously from two cell groups driven by the normal eye (N-sites) (*a*, *c*) and two groups driven by the amblyopic eye (A-sites) (*b*, *d*), respectively. Note that response amplitudes decrease at the higher spatial frequency in both cases, while the relative modulation amplitude of the cross-correlogram increases for the N-N pair but decreases for the A-A pair. (*e*) Cumulative distribution functions of the differences in response amplitudes to low and high spatial frequency gratings of optimal orientation. N-sites, squares ($n = 53$); A-sites, triangles ($n = 35$); abscissa, responses to high spatial-frequency minus responses to low spatial-frequency gratings. Note the similarity of the two distributions ($P > 0.1$). (*f*) Cumulative distribution functions of the differences between relative modulation amplitudes (DRMA) of cross-correlograms computed from responses to high and low spatial-frequency gratings of N-N pairs (squares; $n = 24$) and A-A pairs (triangles; $n = 11$). DRMA values (abscissa) were calculated by subtracting the relative modulation amplitude obtained with the low spatial frequency from that obtained with the high spatial frequency. The difference between the DRMA distributions of N-N pairs and A-A pairs is significant ($P < 0.001$). (From Roelfsema et al. 1994.)

they contribute to synchronization. Our discussion of these mechanisms focuses on activity in the gamma-frequency band (30–80 Hz) because this is the range in which the majority of synchronous activity in the visual cortex has been described. There are three basic mechanisms likely to underlie the generation of oscillatory firing in the visual cortex. The first and most obvious mechanism to consider is oscillatory afferent input. The periodic temporal structure of cortical responses could result from rhythmic input from the lateral geniculate nucleus (LGN) or other thalamic nuclei. Support for this notion has come from studies demonstrating robust oscillatory activity in the frequency range of 30–80 Hz in both the retina and the LGN (Doty and Kimura 1963, Fuster et al. 1965, Laufer and Verzeano 1967, Arnett 1975, Ariel et al. 1983, Munemori et al. 1984, Ghose and Freeman 1992). In both structures, the rhythmic activity is present in a subpopulation of roughly 10–20% of the cells, and it occurs spontaneously, in response to diffuse changes in illumination or specific stimulation of the receptive field (Laufer and Verzeano 1967, Arnett 1975, Robson and Troy 1987, Ghose and Freeman 1992). In some cases, however, neuronal oscillations in the LGN or perigeniculate nucleus are suppressed or not influenced by visual stimuli (Ghose and Freeman 1992, Pinault and Deschenes 1992). In spite of its prevalence, and surprising regularity, it is unlikely that oscillatory activity in the LGN can account for the cortical oscillations and their long-range synchronization. Rather, the data of Sillito et al. (1994) indicate that one form of thalamic synchronization depends on corticofugal influences.

A second mechanism likely to underlie the generation of cortical oscillations relies on intracortical network interactions. In this scenario, cyclical changes in firing probability are thought to arise through synaptic interactions of populations of excitatory and inhibitory neurons (Freeman 1968, 1975; Wilson and Cowan 1972; Bush and Douglas 1991; Wilson and Bower

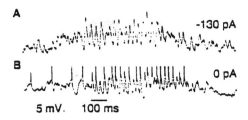

Figure 64.7
Intracellular recording of the response of a complex cell in area 17 of an anesthetized cat to the presentation of an optimally oriented light bar passed over the cell's receptive field. (*a*) Cell hyperpolarized by the injection of −130 pA of current. (*b*) The action potentials have been truncated. (From Jagadeesh et al. 1992.)

1992; Bush et al. 1993). Evidence supporting this hypothesis has come from intracellular recordings in cat striate cortex in vivo (Jagadeesh et al. 1992, Bringuier et al. 1992). These studies have revealed both high (30–60 Hz) and low (10–20 Hz) frequency oscillations of membrane potential closely resembling the properties of neuronal oscillations observed extracellularly (Gray and Singer 1989). The membrane potential oscillations occur during visual stimulation: They are orientation specific, and occur less often in cells receiving monosynaptic input from the LGN (Jagadeesh et al. 1992). Moreover, spike discharges occur on the depolarizing phase of the oscillation, which mirrors the extracellularly observed negativity (figure 64.7) (compare to figure 64.1). When the cells exhibiting these fluctuations are hyperpolarized below the firing threshold by current injection, the visually evoked oscillations increase in amplitude but do not change in frequency (figure 64.7) (Bringuier et al. 1992, Jagadeesh et al. 1992). These data suggest that the rhythmic fluctuations of membrane potential reflect a synchronous pattern of excitatory synaptic input onto the cells that arises in the cortex.

These data do not, however, rule out the possibility that cortical oscillations may arise as a consequence of activity in a subpopulation of cells that are intrinsically oscillatory (Llinas 1988). Support for this conjecture has been obtained from both in vitro and in vivo intracellular recordings. In the former case, a subpopulation of inhibitory interneurons in layer 4 of the rat frontal cortex exhibited subthreshold, voltage-dependent, 10- to 50-Hz oscillations in membrane potential in response to depolarizing current injection (Llinas et al. 1991). These cells, if present in the visual cortex, would be expected to produce rhythmic hyperpolarizing potentials in their postsynaptic targets, a result for which the experimental evidence is currently limited (Ferster 1986). Recent intracellular recordings in vivo from cat striate cortex have revealed a subpopulation of cells that fire in regular repetitive bursts at 20–70 Hz in response to visual stimulation and intracellular depolarizing current injection (McCormick et al. 1993). The firing properties of these cells are very similar to the burst-firing cells observed extracellularly in cat visual cortex (Hubel and Wiesel 1965a, Gray et al. 1990, Gray and Viana Di Prisco 1993), and they are distinct from the previously defined class of intrinsic bursting cells known to be present in layer 5 (Connors 1982, McCormick et al. 1985). Whether these cells are excitatory or inhibitory is unknown, but in either case their activation might serve to drive a local network of cells into a pattern of synchronous oscillation.

Conclusions

Visual scenes are inherently complex and can exist in a nearly infinite combinatorial variety. In spite of this complexity, mammalian species have evolved a virtually unlimited capacity for the rapid recognition of patterned visual information, which suggests that the visual system possesses effective mechanisms to enable the flexible integration of featural information. Anatomical and physiological evidence indicates that the featural attributes of visual images are processed in different parts of the visual cortex. Therefore, the representation of perceptual objects is not likely to take place at a single location but rather to involve the concerted action of large populations of cells distributed throughout the visual cortex. This raises the fundamental question, often referred to as the binding problem, of how the visual system establishes the appropriate relationships among the large number of neurons that respond to the many features in any given visual scene. Such relationships must be specific and yet flexible in order to cope with the combinatorial variety of features constituting visual images.

The experimental results reviewed in this chapter are compatible with the hypothesis that synchronization of neuronal activity on a millisecond time scale may be exploited to link featural information that is represented in different parts of the cortex (Milner 1974; von der Malsburg 1981, 1985). In this view the identification of related features, for example those belonging to the same perceptual object, is achieved by the temporal coincidence of the neuronal discharges evoked by those features. In a distributed network, such as the neocortex, where any given cell contacts any other cell with only a few synapses, but where individual cells receive converging input from many thousands of different cells (Braitenberg and Schüz 1991), synchronization may also be a particularly efficient mechanism to increase the saliency of activity. Thus, synchronization can, in principle, be used to select with high spatial and temporal resolution those activity patterns that belong together and to enhance the effect of this activity so it may be evaluated for further processing. The proposal presented here is that this selection is achieved in a distributed and parallel fashion by the system of corticocortical association fibers. In this context, the function of these connections consists largely of adjusting the timing of discharges rather than modulating discharge rates. Synchronization will of course affect discharge rates by enabling more effective summation than asynchronous inputs.

Hence, modulation of response amplitude and synchronization of discharges can operate as complementary mechanisms for the selection and binding of responses.

In consideration of these functional issues, the fundamental question also arises as to how, at a cellular level, synchrony can be established on a millisecond time scale over the broad range of spatial scales that are required. One possibility is that during development those connections having a conduction velocity appropriate for the generation of synchrony get selectively stabilized. The fact that synchronizing connections are selected according to a correlation rule supports this possibility. Additional temporal patterning of discharges may further facilitate the establishment of synchronous firing. The evidence presented here suggests that this requirement may be met in many instances by discharge patterns in which bursts and pauses follow one another with a certain degree of rhythmicity. The refractory period following a burst will produce a brief period of decreased sensitivity, making synaptic inputs arriving at that time less likely to have an effective influence on the overall pattern of activity.

In this context, the question arises as to why the observed oscillations are so irregular and cover such a broad frequency range (Gray et al. 1992). Functionally, such variation could facilitate the desynchronization of activity and thereby prevent the cortical network from entering global states of synchrony that would be inappropriate for information processing. Furthermore, the number of assemblies that can coexist in the same cortical region increases if the oscillation frequencies are variable, because spurious correlations arising from aliasing effects would be rare and only of short duration. Thus, a broad-banded oscillatory signal appears as a reasonable compromise between several opposing constraints. However, synchronous activity may arise in cortical networks without oscillatory firing, and the presence or absence of a regular oscillatory time structure in single-cell activity neither proves nor disproves that spatially segregated cells discharge in synchrony. Oscillations per se are thus of little diagnostic value for the testing of the temporal correlation hypothesis. The synchronization of activity is the relevant issue.

To directly test the hypothesis that correlated activity contributes to the integration of distributed featural information, experiments are needed in which the dependence of the occurrence and the magnitude of synchronized activity on stimulus configuration and behavioral performance can be assessed. This minimally requires the simultaneous recording of activity from several locations in the brain of awake, behaving animals and the evaluation of temporal correlations of activity at high resolution. With the techniques currently available, the number of recording sites that can be examined simultaneously is bound to remain small, which poses a severe sampling problem. For the brain, a brief sequence of correlated activity may be a highly significant event if it occurs in a large number of cells (Bressler et al. 1993). However, for the experimenter, who can only look at a few cells (most often 2; occasionally as many as 100) (Wilson and McNaughton 1993), such brief synchronous events may pass undetected. They will only be recognized as significant if they recur. Thus, until new techniques become available, the relationships between synchronized neuronal activity and behavior are likely to be detectable only for conditions that maintain synchronization for longer periods of time. This limitation may confine the behavioral conditions suitable for such analyses to problem-solving tasks that are difficult, fraught with ambiguity, and require periods of sustained, focused attention.

Acknowledgments

We thank Francis Crick and Christof Koch for helpful comments on an earlier version of the manuscript. This work was supported by the Max-Planck-Gesellschaft (WS) and grants from the National Science Foundation, the National Eye Institute, the Klingenstein Foundation, and the Sloan Foundation (CMG).

References

Abeles M, ed. 1991. *Corticonics.* Cambridge: Cambridge Univ. Press

Adrian ED. 1950. The electrical activity of the mammalian olfactory bulb. *Electroencephalogr. Clin. Neurophysiol.* 2:377–88

Ahissar E, Vaadia E, Ahissar M, Bergman H, Arieli A, Abeles M. 1992. Dependence of cortical plasticity on correlated activity of single neurons and on behavioral context. *Science* 257:1412–15

Aiple F, Krüger J. 1988. Neuronal synchrony in monkey striate cortex: interocular signal flow and dependency on spike rates. *Exp. Brain Res.* 72:141–49

Alonso A, Garcia-Austt E. 1987. Neuronal sources of theta rhythm in the entorhinal cortex of the rat. II. Phase relations between unit discharges and theta field potentials. *Exp. Brain Res.* 67:502–9

Ariel M, Daw NW, Rader RK. 1983. Rhythmicity in rabbit retinal ganglion cell responses. *Vision Res.* 23:1485–93

Arnett DW. 1975. Correlation analysis of units recorded in the cat dorsal lateral geniculate nucleus. *Exp. Brain Res.* 24:111–30

Bair W, Koch C, Newsome W, Britten K, Niebur E. 1994. Power spectrum analysis of bursting cells in area MT in the behaving monkey. *J. Neurosci.* 14:2870–92

Ballard DH, Hinton GE, Sejnowski TJ. 1983. Parallel visual computation. *Nature* 306:21–26

Basar E. 1988. EEG—dynamics and evoked potentials in sensory and cognitive processing by the brain. In *Dynamics of Sensory and Cognitive Processing by the Brain. Springer Series in Brain Dynamics,* ed. E Basar, 1:30–55. Berlin/Heidelberg/New York: Springer

Basar E, Bullock TH. 1992. *Induced Rhythms in the Brain.* Boston: Birkhaeuser

Baylis GC, Rolls ET, Leonard CM. 1985. Selectivity between faces in the responses of a population of neurons in the cortex in the superior temporal sulcus of the monkey. *Brain Res.* 342:91–102

Blakemore C, Vital-Durand F. 1992. Different neural origins for "blur" amblyopia and strabismic amblyopia. *Ophthalmic Physiol. Opt.* 12

Bland BH, Andersen P, Ganes T. 1975. Two generators of hippocampal theta activity in rabbits. *Brain Res.* 94:199–218

Bouyer JJ, Montaron MF, Rougeul A. 1981. Fast fronto-parietal rhythms during combined focused attentive behaviour and immobility in cat: cortical and thalamic localizations. *Electroencephalogr. Clin. Neurophysiol.* 51:244–52

Bouyer JJ, Montaron MF, Vahnee JM, Albert MP, Rougeul A. 1987. Anatomical localization of cortical beta rhythms in cat. *Neuroscience* 22:863–69

Bragin A, Jandó G, Nádasdy Z, Hetke J, Wise K, Busaki G. 1994. Gamma (40–100 Hz) oscillation in the hippocampus of the behaving rat. *J. Neurosci.* In press

Braitenberg V. 1978. Cell assemblies in the cerebral cortex. In *Lecture Notes in Biomathematics 21, Theoretical Approaches in Complex Systems,* ed. R Heim, G Palm, pp. 171–88. Berlin: Springer

Braitenberg V, Schüz A. 1991. *Anatomy of the Cortex: Statistics and Geometry.* Berlin/Heidelberg/New York: Springer

Bressler SL. 1984. Spatial organization of EEGs from olfactory bulb and cortex. *Electroencephalgr. Clin. Neurophys.* 57:270–76

Bressler SL. 1987. Relation of olfactory bulb and cortex. I. Spatial variation of bulbocortical interdependence. *Brain Res.* 409:285–93

Bressler SL, Coppola R, Nakamura R. 1993. Episodic multiregional cortical coherence at multiple frequencies during visual task performance. *Nature* 366:153–56

Bringuier V, Fregnac Y, Debanne D, Shulz D, Baranyi A. 1992. Synaptic origin of rhythmic visually evoked activity in kitten area 17 neurons. *NeuroReport* 3:1065–68

Bullier J, Munk MHJ, Nowak LG. 1992. Synchronization of neuronal firing in areas V1 and V2 of the monkey. *Soc. Neurosci. Abstr.* 18:11.7

Bush P, Douglas RJ. 1991. Synchronization of bursting action potential discharge in a model network of neocortical neurons. *Neural Comput.* 3:19–30

Bush P, Gray CM, Sejnowski T. 1993. Realistic simulations of synchronization in networks of layer V neurons in cat primary visual cortex. *Soc. Neurosci. Abstr.* 19:359.7

Buzsaki G, Horvath Z, Urioste R, Hetke J, Wise K. 1992. High-frequency network oscillation in the hippocampus. *Science* 256:1025–27

Buzsaki G, Leung LS, Vanderwolf CH. 1983. Cellular bases of hippocampal EEG in the behaving rat. *Brain Res. Rev.* 6:139–71

Callaway EM, Katz LC. 1990. Emergence and refinement of clustered horizontal connections in cat striate cortex. *J. Neurosci.* 10:1134–53

Callaway EM, Katz LC. 1991. Effects of binocular deprivation on the development of clustered horizontal connections in cat striate cortex. *Proc. Natl. Acad. Sci. USA* 88:745–49

Chatrian GE, Bickford RG, Uilein A. 1960. Depth electrographic study of a fast rhythm evoked from the human calcarine region by steady illumination. *Electroencephalgr. Clin. Neurophysiol.* 12:167–76

Connors BW, Gutnick MJ, Prince DA. 1982. Electrophysiological properties of neocortical neurons in vitro. *J. Neurophysiol.* 48:1302–20

Crewther DP, Crewther SG. 1990. Neural sites of strabismic amblyopia in cats: spatial frequency deficit in primary cortical neurons. *Exp. Brain Res.* 79:615–22

Crick F, Koch C. 1990. Towards a neurobiological theory of consciousness. *Semin. Neurosci.* 2:263–75

Desimone R, Schein SJ, Moran J, Ungerleider LG. 1985. Contour, color and shape analysis beyond the striate cortex. *Vision Res.* 24:441–52

DeYoe EA, Van Essen DC. 1988. Concurrent processing streams in monkey visual cortex. *Trends Neurosci.* 115:219–26

Doty RW, Kimura DS. 1963. Oscillatory potentials in the visual system of cats and monkeys. *J. Physiol.* 168:205–18

Eckhorn R, Bauer R, Jordan W, Brosch M, Kruse W, et al. 1988. Coherent oscillations: a mechanism for feature linking in the visual cortex? *Biol. Cybern.* 60:121–30

Eckhorn R, Frien A, Bauer R, Woelbern T, Kehr H. 1993. High Frequency 60–90 Hz oscillations in primary visual cortex of awake monkey. *Neuro Rep.* 4:243–46

Eckhorn R, Schanze T, Brosch M, Salem W, Bauer R. 1992. Stimulus-specific synchronizations in cat visual cortex: multiple microelectrode and correlation studies from several cortical areas. In *Induced Rhythms in the Brain*, ed. E Basar, TH Bullock, pp. 47–82. Boston: Birkhauser

Edelman GM. 1987. *Neural Darwinism: The Theory of Neuronal Group Selection.* New York: Basic Books

Engel AK, König P, Gray CM, Singer W. 1990. Stimulus-dependent neuronal oscillations in cat visual cortex: inter-columnar interaction as determined by cross-correlation analysis. *Eur. J. Neurosci.* 2:588–606

Engel AK, König P, Kreiter AK, Singer W. 1991a. Interhemispheric synchronization of oscillatory neuronal responses in cat visual cortex. *Science* 252:1177–79

Engel AK, König P, Singer W. 1991b. Direct physiological evidence for scene segmentation by temporal coding. *Proc. Natl. Acad. Sci. USA* 88:9136–40

Engel AK, Kreiter AK, König P, Singer W. 1991c. Synchronization of oscillatory neuronal responses between striate and extrastriate visual cortical areas of the cat. *Proc. Natl. Acad. Sci. USA* 88:6048–52

Engel AK, Kreiter AK, Singer W. 1992. Oscillatory responses in the superior temporal sulcus of anesthetized macaque monkeys. *Soc. Neurosci. Abstr.* 18:11.10

Felleman DJ, van Essen DC. 1991. Distributed hierarchical processing in the primate cerebral cortex. *Cerebral Cortex* 1:1–47

Ferster D. 1986. Orientation selectivity of synaptic potentials in neurons of cat primatry visual cortex. *J. Neurosci.* 6:1284–1301

Freeman WJ, ed. 1975. *Mass Action in the Nervous System.* New York: Academic

Freeman WJ. 1968. Analog simulation of prepiriform cortex in the cat. *Math. BioSci.* 2:181–90

Freeman WJ. 1978. Spatial properties of an EEG event in the olfactory bulb and cortex. *Electroencephalogr. Clin. Neurophysiol.* 44:586–605

Freeman WJ. 1987. Analytic techniques used in the search for the physiological basis for the EEG. In *Handbook of Electroencephalography and Clinical Neurophysiology*, ed. A Gevins, A Remond, 3A(Part 2):583–664. Amsterdam: Elsevier

Fujita I, Tanaka K, Ito M, Cheng K. 1992. Columns for visual features of objects in monkey inferotemporal cortex. *Nature* 360:343–46

Fuster JM, Herz A, Creutzfeldt OD. 1965. Interval analysis of cell discharge in spontaneous and optically modulated activity in the visual system. *Arch. Ital. Biol.* 103:159–77

Galambos R, Makeig S, Talmachoff PJ. 1981. A 40-Hz auditory potential recorded from the human scalp. *Proc. Natl. Acad. Sci. USA* 78:2643–47

Gallant JL, Braun J, Van Essen DC. 1993. Selectivity for polar, hyperbolic, and Cartesian gratings in macaque visual cortex. *Science* 259:100–3

Gawne TJ, Richmond BJ. 1993. How independent are the messages carried by adjacent inferior temporal cortical neurons? *J. Neurosci.* 137:2758–71

Gerstein GL, Bedenbaugh P, Aertsen AMHJ. 1989. Neuronal assemblies. *IEEE Trans. Biomed. Eng.* 361:4–14

Ghose GM, Freeman RD. 1992. Oscillatory discharge in the visual system: does it have a functional role? *J. Neurophysiol.* 68:1558–74

Gilbert CD, Wiesel TN. 1983. Clustered intrinsic connections in cat visual cortex. *J. Neurosci.* 35:1116–33

Gilbert CD, Wiesel TN. 1989. Columnar specificity of intrinsic horizontal and corticocortical connections in cat visual cortex. *J. Neurosci.* 97:2432–42

Gochin PM, Miller EK, Gross CG, Gerstein GL. 1991. Functional interactions among neurones in inferior temporal cortex of the awake macaque. *Exp. Brain Res.* 84:505–16

Gray CM. 1993. Rhythmic activity in neuronal systems: insights into integrative function. In *Lectures in Complex Systems. Santa Fe Institute Studies in the Sciences of Complexity*, ed. L Nadel, D Stein, 5:89–161. Santa Fe, NM: Addison-Wesley

Gray CM, Engel AK, König P, Singer W. 1990. Stimulus-dependent neuronal oscillations in cat visual cortex: receptive field properties and feature dependence. *Eur. J. Neurosci.* 2:607–19

Gray CM, Engel AK, König P, Singer W. 1992. Synchronization of oscillatory neuronal responses in cat striate cortex: temporal properties. *Vis. Neurosci.* 8:337–47

Gray CM, König P, Engel AK, Singer W. 1989. Oscillatory responses in cat visual cortex exhibit intercolumnar synchronization which reflects global stimulus properties. *Nature* 338:334–37

Gray CM, Singer W. 1987. Stimulus-specific neuronal oscillations in the cat visual cortex: a cortical functional unit. *Soc. Neurosci. Abstr.* 13:404.3

Gray CM, Singer W. 1989. Stimulus-specific neuronal oscillations in orientation columns of cat visual cortex. *Proc. Natl. Acad. Sci. USA* 86:1698–1702

Gray CM, Skinner JE. 1988. Centrifugal regulation of neuronal activity in the olfactory bulb of the waking rabbit as revealed by reversible cryogenic blockade. *Exp. Brain Res.* 69:378–86

Gray CM, Viana Di Prisco G. 1993. Properties of stimulus-dependent rhythmic activity of visual cortical neurons in the alert cat. *Soc. Neurosci. Abstr.* 19: 359.8

Gross CG, Rocha-Miranda EC, Bender DB. 1972. Visual properties of neurons in inferotemporal cortex of the macaque. *J. Neurophysiol.* 35:96–111

Grossberg S. 1980. How does the brain build a cognitive code? *Psychol. Rev.* 87:1–51

Merigan WH, Maunsell JH. 1993. How parallel are the primate visual pathways? *Annu. Rev. Neurosci.* 16:369–402

Michalski A, Gerstein GL, Czarkowska J, Tarnecki R. 1983. Interactions between cat striate cortex neurons. *Exp. Brain Res.* 51:97–107

Milner P. 1974. A model for visual shape recognition. *Psychol. Rev.* 816:521–35

Montaron M, Bouyer J, Rougeul A, Buser P. 1982. Ventral mesencephalic tegmentum VMT controls electrocortical beta rhythms and associated attentive behaviour in the cat. *Behav. Brain Res.* 6:129–45

Munemori J, Hara K, Kimura M, Sato R. 1984. Statistical features of impulse trains in cat's lateral geniculate neurons. *Biol. Cybern.* 50:167–72

Murthy VN, Aoki F, Fetz FE. 1994. Synchronous oscillations in sensorimotor cortex of awake monkeys and humans, See Pantev et al. 1994, In press

Murthy VN, Fetz EE. 1992. Coherent 25- to 35-Hz oscillations in the sensorimotor cortex of awake behaving monkeys. *Proc. Natl. Acad. Sci. USA* 89:5670–74

Nelson JI, Nowak LG, Chouvet G, Munk MHJ, Bullier J. 1992a. Synchronization between cortical neurons depends on activity in remote areas. *Soc. Neurosci. Abstr.* 18:11.8

Nelson JI, Salin PA, Munk MHJ, Arzi M, Bullier J. 1992b. Spatial and temporal coherence in corticocortical connections: a cross-correlation study in areas 17 and 18 in the cat. *Visual Neurosci.* 9:21–38

Neuenschwander S, Varela FJ. 1993. Visually triggered neuronal oscillations in birds: an autocorrelation study of tectal activity. *Eur. J. Neurosci.* 5:870–81

Nicoll A, Blakemore C. 1993. Single-fiber EPSPs in layer 5 of rat visual cortex in vitro. *NeuroReport* 42:167–70

Nowak LG, Munk MHJ, Chounlamountri N, Bullier J. 1994. Temporal aspects of information processing in areas V1 and V2 of the macaque monkey. See Pantev et al. 1994, In press

Olshausen BA, Anderson CH, Van Essen DC. 1993. A neurobiological model of visual attention and invariant pattern recognition based on dynamic routing of information. *J. Neurosci.* 1311:4700–19

Palm G. 1990. Cell assemblies as a guideline for brain research. *Concepts Neurosci.* 1:133–37

Pantev C, Elbert T, Lutkenhoener B, eds. 1994. *Oscillatory Event-Related Brain Dynamics.* New York: Plenum

Pantev C, Makeig S, Hoke M, Galambos R, Hampson S, Galen C. 1991. Human auditory evoked gamma-band magnetic fields. *Proc. Natl. Acad. Sci. USA* 88:8996–9000

Payne BR. 1993. Evidence for visual cortical area homologs in cat and macaque monkey. *Cerebral Cortex* 3:1–25

Perez-Borja C, Tyce FA, McDonald C, Uihlein A. 1961. Depth electrographic studies of a focal fast response to sensory stimulation in the human. *Electroencephalogr. Clin. Neurophysiol.* 13:695–702

Perkel DH, Gerstein GL, Moore GP. 1967. Neuronal spike trains and stochastic point processes. II. Simultaneous spike trains. *Biophys. J.* 7:419–40

Perrett DI, Mistlin AJ, Chitty AJ. 1987. Visual neurones responsive to faces. *Trends Neurosci.* 10:358–64

Pinault D, Deschenes M. 1992. Voltage-dependent 40 Hz oscillations in reticular thalamic neurons. *Neuroscience* 251:245–258

Price DJ, Blakemore C. 1985. The postnatal development of the association projection from visual cortical area 17 to area 18 in the cat. *J. Neurosci.* 5:2443–52

Raether A, Gray CM, Singer W. 1989. Intercolumnar interactions of oscillatoary neuronal responses in the visual cortex of alert cats. *Eur. Neurosci. Assoc.* 12:72.5

Ribary U, Joannides AA, Singh KD, Hasson R, Bolton JPR, et al. 1991. Magnetic field tomography of coherent thalamocortical 40 Hz oscillations in humans. *Proc. Natl. Acad. Sci. USA* 88:11037–41

Robson JG, Troy JB. 1987. Nature of the maintained discharge of Q, X, and Y retinal ganglion cells of the cat. *J. Opt. Soc. Am. Ser. A* 412:2301–7

Roe AW, Ts'o DY. 1992. Functional connectivity between V1 and V2 in the primate. *Soc. Neurosci. Abstr.* 18:11.4

Roelfsema PR, König P, Engel AK, Sireteanu R, Singer W. 1994. Reduced neuronal synchrony: a physiological correlate of strabismic ambylopia in cat visual cortex. *Eur. J. Neurosci.* In press

Rosenquist AC. 1985. Connections of visual cortical areas in the cat. In *Cerebral Cortex*, ed. A Peters, EG Jones, pp. 81–117. New York: Plenum

Sakai K, Miyashita Y. 1991. Neural organization for the long-term memory of paired associates. *Nature* 354:152–55

Sanes JN, Donoghue JP. 1993. Oscillations in local field potentials of the primate motor cortex during voluntary movement. *Proc. Natl. Acad. Sci. USA* 90:4470–74

Schwarz C, Bolz J. 1991. Functional specificity of the long-range horizontal connections in cat visual cortex: a cross-correlation study. *J. Neurosci.* 11:2995–3007

Sem-Jacobsen CW, Petersen MC, Dodge HW, Lazarte JA, Holman CB. 1956. Electroencephalographic rhythms from the depths of the parietal, occipital and temporal lobes in man. *Electroencephalogr. Clin. Neurophysiol.* 8:263–78

65

Metaphors of Consciousness and Attention in the Brain

Bernard J. Baars

Metaphors and analogies have a long history in scientific thought: for example, the Rutherford planetary analogy for atomic structure, the clockwork metaphor for the solar system, and Harvey's pump metaphor for the heart. A metaphor can be defined as "the application of a word or phrase to an object or concept it does not literally denote, suggesting comparison to that object or concept."[1] Heuristic metaphors are especially useful when the sciences encounter a topic that has no clear precedent, and this is the case with consciousness and attention. A classical metaphor for consciousness has been a "bright spot" cast by a spotlight on the stage of a dark theater that represents the integration of multiple sensory inputs into a single conscious experience, followed by its dissemination to a vast unconscious audience. In cognitive theory, such a theater stage is called a "global workspace,"[2] and implies both convergence of input and divergent dissemination of the integrated content. In this century, features of the theater metaphor have been suggested by neurobiologists from Pavlov to Crick. Indeed, nearly all current hypotheses about consciousness and selective attention can be viewed as variants of this fundamental idea[2–4]; thus, its pros and cons are worth exploring.

The bright spot metaphor was extended in 1984 by Crick: he proposed a "searchlight of attention" metaphor for thalamocortical interaction, specified in terms of testable hypotheses at the cellular level. As Crick wrote,[5]

What do we require of a searchlight? It should be able to sample activity in the cortex and/or the thalamus and decide "where the action is." It should then be able to intensify thalamic input to that region of the cortex, probably by making the active thalamic neurons in that region fire more rapidly than usual. It must then be able to turn off its beam, move to the next place demanding attention, and repeat the process. It seems remarkable, to say the least, that the nature of the re-ticular complex [of the thalamus] and the behavior of the thalamic neurons fit this requirement so neatly.

Crick derived four testable hypotheses from this metaphor and, if this was its only use it could be discarded as having done its job. However, Crick suggested that "there may be at least two searchlights: one for the first visual area and another for all the rest." Thalamocortical searchlights for auditory and somatosensory cortex could be included, perhaps interacting in a mutually inhibitory fashion, so that only one sensory searchlight could be turned on at any time. But humans can be aware of more than sensory inflow; inner speech and visual imagery can compete for access to consciousness. Indeed, recent evidence indicates that inner speech involves speech-production cortex and speech-perception cortex, and that visual-projection areas participate in visual imagery.[6,7] However, humans also have conscious access to ideas that might involve prefrontal activation.[8] Conscious contents also influence motor output, involving prefrontal, motor and anterior cingulate cortex. Because all these cortical regions interact with corresponding thalamic nuclei, the searchlight metaphor could generate testable hypotheses about the role of consciousness and attention in all these parts of the brain.[9,10]

But that is not all: real searchlights are guided to their targets, suggesting executive control, and are useless without an audience to whom the contents in the illuminated spot are disseminated. In the brain, the "audience" could consist of unconscious regions, such as cerebral cortex, hippocampus, basal ganglia and amygdala, that might be activated by conscious contents. The audience for a brain searchlight could also include executive or interpreter systems, such as Gazzaniga's "narrative interpreter" of the left hemisphere,[11] and other executive regions of prefrontal cortex might receive conscious information. Thus searchlight metaphors do not stand alone, but imply a larger framework: a surrounding "theater."

Cognitive models of memory have a similar set of implications: a working memory whose active items are conscious and reportable, under executive control, with an audience of memory systems to receive its contents.[12] "Cognitive architectures" are large-scale simulations that have been developed since the 1950s (refs. 13–16) and have been used to model a range of behavioral tasks from chess-playing to language comprehension, memory retrieval and decision-making. Cognitive architectures resemble theaters, typically receiving input into a narrow "stage" of working memory, interacting with a large "audience" of semantic networks, automatic routines and memory systems. This theoretical tradition has been qualitatively related to consciousness in a framework called "global workspace theory."[2,3] For example, all cognitive architectures treat active elements in working memory as reportable, but reportability is the most widely used operational definition of conscious contents. Elements outside working memory are automatic or in long-term memory, and are therefore unreportable and unconscious. Thus, cognitive architectures seem to reflect the same theater metaphor that is implicit in the searchlight notion.

Theater models are also consistent with proposals for the integration of perceptual features, and for "convergence zones" that combine various inputs into unified neural representations. Damasio[17] has suggested that consciousness might be associated with cortical convergence zones, and theaters exist to allow numerous convergent influences to shape a coherent performance on stage that is then distributed divergently to the audience. Schacter[18] notes that conscious or explicit processes involve integration across multiple dissociable subsystems, which is, metaphorically, what theaters are good for. The widely discussed "binding function" of consciousness involves yet another feature that is compatible with the theater metaphor. Gaz-

zaniga has proposed that conscious experiences involve a "publicity organ" in the "society" of mind, just as a theater allows selected information to be made public.[19] Finally, a vast unconscious "audience" of specialized neuronal assemblies and routines is almost universal in contemporary thinking about the brain.[20–22] In all of these proposals, the fundamental function of the theater architecture is to make possible novel, adaptive interactions between the sensory inflow, motor outflow and a range of knowledge sources in the brain.

The Theater Metaphor: A Misleading Concept or Useful Thinking Tool?

The theater metaphor has encountered criticism from Dennett and Kinsbourne,[4] who agree that it is implicit in much current thinking, but claim that it is "Cartesian" and misleading. A "Cartesian theater" in their view has a "point center" where all sensory input converges, like the pineal gland in Descartes's seventeenth century view of the brain. However, neither Crick's thalamo-cortical searchlight nor cognitive architectures propose a single-point center. Rather, all current proposals involve "binding," "convergence zones," or "working memories" for the integration of conscious input. However, Dennett and Kinsbourne maintain that there is no single place in the brain where "it all comes together," as suggested by Damasio, Crick, and Koch, and by others. However, recent single-cell studies by Sheinberg and Logothetis[23] suggest strong convergence of conscious visual-object information in inferotemporal cortex and the superior temporal sulcus in the macaque. Approximately 90% of visual neurons in these areas respond differentially to the conscious but not the unconscious visual flow in a binocular rivalry task. Lower visual levels show low response rates to both conscious and unconscious rivalling input. Because the anterior temporal lobe integrates many visual features into object representations, it might indeed be a place where conscious visual information comes together.

Other philosophical critics maintain that consciousness could not possibly play the role attributed to it by theater hypotheses, because computers can simulate such hypotheses without consciousness. But the brain does many things differently from computers, and few scientists would rely on computers in lieu of direct evidence on the neurobiology of consciousness. Still other philosophers claim that some aspects of consciousness, such as subjectivity, might be inherently inexplicable. But that implies a misunderstanding of the scientific enterprise. The aim of the theater metaphor is to achieve a modest increase in knowledge. We cannot know today whether or not we will eventually understand a problem like subjectivity, although this might become clearer as more plausible hypotheses are tested. In summary, such philosophical challenges do not invalidate a useful thinking tool.

The criteria for productive metaphors are the same as for other scientific ideas: they should help organize existing evidence, yield testable hypotheses and suggest conceptual clarifications. For example, the terms "consciousness" and "attention" are conflated in much current work, but are they the same thing?[24] An attractive distinction is to limit the term "attention" to selective operations, while applying "consciousness" to events that humans can report. Thus, attention involves the selection of targets for the searchlight to shine on, while consciousness results from illumination of the target. When reading, we do not consciously control eye movements, but we have conscious access to the results of eye movements. Likewise, we might not consciously select a certain conversation at a cocktail party, but we become aware of the results of selective operations. This distinction is already implicit in much research, but it is not applied consistently. In this article, "attention" will be used for selective processes, and "consciousness" for events that can be reported.

In broad terms, the theater metaphor aids the organization of basic evidence, and has yielded new, testable hypotheses.

Evidence for Consciousness

It has been said that there is a lack of firm evidence about consciousness, but there is a large body of relevant findings; this evidence has often been collected under other headings. Relevant evidence comes from any study that treats consciousness as an experimental variable. Crick has pointed out, for example, that before Livingstone and Hubel,[25] single-cell studies of visual cortex rarely compared cortical activity in anesthetized and waking animals (F. H. C. Crick, personal communication). While previous studies had monitored waking visual processes, direct comparisons that allowed consciousness to be studied as a variable were difficult to find. In 1981, Livingstone and Hubel made history by pinching the tail of an anesthetized cat, thereby waking it up, and observing that this caused visual neurons to fire differently. Pinching the tail of an anesthetized cat while recording neuronal responses is one way to manipulate consciousness, but there are many others. For example, comparisons can be drawn between cortically blind and sighted parts of the visual field; between parietal neglect and normal vision; alertness compared with deep sleep, coma and anesthesia; explicit versus implicit knowledge in normal and brain damaged subjects; subliminal versus supraliminal stimulation; immediate versus long-term memory; the attended and unattended stream in dual-input tasks; and novel versus habituated stimuli or automatic skills. In each of these cases consciousness can be treated as an experimental variable.[26-31]

Some knowledge seems so obvious that it is rarely made explicit. We know, for example, that waking consciousness is biologically adaptive. Without it, vertebrates do not feed, mate, reproduce, defend their territory or young, migrate, or carry out any other survival or reproductive activity. Neurophysiologically, consciousness has pervasive effects: its characteristic electrical signature (fast, low-voltage and irregular) can be found throughout the waking brain; and in unconscious states, like deep sleep and coma, slow and coherent waves are equally widely distributed. In these respects, consciousness is not a subtle or hard-to-observe phenomenon: it is hard to ignore.

The Puzzle of Conscious Limited Capacity in a Massively Parallel Brain

The behavioral and brain sciences have presented remarkably different views. Behavioral experiments on humans are used to study conscious input and voluntary motor output. They seem to show a brain that does fairly simple things, like mental arithmetic, slowly, serially, with many errors and a great deal of interference between tasks. Humans cannot perform two conscious tasks at the same time, such as talking freely while driving in traffic. Competition between such tasks depends on the extent to which they are conscious: the more they become habitual and unconscious (through practice), the less they compete.[32] This suggests that consciousness might be responsible for capacity limits.

In contrast, direct brain observation shows a very different system, with vast, orderly forests of neurons, displaying massive parallelism, mostly unconscious in their detailed functioning and with processing capacities so large that they are difficult to estimate; the processing of any given task seems widely distributed across many brain locations.[20–22] The neurobiological view of the brain is therefore quite different from the behavioral one: it is not slow, serial, mostly conscious and limited in capacity, but fast, parallel, largely unconscious and with vast capacity.

Both of these perspectives are accurate; the difference is in which aspects of the brain are observed. Until recently, psychological studies have tended to ignore the massive parallelism of the brain, and many neuroscience experiments have paid relatively little attention to the seriality, slowness, and capacity limits of the conscious stream.

Given that the brain appears massively parallel, why is the conscious component so limited and serial? Would it not be adaptive to be able to do several conscious things at the same time? Certainly human ancestors might have benefited from simultaneously being able to gather food, watch for predators and keep an eye on their offspring. Yet all tasks that require consciousness compete with each other, so that only one can be done well at any given moment. These drawbacks suggest a biological tradeoff. The nervous system might show limited capacity effects when there is competition for the bright spot on the stage of a large, parallel theater, but not when specialized audience members carry out similar functions unconsciously.

Consciousness Creates Access

Consciousness, although limited in capacity at any single moment, does appear to offer a gateway to extensive unconscious knowledge sources in the brain. There is much behavioral evidence for this claim. Consider autobiographical memory, which is believed to involve the hippocampus: the size of long-term episodic memory is unknown, but we do know that by paying attention to as many as 10,000 distinct pictures over several days, without attempting to memorize them, we can spontaneously recognize more than 90% a week later.[33] Remarkable results like this are common when we use recognition probes, that is, asking people to choose between known and new pictures. Recognition probes appear to work because they reinstate the original conscious experience of each picture. With this kind of retrieval the brain does a remarkable job, with little effort. It seems that humans create memories from the stream of perceptual input merely by paying attention, but because we are always paying attention to something, this suggests that autobiographical memory could be very large indeed. Mere consciousness of some event appears to help to store a recognizable memory of it, and when we experience it again, we can distinguish it accurately from millions of other conscious experiences; both episodic storage and retrieval seem to require consciousness.

Another example is the vocabulary of educated English speakers, which contains about 100,000 words. Although we do not use all these words in everyday speech, we can understand them. Each vocabulary item is already quite complex: for example, the *Oxford English Dictionary* devotes 75,000 words to the many different meanings of the single word "set," but all we need to access such complex unconscious domains of knowledge is to become conscious of a word. Conscious exposure to any printed word on this page is sufficient to access its meaning, syntactic role, inner speech phonology, emotional connotations, semantic and sound associates and imagery components, and to trigger automatic inferences. Understanding words seems to require the gateway of consciousness.

The ability to access unconscious knowledge via consciousness also applies to the vast number of automatisms that can be triggered by conscious events, including the automatic inner speech that often accompanies reading; automatic inferences in social judgments; and the automatic transformations of visual patterns on this page into letters, words and phrases. None of these automatisms are conscious in any detail, yet they are triggered by conscious events. This triggering function is hampered when conscious input is degraded by distraction, fatigue, somnolence, sedation or low signal fidelity.[32]

Indeed, it appears that humans can access a great range of brain functions by way of conscious sensory feedback. No one knows directly which groups of vocal-tract muscles they use to say a word, but by way of conscious sensory feedback a wide variety of vocal parameters are controlled. Conscious feedback seems to create spectacular access not only to skeletal muscles, but also, in the short term to autonomic muscu-

lature. Biofeedback control of single neurons and populations of neurons almost anywhere in the brain is well established.[34] To gain control over a single spinal motor unit we monitor its electrical activity, amplify it and play it back over headphones; in half an hour subjects have been able to play drumrolls using a single motor unit isolated from adjacent units. To gain control over alpha waves in occipital cortex we merely sound a tone when alpha is detected in the EEG, and shortly subjects can learn to increase the amount of alpha at will. Consciousness of sensory feedback appears to be a necessary condition for the establishment of biofeedback control, although the neural activities themselves remain entirely unconscious. It is as if consciousness of results creates access to unconscious neuronal systems that are normally inaccessible and autonomous.

Testable Hypotheses

Some anatomical structures could function like the basic elements of a theater. They might integrate, shape, display and disseminate conscious contents, to be received and analyzed by other brain structures, and to receive feedback from them.

Convergence Zones: The "Theater Stage"

Sensory projection areas of the posterior cortex might provide one kind of "theater stage," when "lit up" by attentional activation, thus displaying coherent conscious information to be distributed frontally and subcortically. In the case of visual consciousness, the first cortical projection area, V1, is an essential structure, whose lesioning leads to blindsight, that is, visual knowledge without visual consciousness. Higher visual lesions lead to selective impairment of conscious motion, color or objecthood, and thus we must include the brain areas V1–V5 and finally, IT (inferotemporal cortex) for multiple levels of visual content.[35] Recent single-cell work by Logothetis and colleagues strongly suggests that fully integrated, conscious visual information does not emerge until the anterior pole of the temporal cortex is reached. This can be explained by the neurons in these areas responding to whole objects, combining information from previous levels. The sensory projection areas for audition and the body senses could play similar roles: even abstract conscious contents, such as meaningful ideas, often appear to be mediated by sensory indices such as words, images and sensory metaphors.[36] Recent functional magnetic resonance imaging (fMRI) work suggests that the left prefrontal cortex might play a crucial role in semantic access.[8] Finally, conscious or voluntary control involves frontal cortex, including the anterior cingulate, which seems to "light up" during tasks that require effortful attention.[37]

Multiple Theater Stages

If each sensory area has its own kind of consciousness, in addition to abstract and voluntary kinds of conscious involvement, how do we cope with not just one, but five or more theater stages, over which the spotlight of attention can play? One hypothesis is that the spotlight of attention can switch from visual to auditory, somatosensory, abstract or voluntary cortex in multiples of 100 ms steps.[2,3] Such an arrangement would make it possible for several "stages" to operate together. Each one could broadcast widely to the audience of unconscious networks as soon as the spotlight touches on it. There are other ways to get multiple global workspaces to co-operate and compete, but this is a testable first hypothesis.

Inner Speech, Imagery, and Working Memory

Both auditory and visual consciousness can be activated internally as well as externally. Inner speech is a particularly important source of conscious auditory-phonemic events, and visual imagery is useful for solving spatial problems. They are often taken as the two basic components of cognitive working memory, and are now known

to involve corresponding sensory cortex.[6,7,12,38] Internally generated somatosensory imagery reflects emotional and motivational processes, including feelings of pain, pleasure, hope, fear and sadness.

Selective Attention "Searchlight" Control

How are conscious contents selected? The thalamus is ideally situated for controlling sensory traffic to cortex and, among thalamic nuclei, the reticular nucleus is known to exercise inhibitory modulation over the sensory nuclei. This is indeed an expansion of Crick's 1984 proposal for visual attention.[5] The reticular nucleus operates under dual control of frontal executive cortex and automatic interrupts from areas such as the brain stem, emotional centers like the amygdala and limbic cortex, and pain systems. It is these attentional interrupt systems that presumably allow significant stimuli like one's own name to "break through" into consciousness in a selective listening task, when the name is spoken in the unconscious channel. Interrupt control is quite separate from frontal executive (voluntary) control. Posner[37] suggests that effortful visual attention operates through the anterior cingulate cortex.

Receiving Regions: The "Audience"

Which brain regions receive conscious information? We have already listed some possibilities. Consciousness seems to be needed to access at least four bodies of unconscious knowledge: (1) autobiographical memory, which is believed to require the hippocampus; (2) the lexicon of natural language, thought to involve speech perception areas of both hemispheres; (3) automatic routines that control actions, requiring motor and prefrontal cortex, basal ganglia and cerebellum; and (4) the detailed firing of neurons and neuronal populations by way of sensory feedback. In addition, (5) the amygdala is also known to receive information about visual facial expressions. (6) Area 46 of the prefrontal cortex contains another visual map, and neurons in this area are believed to support one kind of working memory.[39]

Broadcasting of Selected Contents: "Speaking to the Audience"

How is conscious information disseminated? Sensory conscious events from posterior cortex might be broadcast frontally and subcortically. Because there are many spatial maps throughout the brain, the "trade language" of the brain could consist of activated maps co-ordinated by temporal oscillations. High fidelity is important to such broadcasting, which implicates the "labeled line" system of the brain. Labeled line fibers emerging from posterior sensory cortex include corticocortical axon bundles, the arcuate fasciculi and the posterior portions of the corpus callosum. A second major system of high-fidelity transmission operates via the thalamus, including the mediodorsal nuclei that project to prefrontal cortex.

Labeled-line fibers also connect to subcortical structures, including the limbic brain, hippocampi, amygdalae and basal ganglia, all of which are known to have precise spatial maps. Because such connections are typically bidirectional, it seems plausible that labeled line tracts establish activation loops, lasting for up to tens of seconds. Significant conscious events can be renewed by inner speech, by visual imagery, or by conscious emotional feeling states, thus re-initializing such activity loops. Storage of such activated information in long-term memory might occur via NMDA synapses.[40,41]

Unconscious Systems That Shape Conscious Events: "Backstage"

How are conscious contents shaped? Behind the stage in a theater are many people who shape and influence the performance without themselves being visible: they include the playwright, makeup artists and the stage director. There are analogous "contextual" systems in the brain that shape conscious contents while being unconscious. In the visual system, sensory contents seem to be produced by the ventral visual pathway, whereas unconscious contextual systems in the dorsal pathway define a spatial object-centered framework within which the sensory event is defined. There is a major difference between damage to content regions compared with contextual areas: in the case of lesioned content systems such as the ventral pathway, the subject can generally notice a missing aspect of normal experience; for damaged context systems, one no longer knows what to expect. Without a spatial framework for vision, it is hard to define what might be missing. This might be why parietal neglect is so often accompanied by anosognosia, a massive loss of knowledge about one's body space.[42]

Narrative Observer and Executive Systems: The "Stage Director"

How do conscious events influence decision-making and motor control? Gazzaniga[19] describes conditions under which split-brain patients encounter conflict between right and left hemisphere functions. Such patients often use the left hemisphere to talk to themselves, sometimes attempting to force the right hemisphere to obey its commands. When that proves impossible, the left hemisphere might rationalize or reinterpret events. The left-brain "narrative interpreter" receives its own sensory inflow from the right visual field, so that it "observes" a conscious flow of visual information. The right hemisphere might have a parallel executive interpreter that observes its own conscious flow from the left visual field. Although the right-brain observer does not speak, it might be able to deal better with anomaly via irony, jokes and other emotional strategies. Each interpretive system can control its own voluntary motor functions and thus there is an obvious analogy with a stage director, who observes events on stage and orders changes where needed. It is possible that full consciousness does not exist without the participation of such self systems, which might be centered in prefrontal cortex.

Concluding Remarks

Many proposals about brain organization and consciousness reflect a single underlying theme that can be labeled the "theater metaphor." In these views the overall function of consciousness is to provide very widespread access to unconscious brain regions. Such access is needed for global activation, co-ordination and control. The theater metaphor yields testable hypotheses about perceptual binding, thalamocortical interaction, working memory and selective attention, multimodal convergence zones, aspects of hemispheric specialization, and much more.

Selected References

1. *Webster's College Dictionary* (1995), Random House
2. Baars, B. J. (1988) *A Cognitive Theory of Consciousness*, Cambridge University Press
3. Baars, B. J. (1997) *In the Theater of Consciousness: The Workspace of the Mind*, Oxford University Press
4. Dennett, D. C. and Kinsbourne, M. J. (1992) *Behav. Brain Sci.* 15, 183–247
5. Crick, F. H. C. (1984) *Proc. Natl. Acad. Sci. U.S.A.* 81, 4586–4590
6. Kosslyn, S. M. (1988) *Science* 240, 1621–1626
7. Paulesu, E., Frith, D. and Frackowiak, R. S. J. (1993) *Nature* 362, 342–335
8. Gabrieli, J. et al. (1996) *Psychol. Sci.* 7, 278–283
9. Scheibel, A. B. (1980) in *The Reticular Formation Revisited* (Hobson, J. A. and Brazier, M. A., eds), pp. 55–56, Raven Press
10. Newman, J. and Baars, B. J. (1993) *Concepts Neurosci.* 2, 255–290
11. Gazzaniga, M. S. (1995) in *The Cognitive Neurosciences* (Gazzaniga, M. S., ed.), pp. 1391–1400, Bradford/MIT Press
12. Baddeley, A. D. (1992) *Science* 255, 556–559
13. Newell, A. and Simon, H. A. (1972) *Human Problem Solving*, Prentice Hall
14. Anderson, J. R. (1983) *The Architecture of Cognition*, Harvard University Press
15. Newell, A. (1990) *Unified Theories of Cognition*, Harvard University Press
16. Hayes-Roth, B. (1985) *Artif. Intell.* 26, 251–351
17. Damasio, A. R. (1989) *Cognition* 33, 25–62
18. Schacter, D. L. (1990) *J. Clin. Exp. Neuropsychol.* 12, 155–178
19. Gazzaniga, M. S. (1985) *The Social Brain*, Basic Books
20. Geschwind, N. (1979) *Sci. Am.* 241, 180–201
21. Mountcastle, V. B. (1978) in *The Mindful Brain* (Edelman, G. M. and Mountcastle, V. B., eds), pp. 76–122, MIT Press
22. Rumelhart, D. E., McClelland, J. E. and the PDP Research Group (1986) *Parallel Distributed Processing: Explorations in the Microstructure of Cognition, Vol. 1: Foundations*, Bradford/MIT Press
23. Sheinberg, D. L. and Logothetis, N. K. (1997) *Proc. Natl. Acad. Sci. U.S.A.* 94, 3408–3413
24. Baars, B. J. (1997) *Consciousness and Cognition* 6, 363–371
25. Livingstone, M. S. and Hubel, D. H. (1981) *Nature* 291, 554–561
26. Logothetis, N. K. and Schall, J. D. (1989) *Science* 245, 761–763
27. Leopold, D. A. and Logothetis, N. K. (1995) *Nature* 379, 549–553
28. Weiskrantz, L. (1986) *Blindsight: A Case Study and its Implications*, Clarendon Press
29. Stoerig, P. and Cowey, A. (1989) *Nature* 342, 916–918
30. Edelman, G. (1989) *The Remembered Present: A Biological Theory of Consciousness*, Basic Books
31. Baars, B. J. (1993) in *Ciba Symposium on Experimental and Theoretical Studies of Consciousness* (Bock, G. R. and Marsh, J., eds), pp. 282–290, Wiley
32. Shiffrin, R. M., Dumais, S. T. and Schneider, W. (1981) in *Attention and Performance IX* (Long, J. and Baddeley, A., eds), pp. 223–240, Erlbaum
33. Kosslyn, S. M. (1994) *Image and Mind*, Harvard University Press

34. Buchwald, J. S. (1974) in *Operant Conditioning of Brain Activity* (Chase, M. H., ed.), pp. 12–43, University of California Press

35. Zeki, S. (1993) *A Vision of the Brain*, Blackwell Scientific

36. Rosch, E. H. (1975) *J. Exp. Psychol.* 104, 192–233

37. Posner, M. I. (1992) *Curr. Dir. Psychol. Sci.* 11, 11–14

38. Goldman-Rakic, P. (1987) in *Higher Cortical Function: Handbook of Physiology* (Plum, F. and Mountcastle, V., eds), pp. 373–417, American Physiological Society

39. Kandel, E., ed. (1990) *Frontiers in Neurosciences*, Bradford/MIT Press

40. Bisiach, E. and Geminiani, G. (1991) in *Awareness of Deficit after Brain Injury: Clinical and Theoretical Issues* (Prigatano, G. P. and Schacter, D. L., eds), pp. 17–39, Oxford University Press

41. Schacter, D. L. (1990) *Am. Psychol.* 47, 559–569

42. Sperry, R. W. (1966) in *Brain and Conscious Experience* (Eccles, J. C., ed.), pp. 298–313, Springer-Verlag

66

How Does a Serial, Integrated, and Very Limited Stream of Consciousness Emerge from a Nervous System That Is Mostly Unconscious, Distributed, Parallel, and of Enormous Capacity?

Bernard J. Baars

Asking the right question can often help organize and simplify an otherwise overwhelming amount of evidence. This paper asks how a narrowly limited conscious stream emerges from a massively parallel, largely unconscious nervous system. Limited capacity mechanisms associated with consciousness appear to be biologically very costly, and one may reasonably ask what biological benefits could possibly accrue from such basic "architectural" features. "Global Workspace" theory, described below, suggests one reasonable answer, which when compared to others shows a striking amount of agreement as well as some significant differences (Baars 1983, 1988; Baddeley 1992a,b; Crick 1984; Crick and Koch 1990; Dennett 1991; Dennett and Kinsbourne 1992; John 1976; Kinsbourne 1988; Marcel 1983; Norman and Shallice 1986; Posner 1992; Shallice 1978; Damasio 1989; Edelman 1989).

Limited Capacity versus Massive Capacity

There is increasing agreement that large parts of the human nervous system, such as the neocortex, can be viewed as "societies" of separable, very specialized unconscious systems (Dennett and Kinsbourne 1992, Kinsbourne 1988, Marcel 1993). The neurobiological evidence for this view comes from anatomical studies (e.g., Mountcastle 1978), as well as physiological experiments and careful studies of patients with brain damage (e.g., Geschwind 1979, Luria 1980, Gazzaniga 1988). Convergent psychological evidence comes from studies of automaticity due to practice (Shiffrin et al. 1981), from psycholinguistics and memory theory, and from the study of errors and slips (e.g., Baars 1992). The connectionist movement in cognitive science also suggests that small networks which change connection strength as a function of node activity provide elegant and often powerful models of many local phenomena. Purely functional models combining many independent expert systems have been studied for at least two decades. Indeed, computational models of complex human functions like language comprehension, motor control or visual analysis always contain multiple specialized modules. All these sources suggest that the nervous system has a great number of specialized cell populations which can operate in parallel, unconsciously, and with some autonomy.

Paradoxically, an equally impressive body of evidence points to quite a different nervous system. There is strong and reliable support for a mechanism that is serial rather than parallel, internally consistent at any single moment rather than distributed, very limited in capacity, and strongly associated with consciousness.

Evidence for a limited capacity mechanism comes from three major sources. First, selective attention tasks, in which humans can follow only a single dense and coherent flow of information, such as a spoken message or a basketball game, at one time; any other streams of information are unconscious. Second, dual-task phenomena, where the mutual interference and degradation of simultaneous tasks requires consciousness or mental effort (Shallice 1978, Norman and Shallice 1986). Third, immediate memory, consisting of sensory memories and rehearsable short-term memory, with its known capacity limit of seven plus or minus two separate and unrelated items (Baddeley 1992a,b). These three sets of phenomena point to a nervous system that is rather slow, prone to error, unable to perform simultaneous tasks, and quite limited—just the opposite of the parallel distributed system described above.

Limited capacity phenomena are strongly associated with consciousness. Selective attention tasks separate two coherent streams of information into a conscious and an unconscious one. In dual-task paradigms, interference between the two tasks depends upon the extent to which both are conscious: the more the tasks become predictable and automatic, the less they interfere with each other (Shiffrin et al. 1981). Thus, the more skilled we become in driving along a predictable road, the more easily we can carry on a conversation at the same time. Sensory memory always involves conscious information; short-term memory involves inner rehearsal of numbers or words, in which the items are "refreshed" by being made conscious every several seconds. The relationship between consciousness and the limited capacity system is therefore very close.

I have suggested that consciousness *underlies* the limited capacity system (Baars 1988). One of the most explicit models of limited capacity is Baddeley's well-developed notion of "working memory." It has two major content components, the "phonological loop" (for rehearsing verbal items) and the "visuospatial sketchpad" (for using visual imagery in planning, for example) (Baddeley 1992a). There is a great deal of solid empirical evidence for both components. However, contrary to expectation, the phonological loop and the visuospatial sketchpad have recently been found to interfere with each other (Baddeley 1992b). This suggests to Baddeley and others that both of these components are aspects of normal conscious experience. (See Baars 1988, chapter 8, for one model relating working memory to consciousness.)

Consciousness "As Such"

The evidence that bears most directly on the issue of consciousness *as such* compares similar conscious and unconscious phenomena. For example, Libet's (1981) work suggests that somatosensory stimuli are represented in the cortex for a considerable time before they become conscious. The bodily location, and perhaps other parameters, of the stimuli, may exist before the onset of conscious experience. Dennett (1991)

and Dennett and Kinsbourne (1992) have criticized the notion of "onset of conscious experience," but this idea does not have to emerge from a naïve Cartesian theatre. Within rather broad time limits, we can probably specify the onset of perceptual consciousness, as indicated by Libet's work (see Libet 1993).

Another example concerns event-related potentials created by repetitive stimuli which habituate over time, although the habituated representation can be shown to continue after conscious access fades. E. R. John (1976) reports that activity before habituation is widespread throughout a cat's brain, but, after habituation, event-related potentials can be found only in the sensory tract that continues to be stimulated. Recent work with positron emission tomography suggests the same result: that a novel task, of which subjects are conscious in its details, increases metabolic activity all over the brain, whereas the same task performed automatically after practice causes high metabolic activity only locally (Haier 1992).

The remarkable phenomenon of blindsight likewise suggests a natural contrast between visual representations that are conscious and similar representations that are unconscious (Weiskrantz 1988). It is important to distinguish research that compares similar conscious and unconscious events, and therefore tells us about consciousness *as such*, from work that compares different *contents* of consciousness, such as different perceptual experiences, images and inner speech. In comparisons of similar conscious and unconscious phenomena, consciousness is the independent variable (Libet 1981, Baars 1983). On the other hand, if we study the ability of subjects to switch from foveal to non-foveal visual experience, we are not studying consciousness as such, but something that is more accurately called "attention," that is, the *control of access to different conscious contents* (Baars 1988, chapter 8). From this point of view, Posner's important work on "attentional networks" in the brain involves selective or directed attention rather than consciousness (e.g., Posner 1992). Obviously, attention and consciousness are intimately related, but the distinction is vital.

Resolving the Limited Capacity Paradox

The flow of conscious experience is traditionally viewed as a serial *stream*—one that integrates different sources of information, but is limited to a single internally consistent content at any given moment (Baars 1988). But what is this very limited, serial, integrated stream of consciousness doing in an enormous society of parallel and distributed unconscious bioprocessors? Why do people have trouble keeping more than nine items in short-term memory, when an inexpensive calculator can store dozens of long numbers? Over one thousand million years of evolution of nervous systems, why did truly independent conscious streams not develop?

Such questions focus on the functional paradox of limited capacity mechanisms. By any reasonable measure, the conscious stream is biologically very expensive. The human brain consumes about 25% of body glucose and is dependent on an uninterrupted supply of oxygen; because its major input and output functions involve consciousness, a substantial part of this energy investment must go toward supporting limited capacity mechanisms (Lassen et al. 1978). There must also be an evolutionary cost in being limited to a single coherent stream of events at one time. Surely if animals could not be *distracted*, that is, if they could be conscious of multiple streams of events simultaneously, such as guarding against predators, searching for food and interacting with their social group, they would increase their chances for survival and reproduction. But vertebrates can orient to only a single informative flow of events at any given time. What evolutionary benefits could justify such costs?

There is a class of information-processing architectures that have exactly the form described above—that is, they combine a serial stream with a large, parallel, distributed society of processors—which suggests an answer to the question of cost and benefits. These global workspace architectures have been developed by a number of cognitive scientists for purely pragmatic reasons: not primarily as a model of human functioning, but to solve very difficult problems, such as speech analysis, which involve multiple knowledge sources. They are expensive in terms of processing resources, but they justify their cost because they can combine the activities of many different quasi-autonomous "specialists" to solve problems that cannot be solved by any single one (Hayes-Roth 1985). Global workspace architectures consist of collections of specialized processors, integrated by a single memory, whose contents can be broadcast to all the specialists. They are publicity systems in the society of specialists. Input specialists (such as perceptual systems) compete for access to the global workspace; once they gain access, they are able to disseminate a message to the system as a whole. When a problem has a predictable solution, it is handled by a specialized processor. But when novel problems arise, or when new, coherent actions must be planned and carried out, the global workspace becomes necessary (Baars 1983, 1988, 1992).

The Global Workspace theory of conscious experience employs this remarkably simple and useful architecture to explain many pairs of matched conscious and unconscious processes, all bearing on consciousness *as such* (see above). The theory currently consists of a series of seven increasingly adequate models which together are able to account for a vast amount of evidence about perceptual consciousness, unconscious problem-solving, habituation and automaticity, voluntary control of action, the role of intentions and expectations, selective and directed attention, contextual influences on conscious experience, and the adaptive roles of consciousness in the nervous system (Baars 1988). Global Workspace theory is consistent with, but not reducible to, other theories of limited capacity.

A global workspace does not perform executive functions, though it can be used by executive systems (Baars 1988, chapter 9). If the global workspace is a publicity organ in a society of specialists, then executive systems resemble a government, or, more flexibly, a variety of processor coalitions that aim at various times to control access to the global workspace in order to control the society as a whole.

Global workspace architectures are somewhat counterintuitive, because the intelligence of the system does *not* reside in the global workspace, but rather in the experts that provide input to and receive output from it. Take the example of spotting errors in a consciously perceived sentence. We can detect errors at many different levels: in acoustics, phonology, lexical choice, syntax, morphology, semantics and the pragmatic goals of the speaker. We rapidly detect such errors in any conscious sentence, *even though we are not conscious of the many complex rule systems that detect the error*. Thus, the detailed intelligence of the system does not become conscious in error detection.

Global Workspace theory provides a *functional account* of the limited capacity stream of consciousness, because global messages need to reach the whole "society" of processors, so that any arbitrary knowledge source can be related to any other. This is because, in the case of truly novel problems, the particular processor or coalition of processors that may find a solution *cannot be specified in advance*. Perhaps the most impressive example of this ability of the nervous system to access unpredictable sets of processors comes from the extensive literature on conscious feeback in the control of either single neurons or, apparently, any population of neurons (Chase 1974). The feedback signal must always be conscious—we would not expect people or animals to learn feedback tasks if they were distracted, habituated to the feedback signal, or asleep.

Comparisons to Other Models

Global Workspace theory shows a striking amount of agreement with other approaches, as well as some significant differences. It is important to note that the theory defines a *class* of models, rather than just a single one. One can imagine many different instantiations. Mc-Clelland (1986) has shown that connectionist networks can make up a global workspace configuration. It is possible to interpret the brainstem reticular formation as a hierarchy of increasingly global workspaces, culminating in a single high-level workspace corresponding to consciousness (Baars 1988, p. 132). A set of global workspaces corresponding to mutually inhibitory perceptual systems is also attractive for understanding perceptual consciousness (Baars 1988, p. 105; Baars and Newman 1992). In principle, such workspaces could be instantiated in the brain by modulation of rapid, correlated waveforms (as suggested by Crick and Koch 1980), by "multiregional retroactivation" (Damasio 1989), by a "cortical focus" (Kinsbourne 1988), by "re-entrant signalling" (Edelman 1989), or by "multiple drafts" (Dennett 1991, Dennett and Kinsbourne 1992).

However, some important differences should be noted. Approaches to consciousness seem to be separable into those that emphasize the parallel and distributed nature of neural functioning, and those that emphasize limited capacity mechanisms. In the first category are models suggested by Dennett (1991), Dennett and Kinsbourne (1992), Damasio (1989), and John (1976). Models emphasizing limited capacity include those of Baddeley (1992a), Shallice (1978), Norman and Shallice (1986), Crick (1984), and Crick and Koch (1990). The point of this paper is that *both* distributed and limited capacity aspects of consciousness must be accounted for in a single, unified model (cf. Kinsbourne 1988).

A Possible Neural Substrate

Given the defining properties of global workspace systems, we can study the neuroscience literature to see if analogous properties exist in the brain. Two defining properties are (a) competition for input to a neural global workspace, and (b) global distribution of its output (Baars and Newman 1992).

Two neural mechanisms associated with conscious experience (in the sense that their absence results in loss of consciousness) show competition between different input modalities. These are the brainstem reticular formation (Magoun 1962, Hobson and Brazier 1980) and the nucleus reticularis of the thalamus (Scheibel 1980). The reticular formation is thought to modulate the activity of many higher-level neural structures, notably the neocortex; the nucleus reticularis is believed to control thalamic "gatelets" that can open or close sensory tracts on their way to the cortex. Lesions in either structure result in a loss of consciousness.

The problem with both of these systems is that their output bandwidth does not seem to be large enough to carry the information for a conscious visual scene, for example. Further, phenomena like blindsight suggest that primary cortical projection areas are needed for conscious perceptual experiences, because abolition of striate cortex leads to a loss of normal conscious vision without abolishing object representation. The situation can therefore be summarized as follows:

1. Activities in the reticular formation and the nucleus reticularis seem to be necessary but not sufficient for conscious experience;

2. Stimulus representation in primary sensory projection areas also seems to be necessary but not sufficient for conscious perceptual experience (Weiskrantz 1988).

The simplest hypothesis is that *both* components together are necessary *and* sufficient to support conscious perceptual experience. For consciousness of a visual object, like a coffee cup, one plausible account is that a thalamo-cortical feedback loop, along the lines of Edelman's "re-entrant signalling loop" (1989), may be necessary in order to establish a specific cortical focus corresponding to the stimulus (Kinsbourne 1988). Once the loop is established, information from primary visual cortex can be broadcast via massive connections from striate cortex to subcortical mechanisms via the thalamus, and to other cortical areas via massive connections, such as the arcuate fasciculi, long and short association fibres, commissural tracts to the contralateral hemisphere, and possibly through the "feltwork" of layer 1 of the cortex (Baars and Newman 1992). Thus, once the stimulus is maintained long enough in primary sensory cortex, there are massive opportunities for global broadcasting to other parts of the brain.

Summary and Conclusions

Any adequate theory of consciousness must account for both limited capacity, integrative mechanisms and wide-spread, distributed intelligence. Global workspace architectures have both features, are practical for solving problems that need to combine specialized autonomous systems, and provide a natural way to think about consciousness. The global workspace approach discussed here can model perceptual consciousness, conscious components of problem-solving and conscious involvement in action control. This approach resembles other accounts of the role of consciousness in the nervous system, but is not reducible to them. Global workspace architectures can be instantiated in many different ways, but all of them involve competition between global workspace input, and global dissemination of output. Brain structures that are required for normal conscious experiences can carry out these functions.

Acknowledgments

The theoretical framework presented here has been in development since 1978, greatly aided by a Sloan Foundation Cognitive Science Scholar appointment (1979–1980) at the Center for Human Information Processing, University of California at San Diego, and by a Visiting Scientist appointment (1985–1986) at the John D. and Catherine T. MacArthur Foundation Program on Conscious and Unconscious Mental Processes, University of California at San Francisco. I am especially grateful to Donald A. Norman, David Galin, and Katherine McGovern.

References

Baars BJ 1983 Conscious contents provide the nervous system with coherent, global information. In: Davidson R, Schwartz G, Shapiro D (eds) Consciousness and self regulation. Plenum Publishing Corporation, New York, vol 3:45–76

Baars BJ 1988 A cognitive theory of consciousness. Cambridge University Press, New York

Baars BJ 1992 The psychology of human error: implications for the architecture of voluntary control. Plenum Publishing Corporation, New York

Baars BJ, Newman J 1992 A neurobiological interpretation of the Global Workspace theory of consciousness. In: Revonsuo A, Kamppinen M (eds) Consciousness in philosophy and cognitive neuroscience. Hillsdale, NJ: Erlbaum

Baddeley AD 1992a Working memory. Science (Wash DC) 255:556–559

Baddeley AD 1992b Consciousness and working memory. Consci & Cognit 1:3–6

Chase MH (ed) 1974 Operant control of brain activity. University of California Press, Berkeley, CA

Crick FHC 1984 Function of the thalamic reticular complex: the searchlight hypothesis. Proc Natl Acad Sci USA 81:4586–4593

Crick FHC, Koch C 1990 Towards a neurobiological theory of consciousness. Semin Neurosci 2:263–275

Damasio AR 1989 Time-locked multiregional retroactivation: a systems-level proposal for the neural substrates of recall and recognition. Cognition 33:25–62

Dennett D 1991 Consciousness explained. Little, Brown, Boston, MA

Dennett D, Kinsbourne M 1992 Time and the observer: the where and when of consciousness in the brain. Behav Brain Sci 15:175–220

Edelman G 1989 The remembered present: a biological theory of consciousness. Basic Books, New York

Gazzaniga MS 1988 Brain modularity: towards a philosophy of conscious experience: In: Marcel AJ, Bisiach E (eds) Consciousness in contemporary science. Oxford University Press, Oxford

Geschwind N 1979 Specializations of the human brain. Sci Am 241:180–201

Haier RJ 1992 Regional glucose metabolic changes after learning a complex visuospatial/motor task: a positron emission tomography study. Brain Res 570:134–143

Hayes-Roth B 1985 A blackboard architecture of control. Artif Intell 26:251–351

Hobson JA, Brazier MAB 1980 The reticular formation revisited: specifying function for a non-specific system. Raven Press, New York

John ER 1976 A model of consciousness. In: Schwartz G, Shapiro D (eds) Consciousness and self-regulation. Plenum Publishing Corporation, New York, p 6–50

Kinsbourne M 1988 Integrated field theory of consciousness. In: Marcel AJ, Bisiach E (eds) Consciousness in contemporary science. Oxford University Press, Oxford

Lassen NA, Ingvar DH, Skinhøj E 1978 Brain function and blood flow. Sci Am 239:50–59

Libet B 1981 Timing of cerebral processes relative to concomitant conscious experiences in man. In: Adam G, Meszaros I, Banyai EI (eds) Advances in physiological science. Pergamon Press, Oxford

Libet B 1993 The neural time factor in conscious and unconscious events. In: Experimental and theoretical studies of consciousness. Wiley, Chichester (Ciba Found Symp 174) p 123–146

Luria AR 1980 Higher cortical functions in man, 2nd edn. Basic Books, New York (Russian language edition 1969)

Marcel AJ 1983 Conscious and unconscious perception: an approach to the relations between phenomenal experience and perceptual processes. Cognit Psychol 15:238–300

Marcel AJ 1993 Slippage in the unity of consciousness. In: Experimental and theoretical studies of consciousness. Wiley, Chichester (Ciba Found Symp 174) p 168–186

McClelland JL 1986 The programmable blackboard model of reading. In: McClelland JL, Rumelhart DE and the PDP Group (eds) Parallel distributed processing—explorations in the microstructure of cognition, vol 2: Psychological and biological models. MIT Press, Cambridge, MA, p 122–169

Magoun WH 1962 The waking brain, 2nd edn. Thomas Publishers, Springfield, IL

Mountcastle VB 1978 An organizing principle for cerebral function: the unit module and the distributed system. In: Edelman GM, Mountcastle VB (eds) The mindful brain. MIT Press, Cambridge, MA, p 7–50

Norman DA, Shallice T 1986 Attention to action: willed and automatic control of behavior. In: Davidson RJ, Schwartz GE, Shapiro D (eds) Consciousness and self-regulation. Plenum Publishing Corporation, New York, vol 4:1–8

Posner MI 1992 Attention as a cognitive and neural system. Curr Dir Psychol Sci 11:11–14

Scheibel AB 1980 Anatomical and physiological substrates of arousal. In: Hobson JA, Brazier MA (eds) The reticular formation revisited. Raven Press, New York, p 55–66

Shallice T 1978 The dominant action system: an information-processing approach to consciousness. In: Pope KS, Singer JL (eds) The stream of consciousness: scientific investigations into the flow of experience. Plenum Publishing Corporation, New York, p 117–153

Shiffrin RM, Dumais ST, Schneider W 1981 Characteristics of automatism. In: Long J, Baddeley A (eds) Attention and performance IX. Erlbaum Associates, Hillsdale, NJ, p 223–238 (Atten Perform Ser)

Weiskrantz L 1988 Some contributions of neuropsychology of vision and memory to the problem of consciousness. In: Marcel AJ, Bisiach E (eds) Scientific approaches to consciousness. Oxford University Press, Oxford, p 183–199

67 A Neural Global Workspace Model for Conscious Attention

James Newman, Bernard J. Baars, and Sung-Bae Cho

Introduction

Consciousness has been widely portrayed as an intractable or irrelevant problem for cognitive science (e.g., Harnad 1994, Penrose 1994, O'Nuallain et al. 1997). Certainly its serious consideration is a fairly recent development (Jackendorf 1987, Baars 1988, Johnson-Laird 1988, Edelman 1989, Crick and Koch 1990a), although a brief enthusiasm for the subject surfaced, and submerged, three decades ago (Eccles 1966, Penfield 1975). While it is not widely realized, the experimental neuroscience which served as the basis for that earlier enthusiasm is proving increasingly relevant to the present recrudescence of interest in conscious processes (see, e.g., Stryker 1989; Newman 1995a, 1997). Beginning with historical developments in both AI and neuroscience, this paper reviews a growing body of evidence that some of the basic mechanisms underlying consciousness can be modeled, to a first approximation, employing variations upon current neural network architectures (see also Taylor, 1992, 1996; Baars et al. 1998; Newman et al. 1997).

Baars (1983, 1988, 1992, 1994) has developed a set of Global Workspace models, based upon a unifying pattern, and addressing a substantial domain of evidence explicitly related to conscious experience. These models explicate an architecture in which many parallel, non-conscious experts interact via a serial, conscious and internally consistent Global Workspace (GW), or its functional equivalent. GW, or blackboard, architectures were first developed by cognitive scientists in the 1970s and this framework is closely related to the Unified Theories of Cognition of Simon, Newell and Anderson (see Newell 1992).

The HEARSAY model of speech understanding (Reddy et al. 1973) was one of the earliest attempts to simulate a massively parallel/interactive computing architecture. The notion of a global workspace was initially inspired by this architecture, consisting of a large number of knowledge modules, or "local experts," all connected to a single "blackboard," or problem-solving space. Activated experts could compete to post "messages" (or hypotheses) on the blackboard for all the other experts to read. Incompatible messages would tend to inhibit each other, while the output of cooperating experts would gain increasing access to the blackboard until a global solution emerged. Blackboard architectures are relatively slow, cumbersome and error-prone, but are capable of producing solutions to problems too novel or complex to be solved by any extant modular knowledge source. Once such "global solutions" are attained, however, the original problems can be allocated to modular processors for "nonconscious" solution.

McClelland (1986) attested to the significance of this set of models to subsequent developments in cognitive science when he described HEARSAY, not only as "a precursor of the interactive activation model," but "of the approach that underlies the whole field of parallel distributed processing" (p. 122). We consider McClelland's own Programmable Blackboard Model of Reading as a connectionist example of a global workspace architecture, and discuss its applicability to modeling conscious processes in a concluding section.

Another class of models that may turn out to be compatible with GW theory comes from distributed artificial intelligence (DAI), which Durfee (1993) characterizes as the study of "how intelligent agents coordinate their activities to collectively solve problems that are beyond their individual capabilities" (p. 84). He cites examples of DAI applications, such as generic conflict resolution, unified negotiation protocols, and search-based models of coordination/cooperation. DAI applications appear to more closely approximate human interpersonal behaviour than purely logic-driven AI. They require that agents learn to be "knowledgeable and skilled in interacting with others" (p. 86). DAI models would appear to reflect an intelligent balance between competitive self-interest and cooperative problem-solving that is essential to optimizing overall outcomes in complex "social" organizations. This, like GW theory, is consistent with other well-known metaphors in cognitive science, such as Minsky's Society Theory (Minsky 1979) and Gazzaniga's Social Brain (Gazzanigga 1985).

A similar, globally-integrative balancing of priorities appears to characterize the optimal processing of conscious information. Conscious percepts are characterized by unified gestalts of shape, texture, color, location and movement, despite the fact that these contributions to perception are initially processed in parallel areas of the cortex, in both hemispheres. Moreover, conscious intentions are generally single-minded and goal-directed. Of course, conflicts can and do arise, but a central purpose of consciousness seems to be resolving such conflicts (employing both integrative and inhibitory algorithms).

While such global states can be highly adaptive—indeed, are essential to explicit learning—GW theory maintains that the vast majority of cognitive tasks performed by the human brain are automatic, and largely non-conscious (Baars 1988, 1997; Newman and Baars 1993; Newman 1997). Consciousness generally comes in play when stimuli are assessed to be novel, threatening, or momentarily relevant to active schemas or intentions.

The defining properties of stimuli which engage conscious attention (i.e., the global allocation of processing resources) are that they: (1) vary in some significant degree from current expectations; or (2) are congruent with the current, predominant intent/goal of the organism. In contrast, the processing of stimuli which are predictable, routine or over-learned is automatically allocated to non-conscious, highly modularized cognitive systems. (Newman 1995b, p. 691)

Generally, we are conscious of what has the highest relevance to us at that moment. This may be a momentary threat, a sudden insight, a pleasant sensation, and so on (in relaxed moments, there may be no particular focus or intent, simply a stream of associations). Yet, while the range of our awareness is immense (limited only by our most developed cognitive capacities), we contend that the basic mechanism for the allocation of these capacities remains constant under virtually all contingencies; and the basic neural circuitry of that resource-allocation mechanism is reasonably well understood. Indeed, in subsequent sections, we suggest how it might be modeled based upon already existing neural network simulations (McClelland 1985, Hampshire and Waibel 1992, Taylor and Alavi 1993, Llinas et al. 1994).

The relevance of Global Workspace theory extends beyond NN modeling, however. Indeed, it bears upon central philosophical problems in consciousness studies, such as the *homunculus* and Cartesian theater. The two are, of course, related. The image of a "little man in our head" observing and manipulating the play of conscious images is beguiling, but absurd. For who is this strange being lodged in our brains? And who is watching *him*?

In Global Workspace theory the single homunculus is replaced by a large "audience of experts." The "theater of consciousness" then becomes a workspace, with stage (Baars 1997). Almost everyone in an audience has potential access to center stage (although most prefer to simply observe, or exert indirect influences). The focus of conscious activity, at any moment, corresponds to the "work" produced by the most active coalition of experts, or modular processors: whoever has managed to win the competition for "the spotlight." There is no fixed, superordinate observer. Individual modules can pay as much or as little attention as suits them, based upon their particular expertise. At any one moment, some may be dozing in their seats, others busy on stage. In this sense, the global workspace resembles more a deliberative body than a theater audience. Each expert has a certain degree of "influence," and by forming coalitions with other experts can contribute to deciding which issues receive immediate attention and which are "sent back to committee." Most of the work of this deliberative body is done "off stage" (i.e., non-consciously). Only matters of greatest relevance in-the-moment gain access to consciousness.

While the GW is a teaming multiplicity, what is explicitly represented in consciousness is largely coherent and adaptive. The overall workspace serves as a "global integration and dissemination system," in which all experts can participate, but only select coalitions dominate, momentarily, producing an orderly succession of global representations. The stream of consciousness arises out of the operations of the GW system—and, over time, our sense of being a coherent "I" (the memory and intention systems vital to this aspect are beyond the scope of this paper; see Baars et al. 1998; Newman 1997). It is this unitary awareness, not any agent or homunculus, that is globally superordinate. Of course, such a system is prone to inefficiencies and pathological perturbations, but this is consistent with the scientific literature concerning human consciousness (see Baars 1988).

If we are to proceed beyond pleasing metaphors, however, it is necessary to operationalize the GW model in explicit neurocognitive terms. This process begins in the next section. To introduce it, we offer the following working definition:

Consciousness reflects the operations of a global integration and dissemination system, nested in a large-scale, distributed array of specialized bioprocessors; among the various functions of this system are the allocation of processing resources based, first, upon biological contingencies of novelty, need or potential threat and, secondly, cognitive schemas, purposes and plans.

Modeling Global, Competitive Attention

We have introduced the theoretical background for the model. Newman and Baars (1993) and Newman (1997) present detailed accounts of its neural architecture. We would stress, however, that consciousness is a dynamic process, not a static structure. Also, it is not localized to some "brain center," but arises out of the coordinated activities of widely distributed networks of neurons. Resource allocation is integral to these activities. The neural bases of resource allocation, or attention, have been extensively explored (see, e.g., Heilman et al. 1985; Mesulam 1985; Posner and Rothbart 1991; Posner 1994; LaBerge 1990, 1995). But, of course, not all forms of attention are conscious. As an example from AI, McClelland (1986) notes that in simulations of reading, activated modules must be "sticky," that is "interactive activation processes continue in older parts of the programmable blackboard while they are being set up in newer parts as the eye moves along ..." (pp. 150–151). This "stickiness" would seem to entail a type of attention. It normally proceeds quite automatically, however, both in a reading machine and in a literate human being. Only when the process is disrupted by, say, a mis-spelled or unknown word, does that word becomes the focus of our conscious awareness. Normally, we are only conscious of the overall sense of the passage of text, and the images and thoughts it evokes, not particular semantic or syntactical operations. These linguistic processes became second nature to us long ago. Such "particular operations" are hardly trivial aspects of language acquisition, but as Kihlstrom (1987) noted, in humans they tend to be "automatized through experience and thus rendered unconscious" (p. 285).

Conscious awareness clearly involves a higher order of resource allocation, which Newman and Baars (1993) call "global attention." The term "refers to a level of cognitive processing at which a single, coherent stream of information emerges out of the diverse activities of the CNS" (p. 258). The focus of that stream could (under atypical circumstances) be an individual word; but the conscious mind seldom confines itself to the processing of such rudimentary representations. Rather it seems to be decisively biased towards multifaceted, yet unified images. Thus, we are able to perceive a Necker cube as projecting out of a two-dimensional page, alternately to the left, then to the right; but we are curiously incapable of perceiving these two perspectives simultaneously.

The processing load of global attention (like working memory), is both highly chunked and highly restricted (Baars 1988). The non-conscious allocation of processing resources operates under no such constraints. For example, neuroscience has shown that specialized areas in the visual cortex process, in parallel, the contour, movement, color, spatial location, and so forth of a stimulus (LaBerge 1995). Yet our awareness is of a single, coherent object (and often includes tactile, auditory and associative aspects). Thus, neuroscience is faced with the "binding problem" of how these multifarious representations, generated by widely separated areas, are integrated into real-time "objects" of perception (see Crick and Koch 1990a, Newman and Baars 1993).

One would expect the neural mechanism for global attention to be complex, and widely distributed, which it is. But the basic circuitry can be described, to a first approximation, in terms of repeating, parallel loops of thalamo-cortico-thalamic axons, passing through a thin sheet of neurons known as the *nucleus reticularis thalami* (nRt). The loops are formed by long-axoned, excitatory neurons. The neurons of nRt are largely GABAergic, inhibitory neurons. Most, if not all, of the looping axons give off collaterals as they pass through nRt, while nRt neurons themselves project mainly to cells of the particular thalamic nucleus lying directly beneath them. There is an orderly topography to

this array of axon collaterals and underlying thalamic nuclei (Scheibel and Scheibel 1966, Mitrofanis and Guillery 1993). It essentially mirrors, in miniature, the modular architecture of the cortex (see Newman and Baars 1993, LaBerge 1995, Newman 1997 for reviews).

Evidence for the central role of this "thalamocortical circuit" (LaBerge 1995) in attention and consciousness has been accumulating for decades (Jasper 1960, Scheibel 1980, Jones 1985, Steriade and Llinas 1988, Llinas and Pare 1991). Skinner and Yingling (1977) first proposed a neural model for its role in selective attention. Our "wagon wheel" model (next section) represents a synthesis of both the accumulated evidence, and related models (Skinner and Yingling 1977, Scheibel 1980, Crick 1984, Taylor and Alavi 1993, Llinas et al. 1994, LaBerge 1995). These related models vary in their details, as the precise connectivities and physiology of the thalamocortical circuit are not fully worked out.

Most attentional models are based upon conventional simulations of mechanisms such as center-surround inhibition, or winner-take-all (WTA) competitions, among local circuits. Various researchers have described the network of nRt neurons as a mosaic, or array, of neural "gatelets" acting to selectively filter the flow of sensory inputs to the cortex (Skinner and Yingling 1977, Scheibel 1980, Crick 1984). The WTA dynamic may seem analogous to the "competition" posited by GW theory. The problem with such conventional networks is that they are poorly suited to global forms of competition, because prohibitively long-range and geometrically increasing numbers of connections would be required. Moreover, most long-range, reciprocal connections in the CNS are excitatory. Inhibitory effects tend to be local.

Taylor and Alavi (1993), however, have modeled a competitive network for global attention based upon a highly simplified version of the thalamus-NRT-cortex complex. Their model is unique, in that it takes into account the effects of dendro-dendritic interactions throughout nRt.

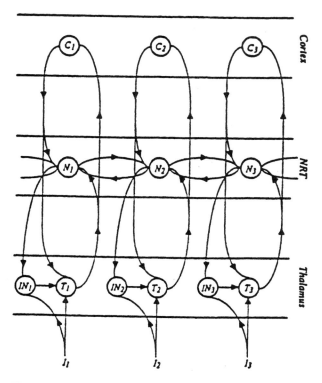

Figure 67.1
The wiring diagram of the main model of the thalamus-NRT-cortex complex. Input I_1 is sent both to the thalamic relay cell T_1 and the inhibitory interneuron IN_1, which latter cell also feeds to T_1. Output from T_1 goes up to the corresponding cortical cell C_1, which returns its output to T_1. Both the axons T_1C_1 and C_1T_1 send axon collaterals to the corresponding NRT cell N_1. There is axonal output from N_1 to IN_1 as well as collaterals to neighbouring NRT cells. There are also dendro-dendritic synapses between the NRT cells (from Taylor and Alavi 1993).

The dendrites of nRt cells project out tangentially within the reticular sheet, bidirectionally. The physiology of information processing in dendritic trees is highly complex, and not well understood (Mel 1994); but Koch and Poggio (1992) review evidence for the dendritic trees playing a role in several types of second-order, multiplicative computations. We will have more to say about this subsequently.

Figure 67.1 (taken from Taylor and Alavi 1993) illustrates three thalamocortical circuits, as well as the nonlinear, dendro-dendritic connections between N1, N2, N3,... within NRT. We would refer the reader to the original paper for a detailed description of the simulations carried out, employing a network of 100 thalamocortical loops. To briefly summarize the results, the addition of dendro-dendritic connections to the looping circuits provided "the basis for a simple version of the global gating model ... that instantiates a form of competition in the spatial wavelength parameters of incoming inputs ..."

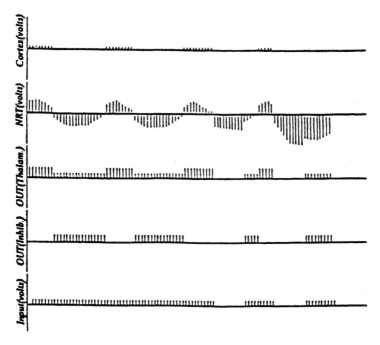

Figure 67.2
One of 15 simulation runs for the thalamus-NRT-cortex model showing full global control with semi-constant spatial input. Note that cortex activity is influenced by the NRT alone (from Taylor and Alavi 1993).

(p. 352). In this version of the model, the entire nRt network oscillates with a wavelength,

with the net strength given by the component of the input with the same wavelength.

The way in which global control arises now becomes clear. Only those inputs which have special spatial wave-length oscillations are allowed through to the cortex, or are allowed to persist in those regions of the cortex strongly connected to the NRT: the thalamus-NRT system acts as a spatial Fourier filter (p. 353).

Simulation runs demonstrated the global, wave-like properties of the competitive model. The overall pattern of activation in cortical units was shown to be exclusively dependent upon the wave pattern spanning across all of the NRT units (figure 67.2). As LaBerge (1995) notes, the actual physiology of nRt gating in alert states remains unclear, but it is firmly established that nRt is the source of global oscillatory activity (at 8–13 Hz) initiating the descent into sleep.

The RN cells are known to inhibit each other, and when inhibition hyperpolarizes an RN cell sufficiently, it produces a rebound burst. In this way a network of connected RN inhibitory cells can spread activity to every cell within the network, apparently without decrement in the intensity of the activity. (p. 184)

Here then, is a plausible circuitry for a global, winner-take-all competition among the large array of specialized cortical processing areas.

Llinas et al. (1994) offer an interesting variation upon this circuitry, in which thalamocortical loops of the "non-specific" intralaminar nuclei operate in parallel with the specific (input) loops described above. The synchronous activation of specific and non-specific loops is postulated to provide a basis for "perceptual unity ... by which different sensory components are gathered into one global image" (p. 251). Their modeling is concerned with high-frequency EEG oscillations (and omits dendro-dendritic connections), yet appears to parallel much of what we discuss above.

When the interconnectivity of these nuclei is combined with the intrinsic properties of the individual neurons, a network for resonant neuronal oscillations emerges in which specific corticothalamic circuits would tend to resonate at 40 Hz. According to this hypothesis, neurons at the different levels, and particularly those in the reticular nucleus, would be responsible for the synchronization of 40-Hz oscillations in distant thalamic and cortical sites ... these oscillations may be organized globally over the CNS, especially as it has been shown that neighboring reticular cells are linked by dendrito-dendritic and intranuclear axon collaterals. (Deschenes et al. 1985; Yen et al. 1985, pp. 253–254)

A Neural Model for Global Resource Allocation

We have introduced a set of convergent models for the basic circuitry of a Global Workspace system involved in the integration and dissemination of the processing resources of the nervous system. This "bare bones" version accounts for how a global, winner-take-all competition might be mediated between various external inputs and cortical modules, to produce "a single, coherent stream of information out of the diverse activities of the CNS" (Newman and Baars 1993). There remains to be explained how the thalamocortical circuit fits in with the second half of our working definition for the conscious system: the allocation of processing resources based, first, upon biological contingencies of

novelty, need or potential threat and, secondly, cognitive schemas, purposes and plans. In keeping with our definition, we will first add a subcortical component for orienting to "novelty, need, or potential threat," and then discuss the much more complex aspects of cortically mediated effects upon the system.

This extended version of the model is schematically illustrated in figure 67.3 as a "wagon wheel," with the thalamus (Th) as its "hub." The reticular nucleus (nRt) corresponds to the metal sleeve fitted around the hub. The upper rim of the wheel represents the cerebral cortex (PFC/S1 ... V1), and closely associated basal ganglia (BG). The lower half shows the major sensory systems and subcortical nuclei whose projections converge upon the thalamus. The outer "spokes" represent the sensory pathways for vision, audition and the bodily senses. These project, in an orderly topography, to modality-specific nuclei in the thalamic "hub." As they ascend towards the thalamus, these pathways give off collaterals to the midbrain reticular formation (MRF) (see also Newman et al. 1997). Scheibel (1980) reviewed three decades of experimental evidence indicating that these midbrain collaterals serve as the basis for an initial "spatial envelope," or global map, of the environment surrounding the animal.

Most reticular [MRF] neurons ... appear multimodal, responding to particular visual, somatic and auditory stimuli, with combinations of the last two stimuli most numerous. The common receptive fields of typical bimodal cells in this array show a significant degree of congruence. For instance a unit responding to stimulation of the hind limb will usually prove maximally sensitive to auditory stimuli originating to the rear of the organism. These twin somatic and auditory maps retain approximate register and overlap the visuotopic map laid down in the ... superior colliculus ... These data might be interpreted to mean that each locus maps a point in the three-dimensional spatial envelope surrounding the organism. Further studies suggest the presence of a deep motor map closely matching and in apparent register with the sensory map. (p. 63)

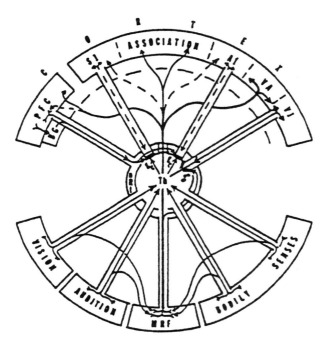

Figure 67.3
"Wagon wheel" model of CNS systems contributing to global attention and conscious perception. A1, primary auditory area; BG, basal ganglia; g$_c$, "closed" nRt gate; g$_o$, "open" nRt gate; MRF, midbrain reticular formation; nRt, nucleus reticularis thalami; PFC, prefrontal cortex; S1, primary somatosensory area; Th, ventral thalamus; V1, primary visual cortex (from Newman et al. 1997).

More recent research has supported Scheibel's portrayal of the superior colliculus as the visual component of what Crick and Koch (1990b) termed a "saliency map" for eye movements, involved in orienting the animal to biologically relevant stimuli. Subsequent findings have both confirmed Scheibel's analysis, and revealed a number of "top-down" projections that modulate activities in MRF. LaBerge (1995) writes:

the superficial area [of the superior colliculus] receives strong cortical inputs from V1, V2 and V3 [primary and secondary visual cortex], the deep layers in the monkey SC receive their main cortical inputs from the posterior parietal area (Lynch et al. 1985), from the

prefrontal areas (Goldman and Nauta 1976), and the frontal eye fields (Leichnetz et al. 1981). The deep layers contain a map of visual space that is stacked adjacent to maps for auditory and somatosensory spaces in a manner that cells corresponding to points in space lie along the same vertical axis (Merideth and Stein 1990). Stimulation of these cells by microelectrodes produces movements of eyes and head ... (LaBerge 1995, p. 145)

LaBerge goes on to describe basal ganglia inputs that "are of particular importance because they tonically inhibit activity in the SC cells." It has long been known that the frontal eye fields, and posterior parietal area "exert strong influences on eye movements and must be considered together with the superior colliculus in accounting for ... orienting of attention" (p. 142). These facts emphasize two key aspects of the "conscious system" we are modeling: (1) it is polymodal, integrating not just visual, auditory and somatosensory inputs, but motor and "higher-order" cortical effects; and (2) it is extended, with input/output relations reaching from the brain stem core to association cortices. Indeed, the general term we have used to describe it elsewhere is the "extended reticular-thalamic activation system" (ERTAS) (Baars 1988; Newman and Baars 1993; Newman 1995a,b, 1997).

The third key aspect of the system (as exemplified by the "wagon wheel" model) is that it converges on the thalamus. We have already discussed this in terms of the thalamocortical circuit, which connects to "virtually every area of the cerebral cortex" (LaBerge 1995, p. 221). Scheibel (1980) described the MRF portion of the system as:

sweep[ing] forward on a broad front, investing the [intralaminar complex of the] thalamus and nucleus reticularis thalami. The investiture is precise in the sense that the sites representing specific zones of the spatial envelope (receptive field) project to portions of the nucleus reticularis concerned with similar peripheral fields via projections from both sensory thalamus and sensory association cortices. (p. 62)

The fact that Scheibel's (1980) "spatial envelope" projects with some topographic precision upon nRt, would appear to enable it to disinhibit particular arrays of nRt gatelets, selectively enhancing the flow of sensory information to the cortex. The "intralaminar complex" (Newman and Baars 1993) is also integral to the ERTAS system, as the non-specific portion of the thalamocortical circuit. It is intralaminar projections which relay MRF activation to the cortex (illustrated by the vertical MRF-Th projection, above which it branches out to all areas of CORTEX). As noted above, Llinas et al. (1994) hypothesize the perceptual unity of consciousness (binding)

to be brought about by the global synchronization of specific and non-specific circuits via nRt. Scheibel (1980) earlier concluded as much concerning the role of this extended activation system in "selective awareness":

From these data, the concept emerges of a reticularis complex [nRt] selectively gating interaction between specific thalamic nuclei and the cerebral cortex under the opposed but complementary control of the brain stem reticular core [MRF] and the frontal granular cortex [PFC]. In addition, the gate is highly selective; thus, depending on the nature of the alerting stimulus or central excitation, only that portion of the nucleus reticularis will open which controls the appropriate subjacent thalamic sensory field. The reticularis gate [thus] becomes a mosaic of gatelets, each tied to some specific receptive zone or species of input. Each is under the delicate yet opposed control of: (a) the specifically signatured sensory input and its integrated feedback from cortex [S1 ... V1]; (b) the reticular core [MRF] with its concern more for novelty (danger?) than for specific details of experience; and (c) the frontal granular cortex-medial thalamic system [PFC/BG] more attuned to upper level strategies of the organism, whether based on drive mechanisms (food, sex) or on still more complex derivative phenomenon (curiosity, altruism). Perhaps here resides the structuro-functional substrate for selective awareness, and in the delicacy and complexity of its connections, our source of knowing, and of knowing that we know. (p. 63)

Here, as well, is a summary description of a neural substrate for the global allocation of the processing resources of the CNS. All that it lacks is the mechanisms for a global competition (Taylor and Alavi 1993) and binding (Llinas et al. 1994) introduced in the previous section. But we must tie the operations of this thalamus-centered system more closely to those of the cortex and basal ganglia, or most of the functions routinely studied by cognitive science have no place in the model. This introduces an exponentially higher level of complexity (one of the hazards of dealing with global systems).

One of the values of GW theory, however, is that it provides a framework for understanding this complexity. First, it holds that the vast majority of cognitive functions are carried out, nonconsciously, via changing arrays of specialized, modular processors. This is reflected, anatomically, in the immense number of cortico-cortical connections in the human brain, outnumbering those with subcortical nuclei by nearly ten to one. Thalamocortical projections are comparatively sparse, but serve at least two essential functions: (1) transmitting sensory inputs to the primary cortical areas (S1, A1, V1, figure 67.3); and (2) providing a means to selectively amplify/synchronize cortex-wide activation (see previous section).

GW theory also reminds us that conscious functions operate upon an information load about the size of working memory. Thus, we are talking of a highly coarse-grained level of processing. In this context, global attention is (at least) a second-order operation, acting upon a highly selective stream of information. All this is to say that a relatively low density of widely distributed, yet highly convergent, circuits could be all that are required to create a conscious system; and these are the very characteristics of the neural model we have described.

However, most neural network modelers take a cortically-centered view of cognition, from which the brain stem functions so far described probably seem rather primitive or trivial (i.e., orienting, controlling eye movements) when compared to cortically mediated processes such as language acquisition, pattern recognition, motor planning, etc. What evidence is there that cortical (and other forebrain systems) depend upon projections to the thalamus for effecting high-level cognitive processes?

Early support for such effects, mediated by prefrontal projections, was provided by animal experiments undertaken by Skinner and Yingling (1977). They found that selective activation of one portion of a fronto-thalamic tract could shut down sensory processing in visual, but not auditory, cortex. Activation of another "spoke" of the prefrontal-thalamic tract shut down auditory

processing, but allowed visual inputs to reach posterior cortex. Skinner and Yingling wrote "This result implies that selective attention emerges via selective inhibition in certain sensory channels that the animal must know in advance are irrelevant to its situation" (p. 54). To inhibit orienting based upon advanced knowledge is clearly a sophisticated use of cognition. Several lines of research have converged in recent years to support this concept. Summarizing the current state of knowledge of prefrontal regulation of subcortical systems, Newman (1997) wrote:

It is now generally accepted that the prefrontal lobes (with the cingulate cortex) constitute an 'executive' over the limbic system mediating such functions as working memory, inhibition of conditioned responses, and goal-directed attention (see Fuster 1980, Goldman-Rakic 1988b, Damasio 1994, Posner 1994). More recent research on the basal ganglia (see reviews by Groenewegen and Berendse 1994, Parent and Hazrati 1995) have suggested that they constitute a "motor programming extension" of the frontal lobes as well—routed through the thalamus. (p. 112–113)

Newman (1997) goes on to cite evidence (Parent and Hazrati 1995) that the BG "extension" (like the thalamocortical loops) sends rich, collateral projections to nRt that effect not only its "gating" of motor programs, but hippocampal-mediated episodic memory functions (see also Newman 1995b).

Finally, we would note that cortico-thalamic projections to nRt and associated specific nuclei are both more topographically precise (Mitrofanis and Guillery 1993) and more pervasive than had once been thought (Jones 1985). Llinas and Pare (1991) estimate that, for every axon the thalamus sends to the cortex, the cortical area it projects to reciprocates with ten. Given the modular architecture of the neocortex, one might reasonably predict that these cortico-thalamic projections exert highly differentiated influences upon the flow of information through the thalamus. Efforts by experimental neuroscience throughout the 1980s to elucidate the precise effects of cortico-thalamic projections were frustratingly inconclusive. But a recent review by Buser and Rougeul-Buser (1995) notes:

The situation has however recently swung back, due to some new and perhaps consistent findings, indicating that the visual cortex appears to have a major action down onto the lateral geniculate nucleus, which may generate thalamic oscillations (Funke and Eyse 1992, McCormick and Krosigk 1992, Krosigk et al. 1993, Sillito et al. 1994). (p. 252)

While additional research is clearly needed, these recent findings suggest that Scheibel's (1980) early model of the converging influences of projections upon a thalamic hub—with the addition of basal ganglia inputs to nRt and the intralaminar complex—remains a viable model for "global attention," including the influences of cortically generated "schemas, purposes and plans." Newman (1997) discusses the contributions of the "cortico-basal ganglia-thalamo-cortical loop" to memory and volitional processes in greater detail. The complexities of this system are beyond the scope of the models presented here, although Monchi and Taylor (1995) and Taylor and Michalis (1995), among others, have developed neural models simulating functions of the BG and hippocampal systems.

What we propose to do instead is present a much simpler, but highly relevant, connectionist model that simulates the sorts of second-order operations one would predict in a GW system employing a gating network to selectively filter and integrate inputs as a function of central knowledge stores. The basic heuristic for this type of model is described in Newman and Baars (1993). It posits that

prefrontal cortex acts as an executive attentional system by actively influencing information processing in the posterior cortex through its effects upon the nucleus reticularis. In this manner, the highly parallel [processing] functions of the posterior cortex are brought into accord with increasingly complex and intentional cognitive schemes generated within the prefrontal regions of the brain. (p. 281)

A defining property of an executive system is that it acts upon other sub-systems, modifying their inputs for its particular purposes. Posterior cortical areas act more like arrays of quasi-autonomous processing modules (or local experts)—the bread and butter of NN simulations. Note that an executive system is not an *essential* requirement for consciousness. That this is the case is illustrated by the literature on extensive damage to the frontal lobes of the brain. PFC damage results in significant deficits in such purposeful activities as: the inhibition of inappropriate responding; switching of response set, planning and monitoring of actions, and so on; but produces little or no alteration in basic mental status. Indeed, many patients with frontal lobe pathology perform at pre-morbid levels on intelligence tests (Walshe 1978, Damasio 1994). In terms of the GW model we have presented, it is not executive attentional processes, but the selective binding of coalitions of active cortical modules via a thalamocortical competition which is the *sine qua non* for the generation of a coherent stream of conscious representations. Examples of these aspects of the GW model have already been offered.

Second-Order Models for Global Gating

Let us return to the "wagon wheel" model illustrated in figure 67.3, and transform its components into a connectionist GW, with an executive system. To simplify things, the network will have only two sensory modules, one for processing auditory (A1) inputs, and one for visual (V1). In order to provide second-order control over processing in both modules, we will add a gating module (nRt) with the same number of units as connections in each sensory module. Each gating unit sends its output to a corresponding connection in A1 and V1. The connections between the gating units and sensory units are multiplicative. As Rummelhart et al. (1986) write about such connections:

if one unit of a multiplicative pair is zero, the other member of the pair can have no effect, no matter how strong its output. On the other hand, if one unit of a pair has value 1, the output of the other passe[s] unchanged to the receiving unit.... In addition to their use as gates [such] units can be used to convert the output level of a unit into a signal that acts like a weight connecting two units. (p. 73)

In this manner, a fully connected gating module can actually program the connection strengths of one or more input modules to process a particular type of input, for example phonemes, or letters, into words. For maximum flexibility, it is preferable that the gating module not have fixed connections either, but simply relay gating (connection strength) information from a central module to which its units are connected. The central module contains (in this case) word-level knowledge needed to program the sensory modules to process words. Another central module might be specialized for knowledge for processing visual scenes or tactile shapes. To complete the system, each programmable input unit sends a corresponding connection to a central module unit.

The highly simplified network just described is really a variation on a Programmable Blackboard Model for Reading developed by McClelland (1985, 1986). Its four modules correspond to those labeled in figure 67.4: a Central Module (PFC); Connection Activation System (PFC-nRt); and two Programmable Modules (A1, V1). The connections described above are shown in figure 67.5 (note: McClelland's modules are identical, and used only for reading (not hearing) words, but theoretically they could be programmed to process *any* type of input).

In the brain, of course, the primary areas (A1, V1, S1) send no direct projections to PFC; but they do send convergent projections (as in figure 67.5) to secondary association areas, which send projections directly to PFC (as well as posterior association areas). Although these feed-forward projections to PFC are less topographically precise (e.g., the receptive fields of visual neurons in the secondary areas are much larger), they maintain a fair degree of parallel distribution, indicating that much of the prefrontal cortex is as modular in its organization as the posterior "association" cortex. Moreover, PFC "modules" reciprocate these parallel, feed-forward projections, although in a more divergent pattern (Goldman-Rakic 1988a, LaBerge 1995). Interestingly, this convergence/divergence pattern is paralleled by the connections in figure 67.5 for the central module.

In the actual prefrontal cortex there are hundreds (if not thousands) of "central modules." Feed-forward inputs allow them to use and store highly processed information from the posterior (sensory) cortex. Of course, feedback (or re-entrant) connections enable PFC to influence processing in the posterior areas as well. But such divergent and indirect feedback pathways are poorly suited to exercising momentary, direct effects upon processing at the input level. Nor could such centrally stored knowledge be employed to guide, or anticipate, how inputs are processed (re the "knowing in advance" Skinner and Yingling (1977) attributed to PFC-Th circuits). This is where direct projections to the primary processing areas (actually the thalamocortical circuit) could prove quite valuable. Instead of the sensory input units (A1-Th; V1-Th) responding based upon fixed connection strengths, a central module could program input modules to process (i.e., pay attention to) particular categories of inputs. McClelland (1986) calls this form of activation "connection information distribution" (CID) and compares its benefits to those of:

the invention of the stored program.... The use of centrally stored connection information to program local processing structures is analogous. It allows the very same processing structures to be programmed to perform a very wide range of different tasks.... [CID] also carries out a form of what is known in production systems as "resolution," binding the right tokens in the blackboard together into higher-order structural patterns. (p. 165)

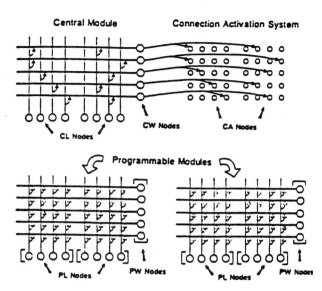

Figure 67.4
A simplified example of a Connection Information Distributor (CID), sufficient for simultaneous bottom-up processing of two two-letter words. The programmable modules consist of the programmable letter (PL) and programmable word (PW) nodes, and programmable connections between them (open triangles). The central module consists of a set of central letter (CL) nodes and a set of central word (CW) nodes, and hard-wired connections between them (filled triangles). The connection activation system includes the central word nodes, a set of connection activator (CA) nodes, and hard-wired connections between them. Connections between the central knowledge system (central module plus connection activation system) and the programmable blackboard are shown in figure 67.6 (from McClelland 1985).

Finally, he notes analogous aspects in the CID's operations to "working memory," a process which has been tied by neuroscientists to a prefrontal/thalamic/hippocampal system (e.g., Fuster 1980, Goldman-Rakic 1988b). These comparisons between the Wagon Wheel and Programmable Blackboard models, of course, have purely heuristic value (although McClelland's (1986) PABLO simulation of his model contained a sufficient programmable blackboard to read lines of text up to 20 characters long). But the use of gating networks to generate useful "higher-order structural patterns" is fairly widespread.

For engineering problems such as object recognition and robot motion control, the concept of combining modular networks using gating connections has been actively exploited to develop highly reliable systems (Jacobs et al. 1991, Hampshire and Waibel 1992, Jacobs and Jordan 1993, Cho and Kim 1995). The key issue in this approach is how to combine the results of the individual networks to give the best estimate of the optimal overall result. Architectures used in this approach consist of two types of networks: an expert and a gating network. Basically, the expert networks compete to learn the training instances, and the gating network facilitates co-

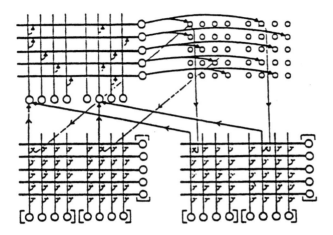

Figure 67.5
Each CA node projects to the corresponding connection in both programmable modules, and each central letter node receives projections from the corresponding programmable letter node in both programmable modules. The inputs to two central letter nodes, and the outputs from two CA nodes are shown (from McClelland 1985).

operation by the overall mediation of this competition. The expert networks may be trained separately using their own preassigned sub-tasks and differing modalities (e.g., vision and touch), or the same modality at different times (e.g., the consecutive 2-D views of a rotating 3-D object). The gating network need only have as many output units as there are expert networks.

To train such a gating network, Hampshire and Waibel (1992) developed a new form of multiplicative connection, which they call the "Meta-Pi" connection. Its function is closely aligned with predecessors described in McClelland (1986). The final output of the overall system is a linear combination of the outputs of the expert networks, with the gating network determining the proportion of each local output in the linear combination. Figure 67.6 illustrates this architecture with three expert networks.

The final output of the overall system is a linear combination of the outputs of the expert networks, with the gating network determining the proportion of each local output in the linear combination. The Meta-Pi gating network allo-

cates appropriate combinations of the expert networks when stimuli are assessed to be novel, while an automatic ("non-conscious") decision process operates in instances where a single expert can execute the task. This coupling of modular, expert networks and gating controls produces new levels of cooperative behavior. The expert networks are local in the sense that the weights in one network are decoupled from the weights in other expert networks. However, there is still some indirect coupling because if some other network changes its weights, it may cause the gating network to alter the responsibilities that get assigned to the expert network.

These examples from engineering applications of multiplicative, gating networks are not based upon the Wagon Wheel model or, for that matter, any specific neural circuitry. Yet Koch (1997) notes:

Multiplication is one of the most common operations carried out in the nervous system (for example, for estimating motion or the time-to-contact with an approaching stimulus). (p. 208)

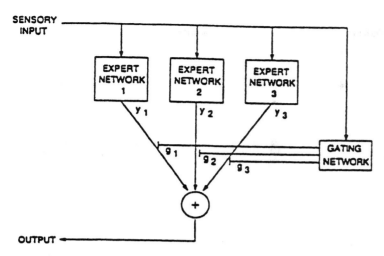

Figure 67.6

Schematic diagram of modular neural networks with three expert networks and a gating network. The output of the entire architecture, denoted by Y, is $Y = g_1y_1 + g_2y_2 + g_3y_3$, where y_i denotes the output of the ith expert network.

We are not aware of any studies of either the axon collateral or dendro-dendritic projections in nRt demonstrating multiplicative properties, but Mel (1994) has modeled such connections in the NMDA-rich dendritic trees of cortical pyramidal cells. He postulates that they perform nonlinear pattern discrimination and correlative operations. Given the role of the bidirectional dendritic trees of nRt cells in globally synchronizing the thalamocortical circuit (Taylor and Alavi 1993, LaBerge 1995), it seems likely that they will eventually be found to have important computational functions as well.

Even if it transpires that synchronous oscillations, not multiplicative connections, are the basis for the "gating" functions of nRt upon the thalamocortical circuit, NN models based upon Meta-Pi connections may still be useful for simulating global workspace systems. The use of Meta-Pi connections has already been extended to synchronous oscillators in modular cortical neural networks. Indeed, computational simulations of phase-locked oscillations characteristic of neurons involved in the "binding" of visual (Grossberg and Somers 1991, Sompolinsky et al. 1991) and auditory (Vibert et al. 1994) features of an attended object have already been extended to synchronous oscillators using Meta-Pi connections. Such oscillatory circuits have also been employed in modeling storage and retrieval in pattern recognition tasks (Yao and Freeman 1990).

In this paper, we have introduced a collection of neuroscience and NN models for attention and binding, resource allocation, and second-order gating, which share important features and parallels with a Neural Global Workspace System for conscious attention (Newman and Baars 1993). While the NN models we have presented only implement partial aspects of the GW system, and even our Wagon Wheel model largely neglects the influences of memory and affective systems upon the stream of consciousness, the outlines of a general framework for understanding conscious processes should be discernable (see Newman 1997 for a fuller account). This is certainly great progress, given the virtual *terra incognita* consciousness has been for most of the history of science.

References

Baars, B. J. (1983). How does a serial, integrated and very limited stream of consciousness emerge out of a nervous system that is mostly unconscious, distributed, and of enormous capacity? In G. R. Brock & J. Marsh (Eds), *CIBA Symposium on Experimental and Theoretical Studies of Consciousness* (pp. 282–290). London: John Wiley and Sons.

Baars, B. J. (1988). *A cognitive theory of consciousness.* Cambridge: Cambridge University Press.

Baars, B. J. (1992). *Experimental slips and human error: Exploring the architecture of volition.* New York: Plemun Press.

Baars, B. J. (1994). A global workspace theory of conscious experience. Baars, B. J. and Newman, J. (1994). A neuro-biological interpretation of a Global Workspace theory of consciousness. In A. Revonsuo and M. Kamppinen (Eds), *Consciousness in philosophy and cognitive neuroscience.* Hillsdale, NJ: Erlbaum.

Baars, B. J. (1997). *In the theatre of consciousness: The workspace of the mind.* Oxford: Oxford University Press.

Baars, B. J., Newman, J. and Taylor, J. G. (1998). Neuronal mechanisms of consciousness: A Relational Global Workspace framework. In S. Hameroff, A. Kaszniak, J. Laukes, and A. Scott (Eds), *Towards a science of consciousness: The second Tucson discussion and debates.* Cambridge, MA: MIT Press.

Buser, P., and Rougeul-Buser, A. (1995). Do cortical and thalamic bioelectric oscillations have a functional role? A brief survey. *Journal of Physiology (Paris), 89,* 249–254.

Cho, S.-B., and Kim, J. H. (1995). Multiple network fusion using fuzzy logic. *IEEE Trans. Neural Networks, 6,* 497–501.

Crick, F. (1984). Function of the thalamic reticular complex: the searchlight hypothesis. *Proceedings of the National Academy of Sciences, USA, 81,* 4586–4590.

Crick, F., and Koch, C. (1990a). Towards a neurobiological theory of consciousness. *Seminars in the Neurosciences, 2,* 263–275.

Crick, F., and Koch, C. (1990b). Some reflections on visual awareness. *Cold Spring Harbor Symposium on Quantitative Biology, 15,* 953–962.

Damasio, A. R. (1994). *Descartes' Error.* New York: G.P. Putnam Sons.

Deschenes, M., Madariage-Domich, A., and Steriade, M. (1985). Dendrodendritic synapses in the cat reticularis thalami nucleus: A structural basis for thalamic spindle synchronization. *Brain Research, 334,* 165–168.

Durfee, E. H. (1993). Cooperative distributed problem solving between (and within) intelligent agents. In P. Rudomin et al. (Eds), *Neuroscience: From neural networks to artificial intelligence* (pp. 84–98). Heidelberg: Springer-Verlag.

Eccles, J. C. (1966). *Brain and conscious experience.* Heidelberg: Springer-Verlag.

Edelman, G. M. (1989). *The remembered present, a biological theory of consciousness.* New York: Basic Books.

Funke, K., and Eyse, U. T. (1992). EEG-dependent modulation of response dynamics of cat dLGN relay cells and the contribution of corticogeniculate feedback. *Brain Research, 573,* 217–227.

Fuster, J. M. (1980). *The prefrontal cortex.* New York: Raven Press.

Gazzanigga, M. S. (1985). *The social brain, discovering the networks of the mind.* New York: Basic Books.

Goldman-Rakic, P. S. (1988a). Changing concepts of cortical connectivity: parallel distributed cortical networks. In P. Rakic and W. Singer (Eds), *Neurobiology of the cortex* (pp. 177–202). Berlin: John Wiley and Sons Ltd.

Goldman-Rakic, P. S. (1988b). The prefrontal contribution to working memory and conscious experience. In O. Creutzfeld and J. Eccles (Eds), *The brain and conscious experience.* Rome: Pontifical Academy.

Groenewegen, H. J., and Berendse, H. W. (1994). The specificity of the "nonspecific" midline and intralaminar thalamic nuclei. *Trends in Neuroscience, 4*(2), 52–58.

Grossberg, S., and Somers, D. (1991). Synchronized oscillations during cooperative feature linking in a cortical model of visual perception. *Neural Networks, 4,* 452–466.

Hampshire II, J. B., and Waibel, A. (1992). The Meta-Pi network: Building distributed knowledge representations for robust multisource pattern recognition. *IEEE Trans. Pattern Analysis and Machine Intelligence, 14*, 751–769.

Harnad, S. (1994). Guest editorial—Why and how we are not zombies. *Journal of Consciousness Studies, 1*(2), 164–168.

Heilman, K. M., Watson, R. T. and Valenstein, E. V. (1985). Neglect and related disorders. In K. M. Heilman and E. V. Valenstein (Eds), *Clinical neuropsychology.* New York: Oxford University Press.

Jackendorf, R. (1987). *Consciousness and the computational mind.* Cambridge, MA: MIT Press.

Jacobs, R. A., Jordan, M. I., Nowlan, S. J., and Hinton, G. E. (1991). Adaptive mixtures of local experts. *Neural Computation, 3*, 79–87.

Jacobs, R. A., and Jordan, M. I. (1993). Learning piecewise control strategies in a modular neural network architecture. *IEEE Trans. Systems, Man, and Cybernetics, 23*, 337–345.

Jasper, H. H. (1960). Unspecific thalamocortical relations. In J. Field, H. W. Magoun and V. E. Hall (Eds), *Handbook of neurophysiology, Vol. 1* (pp. 1307–1322). Washington, DC: American Physiological Society.

Johnson-Laird, P. N. (1988). *The computer and the mind.* Cambridge, MA: Harvard University Press.

Jones, E. G. (1985). *The thalamus.* New York: Plenum Press.

Kihlstrom, J. F. (1987). The cognitive unconscious. *Science, 237*, 285–292.

Koch, C. (1997). Computation and the single neuron. *Nature, 385*, 207–210.

Koch, C., and Poggio, T. (1992). Multiplying with synapses and neurons. In T. McKenna, J. Davis and S. F. Zornetzer (Eds), *Single neuron computation* (pp. 315–345). Boston, MA: Academic Press.

Krosigk, von M., Bal, T., and McCormack, D. (1993). Cellular mechanisms of a synchronized oscillation in the thalamus. *Science, 261*, 361–364.

LaBerge, D. L. (1990). William James symposium: Attention. *Psychological Science, 1*(3), 156–162.

LaBerge, D. L. (1995). *Attentional processing: The brain's art of mindfulness.* Cambridge, MA: Harvard University Press.

Llinas, R. R., and Pare, D. (1991). Commentary: of dreaming and wakefulness. *Neuroscience, 44*(3), 521–535.

Llinas, R., Ribary, U. Joliot, M. and Wang, X.-J. (1994). Content and context in temporal thalamocortical binding. In G. Busaki et al. (Eds), *Temporal coding in the brain* (pp. 251–272). Heidelberg: Springer-Verlag.

McClelland, J. L. (1985). Putting knowledge in its place: A scheme for programming parallel processing structures on the fly. *Cognitive Science, 9*, 113–146.

McClelland, J. L. (1986). The programmable blackboard model of reading. In J. L. McClelland and D. E. Rummelhart (Eds), *Parallel distributed processing*, Vol. 2 (pp. 122–169). Cambridge, MA: MIT Press.

McCormick, D. A., and Krosigk, M. (1992). Corticothalamic activation modulates thalamic firing through glutamate metabotropic receptors. *Proceedings of the National Academy of Science USA, 89*, 2774–2778.

Mel, B. W. (1994). Information processing in dendritic trees. *Neural Computation, 6*, 1031–1085.

Mesulam, M. (1985). *Principles of behavioral neurology.* Philadelphia: F.A. Davis.

Minsky, M. (1979). The society theory. In P. H. Winston and R. H. Brown (Eds), *Artificial intelligence, an MIT perspective, Vol. 1* (pp. 423–450). Cambridge, MA: MIT Press.

Mitrofanis, J., and Guillery, R. W. (1993). New views of the thalamic reticular nucleus in the adult and developing brain. *Trends in Neuroscience, 16*, 240–245.

Monchi, O. and Taylor, J. G. (1995). A model of the prefrontal loop that includes the basal ganglia in solving a recency task. *Proceedings of the International Neural Network Society Annual Meeting*, July 1995. Washington, DC: International Neural Network Society Press.

Newell, A. (1992). SOAR as a unified theory of cognition: Issues and explanations. *Behavioral and Brain Sciences, 15*(3), 464–492.

Newman, J. (1995a). Review: Thalamic contributions to attention and consciousness. *Consciousness and Cognition, 4*(2), 172–193.

Newman, J. (1995b). Reticular-thalamic activation of the cortex generates conscious contents. *Behavioral and Brain Sciences, 18*(4), 691–692.

Newman, J. (1997). Putting the puzzle together: Towards a general theory of the neural correlates of consciousness. *Journal of Consciousness Studies, 4* (1 and 2), 47–66 and 99–120.

Newman, J., and Baars, B. J. (1993). A neural attentional model for access to consciousness: A Global Workspace perspective. *Concepts in Neuroscience, 4*(2), 255–290.

Newman, J., Baars, B. J. and Cho, S.-B. (1997). A neurocognitive model for attention and consciousness. In S. O'Nuallain, P. McKevitt and E. MacAogdin (Eds), *Two sciences of mind: Readings in cognitive science and consciousness*. Philadelphia, PA: John Benjamins of North America.

O'Nuallain, S., McKevit, P. and MacAogdin, E. (1997). *Two sciences of mind: Readings in cognitive science and consciousness*. Philadelphia, PA: John Benjamins of North America.

Parent, A., and Hazrati, L.-N. (1995). Functional anatomy of the basal ganglia. I. The cortico-basal ganglia-thalamo-cortical loop. *Brain Research Reviews, 20*, 91–127.

Penfield, W. (1975). *The mystery of the mind: A critical study of consciousness and the human brain*. Princeton, NJ: Princeton University Press.

Penrose, R. (1994). *Shadows of the mind—In search of the missing science of consciousness*. Oxford: Oxford University Press.

Posner, M. I. and Rothbart, M. K. (1991). Attentional mechanisms and conscious experience. In A. D. Milner and M. D. Rugg (Eds), *The neuropsychology of consciousness* (pp. 11–34). London: Academic Press.

Posner, M. I. (1994). Attention: The mechanisms of consciousness. *Proceedings of the National Academy of Science USA, 91*, 7398–7403.

Reddy, D. R., Erman, L. D., Fennell, R. D., and Neely, R. B. (1973). The Hearsay speech understanding system: An example of the recognition process. *Proceedings of the International Conference on Artificial Intelligence*, 185–194.

Rummelhart, D. E., Hinton, G. E. and McClelland, J. L. (1986). A general framework for parallel distributed processing. In J. L. McClelland and D. E. Rummelhart (Eds), *Parallel distributed processing*, Vol. 1 (pp. 43–76). Cambridge, MA: MIT Press.

Scheibel, M. E., and Scheibel, A. B. (1966). The organization of the nucleus reticularis: A Golgi study. *Brain Research, 1*, 43–62.

Scheibel, A. B. (1980). Anatomical and physiological substrates of arousal: A view from the bridge. In J. A. Hobson and M. A. B. Brazier (Eds), *The reticular formation revisited* (pp. 55–66). New York: Raven Press.

Sillito, A., Jones, H., Gerstein, G., and West, D. (1994). Feature-linked synchronization of thalamic relay cell firing induced by feedback from the visual cortex. *Nature, 369*, 479–482.

Skinner, J. E. and Yingling, C. D. (1977). Central gating mechanisms that regulate event-related potentials and behavior. In J. E. Desmedt (Ed.), *Progress in clinical neurophysiology: Attention, voluntary contraction and event-related cerebral potentials. Vol. 1* (pp. 30–69). Basel: Karger.

Sompolinsky, H., Golomb, D., and Kleinfeld, D. (1991). Cooperative dynamics in visual processing. *Physical Review A, 43*(12), 6990–7011.

Steriade, M., and Llinas, R. R. (1988). The functional states of the thalamus and the associated neuronal interplay. *Physiological Reviews, 68*(3), 649–742.

Stryker, M. P. (1989). Is grandmother an oscillation? *Nature, 338*, 297–337.

Taylor, J. G. (1992). Towards a neural network model of the mind. *Neural Network World, 2*, 797–812.

Taylor, J. G. (1996). A competition for consciousness? *Neurocomputing, 11*, 271–296.

Taylor, J. G. and Alavi, F. N. (1993). Mathematical analysis of a competitive network for attention. In J. G. Taylor (Ed.), *Mathematical approaches to neural networks* (pp. 341–382). Amsterdam: Elsevier Science Publishers B.V.

Taylor, J. G. and Michalis, L. (1995). The functional role of the hippocampus in the organization of memory. *Proceedings of the International Neural Network Society Annual Meeting*, July 1995. Washington, DC: International Neural Network Society Press.

Vibert, J., Pakdaman, K., and Azmy, N. (1994). Interneural delay modification synchronizes biologically plausible neural networks. *Neural Networks, 7*, 589–607.

Walshe, K. W. (1978). *Neuropsychology, A clinical approach*. Edinburgh: Churchill Livingstone.

Yao, Y., and Freeman, W. J. (1990). Model of biological pattern recognition with spatially chaotic dynamics. *Neural Networks, 3*, 153–170.

Yen, C. T., Conely, M., Hendry, S. H. C., and Jones, E. G. (1985). The morphology of physiologically indentified GABAergic neurons in the somatic sensory part of the thalamic reticular nucleus in the cat. *Journal of Neuroscience, 5*, 2254–2268.

68 A Software Agent Model of Consciousness

Stan Franklin and Art Graesser

Global Workspace Theory

Baars's (1988, 1997) Global Workspace theory postulates that human cognition is implemented by a multitude of relatively small, special-purpose processes, almost always unconscious. Coalitions of such processes find their way into a global workspace and thus into "consciousness." From this limited capacity workspace, the message of the coalition is broadcast to all the unconscious processors in order to recruit other processors to join in handling the current novel situation or in solving the current problem. All this takes place under the auspices of various contexts, including goal contexts, perceptual contexts, conceptual contexts, and cultural contexts. Each context is itself a coalition of processes. There is much more to the theory, including attention, learning, action selection, and problem solving.

Baars's Global Workspace theory is a comprehensive theory of both consciousness and general cognition. The theory is appropriately articulated at an abstract, functional, verbal level because of its attempt to account for many cognitive phenomena and empirical findings. Baars's description goes a long way in capturing the cognitive principles and mechanisms at a functional level, but it does not specify all of the mechanisms at the levels of computation and neuroscience. It is the computational level that is the primary focus of the present article. Our goal is to flesh out the computational architectures and mechanisms that are left unspecified in his articulation of Global Workspace theory. At the very least, this article will identify some of the computational issues that must be addressed in any computer implementation of Global Workspace theory.

Autonomous Agents

Conscious Mattie (CMattie) is an autonomous software agent. An autonomous agent (Franklin and Graesser 1997) is a system "situated in" an environment, which senses that environment and acts on it over time in pursuit of its own agenda. It acts in such a way as to possibly influence what it senses at a later time. In other words, it is structurally coupled to its environment (Maturana 1975; Maturana and Varela 1980; Varela, Thompson, and Rosch 1991). Biological examples of autonomous agents include humans and most animals. Nonbiological examples include some mobile robots and various computational agents, including artificial life agents, software agents, and computer viruses. CMattie is an autonomous software agent, designed for a specific clerical task, that "lives" in a real-world UNIX operating system. The autonomous software agent that we are developing is equipped with computational versions of cognitive features, such as multiple senses, perception, short- and long-term memory, attention, planning, reasoning, problem solving, learning, emotions, and multiple drives. In this sense, our software agents are cognitive agents (Franklin 1997a).

We believe that cognitive software agents have the potential to play a synergistic role in both cognitive theory and intelligent software. Minds can be viewed as control structures for autonomous agents (Franklin 1995). A theory of mind constrains the design of a cognitive agent that implements that theory. While a theory is typically abstract and only broadly sketches an architecture, an implemented computational design provides a fully articulated architecture and a complete set of mechanisms. This architecture and set of mechanisms provide a richer, more concrete, and more decisive theory. Moreover, every design decision taken during an implementation furnishes a hypothesis about how human minds work. These hypotheses motivate experiments with humans and other forms of empirical tests. Conversely, the results of such experiments motivate corresponding modifications of the architecture and mechanisms of the cognitive agent. In this way, the concepts and methodologies of cognitive science and of computer science will work synergistically to enhance our understanding of mechanisms of mind (Franklin 1997a), CMattie was designed with this research strategy in mind.

CMattie is designed for the explicit purpose of implementing global workspace theory. Some of the components have already been programmed, whereas others are at the design stage. However, she is far enough along to allow us to address the key question of this paper: how well does CMattie, as a conceptual model, account for the psychological facts that global workspace theory was constructed to explain?

The CM Architecture

Conceptually, CMattie is an autonomous software agent that lives in a UNIX system. CMattie communicates in natural language with seminar organizers and attendees via e-mail, "comprehends" e-mail messages, composes messages, and sends seminar announcements, all without human direction. CMattie is an extension of Virtual Mattie (VMattie) (Franklin et al. 1996; Song and Franklin, forthcoming; Zhang et al. 1998). VMattie, which is currently running in a beta-testing stage, implements an initial set of components of global workspace theory. VMattie performs all of the functions of CMattie, as listed above, but does so "unconsciously" and without the ability to learn and to flexibly handle novel situations. CMattie adds the missing pieces of Global Workspace theory, including computational versions of attention,

associative and episodic memories, emotions, learning, and metacognition.

The computational mechanisms of CMattie incorporate some of the mechanisms of mind discussed at length in *Artificial minds* (Franklin 1995). Each of the mechanisms mentioned required considerable modification, and often extension, so that they would be suitable for use in CMattie. The high-level action selection uses an extended form of Maes's (1990) behavior net. The net is composed of behaviors, drives, and links between them. Activation spreads in one direction from the drives and in the other from CMattie's percepts. The currently active behavior is chosen from those whose preconditions are met and whose activations are over threshold. Lower-level actions are taken by codelets in the manner of the Copycat architecture (Hofstadter and Mitchell 1994, Mitchell 1993). Each codelet is a small piece of code, a little program, that does one thing. Our implementation of Baars's global workspace, discussed in more detail below, relies heavily on the playing field in Jackson's (1987) pandemonium theory. All active codelets inhabit the playing field, and those in "consciousness" occupy the global workspace. Kanerva's (1988) sparse distributed memory (Anwar and Franklin, forthcoming) provides a human-like associative memory for the agent, whereas episodic memory (case-based) follows Kolodner's (1993) model. CMattie's emotion mechanism uses pandemonium theory (McCauley and Franklin 1998). Her metacognition module is based on a fuzzy version of Holland's classifier system (Holland 1986; Zhang, Franklin, and Dasgupta 1998). Learning by CMattie is accomplished by a number of mechanisms. Behavior nets can learn by adjusting the weights on links as in artificial neural networks (Maes 1992). The demons in pandemonium theory become (more) associated as they occur together in the arena (Jackson 1987). The associations that occur automatically in sparse distributed memory constitute learning (Kanerva 1988). CMattie also employs one-trial learning using case-based reasoning (Bogner, Ramamurthy, and Franklin 1999; Kolodner 1993; Ramamurthy, Franklin, and Negatu 1998).

We next turn to a brief account of how the CM architecture uses these mechanisms to model Global Workspace theory. The CM architecture can be conveniently partitioned into more abstract, high-level constructs and lower-level, less abstract codelets. Higher-level constructs, such as behaviors and some slipnet nodes, overlie collections of codelets that actually do their work. In CMattie, Baars's "vast collection of unconscious processes" are implemented as codelets much in the manner of the Copycat architecture or almost equivalently as Jackson's demons. His limited capacity global workspace is a portion of Jackson's playing field, which holds the active codelets. Working memory consists of several distinct workspaces, one for perception, one for composing announcements, two for one-trial learning, and others.

Baars speaks of contexts as "... the great array of unconscious mental sources that shape our conscious experiences and beliefs" (Baars 1997, p. 115). He distinguishes several types, including perceptual contexts, conceptual contexts, and goal contexts. The perceptual context provided by a large body of water might help me interpret a white, rectangular cloth as a sail rather than as a bed sheet. The conceptual context of a discussion of money might point me at interpreting "Let's go down by the bank" as something other than an invitation for a walk, a picnic, or a swim. Hunger might well give rise to a goal context. Contexts in Global Workspace theory are coalitions of codelets. In the CM architecture, high-level constructs are often identified with their underlying collections of codelets and, thus, can be thought of as contexts. Perceptual contexts include particular nodes from a slipnet-type associative memory à la Copycat (similar to a semantic net) and particular templates in workspaces. For example, a message-type node is a perceptual context. A node-type perceptual context becomes active via spreading activation in the slipnet when the node reaches a threshold. Several nodes can be active at once, producing composite perceptual contexts. These mechanisms allow "conscious" experiences to trigger "unconscious" contexts that help to interpret later conscious events. Conceptual contexts also reside in the slipnet, as well as in associative memory. Goal contexts are implemented as instantiated behaviors in a much more dynamic version of Maes's behavior nets. They become active by having preconditions met and by exceeding a time variable threshold. Goal hierarchies are implemented as instantiated behaviors and their associated drives. (My hunger drive might give rise to the goal of eating sushi. The first behavior toward that goal might be walking to my car.) The dominant goal context is determined by the currently active instantiated behavior. The dominant goal hierarchy is one rooted at the drive associated with the currently active instantiated behavior.

Recruitment of coalitions of unconscious processors is accomplished by consciousness codelets, as well as by the associations among the occupants of the global workspace, via pandemonium theory. Always active, consciousness codelets jump into action when problematic situations occur. An example is described below. Attention is what goes into the global workspace from perception and from internal monitoring. It also uses pandemonium theory, but requires an extension of it. Both recruitment and attention are modulated by the various context hierarchies. Learning occurs via several mechanisms: as in pandemonium theory, as in sparse distributed memory, as in behavior nets, by extensions of these, and by other mechanisms. High-level action selection is provided by the instantiated behavior net. At a low level, CMattie follows the Copycat architecture procedure of temperature controlled (here emotionally controlled), parallel terraced scanning. Problem solving is accomplished via conscious recruitment of coalitions of unconscious codelets.

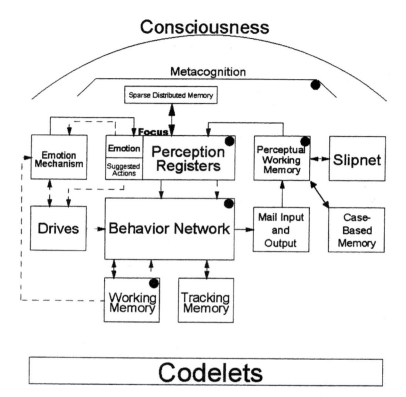

Figure 68.1
Most of the "conscious" Mattie architecture. Solid arrow signifies regular data transfer. Dashed arrow signifies that potential activation of target can occur with data transfer. Solid circle indicates modules where spotlight can shine.

Figure 68.1 gives a functional overview of most of the CMattie architecture. Several important functions, for example, conceptual and behavioral learning, are omitted from the diagram, but not from our discussion. Detailed descriptions of the architecture and mechanisms are given in a series of papers by members of the "Conscious" Software Research Group (Anwar and Franklin, forthcoming; Bogner, Ramamurthy, and Franklin 1999; Franklin 1997b; Franklin et al. 1996; McCauley and Franklin 1998; Ramamurthy et al. 1998; Song and Franklin, forthcoming; Zhang et al. 1998a,b).

CMattie in Action

This section described walks through a typical incoming message through the CM architecture. Suppose CMattie receives the following message from Stan Franklin:

"Dear CMattie, Hope your day hasn't been as busy as mine. Next week Art Graesser will speak to the Cognitive Science Seminar on Kintsch's Comprehension Theory. Have a good one. Stan"

After the message arrives in CMattie's in-box, codelets transfer it to the perceptual workspace

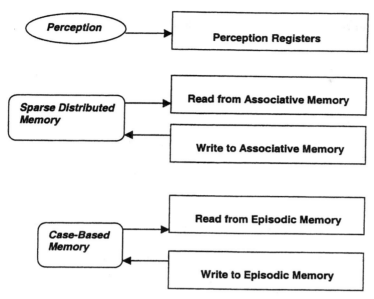

Figure 68.2
The focus.

where other codelets begin the process of making sense of it. Some codelet will recognize "Cognitive Science Seminar" as a known seminar and activate its node in the slipnet. Another will identify "Art Graesser" as a name, possibly a speaker, again activating a node. Other such recognitions will occur. Eventually the slipnet's spreading activation will push some message-type node over threshold, in this case probably the Speaker-Topic message type. Once a tentative message type is identified, a template containing the fields, both mandatory and optional, for that type is placed in the perceptual workspace, and codelets begin to fill in the blanks. If successful, the message is deemed "understood" and its content (meaning) is placed in perception registers inside the focus (see figure 68.2), for use by the rest of the system. That is what is known as the "initial percept."

CMattie will have ignored the first and last sentences of the messages, since their contents

would have triggered no recognition by her codelets. She would have recognized and filled in the following fields: Organizer–Stan Franklin; Seminar Name–Cognitive Science Seminar; Speaker Name–Art Graesser; Title-Kintsch's Comprehension Theory. Each would occupy the appropriate perception register in the focus. Other optional fields, including Date, Day-of-week, Building-Room, and Time, would result in empty registers. VMattie, CMattie's predecessor, does all of this with almost 100% success.

CMattie's understanding of incoming messages is based on her knowledge of surface features that is stored in her slipnet and in her perceptual codelets. It is possible for us to implement this on a computer in real time because of the narrow domain of knowledge in our application. CMattie need be concerned with only a few message types, for example, seminar-initiation, speaker-topic, seminar-conclusion, change-of-time (or day or room), on-mailing-list, off-mailing-list, negative-response, and a few others.

At this point, the perception registers already begin to activate the emotion mechanism. Simultaneously, the associative and episodic memories are read into sets of registers of their own within the focus (see figure 68.2), with the initial percept used as the address to these content-addressable memories. The new contents of the associative memory registers should contain correct default information about the Date, Time, etc., as well as an associated emotion and an associated behavior. Together with the perception register contents, these constitute CMattie's percept from the "sensory stimulus" of the incoming message. All this again activates the emotion mechanism and through consciousness the behavior net. Typically, a new behavior will be selected by the net and a new emotion by its mechanism as well. The behavior, the emotion, and the initial percept augmented by default values are then written from the write registers to both memories. This ends one perceptual cycle.

Consciousness codelets carrying the information of this percept typically form a coalition that falls within the "spotlight of consciousness." This corresponds to the global workspace of Baars's theory. The resulting broadcast results in streams of behaviors being instantiated, eventually leading to an "acknowledge message" being sent to the sender of the message. It would also result in this information being written into the announcement template in the composition workspace. This activation for these behavior streams comes from the drives, is influenced by emotions, and is driven by the percept as extended by memory. A selected behavior will, in turn, activate the codelets in its service. These codelets do the actual work.

CMattie's high-level actions, as produced by streams of several behaviors, include sending an acknowledgement, sending a seminar announcement, sending a reminder, adding to or removing from the mailing list, and a very few others. One of these others sends a warning to seminar organizers whose sessions for the week overlap in time and place. This situation might be discovered by a consciousness codelet comparing the incoming percept as fleshed out from associative memory to the contents returned from the case-based episodic memory. The latter might describe another seminar with overlapping time and place. In this case the consciousness codelet making the discovery would become highly activated and would be gathered into a coalition with other codelets carrying the pertinent information, and this coalition would find its way into the spotlight of consciousness. The resulting global broadcast would awaken a stream of behaviors to send the appropriate warnings.

Accounting for the Facts

When Baars published his recent book describing his Global Workspace theory (1997), he included an appendix that summarized the "major bodies of evidence about conscious experience." That is, he listed a couple dozen psychological findings that "any complete theory [of consciousness] must explain." Global Workspace theory was designed by Baars to explain these "facts." This section reviews these facts and discusses the extent to which CMattie models them.

It is important to acknowledge one of the central arguments that we are making in this article with respect to software and consciousness. We assume that we are simulating consciousness on a computer to the extent that we can simulate the psychological and empirical phenomena that Baars articulates as being the bodies of evidence about conscious experience. He has articulated the facts that have constrained his Global Workspace theory. Similarly, we have developed a conceptual model and, hopefully, a computational system that models these facts and implements the Global Workspace theory. We argue that this is a justifiable method of approaching the problem scientifically. We are not making any strong claims about whether the software is truly aware or whether the awareness in software is equivalent to awareness in humans. We regard such questions as unanswerable or in the provinces of philosophy (ontology, not epistomology). Our present approach will presumably advance the scientific study of consciousness and may be useful to the philosophical debates.

Below-Threshold or Masked Stimulation (p. 170)

An external stimulus can have an impact on unconscious processes without having a direct impact on consciousness. This phenomenon essentially addresses the disassociation between conscious and unconscious experience. For example, suppose that we briefly present the word MONEY for 5 ms and then immediately mask the word with letters XXXXX to cut off stimulus-driven sensing of the word. The brief presentation is sufficient to activate unconscious processors, but not long enough for a coalition of processors to evolve into the conscious spotlight. The brief activation of MONEY can still prime the activation of words that are semantically related to it (e.g., dollars, bank, mint). The activation of semantic associates is accomplished without any participation of consciousness.

CMattie is capable of simulating the unconscious activation of processors. One subset of the codelets in working memory participates in the coalition of codelets that are in the spotlight of consciousness. However, another subset (most of them, in fact) never makes it into the spotlight of consciousness. The strictly unconscious codelets are activated and in turn activate other codelets, but they never become part of a coalition that reaches consciousness. The pertinent example here concerns perceptual codelets working with the slipnet. These unconscious codelets often activate a message-type node that is not chosen for the message in question. The residual activation gives this node a leg up when the next message arrives.

Preperceptual Processes (p. 170)

The unconscious preperceptual processes tap the meaning representation in addition to the surface code and sensations. While people are sleeping, they are not directly attending to the environment. However, the meaning of words spoken by others and the lyrics on the radio can have an impact on the cognitive system. When a word in a language has multiple meanings (e.g., bank is both a region by a body of water and a building that houses money), the relevant meaning of the words is resolved without the need for conscious processing (Kintsch 1998). When the environment is severely degraded (e.g., the fuzzy and warped image when you put on the wrong pair of spectacles), consciousness is needed to generate hypotheses about the objects and features in the environment.

Preperceptual processing in CMattie includes all processing prior to the appearance of information in the perception registers. These processes include meanings of words in addition to the more surface characteristics, such as letters, punctuation marks, and quotes. Local ambiguities are often resolved with respect to the current perceptual context, namely the message type. Unconscious preperceptual hypotheses may occur both before and after the choice of a message type. Issues that cannot be resolved unconsciously eventually make their way into the spotlight of attention.

Postperceptual Representations (p. 170)

Humans habituate to stimulus events that frequently occur in their environment. A new piece of jewelry can be attention demanding for a few minutes after first put on, but we fail to notice it after we have worn it for a few days. We can become habituated to the noisy television or lawnmower. Indeed, sometimes it is the silence that can be distracting whenever we have successfully become habituated to a noisy environment. The deviations from norms and habituated processing command our attention and consciousness.

CMattie has a slipnet of typical knowledge to which the system has been habituated. For example, particular seminars meet at particular times and locations and have a particular organizer. When an e-mail message contains content that is compatible with the slipnet content, then the message can be preperceptually processed unconsciously, that is, without the services of a consciousness codelet and without a global broadcast. However, when the content of the message clashes with the slipnet content, then consciousness needs to be recruited to resolve the discrepancy. These mechanisms are handled naturally by CMattie. One component that is currently being implemented is the process of learning during habituation. We are currently adding this feature as part of CMattie's conceptual learning apparatus. This will be accomplished using episodic memory, implemented by case-based memory (Kolodner 1993). Whenever a particular seminar is held at a particular room, for example, this invariance is induced and the slipnet's content gets updated. The deviations from habituation will be handled by an explanation-based learning mechanism (Mooney 1990, Schank 1986) that induces new concepts, dimensions, and indexes from a set of deviant cases.

Unaccessed Interpretations of Ambiguous Stimuli (p. 171)

Most stimulus events are ambiguous when considered out of context, but are rarely ambiguous when considered in context. For example, the word BANK can refer to a building with money, a region of land by the river, or a type of shot in a basketball game. An adequate cognitive model accurately accounts for the process of resolving the ambiguity when the stimulus is processed in context. When an ambiguous word is being processed during the first 200 ms, all senses of the word are initially activated although only one of the senses is relevant to the context (Kintsch 1998). Later in the processing stream (after 400 ms) the constraints of context prevail and there is convergence on a single sense (except for the rare occasions when two senses equally fit the context). This convergence onto a single sense of a word is normally accomplished unconsciously, but occasionally consciousness does play a role in the disambiguation.

Once again, unconscious interpretations are very much part of the CM architecture. Slipnet nodes retain their increased activation even when they fail to make it into the spotlight of consciousness. One would expect the understanding of ambiguous data to take longer in VMattie, even when the processing is accomplished in parallel. Extra time is of course needed when consciousness is recruited to resolve clashes and contradictions. However, even when consciousness is not involved, extra time is needed to sort out which of the alternative meanings is most compatible with the message type and the remaining content. CMattie will eventually be tested to verify whether ambiguous data actually take longer to process.

The matter of emotional priming (p. 172) is also accounted for. As seen in figure 68.1, CMattie's emotions are influenced by associated memories, drives, and internal perceptual states. They activate drives and these drives in turn activate appropriate streams of behaviors. CMattie will become anxious as the time for an announcement approaches, without all the information being in. She will be annoyed at organizers who fail to respond to her duns. She many be fearful at the possibility of an impending shutdown of the system. The annoyance and the fear result from the actions of emotion codelets. All these emotions serve to direct her attention and to spur her actions. She may, or may not, become conscious of the emotions. But, as in Baars's example, her actions can be primed by prior emotions.

Contextual Constraints on Perception (p. 173)

We often perceive what we expect to see, and many of these expectations are formulated at an unconscious level. Similarly, perceptual experiences in CMattie are often constrained by unconscious factors. The currently chosen message type, most often unconscious, constrains the fields available for perception. For example, with a change-of-time message type as a perceptual context, the "30" in "1:30" would be recognized as part of a time rather than as part of a date (as in "April 30"). Earlier in the process, the unconscious recognition of a day of the week serves to constrain the recognition of a message type. CMattie has no difficulty accounting for these contextual constraints on perception.

Expectations of Specific Stimuli (p. 173)

We frequently have expectations of what will happen next at an abstract level, but we rarely predict what specific stimulus events will occur (Graesser, Singer, and Trabasso 1994; Kintsch 1998). We expect that we will have dinner the next day, but we rarely have precise expectations of what we will eat and how much. Consequently, clashes with expectations can readily be spotted, whereas it is difficult to get humans to be specific in articulating what expectations they are having.

The understanding of messages by CMattie occurs in two stages. First, a candidate message type is selected on the basis of what types of fields (day of week, time, various key words) are recognized by codelets. Then a template for that type of message is moved into the workspace and the codelets attempt to fill in the "blanks." This template implements expectations as to what is to be found, expectations expressed in terms of which classes of codelets are looking for what. The expectations are at an abstract level, awaiting classes of input rather than specific input. For example, speaker name is expected, but

there is no expectation about who the speaker will be. These expectations influence lower-level unconscious actions. However, when the content of the input clashes with the expectations, consciousness needs to be recruited to help resolve the discrepancies. This is accomplished by consciousness codelets and a resulting global broadcast as described above.

The Conscious Side of Imagery (p. 174)

According to Baars, images are "quasi-perceptual events" that occur when there is no external stimulation in any modality. Imagery includes inner speech and emotional feelings in addition to the prototypical case of the mental visual image. Baars claims that the construction of these images is conscious. Consciousness is recruited when we construct in our minds an argument that we hope to have with a member of the family, when we imagine the feelings of revenge after losing a basketball game, and when we imagine the perfect dessert to have after a frustrating day. One of Baars's goals is to explain which of the images are conscious and which are unconscious.

CMattie accommodates conscious imagery in the form of conscious goals, conscious messages under construction, and items from episodic memory. For example, a codelet might note that information on the Complex Systems Seminar is missing and brings this lack to consciousness. This filling of a gap is a constructive process that requires consciousness. An impending shutdown may engender fear in CMattie, which can become conscious by being part of a coalition that makes it into the spotlight.

Memory Images Before Retrieval (p. 174)

Episodic memory is represented in some fashion and this representation is tapped during the process of actively retrieving and reconstructing the memory. For example, suppose that you want to remember what you wore at the last New Year's Eve party. At the initial stage of memory retrieval there is some form of code or representation that is accessed unconsciously. In CMattie, this initial representation typically arises from an incoming message. The resulting percept addresses both sparse distributed memory (Kanerva 1988) and case-based memory (Kolodner 1993). Reconstructive processes subsequently embellish this initial percept and it becomes conscious. On some occasions, humans replay or mentally simulate the fleshed-out image. These are the instances when consciousness must be recruited to play out the image. Thus, features of the representation must be mapped onto a rudimentary spatial coordinate system when visual mental images are reconstructed in the mind's eye (Baddeley 1992, Kosslyn 1994). Similarly, in CMattie a stream of behaviors must be mapped onto a projected temporal coordinate system when a series of episodes is retrieved and envisioned in real time. In these cases, memories can be unconscious for a time and then conscious. The content of the representations is accessible to consciousness, but not the process of retrieval. The spotlight of consciousness may or may not shine on them, depending on the grain size of the spatial or temporal coordinate systems.

CMattie does not currently have the spatial and temporal coordinate systems that are essential for planning and fleshing out mental images. Since she has no spatial senses, a spatial coordinate system, such as the "visual-spatial sketchpad" that is known to exist in the working memory of humans (Baddeley 1992, Shah and Miyake 1999), is not applicable. However, CMattie must learn through dialogue with human organizers. This process will require a temporal coordinate system to track the order of messages in an interchange. Such a system is currently being designed (see Ramamurthy et al. 1998 for a preliminary report).

Currently Unrehearsed Items in Working Memory (p. 175)

Information is preserved in working memory for a short period of time while it is not being rehearsed. The duration of this unrehearsed information in memory varies from 30 s in short-term memory (e.g., remembering a telephone number while you reach for a phone and dial it) to several minutes in working memory. In the latter case, humans are expected to actively monitor two or more tasks simultaneously (e.g., driving and holding a conversation). According to research by Baddeley (1986, 1992), the contents of working memory can be actively maintained or recycled through a visual-spatial sketchpad, through an "articulatory loop," or through an "executive," so working memory does have a number of separate modalities. In the absence of the active recycling of the information in working memory (much of which involves consciousness), there is content that passively resides in working memory for a few seconds or minutes.

The CMattie architecture allows for several different working memories. In each case the spotlight of attention (consciousness) can shine on individual items in a working memory while not shining on the others. For example, suppose that the seminar announcement template occupies one working memory and the Complex Systems Seminar is under scrutiny. Attention could shine on missing information or on an anomaly, but never the missing information and an anomaly at the same time. Both the missing information and the anomaly would occupy working memory, but only one of these would be in consciousness at a time. The contents of consciousness are in working memory, but the working memory contains additional content and is, therefore, not equivalent to consciousness.

Automatic Mental Images (p. 175)

A mental image can fade from consciousness, yet continue to function subsequently in the processing stream. At one point in time, a mental image is constructed on where a restaurant is located and how to get to it. The image guides the path to the restaurant, even though the image has left consciousness while the person is engaged in conversation with a passenger in the car. CMattie allows an image to linger on well after it has exited consciousness. One example was discussed previously. A reminder being sent to the organizer would likely result in consciousness shifting elsewhere, with the template still in place and the codelet that noted the gap still somewhat activated. At the same time, codelets recruited to deal with the missing situation would likely be both active and unconscious. Another example is when consciousness shines on a perceptual gap, such as a missing seminar location. When the default place is found and inserted, processing would continue unconsciously.

Contrasts That Recruit Attention (p. 175)

Attention is known to be captured by contrasts in the environment, such as light versus dark, loud versus silent, and motion versus rest. Our attention is captured by contrasts between our knowledge and what appears in the environment (such as an anomalous object or event). These contrasts in the environment automatically capture our attention when the contrasts are extreme, such as an explosion that occurs in the midst of silence. We have an "orientation reflex" that automatically turns to the source of extremely loud blasts; this is prewired in the organism, not a learned response. However, we can also voluntarily control our attention and this control can supercede attention being controlled by data-driven contrasts in the environment. Factory workers can voluntarily monitor their attention to ignore loud blasts.

CMattie can accommodate attention being controlled by the environment and by its goals. When there is an important event, such as a shutdown message, this data-driven input would capture attention and drive out the old contents of consciousness. However, for this to happen, these involuntary controls over attention would need to be in a class of high-priority events. Regarding the voluntary control over attention, CMattie's attention will focus on a goal (behavior) as it becomes active as a result of the action of the behavior net. Actions that immediately follow are voluntary. CMattie's metacognitive mechanism can also send activation to a behavior, trying to cause a voluntary action, or send activation to a particular coalition of codelets, bringing it to consciousness and constituting voluntary control of attention.

Attended versus Unattended Messages (p. 175)

Baars described attention experiments by Don Norman that involved dichotic listening. A person is presented a different message in each ear and is asked to attend to the message on only one channel (e.g., the left ear). The person can identify the voice quality of the unattended channel, but not the individual words even though they are repeated up to 35 times. The situation described in Norman's study can occur only in an agent with more than one sensory input channel. CMattie currently does not have multiple sensory channels, but it in principle could be expanded to have more than one channel. Other than the matter of there being different channels, this phenomenon is exactly the same as below threshold stimulation (see "Below Threshold or Masked Stimulation"). As discussed earlier, CMattie is capable of simulating the unconscious activation of processors.

Consider the case when two simultaneous messages are sent to CMattie. CMattie attends to and processes one message at a time, so CMattie will attend to message 1 without deeply processing message 2, and vice versa. However, there could be a residue of the unconscious activations of a privileged set of the codelets from the unattended message while the focal message is being processed. This is in fact necessary for processing a critical interrupting message, such as an impending shutdown from the system operator. The metacognitive component is capable of reconstructing whether this residue of unconscious activation of privileged codelets is different from its base rate profile of activations. Any discrepancies will allow CMattie to reconstruct particular characteristics of the unattended message, such as the person who sent the message.

Interruption of, and Influence on, the Attended Stream (p. 176)

As discussed above, a critical message from the system operator can interrupt the process of CMattie's attending to an incoming e-mail message. In this case, the interrupted messages can be attended to later, though as in humans some information may be lost. A more critical incoming message, such as an announcement of an imminent shutdown of the system, can jump the queue to be processed next. This is based on the unconscious perception of a privileged set of features, as discussed in item 12. Once the urgent message is perceived, it interrupts (and takes precedence over) the further processing of the earlier message.

Voluntary versus Involuntary Attention (p. 176)

The spotlight of consciousness may be constructed voluntarily, following an agenda of goals and drives. This occurs when a person drives his automobile along a dangerous mountain pass. Consciousness is directed and explores information that is relevant to the goals and drives. Alternatively, the spotlight of consciousness may be unexpectedly captured by an intense stimulus, such as the load roar of a nearby train. Thus, consciousness fluctuates along the continuum of being goal-driven and stimulus-driven.

CMattie also has its attention being driven by either goals or stimuli. When CMattie is trying to fill in a missing seminar location, these activities are goal-driven. In contrast, when an unexpected shutdown message occurs, there is a stimulus-driven recruitment of consciousness.

Dishabituation of the Orienting Response (p. 176)

Predictable stimuli are accommodated by unconscious mechanisms, whereas unpredictable stimuli require consciousness. When a shutdown message first occurs, the spotlight of consciousness will be recruited by CMattie. However, when a shutdown message routinely occurs at the same time and at the same place, then this invariant feature will be acquired through CMattie's learning mechanisms. The templates and codelets will eventually be updated. At that point, the shutdown message will be handled by unconscious mechanisms.

The CM architecture permits a mechanism for habituation as part of the controller of the spotlight of attention. If a speaker-topic message is perceived that lists the time of the Cognitive Science Seminar as 1:30 on Wednesday, the traditional time, the controller will likely ignore it entirely. The message meaning will routinely come to consciousness, but the time will be ignored. If it lists 3:30 on Wednesday, a codelet will likely pick up the difference and bring the issue to consciousness. A coalition with high activation will be formed of that codelet and other codelets carrying the information concerning that seminar. A message questioning the accuracy of the new time will also be sent to the organizer, to verify the unexpected deviation. Dishabituation will eventually be completed when the memories are updated.

Most Thinking during Problem Solving Is Inexplicit (p. 176)

Humans are not conscious of all stages and representations in problem solving. We are conscious of the beginning state (the representation of what the problem is), the goal state (what we hope to achieve by solving the problem), the landmark keys to the solution, and some of the salient intermediate states (Ericsson and Simon 1980). However, we are not aware of the massive blur of incubation processes, of searches of large spaces, and of the hundreds of intermediate knowledge states in route to the solution.

In CMattie, the spotlight of consciousness drifts to the content that is affiliated with missing parts, contradictions, obstacles to goals, contrasts, anomalies, and other violations of expectations. Consciousness basks in these challenges of the atypical input. These also are precisely the situations in which problem solving occurs. However, the process of activating codelets and behaviors in the behavior network are unconscious and therefore not in the spotlight of consciousness.

Word Retrieval and Question Answering (p. 177)

The answering of a difficult question is a special case of the problem-solving scenario above. CMattie may well be conscious that the seminar name is missing from a particular speaker-topic message. That is, the spotlight is shining on a part of a template in the perceptual work space. Later, CMattie may be again conscious of the completely understood message without having been conscious of the process of retrieving the seminar name. Research on human question answering has revealed that the search of information is unconscious, fast, and executed in parallel, whereas the process of verifying that a fetched answer is correct is conscious, slow, and serial (Graesser, Lang, and Roberts 1991).

Recall from Long-term Memory (p. 177)

The opacity of memory retrieval is built in to the CM architecture. The spotlight does not shine inside of sparse distributed memory nor inside of the episodic memory. It may occasionally shine on some types of slipnet nodes that constitute a conceptual context that could become conscious during metacognitive reflection.

Action Planning and Control (p. 177)

CMattie plans implicitly and unconsciously as a result of the structure and activity flow of her behavior net. For the most part, she does not plan explicitly or consciously. The spotlight of consciousness drifts to the content affiliated with the missing information, the contradictions, the obstacles to goals, the anomalies, and other violations of expectation that arise throughout the course of planning. CMattie is conscious (a) of what the problem or difficulty is, (b) occasionally of internal activities such as an oscillation, (c) of her external actions, and (d) of the eventual solution if one occurs. She is typically unconscious of intermediate steps.

Perceptual Reorganization (p. 178)

CMattie can be expected to exhibit precisely the "conscious–unconscious–conscious" pattern that occurs when we perceive a Necker cube and other ambiguous stimuli. The consciousness–unconscious–consciousness stream of processing occurs when the spotlight recruits additional codelets or behaviors to help in the recognition and categorization of input. CMattie might oscillate between Dr. Garzon being the organizer of the seminar and Dr. Garzon being the speaker on a particular day. CMattie might oscillate when interpreting 430 as a room number or the time of a seminar.

Developing Automaticity with Practice in Predictable Tasks (p. 178)

Though CMattie is capable of learning by adding particular slipnet nodes, codelets, behaviors, and solutions to particular problems (stored in episodic memory), these are one-trial learning episodes rather than learning with practice. CMattie does overlearn and automatize as a particular collection of codelets increases in their mutual associations to the extent that the codelets become one of Jackson's concept codelets and are called to action as a single unit.

Loss of Conscious Access to Visual Information That Nonetheless Continues to Inform Problem Solving (p. 179)

There is nothing analogous to this in CMattie's architecture. Her two senses "see" only incoming e-mail messages and operating system messages. Her mental images consist of parts of templates in working memory or in perceptual registers. These cannot be manipulated spatially, though they will be manipulated temporally. However, unconscious acts do inform problem solving in many ways (see "Unaccessed Interpretations of Ambiguous Stimuli" for an example). Also, it should not be hard to design and build a conscious software agent, capable of rotating visual images in this way, so that the rotation become unconscious after automaticity occurs, but its problem-solving effect continues. The CM architecture allows this in principle, but it is not currently implemented.

Implicit Learning of Miniature Grammars (p. 179)

Again, CMattie's domain does not allow for this phenomenon, but nothing in principle obstructs a conscious software agent from learning grammars implicitly.

Capability Contrasts (p. 179)

This is perforce an empirical matter to be decided when CMattie is up and running. We suspect that all of the capabilities listed in the table will be found as advertised, but this remains to be seen.

Conclusion

So how well does CMattie's architecture account for Baars's collection of psychological facts that serve to constrain theories of consciousness? How well does she implement Global Workspace theory? For current purposes we take these questions to be synonymous. Our conclusion is: quite well, but not perfectly. Almost all the psychological facts are accounted for. Of those that are not, most fail as a consequence of the choice of domain, for example, because CMattie has no visual sense. They do not, in principle, present difficulty for the architecture. The weakest link seems to be a not completely adequate performance in habituation and in acquiring automaticity. Still, our experience with CMattie as a conceptual model shows her to be a useful tool in thinking through cognitive issues.

Suppose we agree that the CMattie architecture implements Global Workspace theory as intended. Can we then conclude that the eventually computational implementation of CMattie, running on a UNIX system, will be conscious in the sense of being in some way sentient? We do not know and know no way of telling. However, we do believe that should any piece of software become sentient, it must be based on some such architecture that provides mechanisms for consciousness and cannot simply depend on complexity to do the trick.

Acknowledgments

The authors were supported in part by NSF Grant SBR-9720314 and by ONR Grants N00014-98-1-0332 and N00014-98-1-0331. This work was carried out with essential cooperation from the "Conscious" Software Research Group including Myles Bogner, Derek Harter, Arpad Kellerman, Lee McCauley, Aregahegn Negatu, Fergus Nolan, Hongjun Song, Uma Ramamurthy, and Zhaohua Zhang.

References

Anwar, A., and Franklin, S. (forthcoming). Sparse distributed memory for "conscious" software agents.

Baars, B. J. (1988). *A cognitive theory of consciousness.* Cambridge: Cambridge Univ. Press.

Baars, B. J. (1997). *In the theater of consciousness.* Oxford: Oxford Univ. Press.

Baddeley, A. D. (1986). *Working memory.* New York: Oxford Univ. Press.

Baddeley, A. D. (1992). Working memory. *Science,* 255, 556–559.

Bogner, M., Ramamurthy, U., and Franklin, S. (1999). "Consciousness" and conceptual learning in a socially situated agent. In K. Dautenhahn (Ed.), *Human cognition and social agent technology.*

Ericsson, K. A., and Simon, H. A. (1980). Verbal reports as data. *Psychological Review,* 87, 215–251.

Franklin, S. (1995). *Artificial minds.* Cambridge, MA: MIT Press.

Franklin, S. (1997a). Autonomous agents as embodied AI. *Cybernetics and Systems* 28(6), 499–520. [Special issue on Epistemological Aspects of Embodied AI]

Franklin, S. (1997b). Global workspace agents. *Journal of Consciousness Studies,* 4(4), 322–234.

Franklin, S., and Graesser, A. (1997). Is it an agent, or just a program?: A taxonomy for autonomous agents. *Intelligent agents III* (pp. 21–35). Berlin: Springer-Verlag.

Franklin, S., Graesser, A., Olde, B., Song, H., and Negatu, A. (1996). *Virtual Mattie—An intelligent clerical agent.* Paper presented at AAAI Fall Shymposium on Embodied AI.

Graesser, A. C., Lang, K. L., and Roberts, R. M. (1991). Question answering in the context of stories. *Journal of Experimental Psychology: General,* 120, 254–277.

Graesser, A. C., Singer, M., and Trabasso, T. (1994). Constructing inferences during narrative comprehension. *Psychological Review,* 101, 371–395.

Holland, J. H. (1986). A mathematical framework for studying learning in classifier systems. In D. Farmer, et al. (Eds.), *Evolution, games and learning: Models for adaption in machine and nature.* Amsterdam: North-Holland.

Hofstadter, D. R., and Mitchell, M. (1994). The copy-cat project: A model of mental fluidity and analogy-making. In K. J. Holyoak and J. A. Barnden (Eds.), *Advances in connectionist and neural computation theory, Vol. 2, Analogical connections.* Norwood, NJ: Ablex.

Jackson, J. V. (1987, July). Idea for a mind. *SIGGART Newsletter,* No. 181 (pp. 23–26).

Kanerva, P. (1988). *Sparse distributed memory.* Cambridge, MA: The MIT Press.

Kintsch, W. (1998). *Comprehension: A paradigm for cognition.* Cambridge: Cambridge Univ. Press.

Kolodner, J. L. (1993). *Case-based reasoning.* Hillsdale, NJ: Erlbaum.

Kosslyn, S. M. (1994). *Image and brain.* Cambridge, MA: MIT Press.

Leung, K. S., and Lin, C. T. (1988). Fuzzy concepts in expert systems. *Computer,* 21(9), 43–56.

Maes, P. (1990). How to do the right thing. *Connection Science,* 1, 3.

Maes, P. (1992). Learning behavior networks from experience. *Proceedings of the first european conference on artificial life,* Paris, December 1991, Cambridge, MA: MIT Press.

Maturana, H. R. (1975). The organization of the living: A theory of the living organization. *International Journal of Man–Machine Studies,* 7, 313–332.

Maturana, H. R., and Varela, F. (1980). *Autopoiesis and cognition: The realization of the living.* Dordrecht: Reidel.

McCauley, T. L., and Franklin, S. (1998). *An architecture for emotion.* Paper presented at AAAI Fall Symposium on Emotional and Intelligent: The Tangled Knot of Cognition.

Mitchell, M. (1993). *Analogy-making as perception.* Cambridge, MA: The MIT Press.

Mooney, R. J. (1990). *A general explanation-based learning mechanism and its application in narrative understanding.* San Mateo, CA: Morgan-Kaufman.

Ramamurthy, U., Franklin, S., and Negatu, A. (1998). Learning concepts in software agents. *From animals to animats IV,* Proceedings of SAB'98, Cambridge, MA: MIT Press (pp. 372–377).

Schank, R. C. (1986). *Explanation patterns: Understanding mechanically and creatively.* Hillsdale, NJ: Erlbaum.

Shah, P., and Miyake, A. (Eds.) (1999). *Working memory*. New York: Cambridge Univ. Press.

Song, H., and Franklin, S. (forthcoming). Action Selection Using Behavior Instantiation.

Varela, F. J., Thompson, E., and Rosch, E. (1991). *The embodied mind*. Cambridge, MA: MIT Press.

Zhang, Z., Franklin, S., Olde, B., Wan, Y., and Graesser, A. (1998a). *Natural language sensing for autonomous agents*. In Proceedings of the IEEE International Joint Symposium on Intelligence and Systems (pp. 374–381).

Zhang, Z., Franklin, S., and Dasgupta, D. (1998b). *Metacognition in software agents using classifer systems*. In Proceedings of the AAAI 98, (82–88).

Index